Fundamentals of
VETERINARY CLINICAL PATHOLOGY

Second Edition

Fundamentals of
VETERINARY CLINICAL PATHOLOGY

Second Edition

Steven L. Stockham • Michael A. Scott

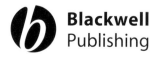

Blackwell
Publishing

Steven L. Stockham, DVM, MS, Diplomate, American College of Veterinary Pathologists (Clinical Pathology); Professor in the Department of Diagnostic Medicine/Pathobiology, College of Veterinary Medicine, Kansas State University, Manhattan, Kansas.

Michael A. Scott, DVM, PhD, Diplomate, American College of Veterinary Pathologists (Clinical Pathology), Assistant Professor in the Department of Pathobiology and Diagnostic Investigation, College of Veterinary Medicine, Michigan State University, East Lansing, Michigan.

Blackwell Publishing Professional
2121 State Avenue, Ames, Iowa 50014, USA

Orders: 1-800-862-6657
Office: 1-515-292-0140
Fax: 1-515-292-3348
Web site: www.blackwellprofessional.com

Blackwell Publishing Ltd
9600 Garsington Road, Oxford OX4 2DQ, UK
Tel.: +44 (0)1865 776868

Blackwell Publishing Asia
550 Swanston Street, Carlton, Victoria 3053, Australia
Tel.: +61 (0)3 8359 1011

First edition, ©2002
Second edition, ©2008

Library of Congress Cataloging-in-Publication Data

Stockham, Steven L.
    Fundamentals of veterinary clinical pathology / Steven L. Stockham, Michael A. Scott.—2nd ed.
        p. ; cm.
Includes bibliographical references and index.
    ISBN-13: 978-0-8138-0076-9 (alk. paper)
    ISBN-10: 0-8138-0076-5 (alk. paper)
    1. Veterinary clinical pathology.   I. Scott, Michael A. (Michael Alan), 1957–   II. Title.
    [DNLM: 1. Animal Diseases–pathology.   2. Clinical Laboratory Techniques–veterinary.
3. Pathology, Veterinary–methods. SF 772.6 S864f 2008]
    SF772.6.S76 2008
    636.089′607–dc22

The last digit is the print number: 9 8 7 6 5 4 3 2

CONTENTS

Preface   *vii*

Acknowledgments   *ix*

1   Introductory Concepts   *3*

2   Leukocytes   *53*

3   Erythrocytes   *107*

4   Platelets   *223*

5   Hemostasis   *259*

6   Bone Marrow and Lymph Node   *323*

7   Proteins   *369*

8   Urinary System   *415*

9   Monovalent Electrolytes and Osmolality   *495*

10   Blood Gases, Blood pH, and Strong Ion Difference   *559*

11   Calcium, Phosphorus, Magnesium, and Their Regulatory Hormones   *593*

12   Enzymes   *639*

13   Liver Function   *675*

14   Glucose, Ketoamines, and Related Regulatory Hormones   *707*

15   Exocrine Pancreas and Intestine   *739*

16   Lipids   *763*

17   Thyroid Function   *783*

18   Adrenocortical Function   *805*

19   Cavitary Effusions   *831*

*   Color plates   *between pages 494 and 495*

Index   *869*

PREFACE

Writing this second edition was motivated by our desire to synthesize and incorporate newer information related to fundamentals of veterinary clinical pathology, and it was driven by the same goals as the first edition: to explain the physiologic, pathologic, and analytical conditions or disorders responsible for abnormal laboratory data, and to do so using consistent terms and a uniform format. Whenever possible, diseases and conditions are grouped by common mechanisms or processes to promote a conceptual understanding of laboratory data that can be generally applied across many species.

The content of the first edition was largely preserved, but the second edition contains additional disorders, diagnostic tests, illustrations, references, and pathophysiologic explanations. There are four major changes: (1) the analytical aspects in Chapter 2 of the first edition are now distributed into their respective chapters on leukocytes, erythrocytes, and platelets (Chapters 2–4), (2) the *Hemostasis* chapter of the first edition is split into two chapters, one focused on nonhemostasis aspects of platelets (Chapter 4) and the other on hemostasis (Chapter 5), (3) a new chapter on cavitary effusions (Chapter 19) focuses on the pathophysiologic processes that create cavitary effusions and relates them to inflammatory, renal, hepatic, electrolyte, protein, and lipoprotein disorders, and (4) the color plate section is revised and expanded to include microscopic images of bone marrow, lymph nodes, and cavitary effusions.

Even though the second edition contains more information than the first, it remains focused on disorders occurring in North America and does not address some of the more specialized aspects of veterinary clinical pathology such as therapeutic drug monitoring and molecular diagnostic assays. Coverage of diagnostic cytology is limited because a second volume would be required to do justice to it. Lastly, material is again restricted mostly to dogs, cats, horses, and cattle because these species provide the basis for a fundamental understanding of veterinary clinical pathology.

Regrettably, we will likely uncover mistakes in the second edition as we did in the first. Corrections for these mistakes will be available at this textbook's Web site (search FVCP Stockham or FVCP Scott), which is linked to the publisher's Web site and the authors' Web sites. Also available in the textbook's Web site are lists of suggested specific objectives that may be used as study guides, and electronic copies of the book's figures available exclusively for educational purposes.

Once again, we found the writing of the second edition to be a great learning experience and hope that our efforts facilitate the learning of others.

ACKNOWLEDGMENTS

FIRST EDITION

Many people directly and indirectly assisted in the writing of this book. We thank our fantastic families for providing the never-ending support for our professional pursuits. We thank our excellent veterinary and graduate students for their active participation in their learning—their questions frequently provided stimuli for finding better explanations, and their answers provided insight into what they were or were not learning. We thank our mentors (Drs. Jan Krehbiel, Doug Weiss, Harold Tvedten, and Julia Stickle) and coresidents at Michigan State University, who provided excellent specialty training. We thank Dr. Jenni Donald, who actively participated in the planning, reviewing, and critiquing of chapters. We also thank the technologists in the Clinical Pathology Laboratory at the University of Missouri, and especially Kathy Curtis, MT (ASCP), for helping us pursue many unanswered questions and for documenting certain abnormalities. We also appreciate the assistance of Howard Wilson and Don Connors during the generation of the plates and figures.

The senior author would not have accepted the challenge of writing this text without the persistent encouragement of a longtime friend, colleague, and excellent teacher—Donald A. Schmidt, DVM, PhD, Diplomate, ACVP, Professor Emeritus. Very few people have the opportunity to work with such a great person who was also one of the pioneers in the specialty of veterinary clinical pathology. His statement that "students must come first, they are the reason we are here" provided the justification for many career decisions. For over 25 years at the University of Missouri, veterinary students (and this senior author) were extremely fortunate to have Dr. Schmidt as a teacher.

The specialty in veterinary clinical pathology grew out of the increased use of laboratory tests in veterinary medicine, was promoted in the early 1960s by a society now known as the American Society for Veterinary Clinical Pathology (ASVCP), and then formalized in the early 1970s by the American College of Veterinary Pathologists (ACVP). The authors extend thanks to the ASVCP and ACVP members (and especially charter members and contemporary colleagues) for their leadership, investigations, and instruction. We have made great advances in our understanding of diseases of domestic mammals in the past 40 years, but there are many facts we do not know and processes we do not understand. The clinical laboratories, their dedicated personnel, and their expanding analytical procedures will play a key role in future advances.

SECOND EDITION

We are still greatly appreciative of the many people who directly or indirectly assisted in the writing of the first edition, and we extend sincere thanks to colleagues, students, and family who supported our efforts to produce the second edition. We appreciate the faculty in our departments and colleges who value the scholarly activities of teaching and the writing of a textbook, and we are especially thankful for the unwavering support of our spouses and for the encouraging feedback offered by veterinary students, residents, and fellow clinical pathologists.

Fundamentals of
VETERINARY CLINICAL PATHOLOGY

Second Edition

Chapter 1

INTRODUCTORY CONCEPTS

Clinical Pathology. 4
Samples. 5
     I.   Blood Samples and Specimens. 5
     II. Urine Samples. 7
     III. Other Body Fluid Samples. 7
Major Types of Laboratory Assays. 7
Significant Figures 9
Units. 10
Reference Intervals. 16
Quality of Laboratory Results 20
     I.   Major Determinants 20
     II. Analytical Properties of Assays. 21
     III. Quality assurance 25
Differences in Laboratory Methods and Their Results. 29
Comparison of Assays. 31
Which Laboratory Do You Use? 35
Evaluating and Validating Laboratory Methods 36
Diagnostic Properties and Predictive Value of Laboratory Assays. 38
Receiver Operating Characteristic (ROC) Curves 45
Herd-based Testing for Cattle. 48

Table 1.1. Abbreviations and symbols in this chapter

$[fT_4]_{ed}$	Free thyroxine concentration by equilibrium dialysis
[x]	x concentration (x = analyte)
BHB	β-Hydroxybutyrate
Ca^{2+}	Calcium
CLSI	Clinical Laboratory Standards Institute
CV	Coefficient of variation
EDTA	Ethylenediaminetetraacetic acid
fCa^{2+}	Free ionized calcium
FN	False negative
FP	False positive
fT_4	Free thyroxine
IFCC	International Federation of Clinical Chemistry
IUPAC	International Union of Pure and Applied Chemistry
K_2EDTA	Dipotassium salt of ethylenediaminetetraacetic acid
K_3EDTA	Tripotassium salt of ethylenediaminetetraacetic acid
Na_2EDTA	Disodium salt of ethylenediaminetetraacetic acid
NCCLS	National Committee for Clinical Laboratory Standards
NEFA	Nonesterified fatty acids (fatty acids)
NIST	National Institute of Standards and Technology
PV(−)	Predictive value of a negative test
PV(+)	Predictive value of a positive test
ROC	Receiver operating characteristic
sd	Standard deviation
SI	Système International d'Unités
T_3	Triiodothyronine
tCa^{2+}	Total calcium
TE_a	Total error allowable
TN	True negative
TP	True positive
TRH	Thyrotropin-releasing hormone
tT_4	Total thyroxine
U	International unit
USD	Usual standard deviation
WRI	Within reference interval

Note: See Table 1.4 for abbreviations of units of measurement and the figure legends for abbreviations unique to figures.

CLINICAL PATHOLOGY

I.   What is clinical pathology?
  A. Definitions[1]
    1. *Pathology* is the "branch of medicine that deals with the basis of disease, especially those structural and functional changes in organs and tissues causing or caused by a disease." In general terms, it is the study of disease.

2. *Clinical pathology* is a "subspecialty of pathology that deals with the use of laboratory methods (clinical chemistry, microbiology, hematology, . . .) for the diagnosis and treatment of disease." In general terms, it is the study of disease in the clinical environment by use of laboratory assays.

B. As currently certified by the American College of Veterinary Pathologists, *veterinary clinical pathologists* are specialists in the disciplines of basic pathology, hematology (study of blood), clinical chemistry (study of physiologic and biochemical reactions), cytology (study of cells), and surgical pathology (study of disease via microscopic analysis of tissue samples obtained during surgery).

C. Veterinary clinical pathologists and other laboratory professionals (medical technologists, medical laboratory technicians, and veterinary technicians) often work in a clinical laboratory that limits its assay "menu" (offered tests) to hematologic assays, clinical chemical assays, urinalysis, and clinical cytologic or histologic examinations. Other assays or diagnostic laboratory procedures are offered by specific laboratories (e.g., microbiology, histopathology, and toxicology) that are supervised by microbiologists, histopathologists, and toxicologists, respectively.

II. Laboratory tests should be used with other diagnostic procedures. Before laboratory tests are used to pursue a possible diagnosis, two diagnostic procedures are imperative: (1) obtain a complete history, and (2) perform a complete physical examination. With knowledge gained from these two basic procedures, a diagnostician can select diagnostic procedures to clarify or classify identified problems. Veterinarians frequently use the laboratory assays in conjunction with other diagnostic methods to identify or classify pathologic states that develop in domestic mammals. Some body systems (e.g., integument, nervous, skeletal, and cardiovascular) are relatively easily evaluated via visual or imaging methods (physical examination, radiography, and ultrasonography), whereas other body systems (e.g., hemic, immune, urinary, and endocrine) are better evaluated by laboratory tests.

III. What are the major reasons for analyzing patient samples via laboratory procedures?
A. To detect an unidentified pathologic state
B. To define, classify, or confirm a pathophysiologic disorder or disease state
C. To eliminate (rule out) a possible cause of the animal's illness
D. To assess changes in a pathologic state either due to natural progression of the disease or because of medical or surgical therapy

SAMPLES

I. Blood samples and specimens
A. Most clinical laboratory assays are designed to detect or quantify substances or cells in blood samples; the substance or cell of interest is called the *analyte*. Obtaining useful results for the analyte requires appropriate samples. Whenever there is doubt about the appropriate sample for a particular test at a particular laboratory, the laboratory should be contacted prior to sample collection. (See Quality of Laboratory Results, section I.A.)
B. Blood
1. Blood and its major components are frequently used as samples for laboratory assays. Blood must be collected and processed properly so that assay results reflect the true composition of blood rather than artifactual changes.

2. Blood is composed of blood cells (erythrocytes, platelets, and five major leukocyte types) and plasma. Blood withdrawn from a blood vessel must immediately be mixed with an anticoagulant to prevent initiation of clot formation and to maintain cells and other components in suspension.

3. Analysis or processing of whole blood must be relatively rapid because the cells die within a few hours, and thus a sample will become unacceptable for analysis. What constitutes adequate sample handling varies with what is to be quantified or evaluated; occasionally, samples must be analyzed within minutes, usually within hours, rarely within days.

C. Plasma

1. Plasma is the fluid component of blood that is harvested after centrifugation of an anticoagulated blood sample. Plasma will contain the anticoagulant that can interfere with some assays.

2. Anticoagulants used for blood sample collection

   a. Calcium-binding agents prevent Ca^{2+} from participating in the formation of a blood clot.

      (1) EDTA (as Na_2EDTA, K_2EDTA, or K_3EDTA)

         (a) EDTA is the preferred anticoagulant for almost all routine hematologic tests, including the complete blood count (CBC) assays.

         (b) EDTA chelates Ca^{2+} and other divalent cations (Mg^{2+}, Cu^{2+}, and Pb^{2+}) but the other anticoagulants do not. A chelating agent wraps around and attaches to the metallic ion in two or more places. EDTA attaches to Ca^{2+} in six places.

      (2) Citrate (as sodium citrate)

         (a) Citrate is the preferred anticoagulant for most tests of the coagulation system. Ca^{2+} is added to the citrated plasma to override the effects of citrate and enable coagulation enzymes to function. Citrate's anticoagulant activity is achieved by its forming an ionic bond with Ca^{2+}.

         (b) Because it has low toxicity, citrate is also preferred for collection of whole blood to be used for transfusions.

      (3) Oxalates (as lithium, ammonium, and potassium salts)

         (a) Oxalate is used for a few laboratory tests; for example, oxalate is the anticoagulant in sodium fluoride tubes that are used for glucose and lactate assays. Generally, oxalates distort morphologic features of leukocytes and erythrocytes and thus are unsuitable for hematologic samples.

         (b) Oxalate's anticoagulant activity is achieved by its forming an ionic bond with Ca^{2+}.

   b. Heparin (as lithium, ammonium, potassium, or sodium salts) activates thrombin (sometimes called antithrombin III), which then inhibits the activity of several coagulation factors (including thrombin). It also forms an ionic bond with Ca^{2+}, but its major action is through antithrombin.

      (1) Used for several special laboratory assays (such as blood gas analysis) and can be used for many clinical chemistry assays

      (2) Major disadvantages

         (a) Alters morphologic features and staining of leukocytes

         (b) Allows clotting as effects are slowly overridden by the coagulation system

         (c) Allows platelet clumps to form

      3. Plasma has two major components.
        a. Water: about 92–95 % of plasma volume; 100 mL of plasma contains 92–95 mL of H_2O.
        b. Solids: about 5–8 % of plasma volume. Most solids are proteins on a weight per volume (weight/volume) basis. Other solids are glucose, urea, electrolytes, and other chemicals.
      4. Generally, the chemical composition of plasma is very similar to interstitial fluid in most tissues. Plasma and interstitial fluid are the extracellular fluids, one intravascular and one extravascular.
    D. Serum
      1. Serum is the fluid component of blood that is harvested after centrifugation of a coagulated (clotted) blood sample. As described in Chapter 5, the clotting involves platelets and coagulation proteins. To get the maximal amount of serum from the clotted sample, centrifugation should not be started prior to the retraction of the clot (which typically takes at least 30 min if a clot activator is not present in the tube). If samples are centrifuged prior to clot retraction, some serum will be trapped in a soft fibrin clot.
      2. Serum has essentially the same composition as plasma except serum does not contain most of the coagulation proteins. The major protein (on a weight/volume basis) that is absent in serum but present in plasma is fibrinogen.
      3. During the clotting process, substances released from cells alter the analyte concentrations in serum. For example, platelets release K^+, and thus serum $[K^+]$ is greater than plasma $[K^+]$ (see Chapter 9).

II.   Urine Samples
    A. Other than blood, urine is the most common sample analyzed by laboratory assays. As with blood, urine must be collected and processed properly so that the assay results reflect the true composition of the product of the urinary system.
    B. To prevent artifactual changes in urine, it should be processed soon after collection. General guidelines for the collection and processing of urine for routine analyses are described in Chapter 8.

III.   Other Body Fluid Samples
    A. Pleural fluid, peritoneal fluid, synovia, and cerebrospinal fluid samples are collected to characterize body cavity effusions, joint diseases, and central nervous system disorders, respectively.
    B. The processing and handling of cavitary fluids are described in Chapter 19.

MAJOR TYPES OF LABORATORY ASSAYS

I.   Many laboratory tests or assays involve the analysis of body fluids (blood, serum, plasma, urine, peritoneal fluid, pleural fluid, cerebrospinal fluid, and synovia), tissue samples, or feces. Most clinical laboratory procedures fall into one of three large groups (examples follow subdivisions); many procedures could be classified into more than one group.
    A. Clinical hematology assays: Most assays are completed on whole blood samples.
      1. Quantitation of cell concentrations in blood: total leukocyte concentration (count), erythrocyte concentration, and platelet concentration

2. Semiquantitation of cell concentrations: calculated absolute leukocyte concentration and platelet estimate from blood film examination
3. Defining or classifying cells by microscopic features: toxic neutrophils, reactive lymphocytes, polychromatophilic erythrocytes, poikilocytes, microcytes, hypochromic erythrocytes, and leukemic cells
4. Assessing the coagulation properties of blood: clotting times and platelet function assays

B. Clinical chemistry assays: Most assays are completed on serum or plasma samples.
   1. Detecting or quantifying the concentration of a chemical substance
      a. Quantitative analysis: Results are close to the true concentration (e.g., serum concentrations of glucose, sodium, protein, creatinine, and urea) and typically are reported with a specific numerical value (see the Significant Figures section).
      b. Semiquantitative analysis: Results are "within the ballpark" (e.g., urine glucose, protein, and bilirubin concentrations by reagent pad chemistry assays) and may be reported as approximate numerical values or in a categorical scale (e.g., 1+, 2 +, or 3 +) that represents ranges of numerical values.
      c. Qualitative analysis: Results indicate that a substance is or is not present (e.g., fat detected microscopically in pleural fluid with a Sudan stain) and are reported as "present" or "absent" or as "positive" or "negative."
   2. Detecting or quantifying the activity of a chemical substance
      a. Quantitative analysis: Results are close to true activity (e.g., measured activities of serum enzymes such as alanine aminotransferase, alkaline phosphatase, lactate dehydrogenase, and creatine kinase).
      b. Qualitative analysis: Results indicate that activity is or is not present (e.g., heme's peroxidase activity or leukocyte esterase in urine).

C. Clinical microscopy
   1. Clinical cytology: The study of cell populations and their microscopic features in an attempt to define or classify abnormal tissue or fluid (e.g., lymph node aspirates to diagnose lymphoma or histoplasmosis, aspirate of a skin tumor to determine whether it is an inflammatory or neoplastic lesion, and analysis of peritoneal fluid to determine if it is a transudate, exudate, or other type of effusion)
   2. Surgical histopathology: The study of frozen or fixed tissue in an attempt to define or classify abnormal tissue (i.e., inflammatory, neoplastic, and toxic disorders) and perhaps establish an etiologic diagnosis
   3. Urine sediment analysis: Microscopic examination of urine to detect or semiquantify the presence of leukocytes, erythrocytes, casts, bacteria, crystals, or other structures
   4. Clinical parasitology: Microscopic analysis of fecal, urine, blood, or other sample to detect ova, larvae, or other microscopic forms of parasites

II. Actual descriptions of the numerous laboratory methods are beyond the scope of this textbook. However, an understanding of basic principles and methods is frequently needed to interpret results of a laboratory assay. Such principles are located in several parts of the textbook.
   A. Chapters 2–5 contain the basic principles and concepts of the common hematologic assays.
   B. Chapter 6 contains the guiding principles and overview of the analysis of bone marrow and lymph nodes, the two major tissues involved in hematopoiesis.

    C. Chapters 7–18 have short sections that describe analytical principles that apply to other individual analytes.

    D. Chapter 19 contains basic principles pertaining to the analysis of cavitary effusions.

SIGNIFICANT FIGURES

I.   Results of many laboratory assays consist of a number, often calculated, accompanied by a unit of measure and reference intervals. The number should be reported to the appropriate number of digits by following three basic rules for reporting significant figures.

    A. Retain only as many significant figures in a result as will give only one uncertain figure. Zero is not a significant figure if it only preserves a space in the number.

    B. When reporting results from multiplications or divisions that use two or more numbers with appropriate significant figures, the final calculated result should have no more significant figures than the number(s) with the fewest significant figures. For $1.23 \times 2.4 = 2.952$, the product should be reported as 3.0.

    C. When reporting results from additions or subtractions that use two or more numbers with appropriate significant figures, the final calculated result should have no more significant figures than the number(s) with the fewest significant figures. For $1.23 + 2.4 = 3.63$, the sum should be reported as 3.6.

II.   It is frequently necessary to round numbers so that only significant figures are reported. The recommended rules for rounding numbers when the last digit is 5 are as follows.

    A. Add 1 to the last retained digit if it is odd (round up).

    B. Do not add 1 to the last retained digit if it is even (round down).

    C. Examples with two significant figures; the third example does not require the rounding rule because 45 is the number to be rounded—not 5.

        1. $1150 \rightarrow 1.2 \times 10^3$

        2. $1250 \rightarrow 1.2 \times 10^3$

        3. $1145 \rightarrow 1.1 \times 10^3$

III.   How many significant figures are in a number? See Table 1.2.

IV.   Using the rules of significant figures for reporting results is one way that laboratory personnel can communicate the known precision of the laboratory's assay result. The first rule of significant figures (see Significant Figures, sect. I.A) is to retain only one uncertain figure. But how is that uncertain figure determined? The following illustrates the process.

    A. One sample is analyzed many times (e.g., 20). The mean and standard deviation of the data are calculated.

    B. For the first assay, the mean value was 125.345 and standard deviation (sd) was 0.578; thus, the interval that represents mean ± 2 sd is 124.189–126.501. With this degree of analytical precision, we are confident that the assay can readily distinguish between 100 and 200 and between 120 and 130, but it may not be able to distinguish consistently between 125 and 126. Thus, we are uncertain of the value in the ones place and should report the measured value to the nearest whole number (e.g., 125).

    C. For the second assay, the mean value was 125.345 and standard deviation was 9.111; thus, the interval that represents mean ± 2 sd is 107.123–143.567. With this degree of analytical precision, we are confident that the assay can readily distinguish between 100 and 200, but it probably cannot reliably distinguish between 120 and 130. Thus, we

Table 1.2. Examples of significant figures

Number	Significant figures	Reason
124	3	All digits imply significance.
124.0	4	The zero was not needed for the whole number. Its addition indicates that it is a significant figure.
120	2 or 3	If the zero is just conserving space, it is not a significant digit. If values are usually reported to the ones place in a particular setting (e.g., 121), then the zero is a significant figure.
120.0	4	The zero in the tenth space indicates it is a significant figure. Thus, the zero in the ones place is also a significant figure.
0.12	2	The zero is only preserving a space and is not a significant figure. It is written by convention so the "." is recognized as a decimal point and not a period, fly dirt, or other extraneous material.
0.02	1	The zero in the tenths place is just conserving space and is not a significant figure.
0.020	2	The zero in the thousandths place indicates it is significant.

        are uncertain of the tens value and should report the measured value to the nearest tens unit (e.g., 130).

D. Understanding significant figures becomes important when laboratory data are interpreted. If one understands that we are uncertain about the last reported significant figure, then it is less likely that a 120 in today's sample and a 130 in tomorrow's sample will be considered a true biologic change. Unfortunately, there are several reasons that all results are not reported this way:

1. It may not be the policy for some laboratories.
2. Analyzers and data management programs may not follow rules of significant figures and may not be modifiable.
3. The appropriate number of places after the decimal point may vary for a particular analyte, depending on the magnitude of the value, but analyzers and software may not allow such variability. An example is shown in Fig. 1.1.

UNITS

I. SI units versus non-SI (conventional) units

A. For several decades, there has been an attempt to switch to a metric system of units throughout the world. Other than the United States, the conversion is mostly complete in a modified practical form. During the 1970s and 1980s, several organizations in the United States attempted to convert members of the medical communities to SI units but had limited success. Because there is a lack of consistent use of the SI unit system, veterinary medical professionals need to be familiar with both SI and non-SI units.

B. In the context of units used for laboratory data, the basic units of measurement are listed in Table 1.3. Many clinical laboratory and professional organizations have agreed to use *liter* as the preferred unit for volume instead of the SI unit of *cubic meter* because such a volume as the latter ($1 \text{ m}^3 = 1000 \text{ L}$) is rarely clinically relevant. Even the use of liter for a volume unit has limited relevance in the clinical laboratory when the sample volume for many assays is less than 0.1 mL.

Measured values
WBC concentration = 21.5×10^9/L
WBC diff. count: 73 % neutrophils, 12 % lymphocytes, 9 % monocytes, 4 % eosinophils, 2 % basophils

Calculations and resultant significant figures
Neutrophils: $(21.5 \times 10^9$/L$) \times 0.73 = 15.695 \times 10^9$/L $= 16 \times 10^9$/L
Lymphocytes: $(21.5 \times 10^9$/L$) \times 0.12 = 2.58 \times 10^9$/L $= 2.6 \times 10^9$/L
For these results: 3 significant figures x 2 significant figures = 2 significant figures

Monocytes: $(21.5 \times 10^9$/L$) \times 0.09 = 1.935 \times 10^9$/L $= 2 \times 10^9$/L
Eosinophils: $(21.5 \times 10^9$/L$) \times 0.04 = 0.86 \times 10^9$/L $= 0.9 \times 10^9$/L
Basophils: $(21.5 \times 10^9$/L$) \times 0.02 = 0.43 \times 10^9$/L $= 0.4 \times 10^9$/L
For these results: 3 significant figures x 1 significant figure = 1 significant figure

However, most computer-based reporting systems will require reporting analyte's value consistenty to a defined decimal point and thus significant figure rules will not be consistently applied.

	Results using significant figure rules	Results using consistent decimal points
Total WBC	21.5×10^9/L	21.5×10^9/L
Neutrophils	$16 \quad \times 10^9$/L	16.0×10^9/L
Lymphocytes	2.6×10^9/L	2.6×10^9/L
Monocytes	$2 \quad \times 10^9$/L	2.0×10^9/L
Eosinphils	0.9×10^9/L	0.9×10^9/L
Basophils	0.4×10^9/L	0.4×10^9/L

Fig. 1.1. Significant figures. The significant figures of the measured and calculated values of a leukogram are provided. However, computer-based reporting systems may not enable the flexibility to report only significant figures. diff., differential; and WBC, white blood cell (leukocyte).

Table 1.3. Examples of measurement in SI units and conventional units

	SI units	Conventional units
Amount of substance	mole (mol)	gram (g)
Length	meter (m)	yard, foot, inch
Mass	kilogram (kg)	pound (lb), grain
Time	second (s)	minute (min), hour (h)
Volume	cubic meter (m^3)	liter (L)

Because the reported units for amount or concentration of substances vary considerably, a veterinary medical professional should know the common abbreviations for the major units (Table 1.4).
  C. The National Institute of Standards and Technology (NIST) provides rules and style conventions for the use of the SI units to reduce ambiguity in scientific communications. Examples of the NIST unit conventions used in this book are in Table 1.5.
  D. Table 1.6 contains the formulas for the conversion of analyte values from non-SI units to SI units; only analytes presented in this textbook are included. The table contains two types of formulas: (1) formulas that show the simple conversion factor that is used

Table 1.4. Common units and abbreviations for laboratory values

				kg	kilogram, 10^3 g
mol	mole	L	liter	g	gram
		dL	deciliter, 10^{-1} L		
mmol	millimole, 10^{-3} mol	mL	milliliter, 10^{-3} L	mg	milligram, 10^{-3} g
μmol	micromole, 10^{-6} mol	μL	microliter, 10^{-6} L	μg	microgram, 10^{-6} g
nmol	nanomole, 10^{-9} mol	nL	nanoliter, 10^{-9} L	ng	nanogram, 10^{-9} g
pmol	picomole, 10^{-12} mol	pL	picoliter, 10^{-12} L	pg	picogram, 10^{-12} g
fmol	femtomole, 10^{-15} mol	fL	femtoliter, 10^{-15} L	fg	femtogram, 10^{-15} g
amol	attomole, 10^{-18} mol	aL	attoliter, 10^{-18} L	ag	attogram, 10^{-18} g

Table 1.5. Examples of NIST[a] style for writing units compared to other styles[b]

Rules	NIST style	Non-NIST
Symbols unaltered in the plural	20 pg	20 pgs
	4 h	4 hrs
Symbols not followed by period unless end of sentence	2 L	2 L.
	6 yr	6 yr.
There is space between the numerical value and unit symbol	10 %	10 %
	37°C	37°C, 37°C
	15 g/dL	15 g/dL

[a] National Institute of Standards and Technology

[b] The NIST system has two styles for a range of numbers; for example, 5 % to 10 % or (5 to 10) %. To save space and to conform to common use in veterinary literature, the numbers will be displayed as follows in this textbook: 5–10 %.

to calculate the numerical value of the SI unit,[2] and (2) formulas that show the conversion of the numerical value and units. When available, the recommended smallest reportable increment of the SI unit is provided.[2] Similar information is contained in the analytical concept sections of each chapter.

II. Amount versus concentration: One important basic concept for interpreting laboratory data is having a clear understanding of what a laboratory test result represents. Besides knowing what is really being measured, it is important to understand what the numbers and units represent. The following examples illustrate the concepts.
   A. A dog acutely lost a large amount of blood because of an injury. Because whole blood including erythrocytes was lost, the number of erythrocytes in the body is decreased. However, because plasma was lost with the erythrocytes, the erythrocyte concentration (number of erythrocytes per volume of blood) in the dog initially will not be decreased, and thus the dog is not initially anemic. After fluid shifts restore plasma volume, the dog will have fewer erythrocytes in its body and a lower erythrocyte concentration in its blood.
   B. You are told that a cat's serum sodium level was increased. Does this mean the cat has more sodium in its body? Well, it might. However, the increased serum sodium concentration might be due to less water in the body, and the amount of sodium may not be increased. In fact, the total amount of sodium in the body could be decreased if there was relatively more water loss than sodium loss.

Table 1.6. Conversion of non-SI units to SI units

Analyte[a]	To convert		Multiply by[b]	Complete conversion formulas	Increment[c]
	From	To			
Acetoacetate	mg/dL	μmol/L	99	mg/dL × 9.9 μmol/mg × 10 dL/L = μmol/L	—
ACTH	pg/mL	pmol/L	0.2202	pg/mL ÷ 4541 pg/pmol × 1000 mL/L = nmol/L	1 pmol/L
Albumin	g/dL	g/L	10	g/dL × 10 dL/L = g/L	1 g/L
Aldosterone	ng/dL	pmol/L	27.74	μg/dL ÷ 360.5 μg/μmol × 1000 nmol/μmol × 10 dL/L = nmol/L	10 pmol/L
β-Hydroxybutyrate	mg/dL	μmol/L	97	mg/dL × 9.7 μmol/mg × 10 dL/L = μmol/L	—
Bile acid (total)	mg/L	μmol/L	2.547	mg/L ÷ 392.6 μg/μmol × 1000 μg/mg = μmol/L	0.2 μmol/L
Bile acid (total)	mg/mL	mmol/L	2.547	mg/mL ÷ 392.6 mg/mmol × 1000 mL/L = mmol/L	0.2 mmol/L
Bt	mg/dL	μmol/L	17.10	mg/dL ÷ 584.8 mg/mmol × 1000 μmol/mmol × 10 dL/L = μmol/L	2 μmol/L
Cholesterol	mg/dL	mmol/L	000.02586	mg/dL ÷ 386.7 mg/mmol × 10 dL/L = mmol/L	0.05 mmol/L
Cl$^-$	mEq/L	mmol/L	1	mEq/L × 1 mmol/mEq = mmol/L	1 mmol/L
Cl$^-$	mg/dL	mmol/L	0.2817	mg/dL ÷ 35.5 mg/mmol × 10 dL/L = mmol/L	1 mmol/L
COP	mmHg	pascals	133.322	mmHg × 133.322 pascals/mmHg = pascals	—
Cortisol	μg/dL	nmol/L	27.59	μg/dL ÷ 362.45 μg/μmol × 1000 nmol/μmol × 10 dL/L = nmol/L	10 nmol/L
Creatinine	mg/dL	μmol/L	88.4	mg/dL ÷ 113.1 mg/mmol × 1000 μmol/mmol ×10 dL/L = μmol/L	10 μmol/L
Cyanocobalamin	pg/mL	pmol/L	0.7378	pg/mL ÷ 1355 pg/pmol × 1000 mL/L = pmol/L	10 pmol/L
fCa^{2+}	mg/dL	mmol/L	0.2495	mg/dL ÷ 40.08 mg/mmol × 10 dL/L = mmol/L	0.01 mmol/L
fCa^{2+}	mEq/L	mmol/L	0.5	mEq/L × 0.5 mmol/mEq = mmol/L	0.01 mmol/L
Fe	μg/dL	μmol/L	0.1791	μg/dL × 0.01791 μmol/μg × 10 dL/L = μmol/L	1 μmol/L
Ferritin	ng/mL	μg/L	1	ng/mL × 1 μg/1000 ng × 1000 mL/L = μg/L	10 μg/L
Fibrinogen	mg/dL	g/L	0.01	mg/dL × g/1000 mg × 10 dL/L = g/L	0.1 g/L

Continues

Table 1.6. Conversion of non-SI units to SI units (Continued)

Analyte[a]	To convert From	To	Multiply by[b]	Complete conversion formulas	Increment[c]
Fibrinogen	mg/dL	μmol/L	0.0294	mg/dL × 0.00294 μmol/mg × 10 dL/L = μmol/L	—
Folate	ng/mL	nmol/L	2.266	ng/mL ÷ 441.3 ng/nmol × 1000 mL/L = nmol/L	2 nmol/L
fT_4	ng/dL	pmol/L	12.87	ng/dL ÷ 777 ng/nmol × 1000 pmol/nmol × 10 dL/L = pmol/L	1 pmol/L
Globulins	g/dL	g/L	10	g/dL × 10 dL/L = g/L	1 g/L
Glucose	mg/dL	mmol/L	0.05551	mg/dL ÷ 180.1 mg/mmol × 10 dL/L = mmol/L	0.1 mmol/L
HCO_3^-	mEq/L	mmol/L	1	mEq/L × 1 mmol/mEq = mmol/L	1 mmol/L
Hgb	g/dL	g/L	10	g/dL × 10 dL/L = g/L	1 g/L
IRG	pg/mL	ng/L	1	pg/mL ÷ 1000 pg/ng × 1000 mL/L = ng/L	10 ng/L
IRI	μU/mL	pmol/L	7.175	μU/mL ÷ 139.4 μU/pmol × 1000 mL/L = pmol/L	5 pmol/L
IRI	μg/L	pmol/L	172.2	μg/L ÷ 5.807 μg/μmol × 1000 pmol/μmol = pmol/L	5 pmol/L
K^+	mEq/L	mmol/L	1	mEq/L × 1 mmol/mEq = mmol/L	0.1 mmol/L
K^+	mg/dL	mmol/L	0.2564	mg/dL ÷ 39 mg/mmol × 10 dL/L = mmol/L	0.1 mmol/L
L-lactate	mg/dL	mmol/L	0.112	mg/dL × 1.11 mmol/mg × 10 dL/L = mmol/L	—
MCHC	g/dL	g/L	10	g/dL × 10 dL/L = g/L	—
Na^+	mEq/L	mmol/L	1	mEq/L × 1 mmol/mEq = mmol/L	1 mmol/L
Na^+	mg/dL	mmol/L	0.4348	mg/dL ÷ 23 mg/mmol × 10 dL/L = mmol/L	1 mmol/L
NEFA	mEq/L	mmol/L	1	mEq/L × mmol/mEq = mmol/L	—
NH_3	μg/dL	μmol/L	0.5871	μg/dL ÷ 17.03 μg/μmol × 10 dL/L = μmol/L	5 μmol/L
NH_4^+	μg/dL	μmol/L	0.5543	μg/dL ÷ 18.04 μg/μmol × 10 dL/L = μmol/L	5 μmol/L
Pi	mg/dL	mmol/L	0.3229	mg/dL ÷ 30.97 mg/mmol × 10 dL/L = mmol/L	0.05 mmol/L
Platelet	#,000/μL	# × 10^9/L	10^9	#,000/μL × 10^6 μL/L = # × 10^9/L	10 × 10^9/L
RBC	# × 10^6/μL	# × 10^{12}/L	10^6	# × 10^6/μL × 10^6 μL/L = # × 10^{12}/L	—

Analyte	Conventional unit	Factor	Conversion	Smallest reportable increment[c]
T_3	ng/dL	0.01536	ng/dL ÷ 651 ng/nmol × 10 dL/L = nmol/L	0.1 nmol/L
T_3	pg/dL	15.36	pg/dL ÷ 651 pg/pmol × 1000 pmol/nmol × 10 dL/L = nmol/L	0.1 nmol/L
tCa^{2+}	mg/dL	0.2495	mg/dL ÷ 40.08 mg/mmol × 10 dL/L = mmol/L	0.02 mmol/L
tCa^{2+}	mEq/L	0.5	mEq/L × 0.5 mmol/mEq = mmol/L	0.02 mmol/L
TIBC	μg/dL	0.1791	μg/dL × 0.01791 μmol/μg × 10 dL/L = μmol/L	1 μmol/L
tMg^{2+}	mg/dL	0.4114	mg/dL ÷ 24.31 mg/mmol × 10 dL/L = mmol/L	0.02 mmol/L
tMg^{2+}	mEq/L	0.5	mEq/L × 0.5 mmol/mEq = mmol/L	0.02 mmol/L
Total protein	g/dL	10	g/dL × 10 dL/L = g/L	1 g/L
Triglyceride	mg/dL	0.01129	mg/dL ÷ 885.7 mg/mmol × 10 dL/L = mmol/L	0.05 mmol/L
TSH	μg/dL	10	μg/dL × 1000 ng/μg ÷ 100 mL/dL = ng/mL	—
tT_4	μg/dL	12.87	μg/dL ÷ 777 μg/μmol × 1000 nmol/μmol × 10 dL/L = nmol/L	1 nmol/L
fT_4	ng/mL	1.287	ng/mL ÷ 777 ng/nmol × 1000 mL/L = nmol/L	1 nmol/L
UN	mg UN/dL	0.3570	mg/dL ÷ 28.01 mg/mmol × 10 dL/L = mmol of urea/L	0.5 mmol/L
Urea	mg urea/dL	0.1665	mg/dL ÷ 60.06 mg/mmol × 10 dL/L = mmol of urea/L	0.5 mmol/L
WBC	#/μL	10^6	#/μL × 10^6 μL/L = # × 10^6/L	—
Xylose	mg/dL	0.06661	mg/dL ÷ 150.1 mg/mmol × 10 dL/L = mmol/L	0.1 mmol/L

[a] ACTH, adrenocorticotropic hormone; Bt, total bilirubin; Cl^-, chloride; COP, colloidal osmotic pressure; Fe, iron; fT_4, free thyroxine; HCO_3^-, bicarbonate; Hgb, hemoglobin; IRG, immunoreactive glucagon; IRI, immunoreactive insulin; K^+, potassium; MCHC, mean cell hemoglobin concentration; Na^+, sodium; NEFA, nonesterified fatty acids; NH_3, ammonia; NH_4^+, ammonium; Pi, inorganic phosphorus; RBC, red blood cell (erythrocyte); SI, Système International d'Unités; T_3, triiodothyronine; tCa^{2+}, total calcium; TIBC, total iron-binding capacity; tMg^{2+}, total magnesium; TSH, thyroid-stimulating hormone; tT_4, total thyroxine; UN, urea nitrogen; and WBC, white blood cell (leukocyte)

[b] *Source:* Lundberg et al.[2]

[c] Recommended smallest reportable increment of the SI unit

    C. You are told that a horse's serum enzyme level was decreased. Does this mean the horse has less of that enzyme? It might. However, it could be that the amount of enzyme (the protein) was not decreased, but the enzyme's activity was inhibited or maybe the structure of the enzyme was defective.

    D. You are told that a cat's reticulocyte percentage is increased. Does this mean that the cat has more reticulocytes in its blood? It might or might not. A percentage is always relative; the same number in the numerator (e.g., number of reticulocytes counted) and a smaller number in the denominator (e.g., total number of erythrocytes counted) will result in an increased percentage.

    E. You are told that the myeloid to erythroid ratio in a cat's marrow is increased. Does the increased ratio mean the cat's marrow contains more myeloid cells, fewer erythroid cells, or both? Or is the ratio increased because the number of myeloid cells is increased more than the increase in erythroid cells? A calculated ratio is always a relative number and must be interpreted accordingly.

    F. You are told that a dog's urine has an increased protein concentration. Because the concentrations of all substances in urine depend on the conservation of water by the kidneys, the increased protein concentration could have resulted from increased water conservation and not increased protein loss via the urinary system.

REFERENCE INTERVALS

I. Reference intervals and their purpose

    A. Results of laboratory tests (laboratory data) on patient samples would be very difficult to interpret without *reference intervals*, which are the results we expect to find in healthy animals. These intervals are used to help detect pathologic states. Other terms that are used as synonyms include *normals*, *normal values*, *normal range*, and *reference range*.

    B. In an attempt to establish uniform usage of terms, the following terms and definitions have been recommended by an Expert Panel of the International Federation of Clinical Chemistry.[3]

       1. *Reference individual*: an animal selected by using defined criteria

       2. *Reference population*: all possible reference individuals

         a. Usually, the number of such individuals is unknown.

         b. In the case of captive wild animals, the total number of animals may be known.

       3. *Reference sample group*: an adequate number of reference individuals selected to represent the reference population

       4. *Reference value*: a value (result) obtained by observation or measurement of a particular substance in a reference individual

       5. *Reference distribution*: the distribution of reference values, which is not necessarily Gaussian (a bell-shaped curve)

       6. *Reference limits*: the lowest value (*lower reference limit*) and the highest value (*upper reference limit*) of the reference interval, as derived from a reference distribution

       7. *Reference interval*: an interval between and including the two reference limits

       8. *Observed value*: a value obtained by observation or measurement that is to be compared to the reference interval

    C. Use of the term *reference range* is discouraged for two reasons.

       1. Statistically, a *range* is the difference between highest and lowest observations; for example, the range is 40 if the highest observation was 50 and the lowest was 10.

2. Some consider a *range* to include all measured values (reference values) from the lowest to the highest (e.g., 10–50). A reference interval does not include all reference values; it contains the values between two reference limits.

D. Using the terms *normal* and *abnormal* to describe laboratory test results can be misleading and is discouraged.

1. A laboratory result can be WRI but still reflect a pathologic process. For example, a serum sodium concentration that is WRI in a dehydrated animal indicates that the animal has lost both water and sodium from its body.

2. Sick animals usually will have some laboratory results that are WRI. Conversely, some apparently healthy animals will have laboratory results outside of the reference interval. Because the laboratory test results for certain diseases overlap between "sick" and "healthy" animals, it is inappropriate to classify a patient as "normal" based just on test results.

3. It is difficult to define "normal" because many variations that may appear to be "abnormal" are caused by physiologic, dietary, environmental, or other nonpathologic factors.

II. Establishment of reference intervals: A complete description of the process of establishing reference intervals is beyond the scope of this book, so readers are referred to other publications.[4,5] The major steps in the process are as follows:

A. Select criteria for reference individuals. Criteria could include species, age, and method of determining health status.

1. Initially, this may seem like a simple task because the criteria define clinically healthy adult animals. Generally, we want to sample a broad group of animals so that the reference interval is useful for a broad group of patients. However, it can become more complex when potentially clinically relevant differences occur because of variations in: (1) breed (e.g., some Akitas have smaller erythrocytes), (2) physiologic state (e.g., milking versus nonmilking cattle or high altitude versus sea level), or (3) nutritional state.

2. Even if a laboratory is successful in establishing reference intervals for adult animals, how about appropriate reference intervals for neonates, nursing animals, or weanlings? Critical assessment of patient values requires that criterion-matched reference intervals be established.

B. Establish a reference sample group. It is preferable to have at least 60 animals that meet selected criteria.

1. Authorities state that at least 120 individuals are needed,[5] but obtaining such numbers is often not accomplished in veterinary medicine. A more realistic number of 60 qualified individuals may be sufficient if a Gaussian distribution is present.[4] Attempts to establish reference intervals with fewer individuals frequently result in weak intervals that are often questioned by clinical observations. A total of 40 reference individuals is a minimum requirement for some methods of establishing reference limits, but the reduced number of individuals probably will not provide the same reference interval as 60 or 120 individuals.

2. Obtaining quality samples from 60 qualified individuals is the most difficult aspect of establishing reference intervals. Typically, samples are collected from animals that are seen because of yearly vaccinations or for elective surgical procedures. Collecting many samples from one kennel, one cattery, one stable, or one herd is typically not recommended because the animals may lack the breed and other physiologic

variations needed for representative reference intervals. For example, reference intervals established for 60 beagles may not be appropriate for healthy dogs of other breeds, but they would be appropriate reference intervals for beagles. Similarly, reference intervals established for cows from one dairy may not be representative of healthy cattle in other dairies or in beef herds.

C. Collect and process the samples. The sample processing should be defined and reflect the processing used for clinical samples. Consideration should be given to the following:

1. Method and site of collection (e.g., jugular versus cephalic vein versus indwelling catheter)
2. Type of sample tube/container or anticoagulant and volume of the sample
3. Storage time and temperature of samples prior to testing

D. Measure or determine the reference values. Analyze the sample for the substance of interest (analyte).

1. This is the most expensive aspect of establishing reference intervals. For example, glucose tests of 60 sera at $5 each cost $300. Since we might measure 20 analytes in sera, with each costing the same amount, $6000 would be spent—and this is for only one species. If the analyses were completed for each major species (bovine, canine, equine, and feline), $24,000 would be spent for the routine chemical assays. A similar amount might be spent for hematologic assays and special assays.
2. This expense is magnified when a laboratory changes laboratory equipment and must establish new reference intervals for a new instrument every 5–7 yr (the expected life span of most instruments).

E. Determine the reference distribution. Apply statistical methods to determine whether data have a Gaussian or a skewed distribution.

1. Many analyte concentrations will fit a normal (Gaussian) distribution, especially those analyte concentrations that are tightly regulated by physiologic systems (e.g., glucose, Na^+, K^+, and fCa^{2+} concentrations).
2. Many analyte concentrations (e.g., serum enzyme activities) will not fit a Gaussian distribution; their data may have positive or negative skewness.

F. Determine reference limits and reference intervals. Use methods to remove outliers (e.g., the range test)[6] and then select the central 95 % of the reference values.

1. Limits may be defined by a stated fraction of reference values that are less than or equal to a certain result. For example, 2.5 % of the values are > 150, and 2.5 % of values are < 50, so the reference limits are 50 and 150. The reference interval would be 50–150.
2. When data have been shown to fit a Gaussian distribution, parametric or nonparametric methods can be used to establish reference limits. Parametric methods generate values that represent the mean ± 2 sd. Nonparametric methods may be more appropriate than parametric methods when the number of reference individuals is low.
3. When the distribution is not Gaussian, the data should either be transformed into a Gaussian distribution, or, more commonly, the data within the top and bottom 2.5 percentiles are removed by nonparametric methods.
4. Figure 1.2 shows the differences between Gaussian and skewed distributions and the reference intervals obtained from such distributions.

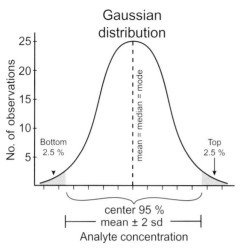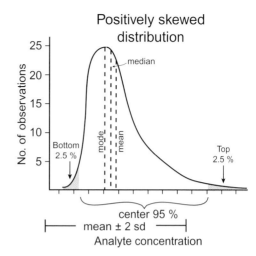

Fig. 1.2. Reference distribution.
- In the **left graph**, the reference values conformed to a Gaussian distribution. If data have this distribution, then mean ± 2 sd will represent the central 95 % of the reference values and thus the reference interval. If values have a Gaussian distribution, the mean, median, and mode values will be equal.
- In the **right graph**, the reference values had positive skewness. If data have this distribution, nonparametric methods are used to determine the central 95 % of the values. If the interval represented by mean ± 2 sd were calculated, the lower reference limit would be below the lowest reference value, and the upper reference limit would exclude more than the top 2.5 % of the reference values. Therefore, mean ± 2 sd would not be an accurate representation of the values expected in healthy animals. The mean, median, and mode values will be different if the reference values have a non-Gaussian distribution.

III. Use of reference intervals
   A. It is important to understand that *most* reference intervals represent results expected in 95 % of the healthy animals (i.e., in 19 of 20 healthy animals).
     1. Therefore, 1 of 20 healthy animals is expected to have a measured value outside of the reference interval. The value that is outside the reference interval but still represents a value from a healthy animal is expected to be close to the reference limits. A marked difference from the reference interval probably represents a pathologic state.
     2. When examining multiple test results for one animal, it is important to remember that this 95 % chance of a value from a healthy animal falling WRI applies to each result separately.
       a. Thus, in a panel of 20 assays, each with a 5 % chance of being outside of the reference interval even without pathologic change, there is a 64 % chance for at least one value to be outside the reference interval (see Reference Intervals, sect. III.A.2.b). With a panel of five results, there is a 23 % chance. However, that value should be close to the lower or upper reference limit. This concept is important when laboratory tests are requested for clinically healthy animals for a yearly health profile or a geriatric profile.
       b. This concept can also be explained using multivariate comparison calculations.[6] Because there is a 95 % (0.95) probability in healthy animals that each result is

WRI, the probability that all "n" values are WRI is 0.95^n, and the probability that not all values are WRI is $1 - 0.95^n$ (where n is the number of observations). Thus, for a panel of 20 test results, $100 \times (1 - 0.95^{20}) = 64\%$, so there is a 64% chance that at least one value is outside the reference interval.

B. Not all reference intervals accurately reflect expected findings in a population of interest. This may be because of such problems as an inadequate procedure of establishing the values, a difference between reference and test populations, or a change in methods or instrumentation by the laboratory without an appropriate change in reference intervals.

C. Laboratories should provide information about their reference values when requested. Such requests are particularly appropriate when first contemplating use of a laboratory. This enables evaluation of how likely it is that the values reflect health in the population of interest. Requested information might include the following:
   1. Number of reference individuals
   2. Ages, breeds, and genders of reference individuals
   3. Criteria for inclusion as a reference individual
   4. Methods for establishing reference intervals

IV. *Reference limits* versus *decision thresholds* (limits)
   A. As defined above (Reference Intervals, sect. I.B.6), *reference limits* are the highest value or lowest value of the reference interval as derived from a reference distribution; a reference interval includes values expected in 95 % of the healthy animals. These values are used diagnostically to help detect pathologic states in ill animals. A patient value that is above or below the reference limits may indicate the presence of a pathologic state.

   B. A *decision threshold* (sometimes called *decision limit* or *cutoff point* or *cutoff value*) is a value that is used to classify a result as positive or negative for a disease or to decide whether to treat or not to treat.[7,8] As described in the section on Diagnostic Properties and Predictive Value of Laboratory Assays, a decision threshold may not be a reference limit. Decision thresholds can also be used to estimate a cost to benefit ratio for diagnostic methods.

   C. The term *decision limit* is also used in the context of a *critical decision limit*, which is a value that is used for making critical therapeutic decisions. For example, a critical decision limit for serum calcium concentration may be 15.0 mg/dL, meaning that aggressive therapy is initiated whenever a serum calcium concentration is greater than 15.0 mg/dL. In contrast, the *upper reference limit* might be 12.0 mg/dL, and a *decision threshold* for a hypercalcemic disorder might be 12.5 mg/dL.

QUALITY OF LABORATORY RESULTS

I. Major determinants: Laboratory test results will be of the most benefit if they are consistently correct from patient to patient, day to day, and month to month. Three major factors determine whether results are valid: (1) quality of sample, (2) quality of analysis, (3) quality of laboratory and patient records. When results are not what a veterinarian expects, he or she might say, "I do not believe those results; there must have been a lab error." When such conclusions are formed, it is important to remember that there are many potential reasons for an erroneous laboratory test result. Errors may be preanalytical, analytical, or postanalytical.

A. A laboratory test result can only be as good as the sample. *Preanalytical errors*, which are relatively common, arise from problems with sample collection and processing. These errors can be minimized with attention to the following:
   1. Sample collection
      a. Properly prepared patient (e.g., the animal should be fasted for at least 8 h prior to collection of most blood samples)
      b. Proper collection technique (e.g., atraumatic venipuncture to minimize hemolysis and activation of clotting proteins and platelets)
      c. Proper collection container (e.g., sterile versus nonsterile or clot tube versus an EDTA tube)
      d. Proper anticoagulants when needed (e.g., EDTA versus heparin, or sodium heparin versus lithium heparin)
      e. Adequate volume for assays (e.g., to obtain 1 mL of serum, a volume of at least 3 mL of blood is usually needed)
   2. Sample handling
      a. Proper labeling of all specimens (e.g., animal identification by name or number, date, and time of collection)
      b. Samples kept at appropriate temperature prior to and after processing, during shipment, or during storage (e.g., 25 °C, 4 °C, or −25 °C)
      c. Prompt processing (e.g., for a labile analyte, process immediately so the analyte does not deteriorate)
B. *Analytical errors* should be minimized by attention to the following:
   1. Method appropriate for species (e.g., an instrument designed to measure the relatively large human erythrocytes may not provide accurate measurement of smaller erythrocytes from the domestic mammals)
   2. Quality of instruments and equipment (i.e., generally "you get what you pay for," but a quality instrument remains a quality instrument only if it is properly maintained)
   3. Quality of reagents (e.g., fresh and within the expiration date, being used according to instructions)
   4. Quality of laboratory technique (e.g., person-to-person variation, training of person, and inherent procedural difficulty)
   5. Quality control program (quality assurance program) (e.g., the laboratory personnel subscribe to and adhere to internal assessment procedures to assure that all parts of the quality analysis of the sample are maintained daily)
C. *Postanalytical errors* can be minimized with attention to the following:
   1. Transcriptional errors minimized (e.g., errors can be made during manual transcription of results to a laboratory report or during keyboard entering of data into computers)
   2. Data presented in a report that is easy to read and thus reduces the likelihood of incorrect interpretation

II. Analytical properties of assays: From the analytical perspective, the best clinical laboratory assay is one that consistently measures the true concentration of the substance and at concentrations that are clinically relevant. When evaluating and comparing laboratory assays, five properties can be assessed:
   A. *Analytical precision*:[9] the ability of an assay to get the same result if a sample is analyzed several times; also called *reproducibility* or *random analytical error* (Fig. 1.3a)

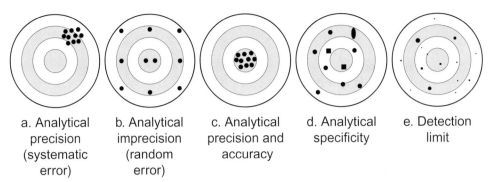

| a. Analytical precision (systematic error) | b. Analytical imprecision (random error) | c. Analytical precision and accuracy | d. Analytical specificity | e. Detection limit |

Fig. 1.3. Illustrations of analytical properties of assays.

a. *Analytical precision (systematic error)*: Because the ten holes in the target are tightly clustered, the target shooter was precise even though consistently inaccurate.

b. *Analytical imprecision (random error)*: Because the holes in the target are evenly distributed, the average of ten shots is exactly in the middle of the target area. Thus, the shooter was statistically accurate but imprecise.

c. *Analytical precision and accuracy*: Because all ten holes in the target are tightly clustered in the middle of the target, the shooter was accurate and precise.

d. *Analytical specificity*: Of the ten holes in the target, seven are round, two are square, and one is oval. Of the ten observations, the shooter probably created seven, and three were created by other factors. Thus, the presence of holes in the target is not specific for the shooter's actions.

e. *Detection limit and analytical sensitivity*: How many holes can you see in the target? The smallest hole that you can reliably detect is the detection limit of your eyes. Analytical sensitivity in this context is the smallest change in hole sizes that your eyes can reliably differentiate. If your eyes can reliably detect the different sizes of all holes, then the sensitivity limit has not been reached. If your eyes can differentiate the changes in the four largest holes but not the other holes, the sensitivity limit is between the fourth and fifth holes. Each shot was made with a bullet whose diameter was 75 % of the previous shot.

1. The need for analytical precision depends on the degree of variation that can be accepted as random variation (error). When management of a case requires that small changes in concentration reflect a biologic change and not analytical variation, an assay needs to have high precision. However, if a wide range of measured values can be accepted, then high precision is not needed.

2. Control solutions are used to assess assay performance. Repeated analysis of control solutions enables assessment of precision.

   a. A control solution contains an analyte's concentration that can be a known specific concentration (like a standard solution), but more frequently the concentration is determined by multiple measurements using the same assay for which precision is being assessed.

   b. If results for a control solution are within acceptable limits, then the assay was probably performed correctly and thus the patient's result is probably valid. Control solution results that are outside acceptable limits suggest instrument malfunction, deteriorated reagents, or poor analytical techniques. The patient's result determined by the same assay may or may not be accurate.

3. Precision is frequently expressed in clinical laboratories by the method's CV (Eq. 1.1).

$$\text{CV (expressed as a percentage)} = \frac{\text{standard deviation}}{\text{mean}} \times 100 \qquad \textbf{(1.1.)}$$

a. A method's CV is determined from replicate analysis within an assay run and between different runs of the same assay.
   (1) A *within-assay CV* represents the random error that is expected when one sample is analyzed multiple times in one run of an assay. If an assay has a poor within-assay CV, the sample's analyte concentration is determined by analyzing the sample in duplicate or triplicate and then calculating a mean concentration.
   (2) A *between-assay CV* represents the random error within one run of the assay plus the error from additional runs of the assay by using the same sample. The within-assay CV will be smaller than the between-assay CV.
b. The clinical relevance of an assay's CV is determined by many factors.
   (1) If critical clinical decisions are made when changes in an analyte's concentration are minimal, then the assay must have a low CV (high precision). Otherwise, the diagnostician would not know if the change in analyte concentration is due to a true change that occurred in the animal or if the change represents analytical error.
   (2) An assay's CV will typically vary with the analyte's concentration. Higher CV values may be found at the lower and upper limits of the assay's analytical range. Within the analytical range, CV values are typically higher at the lower analyte concentrations because CV values are expressed as percentages.
      (a) If an assay has a CV of 10 % at all concentrations, then the assay's standard deviation would be 0.1 mg/dL at an analyte concentration of 1 mg/dL, 1 mg/dL at an analyte concentration of 10 mg/dL, 10 mg/dL at an analyte concentration of 100 mg/dL, etc. Depending on the analyte and the amount of biologic variation, a CV of 10 % can be completely unacceptable analytical variation or be very acceptable.
      (b) If an assay's standard deviation is 10 mg/dL at all concentrations, the assay's CV values would be 50 % at a mean concentration of 20 mg/dL, 10 % at a mean of 100 mg/dL, and 1 % at a mean of 1000 mg/dL.
   (3) Knowing the amount of analytical variation for an assay is helpful when trying to determine whether a change in a patient's data represents analytical variation or a true biologic change. One way to approach this decision is using an assay's USD. *USD* is an average of standard deviation values from 3–6 consecutive months of quality assurance values. If a change in a patient's data is less than twice the USD, the change may be only analytical variation. If a change in patient data samples is greater than three times an assay's USD, then the change is probably due to biologic variation. The *three times USD* is an estimate of significant change limit;[10] a change in data of at least three times the USD is probably a significant biologic change and not simply analytical variation.
      (a) If the USD for sodium concentration at 150 mmol/L is 1.5 mmol/L and a patient's sodium concentration is 150 mmol/L on day 1 and 148 mmol/L on day 2, then the change of 2 mmol/L may be due to

analytical variation since it is less than twice the USD. However, a value of 145 mmol/L on day 2 (a change greater than three times the USD) probably represents a true biologic change.

    (b) If the USD for blood neutrophil concentration is 1000/μL at a neutrophil concentration of 10,000/μL, then neutrophil concentration in a second sample needs to be < 7000/μL or > 13,000/μL to be reliably considered a biologic change if the first sample had a neutrophil concentration of 10,000/μL.

    (4) The CV percentages and USD values may vary considerably between assay methods, and the percentages or values are frequently not known by the diagnostician. However, such information can improve the interpretation of laboratory data because changes can be recognized as potential analytical variation or confidently classified as biologic change.

B. *Analytical accuracy* (IFCC definition):[9] the closeness of the agreement between the measured value of an analyte and its "true" value (Fig. 1.3c)

  1. The methods of establishing the "true" values vary considerably. At times, the true value is established by a reference method (e.g., a method developed by the NIST). If such standards have not been developed, the "true" value might represent the mean concentration determined by numerous observations using an assay that is accepted as the best available.

  2. Typically, accuracy of a clinical assay is assessed by comparison of its results to the results of an accepted reference method, a method that has been accepted by a standardization group as providing a true value. Optimally, the assay that is accepted as the reference method is also precise so that only a few observations are needed to determine the true value (Fig. 1.3c).

  3. Standard solutions

    a. The accuracy of the clinical assay may be assessed by measuring an analyte's concentration in a reference standard solution whose concentration was determined by a reference method.

    b. Reference standard solutions are not the same as calibration standard solutions. Calibration standard solutions are commercially prepared, are used to calibrate an instrument or method, and should closely agree with reference standard solutions.

C. *Analytical specificity*:[9] the ability of an assay to detect only the substance of interest (analyte) or freedom from interfering substances (Fig. 1.3d)

  1. Analytical specificity is related to analytical accuracy because an assay cannot be accurate if a nonspecific reaction is occurring.

  2. The need for analytical specificity varies directly with the likelihood of interfering substances. A serum glucose assay may be designed to react with all hexoses. Such specificity may be acceptable if glucose is the only hexose in serum that is at a sufficient concentration to be detected by the assay. Other glucose assays may be designed to react only with glucose even if other hexoses might be present in the sample.

  3. Substances may interfere with an assay in many ways.

    a. The substance may be very similar chemically, and the assay may react with either the analyte or the interfering substance.

    b. The substance may produce the same response that is detected in the assay system.

        (1) The presence of glucose may be detected when a chemical reaction produces hydrogen peroxide (H_2O_2). A substance may interfere with the assay by having the same oxidizing properties as H_2O_2.

        (2) In spectrophotometric assays, the presence of lipids, bilirubin, or hemoglobin may interfere with light transmission through a sample, and thus the results of the assay are changed by artifactual spectral changes and not by a chemical reaction.

    4. Depending on how a substance interferes with an assay, it may lead either to falsely increased or to falsely decreased concentrations—positive interference or negative interference, respectively.

  D. *Detection limit* (IUPAC definition):[9] the smallest concentration or quantity of an analyte that can be detected with reasonable certainty for a given analytical range (Fig. 1.3e)

    1. An assay's detection limit involves the ability of the assay to differentiate background "noise" from a true change because of the presence of an analyte. The detection limit defines the lowest value of an assay's analytical range; *analytical range* is the range of values over which the assay can provide reliable results.

    2. If an analyte is relatively abundant (e.g., serum Na^+), then a detection limit of 100 mmol/L may be adequate. For substances that are relatively rare (e.g., aldosterone), a detection limit of 100 pmol/L may be needed to be clinically useful.

  E. *Analytical sensitivity* (IUPAC definition):[9] slope of the calibration curve and the ability of an analytical procedure to produce a change in the signal for a defined change of the quantity

    1. In other terms, an assay's analytical sensitivity is how much change of the analyte (concentration, property, etc.) is needed for the assay to detect the change. For example, an assay that can differentiate 50 mg/dL from 51 mg/dL has better analytical sensitivity than an assay that can only differentiate 5.0 g/dL (or 5000 mg/dL) from 5.1 g/dL (5100 mg/dL).

    2. Analytical sensitivity should not be confused with detection limit. The two are related because both relate to small changes in concentration. However, *analytical sensitivity* applies to changes within an assay's analytical range, whereas *detection limit* applies to the lowest limit of the analytical range.

III. Quality assurance

  A. Quality assurance concepts

    1. Every laboratory assay has the potential to produce erroneous results because of a variety of analytical factors (e.g., reagent deterioration, pipetting errors, incubation errors, and electronic interference). To detect errors, every laboratory or clinical practice that analyzes samples should have a quality assurance program that is designed to detect unacceptable errors in its assays and assure that only quality results are generated.

    2. Each laboratory assay has some random analytical error (see Quality of Laboratory Results, sect. II.A). Typically, manual assays have more random errors than do automated methods because people generally cannot reproduce their work as well as a machine can. Variations in results that are caused by random error should have a Gaussian or normal distribution (see Fig. 1.2). With that distribution, 95 % of the results should fall within the interval that is equal to mean ± 2 sd. If the same sample is analyzed 20 times, 19 of 20 results are

expected to be within that interval. But it is also important to recognize that 1 of 20 results is expected to be outside of that interval—even when the assay is performing well!

3. Another key concept in quality assurance programs is that acceptable random error for a clinical assay should be based on what is considered to be a biologically significant change in the result. If within-individual and between-individual biologic variations of a particular analyte are small, and clinical decisions are made when there is only a minor change in a laboratory test result, then the random error of the assay needs to be relatively small. However, if clinical decisions are made only when there is a marked change in a laboratory test result, a larger random error may be acceptable. Two examples illustrate these concepts:

   a. Serum [Na$^+$] in most healthy mammals is near 150 mmol/L. If a patient has a serum [Na$^+$] of 150 mmol/L on day 1 and 160 mmol/L on day 2, most clinicians will conclude that something has happened in the animal to alter the serum [Na$^+$] significantly or that there has been change because of biologic, pathologic, or therapeutic reasons. Therefore, for the serum Na$^+$ assay to be clinically valuable, its acceptable random error definitely needs to be < 10 mmol/L. Otherwise, erroneous decisions may be made because of random analytical error.

   b. Serum [glucose] in most healthy mammals is near 100 mg/dL. If a patient has a serum [glucose] of 100 mg/dL on day 1 and 110 mg/dL on day 2, most clinicians will conclude that such changes are within expected biologic variation; that is, there has not been a change for biologic, pathologic, or therapeutic reasons. Therefore, for the serum glucose assay to be clinically valuable, its acceptable random error can be larger than the random error of the serum Na$^+$ assay.

B. Westgard rules. James O. Westgard, Ph.D., is a leader in the field of quality assurance programs for clinical laboratories. He has developed a system that is designed to decide whether an assay's run (all patient samples assayed at the same time as the control sample) is "in control" or "out of control." Details of this system are beyond the scope of this book, but an excellent Web site explains the key concepts (http://www.westgard.com).

   1. A quality assurance program should be designed so that it detects analytical errors that may be of clinical significance. All measurements contain errors, and the two major types are random error and systematic error. Random error is caused by factors that randomly affect the measurements, such as variations in dispensed volume of reagent or sample. Systematic error is a reproducible inaccuracy that will consistently result in values that are too high or too low. The Westgard system is designed to detect both types of errors.

   2. *Westgard rules* are a series of rules that are applied systematically, either singly or in combinations.[11] This system is applied to the results obtained for control samples that are analyzed concurrently with patient samples. In his abbreviation system, "s" stands for standard deviation.

      a. 1_{2s} rule: A run is rejected when a single control measurement exceeds the mean plus 2s or the mean minus 2s of previous control sample values, or it serves as a warning system to initiate additional inspection of control data.

      b. 1_{3s} rule: A run is rejected when a single control measurement exceeds the mean plus 3s or the mean minus 3s of previous control sample values. This rule is primarily sensitive to random error.

   c. 2_{2s} rule: A run is rejected when two consecutive control measurements exceed the same mean plus 2s or the same mean minus 2s of previous control sample values. This rule is primarily sensitive to systematic error.

   d. R_{4s} rule: A run is rejected when one control measurement in a group exceeds the mean plus 2s and another exceeds the mean minus 2s. This rule is primarily sensitive to random error.

   e. 4_{1s} rule: A run is rejected when four consecutive control measurements exceed the same mean plus 1s or the same mean minus 1s control limit. This rule is primarily sensitive to systematic error.

   f. 10_x rule: A run is rejected when ten consecutive control measurements fall on one side of the mean (this rule is sometimes modified to either an 8_x rule or a 12_x rule). This rule is primarily sensitive to systematic error.

3. Selection of the appropriate Westgard rules to control an assay depends on the analytical precision of the assay and the acceptable random analytical error. The less imprecise the assay is, the more likely it is that a high or low control sample value will truly indicate a problem with the assay and the less stringent the Westgard rules need to be to keep the assay in control. The more imprecise the assay is, the more difficult it is to know whether a high or low control sample value is caused by analytical variation, so more stringent Westgard rules will be required.

4. When an assay's run is rejected, the results for the control samples were unacceptable and thus the results for the patient samples may be erroneous because of an analytical error. When the control sample results are unacceptable, laboratory personnel should isolate the factor that is causing the error. The error could be related to (1) the operator, (2) the protocol, (3) the reagents and materials, or (4) the analyzer. When the problem is found, appropriate corrective actions are taken (e.g., change reagents, clean pipette, or recalibrate the machine), and then the control samples and patient samples are reanalyzed.

5. A common method of monitoring the results of the control samples is to plot them in a Levey-Jennings control chart (Fig. 1.4). However, such plots do not help us decide what is acceptable or unacceptable variation in a clinical laboratory assays.

6. Dr. Westgard has also addressed this issue in his work using concepts of total quality management and Six Sigma Quality Management (http://www.westgard.com/sixsigmabook.html).[12] These concepts have been accepted by some international groups as the preferred quality assurance method. The understanding and application of the Six Sigma Quality Management system requires considerable effort; a few key concepts introduce the topic:

   a. *Sigma* refers to the Greek letter σ, which stands for standard deviation—a statistical index used to express random deviation from the mean (central tendency).

   b. A *sigma* classification for a test refers to its precision relative to the amount of acceptable error (total random and analytical variation that is acceptable). If, based on knowledge of biologic variations, we interpret two values that are within 10 mg/dL of each other at a decision threshold to be the same, then we will consider such error as acceptable or allowable. Thus, the allowable total error (TE_a) for an assay is 10 mg/dL at a decision threshold. Errors of that magnitude or less will not affect interpretation of the results. TE_a must be determined at clinical decision thresholds, the values at which decisions about the presence or absence of disease are made.

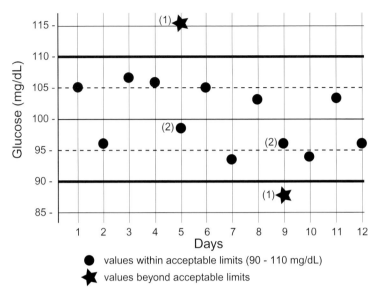

Fig. 1.4. Levey-Jennings control chart for a glucose control solution. Quality assurance data for 12 d of testing are displayed; each day, the measured [glucose] in the control solution is plotted on the chart. Previous analyses established that the acceptable limits for the control solution are 100 ± 10 mg/dL (mean ± 2 sd). On days 5 and 9, the first measured concentration (1) was outside acceptable limits. After corrective actions were taken (e.g., recalibrate, new reagent set, and clean pipette), a second measured concentration (2) was within acceptable limits so values measured in patient samples could then be considered reliable. For some assays, at least two control solutions are analyzed with each set of patient samples, and results of each control solutions are plotted in separate Levey-Jennings control charts. For other assays, control solutions might be analyzed with each shift (e.g., day and night) or each day. The frequency of analyzing control solutions is determined by several factors but with the primary goal of detecting unacceptable assay performance before a patient's result is used for diagnostic or therapeutic decisions.

c. For theoretical assay A with a TE_a of 10 mg/dL, analysis of control solution with an analyte concentration near the decision threshold reveals a standard deviation of 5 mg/dL. Assuming there is no systematic error (*bias*), this assay would be called a *two-sigma* assay because the TE_a divided by its standard deviation is 2. When designing a quality assurance program for this assay, there would be strict criteria established with several control solutions so that unacceptable errors could be detected when present. By random error alone, about 1 of 20 values is expected to be unacceptable.

d. For theoretical assay B, also with a TE_a of 10 mg/dL, analysis of control solution with an analyte concentration near the decision threshold reveals a standard deviation of 2 mg/dL. Assuming there is no systematic error (bias), this assay would be called a *five-sigma* assay because the TE_a divided by its standard deviation is 5. When designing a quality assurance program for this assay, there would be relatively loose criteria established with two control solutions because it is very unlikely that its random error would create changes that are clinically relevant (i.e., less than one unacceptable value per million assays).

   e. In this system, the ideal assay is a *six-sigma* assay because an unacceptable error would occur only 0.002 times per million assays. In a *six-sigma* assay, six standard deviations of variation are within the acceptable tolerance limits of the process.

C. Every clinical laboratory (from large reference laboratories to small in-house laboratories) should have a quality assurance program to monitor the performance of each assay. To do so, several steps must be taken:

   1. There must be a commitment by laboratory staff to use the program.
   2. There must be a financial commitment to the program because the analysis of control samples results in an expense that must be incorporated into the cost of analyzing patient samples.
   3. The laboratory staff needs to decide which assays will be included in the program. Some assays/procedures are very difficult to monitor because there is not a suitable control material (e.g., urinalysis sediment examination). In such situations, other methods may be used for quality assurance (e.g., replicate analysis of the same sample by two people).
   4. Laboratory staff must decide on the appropriate decision criteria for accepting or rejecting a run (or the results for control samples).
   5. For optimal use of quality assurance materials, their use should mirror operation of the instrument for patient samples.
      a. The person who will analyze the patient sample should analyze the control material because one of the most common sources of analytical error is the operator.
      b. The control material should test the entire operation of the analyzer and not just be what is called an *electronic control*, a control that may simply ensure that the instrument's circuitry is functioning without actually running a sample through it.

DIFFERENCES IN LABORATORY METHODS AND THEIR RESULTS

I. Not only do veterinarians face challenges of species variations, they also must deal with the different results generated by different laboratories and different laboratory methods. There are many potential reasons for the differences; some of the differences are due to random errors that are not preventable, others are caused by analytical or systematic errors (bias), and others are because of poor analytical methods that produce inaccurate results.

II. Examples of differences
    A. Figure 1.5 illustrates results of a survey completed by the Veterinary Laboratory Association (VLA) as part of a quality assurance program. For the survey, the VLA distributed aliquots of a pooled serum to laboratories that subscribed to its quality assurance program. After analysis of the distributed sample, each subscribing laboratory sent its results to the association for compilation and analysis. The association then distributed the results of the analyses. The type of program is sometimes referred to as a *proficiency testing* program and can be used to determine the validity of a laboratory's assay. Ideally, the results of an individual laboratory could be compared to the results established by a laboratory that analyzed the same sample by using a recognized reference method. Without such a value, the *proficiency testing* provides a method of periodically monitoring an assay's performance compared to other laboratories.

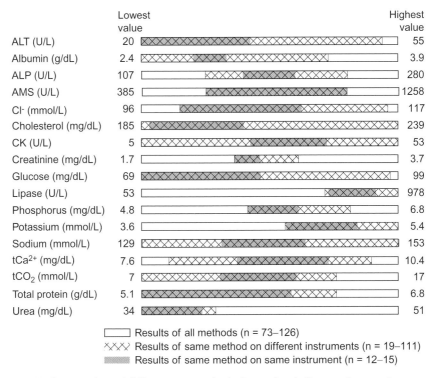

Fig. 1.5. Results from similar and different assay methods that analyzed aliquots of one canine serum sample as part of one survey completed by the Veterinary Laboratory Association (VLA) during 2000. Ranges for most measured analyte concentrations or enzyme activities were extracted from graphs within the survey's report, but data for ALP, AMS, and LPS activities were obtained from the VLA because graphed bars were too small to be reliably interpreted.

- For nearly every measured analyte, the difference between the lowest and highest values would be considered clinically relevant if they represented values obtained from the same animal but different samples.
- The greatest differences occur when different assay methods are used, but frequently there were large differences when the same assay method was used on different machines (e.g., ALT, ALP, AMS, cholesterol, CK, glucose, sodium, and tCa^{2+}).
- For the data used in this figure, the "results of the same method on same instrument" represent data for the same dry chemistry reagent system on the same type of instrument. Even so, the lack of agreement emphasizes the need for the establishment of reference intervals by each laboratory.

ALT, alanine transaminase; ALP, alkaline phosphatase; AMS, amylase; Cl$^-$, chloride; CK, creatine kinase; tCa^{2+}, total calcium; and tCO$_2$, total carbon dioxide.

   B. Careful review of the data in Fig. 1.5 can be disturbing because there are marked differences in the results generated by laboratories. It is beyond the scope of this textbook to describe the possible reasons for the differences in detail. In general, the results may vary because of one or more of the following:
      1. Commercial standard solutions vary and may be poorly calibrated. Although there are strict requirements for development of human assays, there are not the same requirements for veterinary assays.

2. For assays that measure enzyme activity or depend on enzymatic activity within the assay, there can be marked differences in enzyme activity because of different substrates (reagents), reaction temperatures, or pH of assay systems.

3. Even though two laboratories might have the same chemistry instrument and assay method, the laboratories might purchase reagents from different companies. The reagents might have the same constituents but at different concentrations.

C. Because of the potential marked differences in results determined by laboratories, several recommendations are made:

1. Sample collection, processing, and transport should follow policies that minimize the chances of sample damage.

2. Samples should be submitted to *veterinary* laboratories that adhere to stringent quality assurance guidelines.

3. Your patient's results should be compared against appropriate reference intervals established for the same assay method in the same laboratory.

   a. Reference intervals established for another assay can be very misleading. Comparison against reference intervals published in textbooks is discouraged. However, if done, the potential differences due to analytical variation must be considered.

   b. Reference intervals provided by the manufacturer of an instrument should be carefully scrutinized. The manufacturer should provide details about the reference intervals, including the criteria used to select reference individuals, the number of animals in the reference sample group, and the method of determining the reference limits. If the manufacturer's reference intervals are going to be used, then split samples should be analyzed by the manufacturer and your laboratory to ascertain whether there is excellent agreement in the assays' results. Alternatively, samples from 20 healthy animals could be assayed; only 1 of 20 values should fall outside the reference interval if it was based on the central 95 % of the reference population. If more than one value is outside the manufacturer's reference interval, the reference interval may not be appropriate.

4. A good diagnostician detects and confirms abnormalities. If a laboratory result is not consistent with your impression of the case, you should ask the laboratory to repeat the assay or you should submit another sample to confirm a significant abnormality.

5. You should establish a strong professional relationship with your laboratory's personnel. The quality laboratory will strive to provide you quality and timely results. You should strive to provide the laboratory with quality samples.

COMPARISON OF ASSAYS

I.   As described in the previous section (Quality of Laboratory Results, sect. II.B), it is sometimes necessary to compare the results of assays to determine the degree of agreement between two assays. Assays are in agreement when they produce essentially the same result from the same sample.

A. Importantly, results may be strongly correlated but not in agreement. Linear regression can be used to establish a relationship between independent and dependent variables. If two assays are attempting to measure the same analyte, they should have a relationship, but neither measured value is a dependent variable.

B. The methods of comparing assays and guidelines for completing a comparison were recently reviewed.[13]

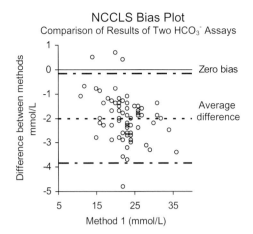

Fig. 1.6. NCCLS and Altman-Bland bias plots. The results were tabulated and entered in a software program (Analyse-it) to generate the bias plots.
- In the NCCLS bias plot, the differences between HCO_3^- concentrations measured by two assays (method 2 − method 1 in this example) are plotted on the y-axis; the concentrations measured by method 1 are plotted on the x-axis. The average difference for all samples is calculated; in this comparison, the average difference is 2 mmol/L (bias, − 2 mmol/L). Lines representing ± 2 sd of the differences are also displayed. The NCCLS bias plot is the preferred plot when a second method is being compared to a reference method or an established method.
- The Altman-Bland bias plot is the same as the NCCLS bias plot except the average of the two measured values (average of method 1 and method 2 concentrations) are plotted on the x-axis. The advantage of the Altman-Bland bias plot is that neither method is considered to be the more accurate method.
HCO_3^-, bicarbonate.

II.   There are four major methods of assessing agreement of assays. It is beyond the scope of this book to address the application of these methods, but veterinarians should be aware of what these methods provide.
   A. Bias plots (Fig. 1.6)
      1. NCCLS or CLSI bias plot (NCCLS is an abbreviation for National Committee for Clinical Laboratory Standards that has been renamed the Clinical Laboratory Standards Institute)
         a. The NCCLS plot displays the degree of agreement between a new method and the old method (or reference method). The values determined by the old/reference method are plotted on the x-axis, and the difference between values determined by the new and old method is plotted on the y-axis. Besides plotting the paired data points, the mean and standard deviations of the differences are also plotted.
         b. The graph displays a positive bias (mean difference > 0) or a negative bias (mean difference < 0), and may indicate either a *constant bias* (a difference between the results that is constant over all values) or a *proportional bias* (a difference between the results that changes proportionately with the magnitude of the result).
      2. The Altman-Bland bias plot is similar but different: the *average* of the two values is plotted on the x-axis and the difference between the two values is plotted on the y-axis. This method does not assume that either the new or the old method is more accurate.

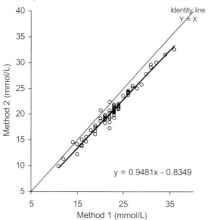
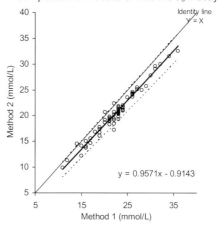

Fig. 1.7. Deming and Passing & Bablok method comparisons. The results were tabulated and entered in a software program (Analyse-it) to generate the comparison graphs. The analysis of the two graphs reveals a mild proportional bias; that is, the absolute difference between the two methods increases at higher concentrations.

- In the Deming method, the results of the two assays are plotted on the y-axis and the x-axis, and a best-fit regression line is drawn and compared to the identity line ($y = x$). The equation for the best-fit line ($y = mx + b$) and associated confidence intervals are used to detect constant bias or proportional bias. In this method of comparison, imprecision of the assays should be normally distributed.
- The Passing and Bablok method comparison is very similar to the Deming method, but the imprecision need not be normally distributed and can have nonconstant variance over the sampling range. The 95 % confidence interval of the best-fit line is also displayed.

HCO_3^-, bicarbonate.

B. Deming method comparison (Fig. 1.7)
1. In the Deming method comparison, the values obtained for a given sample are plotted with the new method on the y-axis and the old (or comparison) method on the x-axis. An equation for the best-fit line ($y = mx + b$) and the 95 % confidence intervals for the slope and y-intercepts are calculated.
   a. A *proportional bias* is detected if the 95 % confidence interval for the slope does not include 1 (i.e., slope of the identity line).
   b. A *constant bias* is detected if the 95 % confidence interval for the y-intercept does not include 0 (i.e., y-intercept of the identity line).
2. The regression equation ($y = mx + b$) has been used to calculate or predict values. If the x value is known, the equation predicts what the y value would be.[14]
   a. Regression analysis is designed for the x value to be an independent variable and the y value to be dependent on x. However, the results of two methods are both independent variables.
   b. Regression analysis to compute a correlation coefficient (r value) is designed to assess the strength of agreement against the null hypothesis of no relationship. It does not make sense that there is no relationship if two assays are designed to measure the same analyte concentration.

      c. The correlation coefficient depends on the range of data in the sample.[15] A large range of data will tend to have a higher correlation than will a small range, even when most values are clustered in a narrow range and a single value stretches the range more broadly.

      d. Figures 1.6 and 1.7 show excellent correlation (r = 0.98) between data sets, but the bias plots illustrate there is a bias between the assays.

    3. In the Deming method, imprecision is allowed in both methods and the variances must be normally distributed (i.e., it is a parametric analysis method). The data from the comparison are improved if the compared data are obtained from duplicate measurements by both methods.

C. Passing and Bablok method comparison (Fig. 1.7)

    1. The Passing and Bablok method is similar to the Deming method in that imprecision is allowed in both methods and their graphs are constructed the same way. However, the Passing and Bablok method does not require that the variances in the data sets have normal distributions (i.e., it is a nonparametric method).

    2. This method also includes a plot to assess linearity. If several data points fall on one side of the identity line, then the relationship between the two methods may not be linear.

D. Kappa agreement (Fig. 1.8)

    1. This method can be used when laboratory results are in a categorical scale such as 1+, 2+, 3+, and 4+ or trace, mild, moderate, and marked. A 2+ value may not be twice that of a 1+, and a 4+ may not be twice the value of a 2+.

    2. The calculated kappa value provides a guide to the degree of agreement. The size or degree of disagreement is not considered with the standard kappa method, but it is with the weighted kappa method.

Comparison of Urine Heme Reactions:
Reflectance Photometric versus Visual Grading

		Reflectance Photometric Grading				
		negative	trace	1	2	3
Visual Grading	negative	25	1	0	0	0
	trace	12	15	3	0	0
	1	0	6	15	1	0
	2	0	0	5	5	1
	3	0	0	0	2	9

Weighted kappa value: 0.78

Interpretation guidelines

Kappa value	Agreement
0.80 – 1.00	Very good
0.60 – 0.79	Good
0.40 – 0.59	Moderate
0.20 – 0.39	Fair
0.00 – 0.19	Poor

Fig. 1.8. Kappa-agreement data for urine heme reaction. After dipping the reaction pad in 100 urine samples, the color changes in a heme-reaction pads were assessed by two methods (reflectance photometry and visual examination) and graded as negative, trace, 1+, 2+, or 3+. The results were tabulated and entered in a software program (Analyse-it) to calculate a weighted kappa value.

III. After the quantitative aspects of the assays are compared, a decision is made as to whether the degree of agreement is acceptable or unacceptable.
    A. Visual inspection of graphed data may reveal that the results differ sufficiently so that the two assays cannot be considered the same. Thus, there would need to be different reference intervals and decision thresholds for the two assays.
    B. Because both assays will inherently not be 100 % precise, some differences are expected even if the assays have excellent agreement. The amount of inherent difference can be assessed by calculating a combined inherent CV.[13]
    C. The acceptability of a new assay can also be assessed using a medical decision chart.[13]

WHICH LABORATORY DO YOU USE?

I. Many factors must be considered before you decide how you will obtain laboratory data for your patients. Basically, there are three major options: in-house laboratory, veterinary reference laboratory, and laboratory in local human hospital. Four major questions must be considered:
    A. How will the results affect the care of the patient?
    B. Can the laboratory consistently provide quality analysis of the sample?
    C. How much will it cost to analyze the sample?
    D. How important is a short turnaround time?

II. In-house laboratory (in a veterinary clinic or hospital)
    A. Advantages
        1. May allow 24 h access to laboratory data
        2. Shorter turnaround times, which are sometimes required for emergency cases
        3. Fresh samples and thus fewer concerns about sample deterioration
    B. Disadvantages
        1. Capital expenditure of several thousand dollars is required and equipment depreciates rapidly.
        2. Need to maintain inventory of reagents and supplies
        3. Need personnel trained to operate and maintain equipment
        4. Need to follow a quality assurance program (You may be legally responsible for documenting quality of laboratory data.)
        5. Typically need high sample volume to generate enough income to cover expenses
        6. Reference intervals typically are provided by the manufacturer of instruments or assay and may or may not be quality reference intervals.
        7. May need to ship a malfunctioning instrument to the manufacturer for repairs and thus need a replacement instrument or backup methods
    C. Excellent in-house testing can be provided, but the quality and value of the results are often inferior to those provided by veterinary reference laboratories. Sources of error include the following:
        1. Inappropriate sample is tested rather than rejected (e.g., because of wrong tube, wrong volume, or interferent present such as lipemia).
        2. Sample processing is inappropriate (e.g., sample not mixed adequately).
        3. Analyzer is not maintained adequately.
        4. Outdated reagents are used.
        5. Personnel do not follow a standard operating procedure.
        6. Control samples are not tested or are not tested frequently enough to trust results.

    7. For hematology, microscopic evaluation is not done, or it is done by someone with less experience than referral laboratory personnel.

III.   Veterinary reference laboratory
    A. Advantages
       1. Laboratory personnel are typically trained to provide quality analysis of veterinary samples and recognize samples that may lead to inaccurate results.
       2. Diagnostic support may be available from veterinary clinical pathologists in the laboratory.
       3. Reference intervals should be appropriate for the species.
       4. Most laboratories have a quality management system in place to help ensure quality results. The system often includes proficiency testing by an external group such that performance can be compared to that of peers.
       5. Many more diagnostic assays are typically available than are available in an in-house laboratory.
       6. The cost for sample analysis is more clearly determined and thus can be charged to the client on a sample-by-sample basis.
    B. Disadvantages
       1. Not all analytes are stable and thus some deteriorate during shipment. Some analytes require special shipping.
       2. Turnaround times vary with location: some are available the same day, and most are available the next day except for special tests. Some laboratories offer courier service and results reported via fax machines or e-mail.

IV.   Laboratory in local human hospital
    A. An advantage is that turnaround times can be within hours.
    B. Disadvantages
       1. Quality reference intervals for veterinary samples may not be established by the laboratory.
       2. Assay methods may not be appropriate for veterinary samples.
       3. Technicians and technologists may not be trained to correctly identify species variations or diseases that are unique to veterinary samples.
       4. Pathologists who specialize in human patients frequently are very interested in helping, but lack the training in the diseases of domestic animals and variations seen in veterinary samples.
       5. The fees charged by laboratories may be relatively high.
    C. Testing in local laboratories that specialize in human medicine should generally be avoided.

EVALUATING AND VALIDATING LABORATORY METHODS[16]

I.   Reasons for evaluating laboratory methods
    A. New or revised laboratory methods may be evaluated for clinical use when the following are true: (1) recent research findings suggest a better approach, (2) newer assays might be more accurate, more precise, less expensive, or less difficult, or (3) an instrument was purchased to replace an outdated or malfunctioning instrument.
    B. A clinical perspective needs to be considered for new or revised laboratory methods. Is the method practical? What are the equipment and space needs? Are personnel trained

for the method? Will it improve patient care at a reasonable cost? Has there been adequate study of the method to prove its clinical value or is the method still in the development stage? Are the requirements for sample collection, processing, and handling practical?

II. What are the sources of analytical error?
   A. Each assay system has it own inherent *random error* (see Quality of Laboratory Results, sect. II.A). Typically, the more precise the assay is, the better it is, but sometimes the most precise methods are too expensive or time consuming.
   B. Besides random error, a method may not provide accurate results because of *systematic error* (bias). For example, the mean concentration of a new method might be consistently 5 mmol/L too high compared to the mean value determined by a reference method.
   C. *Accuracy* is a relative term, and an assay's analytical accuracy is sometimes difficult to assess in a clinical laboratory. An assay's result may be compared against one of two "true" values:
      1. The mean concentration determined by the reference method (a gold standard)
      2. The mean concentration determined by numerous analyses by comparative methods (all laboratories using the same instrument and reagents)
   D. Acceptable analytical performance
      1. The most accurate, precise, specific, or sensitive assay typically is not needed in a clinical environment. However, the assay does need to meet requirements for a clinically useful assay.
      2. Criteria for acceptable performance of clinical assays have been proposed, and they vary considerably among analytes. A hematocrit method might be considered acceptable if it provides results within 6 % of the target value (e.g., 37.6–42.4 % for a hematocrit of 40 %). Or a cortisol method might be considered acceptable if cortisol concentrations are within 25 % of target values.[9,16]

III. Validation methods: After available information has led to a conclusion that a new or revised assay should be evaluated, three stages of validation have been recommended.
   A. Familiarization: This stage includes establishment of a working procedure, initial assessment of the analytical range, and calibration.
   B. Preliminary validation: In this stage, several studies are completed, including within-run replication, interference studies, and recovery studies.
   C. Detailed validation: If initial results are satisfactory, then the final validation includes replication studies, comparison of methods, statistical analyses, determination of acceptable performance criteria, and establishment of reference intervals.

IV. Implementation phase
   A. If results of the validation procedures indicate that the assay will be used in the laboratory, then it needs to be incorporated into the daily routine of the laboratory, including equipment maintenance, reagent inventory, and a quality assurance program.
   B. When the assay is finally ready for clinical use, clinicians are notified of its availability, expected precision at major decision thresholds, and characteristics of reference intervals.

DIAGNOSTIC PROPERTIES AND PREDICTIVE VALUE OF LABORATORY ASSAYS

I.   As mentioned earlier, a frequent purpose of analyzing a patient's sample is to detect or confirm the presence of a disease state. But if a laboratory test result is outside the reference interval, how likely is it that the patient has a certain disorder? Similarly, if a laboratory test result is WRI, how certain are we that the animal doesn't have a certain disease or pathologic state? The following information is an introduction to the diagnostic value of laboratory assays and the predictive value theory, which involve concepts or procedures that are used to answer these questions.

II. There are four classifications of test results relative to the presence or absence of a disease:
     A. TP (true positive): a result that correctly identified a patient as having a specified disease
     B. TN (true negative): a result that correctly identified a patient as not having a specified disease
     C. FP (false positive): a result that incorrectly identified a patient as having a specified disease
     D. FN (false negative): a result that incorrectly identified a patient as not having a specified disease

III. To classify test results into one of the four categories, two factors must be known:
     A. What criterion is used to separate a positive from a negative result? Is it a positive result when the result is above the appropriate reference interval? Or is it a positive result when the value exceeds a certain decision threshold that could be within or outside of the reference interval?
     B. What determines whether an animal has the disease of interest? That is, what is the gold standard that allows us to say that the animal definitely does or does not have the disease? For many spontaneous diseases, there may not be a pure gold standard, and thus the diagnostic value data must be considered to be relative to an imperfect standard.

IV. After test results are appropriately classified as TP, TN, FP, or FN, several calculations are made in an attempt to characterize the diagnostic properties or predictive value of the assay.
     A. *Diagnostic sensitivity*
         1. Definition: the frequency with which a test is positive in patients that have the disease of interest (Eq. 1.2a)
         2. A test that has high diagnostic sensitivity is a good one for screening for the presence of a disease because the test has very few FN results. If the animal has the disease, there is a high probability that the test will be positive.
         3. Diagnostic sensitivity must be differentiated from analytical sensitivity.

$$\text{Diagnostic sensitivity (as \%)} = \frac{\text{number of true positive}}{\text{number with specified disease}} = \frac{\text{TP \#}}{\text{TP \# + FN \#}} \times 100 \qquad \textbf{(1.2a.)}$$

$$\text{Diagnostic specificity (as \%)} = \frac{\text{number of true negative}}{\text{number without specified disease}} = \frac{\text{TN \#}}{\text{TN \# + FP \#}} \times 100 \qquad \textbf{(1.2b.)}$$

$$\text{Diagnostic accuracy (as \%)} = \frac{\text{number correctly classified}}{\text{number of animals in study}} = \frac{\text{TP \# + TN \#}}{\text{TP \# + FP \# + TN \# + FN \#}} \times 100$$

(1.2c.)

$$\text{Predictive value of positive test (as \%)} = \frac{\text{number of true positive}}{\text{all positive results}} = \frac{\text{TP \#}}{\text{TP \# + FP \#}} \times 100 \quad \textbf{(1.2d.)}$$

$$\text{Predictive value of negative test (as \%)} = \frac{\text{number of true negative}}{\text{all negative results}} = \frac{\text{TN \#}}{\text{TN \# + FN \#}} \times 100 \quad \textbf{(1.2e.)}$$

    B. *Diagnostic specificity*
       1. Definition: the frequency with which a test is negative in patients that do not have the disease of interest (Eq. 1.2b)
       2. A test that has high diagnostic specificity can be a good one for confirming that an animal has a disease because the test has very few FP results. If the result is positive, there is a high probability that the animal will have the disease.
       3. Diagnostic specificity must be differentiated from analytical specificity.
    C. *Diagnostic accuracy*
       1. Definition: the frequency with which a test correctly classifies an animal as having or not having the disease (Eq. 1.2c)
       2. A test has high diagnostic accuracy when it has relatively few FP and FN results compared to TP and TN results.
    D. PV(+), the predictive value of a positive test, *positive predictive value*
       1. Definition: the probability that a positive test result indicates that the animal has the disease (Eq. 1.2d)
       2. A test that has a high PV(+) is one that has very few FP compared to TP results. Thus, a positive test result strongly suggests the presence of the disease.
    E. PV(−), the predictive value of a negative test, *negative predictive value*
       1. Definition: the probability that a negative test result indicates that the animal does not have the disease (Eq. 1.2e)
       2. A test that has a high PV(−) is one that has very few FN compared to TN results. Thus, a negative test result strongly suggests the absence of the disease.

V. Basic concepts of predictive values. Three major questions are considered when the diagnostic properties of an assay are evaluated:
    A. What is the prevalence of the disease in the studied population? The effect of prevalence is illustrated in Fig. 1.10. Basically, when the disease prevalence is very low, it is more likely that there will be FP results. Conversely, when the disease prevalence is very high, it is more likely that there will be FN results.
    B. What method is used as the gold standard for establishing the presence or absence of disease? Having an excellent gold standard is sometimes very difficult for spontaneous diseases and thus comparison against a poor gold standard may lead to questionable results. Also, consider this question: What would be the results of a comparison study if the new assay is actually better than the existing gold standard?

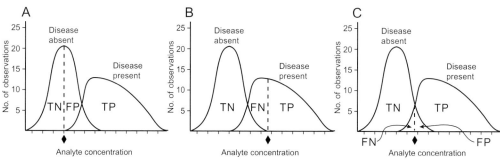

$\blacklozenge$ = decision threshold

Fig. 1.9. Effects of different decision thresholds on classifying test results. In these examples, the distribution of observed values in the animals without the disease appears to be Gaussian; such a distribution may or may not be true in real studies. The distribution of data in the diseased group is not Gaussian; typically, such data are not Gaussian but may not be skewed as shown in this example.

A. The decision threshold is near the mean analyte concentration found in the animals without the disease. With such a decision threshold,
- The diagnostic sensitivity would be 100 % because there are no FN results.
- The diagnostic specificity would be 50 % because there are equal numbers of TN and FP results.
- The diagnostic accuracy would be poor because of the many FP results.
- The PV(+) would be poor because of the many FP results.
- The PV(−) would be 100 % because there are no FN results.

B. The decision threshold is at the highest value found in the animals without the disease.
- The diagnostic sensitivity would be poor (about 60 %) because there are relatively many FN results.
- The diagnostic specificity would be 100 % because there are no FP results.
- The diagnostic accuracy would be poor because of the many FN results.
- The PV(+) would be 100 % because there are no FP results.
- The PV(−) would be poor because there are many FN results.

C. The decision threshold is at a concentration where the least overlap between the groups occurs.
- This decision threshold represents a compromise to obtain the best combination of diagnostic sensitivity and diagnostic specificity and provides the best diagnostic accuracy because there are relatively few FP and FN results.
- The values for PV(+) and PV(−) would be high but not 100 %.

    C. What is going to be the decision threshold that separates a positive result from a negative result? Extensive evaluation of an assay is sometimes needed to find the best decision threshold. The effects of changing the decision threshold are illustrated in Fig. 1.9.

VI.   Application and interpretation of predictive value concepts
    A. The clinical value of the calculated diagnostic properties is influenced by the prevalence of a disease. For examples A and B in Fig. 1.10, assume the diagnostic sensitivity of a test is 90 % and its diagnostic specificity is 80 %.
       1. In example A of Fig. 1.10, with a disease prevalence of 30 %:
          a. The PV(+) is 66 %; for all positive test results, 66 % will be TP results.
          b. The PV(−) is 95 %; for all negative test results, 95 % will be TN results.
       2. In example B of Fig. 1.10, with a disease prevalence of 1 %:
          a. The PV(+) is 4.3 %; for all positive test results, 4.3 % will be TP results.
          b. The PV(−) is 99.9 %; for all negative test results, 99.9 % will be TN results.

Example A – 30 % disease prevalence

Step 1	Disease present		Disease absent	
Positive test	(TP)	270	(FP)	140
Negative test	(FN)	30	(TN)	560
Totals		300		700

Step 2	Disease present		Disease absent		Totals
Positive test	(TP)	270	(FP)	140	410
Negative test	(FN)	30	(TN)	560	590
Totals		300		700	1000

Step 3

$$\text{Predictive value of positive test (as \%)} = \frac{\text{TP \#}}{\text{TP \# + FP \#}} \times 100 = \frac{270}{410} \times 100 = 66 \text{ \%}$$

$$\text{Predictive value of negative test (as \%)} = \frac{\text{TN \#}}{\text{TN \# + FN \#}} \times 100 = \frac{560}{590} \times 100 = 95 \text{ \%}$$

Example B – 1 % disease prevalence

Step 1	Disease present		Disease absent	
Positive test	(TP)	9	(FP)	198
Negative test	(FN)	1	(TN)	792
Totals		10		990

Step 2	Disease present		Disease absent		Totals
Positive test	(TP)	9	(FP)	198	207
Negative test	(FN)	1	(TN)	792	793
Totals		10		990	1000

Step 3

$$\text{Predictive value of positive test (as \%)} = \frac{\text{TP \#}}{\text{TP \# + FP \#}} \times 100 = \frac{9}{207} \times 100 = 4.3 \text{ \%}$$

$$\text{Predictive value of negative test (as \%)} = \frac{\text{TN \#}}{\text{TN \# + FN \#}} \times 100 = \frac{792}{793} \times 100 = 99.9 \text{ \%}$$

Fig. 1.10. Examples of diagnostic properties of assays. For each example, the values for diagnostic sensitivity and specificity are 90 % and 80 %, respectively.

- *In example A*, we discovered (via a gold standard) that 30 % of 1000 dogs have the disease. Based on the prevalence, what is the test's positive predictive value? What is the test's negative predictive value?
  - *Step 1*: Construct a table from the available information. Because 30 % of the dogs have the disease, 300 dogs have the disease and 700 dogs do not. As the diagnostic sensitivity is 90 %, then 90 % (270) of the 300 diseased dogs will have a positive test result (TP) and 30 will have a negative test result (FN). Because the diagnostic specificity is 80 %, then 80 % (560) of 700 dogs will have negative results (TN) and 140 will have a positive result (FP).
  - *Step 2*: Add the values for the number of positive and negative results.
  - *Step 3*: Calculate the positive predictive value and negative predictive value by using the Eq. 1.1 formulas.
- *In example B*, we discovered (via a gold standard) that 1 % of 1000 dogs have the disease. Based on the prevalence, what is the test's positive predictive value? What is the test's negative predictive value?
  - *Step 1*: Construct a table from the available information. Because 1 % of the dogs have the disease, ten dogs have the disease and 990 dogs do not. Because the diagnostic sensitivity is 90 %, 90 % (nine) of the ten diseased dogs will have a positive test result (TP) and 10 % (one) will have a negative test result (FN). Because the diagnostic specificity is 80 %, 80 % (792) of 990 dogs will have negative results (TN) and 198 will have a positive result (FP).
  - *Step 2*: Add the values for the number of positive and negative results.
  - *Step 3*: Calculate the positive predictive value and negative predictive value by using the Eq. 1.1 formulas.

3. By comparing the results of the two examples, these conclusions are formed:
    a. As the prevalence of the disease dropped from 30 % to 1 %, the PV(+) decreased from 66 % to 4.3 %. Thus, the PV(+) is less when the prevalence of the disease is lower.
    b. As the prevalence of the disease dropped from 30 % to 1 %, the PV(−) increased from 95 % to 99.9 %. Thus, the PV(−) is greater when the prevalence of the disease is lower.

B. The predictive value concepts are used to compare the diagnostic value of two laboratory tests. To illustrate this application, data were extracted from an article that compared the diagnostic value of serum $[tT_4]$ and $[fT_4]_{ed}$ for diagnosing feline hyperthyroidism.[17] As described in Chapter 17, serum $[tT_4]$ and $[fT_4]_{ed}$ may increase in sera of cats with hyperthyroidism, but other factors can influence $[tT_4]$ and $[fT_4]_{ed}$.
    1. Gold standard for this study
        a. Cats were classified as having hyperthyroidism by using the following clinical or laboratory findings:
            (1) Clinical signs consistent with hyperthyroidism
            (2) Palpable thyroid nodule
            (3) Good clinical response to treatment for hyperthyroidism
            (4) Basal $[tT_4]$ increased or basal $[tT_4]$ not increased, but positive results of triiodothyronine-suppression or thyrotropin-releasing hormone-stimulation test
        b. Cats were classified as not having hyperthyroidism if they did not meet hyperthyroidism criteria. These cats had clinical signs suggestive of hyperthyroidism (e.g., weight loss, vomiting, diarrhea, and polyuria), but none had a palpable thyroid mass, none had increased $[tT_4]$, and all had a diagnosis other than hyperthyroidism.
    2. Classification of results
        a. tT_4 results were classified as positive if $[tT_4]$ was > 48 nmol/L. fT_4 results were classified as positive if $[fT_4]_{ed}$ was > 51 pmol/L. Decision thresholds represented the upper reference limits determined from 172 healthy cats.
        b. Results were classified as negative if they did not meet positive criteria.
    3. Based on these criteria for the 1138 cats,
        a. 917 cats had hyperthyroidism. Of these, 837 had an increased $[tT_4]$ and 903 had increased $[fT_4]_{ed}$.
        b. 221 cats did not have hyperthyroidism. Of these, none had increased $[tT_4]$ and 14 had increased $[fT_4]_{ed}$.
    4. From the data provided, tables were constructed to show the classification of test results. From the tabulated data, the diagnostic properties and predictive values of $[tT_4]$ and $[fT_4]_{ed}$ were calculated (Fig. 1.11).
    5. Based on the evaluation of reported data and application of the aforementioned gold standard and decision thresholds, these conclusions can be drawn:
        a. Serum $[fT_4]_{ed}$ had better diagnostic sensitivity (98 %) than did serum $[tT_4]$ (91 %) for detecting feline hyperthyroidism. Thus, serum $[fT_4]_{ed}$ would be a better screening test for hyperthyroidism; that is, more cats with hyperthyroidism will have increased $[fT_4]_{ed}$ than increased $[tT_4]$.
        b. Serum $[tT_4]$ had better diagnostic specificity (100 %) than did serum $[fT_4]_{ed}$ (94 %). Thus, an increased serum $[tT_4]$ is more indicative of feline hyperthyroidism than is an increased serum $[fT_4]_{ed}$; that is, $[tT_4]$ had fewer FP results.

[tT$_4$] in feline sera

	Hyperthyroidism present	Hyperthyroidism absent	Totals
Positive test	(TP) 837	(FP) 0	837
Negative test	(FN) 80	(TN) 221	301
Totals	917	221	1138

$$\text{Diagnostic sensitivity (as \%)} = \frac{TP\#}{TP\# + FN\#} \times 100 = \frac{837}{917} \times 100 = 91\ \%$$

$$\text{Diagnostic specificity (as \%)} = \frac{TN\#}{TN\# + FP\#} \times 100 = \frac{221}{221} \times 100 = 100\ \%$$

$$\text{Diagnostic accuracy (as \%)} = \frac{TP\# + TN\#}{TP\# + FP\# + TN\# + FN\#} \times 100 = \frac{1058}{1138} \times 100 = 93\ \%$$

$$\text{Predictive value of postive test (as \%)} = \frac{TP\#}{TP\# + FP\#} \times 100 = \frac{837}{837} \times 100 = 100\ \%$$

$$\text{Predictive value of negative test (as \%)} = \frac{TN\#}{TN\# + FN\#} \times 100 = \frac{221}{301} \times 100 = 73\ \%$$

[fT$_4$]$_{ed}$ in feline sera

	Hyperthyroidism present	Hyperthyroidism absent	Totals
Positive test	(TP) 903	(FP) 14	917
Negative test	(FN) 14	(TN) 207	221
Totals	917	221	1138

$$\text{Diagnostic sensitivity (as \%)} = \frac{TP\#}{TP\# + FN\#} \times 100 = \frac{903}{917} \times 100 = 98\ \%$$

$$\text{Diagnostic specificity (as \%)} = \frac{TN\#}{TN\# + FP\#} \times 100 = \frac{207}{221} \times 100 = 94\ \%$$

$$\text{Diagnostic accuracy (as \%)} = \frac{TP\# + TN\#}{TP\# + FP\# + TN\# + FN\#} \times 100 = \frac{1110}{1138} \times 100 = 98\ \%$$

$$\text{Predictive value of postive test (as \%)} = \frac{TP\#}{TP\# + FP\#} \times 100 = \frac{903}{917} \times 100 = 98\ \%$$

$$\text{Predictive value of negative test (as \%)} = \frac{TN\#}{TN\# + FN\#} \times 100 = \frac{207}{221} \times 100 = 94\ \%$$

Fig. 1.11. Analysis of the diagnostic properties of serum [tT$_4$] and [fT$_4$]$_{ed}$. The source of the data for this figure is explained in the text. Also, conclusions from the analyses are presented in the text.
- [tT$_4$] data
  - From the data provided, a table was constructed to show the classification of test results.
  - From the tabulated data, the diagnostic properties and predictive values of serum [tT$_4$] were calculated.
- [fT$_4$]$_{ed}$ data: The same procedures were completed.

    c. Serum $[fT_4]_{ed}$ had better diagnostic accuracy (98 %) than did serum $[tT_4]$ (93 %). Thus, if only $[tT_4]$ or $[fT_4]_{ed}$ can be determined, serum $[fT_4]_{ed}$ has a better chance of correctly classifying the cat as having or not having hyperthyroidism. However, measuring $[fT_4]_{ed}$ is more expensive than measuring $[tT_4]$.

    d. The PV(+) for increased $[tT_4]$ was 100 %, and it was 98 % for $[fT_4]_{ed}$.

    e. The PV(–)s for $[tT_4]$ and for $[fT_4]_{ed}$ were 73 % and 94 %, respectively. These results indicate that a $[fT_4]_{ed}$ that is WRI would strongly suggest that a cat does not have hyperthyroidism because there were very few FN results.

    f. Note that the results of such studies may vary with different assays, different populations, different gold standards, and different decision thresholds.

       (1) $[tT_4]$ was used to determine the presence or absence of hyperthyroidism. The gold standard used (or method of establishing the presence of hyperthyroidism) in the study is considered an excellent method of establishing the presence of feline hyperthyroidism, but it would have been interesting to learn whether the diagnostic value data for $[tT_4]$ would change if $[tT_4]$ had not been used to help determine the presence or absence of hyperthyroidism.

       (2) Most cats in the study had been referred to specialists for treatment of hyperthyroidism. Thus, there was a high prevalence of hyperthyroidism in the study's population. A high prevalence increases the PV(+) of diagnostic tests and lowers the PV(–). Accordingly, the predictive values of $[tT_4]$ and $[fT_4]_{ed}$ would probably be different in a nonreferral veterinary practice.

VII. Application of the aforementioned methods to evaluate and compare diagnostic methods requires careful planning, appropriate choices of the animal populations (diseased versus nondiseased), and availability of an excellent gold standard.

    A. A deficiency in the diagnostic properties and predictive value theories is that a positive result is given the same weight or importance if the value is only slightly increased or if it is extremely increased. Such a weighting process (i.e., lack of weighting) frequently is not appropriate in the clinical decision process.

    B. After a diagnostic test (assay) has been thoroughly studied, six criteria should be fulfilled before the diagnostic properties (predictive value, diagnostic accuracy, etc.) are transferred to another clinical setting:[18]

      1. The definition of the disease is constant, and the diagnostic criteria are applied in the same way such that two dogs with the same abnormalities in two different settings would be diagnosed with the same disorder.

      2. The same test is used. As described in earlier sections, there may not be complete agreement between two analytical assays even if the same instrument and reagents are used.

      3. The decision thresholds between categories of test results are constant; that is, two different observers should agree on results that are *positive* and on results that are *negative*.

      4. The distribution of test results in the disease group is constant; that is, the data should have the same average and same distribution curve. It may be difficult to fulfill this criterion—perhaps animals are presented early in an illness in one location, but, in another location, animals are not presented until the animals are severely ill. Data for animals with a mild disease will probably be different from those of a group with severe disease.

5. The distribution of test results in the nondisease group is constant; that is, the data should have the same average and same distribution curve. It may be difficult to fulfill this criterion—certain *FP* disorders may be rare in a primary care clinic but very common in a referral clinic.

6. The ratio of disease to nondisease (pretest probability) is constant. Again, this criterion may be difficult to fulfill—certain disorders may be rare in a primary care clinic but very common in a referral clinic.

RECEIVER OPERATING CHARACTERISTIC (ROC) CURVES[19,20]

I. ROC curves were originally developed to assess the ability of radar images to detect enemy aircraft in World War II, and therefore to assess the ability to detect true signals from background noise. In the context of laboratory tests, the ROC curves display the relationship between a TP rate and a FP rate.

A. *TP rate* is equal to diagnostic sensitivity expressed as a decimal. For example, when the diagnostic sensitivity is 90 %, the TP rate is 0.9; results are positive in nine of ten diseased animals.

B. *FP rate* is equal to 1 minus the diagnostic specificity expressed as a decimal. For example, when the diagnostic specificity is 70 %, the FP rate is $1 - 0.7 = 0.3$, and three of ten nondiseased animals would have an FP result. When the diagnostic specificity is 100 %, there would be no FP results and thus the FP rate would be 0.0.

C. Figure 1.12 shows theoretical results from the comparison of two assays: assay A and assay B.

II. The clinical value of the comparison of diagnostic procedures by ROC curves depends on many factors. Major issues to be addressed include the following:

A. The assays should be analytically valid and applicable to clinical investigations.

B. Selection of the comparison groups should be clinically relevant. Both groups should have similar clinical features (e.g., both have polyuria, vomiting, or anemia) so that the ability of the assays to differentiate disorders is evaluated. Conversely, comparison of a sick group versus a healthy group is probably not appropriate or needed (the animal was defined as healthy without laboratory tests).

C. The accuracy of the comparison is very dependent on the accuracy of the gold standard procedure that is used to differentiate disease-present from disease-absent groups. As there are very few "pure gold" procedures, results of the comparison need to be interpreted accordingly.

D. ROC curves can be used to compare the diagnostic accuracy of assays.

1. A visual inspection of Fig. 1.12 reveals that the ROC curve for assay A is closer to the top left corner than assay B, and thus assay A has better diagnostic accuracy than assay B.

2. A more objective comparison can be accomplished by calculating the area under the curve for each assay.[21,22] However, these values should be interpreted carefully if the shapes of the ROC curves differ.

E. ROC curves can be used to help establish a decision threshold to rule in or rule out a diagnosis (Fig. 1.13).[23] Other than being used to establish decision thresholds, Fig. 1.13 also provides information that should be considered when interpreting the test results of assay C.

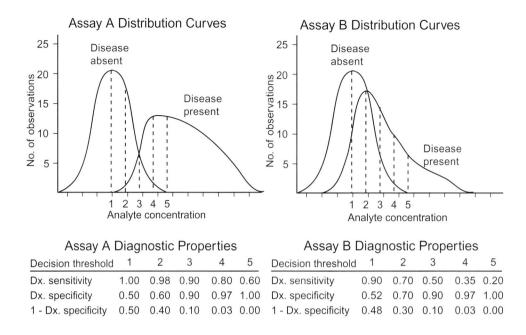

Assay A Diagnostic Properties

Decision threshold	1	2	3	4	5
Dx. sensitivity	1.00	0.98	0.90	0.80	0.60
Dx. specificity	0.50	0.60	0.90	0.97	1.00
1 - Dx. specificity	0.50	0.40	0.10	0.03	0.00

Assay B Diagnostic Properties

Decision threshold	1	2	3	4	5
Dx. sensitivity	0.90	0.70	0.50	0.35	0.20
Dx. specificity	0.52	0.70	0.90	0.97	1.00
1 - Dx. specificity	0.48	0.30	0.10	0.03	0.00

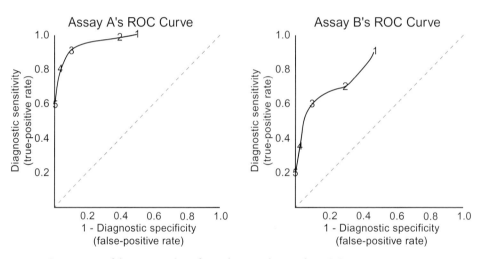

Fig. 1.12. Comparison of diagnostic value of two theoretical assays by ROC curves.

- The initial step of the evaluation is the analysis of samples from two groups of animals (disease present and disease absent) by the two assays. The presence or absence of disease is established by a gold standard procedure.
- The data are plotted to obtain the distribution curves (top curves in figure). To gather data for the ROC curve, multiple decision thresholds are selected that will provide different diagnostic sensitivity and specificity values. The decision thresholds are then used to classify actual measured concentrations as being TP, FP, TN, or FN results. For the illustration in the top graphs, five decision thresholds were selected, and the dashed lines represent the separation of positive and negative results at each decision threshold.
- From the classified data, the diagnostic sensitivity (TP rate) and specificity values are calculated for each decision threshold. (For this illustration, the number of animals in both groups were estimated from the graphs with an assumption that the total number in each group was equal.) The FP rate is calculated by subtracting diagnostic specificity from 1.
- The decimal fractions for TP rate and FP rate are plotted (bottom graphs). The 45° dashed line represents the ROC curve that would be obtained by random classification (e.g., flipping a coin to classify animals as disease present or disease absent). The best ROC curve approaches the top left corner of the graph where nearly all positive results are TP results. In this comparison, assay A is a better diagnostic procedure than assay B for detecting a certain disease.

Dx., diagnostic.

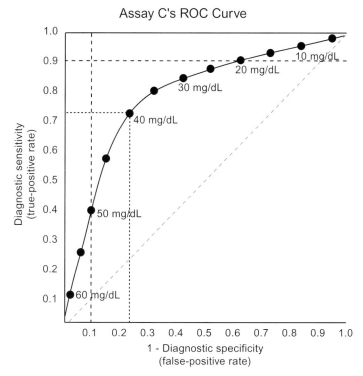

Fig. 1.13. Selecting decision thresholds with ROC curves. In this theoretical assay C, the analyte concentrations are plotted on the ROC curve for assay C.

- The top-leftmost point provides the best balance between diagnostic sensitivity and diagnostic specificity and is often chosen as a decision threshold to conclude that a patient has a particular condition. Values of > 40 mg/dL would be considered evidence of the disease. With this decision threshold, the assay would have a diagnostic sensitivity of 73 % and a diagnostic specificity of 78 %.
- For use as a screening test, one might choose to set the decision threshold for disease at 20 mg/dL, accepting only 10 % FNs (i.e., 90 % diagnostic sensitivity). Values of > 20 mg/dL would suggest the presence of the disease. With this decision threshold, the assay would have a high diagnostic sensitivity (90 %), but a diagnostic specificity of only 37 %.
- For a confirmatory test, the decision threshold for disease may be set at 50 mg/dL to accept only 10 % FPs (i.e., 90 % diagnostic specificity, or an FP rate = 1.0 − 0.9 = 0.1). Values of > 50 mg/dL suggest that the animal has the disease. With this decision threshold, the diagnostic specificity would be high (90 %), but the diagnostic sensitivity would be only 40 %.
- One could also use the ROC curve to determine upper and lower decision thresholds. A value of 20 mg/dL might be chosen as the lower decision threshold, so animals with values of < 20 mg/dL would be considered likely not to have the disease. A value of 50 mg/dL might be chosen as the upper decision threshold, so animals with values of > 50 mg/dL would be considered likely to have the disease.
- Based on this theoretical example, what would be the decision thresholds if you decide to accept 5 % FNs and 5 % FPs?

1. Consider a patient with clinical signs suggestive of the disease of interest and an assay C result of 40 mg/dL
   a. At 40 mg/dL, assay C has a FP rate near 0.22, or a diagnostic specificity of 78 %. In other words, of 100 dogs that do not have the disease of interest, about 22 will have an analyte concentration of > 40 mg/dL (22 % of those without the disease classified as diseased). Therefore, the patient may or may not have the disease, but disease is more likely than not.
   b. At 40 mg/dL, assay C has a TP rate near 0.73, or a diagnostic sensitivity near 73 %. So, of 100 dogs that do have the disease of interest, 73 will have an analyte concentration of > 40 mg/dL (73 % of those with the disease classified as diseased). Therefore, despite a value that is not > 40 mg/dL, the patient may still have the disease because 27 % of patients with the disease have values of 40 mg/dL or less.
   c. This example emphasizes that for many diagnostic tests, animals with and without the disease of interest may have the same assay result.
2. Another key concept related to this illustration is that each ROC curve represents the results obtained from one sampling of the defined populations by using one assay as it compares to one gold standard. Another sampling using the same selection criteria, the same assay, and the same gold standard probably will not produce the same ROC curve.

F. Factors other than the probability of correctly classifying an animal as having or not having a disease can influence where decision thresholds are established:
   1. If the mortality rate is very high for a disease that is not treated promptly, the decision threshold may be changed so that there are fewer false negatives.
   2. If the disease is known to cause pain or unreasonable discomfort, the decision threshold may be changed so that there are fewer false negatives.
   3. If the treatment is known to have severe side effects, the decision threshold may be changed so that there are fewer false positives.
   4. If the financial cost of a certain diagnosis is great, the decision threshold may be changed so that there are fewer false positives.

HERD-BASED TESTING FOR CATTLE

I. Other than using results of laboratory assays to help detect or establish the presence of pathologic states in individual animals, clinical laboratory assays also are used to evaluate the nutritional and metabolic status of groups of cattle. These evaluations should complement other management tools such as ration evaluation, milk composition analysis, and body condition scoring. The goal is to detect subclinical laboratory abnormalities that reflect correctible nutritional management practices so that changes can be instituted prior to adverse clinical and economic consequences. Metabolic profiling may be most applicable to large herds where (1) adequate sample sizes are available, (2) costs are diluted across more animals, and (3) correcting a suboptimal nutritional state could translate into considerable economic savings.

II. The approach to group testing differs in several ways from individual animal testing with diagnostic profiles.[24–27]
   A. Emphasis is placed on evaluating and monitoring subclinical rather than clinical disease. Clinically ill cattle are excluded from herd-based testing because their results may be indicative of an individual disease problem rather than a herd problem.

B. Individuals to be tested must belong to defined groups of similar age and lactation stage under similar environmental conditions and nutritional management (e.g., prefreshening cows and postcalving cows). Specific group trends or abnormalities may not be apparent if inclusion criteria are too broad, thus allowing a greater degree of physiologic variation.

C. Useful information requires adequate group representation and therefore an adequate sample size for the group of interest. Sampling multiple animals from a defined group helps reduce variation unrelated to nutritional state.

1. Sample sizes of 7–12 have been advocated as reasonable pools to provide useful information for most purposes, regardless of herd size. However, greater numbers of test individuals would provide results with tighter confidence limits and may be necessary to adequately represent target groups in large herds.

2. Herd size may limit the number of animals in a relevant group that can be tested at one time (e.g., too few prefresh cows). However, useful information may be obtained in these groups by testing over time as animals enter the group. Interpretation must then include considerations of temporal variables.

3. Economic pressures encourage smaller test groups and pooling of samples, but pooling may be undesirable.

   a. In one study, 5 of 21 analytes (including tCa^{2+} and BHB concentrations) had pooled mean values that differed from mean values of the individual animals in some pools.[28]

   b. Unexpected marked abnormalities in one or more samples may bias the pooled results, especially if unequal volumes of sample from each individual are used.

   c. Individual animal data cannot be generated, so only mean values rather than ranges of values or proportions of abnormal results above or below a decision threshold can be assessed (see Herd-based Testing for Cattle, sect. III).

D. Analytes measured by herd-based metabolic profiling tests should reflect metabolic/nutritional status. Typically, they are not tightly regulated by hormonal or other physiologic factors. For example, metabolic pathways attempt to maintain glucose concentration within a certain range even if there is a marked difference in the intake of carbohydrates; thus, serum [glucose] is not a good analyte for assessing carbohydrate intake or digestibility. In contrast, plasma [BHB] is not tightly regulated, and increased concentrations reflect a deficient energy status. Even if analytes meet this criterion, it is also important that analytical variation is small compared to changes caused by altered nutritional states. Examples of tests and results that may be useful include the following:

1. Low blood hematocrit values in the first 8 wk of lactation suggest the need to evaluate energy and protein nutrition.

2. Serum [urea] at any lactation stage is an assessment of ruminal balance of energy and available protein.

3. High serum β-hydroxybutyrate (BHB) concentration at about 5–50 d into lactation is associated with suboptimal energy and glucose balance and, clinically, reduced milk production, increased clinical ketosis, displaced abomasums, and reduced fertility. Samples should be collected at a consistent time relative to feeding; for example, 4–5 h after the first meal of the day, when rumen butyric acid production is high.

4. High serum or plasma nonesterified fatty acid (NEFA) concentrations in prefresh dry cows in the last month of gestation (especially 2–14 d prior to calving) are evidence of a negative energy balance. Samples should be collected shortly before feeding time. One can draw and freeze multiple samples and send those that fulfill the 2- to 14-d precalving criterion once this is known.

     5. Low serum [tCa^{2+}] 12–24 h after calving by multiparous cows indicates clinical or subclinical parturient hypocalcemia.

III. Interpretation
  A. Abnormalities in herd-based test results must be interpreted with attention to all the variables that can affect them, not just nutritional factors. Other factors include preanalytical sample variation, analytical variation, biological variation, circadian/prandial variation, seasonal variation, variation in physiologic states, occurrence of pathological states, and other environmental and management factors. Most of these variations are controlled by careful group selection criteria and appropriate procedures for sample collection, processing, and analysis.
  B. Most herd-based test results will fall within diagnostic reference intervals because the sampled individuals lack clinical signs of disease. Therefore, a different set of interpretive guidelines is necessary to detect subclinical abnormalities. Currently, interpretive guidelines are suggested recommendations by experts in the field based on experience and research. Given the interlaboratory variability in assay results, it is not clear to the authors how widely applicable specific recommendations are.
  C. Data have been evaluated in several ways.
    1. Mean herd values may be compared to mean values of reference herds. When metabolic profiling was first described, the reference interval for an analyte was defined as the mean of its means for reference herds, ± 2 sd. However, these herd reference intervals are not readily available because of the expense of testing and difficulties identifying suitable reference herds.
    2. Mean herd values may be compared to an established expected mean result for the analyte and group of interest. For example, it has been suggested that mean urine pH should be 6.0–7.0 in prefresh cows fed anions to help prevent milk fever. A mean pH of 6.0–7.0 supports appropriate acidification of the group. When the herd's mean ± an uncertainty interval does not include 6.0–7.0, a herd's urine pH is considered inappropriate. When the herd's mean value is not 6.0–7.0, but the mean ± uncertainty interval overlaps this target, the results are considered borderline. A 75 % confidence interval has been suggested as a useful guide for metabolic profiling and a reasonable compromise between 95 % confidence and practicality.
    3. The percentage of individual results above or below an established decision threshold may be calculated and compared to what is considered an acceptable percentage of high or low values. A percentage (± uncertainty interval) greater than the accepted percentage signals a problem. A percentage and confidence interval overlapping with the accepted percentage is a borderline result. Decision thresholds may be somewhat artificial in that the risk for some conditions increases continuously with the magnitude of the analyte (e.g., NEFA concentration and displaced abomasums).
    4. Others have suggested using process control charts to graphically monitor changes of an analyte in a particular group over time. A running graph of mean values and high-low ranges of individual values can be plotted over time to evaluate for group changes that signal problems. Fluctuations must be assessed relative to established limits to determine when action should be taken.
  D. Just as diagnostic testing reference intervals are often imperfect, recommendations for analytes used in herd-based metabolic profiling are also imperfect. However, this does not prevent the acquisition of useful information.

References

1. Bennington JL. 1984. *Saunders Dictionary and Encyclopedia of Laboratory Medicine and Technology*. Philadelphia: WB Saunders.
2. Lundberg GD, Iverson C, Radulescu G. 1986. Now read this: The SI units are here. J Am Med Assoc 255:2329–2339.
3. Saris NE, Gräsbeck R, Siest G, Wilding P, Williams GZ, Whitehead TP. 1979. Provisional recommendation on the theory of reference values (1978). Clin Chem 25:1506–1508.
4. Lumsden JH. 2000. Reference values. In: Feldman BF, Zinkl JG, Jain NC, eds. *Schalm's Veterinary Hematology*, 5th edition, 12–15. Philadelphia: Lippincott Williams & Wilkins.
5. Solberg HE. 1983. The theory of reference values. Part 5: Statistical treatment of collected reference values—Determination of reference limits. J Clin Chem Clin Biochem 21:749–760.
6. Solberg HE. 1999. Establishment and use of reference values. In: Burtis CA, Ashwood ER, eds. *Tietz Textbook of Clinical Chemistry*, 3rd edition, 336–356. Philadelphia: WB Saunders.
7. Metz CE. 1978. Basic principles of ROC analysis. Semin Nucl Med 8:283–298.
8. Eraker SA, Eeckhoudt LR, Vanbutsele RJ, Lebrun TC, Sailly JC. 1986. To test or not to test—to treat or not to treat: The decision-threshold approach to patient management. J Gen Intern Med 1:177–182.
9. Koch DD, Peters T Jr. 1999. Selection and evaluation of methods. In: Burtis CA, Ashwood ER, eds. *Tietz Textbook of Clinical Chemistry*, 3rd edition, 320–335. Philadelphia: WB Saunders.
10. Passey RB. 1996. Quality control for the clinical chemistry laboratory. In: Kaplan LA, Pesce AJ, eds. *Clinical Chemistry: Theory, Analysis, and Correlation*, 3rd edition, 382–401. St Louis: CV Mosby.
11. Westgard JO, Barry PL, Hunt MR, Groth T. 1981. A multi-rule Shewhart chart for quality control in clinical chemistry. Clin Chem 27:493–501.
12. Westgard JO. 2006. *Six Sigma Quality Design and Control*, 2nd edition. Madison, WI: Westgard QC.
13. Jensen AL, Kjelgaard-Hansen M. 2006. Method comparison in the clinical laboratory. Vet Clin Pathol 35:276–286.
14. Glantz SA. 2001. *Primer of Biostatistics*, 5th edition. New York: McGraw-Hill.
15. Stöckl D, Dewitte K, Thienpont LM. 1998. Validity of linear regression in method comparison studies: Is it limited by the statistical model or the quality of the analytical input data? Clin Chem 44:2340–2346.
16. Lumsden JH. 2000. Laboratory test method validation. Rev Med Vet 151:623–630.
17. Peterson ME, Melián C, Nichols R. 2001. Measurement of serum concentrations of free thyroxine, total thyroxine, and total triiodothyronine in cats with hyperthyroidism and cats with nonthyroidal disease. J Am Vet Med Assoc 218:529–536.
18. Irwig L, Bossuyt P, Glasziou P, Gatsonis C, Lijmer J. 2002. Designing studies to ensure that estimates of test accuracy are transferable. BMJ 324:669–671.
19. Shultz EK. 1999. Selection and interpretation of laboratory procedures. In: Burtis CA, Ashwood ER, eds. *Tietz Textbook of Clinical Chemistry*, 3rd edition, 310–319. Philadelphia: WB Saunders.
20. Dawson-Saunders B, Trapp RG. 2000. Evaluating diagnostic procedures. *Basic and Clinical Biostatistics*, 2nd edition, 232–247. Norwalk, CT: Appleton & Lange.
21. Huguet J, Castiñeiras MJ, Fuentes-Arderiu X. 1993. Diagnostic accuracy evaluation using ROC curve analysis. Scand J Clin Lab Invest 53:693–699.
22. Boyd JC. 1997. Mathematical tools for demonstrating the clinical usefulness of biochemical markers. Scand J Clin Lab Invest Suppl 227:46–63.
23. Fischer JE, Bachmann LM, Jaeschke R. 2003. A readers' guide to the interpretation of diagnostic test properties: Clinical example of sepsis. Intensive Care Med 29:1043–1051.
24. Herdt TH. 2000. Variability characteristics and test selection in herd-level nutritional and metabolic profile testing. Vet Clin North Am Food Anim Pract 16:387–403.
25. Oetzel GR. 2004. Monitoring and testing dairy herds for metabolic disease. Vet Clin North Am Food Anim Pract 20:651–674.
26. Herdt TH, Dart B, Neuder L. 2001. Will large dairy herds lead to the revival of metabolic profile testing? In: Smith RA, ed. *34th Annual Conference of American Association of Bovine Practitioners*, 27–34. Stillwater, OK: American Association of Bovine Practitioners.
27. Oetzel GR. 2005. Herd-based testing for the preventive medicine practice. In: Smith RA, ed. *38th Annual Conference of American Association of Bovine Practitioners*, 133–138. Stillwater, OK: American Association of Bovine Practitioners.
28. Tornquist SJ, Van Saun RJ. 1999. Comparison of biochemical parameters in individual and pooled bovine sera. Vet Pathol 36:487 (abstract).

Chapter 2

LEUKOCYTES

Physiologic Processes Involving Leukocytes. 54
Analytical Principles and Methods. 60
    I. Complete Blood Count (CBC) 60
    II. Leukogram. 62
    III. Principles of Determining Leukocyte Concentrations. 62
    IV. Relative versus Absolute Changes in Leukogram Results 69
Abnormal Leukocyte Concentrations in Blood 70
    I. Abnormal Neutrophil Concentrations. 70
    II. Abnormal Lymphocyte Concentrations 81
    III. Abnormal Monocyte Concentrations 85
    IV. Abnormal Eosinophil Concentrations. 86
    V. Abnormal Basophil Concentrations 88
    VI. Abnormal Mast Cell Concentrations. 88
Leukogram Patterns. 90
Abnormal Morphologic Features of Leukocytes. 92
    I. Changes Associated with Inflammatory Diseases. 92
    II. Leukocytes That Contain Miscellaneous Inclusions 94
    III. Organisms in Leukocytes. 95
    IV. Leukocyte Agglutination/Aggregation 98
    V. Hereditary Disorders That Have Leukocyte Inclusions 99
Other Nonneoplastic Leukocyte Disorders 100

Table 2.1. Abbreviations and symbols in this chapter

[x]	x concentration (x = analyte)
ASVCP	American Society for Veterinary Clinical Pathology
BFU-E	Blast-forming unit–erythroid
BLV	Bovine leukemia virus
C5a	Complement, fragment 5a
CBC	Complete blood count
CFU-Baso	Colony-forming unit–basophil
CFU-E	Colony-forming unit–erythroid
CFU-Eo	Colony-forming unit–eosinophil
CFU-G	Colony-forming unit–granulocyte
CFU-GM	Colony-forming unit–granulocyte/macrophage
CFU-M	Colony-forming unit–monocyte
CFU-Mast	Colony-forming unit–mast cell
CFU-Meg	Colony-forming unit–megakaryocyte
CLP	Circulating lymphocyte pool
CNP	Circulating neutrophil pool
EDTA	Ethylenediaminetetraacetic acid
FeLV	Feline leukemia virus
f-MLP	n-Formylmethionine leucyl–phenylalanine
G-CSF	Granulocyte colony–stimulating factor
GM-CSF	Granulocyte/macrophage colony–stimulating factor
IgE	Immunoglobulin E
IL-x	Interleukins (x for Arabic numbers)
INFγ	Interferon gamma
LTB$_4$	Leukotriene B$_4$
MatNP	Maturation neutrophil pool
MLP	Marginated lymphocyte pool
MNP	Marginated neutrophil pool
MPS	Mucopolysaccharidosis
nRBC	Nucleated erythrocyte (nucleated red blood cell)
PAF	Platelet-activating factor
ProNP	Proliferation neutrophil pool
SNP	Storage neutrophil pool
TNFα	Tumor necrosis factor alpha
TNFβ	Tumor necrosis factor beta
TNP	Tissue neutrophil pool
URL	Upper reference limit
WBC	White blood cell (leukocyte)
WRI	Within the reference interval

PHYSIOLOGIC PROCESSES INVOLVING LEUKOCYTES

I. *Leukon*: all leukocytes in an animal, including leukocyte precursors, leukocytes in blood and lymph vessels, and tissue leukocytes
   A. Bone marrow contains precursors for neutrophils, eosinophils, basophils, monocytes, lymphocytes, and mast cells (considered tissue leukocytes).

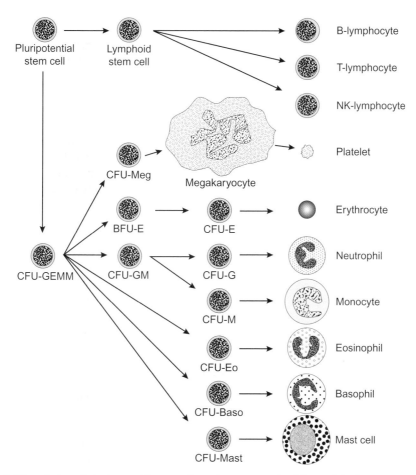

Fig. 2.1. Differentiation of pluripotential stem cells to the committed cell lines of the hematopoietic system. Major features of the hematopoietic system include the following: (1) Proliferation of myeloid and lymphoid cells classically occurs in marrow and other lymphoid tissues, respectively. (2) Seven nonlymphoid cell types and three major types of lymphoid cells are produced by the system. In this figure, all cells are part of the leukon except those of the erythrocyte and platelet lineage.

CFU-GEMM, colony-forming unit–granulocyte, erythrocyte, monocyte, megakaryocyte.

1. Leukopoiesis is part of hematopoiesis, which is a complex system involving stem cells that are capable of self-renewal or differentiation toward a committed cell line (Fig. 2.1).
2. Stem cells look like small lymphocytes via light and transmission electron microscopy and are present in blood and other tissues, including bone marrow, spleen, and liver.
3. Specific stimuli and regulators govern leukocyte differentiation and production.
B. Lymph nodes, spleen, and thymus contain precursors for B-lymphocytes, T-lymphocytes, and null-lymphocytes.
C. Leukocytes in blood are in transit from sites of production to sites of function or destruction.

D. Tissue leukocytes
   1. Granulocytes (neutrophils, eosinophils, and basophils) perform their roles in host defense and die.
   2. Lymphocytes may undergo blastogenesis, return to blood via lymphatic vessels, or die.
   3. Monocytes transform into histiocytes or macrophages that are capable of mitosis, perform their host defense functions, and die.
   4. Mast cell precursors differentiate into tissue mast cells, perform their roles in host defense, and die. Subsets are known.

II.   Neutrophil pools and kinetics (movement of neutrophils) (Fig. 2.2)

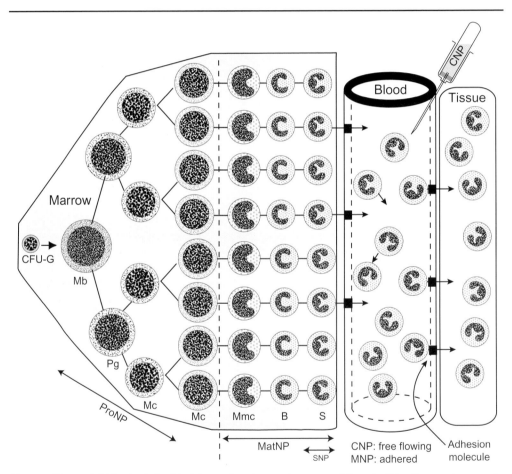

Fig. 2.2. Neutrophil kinetics in health. Marrow has three major neutrophil pools: (1) self-renewal stem cells (CFU-G); (2) ProNP, or mitotic pool, that contains myeloblasts (Mb), progranulocytes (Pg), and myelocytes (Mc); and (3) MatNP, or postmitotic pool, that contains metamyelocytes (Mmc), band neutrophils (B), and segmented neutrophils (S). A SNP is within the MatNP and contains segmented neutrophils. When neutrophils leave the marrow and enter blood, they distribute between the MNP and CNP. After neutrophils bind to adhesion proteins on endothelial cells, they migrate into tissues to form the TNP. In the TNP, the neutrophils perform their protective functions and die.

A. Marrow neutrophils
   1. IL-1, IL-3, IL-6, GM-CSF, and G-CSF stimulate CFU-G to differentiate into the neutrophilic cell line and to enter the ProNP (mitotic pool).
   2. Myeloblasts, progranulocytes (promyelocytes), and myelocytes divide and mature in the ProNP. Programmed cell death occurs in the myelocyte stage to limit neutropoiesis in health. During enhanced neutropoiesis, fewer cells die in this stage, and thus more enter the MatNP (postmitotic pool). In healthy mammals, neutrophil precursors are in this pool for about 3 d.
   3. In the MatNP, metamyelocytes mature to band neutrophils and then to segmented neutrophils. Segmented neutrophils that are ready for release to marrow sinusoids are in a subpool called SNP (storage neutrophil pool). Neutrophilic cells are in the MatNP for 2–3 d in dogs and for 4–6 d in people. The MatNP:ProNP ratio is about 4–6, meaning that the number of cells in the MatNP is 4–6 times the number of cells in the ProNP.
   4. In health, segmented neutrophils are released from the MatNP to marrow sinuses and then to peripheral blood. Neutrophil-releasing factors include chemoattractants (C5a, IL-8, f-MLP, LTB_4, and PAF) and cytokine leukocytosis factors (IL-1, IL-6, TNFα, TNFβ, G-CSF, and GM-CSF).
B. Blood neutrophils
   1. In health, neutrophils have a blood half-life of about 5–10 h before they enter tissues.
   2. Blood neutrophils are distributed into two pools as determined by their location in vessels.
      a. Neutrophils that are free flowing in blood (and thus collected in blood samples) are in a CNP (circulating neutrophil pool).
      b. Neutrophils that temporarily adhere to endothelial cells are in the MNP (marginated neutrophil pool), which is located primarily in small capillaries and veins in which neutrophils have the most opportunity to contact endothelial cells. After adhesion, neutrophils may break loose and reenter the CNP or migrate into the TNP.
         (1) Inflammatory cytokines (including IL-1 and TNF from macrophages and IFNγ from lymphocytes) stimulate endothelial cells to produce and express adhesion proteins (selectins) that mediate migration and "rolling."
         (2) Endogenous chemical mediators, including LTB_4 and PAF, activate neutrophils, leading to expression of high-affinity membrane integrins, which bind to endothelial cell receptors that mediate the process of migration into tissues.
      c. In most mammals, the MNP:CNP ratio is near 1. In cats, the ratio is 3.[1]
      d. Major processes that influence measured blood neutrophil concentrations
         (1) Production
            (a) Stem cell proliferation and differentiation
            (b) Effectiveness of maturation in the myelocyte stage
         (2) Release from marrow: The oldest or most mature neutrophils preferentially leave the marrow.
         (3) Distribution of neutrophils between the CNP and MNP
         (4) Migration from blood to tissues: Compared to immature neutrophils, mature segmented neutrophils have more potential to emigrate to tissue.

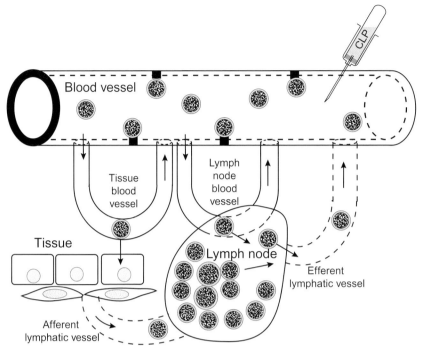

Fig. 2.3. Lymphocyte kinetics in health. Lymph nodes and other primary lymphoid tissues are sites of lymphocyte production but also potential destinations of blood lymphocytes. Blood lymphocytes are distributed between marginal and circulating pools and may enter lymphoid organs or nonlymphoid tissues. Lymphocytes that enter nonlymphoid tissue may remain or may enter the afferent lymphatic vessels and be transported to regional lymph nodes and then perhaps to blood via the thoracic duct.

    C. Tissue neutrophils
       1. Chemotactic substances such as C5a, IL-8, LTB$_4$, and PAF promote neutrophil migration to specific sites. Once in tissue, neutrophils generally do not return to blood.
       2. In the absence of disease, most of an animal's neutrophils die in respiratory and alimentary tissues.

III. Lymphocyte pools and kinetics (Fig. 2.3)
    A. Lymph nodes and other lymphoid tissues
       1. Mediators stimulate differentiation and proliferation of B-lymphocytes and T-lymphocytes.
       2. Lymphocytes leave lymph nodes via efferent lymphatic vessels and enter blood via the thoracic duct.
    B. Blood lymphocytes
       1. Like neutrophils, lymphocytes are distributed into two pools: CLP and MLP. Most lymphocytes in blood are T-lymphocytes.
       2. From blood, lymphocytes enter lymph nodes and other tissues.

    C. Lymphocytes in lymph nodes
      1. Lymphocytes migrate to lymph node cortices via specialized postcapillary venules (high endothelial venules). They then migrate through lymph nodes, exit via efferent lymphatic vessels, and return to blood.
      2. About 25 % of blood lymphocytes enter lymph nodes each day through postcapillary venules, which have unique tall endothelial cells and receptors.
    D. Lymphocytes in other tissues
      1. Lymphocytes emigrate to tissues to perform functions. There they may undergo blastogenesis, enter lymphatic vessels to return to blood, or die.
      2. Like neutrophils, migration to tissues involves lymphocyte chemotaxis and binding to endothelial cell receptors.
    E. Major processes that influence measured blood lymphocyte concentrations
      1. Production
        a. Stem cell proliferation and differentiation
        b. Blastogenesis
      2. Distribution of lymphocytes between the CLP and the MLP
        a. Migration from blood to lymph nodes and other tissues
        b. Migration from lymph nodes via efferent lymphatic vessels to blood
    F. Lymphocyte life span varies from hours to years.

IV. Monocyte pools and kinetics
    A. Monocytes and neutrophils share a common bipotential stem cell (CFU-GM) that is stimulated to differentiate by inflammatory cytokines.
    B. Monocytes develop from monoblasts and promonocytes. When released from marrow, monocytes distribute between marginated and circulating pools.
    C. Like other leukocytes, monocytes emigrate to tissues after binding to endothelial cells. Once in tissues, monocytes may differentiate into cells of the mononuclear phagocyte system: macrophages (including Kupffer cells, alveolar macrophages, and type A synoviocytes), microglial cells, or dendritic cells.
      1. The resting macrophage is sometimes called a histiocyte or fixed macrophage.
      2. Dendritic cells are antigen-presenting cells. Examples include the Langerhans cells of the skin and interdigitating cells in lymph nodes.

V. Eosinophil pools and kinetics
    A. Eosinopoiesis is stimulated by specific mediators, including IL-5 (eosinophil differentiation factor) and GM-CSF from mast cells, macrophages, and lymphocytes.[2]
    B. Marginated and circulating blood eosinophils remain in blood from minutes to hours and die in tissues (the duration in tissues not established but may be weeks or longer).
    C. Eosinophils have phagocytic and bactericidal properties, inactivate mediators from mast cells, and attack larval and adult stages of a few parasites.

VI. Basophil pools and kinetics
    A. Basophils originate in bone marrow, where their production and differentiation is controlled by IL-3 and other cytokines.
    B. The marrow transit time of basophils is at least 2.5 d, their circulating half-life is about 6 h, and they may survive for as long as 2 wk in tissues.
    C. Basophil emigration to tissues is promoted by IL-1, TNFα, and endotoxin and is similar to the process used by neutrophils. Basophils are activated by IL-3 and IgE

binding. Basophil granules contain substances that promote hypersensitivity inflammatory reactions and attract eosinophils.

VII. Mast cell kinetics
    A. Mast cell precursors are found in marrow and are derived from a committed stem cell that is different from the basophil's committed stem cell.
    B. Undifferentiated but committed mast cells leave marrow and circulate in blood but are recognized only by special methods that are not used clinically. Finding differentiated mast cells in the blood of domestic mammals is considered a pathologic state.
    C. Once in tissues, mast cell precursors differentiate into mast cells, undergo mitosis, or die. Mast cells play roles in hypersensitivity reactions, fibrosis, and other inflammatory responses in tissues. Mast cells are considered long-lived cells.

ANALYTICAL PRINCIPLES AND METHODS

I. Complete blood count (CBC)
    A. Numerical and microscopic data of blood leukocytes are components of mammalian CBC results. The primary purposes of the CBC are to screen the hemic system for abnormalities or its response to a disease and to confirm or define the presence of a hematologic disorder.
    B. Major components of the CBC
        1. *Leukogram* (meaning "leukocyte picture"): results of laboratory assays and calculated data that characterize the leukocytes in blood
        2. *Erythrogram* (meaning "erythrocyte picture"): results of laboratory assays and calculated data that characterize the erythrocytes in blood (see Chapter 3)
        3. *Thrombogram* (meaning "platelet picture"): results of laboratory assays and calculated data that characterize the platelets in blood (see Chapter 4)
    C. Basic information obtained from the results of a CBC
        1. If CBC results are WRI, the net effect of a disease on the hematopoietic system has been minimal.
        2. If a cell concentration is increased, the disease is causing at least one of the following:
            a. Increased production of that cell type
            b. A shift of that cell type from a storage or noncirculating pool to circulating blood
            c. An increased circulating life span of the cell type because the rate of cell loss to tissues or rate of cell death is decreased
        3. If a cell concentration is decreased, the disease is causing at least one of the following:
            a. Decreased production of that cell type
            b. A shift of that cell type from the circulation to a noncirculating pool
            c. Decreased circulating life span of the cell type
        4. If morphologic features of a given cell type are abnormal, either (1) a defect in hematopoiesis has caused the production of abnormal cells, or (2) morphological abnormalities have been acquired as the cells circulate in the body.
    D. Blood sample for leukocyte evaluation
        1. Blood is collected into a tube containing either K_2EDTA or K_3EDTA and immediately mixed by slowly inverting the tube at least ten times. To obtain complete and accurate results, the sample must be free of clots and platelet clumps.

2. Stability of cells: [WBC] is usually considered to be stable for several hours at 25 °C and for up to 24 h at 4 °C.

E. Microscopic examination of stained blood films

1. Microscopic examination of a stained blood film should always be a part of a CBC, even if an instrument provides an automated leukocyte differential count. A detailed description of the preparation, staining, and examination of the blood film is beyond the scope of this chapter. The basic components of the processes are as follows:

    a. A blood film is made to obtain an even distribution of cells and an adequate *"counting window"* (i.e., that part of the smear where there is a monolayer of erythrocytes that occasionally touch each other and where nuclear and cytoplasmic features of leukocytes are distinct). Cells will be separated more in the counting window of blood films from anemic individuals.

    b. The air-dried blood film is stained with a Romanowsky-type stain (e.g., Wright, Wright-Giemsa, Diff-Quik, or Quik-Dip) that provides differential staining of cells.

    c. A blood film examination includes scanning with 4× or 10× objectives and more critical evaluation with high-dry (40×) or oil objectives (40×, 50×, or 100×).

        (1) Are the cells evenly distributed and properly stained?

        (2) Are there abnormal large structures in the blood (frequently concentrated in the feathered edge) such as microfilaria, platelet clumps, macrophages, epithelial cells, endothelial cells, or megakaryocytes? If so, record their presence.

        (3) Do the erythrocyte and leukocyte densities correspond with the known cell concentrations in the sample? If not, check the accuracy of the cell concentrations.

        (4) Estimate the platelet density in several 1000 × oil fields and compare with the expected values. Record the presence of giant or shift platelets (platelets larger than erythrocytes in most species) or platelet inclusions.

        (5) Evaluate erythrocytes for abnormal shapes, sizes, colors, inclusions, or associated organisms.

        (6) Complete a leukocyte differential count (see Analytical Principles and Methods, sect. III.E) and record it. Evaluate the observed leukocytes for morphologic abnormalities and record the findings.

2. Microscopic examination of a stained blood film is especially important in sick patients and those with abnormal concentrations of leukocytes, erythrocytes, or platelets. Defects found in the blood cells are described in Chapters 2–4.

F. Staining of blood cells

1. *Romanowsky stains*, which are the best for staining blood cells, were described by Romanowsky (1891) as a combination of eosin and methylene blue to produce a spectrum of colors from blue to reddish orange, depending on the pH of the cell's content.

    a. *Wright stain* is a combination of eosin and oxidized methylene blue. The oxidized methylene blue stains are called *azure dyes*.

    b. Other Romanowsky stains include Giemsa, Wright-Giemsa, and Wright-Leishman, which are various combinations of azure dyes and eosin.

    c. Generally when stated or written, "Wright" stain refers to a Romanowsky-type stain and not the original Wright stain.

    2. What are the contents of cells that are stained?
       a. Acidic structures (e.g., DNA and RNA) attract the basic azure dyes, which stain structures various colors from purple to blue.
       b. Alkaline structures (e.g., hemoglobin, and eosinophil granules) attract the acidic eosin dye and stain structures from red or pink to orange.
    3. Terms used to describe colors or staining properties
       a. *Neutrophilic*: *neutro* (neither alkaline nor acidic) plus *philic* ("loving")
       b. *Eosinophilic*: loves eosin (acidic) dye; will be red to orange
       c. *Basophilic*: loves basic (alkaline and azure) dyes; will be blue to purple
       d. *Azurophilic*: loves azure dye; will have a blue to purple to reddish purple to pink color depending on the substance's pH

II.   Leukogram
    A. Morphologic (microscopic) evaluation
      1. A microscopic evaluation of stained leukocytes is an important part of the leukogram, especially when there is a leukocytosis or leukopenia. It helps confirm or refute automated quantitative results, and provides additional diagnostic and prognostic information that cannot be obtained without microscopy.
      2. Later sections of this chapter describe the clinical significance of leukocytes with abnormal nuclei, cytoplasms, sizes, inclusions, or other features. Besides those changes associated with pathologic states, in vitro changes caused by poor sample handling can make accurate identification of leukocytes nearly impossible.
    B. [WBC]
      1. *[WBC]* is the number of leukocytes per unit volume of blood (in clinical jargon, commonly referred to as *WBC count*). The [WBC] by itself is of limited value without assessing the concentrations of each type of leukocyte.
      2. By some methods, the [WBC] actually is a total nucleated cell concentration. If it is, the [WBC] must be corrected when nRBCs are present (see corrected [WBC] in Eq. 2.1).
      3. Unit conversion: $\#/\mu L \times 10^6 \; \mu L/L = \# \times 10^6/L$ (SI unit)
    C. Differential leukocyte count
      1. A *differential leukocyte count* is a method of determining the relative numbers (or the percentages) of the leukocytes in blood.
      2. Raw data are reported as percentages (e.g., 80 % neutrophils). These percentages plus the [WBC] are used to calculate the concentrations of each type of leukocyte in a blood sample.

III. Principles of determining leukocyte concentrations
    A. Hemocytometer method
      1. A hemocytometer (Fig. 2.4) is used to determine [WBC] by diluting the blood (usually with the Unopette system) and then dispensing the diluted blood into the hemocytometer chambers formed beneath a cover glass. The leukocyte diluent contains a lysing agent that ruptures the erythrocytes so they do not interfere with the nucleated cell enumeration.
      2. The chamber is examined with a microscope, and leukocytes are counted within the 0.9 μL volume of fluid demarcated by the nine large squares. To obtain a leukocyte concentration, the number of leukocytes counted is first multiplied by 1.1 to

Hemocytometer

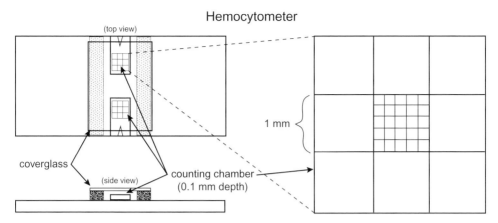

Fig. 2.4. Hemocytometer. The hemocytometer has two components: the thicker glass with special grids on each side and a cover glass. Each grid has nine 1 mm² squares used for leukocyte counting, and each central square is divided into 25 smaller squares that are used for erythrocyte and platelet counting. The distance between the grid surface and the coverslip is 0.1 mm; thus, the volume of the space above the grid is 0.9 mm³ (0.9 µL).

calculate a concentration in the diluted blood. This product is then multiplied by the dilution factor (e.g., 100) to calculate the [WBC] in the blood.

3. Counts should be done in both chambers of the hemocytometer, and the mean of the two values should be used. Markedly different values on the two sides suggest uneven sample distribution and potential error.

B. Impedance cell counters (e.g., Coulter counters, Baker System, Cobas Minos ST-Vet, Mascot Multispecies Hematology System, CELL-DYN, and Heska CBC-Diff Veterinary Hematology System)

1. Basic principles (Fig. 2.5)

   a. When a nonconductive particle (e.g., cell) passes through an aperture, it creates an electrical interference in a current that is flowing through a conductive liquid.

   b. The number of particles detected within a defined volume of diluted blood represents a cell (particle) concentration. The degree of interference depends on the apparent volume (and possibly shape) of the particle, and apparent volumes are used to differentiate particles. The volume of each particle is recorded so that an average volume can be calculated.

   c. Most impedance cell counters are designed to evaluate human blood cells and need to be modified to evaluate domestic mammal blood. Erythrocytes of some species (e.g., goats, sheep, and some horses) are too small to be reliably detected. Also, large platelets (as commonly seen in cats) may be counted as erythrocytes instead of platelets. Lysing solutions and procedures may also need modification because of species differences in susceptibility to cell lysis.

2. Typically, blood is processed along two paths.

   a. Erythrocyte path: mean cell volume, [RBC], and platelet concentrations are determined in diluted blood.

   b. Leukocyte path

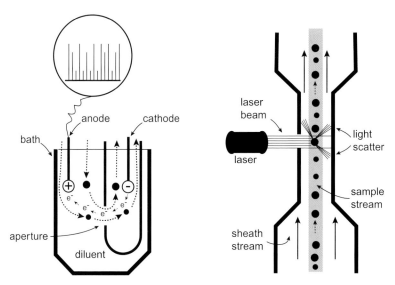

Fig. 2.5. Schematic representation of cell counting principles.

Left: Impedance principle: Blood cells (*solid circles*) suspended in an isotonic diluent enter a bath, pass through a small aperture (about 100 μm diameter), and then leave the bath (flow shown by *dotted arrows*). Concurrently, electrons (e⁻) are moving from a cathode, through the aperture, to an anode. When a cell passes through the aperture, it displaces electrons and interrupts the current briefly, thus creating a voltage peak than can be viewed via an oscilloscope (*top*). Each voltage peak represents a cell (a particle) passing through the aperture; the height of the peak corresponds primarily to the volume of the cell. Particles within a certain impedance range are considered erythrocytes, particles in a lower range are considered platelets, and other particles are not recognized as cells (if the instrument has a "voting out" program). The mean cell volume represents the average volume detected within the erythrocyte range. The erythrocyte concentration represents the number of particles (within the erythrocyte range) per volume. Another bath is used for determining leukocyte concentration. After addition of lysing agent to remove erythrocytes and platelets, the leukocyte nuclei and fluid pass through an aperture and the instrument considers those particles to be leukocytes.

Right: Flow cytometry principle: Blood cells suspended in an isotonic diluent are injected into a special flowing fluid. The fluid dynamics in the system create a sheath around the diluent to form a sample stream. Cells in the sample stream pass through a laser beam, mostly one at a time. Each cell scatters the light in different directions, depending on the cell's size and contents. Sensors detect the scattered light at various locations. Computer programs analyze the data from the sensors to determine which cell has passed through the laser beam.

    (1) The [WBC] and the blood [hemoglobin] are determined in diluted blood after cells (leukocytes, erythrocytes, and platelets) are lysed but nuclei remain as particles.

    (2) In classic impedance methods, the [WBC] is really a total nucleated cell concentration because the nuclei from leukocytes and nucleated erythrocytes are not differentiated.

  C. Optical or laser flow cell cytometers (e.g., CELL-DYN instruments, ADVIA, and IDEXX LaserCyte Hematology Analyzer)

    1. Basic principle (Fig. 2.5)

    a. Laser light is scattered when it hits a cell. The type of scatter depends on cell size, internal structure, granularity, and surface structure, and these features are used to differentiate cells.

    b. Instruments may be able to differentiate the major leukocytes, but computer programs must be specific for each species. Abnormal and some normal leukocytes may not be correctly classified.

2. Some instruments (e.g., CELL-DYN) use both impedance methods and optical methods to determine results: the white cell impedance count (WIC) and the white cell optical count (WOC). When the WIC and WOC disagree (e.g., when nRBCs are present), an error message is generated by the instrument.

3. The ADVIA uses a combination of methods to determine a [WBC] and concurrently a differential leukocyte count.

    a. Peroxidase channel: After lysis of erythrocytes, blood leukocytes are exposed to H_2O_2 and a chromogen (4-chloro-1-naphthol). Leukocytes with peroxidase activity (i.e., neutrophils, eosinophils of some species, and monocytes) initiate reactions that produce a black precipitate in those cells. The leukocytes (stained and unstained) then pass through a beam of tungsten light, and sensors detect increased light absorbance (due to stained cells) and light scatter (due to the size of cells). The peroxidase channel provides a [WBC] and percentages of eosinophils (3+ peroxidase), neutrophils (2+ peroxidase), monocytes (1+ peroxidase), lymphocytes (small, negative peroxidase), and large unstained cells (large, negative peroxidase). Because cat eosinophils lack peroxidase activity, they must be classified by using a special stain (oxazine 750) that is also used for detecting reticulocytes. Eosinophils of some greyhounds, Great Danes, and other dogs have low peroxidase activity and are misclassified as monocytes. Basophils are not accurately classified in domestic species.

    b. Basophil channel: By using a different lysing agent, erythrocytes and leukocytes other than basophils (in human samples) are lysed, and then the fluid passes through a laser beam. Light scatter is used to differentiate particle sizes (intact human basophils versus other cell nuclei) and nuclear density or lobularity. The basophil channel provides a [WBC] and percentages of minimally lobulated cells (lymphocytes, monocytes, immature granulocytes, and blastic cells), basophils (in human samples), and polymorphonuclear cells (neutrophils and eosinophils). Canine and feline basophils are not detected by the basophil channel.

    c. If there are erythrocytes that are resistant to lysis, the [WBC] of the peroxidase channel will be falsely increased, but the basophil channel [WBC] should be accurate. The presence of nucleated erythrocytes is suggested if the "polymorphonuclear cell" concentration from the basophil channel is greater than the sum of the neutrophils and eosinophil concentrations from the peroxidase channel (except in cats, because their eosinophils lack peroxidase activity).

    d. In contrast to the microscopic differential leukocyte count, this electronic differential count differentiates thousands of leukocytes, and thus sampling error is typically not a problem. However, the electronic methods must be species specific and may not be accurate when atypical cells (e.g., toxic neutrophils, and reactive lymphocytes) are present. Automated differential counts may be considered reliable when cell populations are clearly separated as indicated by certain defined criteria.

D. Quantitative buffy coat (QBC) analysis[3,4] (QBC VetAutoread)

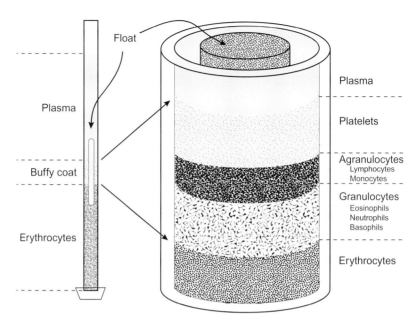

Fig. 2.6. Schematic representation of IDEXX QBC VetTube after centrifugation of whole blood. Centrifugal forces separate the components of blood into five layers (plasma, platelets, agranulocytes, granulocytes, and erythrocytes) based on their relative densities. The buffy coat (composed of platelets and leukocytes) is expanded by a float that has a density similar to buffy coat cells. Layers are recognized by use of fluorescence markers for DNA, RNA, and lipoprotein, and the thickness of each cell layer is used to derive cell concentrations (see the text).

1. A special capillary tube that contains a plastic cylinder or float is used. Because of the cylinder's density, it will float in the region of the buffy coat cells with centrifugation. Because of the cylinder's diameter, the length of the buffy coat is expanded around the float (Fig. 2.6). Fluorescence is used to differentiate cell layers on the basis of lipoprotein, RNA, and DNA contents.

2. If the quantity of blood that is put into the capillary tube is constant and the mean volumes of each cell type are relatively constant, then the concentration of a given cell type will correlate with the thickness of the layer for that cell type. Based on these assumptions, the thickness of a layer is multiplied by a conversion factor to obtain an approximate cell concentration.

3. Results generated by the IDEXX QBC VetAutoread hematology system and the basic principles of each evaluation
   a. Total [WBC] is calculated by adding the granulocyte and combined lymphocyte/monocyte concentrations.
   b. Granulocyte concentration is determined by the thickness of the cell layer with characteristic DNA and RNA/lipoprotein fluorescence for granulocytes. An eosinophil concentration may be reported for dogs and cattle because their eosinophils show detectably more RNA/lipoprotein fluorescence than do their neutrophils and basophils.

     c. Lymphocyte/monocyte concentration is determined by the thickness of the cell layer above the granulocyte layer that has the DNA fluorescence characteristic of lymphocytes and monocytes.

   4. The accuracy of the partial leukocyte differential count depends on the staining reactions of the leukocytes and their densities. Atypical staining or densities will result in erroneous values.

E. Differential leukocyte count by microscopy

   1. A microscopic differential leukocyte count is done by differentiating 100 or more consecutive leukocytes on a stained blood film. Results of the differential count are percentages. A differential leukocyte count should be done in a blood film's counting window. This region is where the leukocytes lie flat enough for their nuclear and cytoplasmic features to be distinct, and where erythrocytes form a monolayer and occasionally touch each other (cells will be more widely spread in samples from anemic patients).

   2. This differential leukocyte count is only an estimate of the leukocyte percentages in a blood sample because of two major factors.

     a. Sampling error: In the microscopic differential count, only a small percentage of all leukocytes in a blood sample are differentiated; the differentiated cells may not be representative. This sampling error can be reduced if more leukocytes are included in the differential count, but this process also requires more time. As a rule of thumb, the count should differentiate 100 leukocytes for every 10,000 leukocytes/μL to obtain representative percentages.

     b. Identification accuracy: A skilled laboratory technologist/technician should be able to identify most leukocytes accurately during the microscopic examination of mammalian blood, but it can be very difficult to classify the leukocytes in some samples; for example, toxic neutrophils versus monocytes, and atypical lymphocytes versus monocytes.

   3. Accuracy and precision of the microscopic leukocyte differential count

     a. Assuming proper sample collection and handling and that cells are identified correctly, the accuracy and precision of the leukocyte percentages are determined by the number of leukocytes included in the differential count and the actual leukocyte percentage in the blood. A confidence interval table of leukocyte differential counts has been generated (Table 2.2) that addresses those two factors.[5]

     b. Evaluation of the data in Table 2.2 reveals several key concepts.

       (1) The confidence interval becomes smaller as the number of cells in the differential count increases. However, it is not practical to do a 1000-cell microscopic differential count in most blood films.

       (2) The confidence intervals are large enough (especially for the 100-cell count) to yield considerable uncertainty in the results (Table 2.3). Thus, the blood of an animal may have exactly the same leukocyte concentrations on 2 different days, but the differential leukocyte counts may differ considerably simply because of encountering different cells during the differential cell counts.

     c. The *absolute* or calculated concentrations of the leukocytes are much better values to interpret compared to the differential count percentages, but the absolute concentrations should be considered estimates in most CBC results, and thus differences (compared to reference intervals or compared to serial results) should be interpreted accordingly.

Table 2.2. The 95 % confidence limits[a] for percentages obtained in differential leukocyte counts[b,c]

α[e]	Number differentiated[d]						α	Number differentiated					
	100		200		1000			100		200		1000	
0	0	4	0	2	0	1	10	4	18	6	16	8	13
1	0	6	0	4	0	2	15	8	24	10	21	12	18
2	0	8	0	6	1	4	20	12	30	14	27	17	23
3	0	9	1	7	2	5	25	16	35	19	32	22	28
4	1	10	1	8	2	6	30	21	40	23	37	27	33
5	1	12	2	10	3	7	35	25	46	28	43	32	39
6	2	13	3	11	4	8	40	30	51	33	48	36	44
7	2	14	3	12	5	9	45	35	56	38	53	41	49
8	3	16	4	13	6	10	50	39	61	42	58	46	54
9	4	17	5	15	7	11	80	70	88	73	86	77	83

[a] Confidence intervals for the actual percentage of a given leukocyte if the specified number of cells were differentiated and the observed percentage was α.

[b] *Source*: Rümke[5]

[c] If observed percentage x is greater than 50 %, then confidence limits are obtained by subtracting the confidence limits of (100 − x) from 100. For example, if x = 80 % in a 100-cell count, then the confidence limits for 20 (100 − x) are subtracted from 100 (100 − 30 or 100 − 12) to give reference limits of 70 % and 88 %, respectively.

[d] Number (100, 200, or 1000) of leukocytes differentiated in a blood film

[e] α is the percentage of a given leukocyte found in a differential count.

Table 2.3. Potential differences in absolute leukocyte concentrations due to random error of microscopic differential leukocyte counts if the total leukocyte concentration was $20.0 \times 10^3/\mu L$

	Low confidence limit values		Actual values		High confidence limit values		Canine reference interval
	%[a]	$\times 10^3/\mu L$	%[b]	$\times 10^3/\mu L$	%[a]	$\times 10^3/\mu L$	$\times 10^3/\mu L$
Neutrophils	70	14.0[c]	80	16.0[c]	88	17.6[c]	3.0–11.5
Neutrophils	30	6.0	40	8.0	51	10.2	3.0–11.5
Eosinophils	4	0.8	10	2.0[c]	18	3.6[c]	0.1–0.8
Eosinophils	0	0.0[d]	0	0.0[d]	4	0.8	0.1–0.8

[a] Percentages for the confidence limits obtained from Table 2.2.

[b] The actual percentage is determined by examining all of the leukocytes in the blood film.

[c] The calculated concentration is above the reference interval.

[d] The calculated concentration is below the reference interval.

    F.   Correction of [WBC] for the presence of nucleated erythrocytes (nRBCs) if the [WBC] is really a total nucleated cell concentration

          1. Microscopic and some electronic methods determine [WBC] by counting nucleated cells or nuclei (either of leukocytes or nRBCs). By these methods, a measured [WBC] represents the sum of nucleated cell concentrations (leukocytes + nRBCs).

2. If nRBCs are observed during the examination of the blood film, they are enumerated by counting the number of nRBCs seen while 100 leukocytes are differentiated and counted. The conventional method of recording the number of nucleated erythrocytes is the number of nRBCs/100 WBCs (e.g., 10 nRBCs/100 WBCs).

3. Rule of thumb: If there are 10 or more nRBCs/100 WBCs, the measured [WBC] is corrected for the presence of nRBCs. The error in the measured [WBC] is usually clinically insignificant when there are fewer than 10 nRBCs/100 WBCs. However, the correction may be done with fewer than 10 nRBCs/100 WBCs.

4. Basis of corrected [WBC] equation (Eq. 2.1)

$$\text{corrected [WBC]} = \text{measured [WBC]} \times \frac{100}{100 + \#\text{nRBC}/100\text{WBC}} \qquad \textbf{(2.1.)}$$

Example: measured [WBC] = 20,000/µL, nRBC = 25/100 WBC

$$\text{corrected [WBC]} = 20,000/\mu L \times \frac{100}{100 + 25} = 20,000/\mu L \times \frac{100}{125} = 16,000/\mu L$$

    a. While 100 leukocytes were counted, 25 nRBCs were also counted. Thus, there were actually 100 leukocytes out of a total of 125 nucleated cells. Therefore, 100 of 125 nucleated cells (4 of 5) must be leukocytes.

    b. If the measured [WBC] was $20.0 \times 10^3/\mu L$, then 4 of 5 of the nucleated cells were leukocytes, and thus the corrected [WBC] is 16.0×10^3 leukocytes/µL.

5. The concentrations of the individual types of leukocytes are calculated after calculation of a corrected [WBC].

IV. Relative versus absolute changes in leukogram results

  A. Except for the centrifugation method, the leukocyte concentrations are calculated by multiplying the total leukocyte concentration by the percentages obtained from the differential count. These calculated concentrations are used to detect *absolute* changes in the leukogram, but it is important to understand that these calculated concentrations can only be as accurate as the values used to calculate them.

  B. Relative changes in leukocyte populations may not reflect true changes.

    1. As shown in Table 2.4, detection of true changes in a leukocyte population should be based on evaluation of the calculated *concentrations* of the individual leukocyte types.

    2. If a leukocyte percentage is increased or decreased compared to reference intervals, the finding can be described as a relative change; that is, relative neutrophilia or relative lymphopenia. However, such descriptions are not recommended because they can be confused with true changes in leukocyte concentrations. For example, dog 2 in Table 2.4 has a relative neutropenia, but the results actually indicate the dog has a neutrophilia (the neutrophil concentration is above the reference interval). When interpreting dog 2's CBC results, one should consider potential causes of a neutrophilia, not of a neutropenia.

  C. The concepts of relative changes are presented to clarify why they should not be used when interpreting a leukogram. In all other sections of this book, terms used to describe leukogram findings refer to absolute changes; that is, abnormal concentrations rather than abnormal percentages.

Table 2.4. Relative versus absolute changes in leukocyte values in CBC results

	Units	Dogs 1[a]	2[b]	3[c]	4[d]	Reference interval
Neutrophils	%	30	30	70	70	60–80
Lymphocytes	%	70	70	30	30	20–35
WBCs	$\times 10^3/\mu L$	2.0	50.0	2.0	50.0	6.0–17.0
Neutrophils	$\times 10^3/\mu L$	0.6	15.0	1.4	35.0	3.0–11.5
Lymphocytes	$\times 10^3/\mu L$	1.4	35.0	0.6	15.0	1.0–4.0

[a] Based on percentages, relative neutropenia and relative lymphocytosis are present. There is a high lymphocyte percentage because of an absolute neutropenia.

[b] Dog 2: Based on percentages, relative neutropenia and relative lymphocytosis are present. There is a low neutrophil percentage because of the marked absolute lymphocytosis. A mild absolute neutrophilia is also present.

[c] Dog 3's leukocyte percentages are within reference intervals. The dog has an absolute neutropenia and absolute lymphopenia.

[d] Dog 4's leukocyte percentages are within reference intervals. The dog has an absolute neutrophilia and an absolute lymphocytosis.

ABNORMAL LEUKOCYTE CONCENTRATIONS IN BLOOD

I.   Abnormal neutrophil concentrations
    A. Left shift
        1. A *left shift* (shift to the left) is an increased concentration of nonsegmented neutrophils (usually bands) in blood. When there is great demand for neutrophils in tissues, younger stages (metamyelocytes, myelocytes, and rarely progranulocytes) may be present in the left shift.
            a. Left shifts occur when release of neutrophils from marrow diminishes the SNP, and younger cells are then released from the MatNP. The capability of neutrophils to respond to stimuli and migrate increases as they mature; thus, segmented neutrophils respond first and immature forms respond later.
            b. Because it usually occurs in response to relatively intense, often acute inflammatory stimuli, a left shift is frequently considered the hallmark of acute inflammation. Such inflammation is typically caused by infectious agents (e.g., pyogenic bacteria, or fungi) but can be caused by noninfectious disorders (e.g., necrosis, immune-mediated disease, or neoplasia). Glucocorticoid hormones and endotoxins also stimulate release of neutrophils and thus may cause a mild left shift.
        2. Left-shift classifications
            a. Severity: Two different features might be considered when describing the severity of a left shift. Since the terms can describe different findings, one must be careful in interpreting or using the terms.
                (1) Immaturity of neutrophils in the left shift: bands (1+ or slight); band and metamyelocytes (2+ or moderate); and band, metamyelocytes, and myelocytes (3+ or marked)[6]
                (2) Magnitude of nonsegmented neutrophil concentrations: mild ($< 1.0 \times 10^3/\mu L$), moderate (1.0–$10.0 \times 10^3/\mu L$), and marked ($> 10.0 \times 10^3/\mu L$). Ranges are provided as examples and such guidelines vary with species.

    b. Regenerative versus degenerative left-shift classifications
      (1) When first described by Dr. O.W. Schalm (father of veterinary hematology), specific criteria for classifying left shifts were not provided.[6]
        (a) A regenerative left shift is "characterized by a leukocytosis due to neutrophilia and with the appearance of immature neutrophils in peripheral blood" (p. 272).
        (b) In a degenerative left shift, "total leukocyte count remains within the normal range or is only slightly elevated, while the occurrence of young granulocytes in the circulation is prominent" (p. 272).
      (2) In the 1986 edition of *Schalm's Veterinary Hematology*, these states are described as follows:[7]
        (a) "Regenerative left shift is characterized by a leukocytosis due to neutrophilia and with the appearance of immature neutrophils in peripheral blood. . . . In the typical regenerative left shift, the proportion of various immature neutrophils is orderly and follows a pyramidal distribution, with the most immature cell being the least numerous. Usually the mature neutrophils outnumber the immature cells" (p. 824).
        (b) "The main feature of a degenerative left shift is the occurrence of young neutrophilic granulocytes in the circulation in numbers exceeding mature neutrophils. The WBC count is often suggestive of leukopenia, but it may sometimes be within the normal range or, rarely, elevated" (p. 824).
        (c) These descriptions allow for the classification of most left shifts. However, a neutropenia with mature forms exceeding immature forms does not fall within the classifications but has been considered by some to be a degenerative left shift.
      (3) Clinical significance
        (a) A regenerative left shift indicates that a neutrophil response to the inflammatory state is appropriate and, at the time of sampling, neutrophil production and release are adequately responding to the demand.
        (b) A degenerative left shift suggests that neutrophil production and release are not adequately responding to the demand.
      (4) Samplings from multiple days will better characterize the neutrophil response. If the regenerative left shift persists, then neutropoiesis is regenerating a replacement population of neutrophils that are being used in tissues to fight the invader. If it progresses to a degenerative left shift or if a degenerative left shift persists, then there is inadequate neutropoiesis and the animal's condition is probably deteriorating (or degenerating).

B. A *right shift* (shift to the right) is an increased concentration of hypersegmented neutrophils in blood. Hypersegmented neutrophils have five or more nuclear lobes and usually indicate older cells that have aged in blood because of increased circulation time. The presence of hypersegmented neutrophils in blood is typically recorded as a comment in the CBC results and not as a separate part of a leukocyte differential count.

    1. Glucocorticoid hormones (endogenous or exogenous) decrease emigration of neutrophils to tissue by down-regulating adhesion molecules and thus can cause a right shift.

Table 2.5. Diseases and conditions that cause neutrophilia

Inflammatory neutrophilia
   *Infections: bacterial, fungal, viral, protozoal
   *Immune hemolytic anemia
   *Necrosis: hemolysis, hemorrhage, infarcts, burns, neoplasia, sterile inflammation
   Sterile foreign body
Steroid neutrophilia
   *Stress (physical or neurogenic)
   Hyperadrenocorticism
   *Glucocorticoid therapy
   Adrenocorticotropic hormone administration
Physiologic (shift) neutrophilia
   *Fight-or-flight response: excitement, fright, pain, exercise, anxiety
   Catecholamine injections: epinephrine or norepinephrine
Chronic neutrophilic leukemia
Paraneoplastic neutrophilia
Others or unknown mechanisms
   Neutrophilia of leukocyte adhesion deficiency
   G-CSF administration
   Estrogen toxicosis (early)

  * Relatively common disease or condition

    2. Other causes of a right shift: Poodle marrow dyscrasia,[8] FeLV-associated myelodyscrasia,[9] equine idiopathic hypersegmentation,[10,11] vitamin B_{12} deficiency in giant schnauzers with an inherited malabsorption syndrome,[12] folate deficiency in a cat,[13] occasionally chronic inflammatory diseases, and in vitro aging due to delayed analysis.
  C. Neutrophilia (increased measured blood neutrophil concentration) (Table 2.5)
    1. Acute inflammatory neutrophilia
      a. This neutrophilia results from changes in neutrophil kinetics that are caused by acute inflammatory mediators. The net result is an increased CNP that may contain a left shift (Fig. 2.7B).
        (1) Release from SNP occurs within hours after onset of inflammation and causes initial neutrophilia if release exceeds neutrophil emigration to inflamed tissue.
        (2) Release from MatNP causes a left shift and occurs after reduction or depletion of SNP.
        (3) Increased production from the myelocyte stage: It takes 2–4 d before effects are seen in peripheral blood.
        (4) Increased production via stem cells: This will lead to granulocytic hyperplasia. It takes about 5 d before effects are seen in peripheral blood.
      b. *Acute* refers to the type of inflammatory reaction and *not* the duration of the disease. The acute inflammatory pattern can be seen in an animal with a prolonged inflammatory state if there remains an active need for neutrophils in the inflamed tissue.
      c. Inflammatory mediators must enter systemic blood and stimulate marrow cells for a neutrophilia to develop.

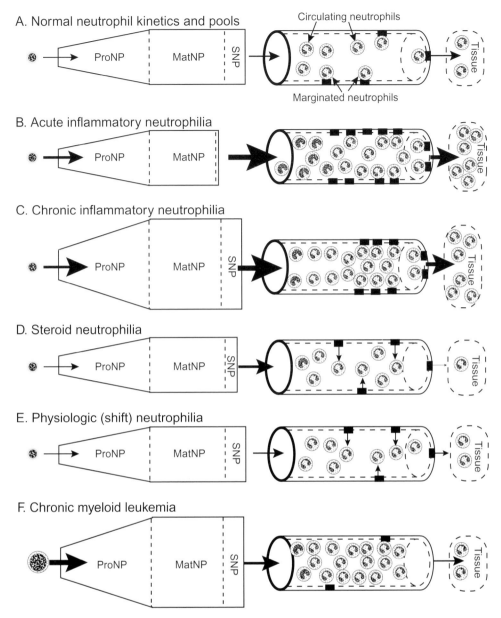

Fig. 2.7. Neutrophilia kinetics.

A. Neutrophil kinetics in health (a reduced version of Fig. 2.2).

B. Acute inflammatory neutrophilia: Neutrophilia occurs because the release of neutrophils from the marrow exceeds the migration of neutrophils to the inflamed tissue. A left shift is created by the release of band neutrophils from the MatNP.

C. Chronic inflammatory neutrophilia: Neutrophilia occurs because the release of neutrophils from the marrow exceeds the migration of neutrophils to the inflamed tissue. A left shift may not be present because granulocytic hyperplasia maintains the SNP.

D. Steroid neutrophilia: Neutrophilia occurs because of a shift of neutrophils from the MNP to the CNP, decreased migration of neutrophils to tissue, and release of neutrophils from the SNP and sometimes the MatNP.

E. Physiologic (shift) neutrophilia: Neutrophilia occurs because of the shift of neutrophils from the MNP to the CNP.

F. Chronic myeloid leukemia: Neutrophilia occurs because of an uncontrolled proliferation of a clone of neoplastic neutrophil precursors. Acute myelogenous leukemia may create a leukocytosis, but the neoplastic cells may not be easily recognized as being of neutrophil lineage.

Table 2.6. Species differences in the magnitude of inflammatory neutrophilia

	Reference intervals	Common magnitude	Occasional magnitude	Uncommon magnitude
Dogs	3.0–11.0[a]	12.0–30.0	30.0–60.0	> 60.0
Cats	2.0–12.5	13.0–25.0	25.0–40.0	> 40.0
Horses	2.2–8.6	9.0–20.0	20.0–30.0	> 30.0
Cattle	0.6–4.0	4.0–10.0	10.0–20.0	> 20.0

[a] Neutrophil concentrations are expressed $\times 10^3/\mu L$ of blood.

(1) A neutrophilia is expected if there is substantial acute inflammation of subcutaneous tissues or internal tissues (respiratory tract, pancreas, peritoneal or pleural cavity, and occasionally uterus, liver, or intestine), because mediators can easily access systemic blood.

(2) Inflammation of brain, spinal cord, superficial cutaneous lesions, and lower urinary tract may not cause a neutrophilia, because mediators are lost (to urine or skin) or do not leave the protected environment (brain or spinal cord).

d. The magnitude of inflammatory neutrophilias varies among species, and thus interpretation of specific concentrations differs among species (Table 2.6).

e. The inflammatory bovine neutrophilia results primarily from increased production (granulocytic hyperplasia) and not from release of stored neutrophils, because cattle have a small SNP.

f. The term *leukemoid response* has been used to describe any extreme inflammatory leukocytosis that is leukemia-like but proven not to be leukemic. The term can be applied only retrospectively.

(1) Classically, disorders associated with a marked inflammatory neutrophilia included focal suppurative lesions (e.g., canine pyometra, pleuritis or pyothorax, peritonitis, prostatitis, pneumonia, and abscesses) and hemolytic anemia (especially immune mediated).

(2) Other disorders recognized as causing an extreme inflammatory neutrophilia include canine rectal neoplasms,[14] canine pulmonary neoplasms,[15] canine babesiosis,[16] and canine hepatozoonosis caused by *Hepatozoon americanum*.

g. An animal that has an acute inflammatory neutrophilia usually has a lymphopenia, often an eosinopenia, and occasionally a monocytosis or toxic neutrophils. In dogs, a mastocytemia may be found.

2. Chronic inflammatory neutrophilia

a. This neutrophilia results from changes in neutrophil kinetics when an inflammatory process continues for at least a week during which inflammatory mediators stimulate development of granulocytic hyperplasia (Fig. 2.7C). If the SNP is replenished, segmented neutrophils are released instead of band neutrophils, and thus the left shift diminishes. In addition, other defense mechanisms become active, and thus the need for neutrophils in tissues may diminish. However, if the inflammatory stimulus is more intense, a left shift may persist, or a chronic inflammatory pattern may never be reached. In these disorders, there is increased production of neutrophils because of granulocytic hyperplasia and increased neutrophil release from SNP in response to inflammatory mediators. When the rate of neutrophil release from marrow is greater than the rate of neutrophil margination and emigration to tissues, a neutrophilia develops.

b. *Chronic* indirectly refers to the duration of the disease; the inflammatory process has persisted long enough to result in granulocytic hyperplasia.

c. When an animal has a chronic inflammatory neutrophilia, other leukocyte abnormalities may include lymphocytosis (with or without reactive lymphocytes), monocytosis, eosinophilia, basophilia, a left shift, a right shift, and toxic neutrophils.

3. Steroid (stress) neutrophilia

a. This neutrophilia results from changes created by the effects of endogenous or exogenous glucocorticoids on neutrophil kinetics (Fig. 2.7D). Although this neutrophilia is frequently called a *stress neutrophilia*, it should not be confused with the *physiologic (shift) neutrophilia* caused by the stress-induced release of catecholamines.

(1) Neutrophils shift from the MNP to the CNP because the production of adhesion molecules is down-regulated.

(a) This process can potentially double the measured neutrophil concentrations in canine, equine, and bovine blood. Greater increases in measured neutrophil concentrations may occur in feline blood because of the larger feline MNP.

(b) Because of this shift, fewer neutrophils emigrate to tissues, and thus neutrophils have an increased circulating life span. The older neutrophils may become hypersegmented.

(2) Increased release of neutrophils from marrow: Mostly segmented neutrophils are released, but glucocorticoids may cause release of band neutrophils and thus a mild left shift.

b. Classic steroid leukograms are seen most frequently in dogs, where they consist of a mature neutrophilia (2–4 × URL), lymphopenia, monocytosis, and eosinopenia.[7] The magnitude of neutrophilia varies with different glucocorticoids and dosages. The effects on neutrophil kinetics diminish with chronic elevations in glucocorticoids.

c. Blood may have a mild left shift (typically band neutrophils < 1000/μL), a right shift, or no shift.

d. Typical glucocorticoid effects differ among species of animals (Table 2.7).

Table 2.7. Expected leukocyte concentrations in animals with steroid leukograms

Leukocyte concentrations	Dogs	Cats	Horses	Cattle
Total WBCs (× 10³/μL)	15.0–35.0	20.0–30.0	15.0–20.0	8.0–18.0
Segmented neutrophil	↑	↑	↑	WRI–↑
Band neutrophil	WRI–slight ↑	WRI	WRI	WRI
Lymphocyte	↓	↓–WRI	↓–WRI	↓
Monocyte	WRI–↑	WRI–↑	WRI	↓–WRI
Eosinophil	↓[a]	WRI[b]	WRI[b]	↓–WRI

[a] Decreased eosinophil concentrations in routine CBC results are typically not reliable because of the imprecision of leukocyte differential counts; also, lower reference limit may be 0/μL

[b] Eosinopenia is not typically recognized because the lower reference limit for eosinophils is 0/μL.

4. Physiologic (shift) neutrophilia
   a. This neutrophilia results from effects of catecholamines (typically associated with fear, excitement, and exercise) that cause a shift from the MNP to the CNP (Fig. 2.7E). The shift may be caused by the change in fluid dynamics that results from increased blood flow rate, especially in lungs.[17] Neutrophil adherence to endothelial cells may also be reduced.[18]
   b. The magnitude of neutrophilia may be up to twice the URL for canine, equine, and bovine blood, and potentially up to 3–4 × URL for a cat because of a cat's larger MNP.
   c. It is seen most frequently in healthy animals and mostly in cats. Leukocyte concentrations return to reference intervals relatively fast (within an hour) if the stimulus disappears.
   d. Because the increased blood flow rate alters kinetics of other leukocytes, there also may be increased concentrations of other leukocytes, especially lymphocytes. The entire response results in a physiologic leukocytosis.
5. Chronic myeloid leukemia (Table 6.5)
   a. Neutrophilia is caused by a clonal proliferation of neutrophils. To be recognized as a neutrophilia, the cells would be well-differentiated neutrophils in a chronic myeloid leukemia; this condition is difficult to differentiate from nonneoplastic neutrophilias. There may be an extreme leukocytosis with a left shift that is more apparent in the bone marrow (Fig. 2.7F).
   b. In acute myeloid leukemia, the cells would be immature granulocyte precursors that may not be classified as neutrophils in leukogram results.
6. Paraneoplastic neutrophilic leukocytosis
   a. Neoplastic tissues produce G-CSF or a similar substance that stimulates neutropoiesis. The neutrophil concentrations of the blood may resemble either an acute or a chronic inflammatory neutrophilia.
   b. Canine neoplasms associated with extreme neutrophilic leukocytoses include rectal adenomatous polyp,[19] renal tubular carcinoma,[20] and metastatic fibrosarcoma.[21]
7. Other conditions or unknown mechanisms
   a. Neutrophilia of leukocyte adhesion deficiency in cattle and dogs (see details in the Other Nonneoplastic Leukocyte Disorders section)
   b. Neutrophilia induced by G-CSF administration
   c. Neutrophilia of estrogen toxicosis: Neutrophilia occurs 2–3 wk after estradiol injections.[22]
D. Neutropenia (decreased measured blood neutrophil concentration) (Table 2.8)
   1. Inflammatory neutropenia (Fig. 2.8B)
      a. Typically, this neutropenia occurs during an overwhelming or severe acute inflammatory disease. If associated with endotoxemia, margination of neutrophils may be a dominant change in neutrophil kinetics.
      b. Neutropenia results when margination in vessels or emigration of neutrophils to inflamed tissue exceeds the release of neutrophils from marrow.
         (1) Cytokines and chemoattractants stimulate margination and emigration of large numbers of neutrophils to inflamed tissue. This movement may occur within hours of introduction of an infectious agent. Cytokines also stimulate increased production of neutrophils, but the blood changes caused by this stimulation are not expected for at least 2 d.

Table 2.8. Diseases and conditions that cause neutropenia

Inflammation
   *Overwhelming bacterial infections: equine salmonellosis
   *Some viral infections: canine and feline parvovirus, equine influenza
   *Variety of inflammatory states in cattle: mastitis, pneumonia
Peripheral destruction
   Immune-mediated neutropenia
   Hemophagocytic syndromes
Granulocytic hypoplasia
   *Infectious: parvovirus (dogs and cats), FeLV, *Toxoplasma*, *Ehrlichia*
   Neoplastic: primary or metastatic
   Toxic
     *Predictable: estrogen, chemotherapeutic drugs, chloramphenicol (cats)
     Idiosyncratic: phenylbutazone, bracken fern, griseofulvin
   Marrow necrosis
   Myelofibrosis
Ineffective production
   Immune-mediated neutropenia
   Diphenylhydantoin and phenylbutazone toxicosis (suspected in animals)
   Chronic idiopathic neutropenia (G-CSF deficiency)
Cyclic hematopoiesis
   Cyclic hematopoiesis of grey collies
   Cyclic hematopoiesis associated with FeLV

* A relatively common disease or condition
Note: Lists of specific disorders or conditions are not complete but are provided to give examples. Some dogs of the Belgian Tervuren breed have lower neutrophil concentrations than reference intervals for most dogs.[130]

    (2) Neutrophil-releasing factors stimulate a sudden release of neutrophils from the SNP. After the SNP is depleted, cells in the MatNP are released, and thus a left shift is typically present. However, there may not be a left shift even with the release of cells from the MatNP, because the total measured neutrophil concentration may be less than the URL for the band neutrophil concentration. If bone marrow is examined during the illness, cell populations reflect the changes in the leukon.
      (a) Early: depletion of SNP and possibly decreased MatNP
      (b) 2–3 d: increased ProNP without increased MatNP
      (c) 5–7 d: granulocytic hyperplasia from increases in both ProNP and MatNP
  c. Inflammatory neutropenia is common in adult cattle because they have a relatively small SNP. Once there is a demand for neutrophils, there is not a sudden release of neutrophils from bone marrow to create a neutrophilia. Also, experimental data indicate that it takes longer for cattle to generate neutrophils once the reserve pool is depleted.[23]
    (1) The following sequence is the expected bovine response with acute inflammation induced by introduction of *Enterobacter aerogenes* into lactating quarters.[7]

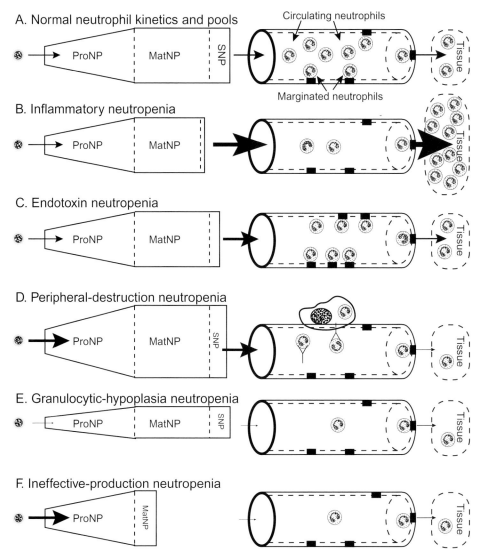

Fig. 2.8. Neutropenia kinetics.

A. Neutrophil kinetics in health (a reduced version of Fig. 2.2).

B. Inflammatory neutropenia (overwhelming tissue demand): Neutropenia occurs because the margination and migration of neutrophils into the inflamed tissues exceed the release of neutrophils from marrow.

C. Endotoxin neutropenia: Neutropenia occurs because endotoxins stimulate the margination of neutrophils (sequestration of neutrophils in the MNP). With the concurrent inflammatory response, a variety of changes in neutrophil kinetics are possible. Endotoxins may also affect marrow cells to cause increased release of neutrophils (see the text).

D. Peripheral destruction neutropenia: Neutropenia occurs because neutrophils are being destroyed by macrophages, perhaps because of antineutrophil antibodies. If persistent, granulocytic hyperplasia will develop.

E. Granulocytic hypoplasia neutropenia: Neutropenia occurs because neutrophil production is decreased.

F. Ineffective production neutropenia: Neutropenia occurs because a disorder prevents an orderly maturation of neutrophil precursors in the marrow and thus neutrophil production is decreased. This may occur at different stages of neutrophil maturation. It may be caused by immune-mediated cell destruction in some cases.

       (a) Initial neutropenia (within 6 h)
       (b) Significant left shift (by 24 h)
       (c) Nadir of neutropenia (by 31 h)
    (2) The severity of the neutropenia typically will be greater in bacteremic than nonbacteremic cattle with mastitis.[24]

2. Neutropenia caused by endotoxemia (Fig. 2.8C)
   a. Whenever an infection with Gram-negative organisms causes an endotoxemia, endotoxins initiate changes in the leukon.
   b. This neutropenia occurs because endotoxins cause the rapid shift of neutrophils from the CNP to the MNP. This effect lasts for 1–3 h after a single exposure. Endotoxins also induce the release of inflammatory mediators (e.g., TNF and IL-1) that promote the adhesion of neutrophils to endothelial cells. Concurrent activation of the neutrophils may cause oxidative damage to endothelial cells.[25]
   c. Because of several factors, a neutropenia may no longer be present when a veterinarian examines an endotoxemic animal.
    (1) Endotoxins stimulate release of neutrophils from bone marrow in about 8–12 h.
    (2) Endotoxins stimulate increased production of neutrophils, which affects blood neutrophil concentrations in about 3–5 d.
    (3) Other inflammatory mediators may concurrently alter neutrophil kinetics.
   d. Most studies of endotoxin-induced changes in neutrophil kinetics involved injection of endotoxins. In spontaneous infections, other mediators are probably also altering neutrophil movement.

3. Peripheral destruction neutropenia (Fig. 2.8D)
   a. Immune-mediated neutropenia[26,27]
    (1) Antineutrophil antibodies bind to neutrophils that are then destroyed by the mononuclear phagocytic system.
    (2) Factors that induce the pathologic process are not established in domestic mammals.
    (3) Animals may be responsive to glucocorticoid therapy or other immunosuppressive agents.[28]
    (4) Examination of marrow may reveal granulocytic hyperplasia.
   b. Neutropenia of hemophagocytic syndrome[29–31]
    (1) Neutropenia may be one of multiple cytopenias associated with phagocyte hyperplasia.
    (2) In people, the acquired syndromes are associated with a variety of infectious and neoplastic states.[32]

4. Granulocytic hypoplasia neutropenia (decreased-production neutropenia) (Fig. 2.8E)
   a. Granulocytic hypoplasia occurs when either stem cells or cells of the marrow microenvironment are damaged. The hypoplasia causes decreased neutrophil production.
   b. This form of neutropenia is usually differentiated from other neutropenias by persistence of neutropenia (usually without a left shift, though secondary infections may cause left shifts) and bone marrow examination findings of granulocytic hypoplasia. Typically, maturation within the neutrophilic cell line is complete and orderly. Because the disease may damage other cell lines in the marrow, concentrations of other blood cells (e.g., erythrocytes or platelets) may

be decreased. There may not be a lymphopenia, because lymphopoiesis in other lymphoid tissues may not be impaired.

   c. Chemotherapeutic agents can be cytotoxic to many rapidly dividing cells, including neutrophil precursors. Thus, neutropenia can result from the administration of chemotherapeutic agents such as vincristine, doxorubicin, cyclophosphamide, cisplatin, and carboplatin. The onset of the neutropenia depends on several factors but typically occurs 7–10 d after the last dose.

5. Ineffective production neutropenia (neutropenia of ineffective neutropoiesis) (Fig. 2.8F)

   a. Ineffective production occurs when neutrophil precursors are defective or damaged and die before they are released from marrow.

   b. Lack of an orderly maturation sequence in marrow samples suggests there is a maturation arrest (e.g., hyperplasia up to one stage and then hypoplasia after that stage). There also may appear to be a failure to release (i.e., the animal may have a persistent neutropenia and a concurrent granulocytic hyperplasia in the marrow). These patterns occur in some dogs in which immune-mediated neutropenia is suspected[28] and parallels findings in some dogs with marrow-directed immune-mediated anemia.

   c. Ineffective neutropoiesis is characterized by a persistent neutropenia (with little or no left shift) concurrent with marrow hyperplasia prior to the defective stage. A monocytosis may be present because stimulation of CFU-GM results in more cells differentiating toward monocytes and neutrophils. Lymphocyte concentrations typically are WRI.

   d. Chronic idiopathic neutropenia was reported in a rottweiler that had a G-CSF deficiency.[33] The dog's marrow had granulocyte and mononuclear cell populations indicative of a maturation arrest. The findings suggested that G-CSF was needed for terminal neutrophil differentiation.

6. Cyclic hematopoiesis

   a. Canine cyclic hematopoiesis (cyclic neutropenia)[34]

     (1) Canine cyclic hematopoiesis is a hereditary disorder of grey collies and grey collie crosses. Its diagnostic features are caused by 11 d to 14 d cycles of neutrophil, erythrocyte, platelet, and monocyte production that result from cyclic differentiation of stem cells toward committed stem cells. The cycle of neutrophil production is out of synchrony with the other cycles.

     (2) Affected dogs are susceptible to infections because of recurrent neutropenia and usually grow ill prior to 6 mo of age. Anemia is usually mild because the life span of erythrocytes is longer than the 11- to 14-d cycles. A thrombocytosis may be present, and defective platelet function has been described.

     (3) People with cyclic neutropenia have mutations in the gene that encodes the serine proteinase neutrophil elastase. Mutations to this gene were not detected in affected dogs.

     (4) Affected dogs do have defects in the intracellular trafficking of neutrophil elastase such that it becomes incorporated into the plasma membrane rather than into granules. These dogs have a decreased production of the β-subunit of *adaptor protein complex 3* (AP3), which is a cargo protein for neutrophil elastase.[35] It is hypothesized that transmembrane elastase degrades unknown local target protein(s) important in hematopoiesis (e.g., hematopoietic

Table 2.9. Diseases and conditions that cause lymphocytosis

Chronic inflammation
  *Bacterial infections, especially anaplasmal (e.g., *Ehrlichia canis*)
  Fungal infections, primarily systemic
  Viral infections: FeLV, BLV, equine infectious anemia virus
  Protozoal infections, especially babesial and theilerial
Physiologic (shift) lymphocytosis
  *Fight-or-flight response: excitement, fright, pain, exercise, anxiety
  Catecholamine injections: epinephrine or norepinephrine
Lymphoproliferative disorders
  *Lymphoma (BLV, FeLV, and idiopathic), leukemic phase
  Lymphoid leukemia
  Persistent lymphocytosis of cattle (BLV)
Hypoadrenocorticism

* A relatively common disease or condition
Note: Lists of specific disorders or conditions are not complete but are provided to give examples. Puppies, kittens, and foals have higher lymphocyte concentrations than do mature animals of the respective species.

cytokines or receptors), resulting in decreased hematopoiesis. When neutropenia develops, there is less elastase-induced inhibition of hematopoiesis, thus allowing a new wave of progenitors to develop until the cycle repeats.
  b. Cyclic hematopoiesis associated with FeLV infection[36]

II. Abnormal lymphocyte concentrations
  A. Lymphocytosis (increased measured blood lymphocyte concentration) (Table 2.9)
    1. Chronic inflammatory lymphocytosis (Fig. 2.9B)
      a. This lymphocytosis is caused by increased lymphopoiesis in response to chronic antigenic or cytokine stimulation. Reactive lymphocytes may be seen.
      b. Lymphocytosis is part of a hyperplastic lymphoid system. There may be concurrent enlarged lymph nodes or lymphoid hyperplasia in other tissues.
      c. Lymphocytosis is usually mild to moderate (2–$3 \times$ URL). Occasionally there will be a marked lymphocytosis ($> 30.0 \times 10^3/\mu$L in dogs).
      d. Concurrent leukogram abnormalities commonly include a neutrophilia (mature, perhaps with right shift or left shift) and/or a monocytosis and occasionally an eosinophilia and/or basophilia.
    2. Physiologic (shift) lymphocytosis (Fig. 2.9C)
      a. This lymphocytosis is caused by shifting of lymphocytes from the MLP to the CLP (especially from the spleen) that is promoted by exogenous or endogenous catecholamines. The lymphocyte shift is probably mediated through both increased blood flow rate and decreased lymphocyte adherence to endothelium.[18]
      b. The magnitude of lymphocytosis may be up to $2 \times$ URL, and the lymphocytosis usually lasts minutes to hours.
      c. Morphologic changes in lymphocytes are not expected, but there are data to indicate that the catecholamine effect is mostly on natural killer cells, which may appear as granular lymphocytes (also called large granular lymphocytes).[18]

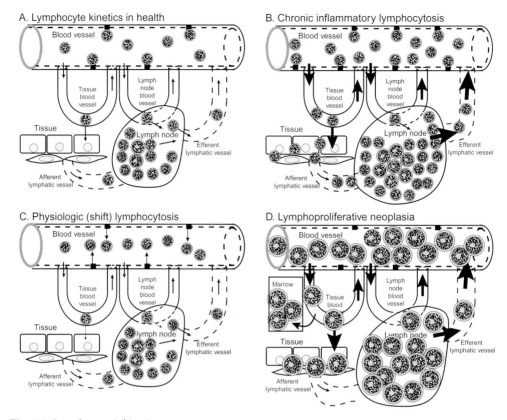

Fig. 2.9. Lymphocytosis kinetics.
A. Lymphocyte kinetics in health (a reduced version of Fig. 2.3).
B. Chronic inflammatory lymphocytosis: Lymphocytosis occurs because of increased lymphopoiesis associated with the immune response to the inflammatory agent. The lymphocytosis is a part of lymphoid hyperplasia.
C. Physiologic (shift) lymphocytosis: Lymphocytosis occurs because of the shift of lymphocytes from the MLP to the CLP.
D. Lymphoproliferative neoplasia: A lymphoid leukemia results from an uncontrolled proliferation of a lymphoid cell clone. This figure illustrates the leukemic manifestation of lymphoma; see the text for other lymphoid leukemias.

       d. As with shift neutrophilia, shift lymphocytosis is seen most frequently in cats, young horses, and healthy animals.
  3. Lymphoproliferative disorders (Table 6.5 and Fig. 2.9D)
       a. This lymphocytosis usually is caused by a neoplastic proliferation of lymphoid cells in lymph nodes, bone marrow, or other tissues.
       b. BLV and FeLV are known to induce neoplastic transformation of lymphocytes, but not all forms of lymphoid neoplasia in cats and cattle are caused by these viruses. Causes of lymphoid neoplasia in other domestic mammals are not known.
       c. BLV infections may also induce a persistent polyclonal B-cell lymphocytosis without the other features of lymphoid neoplasia (e.g., blast transformation, and tissue manifestations of lymphoma).

  d. In domestic mammals, lymphoid leukemias usually represent the leukemic manifestations of lymphoma; that is, the neoplasia started in the lymph nodes (or other lymphoid tissues) and spread to the blood.

  e. Leukemia is classically characterized by a marked or extreme lymphocytosis with many lymphocytes having abnormal or "immature" morphologic features. The diagnosis is easiest if both criteria are present and difficult when they are not.

 4. Lymphocytosis of hypoadrenocorticism (Addison's disease)

  a. This lymphocytosis may be caused by an absence of glucocorticoid hormones, which normally inhibit lymphocyte production or alter lymphocyte distribution in the body.

  b. Dogs with hypoadrenocorticism may have a lymphocytosis. *Always* think of hypoadrenocorticism if an obviously stressed dog has a neutropenia and lymphocytosis (stress should cause the opposite—neutrophilia and lymphopenia), especially in azotemic dogs.

  c. The classic leukogram of hypoadrenocorticism consists of a low-normal to decreased neutrophil concentration, high-normal to increased lymphocyte concentration, a normal monocyte concentration, and a high-normal to increased eosinophil concentration.

 5. "Lymphocytosis" of young animals

  a. Puppies, kittens, calves, and foals have greater blood lymphocyte concentrations than do adult animals. Lymphocyte concentrations in cattle increase until about 1 yr of age, and then gradually decrease over the years in adults.[7]

  b. Compared to adult reference intervals, the apparent lymphocytosis may be up to $2 \times$ URL.

B. Lymphopenia (decreased measured blood lymphocyte concentration) (Table 2.10)

 1. Acute inflammatory lymphopenia (Fig. 2.10A)

  a. This lymphopenia is caused by changes in lymphocyte kinetics stimulated by acute inflammatory mediators that reduce the CLP.[37]

Table 2.10. Diseases and conditions that cause lymphopenia

Acute inflammation
 *Acute bacterial infections
 *Acute viral infections
 Endotoxemia
Steroids
 *See the list for steroid neutrophilia in Table 2.5
Depletion
 Lymphoid effusion: chylothorax, and feline cardiomyopathy
 Loss of lymph: alimentary lymphoma, enteric neoplasms, granulomatous enteritis, paratuberculosis, protein-losing enteropathy, lymphangiectasia, ulcerative enteritis
Lymphoid hypoplasia or aplasia
 Immunosuppressive drugs or whole body irradiation
 Destruction of lymphoid tissues: multicentric lymphoma, generalized lymphadenitis
 Combined immunodeficiency of horses (Arabian and Appaloosa) and dogs (basset hound, Cardigan Welsh corgi, and Jack Russell terrier)
 Thymic aplasia of black-pied Danish cattle

---

* A relatively common disease or condition
Note: Lists of specific disorders or conditions are not complete but are provided to give examples.

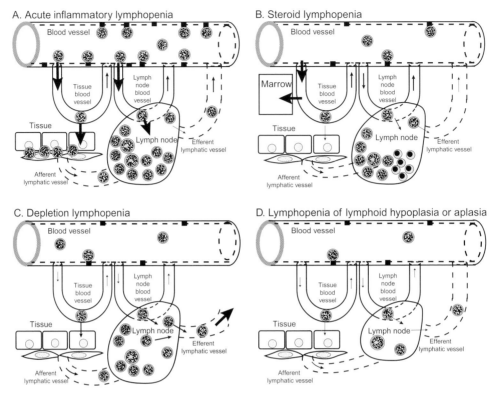

Fig. 2.10. Lymphopenia kinetics.

A. Acute inflammatory lymphopenia: Lymphopenia occurs because of (1) increased migration of lymphocytes to inflamed tissue, (2) homing of lymphocytes to lymphoid tissues, and (3) decreased movement of lymphocytes from lymph nodes back to blood.

B. Steroid lymphopenia: Soon after administration of glucocorticoids, lymphopenia occurs because of the movement of lymphocytes to lymphoid tissues and decreased efflux of lymphocytes from lymph nodes. With persistent administration, glucocorticoids can become lymphotoxic and thus destroy lymphocytes in lymph nodes and other tissues.

C. Depletion lymphopenia: Lymphopenia occurs because lymphocytes are lost from the vascular system with a loss of lymph or lymph-rich fluid.

D. Lymphopenia of lymphoid hypoplasia or aplasia: Lymphopenia occurs because of decreased lymphocyte production.

---

    (1) Increased margination and emigration of lymphocytes to inflamed tissue

    (2) Homing of lymphocytes to lymph nodes by increasing the rate of migration through postcapillary high endothelial cells

    (3) Reducing the rate of lymphocytes leaving lymph nodes via efferent lymphatic vessels

  b. Most acute inflammatory leukograms with neutrophilia or neutropenia also have lymphopenia. Disappearance of lymphopenia is generally considered a good prognostic sign.

  c. Historically, lymphopenia was considered to be caused by the stress associated with acute inflammation rather than caused by the inflammatory process itself.

The stress of an illness may induce the lymphopenia, but documentation of such a pathogenesis was not found.

2. Steroid (stress) lymphopenia (Fig. 2.10B)
   a. This lymphopenia is caused by the changes in lymphocyte kinetics caused by endogenous or exogenous glucocorticoids.
      (1) Immediate: shift of lymphocytes from the CLP to other pools. Once the effects of the glucocorticoids diminish, the lymphocytes return to blood. Some reports indicate the lymphopenia is caused by decreased efflux of lymphocytes from lymph nodes,[38] whereas other data indicate a redistribution to bone marrow.[39,40]
      (2) Later: Lymphotoxic effects cause lymphoid hypoplasia and thus decreased lymphopoiesis. Sensitivity of lymphocytes to glucocorticoids varies with the species and also with the stage of lymphocyte development.[41]
   b. Typical causes are the same as mentioned for steroid neutrophilia, and it is usually considered the most common lymphopenia in all species. The severity and duration of lymphopenia are generally proportional to dose and/or duration of increased glucocorticoids.
3. Depletion lymphopenia (Fig. 2.10C)
   a. This lymphopenia is produced by a loss of lymphocytes from the body via a loss of lymphocyte-rich lymph or because of an incomplete lymphocyte circulation pathway (e.g., repeated removal of chylothoracic fluid from a cat).
   b. Disorders that cause this lymphopenia are not common.
4. Lymphopenia of lymphoid hypoplasia or aplasia (Fig. 2.10D)
   a. This lymphopenia is caused by either congenital or acquired lymphoid hypoplasia or aplasia that decreases lymphocyte production.
   b. Because most blood lymphocytes are T-lymphocytes, selective aplasia of T-lymphocytes will cause a more severe lymphopenia than will a selective aplasia of B-lymphocytes.
5. Lymphopenia of lymphoma
   a. Lymphopenia is common in animals with lymphoma.
   b. The lymphopenia may be caused by decreased production (damage to lymph nodes) or altered lymphocyte kinetics (disrupted circulation patterns).

III. Abnormal monocyte concentrations
   A. Monocytosis (increased measured blood monocyte concentration) (Table 2.11)
      1. Inflammatory monocytosis
         a. Acute and chronic inflammatory diseases may cause monocytosis by cytokine stimulation of monocyte production and release.
         b. Monocytosis generally reflects a need for macrophages in diseased tissue or blood.
      2. Steroid (stress) monocytosis
         a. Glucocorticoid hormones or drugs are a common cause of monocytosis in dogs and cats, but they cause minimal to no changes in horses and cattle.
         b. Monocytosis is probably caused by a shift in monocytes from a marginated pool to a circulating pool.
      3. Neoplastic monocytosis (monocytic leukemia)
         a. This is typically characterized by a marked monocytosis. Monocytes may appear abnormal or relatively normal, but when atypical and immature, they would probably not be categorized as monocytes.

Table 2.11. Diseases and conditions that cause monocytosis

Inflammation
  *Infections: bacterial (including anaplasmal and rickettsial), fungal, protozoal
  *Necrosis: hemolysis, hemorrhage, neoplasia, infarction, trauma
Steroids
  *Stress (physical or neurogenic)
   Hyperadrenocorticism
  *Glucocorticoid therapy
   Adrenocorticotropic hormone administration
Neoplasia: monocytic leukemia
Secondary to immune-mediated neutropenia
Cyclic hematopoiesis
G-CSF administration

* A relatively common disease or condition
Note: Lists of specific disorders or conditions are not complete but are provided to give examples.

      b. This is a relatively uncommon form of leukemia when compared to granulocytic and lymphoid leukemias.
    4. Secondary to immune-mediated neutropenia: Because neutrophils and monocytes share a common bipotential stem cell, there may be increased monocytopoiesis when there is ineffective neutropoiesis.
    5. Cyclic hematopoiesis: Mild monocytosis may occur during neutropenic cycles and herald increases in blood neutrophil concentrations.
    6. G-CSF: This may be administered to promote neutropoiesis, but it will also promote monocytopoiesis.
  B. Monocytopenia: This is difficult to document because healthy domestic mammals may have relatively few blood monocytes. Monocytopenia is not considered a diagnostic problem.

IV.   Abnormal eosinophil concentrations
  A. Eosinophilia (increased measured blood eosinophil concentration)
    1. Most eosinophilias appear to be related to eosinophil anti-inflammatory functions or to the attraction of eosinophils to tissues after mast cell or basophil degranulation.
    2. An eosinophilia suggests the possibility of many disease states (Table 2.12).
      a. In the hypersensitivity disorders, typically there are clinical signs associated with the involved tissues; for example, pruritus with flea bite or staphylococcal dermatitis.
      b. Both internal and external parasites are frequently blamed for an eosinophilia, but many animals with similar parasitic infections do not have an eosinophilia. Persistent mild eosinophilia is occasionally seen in clinically healthy mammals in which parasitism or other subclinical disease cannot be detected. When an eosinophilia is caused by a parasitic infection, it is likely a reaction to a parasite (adult or larva) in tissues and not in the blood or the lumen of the intestines. Organisms that infect blood cells (e.g., hemic *Mycoplasma*, *Babesia*, *Cytauxzoon*, and *Hepatozoon*) are not expected to cause an eosinophilia.
      c. Eosinophilia has been associated with inflammation in a variety of mast cell–rich tissues, although establishing a direct causal relationship may be difficult.

Table 2.12. Diseases and conditions that cause eosinophilia

Hypersensitivity (allergic) disorders
    *Flea-bite dermatitis
    Hypersensitivity to staphylococcal or streptococcal proteins
    Milk allergy in ruminants
    Asthma and eosinophilic respiratory disorders
Parasitism
    Ectoparasites
    *Heartworms
    *Tissue nematodes, trematodes, and protozoa
        Dogs: *Dirofilaria, Acanthocheilonema (Dipetalonema), Spirocerca, Strongyloides,*
          Trichuris, and *Paragonimus* infections; larval migration of hookworms and
          roundworms; *Habronema*
        Cats: *Paragonimus, Aeleurostrongylus*
        Horses: *Strongyloides*
        Cattle: *Sarcocystis*
*Mast cell degranulation caused by inflammation: cutaneous, respiratory, intestinal,
    genital, urinary
Hypoadrenocorticism
Idiopathic eosinophilic conditions
    *Dog: eosinophilic myositis, eosinophilic gastroenteritis, eosinophilic panosteitis,
        eosinophilic pneumonitis, eosinophilic granuloma complex in Siberian huskies
    *Cat: eosinophilic granuloma complex, eosinophilic enteritis, hypereosinophilic syndrome
    Paraneoplastic eosinophilia (including mast cell neoplasms)
Eosinophilic leukemia

* A relatively common disease or condition
Note: Lists of specific disorders or conditions are not complete but are provided to give examples.

       d. Eosinophilia is found in some dogs with hypoadrenocorticism. The pathogenesis
          probably involves the lack of cortisol.
       e. There are several idiopathic eosinophilic conditions (Table 2.12). Typically, there
          are clinical signs associated with the involved tissues.
       f. Idiopathic hypereosinophilic syndrome is occasionally found in cats, dogs, and
          horses.[42–45]
         (1) The syndrome is characterized by persistent marked eosinophilia of undeter-
             mined cause, lack of immature myeloid precursors in blood suggestive of
             leukemia, and eosinophilic infiltration of tissues. Differentiation from
             eosinophilic leukemia is not clear, but animals classified as having hyper-
             eosinophilic syndrome tend not to have anemias, thrombocytopenias, or
             neutropenias.[46]
         (2) There is not an established threshold at which an *eosinophilic* syndrome
             becomes a *hypereosinophilic* syndrome, but most will consider eosinophil
             concentrations $> 20.0 \times 10^3/\mu L$ to be *hypereosinophilic*.
     3. Paraneoplastic eosinophilia
       a. Mast cell neoplasms and adjacent tissues frequently contain eosinophils because
          of chemoattractants released from mast cells. There may be a concurrent
          eosinophilia.

Table 2.13. Diseases and conditions that cause eosinopenia

*Steroids (see Table 2.5)
*Acute inflammation
 Diseases causing a hypoplastic to aplastic marrow

    * A relatively common disease or condition
    Note: Low eosinophil concentrations in routine CBC results may not be reliable because of the imprecision of leukocyte differential counts and sometimes a lower reference limit of 0/μL.

        b. Eosinophilia may also be linked to other neoplasms. The eosinophilia may be caused by the release of eosinophilia-inducing factors (e.g., interleukin 5). Paraneoplastic eosinophilias have been reported in dogs, cats, and horses:[47] dogs—T-cell lymphoma, thymoma, mammary carcinoma, oral fibrosarcoma, and rectal adenomatous polyp; cats—transitional cell carcinoma, T-cell lymphoma, and alimentary lymphoma; and horses—intestinal lymphoma.
    4. Eosinophilic leukemia (Table 6.5): This form of chronic myeloproliferative disease is very uncommon. In cats, it has been linked to a retroviral infection.[48]
  B. Eosinopenia (decreased measured blood eosinophil concentration)
    1. By itself, eosinopenia is of little diagnostic significance. However, eosinopenia may be part of either an acute inflammatory or steroid leukogram (Table 2.13).
    2. Because eosinophil concentrations in healthy animals are typically low, and a calculated eosinophil concentration in CBC results may not be accurate, the observed eosinopenia in CBC results may not truly represent a pathologic state. Also, reference intervals for eosinophil concentrations in some species may have 0/μL as the lower reference limit.

V.   Abnormal basophil concentrations
  A. Basophilia (increased measured blood basophil concentration)
    1. Only substantial or persistent mild increases in basophil concentrations above 200–300/μL should be considered definitive basophilias, because of the imprecision of leukocyte differential counts (especially when dealing with a minority cell population).
    2. A cause of basophilia may not be apparent but can be associated with allergic, parasitic, and neoplastic states (Table 2.14).
  B. Basopenia (decreased blood basophil concentration): This cannot be documented with routine leukocyte differential counts because basophil concentrations are typically very low in domestic mammals. Basopenia is not known to be clinically significant.

VI.   Abnormal mast cell concentrations
  A. Mastocytemia (mast cells detected in peripheral blood)
    1. Finding one mast cell in a blood film or buffy coat preparation of domestic mammals is considered to indicate the presence of mastocytemia. The term *mastocytemia* is preferred over *mastocytosis* because mastocytosis may refer to increased mast cell numbers in tissues other than blood. Either term may refer to neoplastic or nonneoplastic mast cell populations.
    2. Disorders that may cause a mastocytemia (Table 2.15)
        a. Mastocytosis in cats occurs in two forms, systemic and splenic, and mastocytemia may be seen in either.[49-53]

Table 2.14. Diseases and conditions that cause basophilia

Allergic reactions (immediate or delayed)
    Drugs, foods, inhalants, and insect stings or bites
Parasitism
    Fleas
    Gastrointestinal parasites such as nematodes
    *Vascular parasites such as *Dirofilaria immitis* and *Acanthocheilonema* (*Dipetalonema*)
       reconditum
Neoplasia
    Basophilic leukemia
    Mast cell neoplasia
    Feline myeloproliferative diseases
    Lymphomatoid granulomatosis
    Essential thrombocythemia
    Polycythemia vera

  * A relatively common disease or condition
  Note: Lists of specific disorders or conditions are not complete but are provided to give examples.

Table 2.15. Disorders reported to be associated with mastocytemia

Neoplastic disorders
    Cutaneous mast cell neoplasms
    Visceral mast cell neoplasia
    Mast cell leukemia
Nonneoplastic disorders in dogs
    *Inflammatory
        Enteritis, especially parvovirus
        Fibrinous pericarditis and pleuritis
        Bacterial peritonitis
        Aspiration pneumonia
        Acute pancreatic necrosis
        Immune hemolytic anemias
        Renal failure associated with acute inflammation
        Skin diseases: flea-bite hypersensitivity, atopy, sarcoptic mange, and food allergy; some
          with secondary pyoderma
Hemorrhage secondary to hemophilia in dogs
Gastric torsion in dogs

  * A relatively common disease or condition

    b. Cutaneous mastocytoma, which is a common neoplasm of dogs, may spread to blood and hemic organs.[54]
    c. Mast cell leukemias are rare.
    d. Several nonneoplastic mastocytemia disorders have been reported in dogs (Table 2.15). Most such disorders are associated with acute inflammatory diseases.[55–58]
  3. Some articles that describe mastocytemic animals report the number of mast cells found per blood film. This *number per blood film* should be considered descriptive

and not quantitative because the amount of blood examined is not constant or is unknown. For example, finding 30 mast cells per slide on day 1 and 15 mast cells per slide on day 2 should not be interpreted that the animal is responding to treatment, because perhaps a smaller drop of blood was used on day 2 or perhaps the quality of blood film on day 2 prevented a complete examination.
   B. Because no mast cells are expected in the blood of healthy domestic mammals, decreased concentrations do not occur.

LEUKOGRAM PATTERNS

   I. Although each type of leukocyte is unique, alterations in blood leukocyte concentrations frequently occur in predictable patterns that are summarized in Table 2.16. The characteristic features of most patterns are seen in all domestic mammals, but there are significant species differences.
   A. Dogs
      1. Typically, dogs have the most pronounced acute inflammatory leukocytosis.
      2. The classic steroid or "stress" pattern is probably most common in dogs.
   B. Cats
      1. Higher MNP:CNP ratios plus their *fight-or-flight* responses make them more prone to a physiologic leukocytosis.
      2. FeLV-induced changes create alterations in cell concentrations and appearance.
   C. Horses
      1. Horses frequently have little to no neutrophilia or little to no left shift during inflammatory states.
      2. A pronounced left shift is uncommon unless toxic changes are present.
   D. Cattle
      1. Common acute inflammatory states in adult cattle (such as mastitis or pneumonia) cause an inflammatory neutropenia because of the relatively small neutrophil storage pool, but neutrophilia may occur in calves with acute inflammation and in adults with chronic suppurative diseases.
      2. Inflammatory states can cause marked lymphocyte atypia that can be very difficult to differentiate from neoplastic changes.

   II. Hemic neoplasia
   A. Leukogram patterns in animals with hemic neoplasia are extremely variable.
      1. Extreme leukocytosis due to numerous poorly differentiated cells is indicative of an acute leukemia. Occasionally, the initial microscopic findings suggest the poorly differentiated cells are of leukocyte lineage, but additional testing establishes the neoplastic cells to be of erythroid or megakaryocytic lineage.
      2. Extreme leukocytosis due to numerous well-differentiated cells is suggestive of chronic leukemia, but a marked inflammatory leukogram must be excluded.
      3. Low numbers of atypical cells in peripheral blood, particularly if accompanied by cytopenias, suggests the need to examine bone marrow, lymph nodes, or spleen for the source of the atypical cells. Hemic neoplasia may be prominent in the bone marrow, lymph nodes, or spleen when it is not obvious in the blood.
      4. Marked inappropriate rubricytosis is an indication for bone marrow examination to evaluate for hemic neoplasia of erythroid origin (typically in cats).
      5. Hemic neoplasia may be present without any alterations in CBC results.

Table 2.16. Major leukogram patterns (see the text for species differences, especially for cattle)

Leukogram pattern	Total WBCs	Segmented neutrophil	Nonsegmented neutrophil	Lymphocyte	Monocyte	Eosinophil
Acute inflammatory	↑	↑	↑	→	WRI–↑	↓–WRI
Chronic inflammatory	↑	↑	WRI–↑	WRI–↑	WRI–↑	WRI
Steroid leukocytosis	↑	↑	WRI–slight ↑	→	↑	→
Physiologic leukocytosis	↑	↑	WRI	↑	WRI–↑	WRI
Acute overwhelming inflammatory	→	→	WRI–↑	→	WRI	↓–WRI
Acute inflammatory with endotoxemia	→	→	WRI–↑	→	WRI	↓–WRI
Granulocytic hypoplasia	→	→	WRI	WRI	WRI	WRI
Ineffective neutropoiesis	→	→	WRI	WRI	WRI–↑	WRI
Hypoadrenocorticism	WRI	↓–WRI	WRI	WRI–↑	WRI	WRI–↑
Hemic neoplasia	↑↑↑[a]	?	?	?	?	?

[a] The neoplastic cell line is expected to be increased. Other cell lines typically are WRI or decreased.

B. Light-scatter patterns produced by some hematology analyzers (e.g., the CELL-DYN 3500) may provide clues as to the type of hemic neoplasia present. This is because neoplastic cells often have similar light-scatter properties as their nonneoplastic counterparts.[59] However, such findings are typically not definitive.

C. Multiple methods are used to characterize neoplastic hemic cells in an attempt to establish their lineage. Other than the microscopic examination of routinely stained blood, marrow, or lymph node samples, several other methods are used to evaluate cells (see Chapter 6).

    1. Enzyme cytochemistry or histochemistry

    2. Immunocytochemistry or immunohistochemistry

    3. Immunophenotyping via flow cytometry

    4. Antigen receptor gene rearrangement assays to detect clonal cell populations

III. Recognizing a leukogram pattern aids in the understanding of an animal's illness. However, not all disorders will produce classic patterns, concurrent processes can complicate patterns, and some patterns overlap considerably. All leukogram results may even be within reference intervals when the animal has an inflammatory or even infectious disease.

ABNORMAL MORPHOLOGIC FEATURES OF LEUKOCYTES

I. Changes associated with inflammatory diseases

A. Toxic neutrophil (Plate 1A–C [for all plates, see the color section of this book])

    1. *Toxic neutrophils* are neutrophils with any or all of the following characteristics that are called *toxic changes*.

        a. *Foamy cytoplasm* is cytoplasmic clearing due to dispersed organelles. (Note: Similar cytoplasmic appearance may be caused by in vitro changes related to sample deterioration. The foamy vacuolization should not be confused with the clear, discrete vacuoles that develop in neutrophils exposed to EDTA for a few hours.)[60]

        b. *Diffuse cytoplasmic basophilia* is retention or persistence of cytoplasmic RNA during maturation. If cytoplasmic basophilia is caused by toxic change, it should be present in both segmented and nonsegmented neutrophils. Cytoplasmic basophilia in only the nonsegmented stages may reflect the immaturity of the cell and not a toxic change.

        c. *Cytoplasmic Döhle's inclusion bodies* (focal cytoplasmic basophilia, also referred to as Döhle bodies) are irregular, round to angular, blue-grey cytoplasmic structures that are aggregates of rough endoplasmic reticulum that contain RNA.

        d. *Asynchronous nuclear maturation* occurs in nuclei that have finely granular lobes (suggesting immaturity) separated by filaments or pronounced indentations (suggesting maturity).

        e. *Giant neutrophils* are larger neutrophils that are released from marrow because of asynchronous cellular maturation

        f. Hyalinized nuclei have been considered a toxic change but may also represent deterioration or autolysis.

        g. *Toxic granules* are primary granules that are still visible in the later stages (usually not seen after the progranulocyte stage). They are uncommon in domestic mammals and seen mostly in horses.

    2. These structural changes in neutrophils represent maturation defects that occur during rapid neutropoiesis.

3. Apparently healthy cats may have neutrophils with Döhle's inclusion bodies. Therefore, feline Döhle's inclusion bodies without other toxic changes generally are not reported as a toxic change in cats unless they are frequent and prominent (a subjective interpretation).

4. Neutrophils with toxic changes are commonly associated with severe bacterial infections but can be found in noninfectious states,[61] after G–CSF administration, in turpentine-induced inflammation,[62] and in dyscrasias induced by cefonicid or cefazedone.[63] However, it should be noted that just the presence of a left shift is not a toxic change.

5. Toxic changes can be graded based on types and degrees of toxic changes, but classification systems have not been standardized. Probably the more severe the toxic changes are, the more severe the inflammatory state is in the animal. Severe toxic change has been associated with poorer prognosis.[61]

6. Toxic neutrophils (especially band and metamyelocyte stages) can be confused with some monocytes.

   a. If a cell is a toxic band, similar toxic changes should be present in segmented neutrophils.

   b. If a cell is a monocyte, it should be distinguishable from a segmented neutrophil that has the clear to pale pink cytoplasm.

   c. In some cases, immature toxic neutrophils cannot be reliably distinguished from monocytes on a Wright-stained blood film. In these cases, accuracy of a leukocyte differential count may not be as important as recognizing that left shifts and toxic changes indicate that animals have severe inflammatory diseases.

B. Giant neutrophils (Plate 1C)

   1. *Giant neutrophils* are segmented or band neutrophils with a diameter of 14–20 μm. They are larger than typical blood neutrophils, with diameters of 11–13 μm. They probably form because of a skipped cell division in neutropoiesis.

   2. Giant neutrophils may be associated with increased neutropoiesis caused by inflammation, in which case they represent a toxic change. They are seen most commonly in cats.

   3. They also are seen in the poodle marrow dyscrasia, FeLV infections, and after administration of chemotherapeutic drugs that inhibit cell division.

C. Hypersegmented neutrophils (Plate 1D)

   1. *Hypersegmented neutrophils* have a nucleus with five or more definitive lobes separated by filaments.

   2. They typically represent old neutrophils and are seen with increased blood concentrations of glucocorticoids (see Abnormal Leukocyte Concentrations in Blood, sect. I.C.3). The aging effect can also be seen as an in vitro artifact of delayed sample analysis. Their cause is unknown in horses with idiopathic neutrophil hypersegmentation.

   3. They may occur with myelodysplastic syndromes or leukemias involving the neutrophil series and are also seen in the poodle marrow dyscrasia. Giant hypersegmented neutrophils have been observed in dogs after cyclophosphamide treatments (authors' observation) and experimentally in rats.[64]

D. Reactive lymphocytes (Plate 1E–H)

   1. *Reactive lymphocytes* (plasmacytoid lymphocytes, immunocytes, and virocytes) represent either stimulated T-lymphocytes or B-lymphocytes and can be found in

the blood of animals with a variety of acute and chronic inflammatory diseases. Reactive lymphocytes, which are more common in chronic than acute inflammatory states, can be found in most blood samples, but an increased number of them can indicate an inflammatory disease. They are common in young animals.

2. Reactive lymphocytes may have a variety of structural features that are considered to be reactive changes: an increased amount of cytoplasm; an enhanced cytoplasmic basophilia; a perinuclear halo; a prominent focal Golgi zone; and eccentric, enlarged, cleaved, convoluted, lobulated, or bilobed nuclei. The most consistent changes are an increased amount of cytoplasm and an increased cytoplasmic basophilia; a relatively large amount of cytoplasm without basophilia is not clear evidence of reactive change. Granular lymphocytes (large granular lymphocytes) typically have more cytoplasm than other lymphocytes and should not be considered reactive individually, but an increased concentration of granular lymphocytes may indicate a reactive process.

3. Reactive hyperplasia can result in medium and large lymphocytes and lymphoid cells with mitotic nuclei in the peripheral blood.

4. Individual reactive lymphocytes can be impossible to distinguish from neoplastic lymphoid cells, especially in cattle. The more pleomorphic the cells are, the more likely they represent neoplasia and not hyperplasia.

E. Changes in monocytes associated with inflammation (Plate 1I)

1. Monocytes can have increased cytoplasmic basophilia and hyperchromatic nuclei. Such *reactive monocytes* are seen in some inflammatory diseases, especially systemic fungal diseases and immune-mediated disorders. During microscopic examinations, they can be confused with typical and reactive lymphocytes.

2. Monocytes can also acquire the features of macrophages, with abundant grey to blue-grey cytoplasm, with or without vacuoles, and large round to oval nuclei. Cells with this appearance are usually associated with systemic infections such as histoplasmosis, ehrlichiosis, or leishmaniasis.

II. Leukocytes that contain miscellaneous inclusions

A. Sideroleukocyte (Plate 1J)

1. A *sideroleukocyte* is a neutrophil or monocyte containing hemosiderin. On Wright-stained blood films, hemosiderin is a blue-green or yellow-brown pigment. Its presence can be confirmed with an iron stain (Prussian blue).

2. Sideroleukocytes are rarely found but can be seen with hemolytic anemias (e.g., equine infectious anemia or immune-mediated hemolytic anemia) and after transfusion. The hemosiderin in blood leukocytes may represent hemosiderin engulfed by those cells while they were in a spleen or other tissues.[65]

B. Erythrophage (Plate 1K)

1. An *erythrophage* is typically a monocyte or neutrophil that has engulfed an erythrocyte.

2. It is occasionally seen in immune hemolytic anemias such as idiopathic immune hemolytic anemia in dogs, equine infectious anemia, and neonatal isoerythrolysis.

C. Lupus erythematosus (LE) cell

1. A *LE cell* is a neutrophil that engulfed nuclear antigen-antibody complexes. With a Wright stain, this material appears as pink or pale blue homogeneous inclusions of variable sizes. New methylene blue staining produces more prominent LE inclusions with homogeneous staining.

    2. Rarely seen in domestic mammals even in the LE cell test designed to produce the cell in vitro.

  D. Neutrophils containing mast cell granules: Rarely, blood and marrow neutrophils contain mast cell granules. In one described case, the cat had splenic mastocytosis and rare intact mast cells in the peripheral blood.[66]

III. Organisms in leukocytes

  A. Bacteria other than those in the family *Anaplasmataceae*

    1. Rarely, bacteria may be found within neutrophils of bacteremic patients (Plate 1L).

    2. When these bacteria are found in blood, one must attempt to determine whether the bacteria represent a bacteremia or a sample contaminated with bacteria.

  B. Bacteria in the family *Anaplasmataceae* (order Rickettsiales): Morulae of *Ehrlichia* spp. and *Anaplasma* spp. (Plate 2A–C)

    1. For many years, anaplasmal agents that infected leukocytes were classified within the genus of *Ehrlichia*. Molecular diagnostic methods and 16S rRNA analyses resulted in the reclassification of several organisms that previously were considered ehrlichial agents. Some have been moved to the *Anaplasma* genus; others to *Neorickettsia*. The appropriateness of a nomenclature system purely dependent on such genetic sequences has been questioned.[67]

    2. These agents can invade and multiply in the blood leukocytes of many species (Table 2.17). The host range of the monocytic anaplasmal species tends to be limited, but the granulocytic forms are not as host specific.

    3. Anaplasmal species that infect domestic mammals are usually considered separate from those that infect people (*Ehrlichia chaffeensis* and *Neorickettsia sennetsu*), but human isolates have been found that could not be distinguished from *E. ewingii* by nuclei acid sequencing and polymerase chain reaction (PCR) testing.[68,69] Also, agents previously thought to be separate species (*E. equi*, *E. phagocytophila*, and human granulocytic ehrlichia) are now considered to be one organism—called *Anaplasma phagocytophilum*.[70,71]

    4. *Ehrlichia* spp. and the leukocytic *Anaplasma* spp. are located in cytoplasmic vacuoles. The resulting clusters of organisms (2 to > 20) are called *morulae*, which typically have diameters of 1.5–4.0 μm and stain pale to dark blue-grey with a Wright stain. In granulocytic forms, there may be more than one morula per leukocyte. Morulae should not be confused with Döhle's inclusion bodies, platelets lying on leukocytes, or blebs of nuclear membrane.

  C. Canine distemper inclusions (Plate 2D)

    1. Inclusions appear as monomorphic or pleomorphic, red to purplish red or pale blue, cytoplasmic inclusions found in neutrophils, monocytes, lymphocytes, and erythrocytes (see Chapter 3). Quick stains (e.g., Diff-Quik) stain the viral particles better than do traditional Romanowsky stains (e.g., Wright or Wright-Giemsa), which typically produce pale blue inclusions.

    2. They probably occur in the early viremic stage and before clinical illness. They are rarely observed in the United States.

  D. *Hepatozoon americanum* (Plate 2E)[72,73]

    1. This is a protozoon whose gametocytes infect canine neutrophils and monocytes. Prior to 1997, the North American organism was classified as *H. canis*.[72] In North America, it is found mostly in the Southern or Gulf Coast states. Clinical signs of

Table 2.17. Major anaplasmal species that infect leukocytes of domestic mammals[a]

Genogroup	Anaplasmal species	Disease name	Hosts (common listed first)	Cells infected	Frequency of finding morulae in blood leukocytes
I	*E. canis*	Canine ehrlichiosis (tropical pancytopenia)	Dogs	Monocyte, lymphocyte	Reported to be in 25–30 % of cases[131] but are rarely found in more recently diagnosed cases
I	*E. ewingii*	Canine granulocytic ehrlichiosis	Dogs People	Neutrophil, eosinophil, very rarely monocytes	0.1–10 % of neutrophils in first few days of illness; rare thereafter
II	*A. phagocytophilum*[b]	Equine ehrlichiosis, tick fever and bovine ehrlichiosis	Horses Dogs Cattle Sheep Goats	Neutrophil, eosinophil; Neutrophil, eosinophil	1–50 % of neutrophils in first few days of illness; 7.5–30 % of leukocytes 5–10 d after infection[132]
III	*Neorickettsia risticii*[c]	Equine monocytic ehrlichiosis and Potomac horse fever	Horses Dogs Cats	Monocyte	Very rare

[a] This table includes organisms in the family *Anaplasmataceae* (order Rickettsiales) that infect domestic mammalian leukocytes. Other anaplasmal agents infect other cells; for example, *Anaplasma platys* (basonym: *Ehrlichia platys*) infects canine platelets.

[b] Basonyms: *Ehrlichia equi* and *Ehrlichia phagocytophila*

[c] Basonym: *Ehrlichia risticii*

infected dogs include fever, pain, lameness, and ocular discharge. The illness is severe, and the prognosis is guarded.

2. Finding gametocytes of *H. americanum* in blood leukocytes is very uncommon in clinical cases; when present in peripheral blood, there is typically a very low percentage of infected leukocytes. Gametocytes are oval to elliptical, pale blue, and are about 9 μm × 4 μm. They may fill a cell's cytoplasm and cause peripheral displacement of the cell's nucleus. The organism may escape from the cell and leave a nonstaining area surrounded by a capsule.

3. Encysted forms of the protozoa are common in skeletal muscle, and a skeletal muscle biopsy is one method of confirming a diagnosis.

4. Common laboratory data in clinical cases include neutrophilic leukocytosis (sometimes extreme or leukemoid), a normocytic normochromic nonregenerative anemia, thrombocytosis, increased serum alkaline phosphatase activity, and hypoglycemia (which may be caused by glucose consumption by leukocytes in vitro), hypoalbuminemia, and corresponding hypocalcemia. There is poor cross-reactivity between *H. americanum* antibodies and *H. canis* antibodies.

E. *Hepatozoon canis*[73]

1. This is a protozoon whose gametocytes infect canine neutrophils and monocytes. It is found in dogs of Europe, Asia, Africa, and South America and possibly in Brazilian cats.

2. Infected dogs frequently lack obvious clinical signs but can be febrile and lethargic. In contrast to *H. americanum*, gametocytes may be commonly found in the blood leukocytes; sometimes a high percentage of the neutrophils and monocytes are infected. Via light microscopy, the gametocytes are very similar to those of *H. americanum* except that *H. canis* structures are a little longer ($\approx$ 11 μm). Encysted forms of the protozoa are rare in skeletal muscle.

3. In Brazil, a very low percentage of infected leukocytes can be found in dogs infected with *H. canis* (or a very similar organism).[74–76] A nearly identical organism has been found in domestic cats.[77,78]

F. *Histoplasma capsulatum* (Plate 2F)

1. The yeast phase of *H. capsulatum* can be found singly or multiply in the cytoplasm of monocytes (or macrophages), neutrophils, and occasionally eosinophils of peripheral blood. Cells containing *Histoplasma* can usually be more easily found at the feathered edge of blood films (because larger cells are concentrated in the feathered edge) or on buffy coat preparations.

2. The organisms are round to oval, about 2–4 μm long, with a prominent cell wall. Their internal structures are commonly eccentric and stain pale blue and/or dark pink to purple.

3. When found in blood, the infection has advanced to disseminated histoplasmosis, and organisms can typically be found in macrophages of bone marrow, spleen, liver, lymph nodes, and other tissues.

G. *Leishmania* spp. (Plates 9I and 10H)

1. *Leishmania* is a kinetoplastid protozoon that is found primarily in Mediterranean, Central American, and South American countries. However, it has been found in research colonies in Ohio and Oklahoma,[79,80] in Texas and Maryland dogs,[81,82] and in dogs from other Southeastern states.[83]

2. Organisms (amastigotes), which appear as oval to teardrop structures in macrophages, are 2–3 μm long with eccentric reddish nuclei and small cytoplasmic red

bars (kinetoplasts). *Leishmania* amastigotes must be differentiated from amastigotes of *T. cruzi* and the yeast form of *Histoplasma*, which is about the same size and has a thicker cell wall but does not have a kinetoplast.

3. Macrophages laden with amastigotes are usually numerous in bone marrow, lymph nodes, spleen, and liver.

H. *Trypanosoma cruzi*

1. Two species of *Trypanosoma* are found in the United States: *Trypanosoma cruzi* and *T. theileri* (basonym: *T. americanum*). *Trypanosoma cruzi* infects dogs in the Americas and causes Chagas disease.[84,85] Trypomastigotes may be present in blood. *Trypanosoma theileri* infects cattle in the United States, Canada, and Australia and is typically not considered to be a pathogen. The flagellated trypomastigotes can be numerous in bovine blood.

2. Like *Leishmania*, *T. cruzi* is a kinetoplastid, so the amastigotes of these protozoa are similar microscopically. Amastigotes of neither are expected to be found in blood samples, but both can be found in macrophages of lymph nodes. However, amastigotes were found in buffy coat preparations of a puppy with trypanosomiasis; the blood also contained many trypomastigotes.[86]

I. *Mycobacterium* spp. (Plate 2G and H)

1. Rarely, a mycobacterial infection may become systemic and mycobacterial organisms will be found in peripheral blood neutrophils or monocytes.

2. Mycobacterial bacilli are unique in that they do not stain with a Wright stain (negative staining reaction) and thus appear as clear bacterial rods within neutrophils or macrophages.

J. *Sarcocystis* spp.

1. Large oval merozoites of *Sarcocystis* can be found in bovine mononuclear cells during experimental infections.[87,88] Merozoites are about 3–4 μm × 10–12 μm and contain azurophilic nuclear material.

2. The hematogenous merozoite is not a reported observation during natural infections.

K. *Toxoplasma gondii* (Plate 2I)

1. Tachyzoites of *Toxoplasma gondii* are rarely found in blood neutrophils and monocytes of dogs and cats with acute toxoplasmosis.

2. They are more common in macrophages of infected tissues (lung and intestine).

IV. Leukocyte agglutination/aggregation

A. Occasionally, small aggregates of 3–15 leukocytes are found with the body of a well-prepared blood film. Typically they are mixtures of neutrophils and small lymphocytes with fewer eosinophils and monocytes. They should be suspected when leukocytes are distributed in relatively dense streaks at the transition between the monolayer area and the feathered edge of the blood film, running parallel with the long axis of the smear. These streaks are aggregates that have been disrupted. The body and the thick end of the smear should be inspected to confirm leukoagglutination. The diagnostic significance of the finding is not established, but a few points should be considered when they are seen. They should not be confused with the groups of leukocytes that tend to concentrate across the feathered edge of a blood film due to the smearing technique.

B. The published studies of leukocyte aggregation are for human samples. The aggregation of neutrophils might depend on the presence of EDTA and temperature. The aggregation may or may not occur in citrated or heparinized samples.[89,90] When aggregation was seen in room temperature samples but not in samples kept at 37 °C, the neutrophil aggregation was due to an IgM.[91]

    C. A major reason for recognizing leukocyte agglutination is that the measured leukocyte concentrations can be erroneous. The aggregated leukocytes may not be enumerated correctly by the instruments that use impedance or laser methods if the leukocytes do not break apart in the diluent, and thus the total leukocyte concentration would be lower than the true value (i.e., pseudoleukopenia). The aggregated leukocytes may be poorly distributed in a blood film, and thus the differential leukocyte count may be inaccurate if one type of leukocyte is preferentially aggregated.

    D. Leukocyte aggregates have been seen in canine and equine blood (authors' observations) and, in some samples, the aggregation was EDTA dependent (i.e., seen in EDTA samples but little to none seen in citrate samples). Aggregation increased with lower sample temperature and with increased storage time. The authors are not aware of published investigations of neutrophil or lymphocyte aggregations for domestic mammals, but such occurrences are mentioned in veterinary textbooks.[92]

V.   Hereditary disorders that have leukocyte inclusions (rare)

    A. Chédiak-Higashi syndrome[93]

      1. This is a hereditary disorder of blue-smoke Persian cats, Hereford cattle, other nondomestic mammals, and people.

      2. Diagnostic features include large specific granules in cytoplasms of neutrophils, eosinophils, and basophils. Abnormal granules reflect fusion of granules (lysosomes).

    B. GM_1 gangliosidosis[94,95]

      1. This hereditary disorder of Friesian cattle, Siamese and Korat cats, English springer spaniels, mixed-breed beagles, Portuguese water dogs, and Shiba Inus is caused by a deficiency of β-galactosidase.

      2. Diagnostic features include small, distinct, clear cytoplasmic vacuoles in lymphocytes in Wright-stained blood films.

    C. GM_2 gangliosidosis[96–100]

      1. This is a hereditary disorder of Yorkshire pigs, German shorthaired pointers, golden retrievers, and cats that is caused by a deficiency of β-hexosaminidase.

      2. Diagnostic features include dark blue granules in neutrophils and prominent azurophilic granulation or vacuolization in lymphocytes.

    D. Hereditary anomaly of neutrophil granulation in Birman cats[101]

      1. This anomaly is an autosomal recessive trait in purebred Birman cats.

      2. Diagnostic features include prominent fine eosinophilic granulation in the cytoplasms of neutrophils that must be differentiated from toxic granules and inclusions of MPS type VI. Ultrastructural morphologic features of granules are normal.

    E. MPS type I[102,103]

      1. This is a hereditary disorder in domestic cats, dogs, and people that is caused by a deficiency of α-L-iduronidase.

      2. In some studies, leukocytic cytoplasmic inclusions were seen via transmission electron microscopy but not in routine light microscopy. Others have found that feline neutrophils have abnormal cytoplasmic granulation (small pink granules).

    F. MPS type IIIB[104]

      1. This is a hereditary disorder in schipperkes that is caused by a deficiency of lysosomal glycosidase *N*-acetyl-α-ᴅ-glucosaminidase (α-*N*-acetylglucosaminidase).

    2. Blood lymphocytes and marrow macrophages, lymphocytes, and plasma cells were described as having abnormal dark-staining granulation.

G. MPS type VI[105]

    1. This is a hereditary disorder in Siamese cats, domestic shorthair cats, and dachshunds that is caused by a deficiency of arylsulfatase B.

    2. Diagnostic features include the presence of large reddish purple granules in neutrophils that should not be confused with toxic granules (toxic neutrophils have other toxic changes). Cytoplasmic inclusions (granules) represent an accumulation of mucopolysaccharide.

H. MPS type VII[106–108]

    1. This is a hereditary disorder caused by a deficiency of β-glucuronidase.

    2. Neutrophils of dogs and cats with MPS type VII have inclusions like those found in MPS type VI.

I. Fucosidosis[109]

    1. This is caused by a deficiency of α-L-fucosidase, an enzyme in glycoprotein metabolism.

    2. Lymphocytes of dogs with fucosidosis have cytoplasmic vacuoles.

J. Other storage diseases have been recognized in domestic mammals, but leukocyte abnormalities have not been seen in these. These include MPS type IIIA in wirehaired dachshunds[110] and a New Zealand huntaway dog.[111]

OTHER NONNEOPLASTIC LEUKOCYTE DISORDERS

I. Leukocyte adhesion deficiency (LAD)[112]

A. LAD has been recognized in Irish red and white setters and in Holstein cattle; the disorders are referred to as canine LAD (CLAD) and bovine LAD (BLAD). Both disorders are caused by defects in the integrin CD18 molecule that result from single nucleotide substitutions that are different in the two species. The defect prevents formation of functional CD11/CD18 complexes, which are needed for adherence, migration, and aggregation of leukocytes.

B. Dogs with CLAD have a persistent neutrophilia beginning as pups and have a concurrent granulocytic hyperplasia in marrow.[113,114] They have an increased susceptibility to infections. Before the specific defect was established, the disorder was called *canine granulocytopathy syndrome*. A PCR assay was developed to detect dogs with CLAD.[115]

C. Cattle with BLAD have a marked neutrophilia and recurrent infections.[116,117] PCR assays are commercially available to detect cattle with BLAD.

II. Bone marrow dyscrasia of poodles[118]

A. This is a hereditary disorder seen in miniature and toy poodles. The developmental defect in cell production is not known, and there is not a clinical problem associated with the syndrome.

B. Diagnostic features of the syndrome

    1. Hypersegmented or giant neutrophils

    2. Macrocytic normochromic erythrocytes without anemia or reticulocytosis. Their mean cell volumes usually are 80–110 fL (in most unaffected dogs, 60–77 fL), their mean cell hemoglobin concentrations are usually WRI, and their mean cell hemoglobin values are increased (compared to those of most unaffected dogs).

III. Idiopathic hypersegmented neutrophils of horses[10,11]
   A. The diagnostic feature of this syndrome is hypersegmented neutrophils and has been described in two horses of the quarter horse breed. In one report, neutrophil nuclei had 3–11 definitive lobes separated by filaments, and about 70 % of nuclei had 7–10 lobes. Other cases have been similar.
   B. Hypersegmentation is not associated with the common causes of hypersegmentation; that is, hyperadrenocorticism (Cushing's disease) and exogenous glucocorticoids. The cause of the syndrome has not been determined. The possibility that hypersegmentation is caused by vitamin B_{12} or folate deficiency has not been excluded. Clinical significance is not known.

IV. Pelger-Huët anomaly[119–123]
   A. This is a hereditary disorder that occurs in several breeds of dogs, domestic shorthair cats, and in Arabian horses. Most clinical cases involve heterozygotes for the anomaly; a homozygotic kitten was stillborn.[120]
   B. The disorder is characterized by hyposegmentation of neutrophil, eosinophil, and basophil nuclei. The nuclei are round, oval, spectacle shaped, or occasionally have partial segmentation. The nuclear chromatin may appear hyperchromatic or normo-chromatic but lacks the paler appearance of typical band neutrophils (Plate 2J–L). The various nuclear shapes can be graded (round or oval to two or more lobes) to characterize the degree of hyposegmentation.[123,124]
   C. Decreased lobulation of monocyte nuclei has been described, but recognizing the change requires a grading system that is not commonly used.[125]
   D. Pelger-Huët neutrophils should not be classified as band neutrophils (or younger forms), because such classifications will result in a left shift and thus indicate an inflammatory disease.

V. Pseudo–Pelger-Huët neutrophils and eosinophils
   A. Pseudo–Pelger-Huët neutrophils are seen in cows,[126] occasionally in dogs with severe inflammation, and in cats with FeLV-induced myeloid leukemia.[127] The transient defect represents asynchronous neutrophil maturation; some neutrophils look like Pelger-Huët cells, but others do not. Usually other toxic changes are present with severe inflammation.
   B. Pseudo–Pelger-Huët eosinophils have been described in cattle and a horse.[45,126] In cattle, they were found concurrent with pseudo–Pelger-Huët neutrophils. In the horse, they were found concurrent with a marked extreme inflammatory eosinophilia.

VI. Nonstaining eosinophil granules (grey eosinophils) of dogs[128,129]
   A. Canine eosinophils typically contain numerous round eosinophilic granules of varying diameters, along with a few cytoplasmic "vacuoles." In some breeds (especially grey-hounds, but also golden retrievers and Shetland sheepdogs), the eosinophils contain either poorly stained granules, or the nonstaining granules appear as cytoplasmic vacuoles that sometimes have central foci of eosinophilic staining. The cytoplasms of these "agranular" canine eosinophils sometimes appear grey and thus the name grey eosinophils. Altered staining represents a modified chemical composition; the altered composition is associated with ultrastructural changes (authors' unpublished data).
   B. There is no known clinical or pathologic significance to the presence or absence of these eosinophils other than the potential for incorrectly identifying the cells.

1. Microscopically, they are sometimes incorrectly identified as toxic neutrophils or monocytes.
2. Affected eosinophils also have low peroxidase activity and are usually misclassified as monocytes when analyzed in the peroxidase channel of the ADVIA (see the Analytical Principles and Methods Sect. III.C.3) (authors' unpublished data). Some greyhounds' eosinophils contain eosinophilic granules but lack peroxidase and are therefore also misclassified by the ADVIA.

References

1. Prasse KW, Kaeberle ML, Ramsey FK. 1973. Blood neutrophilic granulocyte kinetics in cats. Am J Vet Res 34:1021–1025.
2. McEwen BJ. 1992. Eosinophils: A review. Vet Res Commun 16:11–44.
3. Brown SA, Barsanti JA. 1988. Quantitative buffy coat analysis for hematologic measurements of canine, feline, and equine blood samples and for detection of microfilaremia in dogs. Am J Vet Res 49:321–324.
4. Levine RA, Hart AH, Wardlaw SC. 1986. Quantitative buffy coat analysis of blood collected from dogs, cats, and horses. J Am Vet Med Assoc 189:670–673.
5. Rümke CL. 1959. Variability of results in differential cell counts on blood smears. Triangle 4:154–158.
6. Schalm OW. 1961. *Veterinary Hematology*, 1st edition. Philadelphia: Lea & Febiger.
7. Jain NC. 1986. *Schalm's Veterinary Hematology*, 4th edition. Philadelphia: Lea & Febiger.
8. Schalm OW. 1976. Erythrocyte macrocytosis in miniature and toy poodles. Canine Pract 3:55–57.
9. Raskin RE, Krehbiel JD. 1985. Myelodysplastic changes in a cat with myelomonocytic leukemia. J Am Vet Med Assoc 187:171–174.
10. Prasse KW, George LW, Whitlock RH. 1981. Idiopathic hypersegmentation of neutrophils in a horse. J Am Vet Med Assoc 178:303–305.
11. Ramaiah SK, Harvey JW, Giguère S, Franklin RP, Crawford PC. 2003. Intravascular hemolysis associated with liver disease in a horse with marked neutrophil hypersegmentation. J Vet Intern Med 17:360–363.
12. Fyfe JC, Jezyk PF, Giger U, Patterson DF. 1989. Inherited selective malabsorption of vitamin B_{12} in giant schnauzers. J Am Anim Hosp Assoc 25:533–539.
13. Myers S, Wiks K, Giger U. 1995. Macrocytic anemia caused by naturally-occurring folate deficiency in the cat. Vet Pathol 32:547 (abstract).
14. Knottenbelt CM, Simpson JW, Chandler ML. 2000. Neutrophilic leucocytosis in a dog with a rectal tumour. J Small Anim Pract 41:457–460.
15. Tomlinson MJ, Jennings PB, Wendt JB, Meriwether WA, Crumrine MH. 1973. Adenocarcinoma of the lung with secondary pericardial effusion and leukemoid response in a dog. J Am Vet Med Assoc 163:257–258.
16. Lobetti RG. 1995. Leukaemoid response in two dogs with *Babesia canis* infection. J S Afr Vet Assoc 66:182–184.
17. Foster NK, Martyn JB, Rangno RE, Hogg JC, Pardy RL. 1986. Leukocytosis of exercise: Role of cardiac output and catecholamines. J Appl Physiol 61:2218–2223.
18. Benschop RJ, Rodriguez-Feuerhahn M, Schedlowski M. 1996. Catecholamine-induced leukocytosis: Early observations, current research, and future directions. Brain Behav Immun 10:77–91.
19. Thompson JP, Christopher MM, Ellison GW, Homer BL, Buchanan BA. 1992. Paraneoplastic leukocytosis associated with a rectal adenomatous polyp in a dog. J Am Vet Med Assoc 201:737–738.
20. Lappin MR, Latimer KS. 1988. Hematuria and extreme neutrophilic leukocytosis in a dog with renal tubular carcinoma. J Am Vet Med Assoc 192:1289–1292.
21. Chinn DR, Myers RK, Matthews JA. 1985. Neutrophilic leukocytosis associated with metastatic fibrosarcoma in a dog. J Am Vet Med Assoc 186:806–809.
22. Gaunt SD, Pierce KR. 1986. Effects of estradiol on hematopoietic and marrow adherent cells of dogs. Am J Vet Res 47:906–909.
23. Valli VE, McSherry BJ, Robinson GA, Willoughby RA. 1969. Leukopheresis in calves and dogs by extracorporeal circulation of blood through siliconized glass wool. Res Vet Sci 10:267–278.
24. Wenz JR, Barrington GM, Garry FB, Dinsmore RP. 1999. Differentiation of bacteremic and non-bacteremic cows with acute coliform mastitis. In: Proceedings of the 17th ACVIM Forum, Chicago, 693.
25. Wagner JG, Roth RA. 1999. Neutrophil migration during endotoxemia. J Leukoc Biol 66:10–24.
26. Chickering WR, Prasse KW. 1981. Immune mediated neutropenia in man and animals: A review. Vet Clin Pathol 10:6–16.

27. Jain NC, Vegad JL, Kono CS. 1990. Methods for detection of immune-mediated neutropenia in horses, using antineutrophil serum of rabbit origin. Am J Vet Res 51:1026–1031.

28. Perkins MC, Canfield P, Churcher RK, Malik R. 2004. Immune-mediated neutropenia suspected in five dogs. Aust Vet J 82:52–57.

29. Hirsch VM, Mitcham SA, Dunn JK. 1983. Multiple cytopenias associated with monocytic proliferation in a dog. Vet Clin Pathol 13:16–20.

30. Stockhaus C, Slappendel RJ. 1998. Haemophagocytic syndrome with disseminated intravascular coagulation in a dog. J Small Anim Pract 39:203–206.

31. Walton RM, Modiano JF, Thrall MA, Wheeler SL. 1996. Bone marrow cytological findings in 4 dogs and a cat with hemophagocytic syndrome. J Vet Intern Med 10:7–14.

32. Tsuda H. 1997. Hemophagocytic syndrome (HPS) in children and adults. Int J Hematol 65:215–226.

33. Lanevschi A, Daminet S, Niemeyer GP, Lothrop CD Jr. 1999. Granulocyte colony–stimulating factor deficiency in a rottweiler with chronic idiopathic neutropenia. J Vet Intern Med 13:72–75.

34. Campbell KL. 1985. Canine cyclic hematopoiesis. Compend Contin Educ 7:57–62.

35. Horwitz M, Benson KF, Duan Z, Li FQ, Person RE. 2004. Hereditary neutropenia: Dogs explain human neutrophil elastase mutations. Trends Mol Med 10:163–170.

36. Swenson CL, Kociba GJ, O'Keefe DA, Crisp MS, Jacobs RM, Rojko JL. 1987. Cyclic hematopoiesis associated with feline leukemia virus infection in two cats. J Am Vet Med Assoc 191:93–96.

37. Imhof BA, Dunon D. 1995. Leukocyte migration and adhesion. Adv Immunol 58:345–416.

38. Bloemena E, Weinreich S, Schellekens PTA. 1990. The influence of prednisolone on the recirculation of peripheral blood lymphocytes in vivo. Clin Exp Immunol 80:460–466.

39. Fauci AS. 1975. Mechanisms of corticosteroid action on lymphocyte subpopulations. I. Redistribution of circulating T and B lymphocytes to the bone marrow. Immunology 28:669–680.

40. Sackstein R, Borenstein M. 1995. The effects of corticosteroids on lymphocyte recirculation in humans: Analysis of the mechanism of impaired lymphocyte migration to lymph node following methylprednisolone administration. J Invest Med 43:68–77.

41. Claman HN. 1972. Corticosteroids and lymphoid cells. N Engl J Med 287:388–397.

42. Aroch I, Perl S, Markovics A. 2001. Disseminated eosinophilic disease resembling idiopathic hypereosinophilic syndrome in a dog. Vet Rec 149:386–389.

43. Center SA, Randolph JF, Erb HN, Reiter S. 1990. Eosinophilia in the cat: A retrospective study of 312 cases (1975 to 1986). J Am Anim Hosp Assoc 26:349–358.

44. Sykes JE, Weiss DJ, Buoen LC, Blauvelt MM, Hayden DW. 2001. Idiopathic hypereosinophilic syndrome in 3 rottweilers. J Vet Intern Med 15:162–166.

45. Latimer KS, Bounous DI, Collatos C, Carmichael KP, Howerth EW. 1996. Extreme eosinophilia with disseminated eosinophilic granulomatous disease in a horse. Vet Clin Pathol 25:23–26.

46. Weller PF, Bubley GJ. 1994. The idiopathic hypereosinophilic syndrome. Blood 83:2759–2779.

47. Marchetti V, Benetti C, Citi S, Taccini V. 2005. Paraneoplastic hypereosinophilia in a dog with intestinal T-cell lymphoma. Vet Clin Pathol 34:259–263.

48. Lewis MG, Kociba GJ, Rojko JL, Stiff MI, Haberman AB, Velicer LF, Olsen RG. 1985. Retroviral-associated eosinophilic leukemia in the cat. Am J Vet Res 46:1066–1070.

49. Madewell BR, Gunn C, Gribble DH. 1983. Mast cell phagocytosis of red blood cells in a cat. Vet Pathol 20:638–640.

50. Weller RE. 1978. Systemic mastocytosis and mastocytemia in a cat. Mod Vet Pract 59:41–43.

51. Confer AW, Langloss JM. 1978. Long-term survival of two cats with mastocytosis. J Am Vet Med Assoc 172:160–161.

52. Guerre R, Millet P, Groulade P. 1979. Systemic mastocytosis in a cat: Remission after splenectomy. J Small Anim Pract 20:769–772.

53. Liska WD, MacEwen EG, Zaki FA, Garvey M. 1979. Feline systemic mastocytosis: A review and results of splenectomy in seven cases. J Am Anim Hosp Assoc 15:589–597.

54. O'Keefe DA, Couto CG, Burke-Schwartz C, Jacobs RM. 1987. Systemic mastocytosis in 16 dogs. J Vet Intern Med 1:75–80.

55. Stockham SL, Basel DL, Schmidt DA. 1986. Mastocytemia in dogs with acute inflammatory diseases. Vet Clin Pathol 15:16–21.

56. McManus P. 1997. Canine mastocytemia and marrow mastocytosis: Disease associations, incidence and severity. Vet Pathol 34:474 (abstract).

57. Cayatte SM, McManus PM, Miller WH Jr, Scott DW. 1995. Identification of mast cells in buffy coat preparations from dogs with inflammatory skin diseases. J Am Vet Med Assoc 206:325–326.

58. McManus PM. 1999. Frequency and severity of mastocytemia in dogs with and without mast cell tumors: 120 cases (1995–1997). J Am Vet Med Assoc 215:355–357.

59. Fernandes PJ, Modiano JF, Wojcieszyn J, Thomas JS, Benson PA, Smith R III, Avery AC, Burnett RC, Boone LI, Johnson MC, Pierce KR. 2002. Use of the Cell-Dyn 3500 to predict leukemic cell lineage in peripheral blood of dogs and cats. Vet Clin Pathol 31:167–182.

60. Gossett KA, Carakostas MC. 1984. Effect of EDTA on morphology of neutrophils of healthy dogs and dogs with inflammation. Vet Clin Pathol 13:22–25.

61. Aroch I, Klement E, Segev G. 2005. Clinical, biochemical, and hematological characteristics, disease prevalence, and prognosis of dogs presenting with neutrophil cytoplasmic toxicity. J Vet Intern Med 19:64–73.

62. Gossett KA, MacWilliams PS. 1982. Ultrastructure of canine toxic neutrophils. Am J Vet Res 43:1634–1637.

63. Bloom JC, Lewis HB, Sellers TS, Deldar A, Morgan DG. 1987. The hematopathology of cefonicid- and cefazedone-induced blood dyscrasias in the dog. Toxicol Appl Pharmacol 90:143–155.

64. Kotelnikov VM, Pogorelov VM, Berger J, Kozinets GI. 1988. Cyclophosphamide induced generation of giant hypersegmented granulocytes in rat bone marrow: Cell cycle distribution and silver nucleolar staining. Folia Haematol (Leipz) 115:737–745.

65. Gaunt SO, Baker DC. 1986. Hemosiderin in leukocytes of dogs with immune-mediated hemolytic anemia. Vet Clin Pathol 15:8–10.

66. Casimire-Etzioni AL, Raskin RE, Langohr I, Brenner D. 2005. Mastocytosis with phagocytized mast cell granules. (unpublished case report, ASVCP slide set)

67. Uilenberg G, Thiaucourt F, Jongejan F. 2004. On molecular taxonomy: What is in a name? Exp Appl Acarol 32:301–312.

68. Buller RS, Arens M, Hmiel SP, Paddock CD, Sumner JW, Rikihisa Y, Unver A, Gaudreault-Keener M, Manian FA, Liddell AM, Schmulewitz N, Storch GA. 1999. *Ehrlichia ewingii*, a newly recognized agent of human ehrlichiosis. N Engl J Med 341:148–155.

69. Sumner JW, Storch GA, Buller RS, Liddell AM, Stockham SL, Rikihisa Y, Messenger S, Paddock CD. 2000. PCR amplification and phylogenetic analysis of *groESL* operon sequences from *Ehrlichia ewingii* and *Ehrlichia muris*. J Clin Microbiol 38:2746–2749.

70. Massung RF, Owens JH, Ross D, Reed KD, Petrovec M, Bjoersdorff A, Coughlin RT, Beltz GA, Murphy CI. 2000. Sequence analysis of the *ank* gene of granulocytic ehrlichiae. J Clin Microbiol 38:2917–2922.

71. Chae JS, Foley JE, Dumler JS, Madigan JE. 2000. Comparison of the nucleotide sequences of 16S rRNA, 444 *Ep-ank*, and *groESL* heat shock operon genes in naturally occurring *Ehrlichia equi* and human granulocytic ehrlichiosis agent isolates from Northern California. J Clin Microbiol 38:1364–1369.

72. Vincent-Johnson NA, Macintire DK, Lindsay DS, Lenz SD, Baneth G, Shkap V, Blagburn BL. 1997. A new *Hepatozoon* species from dogs: Description of the causative agent of canine hepatozoonosis in North America. J Parasitol 83:1165–1172.

73. Vincent-Johnson NA. 2003. American canine hepatozoonosis. Vet Clin North Am Small Anim Pract 33: 905–920.

74. Rubini AS, Paduan KS, Cavalcante GG, Ribolla PEM, O'Dwyer LH. 2005. Molecular identification and characterization of canine *Hepatozoon species* from Brazil. Parasitol Res 97:91–93.

75. Paludo GR, Dell'Porto A, de Castro e Trindade AR, McManus C, Friedman H. 2003. *Hepatozoon* spp.: Report of some cases in dogs in Brasília, Brazil. Vet Parasitol 118:243–248.

76. Forlano MD, Teixeira KR, Scofield A, Elisei C, Yotoko KS, Fernandes KR, Linhares GF, Ewing SA, Massard CL. 2007. Molecular characterization of *Hepatozoon* sp. from Brazilian dogs and its phylogenetic relationship with other *Hepatozoon* spp. Vet Parasitol 145:21–31.

77. Rubini AS, dos Santos Paduan K, Perez RR, Ribolla PEM, O'Dwyer LH. 2006. Molecular characterization of feline *Hepatozoon* species from Brazil. Vet Parasitol 137:168–171.

78. Perez RR, Rubini AS, O'Dwyer LH. 2004. The first report of *Hepatozoon* spp. (*Apicomplexa, Hepatozoidae*) in domestic cats from São Paulo state, Brazil. Parasitol Res 94:83–85.

79. Swenson CL, Silverman J, Stromberg PC, Johnson SE, Wilkie DA, Eaton KA, Kociba GJ. 1988. Visceral leishmaniasis in an English foxhound from an Ohio research colony. J Am Vet Med Assoc 193:1089–1092.

80. Anderson DC, Buckner RG, Glenn BL, MacVean DW. 1980. Endemic canine leishmaniasis. Vet Pathol 17:94–96.

81. Gustafson TL, Reed CM, Long TM, McGreevy PB, Pappas MG. 1984. Cutaneous leishmaniasis acquired in Texas. J Am Vet Med Assoc 185:328 (abstract).

82. Eddlestone SM. 2000. Visceral leishmaniasis in a dog from Maryland. J Am Vet Med Assoc 217:1686–1688.

83. Enserink M. 2000. Infectious diseases: Has leishmaniasis become endemic in the U.S.? Science 290:1881–1883.

84. Fox JC, Ewing SA, Buckner RG, Whitenack D, Manley JH. 1986. *Trypanosoma cruzi* infection in a dog from Oklahoma. J Am Vet Med Assoc 189:1583–1584.

85. Barr SC, Van Beek O, Carlisle-Nowak MS, Lopez JW, Kirchhoff LV, Allison N, Zajac A, de Lahunta A, Schlafer DH, Crandall WT. 1995. *Trypanosoma cruzi* infection in Walker hounds from Virginia. Am J Vet Res 56:1037–1044.

86. Russell KE, Barnhart KF, Fryer JS, Craig TM. 2002. Buffy coat smear from a puppy. Vet Clin Pathol 31:9–12.

87. Fayer R. 1979. Multiplication of *Sarcocystis bovicanis* in the bovine bloodstream. J Parasitol 65:980–982.

88. Fayer R, Leek RG. 1979. *Sarcocystis* transmitted by blood transfusion. J Parasitol 65:890–893.

89. O'Connor BM, Shastri KA, Logue GL. 1991. Spurious neutropenia: Ethylenediaminetetraacetate-dependent in vitro neutrophil agglutination. NY State J Med 91:455–456.

90. Lesesve JF, Haristoy X, Thouvenin M, Latger-Cannard V, Buisine J, Lecompte T. 2000. Pseudoleucopenia due to in vitro leukocyte agglutination polynuclear neutrophils: Experience of a laboratory, review of the literature and future management. Ann Biol Clin (Paris) 58:417–424.

91. Bizzaro N. 1993. Granulocyte aggregation is edetic acid and temperature dependent. Arch Pathol Lab Med 117:528–530.

92. Thrall MA, Baker DC, Campbell TW, DeNicola D, Fettman MJ, Lassen ED, Rebar AH, Weiser G. 2004. *Veterinary Hematology and Clinical Chemistry.* Philadelphia: Lippincott Williams & Wilkins.

93. Prieur DJ, Collier LL. 1978. Chédiak-Higashi syndrome. Am J Pathol 90:533–536.

94. Saunders GK, Wood PA, Myers RK, Shell LG, Carithers R. 1988. GM_1-gangliosidosis in Portuguese water dogs: Pathologic and biochemical findings. Vet Pathol 25:265–269.

95. Yamato O, Endoh D, Kobayashi A, Masuoka Y, Yonemura M, Hatakeyama A, Satoh H, Tajima M, Yamasaki M, Maede Y. 2002. A novel mutation in the gene for canine acid beta-galactosidase that causes GM1-gangliosidosis in Shiba dogs. J Inherit Metab Dis 25:525–526.

96. Singer HS, Cork LC. 1989. Canine GM_2-gangliosidosis: Morphologic and biochemical analysis. Vet Pathol 26:114–120.

97. Kosanke SD, Pierce KR, Bay WW. 1978. Clinical and biochemical abnormalities in porcine GM_2-gangliosidosis. Vet Pathol 15:685–699.

98. Yamato O, Matsuki N, Satoh H, Inaba M, Ono K, Yamasaki M, Maede Y. 2002. Sandhoff disease in a golden retriever dog. J Inherit Metab Dis 25:319–320.

99. Yamato O, Satoh H, Matsuki N, Ono K, Yamasaki M, Maede Y. 2004. Laboratory diagnosis of canine G_{M2}-gangliosidosis using blood and cerebrospinal fluid. J Vet Diagn Invest 16:39–44.

100. Yamato O, Matsunaga S, Takata K, Uetsuka K, Satoh H, Shoda T, Baba Y, Yasoshima A, Kato K, Takahashi K, Yamasaki M, Nakayama H, Doi K, Maede Y, Ogawa H. 2004. G_{M2}-gangliosidosis variant 0 (Sandhoff-like disease) in a family of Japanese domestic cats. Vet Rec 155:739–744.

101. Hirsch VM, Cunningham TA. 1984. Hereditary anomaly of neutrophil granulation in Birman cats. Am J Vet Res 45:2170–2174.

102. Shull RM, Helman RG, Spellacy E, Constantopoulos G, Munger RJ, Neufeld EF. 1984. Morphologic and biochemical studies of canine mucopolysaccharidosis I. Am J Pathol 114:487–495.

103. Haskins ME, Aguirre GD, Jezyk PF, Desnick RJ, Patterson DF. 1983. The pathology of the feline model of mucopolysaccharidosis I. Am J Pathol 112:27–36.

104. Ellinwood NM, Wang P, Skeen T, Sharp NJH, Cesta M, Decker S, Edwards NJ, Bublot I, Thompson JN, Bush W, Hardam E, Haskins ME, Giger U. 2003. A model of mucopolysaccharidosis IIIB (Sanfilippo syndrome type IIIB): *N*-acetyl-α-ᴅ-glucosaminidase deficiency in Schipperke dogs. J Inherit Metab Dis 26:489–504.

105. Haskins ME, Jezyk PF, Desnick RJ, Patterson DF. 1981. Mucopolysaccharidosis VI. Am J Pathol 105:191–193.

106. Haskins ME, Desnick RJ, DiFerrante N, Jezyk PF, Patterson DF. 1984. β-Glucuronidase deficiency in a dog: A model of human mucopolysaccharidosis VII. Pediatr Res 18:980–984.

107. Schultheiss PC, Gardner SA, Owens JM, Wenger DA, Thrall MA. 2000. Mucopolysaccharidosis VII in a cat. Vet Pathol 37:502–505.

108. Silverstein Dombrowski DC, Carmichael KP, Wang P, O'Malley TM, Haskins ME, Giger U. 2004. Mucopolysaccharidosis type VII in a German shepherd dog. J Am Vet Med Assoc 224:553–557.

109. Keller CB, Lamarre J. 1992. Inherited lysosomal storage disease in an English springer spaniel. J Am Vet Med Assoc 200:194–195.

110. Jolly RD, Ehrlich PC, Franklin RJM, Macdougall DF, Palmer AC. 2001. Histological diagnosis of mucopolysaccharidosis IIIA in a wire-haired dachshund. Vet Rec 148:564–567.

111. Yogalingam G, Pollard T, Gliddon B, Jolly RD, Hopwood JJ. 2002. Identification of a mutation causing mucopolysaccharidosis type IIIA in New Zealand Huntaway dogs. Genomics 79:150–153.

112. Gu YC, Bauer TR Jr, Ackermann MR, Smith CW, Kehrli ME Jr, Starost MF, Hickstein DD. 2004. The genetic immunodeficiency disease, leukocyte adhesion deficiency, in humans, dogs, cattle, and mice. Comp Med 54:363–372.

113. Debenham SL, Millington A, Kijas J, Andersson L, Binns M. 2002. Canine leucocyte adhesion deficiency in Irish red and white setters. J Small Anim Pract 43:74–75.

114. Trowald-Wigh G, Håkansson L, Johannisson A, Norrgren L, Hard af Segerstad C. 1992. Leucocyte adhesion protein deficiency in Irish setter dogs. Vet Immunol Immunopathol 32:261–280.

115. Verfaillie T, Verdonck F, Cox E. 2004. Simple PCR-based test for the detection of canine leucocyte adhesion deficiency. Vet Rec 154:821–823.

116. Nagahata H. 2004. Bovine leukocyte adhesion deficiency (BLAD): A review. J Vet Med Sci 66:1475–1482.

117. Müller KE, Bernadina WE, Kalsbeek HC, Hoek A, Rutten VP, Wentink GH. 1994. Bovine leukocyte adhesion deficiency: Clinical course and laboratory findings in eight affected animals. Vet Q 16:27–33.

118. Canfield PJ, Watson ADJ. 1989. Investigations of bone marrow dyscrasia in a poodle with macrocytosis. J Comp Pathol 101:269–278.

119. Feldman BF, Ramans AU. 1976. The Pelger-Huët anomaly of granulocytic leukocytes in the dog. Canine Pract 3:22–30.

120. Latimer KS, Rowland GN, Mahaffey MB. 1988. Homozygous Pelger-Huët anomaly and chrondrodysplasia in a stillborn kitten. Vet Pathol 25:325–328.

121. Latimer KS, Rakich PM, Thompson DF. 1985. Pelger-Huët anomaly in cats. Vet Pathol 22:370–374.

122. Gill AF, Gaunt S, Sirninger J. 2006. Congenital Pelger-Huët anomaly in a horse. Vet Clin Pathol 35:460–462.

123. Grondin TM, Dewitt SF, Keeton KS. 2007. Pelger-Huët anomaly in an Arabian horse. Vet Clin Pathol 36:306–310.

124. Latimer KS, Duncan JR, Kircher IM. 1987. Nuclear segmentation, ultrastructure, and cytochemistry of blood cells from dogs with Pelger-Huët anomaly. J Comp Pathol 97:61–72.

125. Latimer KS, Duncan JR, Kircher IM. 1987. Morphology and cytochemistry of canine Pelger-Huët blood cells. Vet Clin Pathol 16:9 (abstract).

126. Osburn BI, Glenn BL. 1968. Acquired Pelger-Huët anomaly in cattle. J Am Vet Med Assoc 152:11–16.

127. Toth SR, Onions DE, Jarrett O. 1986. Histopathological and hematological findings in myeloid leukemia induced by a new feline leukemia virus isolate. Vet Pathol 23:462–470.

128. Jones RF, Paris R. 1963. The greyhound eosinophil. J Small Anim Pract 4(Suppl):29–33.

129. Iazbik MC, Couto CG. 2005. Morphologic characterization of specific granules in greyhound eosinophils. Vet Clin Pathol 34:140–143.

130. Greenfield CL, Messick JB, Solter PF, Schaeffer DJ. 1999. Leukopenia in six healthy Belgian Tervuren. J Am Vet Med Assoc 215:1121–1122.

131. Troy GC, Vulgamott JC, Turnwald GH. 1980. Canine ehrlichiosis: A retrospective study of 30 naturally occurring cases. J Am Anim Hosp Assoc 16:181–187.

132. Pusterla N, Huder J, Wolfensberger C, Braun U, Lutz H. 1997. Laboratory findings in cows after experimental infection with *Ehrlichia phagocytophila*. Clin Diagn Lab Immunol 4:643–647.

Chapter 3

ERYTHROCYTES

Physiologic Processes 110
Analytical Principles and Methods. 120
   I.   Complete Blood Count. 120
   II.   Erythrogram 120
   III.   Methods. 124
Morphologic Features of Erythrocytes: Clinical Significance and Pathogeneses 135
   I.   Assessment. 135
   II.   General Features. 136
   III.   Erythrocyte Color 137
   IV.   Erythrocyte Organisms 138
   V.   Inclusions Other Than Organisms 138
   VI.   Abnormal Erythrocyte Volume 142
   VII. Abnormal Erythrocyte Shape 143
Anemia 151
   I.   General Information. 151
   II.   Classifications of Anemias. 151
        A. Classification by Marrow Responsiveness 151
        B. Classification by Erythrocyte Indices. 153
        C. Pathophysiologic Classification 158
Nonregenerative Anemias. 159
   I.   General Concepts 159
   II.   Disorders That Cause Nonregenerative Anemias. 160
Blood Loss Anemias 167
   I.   Causes of Blood Loss. 167
   II.   Classifications Based on Duration and Location. 167
Hemolytic Anemias 170
   I.   Concepts and Classifications. 170
   II.   Hemolytic Disorders and Diseases. 176
        A. Immune Hemolytic Anemias (Not Associated with Infections) 176
        B. Infectious Hemolytic Anemias. 181
        C. Erythrocytic Metabolic Defects (Acquired or Inherited) 186
        D. Erythrocyte Fragmentation in Blood Creating Schizocytes,
           Keratocytes, or Acanthocytes 191
        E. Hemolytic Disorders of Other or Unknown Pathogeneses. 191
Erythrocytosis and Polycythemia. 193
   I.   Terms and Concepts 193
   II.   Erythrocytotic Disorders and Conditions. 193
Other Erythrocyte Disorders 198
   I.   Methemoglobinemia 198
   II.   Cytochrome-b_5 Reductase (Cb_5R) Deficiency. 199
   III.   Familial Methemoglobinemia Associated with GR Deficiency
        in a Horse 199
   IV.   Hereditary Stomatocytosis 199
   V.   Hereditary Band 3 Deficiency in Japanese Black Cattle. 200
   VI.   Hereditary Elliptocytosis of Dogs Due to Protein Band 4.1
        Deficiency 200
   VII. Elliptocytosis in a Mixed-breed Dog Due to Mutant Spectrin. 200

VIII. Spectrin Deficiency in Dutch Golden Retrievers 201
IX. Megaloblastic Anemia 201
X. Sideroblastic Anemia in Dogs. 202
XI. Distemper Inclusions in Dogs 202
Laboratory Methods for Assessing Iron (Fe) Status. 202
I. Serum [Fe]. 202
II. TIBC and UIBC 205
III. Percent Transferrin Saturation (% Saturation) 206
IV. Stainable Fe in Macrophages of Marrow, Spleen, or Liver 207
V. Serum Ferritin Concentrations 207
VI. Reticulocyte Hgb content (CHr) and volume (MCVr) 208
VII. Comparative Fe Profile Results. 208
Blood Typing and Crossmatching 208
Methods for Detecting Erythrocyte Surface Antibody or Complement 211

Table 3.1. Abbreviations and symbols in this chapter

[x]	x concentration (x = analyte)
2,3-DPG	2, 3-Diphosphoglycerate
AID	Anemia of inflammatory disease
ATP	Adenosine triphosphate
Bc	Conjugated bilirubin
Bu	Unconjugated bilirubin
C3	Complement protein 3
Cb_5R	Cytochrome-b_5 reductase
CBC	Complete blood count
CH	Cell (corpuscular) hemoglobin content mean
CHCM	Cell (corpuscular) hemoglobin concentration mean
CHCMr	Cell (corpuscular) hemoglobin concentration mean of reticulocytes
CHDWr	Cell (corpuscular) hemoglobin distribution width of reticulocytes
CHr	Cell (corpuscular) hemoglobin content mean of reticulocytes
CRP	Corrected reticulocyte percentage
DEA	Dog erythrocyte antigen
DNA	Deoxyribonucleic acid
ECF	Extracellular fluid
EDTA	Ethylenediaminetetraacetic acid
EIAV	Equine infectious anemia virus
Epo	Erythropoietin
ESAIg	Erythrocyte surface-associated immunoglobulin
FAD	Flavin adenine dinucleotide
Fe	Iron, either Fe^{2+} or Fe^{3+}
Fe^{2+}	Ferrous iron
Fe^{3+}	Ferric iron
FeLV	Feline leukemia virus
G6PD	Glucose-6-phosphate dehydrogenase
GR	Glutathione reductase
GSH	Glutathione

Table 3.1. *continued*

HC	Hemoglobin concentration (in individual erythrocytes)
HCO_3^-	Bicarbonate
Hct	Hematocrit
HDW	Hemoglobin concentration distribution width
HDWr	Hemoglobin concentration distribution width of reticulocytes
Hgb	Hemoglobin (iron in Fe^{2+} state)
Hgb-Fe^{3+}	Methemoglobin
Hgb_{delta}	Hemoglobin delta (measure of free plasma [Hgb] by ADVIA)
IgA	Immunoglobulin A
IgG	Immunoglobulin G
IgM	Immunoglobulin M
IL-x	Interleukin 1, 6, 8
IMHA	Immune-mediated hemolytic anemia
MCH	Mean cell hemoglobin
MCHC	Mean cell hemoglobin concentration
MCV	Mean cell volume
MCVr	Mean cell volume of reticulocytes
NADH	Reduced nicotinamide adenine dinucleotide
NADPH	Reduced nicotinamide adenine dinucleotide phosphate
NI	Neonatal isoerythrolysis
NMB	New methylene blue
nRBC	Nucleated erythrocyte
P_aCO_2	Partial pressure of carbon dioxide in arterial blood
P_aO_2	Partial pressure of oxygen in arterial blood
PCR	Polymerase chain reaction
PCV	Packed cell volume
PFK	Phosphofructokinase
pH	$-\log [H^+]$
PK	Pyruvate kinase
RBC	Red blood cell (erythrocyte)
RC	Reticulocyte concentration
RDW	Red cell distribution width
RDWr	Red cell distribution width of reticulocytes
RMT	Reticulocyte maturation time
RNA	Ribonucleic acid
RP	Reticulocyte percentage
SI	Système International d'Unités
TIBC	Total iron-binding capacity
TNF	Tumor necrosis factor
UIBC	Unbound iron-binding capacity
WBC	White blood cell (leukocyte)
WRI	Within the reference interval

Note: See the figure legends for abbreviations that are unique to the figures.

PHYSIOLOGIC PROCESSES

I.   *Erythron*: all erythroid cells in an animal, including precursors and erythrocytes in blood
     vessels and sinuses of spleen, liver, and marrow (Fig. 3.1)
     A. Erythrocyte precursors
         1. Erythropoiesis is part of hematopoiesis, which is a complex system involving stem
            cells and cytokines (see Fig. 3.1). Several cytokines work synergistically with Epo to
            stimulate the replication and differentiation of blast-forming unit–erythroid (BFU-
            E) to committed stem cells (e.g., colony-forming unit–erythroid or CFU-E), which
            respond to Epo either by dividing or by differentiating toward rubriblasts. Epo
            inhibits apoptosis.
         2. Epo is produced mostly by the fetal liver and the adult kidney.[1,2] Renal peritubular
            interstitial cells produce Epo in response to renal hypoxia. Renal hypoxia may be

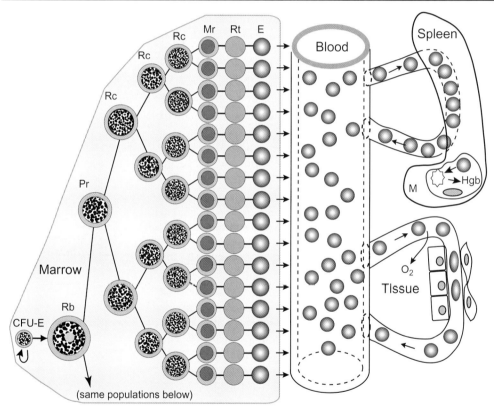

Fig. 3.1. Erythrocyte kinetics in health: The erythron contains three major pools: erythrocyte precursors
(mostly in marrow), blood erythrocytes, and splenic erythrocytes. After stimulation by Epo, colony-forming
unit–erythroid cells (CFU-E) differentiate into rubriblasts (Rb) and the precursors proliferate (via mitosis)
and mature until erythrocytes (E) are formed. An orderly maturation process produces a pyramidal
distribution of erythroid cell populations (only the top half is shown). After release to the blood, erythrocytes circulate in the vascular system to transport O_2 to tissues. A reserve pool of erythrocytes is sequestered
in the spleen of most mammals. Senescent erythrocytes are destroyed by macrophages.

   Mφ, macrophage; Mr, metarubricyte; Pr, prorubricyte; Rc, rubricytes; and Rt, reticulocyte.

caused by anemia, poor oxygenation of blood (e.g., high altitude or pulmonary disease), or poor renal perfusion.

3. After a CFU-E differentiates into a rubriblast, two major cell processes occur.
   a. Cells undergo mitoses to produce more and smaller cells. Evidence suggests that as [Hgb] increases in the developing cell, DNA synthesis decreases and thus fewer mitoses occur.[3]
   b. Cells produce messenger ribonucleic acid (mRNA) for synthesis of Hgb and cytoskeletal proteins.
4. In the later stages of mammalian erythropoiesis, a metarubricyte nucleus is extruded and engulfed by a macrophage. The resulting anucleate cell is a *reticulocyte* when stainable RNA is still present.
5. When a nucleated erythrocyte loses its nucleus and ability to produce mRNA for protein synthesis, it soon loses the ability to produce Hgb and enzymes. The activities of erythrocytic enzymes are greatest in young erythrocytes and decrease slowly with age. Mitochondria deteriorate so that glycolysis becomes the ATP-producing pathway in most animals (except pigs, which use an alternate energy pathway involving inosine).

B. Blood erythrocytes
1. Major features of erythrocytes in different species are compared in Table 3.2.
2. Erythrocyte destruction in health (senescence)
   a. About 250 million erythrocytes die per hour per kg body weight.
   b. Old erythrocytes have very little metabolic machinery (enzymes) to keep themselves functional and deformable. Near death, they may become more rigid, spheroid, and less capable of passing through sinuses.
   c. Age-related changes in erythrocyte membranes expose antigens that are bound by naturally occurring antibodies that may mediate erythrocyte destruction.[4,5]

C. Splenic erythrocytes
1. Spleens of dogs, horses, and cattle have sinusoids and red pulp that are full of erythrocytes; for example, 50–60 % of a horse's erythrocytes can be within its spleen. Damaged or less deformable erythrocytes are removed by macrophages that are adjacent to sinusoids or present in the red pulp. When splenic contraction occurs, erythrocytes are forced into the systemic blood.

Table 3.2. Comparison of typical blood erythrocytes in mature healthy animals

	Dogs	Cats	Horses	Cattle
Reticulocyte concentration ($\times 10^3/\mu L$)	50	40[a]	0	0
RBC concentration ($\times 10^6/\mu L$)	7	7–8	9	7
RBC life span (d)	100	70	150	150
RBCs in blood[b] ($\times 10^{12}$)	5.6	2.2	450	280
RBC diameter (μm)	7	6	5–6	5–6
RBC volume (fL)	70	45	45	50
RBC central pallor	Prominent	Mild	None to mild	Mild to moderate

[a] Counting only aggregate reticulocytes
[b] Estimates are based on 40 mL blood/lb body weight and average-sized animals.
Note: All numbers represent approximate averages to illustrate similarities and differences. They are not reference intervals.

2. Cat spleens are thought to have closed circulation (blood does not flow through red pulp), which is less efficient at removing damaged erythrocytes. They also do not have large reserve erythrocyte pools.

3. Most metarubricytes and reticulocytes that are released from marrow each day are temporarily trapped in mammalian spleens (except for cats).

II. Erythrocyte kinetics
   A. A blood [erythrocyte] is established by the relative rates of erythrocyte production, shifting of erythrocytes to and from splenic sinuses, and erythrocyte destruction.
   B. Erythrocyte production depends on the degree and duration of Epo stimulus and the capability of precursor cells to respond to Epo.

III. Hgb: structure, function, synthesis, and degradation
   A. Hgb structure
      1. *Hgb* is a tetramer with each globin linked to a separate heme that binds O_2; its relative molecular mass is near 64,000. Globins are polypeptides and, in mature healthy mammals, each Hgb molecule contains two α-chains and two β-chains. Approximately 95 % of an erythrocyte is Hgb on a dry weight basis.
         a. Rates of synthesis of heme and globin are balanced and regulated by each other. If a precursor has very little heme and Fe^{2+} is available, heme and globin synthesis should increase.
         b. If synthesis of a globin chain is decreased, an animal has a thalassemia.
         c. If gene mutations produce abnormal amino acid sequences in the globins, an animal has a hemoglobinopathy.
      2. Fe in heme is in the ferrous state (Fe^{2+}) and is kept in the reduced state by enzymatic reactions catalyzed by Cb_5R (NADH-methemoglobin reductase, commonly called just methemoglobin reductase) and NADPH diaphorase (NADPH-methemoglobin reductase).
      3. Amino acids in the globin chains are maintained in a reduced state by reductive reactions involving GR and catalase.
   B. Hgb function (Fig. 10.3)
      1. Hgb (with Fe^{2+}) transports O_2 from lungs to tissues. In health, Hgb is 100 % saturated with O_2 in arterial blood. Hgb-Fe^{3+} does not transport O_2.
      2. Hgb plays two major roles in the transport of CO_2 from tissues to lungs.
         a. When CO_2 diffuses into erythrocytes, carbonic anhydrase catalyzes its reaction with H_2O to form H^+ and HCO_3^-. Hgb acts as a buffer ($H^+ + Hgb^- \rightarrow HHgb$) to remove the H^+, and HCO_3^- diffuses from the cell to the plasma. The buffering of H^+ by Hgb facilitates the additional conversion of CO_2 to HCO_3^-. When erythrocytes return to lungs, reactions are reversed and CO_2 is released for expiration. About 70 % of the CO_2 formed in tissues is transported to lungs via this system.
         b. When CO_2 diffuses into erythrocytes, some binds with Hgb to form carbaminohemoglobin. About 20 % of the CO_2 formed in tissues is transported to lungs via this system.
   C. Hgb synthesis
      1. This occurs in erythrocyte precursors (rubriblasts through reticulocytes) in a series of reactions (Fig. 3.2).

Hemoglobin Synthesis in Erythrocyte Precursors

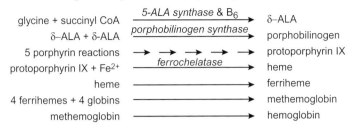

Hemoglobin Degradation in Macrophages

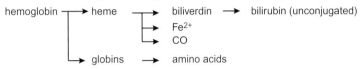

Fig. 3.2. Hemoglobin synthesis and degradation.
- Hgb synthesis in erythrocyte precursors: The synthesis of Hgb has three major stages: (1) a series of porphyrin reactions, (2) incorporation of Fe^{2+} into protoporphyrin IX to form heme, and (3) binding of four ferriheme and four globin molecules to form hemoglobin.
- Hemoglobin degradation in macrophages: In health, senescent erythrocytes are engulfed by macrophages and heme is split from globin chains. Heme is degraded to bilirubin, Fe^{2+}, and carbon monoxide (CO). The globin chains are degraded to amino acids.

---

2. 5-Aminolevulenic acid synthase is the major rate-limiting enzyme. It requires vitamin B_6 (pyridoxine) as a cofactor, and is inhibited by greater heme concentrations.
3. 5-Aminolevulenic acid synthase, porphobilinogen synthase, ferrochelatase, and coproporphyrinogen oxidase are inhibited by lead.
    a. In lead toxicity, inhibition of these enzymes leads to greater concentrations of heme precursors in erythrocytes. Collectively, porphobilinogen through protoporphyrin IX are called *porphyrins*.
    b. *Porphyria*, which is a condition in which concentrations of porphyrins in erythrocytes, plasma, or urine are increased, can be acquired (as in lead toxicity) or congenital. Animals with porphyria are prone to photosensitivity.
4. The maturation rate of erythrocyte precursors is affected by [Hgb] in their cytoplasms. If Hgb synthesis is incomplete, additional mitoses during a cell's development will produce smaller erythrocytes.[3]
D. The type of Hgb synthesized in an individual can vary with the animal's age and health. In people, there are three major types: (1) embryonal with mostly two α- and two ε-globins, (2) fetal with two α- and two γ-globins, and (3) adult with mostly two α- and two β-globins. Embryonal Hgb is replaced by adult Hgb during fetal development in dogs, cats, and horses; these animals do not have fetal Hgb. Neonatal ruminants are thought to have a mixture of fetal Hgb (with two α- and two βF-globins) and adult Hgb but only adult Hgb (with two α- and two βA-globins) after a few postnatal months.[6]

E. Hgb degradation and bilirubin metabolism: After erythrocyte death in macrophages of spleen, liver, or marrow, Hgb is degraded to Bu, amino acids, and Fe (Figs. 3.2 and 3.3). Bu and Bc are excreted or degraded, whereas the amino acids and Fe are recycled.

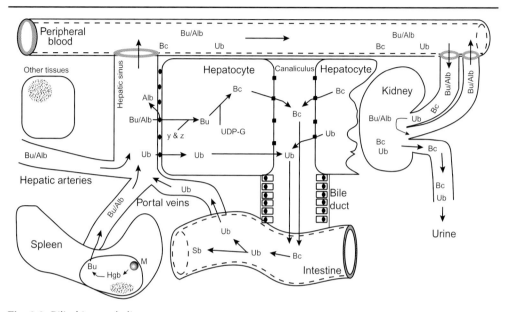

Fig. 3.3. Bilirubin metabolism.

- In health, erythrocyte destruction in macrophages of spleen, liver, or marrow results in Bu formation. Small and usually clinically insignificant amounts of Bu are formed from heme degradation associated with ineffective erythropoiesis and degradation of other heme-containing molecules (catalase, peroxidase, and cytochromes). As Bu leaves a macrophage, it forms a noncovalent association with albumin and is transported to hepatocytes. Bu is relatively water insoluble prior to binding to albumin (Alb).
- When Bu enters the liver and its protein-permeable sinuses, it probably binds to hepatocyte membrane receptors of the organic anion transport polypeptide (OATP) family, enters hepatocytes without albumin, and binds to Y-protein (ligandin, also called glutathione transferase) or Z-protein (fatty acid–binding protein). Bu probably enters hepatocytes by a passive but facilitated process; binding proteins enhance the process by reducing the efflux of Bu back to the sinusoidal plasma.
- Within hepatocytes, Bu diffuses to the endoplasmic reticulum, where it is conjugated with glucuronide (> 60 % with glucose in horses) to form bilirubin monoglucuronide or bilirubin diglucuronide, collectively called Bc. It then diffuses to the canalicular membrane.
- Bc is transported from the hepatocytes into the canaliculi (the rate-limiting step in bilirubin excretion) by an energy-dependent transport system for organic anions other than bile acids. The primary transporter is probably the multidrug resistance protein 2 (MRP2), also called the canalicular multispecific organic anion transporter (cMOAT).
- Bc in bile enters the intestine and is degraded to urobilinogen (colorless), which can be passively absorbed in the intestine and then enter the hepatocytes for excretion in the bile, or bypass the liver and be excreted in the urine. Urobilinogen can also be degraded to stercobilinogen (dark brown) and excreted in feces.
- If Bc escapes the hepatocytes and enters the blood, it can pass through a glomerulus and be excreted in the urine. Because albumin does not pass through the glomerular filtration barrier of most mammals, Bu/ Alb does not enter urine in those animals.

Bu/Alb, Bu associated with albumin; Mɸ, macrophage; Sb, stercobilinogen; Ub, urobilinogen; and UDP-G, uridine diphosphoglucoronide.

IV. Fe
   A. Total body Fe is distributed in three major sites in health: (1) about 50–70 % in erythrocyte Hgb, (2) about 25–40 % in storage, and (3) the remainder in other molecules (e.g., myoglobin, cytochromes, and enzymes).[7]
   B. Physiologic processes or concepts (Fig. 3.4)
   C. The intestinal absorption and cellular release of Fe are regulated by *hepcidin*, a small peptide hormone that is synthesized primarily by hepatocytes. Canine hepcidin has a molecular structure similar to that of human hepcidin.[8] When hepcidin binds to membrane ferroportin (a protein involved in Fe export from vertebrate cells) on the basolateral membranes of small intestinal villus enterocytes, the ferroportin is internalized and the cell loses its ability to export Fe from the cell to the circulation. Accumulated intracellular Fe inhibits the expression of divalent metal transporter 1 and ferric reductase (duodenal cytochrome *b*) on the brush border, so Fe absorption into the cell is also decreased. The synthesis of hepcidin is influenced by hypoxia, Fe availability, and IL-6.[9]
     1. When hepatocytes detect hypoxia, the decreased formation of hepcidin causes a lower [hepcidin] and thus increases the availability of Fe for erythropoiesis; that is, the increased movement of Fe from enterocytes to plasma and increased release of Fe from macrophages to plasma through a similar mechanism.
     2. Fe loading by diet or transfusion increases the formation of hepcidin, whereas Fe deficiency decreases its formation.
     3. During inflammation, cytokines are released, including IL-6. IL-6 promotes the synthesis of hepcidin; it binds to ferroportin which is then internalized. Thus the amount of ferroportin available for the export of Fe from cells (including macrophages) is reduced. This process tends to sequester Fe in macrophages, and thus it is less available for erythropoiesis and for infectious agents.

V. Mature erythrocyte metabolism (Fig. 3.5)
   A. Glucose is the major energy source for mature erythrocytes in most species.
   B. Pig erythrocytes lack a functional glucose transporter and use inosine instead of glucose.

VI. Reticulocytes
   A. *Reticulocytes* are nonnucleated, immature erythrocytes with stainable cytoplasmic RNA.
     1. When erythrocytes are incubated with NMB prior to the making of a blood film, the NMB precipitates and stains the RNA and mitochondria to yield punctate or reticulated (hence the term *reticulocyte*) basophilic structures.
     2. On a Wright-stained blood film, the RNA will give the polychromatophilic erythrocyte its blue or basophilic tinctorial properties. Not all reticulocytes have enough RNA to be detected on a Wright-stained blood film.
   B. The life spans of circulating reticulocytes of nonanemic dogs and people are 1–2 d, after which the cells are mature erythrocytes. The life spans of cat reticulocytes are more variable. In health, cattle and horses do not have circulating polychromatophilic erythrocytes, because maturation is more complete in the bone marrow. However, some hematology analyzers detect low concentrations of reticulocytes in horses.[10]
   C. Types of reticulocytes
     1. In most species, any nonnucleated erythrocyte that contains RNA (stainable with NMB, other vital stains, or Wright stains) is called a *reticulocyte*.

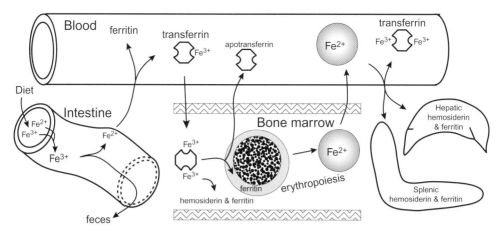

Fig. 3.4. Fe kinetics in healthy animals.

- Absorption: Diets of domestic mammals may contain Fe^{2+} or Fe^{3+}. Ingested Fe^{3+} is converted to Fe^{2+} by ferric reductase (duodenal cytochrome *b* or Dcyt *b*), a surface enzyme, prior to entering enterocytes via divalent metal transporter 1 (DMT1). If there are low intracellular concentrations of hepcidin, there is increased synthesis of ferroportin, which, in conjunction with hephaestin, a copper-containing Fe oxidase related to ceruloplasmin, transports the Fe^{2+} to plasma transferrin in the form of Fe^{3+}. Apoferritin in mucosal epithelial cells binds to Fe^{3+} to form mucosal ferritin, which appears to be lost into the intestine when mucosal cells are sloughed. In most mammals, the rate of intestinal absorption is influenced by the need for Fe by the body; that is, if Fe is needed, more Fe is absorbed. In healthy adults, the amount of Fe absorbed per day is a very small percentage of total body Fe stores.

- Transport: Nearly all Fe in plasma is bound to apotransferrin, a transport protein (β-globulin) produced by hepatocytes. When Fe is bound to apotransferrin, the complex is called transferrin. Transferrin carries Fe^{3+} to and from tissues (for use by cells or for storage). In health, about one-third of transferrin's Fe-binding sites are occupied by Fe. Many cells have transferrin receptors but especially marrow erythroid cells and hepatocytes.

- Use in erythroid cells: After transferrin binds to and enters erythroid precursors, Fe^{3+} dissociates from apotransferrin and binds to cytoplasmic apoferritin (to form ferritin) or is incorporated into heme (Fe^{2+}) and then hemoglobin. Most apotransferrin escapes degradation and is returned to plasma. In health, about 50–70 % of total body Fe is within erythrocytes.

- Storage: Fe^{3+} is stored in two protein-Fe complexes: ferritin (plasma and tissue) and hemosiderin (tissue macrophages). In health, about 25–40 % of total body Fe is within storage forms. Young animals (especially neonates) have low amounts of stored Fe.
  - Ferritin consists of apoferritin complexed with Fe^{3+} and is a relatively soluble, mobile source of Fe^{3+}. There are several forms of apoferritin because of various combinations of H or L subunits. Plasma ferritin is a glycosylated polymer that is relatively Fe poor. Tissue ferritin, which is nonglycosylated and relatively Fe rich, is produced by many cells, primarily macrophages, hepatocytes, intestinal mucosal epithelial cells, and erythroid precursors. Synthesis of apoferritin by hepatocytes and macrophages is increased by inflammation (apoferritin is a positive acute-phase protein) and when Fe storage is increased.
  - Hemosiderin is a relatively insoluble, poorly mobile source of Fe^{3+} and represents the major storage form of Fe. Hemosiderin is a complex of protein and Fe oxides that is found primarily in lysosomes of macrophages in the spleen, liver, and marrow of most mammals. A healthy cat's marrow does not have enough hemosiderin to be detected by routine staining methods.

- Tissue forms: A relatively small quantity of Fe is present in myoglobin, catalase, peroxidases, and cytochromes.

2. In cats, reticulocytes stained by NMB may be classified by two systems.
   a. The more commonly used system differentiates reticulocytes into punctate and aggregate forms.[11] The degree of polychromasia seen on a Wright-stained smear tends to correlate with the aggregate RP.[12]
      (1) *Punctate*: cells with two to six small granules of reticulum
      (2) *Aggregate*: cells with large aggregates of reticulum
   b. Type I, II, and III reticulocytes[13,14]
      (1) *Type I* (lightly reticulated, oldest form): Cells are uniform in size and stain light green with faint blue stippling. Their circulating life span is 3 d, and the maximum concentration occurs about 10–12 d after the onset of anemia.
      (2) *Type II* (moderately reticulated): Cells vary somewhat in size and stain light green with large dark granules. Their circulating life span is about 12 h, and the maximal concentration occurs about 4 d after the onset of anemia.
      (3) *Type III* (heavily reticulated, youngest form): Cells generally are larger than nonreticulated cells and have blue-green cytoplasm and a heavy dark blue granular network. Their circulating life span is 12 h, and the maximal concentration occurs about 4 d after the onset of anemia.
   D. Reticulocytosis: increased RC, CRP, or polychromasia
   1. A reticulocytosis is the best semiquantitative evidence of increased erythropoiesis (in species other than horses).
      a. Cattle: After acute blood loss, a reticulocytosis is expected within 3–4 d, and peak production is expected in 7–14 d. A few large or shift reticulocytes may be seen in the blood before a reticulocytosis is present.[15]
      b. Dogs: The response after acute blood loss is not clearly established but is generally reported to mimic the bovine pattern. Some report that the peak response can be seen prior to 7 d.
      c. Cats: The acute removal of erythrocytes by repeated phlebotomies to create a Hct of 50 % of baseline in five cats resulted in the following:[12]
         (1) An aggregate reticulocytosis occurred by day 2, peaked at day 4, and returned to baseline by day 9, even though the cats were still anemic (Hct in the low 20s).
         (2) A slight punctate reticulocytosis was present by day 1, a peak reticulocytosis occurred from days 7 through 14, and punctate RP did not return to baseline until after Hct returned to prephlebotomy values (after 3 wk).
      d. Horses: They very rarely have circulating polychromatophilic erythrocytes. The clinical value of automated reticulocyte concentrations in assessing equine anemias is investigational.
   2. The degree of increased polychromasia should correspond to the degree of reticulocytosis in dogs and cattle and to aggregate reticulocytosis in cats.

VII. Blood groups or types
   A. General concepts
   1. Erythrocytes can be grouped into different blood groups or types based on the presence or absence of erythrocyte surface antigens, which are sometime called

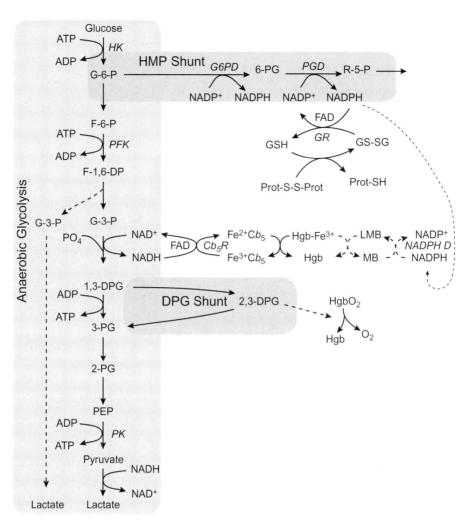

Fig. 3.5. Major biochemical reactions in erythrocytes.

- Anaerobic glycolysis (also known as the Embden-Meyerhof pathway) provides the biochemical skeleton for erythrocyte metabolism and generates ATP and NADH. Because of the split of F-1,6-DP into two molecules of G-3-P for two parallel pathways, glycolysis consumes two molecules of ATP and produces four molecules of ATP. PFK is the rate-limiting enzyme, and its activity is enhanced by alkalemia and reduced by acidemia. PK catalyzes the last reaction, resulting in a net ATP production via anaerobic glycolysis. NADH is used to reduce Hgb-Fe^{3+}.
- The hexose monophosphate shunt (also known as the pentose shunt and the pentose phosphate pathway) generates NADPH that is used to keep GSH in a reduced state in a reaction catalyzed by GR (with cofactor FAD). GSH and NADPH are the major reducing agents in erythrocytes and are used to maintain Hgb and other proteins in a functional reduced state. G6PD is the rate-limiting enzyme of the shunt. R-5-P, which is also formed from inosine in pig erythrocytes, can undergo a series of reactions yielding F-6-P and G-3-P for glycolysis.
- Cb_5R uses FAD and NADH to catalyze the conversion of two molecules of Fe^{3+}Cb_5 to two molecules of Fe^{2+}Cb_5. The Fe^{2+}Cb_5 reduces Hgb-Fe^{3+} to Hgb in a nonenzymatic reaction. Because of the second reaction, Cb_5R is sometimes called methemoglobin reductase (or NADH methemoglobin reductase)
- NADPH D also catalyzes conversion of Hgb-Fe^{3+} to Hgb and thus is another methemoglobin reductase. However, this is a very minor reaction in physiologic states and requires an electron acceptor. Therapeutically, MB can be used as the electron acceptor and is converted to LMB; LMB then reacts nonenzymatically to reduce Hgb-Fe^{3+} to Hgb.

118

blood-group factors. Nearly all blood-group factors are determined by genetics, and each species has different antigens. In people, blood-group factors may function as membrane transporters, receptors, ligands, or structural proteins.

2. A variety of nomenclature systems have been used for some blood types. These are the more common systems used

B. In dogs, at least a dozen blood groups have been described, and nine are currently named using the *dog erythrocyte antigen* prefix: *DEA*. The blood groups that have most clinical relevance are DEA 1.1 and DEA 1.2, which are also called type A1 and A2, respectively. Incidences vary with the breed, but about 50 % of dogs in the United States have DEA 1.1 and 20 % have DEA 1.2.

C. Cats have one blood-group system, the *AB system*, that has three blood phenotypes: type A, type B, and type AB. Type A is the most common in cats (> 90 % in nearly all breeds), and those cats have a natural anti-(B hemagglutinin) antibody. Type B is rare in many breeds but relatively common (25–50 %) in a few (e.g., Devon rex, Cornish rex, and exotic and British shorthair), and those cats have a natural anti-(A hemagglutinin) antibody. Type AB cats are rare (< 1 % of cats) and lack natural antibodies against blood-type antigens.

D. The blood-group systems of horses are relatively complex, with over 30 identified blood factors belonging to at least the seven blood systems that have been recognized by the International Society for Animal Genetics: A, C, D, K, P, Q, and U. Blood types are described by a capital letter to denote the system, and a lowercase letter to denote the specific factor; for example, Qa, Qb, and Qc. The incidence of some blood types varies markedly among breeds. Factors Aa, Ac, Ca, and Qa have particular clinical relevance. Horses that lack Aa, Ac, or Ca may have natural anti-Aa, anti-Ac, or anti-Ca antibodies, so plasma donors should be positive for these factors so that the natural antibodies are not present. Types Aa and Qa are commonly associated with neonatal isoerythrolysis. Mares may develop anti-Qa antibodies after foaling a type Qa foal.

Fig. 3.5. *continued*

• The diphosphoglycerate (DPG) shunt (also known as the Rapaport-Luebering cycle) provides 2,3-DPG at the expense of ATP production; 2,3-DPG decreases Hgb affinity for O_2 and thus promotes O_2 delivery to tissues. Species vary in the 2,3-DPG content of their erythrocytes: Concentrations are high in dogs and horses but very low in cattle and cats.[250]

1,3-DPG, 1,3-diphosphoglycerate; 2,3-DPG, 2,3-diphosphoglycerate; 2-PG, 2-phosphoglycerate; 3-PG, 3-phosphoglycerate; 6-PG, 6-phosphogluconate; ADP, adenosine diphosphate; ATP, adenosine triphosphate; Cb_5R, cytochrome-b_5 reductase; DPG, diphosphoglycerate; F-1,6-DP, fructose-1,6-diphosphate; F-6-P, fructose-6-phosphate; $Fe^{2+}Cb_5$, ferrocytochrome b_5; $Fe^{3+}Cb_5$, ferricytochrome b_5; G-3-P, glyceraldehyde-3-phosphate; G-6-P, glucose-6-phosphate; G6PD, glucose-6-phosphate dehydrogenase; GSH, glutathione, reduced; GS-SG, glutathione disulfide; Hgb, deoxyhemoglobin; Hgb-Fe^{3+}, methemoglobin; Hgb-O_2, oxyhemoglobin; HK, hexokinase; HMP, hexose monophosphate; LMB, leukomethylene blue; MB, methylene blue; NAD^+, nicotinamide adenine dinucleotide; NADH, reduced nicotinamide adenine dinucleotide; $NADP^+$, nicotinamide adenine dinucleotide phosphate; NADPH D, NADPH dehydrogenase; NADPH, reduced nicotinamide adenine dinucleotide phosphate; PEP, phosphoenolpyruvate; PFK, 6-phosphofructokinase; PGD, phosphogluconate dehydrogenase; PK, pyruvate kinase; PO_4, phosphate; Prot-SH, protein with reduced sulfhydryl groups; Prot-S-S-Prot, protein with disulfide bridges; and R-5-P, ribulose-5-phosphate.

E. The blood-group systems of cattle are very complex, with over 700 known blood-group factors in at least 11 blood systems. With this degree of genetic diversity, it is essentially impossible to find two cattle with the same blood type.

ANALYTICAL PRINCIPLES AND METHODS

I.   Complete blood count (CBC): Major concepts pertaining to a CBC are in Chapter 2 (Analytical Principles and Methods, sect. I).

II. Erythrogram
   A. Morphologic evaluation
       1. A microscopic evaluation of stained erythrocytes is an important part of the erythrogram, especially when anemia is present.
       2. In the Morphologic Features of Erythrocytes section, the clinical significance of erythrocytes with abnormal colors, sizes, shapes, inclusions, or other features is described.
   B. Hct (synonym, PCV): *hemato-* ("blood") *-crit* (denoting "separation")
       1. *Hct* is the percentage of blood volume filled by erythrocytes and therefore a measure of the O_2-carrying capacity of the blood. If there are 100 mL of blood with a Hct of 45 %, then erythrocytes occupy 45 mL.
       2. A Hct will accurately reflect the [RBC] in a blood sample if the MCV is WRI.
       3. A Hct will accurately reflect the blood [Hgb] in a sample if the MCHC or CHCM is WRI.
       4. Unit: vol % (commonly just %); and 40 vol % = 0.40 (the SI expression is a unitless decimal fraction)
   C. Blood [Hgb]
       1. The *blood [Hgb]* is the grams of Hgb per 100 mL of blood. Essentially all Hgb in blood is in erythrocytes except in a few pathologic states (e.g., intravascular hemolysis causing hemoglobinemia) or after treatment with Hgb-based O_2 carriers (e.g., Oxyglobin).
       2. The blood [Hgb] will accurately reflect the [RBC] and Hct if the MCHC (or CHCM) and MCV are WRI and hemoglobinemia is not present. The blood [Hgb] is a more direct measure of blood's O_2-carrying capacity than is Hct or the [RBC].
       3. Unit conversion: g/dL × 10 dL/L = g/L (SI unit, nearest 1 g/L)[16]
   D. [RBC]
       1. The *[RBC]* is the number of erythrocytes per unit volume of blood (in clinical jargon, commonly referred to as *RBC count*).
       2. The [RBC] will accurately reflect Hct and the blood [Hgb] if the MCV and MCHC (or CHCM) are WRI. The [RBC] is used to calculate MCH and can be used to calculate the MCV if the MCV is not directly measured.
       3. Unit conversion: (# × 10^6/μL) × 10^6 μL/L = # × 10^{12}/L (SI unit)
   E. Wintrobe's erythrocyte indices: MCV, MCHC, and MCH
       1. The *Wintrobe's erythrocyte indices* are three values that are used to characterize erythrocytes in peripheral blood. The MCHC (or CHCM) and MCV are used to classify anemias (see Anemia, sect. II.B).
           a. *MCV* is the volume per average erythrocyte expressed in femtoliters (fL) or cubic micrometers (μm^3).

b. *MCHC* is the cellular Hgb concentration per average erythrocyte expressed as grams of Hgb per 100 mL of erythrocytes (g/dL); g/dL × 10 dL/L = g/L (SI unit)

c. *MCH* is the quantity of Hgb per average erythrocyte expressed in picograms (pg).

2. In most blood specimens, not all erythrocytes are the same (i.e., the erythrocytes have different volumes, Hgb concentrations, and Hgb contents). It is important to remember that the MCV, MCHC, and MCH represent the averages for all erythrocytes in the sample.

3. Relationship of indices

a. Because the MCH represents how much Hgb is in an average erythrocyte, and the MCV represents the volume of an average erythrocyte, the MCHC of an average erythrocyte can be calculated by dividing the MCH by the MCV (Eq. 3.1a).

$$MCHC = \frac{MCH}{MCV} \qquad\qquad\qquad \textbf{(3.1a.)}$$

Example: MCH = 20 pg, MCV = 60 fL

$$MCHC = \frac{20 \text{ pg}}{60 \text{ fL}} = \frac{20 \times 10^{-12} \text{ g}}{60 \times 10^{-15} \text{ L}} = \frac{20,000 \times 10^{-15} \text{ g}}{60 \times 10^{-15} \text{ L}} = 333 \text{ g/L} = 33.3 \text{ g/dL}$$

$$MCV = \frac{\text{Hct} \times 10}{[\text{RBC}]} \quad MCHC = \frac{[\text{Hgb}] \times 100}{\text{Hct}} \quad MCH = \frac{[\text{Hgb}] \times 10}{[\text{RBC}]} \qquad \textbf{(3.1b.)}$$

$$\text{Hct} = \frac{MCV \times [\text{RBC}]}{10} \qquad\qquad\qquad \textbf{(3.1c.)}$$

b. When originally described by Wintrobe, the indices represented the calculated interrelationships of three measured values: Hct (reported as a %), blood [Hgb] (reported as g/dL), and [RBC] (reported as $10^6/\mu$L) (Eq. 3.1b).

4. The Wintrobe formulas are used to calculate some of the results generated by impedance and light-scatter cell counters.

a. Hct is calculated from the measured MCV and [RBC] (Eq. 3.1c).

b. MCHC is calculated from the measured blood [Hgb] and calculated Hct (Eq. 3.1b).

c. MCH is calculated from the measured blood [Hgb] and measured [RBC] (Eq. 3.1b).

5. Relationship of blood [Hgb] and MCHC

a. Sample 1: Hct = 50 % and blood [Hgb] = 15 g/dL

(1) If you have 100 mL of blood with a Hct of 50 % and a blood [Hgb] of 15 g/dL (grams of Hgb per 100 mL of blood), then you have 50 mL of erythrocytes, 50 mL of plasma, and 15 g of Hgb in the erythrocytes.

(2) Therefore, you have 15 g of Hgb per 50 mL of erythrocytes, or 30 g of Hgb per 100 mL of erythrocytes, and thus the MCHC = 30 g/dL.

b. Sample 2: Hct = 33 % and blood [Hgb] = 10 g/dL

(1) If you have 100 mL of blood with a Hct of 33 % and a blood [Hgb] of 10 g/dL (grams of Hgb per 100 mL of blood), then you have 33 mL of erythrocytes, 67 mL of plasma, and 10 g of Hgb in the erythrocytes.

       (2) Therefore, you have 10 g of Hgb per 33 mL of erythrocytes, or 30 g per 100 mL of erythrocytes, and thus the MCHC = 30 g/dL.

    c. Relationship of Hgb and Hct (with conventional units)

       (1) When the MCHC is 33.3 g/dL, the blood [Hgb] numerical value will be one-third of the Hct numerical value (e.g., Hgb = 15 g/dL and Hct = 45 %, or Hgb = 8 g/dL and Hct = 24 %).

       (2) Because MCHC values in most blood samples are about 32–36 g/dL, the Hgb numerical value typically will be about one-third of the Hct numerical value.

  6. RDW

    a. The RDW is a calculated value (usually expressed as a percentage) that reflects the amount of variation in the erythrocyte volumes (see Morphologic Features of Erythrocytes, sect. VI).

    b. It typically represents the coefficient of variation of the erythrocyte volumes that are used to determine the MCV, and is calculated from the MCV and standard deviation of the MCV; that is, (standard deviation of MCV ÷ MCV) × 100.

    c. Increased RDW reflects increased anisocytosis.

  7. The Bayer Technicon and ADVIA analyzers calculate the MCHC as just described but also measure the [Hgb] of each individual erythrocyte by analysis of Hgb-induced light scatter. This provides the following additional erythrogram results for the ADVIA:

    a. *CHCM* is the average of the cellular Hgb concentration measured in each erythrocyte, with the same concentration and units as the MCHC but determined directly by light scatter.

       (1) The CHCM is unaffected by most of the spectral interferences that can cause a falsely increased MCHC.

       (2) Heinz bodies will falsely increase the CHCM because of altered light scatter.[17]

    b. *CH* is the average Hgb content of erythrocytes, as is MCH, but it is the mean Hgb content of individual cells as calculated from direct measurements of each cell's volume and Hgb concentration.

    c. *HDW* reflects the amount of variation in the erythrocyte Hgb concentration. It is the coefficient of variation of the Hgb concentrations measured in each erythrocyte. Increased HDW is called *anisochromasia*.

F. nRBCs

  1. The nRBCs observed during the examination of a blood film are enumerated by counting the number of nRBCs seen while 100 (or more) leukocytes are differentiated and counted. The conventional method of recording the number of nucleated erythrocytes is number of nRBCs/100 WBCs (e.g., 10 nRBCs/100 WBCs).

  2. Manual and some electronic methods determine the [WBC] by counting nucleated cells or nuclei (either of leukocytes or nRBCs). By these methods, a *measured [WBC]* represents the sum of nucleated cell concentrations (leukocytes plus nRBCs), and correction of the measured [WBC] is necessary to obtain a more accurate [WBC].

  3. A [nRBC] can be calculated from the measured [WBC], the corrected [WBC], or both.

(1) The most direct method is shown in Eq. 3.2a.

$$[nRBC] = measured\,[WBC] \times \frac{\#\,nRBC/100WBC}{100 + \#\,nRBC/100WBC} \qquad \textbf{(3.2a.)}$$

Example: measured [WBC] = 20,000 / μL, nRBC = 25/100 WBC

$$[nRBC] = 20,000/\mu L \times \frac{25}{125} = 4,000/\mu L$$

$$[nRBC] = corrected\,[WBC] \times \frac{\#\,nRBC}{100\,WBC} \qquad \textbf{(3.2b.)}$$

Example: corrected $[WBC] = 16,000/\mu L$, nRBC = 25/100 WBC

or $\dfrac{25\,nRBC}{100\,WBC}$

$$[nRBC] = \frac{16,000\,WBC}{\mu L} \times \frac{25\,nRBC}{100\,WBC} = \frac{4,000\,nRBC}{\mu L} = 4,000/\mu L$$

$$[nRBC] = measured\,[WBC] - corrected\,[WBC] \qquad \textbf{(3.2c.)}$$

(2) A [nRBC] can be calculated from the corrected [WBC] (see Eq. 2.1) by using Eq. 3.2b.

(3) If the corrected [WBC] and measured [WBC] are known, the [nRBC] is easily calculated by using Eq. 3.2c.

4. The conventional method of reporting the enumeration of nRBCs in blood is relative to 100 leukocytes. This method is useful for correcting a measured [WBC] but may give a false impression of the number of nRBCs in blood.
    For example, two blood samples each have 50 nRBCs/100 WBCs. If one sample has a [WBC] of 50,000/μL and the second sample has a [WBC] of 500/μL, then the [nRBC] in the first sample is 100 times as great as the [nRBC] in the second sample. Therefore, reporting the [nRBC] instead of the conventional method will provide a more consistent indication of the degree of rubricytosis.

G. Reticulocytes
    1. Enumeration of reticulocytes in blood can be an important aspect of an erythrogram, especially in anemic dogs, cats, and cattle.
    2. These are the three common methods of enumerating blood reticulocytes:
        a. The *reticulocyte concentration* (RC) is the concentration of reticulocytes in blood expressed as the number of reticulocytes per μL (or L) of blood. The RC is the preferred method for evaluating marrow response to anemia. The RC is also called the reticulocyte count.
        b. The *reticulocyte percentage* (RP) is the percentage of erythrocytes that are reticulocytes in a blood sample. For example, if there are 10 reticulocytes per 1000 erythrocytes, then the RP is 1.0 %. The RP is also called the reticulocyte count.
        c. The *corrected reticulocyte percentage* (CRP) is a calculated percentage that represents the RP if the animal were not anemic but had the same RC (see the following sect. III.K).

III. Methods
  A. Microhematocrit
    1. One of the easiest, most accurate, and most reproducible methods of assessing [erythrocyte] in blood is by the centrifuged microhematocrit.
    2. When first described, the term *hematocrit* (Hct) was the name of the procedure used to separate blood into its major components: packed erythrocytes, buffy coat layer, and plasma. With common use of the procedure, Hct started to indicate the major result of the procedure (i.e., Hct or PCV). When a small capillary tube was introduced for the procedure, it became the *microhematocrit* method to differentiate it from the larger Wintrobe Hct tubes. Today, the terms *hematocrit* and *packed cell volume* are frequently used as synonyms. However, some people differentiate the centrifuged microhematocrit from the calculated Hct by referring to the former as the PCV or spun Hct and to the latter as the Hct or calculated Hct.
    3. High-speed centrifugation (about 13,000 × g) of blood in a microhematocrit tube separates the blood cells into layers based on the density of cells. The buffy coat layer contains platelets, lymphocytes, monocytes, eosinophils, neutrophils, basophils, and nucleated erythrocytes (listed from least to most dense). The buffy coat cells typically occupy about 0.5–1.0 % of the blood volume. The erythrocytes are below the buffy coat.
    4. Because of potential inaccuracies of measuring the [RBC] and MCV, which are used for the calculated Hct, the microhematocrit tube method (centrifuged or spun) is generally considered the gold standard for determining the blood Hct.
    5. Erroneous microhematocrit results can be produced by the following:
      a. Inadequate mixing of blood before the microhematocrit tubes are filled could produce either falsely high or falsely low Hcts.
      b. With an inadequate volume of blood in the EDTA tube, the hypertonic salt shrinks the erythrocytes and thus gives a falsely low Hct.
      c. Inadequate centrifugation may cause a falsely high Hct because plasma remains within the loosely packed erythrocytes.
      d. Misreading of the Hct, including misidentifying the interface between erythrocytes and buffy coat, may result in erroneous values.
    6. Use of the microhematocrit also enables visual subjective evaluation of plasma for hemolysis, lipemia, and icterus.
  B. Impedance cell counters
    1. The basic principles of impedance counters are described in Analytical Principles and Methods, sect. III.B, in Chapter 2. Most impedance counters measure MCV, blood [Hgb], and [RBC]. From those measurements, most instruments calculate Hct, MCHC, MCH, and RDW (see Eq. 3.1 for the Wintrobe equations).
    2. Impedance cell counters may not be able to determine erythrocyte features accurately because an animal's erythrocytes are too small (e.g., in sheep and goats) or because its erythrocytes and platelets have similar volumes.
    3. For most samples, a properly adjusted and calibrated impedance cell counter can provide reliable data for these cells if clots and platelet clumps are not present.[18,19]
      a. For canine blood, most counters can typically differentiate erythrocytes and platelets and thus can provide reliable erythrocyte and platelet data. However, numerous large platelets or small erythrocytes (e.g., in Fe deficiency) can result in false data.

b. For feline blood, most counters cannot reliably differentiate erythrocytes and platelets because of the overlap in cell volumes. Because the instrument classifies large platelets as erythrocytes, the [platelet] is falsely low. Because of relative numbers, the degree of inaccuracy in the erythrocyte data is typically low except when there is a marked anemia.

c. For equine blood, most counters can typically differentiate erythrocytes and platelets and thus can provide reliable erythrocyte and platelet data. The major exception is when the MCV approaches 30 fL (seen primarily in foals).

d. For bovine blood, most counters can typically differentiate erythrocytes and platelets and can provide reliable erythrocyte data. However, the platelet volumes are so low that the [platelet] may be falsely decreased.

C. Optical or laser flow cell cytometers (e.g., CELL-DYN, Bayer Technicon H1, ADVIA, and Sysmex)

1. Basic principles (see Chapter 2, especially Fig. 2.5). The flow cytometric aspects of the CELL-DYN are used in addition to impedance to evaluate leukocytes, whereas the ADVIA uses only flow cytometric methods to evaluate leukocytes, erythrocytes, and platelets.

2. The ADVIA uses unique optical methods of evaluating erythrocytes and reticulocytes. With a special diluent, erythrocytes are isovolumetrically sphered before they pass through a laser beam in which they scatter light. Sphered cells scatter light in a more predictable way. The instrument assesses properties of each erythrocyte to measure or calculate results.

a. As an erythrocyte or platelet passes through the laser beam, its presence is detected by light scatter. The low light scatter (2–3°) is used to determine a cell's volume, whereas high light scatter (5–15°) is used to determine the cell's refractive index. The refractive index is used to differentiate erythrocytes and platelets (platelets have lower refractive indices than erythrocytes) and to determine the Hgb concentration in individual erythrocytes (a greater erythrocyte [Hgb] causes a greater refraction of light).

b. From the data gathered as each erythrocyte passes through the flow cytometer, the following erythrocyte features are measured or calculated:

(1) *V* is the volume of individual erythrocytes.

(2) *MCV* is the average of the individually measured erythrocyte volumes.

(3) *RDW* is the coefficient of variation of the individual erythrocyte volumes.

(4) *[RBC]* is the number of erythrocytes detected in a given blood volume.

(5) *Hct* is the percentage of blood volume occupied by erythrocytes as determined from MCV and [RBC] data (see Eq. 3.1C).

(6) *HC* is the Hgb concentration in individual erythrocytes.

(7) *CHCM* is the average Hgb concentration in erythrocytes (mean of HC values).

(8) *HDW* is the standard deviation of HC values.

(9) *CH* is the average amount of Hgb in erythrocytes. The amount of Hgb in individual erythrocytes is calculated from each cell's HC and V (i.e., pg/fL × fL = pg).

c. Data from erythrocyte analysis can be graphically displayed by the instrument. For example, an erythrocyte cytogram is constructed from the volumes (V) and the [Hgb] in individual erythrocytes (HC) (Fig. 3.6). The displayed data provide

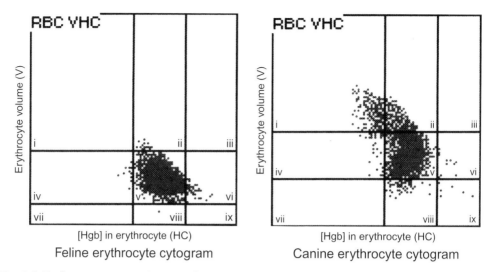

Fig. 3.6. Erythrocyte cytograms (ADVIA) from a healthy cat and an anemic dog: The volume (V) and Hgb concentration (HC) of each erythrocyte (RBC) is graphically displayed in an RBC VHC (volume hemoglobin concentration) grid (tic-tac-toe display). In these cytograms, most erythrocytes are within section *v*, indicating they are normochromic normocytes. Macrocytes are displayed in regions *i*, *ii*, and *iii*; microcytes are in regions *vii*, *viii*, *ix*; hypochromic erythrocytes are in regions *i*, *iv*, and *vii*; and hyperchromic erythrocytes are in regions *iii*, *vi*, and *ix*. Shifts in the erythrocyte distribution represent changes in erythrocyte populations.

- A healthy cat: There are no erythrocyte population shifts from the central normochromic normocyte region (region *v*). Erythrocyte indices from this nonanemic cat were WRIs.
- A dog with regenerative anemia (Hct = 28 % and reticulocytes = $266 \times 10^3/\mu L$): A population of erythrocytes extends into region *i*. This pattern is typical of regeneration because immature erythrocytes are hypochromic macrocytes. The shift may be noted prior to changes in MCV, MCHC, and CHCM because those values reflect the mean values of the erythrocytes. This anemic dog had a mildly increased MCV, mildly decreased MCHC and CHCM, and moderately increased RDW and HDW.

Differences in grid placement reflect different expected erythrocyte indices for cats compared to dogs.

a visual representation of the morphologic classification of erythrocytes (see Anemia, sect. II.B).

d. A dye (oxazine 750) that stains cellular RNA can be used with the special diluent to differentiate reticulocytes from mature erythrocytes by absorbance spectroscopy. The dye interacts with RNA in reticulocytes, which are then identified by their increased light absorption. With this differentiation, the instrument can be used to determine average Hgb content and average cell volumes of mature erythrocytes and reticulocytes separately. The reticulocyte features generated by the ADVIA include the following:

(1) *#RETIC* is the number of reticulocytes detected in a given volume (same as RC).

(2) *MCVr* is the average of the individually measured reticulocyte volumes.

(3) *CHCMr* is the average Hgb concentration in reticulocytes.

(4) *RDWr* is the coefficient of variation of the individual reticulocyte volumes.

(5) *HDWr* is the standard deviation of Hgb concentrations in individual reticulocytes.

(6) *CHr* is the average amount of Hgb in reticulocytes.

(7) *CHDWr* is the distribution width of Hgb concentration in individual reticulocytes (values used for calculating CHr).

e. Like the other instruments, the ADVIA lyses erythrocytes and uses the cyanmethemoglobin (or alternate chemical) method to determine the total blood [Hgb]. With this blood [Hgb] and other data, it calculates the following:

(1) MCHC using the blood [Hgb] and the blood Hct (see Eq. 3.1b): The MCHC should agree with the CHCM if the measured values are accurate and free Hgb is not in the blood's plasma.

(2) MCH using the blood [Hgb] and the blood [RBC] (see Eq. 3.1b): The MCH should agree with the CH if the measured values are accurate and free Hgb is not in the blood's plasma.

f. The ADVIA also determines the [Hgb] contributed by erythrocytes but not plasma by using a calculation involving the CHCM, [RBC], and MCV. The difference between this blood [Hgb] and the blood [Hgb] obtained from the cyanmethemoglobin method is the plasma [Hgb], referred to as Hgb_{delta}. Hgb_{delta} may be increased with intravascular hemolysis, with in vitro hemolysis, or after infusion of Hgb-based O_2 carriers (e.g., Oxyglobin).

D. Quantitative buffy coat (QBC) analysis

1. Major concepts that pertain to the QBC analysis are described in Analytical Principles and Methods, sect. III.D, in Chapter 2. Erythrogram data generated by the QBC analyzer include the Hct, blood [Hgb], MCHC, and RP for dogs and cats. The presence of nRBC may be noted in some samples.

2. The QBC Hct is obtained by centrifugation, and the result should agree with the result obtained by the microhematocrit method.

3. The QBC MCHC is an estimate and is determined by the relationship between the MCHC and the density of the erythrocytes. The lower the MCHC is, the less dense the erythrocytes are.

a. The analyzer measures the erythrocyte density by determining the depth of the plastic float in the erythrocyte layer. A lower erythrocyte density allows the float to penetrate further into the erythrocyte layer. Once the density is determined, the instrument calculates a QBC MCHC.

b. Platelet clumps or blood clots in the sample can accumulate above or below the plastic float and thus alter the depth of the float in the erythrocyte layer. In such samples, the QBC MCHC could be either falsely decreased (if platelets or clots pushed the float down into the erythrocytes) or falsely increased (if platelets or clots prevented the float from sinking).

4. The QBC blood [Hgb] is calculated from the QBC Hct and the QBC MCHC by using a Wintrobe index formula (Eq. 3.1b).

a. If the QBC MCHC is falsely decreased, the QBC blood [Hgb] will be falsely decreased.

b. If the QBC Hct is falsely decreased, the QBC blood [Hgb] will be falsely decreased.

5. RP is based on increased RNA fluorescence at the top of the erythrocyte layer, and the presence of nRBCs is suggested by increasing DNA fluorescence toward the top of the erythrocyte layer.

E. [RBC] by the hemocytometer method
 1. A hemocytometer can be used to measure a [RBC] in blood. Blood is diluted (usually in a Unopette system), and then the diluted blood is used to charge the hemocytometer chamber (Fig. 2.4). A microscope is used to enumerate the erythrocytes, and then a [RBC] is calculated.
 2. Determination of the [RBC] by the hematocytometer method is typically imprecise and thus is not recommended for routine assessment of [RBC].

F. Hct and blood [Hgb] determined by conductivity
 1. Some electrochemical instruments that are designed to measure blood gas analytes (e.g., Po_2, Pco_2, and pH; see Table 10.1 for abbreviations) or electrolytes (e.g., Na^+, K^+, and Cl^-) will also generate a Hct and blood [Hgb] as part of their profile results.
 2. The Hct is determined by measuring the electrical conductivity of the blood and then converting that value to a Hct, based on an inverse relationship between conductivity and blood cell concentration; that is, electrical conductivity of blood decreases with greater blood cell concentration. Because the [RBC] is typically much greater than the [WBC] or [platelet], a blood sample's conductivity depends primarily on the [RBC]. As the [RBC] and Hct are strongly correlated, a blood sample's conductivity changes inversely with its Hct. Some analyzers correct for changes in electrolyte concentrations.
 3. For some analyzers, the Hct that is derived via conductivity is converted to a blood [Hgb] by using Wintrobe's MCHC formula (Eq. 3.1b) and an assumed MCHC (e.g., 33 g/dL). If the blood sample's MCHC is not 33 g/dL, then the conversion yields an incorrect blood [Hgb].
 4. Other instruments (e.g., NOVA CCX) determine the Hct by conductivity and determine the blood [Hgb] by adjusting the conductivity data based on a photometric measurement of the percentage of Hgb saturation with O_2 (So_2; see the Analytical Concepts Sect. I.A.5, in Chapter 10).
 5. The Hct and blood [Hgb] derived by conductivity should be considered estimates. Any change in the blood that alters its conductivity will alter that derived Hct and blood [Hgb]; for example, marked leukocytosis yields a falsely increased Hct, and marked hypoproteinemia yields a falsely decreased Hct.

G. Blood [Hgb]
 1. Blood [Hgb] has been measured by photometric methods for many years. In a variety of current blood analyzers, the blood [Hgb] is typically measured by a cyanmethemoglobin assay using spectrophotometry. Because of concerns of working with or disposing of minute amounts of cyanide, other methods have been developed. High concentrations of cells or the presence of particles that interfere with light transmission may result in a falsely increased blood [Hgb] for that sample (see Anemia, sect. II.B.12).
 2. Portable hemoglobinometers have been used for many decades for measuring blood [Hgb]. The Spencer hemoglobinometer was battery powered and, with proper techniques, provided a good estimate of blood [Hgb].[13] More recently, another portable hemoglobinometer was developed (HemoCue AB). It determines the blood [Hgb] by measuring the absorbance of azide methemoglobin at two wavelengths. Evaluation at two wavelengths may decrease the false increases caused by spectral interference. It has been shown to have good agreement with blood [Hgb] measured by cyanmethemoglobin spectrophotometry.[20]

Table 3.3. Potential effects of selected sample and patient conditions on hematocrit (Hct) and values used to calculate Hct

Condition	Spun Hct[a]	Calc. Hct[b]	MCV[c]	[RBC]	Cond. Hct[d]
Inadequate mixing	↓, ↑	↓, ↑	—[e]	↓, ↑	↓, ↑
Excess EDTA shrinks RBCs in blood	↓	—	↑[f]	—	↓
Clots in sample	↓, ↑	↓	—	↓	↓
In vitro hemolysis	↓	↓	—	↓	↓
Inadequate centrifugation	↑	NA[g]	NA	NA	NA
Agglutination	—	↓	↑	↓	NA
Very small erythrocytes	—	↓, ↑	↑	↓	—
Hyponatremia	—	↓	↓	—	↑
Hypernatremia	—	↑	↑	—	↓
Leukocytosis	—	—	—	—	↑
Thrombocytosis (marked)	—	↑	↓	↑	↑
Hyperproteinemia (marked)	—	—	—	—	↑
Hypoproteinemia	—	—	—	—	↓

[a] Spun Hct is the Hct determined by centrifugation, either the microhematocrit method or the QBC method.

[b] Calc. Hct is the Hct calculated by impedance cell counters after measuring MCV and [RBC].

[c] MCV measured by impedance or light scatter

[d] Cond. Hct is the Hct determined by electrochemical instruments that measure the conductivity of blood.

[e] —, No effect

[f] This is a potential effect with excess K_2EDTA and the Technicon analyzer. The effect is not seen with most other instruments (see the text).

[g] NA, not applicable

3. The LaserCyte Hematology Analyzer determines blood [Hgb] by measuring the transmittance of light from two light-emitting diodes: one for whole blood and one for hemolyzed blood.

H. Differences in erythrocyte data determined by centrifugation, impedance, optical, and conductivity methods

1. A Hct properly determined by centrifugation of microhematocrit tubes is considered the best method of assessing blood [erythrocyte] in domestic animals. As a quality assurance method, the centrifuge Hct (often called *spun Hct*) can be compared to the Hct calculated by impedance counters (calculated Hct) or by conductivity methods (conductivity Hct). Discrepancies among Hct values can be caused by a variety of factors (Table 3.3). As a rule of thumb, calculated Hct and spun Hct should agree with each other within 3 percentage points; for example, if a spun Hct is 38 %, a calculated Hct of 35–41 % should be obtained.

2. Inadequate mixing of blood prior to filling a microhematocrit tube can cause an erroneous Hct. Erythrocytes tend to settle if the anticoagulated blood is left standing in a tube rack, especially with pronounced rouleaux.

   a. Filling the microhematocrit tube with the top portion of that blood will yield a falsely decreased Hct by any method, whereas filling with the bottom portion will yield a falsely increased Hct.

b. The Hct values may differ between methods because the blood was properly mixed prior to one assay but not the other.

3. Collecting or transferring an inadequate amount of blood into an EDTA tube (e.g., 0.5 mL of blood into a tube designed for 3 mL of blood) results in a relative excess amount of EDTA. The excess EDTA creates hypertonic plasma and erythrocytes shrink because of osmosis; the smaller erythrocytes occupy less volume, and thus a spun Hct is falsely decreased. However, when these erythrocytes are suspended in an isotonic diluent prior to impedance counting, they quickly gain volume, and thus the calculated Hct may not be affected. The conductivity Hct may be falsely decreased because the greater concentration of cations and anions from the anticoagulant will increase the conductivity.

4. The presence of small clots can have adverse affects on all methods of determining Hct. The clotting removes erythrocytes from suspension, and thus the Hct on the remaining nonclotted blood will be falsely decreased. However, very small clots could enter the microhematocrit tube and result in incomplete erythrocyte packing and thus falsely increase spun Hct. The effects of clots are less predictable with impedance and conductivity methods because the clots may not allow proper sampling by the instrument or may plug the small orifices or tubing.

5. All three Hct methods will yield falsely decreased Hct if erythrocytes were lysed during blood collection or handling; the Hct may be correct for the sample but the sample is not representative of the animal's blood. Mild hemolysis would have a minimal effect, but gross hemolysis would create larger errors.

6. A spun Hct will be falsely increased if centrifugation of the microhematocrit tube is inadequate because of an inadequate g-force or inadequate time of centrifugation. The spun Hct does include a very small amount of trapped plasma (< 3 % error; e.g., < 1.2 % increase due to trapped plasma at Hct of 40 %), but poor centrifugation would leave more plasma mixed with the packed erythrocytes.

7. The presence of agglutinated erythrocytes (either autoagglutination or agglutination induced by heparin) can falsely decrease the [RBC] determined by impedance because of two factors: (1) clustered erythrocytes are counted as one large erythrocyte, and (2) in some instruments the "large erythrocyte" is considered too large for an erythrocyte and is electronically excluded during the counting. Depending on the size of the erythrocyte cluster and the instrument's size limits for inclusion, the MCV determined might be sufficiently erroneous to give a false calculated Hct (i.e., the falsely decreased [RBC] times a falsely increased MCV may yield a nearly correct calculated Hct).

8. Some erythrocytes of animals (e.g., sheep, goats, and young horses) may be too small to be recognized as erythrocytes by impedance. If the smaller erythrocytes are not included in the MCV determination, the instrument will generate a falsely increased MCV. Concurrently, the [RBC] will be falsely decreased. Because the calculated Hct is the product of the MCV and [RBC], the calculated Hct could be falsely increased or decreased depending on which of the measured values has the greatest error.

9. When an animal has a persistent and marked decrease in plasma osmolality (because of hyponatremia and hypochloremia), the osmolality within erythrocytes also decreases. When those erythrocytes are placed in an isotonic diluent prior to impedance counting, the erythrocytes shrink as H_2O moves from the cells via osmosis.[21] Thus, the MCV measured is falsely decreased, and thus the Hct calculated is falsely decreased. The opposite osmosis occurs when an animal has a

persistent and marked plasma hyperosmolality and thus the calculated Hct is falsely increased.[21] The conductivity Hct may also be affected by marked changes in plasma [Na$^+$] and [Cl$^-$], although analyzers may be designed to correct for such abnormalities; that is, hyponatremic and hypochloremic samples may have less conductivity, which results in a greater conductivity Hct.

10. Autologous blood transfusions may cause a falsely decreased conductivity Hct. In a study using an infusate containing washed patient's erythrocytes in saline, the infusate's greater electrolyte concentrations and lower protein concentrations (compared to plasma) increased its conductivity and thus resulted in a falsely low conductivity Hct; the infusate's spun Hct was near 51 %, but the infusate's conductivity Hct was near 37 %.[22] If a large portion of a patient's blood volume is from administered infusate, then a patient's conductivity Hct could be falsely decreased.

11. The presence of marked leukocytosis, marked thrombocytosis, or marked hyper-proteinemia can reduce the conductivity of blood and thus cause a falsely increased conductivity Hct. If the impedance cell counter cannot differentiate platelets from erythrocytes and thrombocytosis is marked, the measured [RBC] will be falsely increased and probably the MCV will be falsely decreased. If the error in the [RBC] is greater than the MCV error, then the calculated Hct will be falsely increased.

12. Marked hypoproteinemia will increase the conductivity of blood, and thus the conductivity Hct will be falsely decreased.

13. The MCV may be decreased by in vitro events or phenomena in addition to the aforementioned effects of osmolality.
    a. A falsely decreased MCV may occur when an electronic cell counter cannot differentiate large platelets from erythrocytes. This is primarily a problem when there is a marked thrombocytosis and a concurrent marked anemia.[23]
    b. Such erroneous results can be suspected or recognized by other findings.
       (1) The red cell distribution width is increased.
       (2) Microscopic examination of the blood does not confirm the presence of a microcytosis but does identify marked thrombocytosis.
       (3) The MCH will be falsely low (assuming the blood [Hgb] is correct) because the [RBC] will be falsely increased.
       (4) The calculated Hct might be correct, depending on the measured values; that is, a falsely low MCV times a falsely increased [RBC] could provide a calculated Hct that is close to a spun Hct.

I. Reticulocyte concentration (RC) (also called *absolute reticulocyte count*)
    1. The *RC* is the concentration of reticulocytes in blood expressed as number of reticulocytes per μL (or L) of blood.
    2. RC equation (Eq. 3.3a):

$$RC = RP \times [RBC] \tag{3.3a.}$$

$$CRP = RP \times \frac{\text{patient's Hct}}{\text{average Hct for species}} \tag{3.3b.}$$

$$RPI = \frac{CRP}{RMT} \tag{3.3c.}$$

J. Reticulocyte percentage (RP) (sometimes called *reticulocyte count*)

1. The *RP* is the percentage of erythrocytes that are reticulocytes. For example, if there are 10 reticulocytes per 1000 erythrocytes, the RP is 1.0 %.

2. It is used to calculate RC or CRP. It indicates nonregenerative anemia if not increased and possible regenerative anemia if increased

3. Percentages may be affected by agglutination.

4. Basics of procedures

   a. Manual (microscopic) procedure

      (1) Equal volumes of blood and NMB stain are mixed and kept at room temperature for at least 15 min. NMB is a vital stain (i.e., it stains living cells) that penetrates erythrocytes and stains (and precipitates) cytoplasmic RNA. A smear of the blood-NMB mixture is made and air-dried for microscopic examination.

      (2) The number of reticulocytes observed while counting 1000 nonnucleated erythrocytes is recorded. For cats, some laboratories count only the aggregate reticulocytes, whereas other laboratories count aggregate and punctate reticulocytes and report both.

   b. Automated techniques

      (1) QBC-VetAutoread: Canine QBC RP is estimated by determining the thickness of RNA fluorescent cells that are at the top of the erythrocyte layer and below the granulocyte layer.

      (2) Flow cytometric methods

         (a) In some CELL-DYN analyzers (e.g., 3200 and 3700) and after staining with NMB and sphering in a special diluent, reticulocytes are enumerated by a unique light scatter created from precipitated ribosomal RNA. RP is determined by the percentage of erythrocytes with the light-scattering property. Fluorescence rather than light-scatter methods are used with the CELL-DYN 4000.[24]

         (b) In some flow cytometers and after staining reticulocytes with a fluorescent nucleic acid–binding dye (thiazole orange), erythrocytes pass through the instrument that identifies fluorescent and nonfluorescent cells. RP is determined by the percentage of erythrocytes that are fluorescent.

         (c) The ADVIA uses a different stain (oxazine 750) to differentiate reticulocytes from mature erythrocytes (see Analytical Principles and Methods, sect. III.C.2.d). It also has the ability to classify reticulocytes as *most immature (high absorption)*, *intermediate (medium absorption)*, or *most mature (low absorption)* reticulocytes based on their staining intensity (the most immature have the greatest staining and therefore greatest light absorption).

         (d) RC and RP may be affected by agglutination.

5. An increased RP does not always indicate the presence of a reticulocytosis, especially in moderate to severe anemias, because a relative increase may be due to a decrease in the concentration of mature erythrocytes rather than to an increase in the concentration of reticulocytes. Table 3.4 provides examples of RP data. Conversely, a marrow may be responding to a mild anemia without generating an increased RP because the reticulocytes mature in the marrow before release, and thus reticulocytosis is not seen but the Hct steadily increases. The circulating life spans of reticulo-

Table 3.4. Evaluation of reticulocyte data

Canine	Units	Reference intervals	Dog 1[a]	Dog 2[b]	Dog 3[c]		
Hct	%	37–55	15	15	15		
RP	%	0.0–1.0	2.0	9.0	0.0		
CRP	%	0.0–1.0	0.7	3.0	0.0		
[RBC]	$\times 10^6/\mu L$	5.5–8.5	2.0	2.0	2.0		
RC	$\times 10^3/\mu L$	0–80	40	180	0		

Feline	Units	Reference intervals	Cat 1[d]	Cat 2[e]	Cat 3[f]	Cat 4[g]	Cat 5[h]
Hct	%	24–45	12	12	24	12	12
RP (aggregate)	%	0.0–1.0	6.0	2.0	0.6	1.2	0.1
RP (punctate)	%	0.0–10.0	30.0	30.0	30.0	6.0	1.0
CRP (aggregate)	%	0.0–1.0	2.0	0.7	0.4	0.4	< 0.1
CRP (punctate)	%	0.0–10.0	10.0	10.0	20.0	2.0	0.3
[RBC]	$\times 10^6/\mu L$	5.0–10.0	2.0	2.0	4.0	2.0	2.0
RC (aggregate)[i]	$\times 10^3/\mu L$	0–80	120	40	24	24	2
RC (punctate)[i]	$\times 10^3/\mu L$	5–500	600	600	1200	120	20

[a] Dog 1: Evidence of increased erythrocyte production is not present. If the marrow is currently responding to the anemia, it is not reflected by the blood reticulocytes. The RP is increased because fewer erythrocytes, rather than more reticulocytes, are in the blood; that is, RP is increased because the [reticulocyte] is WRI and the [RBC] is decreased.

[b] Dog 2: There is evidence of increased erythrocyte production, and the marrow is currently responding to the anemia. The RP is increased because fewer erythrocytes and more reticulocytes are in the blood than there are in health; that is, the RP is increased because the [reticulocyte] is increased and the [RBC] is decreased.

[c] Dog 3: There is not evidence of increased erythrocyte production. As reticulocytes were not seen, decreased production of erythrocytes may be one reason for the anemia. Or, it could be too early (< 3–4 d) for a reticulocyte response.

[d] Cat 1: There is evidence of increased erythrocyte production. The aggregate reticulocytosis indicates increased erythropoiesis in the past 3–6 d (approximately). The punctate reticulocytosis (↑ punctate RC) is consistent with the aggregate response and may persist for 1–3 wk after initial stimulus. In this case, the punctate CRP is a borderline percentage and thus difficult to interpret by itself.

[e] Cat 2: The duration of the anemia must be known to interpret the results. If the onset of anemia was within the past 2–3 d, then the results are consistent with the punctate reticulocytosis that occurs before an aggregate reticulocytosis. If the anemia has been present longer, the aggregate CRP and RC indicate a poor regenerative response.

[f] Cat 3: The magnitude of the punctate reticulocytosis indicates an Epo stimulus occurred at least 7–10 d ago and erythroid hyperplasia is present (resolving anemia). Absence of an aggregate reticulocytosis suggests that there is no longer an increased release of aggregate reticulocytes.

[g] Cat 4: Evidence of increased erythrocyte production is not present despite an increased aggregate RP. Decreased production of erythrocytes is probably at least one reason for the anemia if there has been sufficient time for a marrow response.

[h] Cat 5: Evidence of increased erythrocyte production is not present. Decreased production of erythrocytes is probably contributing to the anemia, as the reticulocyte concentrations are WRI or decreased.

[i] Reference intervals for reticulocyte concentrations are based on data from the microscopic analysis of blood samples from 45 healthy cats (M.A.S. unpublished data).

cytes and the relationships between marrow stimulus and marrow responses (see Physiologic Processes, sect. VI) need to be considered when blood reticulocyte data are interpreted.

6. Microscopic determination of RP has relatively poor analytical precision. Therefore, RP should be considered an estimate. Values that are calculated using the microscopic RP (i.e., RC, CRP, and RPI) should also be considered estimates.

7. The degree of increased polychromasia should correspond to the increase in RP (except for feline punctate reticulocytes).

K. Corrected reticulocyte percentage (CRP) (also called *absolute reticulocyte percent* and *absolute % reticulocyte count*)

1. Calculation of CRP converts RP to a percentage that would estimate the RP if the animal were not anemic. This is necessary for appropriate interpretation of RP if RC is not calculated. If reticulocyte production was unchanged but anemia developed due to loss or destruction of mature erythrocytes, the RP would be increased because of a decrease in total erythrocytes, not because of increased reticulocyte production and release. The CRP determines whether the increased RP is enough to show regeneration or whether the increased RP is only due to the anemia.

2. The CRP equation is Eq. 3.3b. The CRP is needed only if the RP is increased and anemia is present.

3. In theory, the reference interval for CRP should be the same as the RP reference interval. Therefore, if a CRP is greater than the reference interval for RP, there is a reticulocytosis.

4. Just as the RP must be corrected for the severity of the anemia, the degree of increased polychromasia needs to be interpreted with knowledge of the Hct when the degree of polychromasia is reported based on visual inspection of microscopic fields containing somewhat standardized erythrocyte numbers (see Morphologic Features of Erythrocytes, sect. I.A)

L. Reticulocyte production index (RPI) (also called *corrected reticulocyte count* and *reticulocyte index*)

1. During accelerated erythropoiesis, younger reticulocytes (called *shift reticulocytes*) may be released. In comparison to older reticulocytes, they may have longer circulating life spans before becoming mature erythrocytes. Thus, the CRP may be increased because of the increased life span of reticulocytes and not necessarily increased production. Some people recommend the CRP be adjusted for the prolonged life spans by calculating the RPI.

2. Equation for RPI (Eq. 3.3c).

   a. Application of the RPI requires that a RMT be known for each species in health and during accelerated erythropoiesis. RMT values frequently written for human reticulocytes are as follows: When Hct = 45 %, RMT = 1.0 d; Hct = 35 %, RMT = 1.5 d; Hct = 25 %, RMT = 2.0 d; and Hct = 15 %, RMT = 2.5 d.

   b. Very few RMT values for domestic animals are available.

      (1) In healthy dogs, reported values include a mean of 31 h, with an interval of 19–43 h.[14] Values for anemic dogs are not known but probably are longer and thus RMTs in anemic dogs are probably different from RMTs in anemic people.

      (2) In cats, reported RMTs (as reticulocyte life span) are about 12 h for Type III reticulocytes and 3.5 d for Type I + II reticulocytes, and thus use of the human RMT values is not appropriate for calculating a feline RPI.

   3. Until the validity and clinical value of the RPI is established, the CRP or RC should
      be used to assess regenerative status. When interpreting the CRP and RP in an
      anemic animal, the possibility of a longer RMT should be considered.
   4. Evaluation of reticulocyte percentages and concentrations is presented in Table 3.4.

MORPHOLOGIC FEATURES OF ERYTHROCYTES: CLINICAL SIGNIFICANCE
AND PATHOGENESES

I.   Assessment: Morphologic features of erythrocytes are evaluated as part of a routine CBC or
     as a separate procedure. For abnormalities in size, shape, and color, relative quantities of
     each abnormality per 100× objective microscope field are usually reported on a 3- or 4-plus
     scale. This microscopic assessment is subjective because of varied regions selected for
     evaluation, varied criteria for categorizing abnormalities, and varied grading systems. These
     are the two major methods of selecting microscopic fields for assessment:
     A. By number of erythrocytes in field (provides an estimate relative to erythrocytes in
        blood)
        1. If the features are always evaluated in regions of the blood film where erythrocytes
           occasionally touch one another but do not overlie one another, then the evaluation
           will be done in thicker areas of blood films from anemic animals as compared to
           nonanemic animals. With this approach, the number of erythrocytes per microscope
           field stays somewhat similar, but the volume of blood assessed per field is greater
           with anemia because more fluid volume was deposited in thicker regions of the
           smear. An increase in an abnormality reflects an increased percentage of that
           abnormality; for example, "1+ polychromasia" in an anemic animal would be a
           relative increase (similar to increased RP) and not good evidence of a regenerative
           response without the anemia being considered.
        2. The assessment can also be adjusted based on number of erythrocytes per field. If a
           1+ grade is based on finding six poikilocytes in a field of 300 erythrocytes, then a
           1+ grade would be given if there were three poikilocytes in a field of 150 erythro-
           cytes. This method is also a relative system, so interpretation must include the
           severity of anemia.
        3. Some grading systems have different grades based on the blood Hct. For example,
           the 1+ grade of poikilocytes (as just discussed) would apply if the Hct is 40 %, but
           six poikilocytes in a field of 150 erythrocytes would be a 1+ grade if the Hct is
           20 % (similar to the CRP system).
     B. By thickness of blood film area (provides an estimate of the concentration in blood)
        1. If the features are evaluated in areas of the smear that are always of about the same
           thickness and therefore contain similar blood volumes per field, there will be fewer
           and more separated erythrocytes in evaluated fields of blood from anemic animals.
           With this approach, an increase in an abnormality would more closely reflect an
           increased concentration of that abnormality; "1+ polychromasia" would reflect a
           regenerative response (more reticulocytes per volume of blood).
        2. This method does not require uniform methods of preparing blood films, but does
           require recognition of areas of similar smear thickness. This is typically based on the
           subjective appearance of the cells which "ball up" in thicker areas, lie flat in appro-
           priate areas, and are broken in areas that are too thin. The location of these areas on
           a blood film will vary with the sample and technique (e.g., protein concentration
           and length of blood film).

II. General features
   A. *Discocytes*: Mature erythrocytes of each domestic mammalian species are disks with different degrees of biconcavity that creates a central pallor (Table 3.2). When these erythrocytes have normal volumes, they are called *normocytes*.
   B. *Rouleau, rouleaux* (pl.) (French for "roll" or "rolls"): a linear branching or nonbranching aggregate of erythrocytes resembling a "stack of coins" (Plate 3A [for all plates, see the color section of this book])
      1. Common in some species (especially horses and cats)
      2. Its formation involves charge interactions between erythrocyte membranes and plasma macromolecules and is therefore affected by erythrocyte factors (shape and membrane composition), albumin factors (glycation), globulin factors (charge, size, and number), lipid content of plasma and perhaps erythrocyte membranes, pH (affects cell and protein charges), and exogenous macromolecules (dextrans).[25]
      3. Increased rouleaux tend to occur if there is hyperglobulinemia or hyperfibrinogenemia. An increase in rouleaux is evident when they extend to near the feathered edge of a blood film and thus reduce the width of the effective monolayer area.
      4. Rouleaux may occur in vivo and contribute to blood hyperviscosity, thus decreasing effective blood flow and tissue oxygenation.
   C. *Agglutination*: aggregation or clumping of erythrocytes into grapelike clusters (Plate 3B)
      1. Autoagglutination is seen in some immune hemolytic anemias, in cold agglutinin disorders, and occasionally in animals without evidence of hemolysis. The *agglutinin* (a substance causing the agglutination) is typically a *cold antibody*; that is, an antibody that has maximal activity at 4–20 °C.
      2. The erythrocyte clusters formed by autoagglutination must be differentiated from rouleaux, which classically appear as stacks of erythrocytes but can appear as piles or fallen stacks of coins. When examined macroscopically in a tube or as a drop on a slide, blood containing the agglutinated erythrocytes or rouleaux has a fine to coarse granular appearance.
      3. One method to differentiate agglutination from rouleaux is the saline dilution (dispersion) test, in which blood is diluted with saline and a wet preparation of the diluted blood is examined (Plate 7A–C). Microscopic examination may lead to the false conclusion that agglutination is present.
         a. This test is appropriate when clumping is apparent, but it is not indicated to look for agglutination when clumping is not apparent.
         b. Rouleaux should disperse into individual erythrocytes when the plasma [total protein] is lowered by dilution of blood with saline. A dilution of 1 part blood to 1 part saline (1:2 dilution) will often disperse rouleaux, but occasionally greater dilutions (1 part blood to 9 parts saline) are needed to disperse rouleaux. At least 1 part blood to 3 parts saline (1:4 dilution) is recommended as a starting point.
         c. The erythrocyte clusters of autoagglutination do not disperse with saline dilution (but there may be fewer clusters because of dilution).
      4. Heparin may induce agglutination of equine erythrocytes.
      5. Agglutination may interfere with the electronic or optical evaluation of erythrocytes when groups of erythrocytes pass through the counting chamber as "large cells." In such cases, the measured MCV and [erythrocyte] are erroneous (unless programs exclude outlier values), as are the values calculated from those measured values. Automated RCs may also be unreliable.
   D. Rubricytosis (also known as metarubricytosis or normoblastemia) (Plate 3C)

1. *Rubricytosis* is an increased concentration of nRBCs in blood. Usually, most are metarubricytes, a few may be rubricytes, and younger precursors are rarely seen.
2. Rubricytosis is common in regenerative anemias (i.e., appropriate rubricytosis) but may be seen also in nonregenerative anemias and in nonanemic animals without reticulocytosis (inappropriate rubricytosis). Therefore, rubricytosis should not be considered a consistently reliable indicator of a responsive marrow.
   a. *Appropriate rubricytosis* is rubricytosis concurrent with regenerative anemia (with reticulocytosis). The nRBCs are released as a response to increased Epo stimulus.
      (1) It occurs during accelerated erythropoiesis. Not only is the release of reticulocytes increased, but so is the release of nRBCs to blood.
      (2) It is seen in regenerative anemias of dogs, cats, cattle, and pigs, and seen occasionally in horses.
   b. *Inappropriate rubricytosis* is rubricytosis in the absence of reticulocytosis; for example, concurrent with nonregenerative anemia or in the absence of anemia.
      (1) It occurs primarily when there is a loss of the finely controlled release of nRBCs from marrow or other erythropoiesis sites: nRBCs escape from marrow or other erythropoiesis sites without nuclear extrusion and before maturing to reticulocytes.
      (2) Disorders or conditions that cause inappropriate rubricytosis
         (a) Marrow damaged by necrosis, inflammation, endotoxemia, hemic or nonhemic neoplasia, or hypoxia: Nucleated erythrocytes gain entrance into marrow sinuses through damaged sinusoidal endothelium.
         (b) Extramedullary hematopoiesis (especially splenic): This may allow release of cells before nuclear extrusion.
         (c) Splenic contraction: Splenic blood contains nucleated erythrocytes that are completing maturation.
         (d) Splenectomy: The few nRBCs that are normally released from marrow are not "caught" by the spleen.
         (e) Lead poisoning in dogs, perhaps the result of damage to marrow sinuses
         (f) Bone marrow dyscrasia in poodles with macrocytosis (see Other Nonneoplastic Leukocyte Disorders, sect. II, in Chapter 2)[26]

III. Erythrocyte color
   A. *Central pallor* refers to the pale central region of an erythrocyte that is due to the relative thinness of the area created by the cell's biconcave shape.
      1. Increased central pallor is usually indicative of hypochromasia.
      2. Decreased central pallor usually indicates abnormally shaped erythrocytes (poikilocytes, including spherocytes). It is also commonly seen near a blood film's feathered edge because of artifactual distortion of erythrocyte shape.
   B. A *ghost cell* is an extremely pale-staining erythrocyte consisting primarily of cell membrane with only a small amount of residual peripheral cytoplasmic Hgb (Plate 3D).
      1. Ghost cells are usually formed during complement-mediated intravascular hemolysis. Membrane attack complexes form membrane pores through which Hgb leaks out.
      2. Ghost cells may form in vitro as a result of smearing trauma. These artifactual ghost cells are often distorted.
   C. A *hypochromic erythrocyte* is a poikilocyte with increased central pallor and more faintly stained Hgb than usual (Plate 3E).

1. *Hypochromasia* is an increased number of hypochromic erythrocytes, which may be reflected by a decreased MCHC and CHCM if the hypochromic population is large enough.
2. Hypochromic erythrocytes result from a decreased intracellular Hgb concentration. When visually evident, they usually are associated with Fe deficiency. However, hypochromasia based on the MCHC or CHCM alone (without microscopically apparent hypochromic erythrocytes) is usually associated with the incomplete Hgb synthesis of immature erythrocytes (i.e., regenerative anemias).
3. Hypochromic erythrocytes of Fe deficiency are typically microcytes and leptocytes. They are prone to structural changes such as irregular membranes, loss of circular shape, and fragmentation.

D. A *polychromatophilic erythrocyte* (*polychromatophil*) is a nonnucleated, immature erythroid cell (reticulocyte) with enough cytoplasmic RNA to stain with a Wright stain (Plate 3C).
   1. Polychromatophilic erythrocytes would be aggregate reticulocytes after vital staining with NMB. A cell's *polychromasia* (many colors) is the result of its cytoplasmic RNA (basophilic staining) and Hgb content (eosinophilic staining).
   2. If the concentration of polychromatophilic erythrocytes in blood is increased, there is *increased polychromasia* that reflects accelerated erythropoiesis. However, a subjective assessment of polychromatophilic erythrocytes in blood films may reflect the percentage or the concentration of polychromatophilic erythrocytes, depending on how it is done (see Morphologic Features of Erythrocytes, sect. I). If assessed as a percentage, the increase should be interpreted as for a RP, in light of the degree of anemia.
   3. Note in the preceding two paragraphs that *polychromasia* can refer to the appearance of an individual erythrocyte (i.e., a cell with polychromasia) or a population of erythrocytes (i.e., increased polychromasia).

E. A *reticulocyte* is a nonnucleated, immature erythroid cell with stainable cytoplasmic RNA (Plate 3F and G).
   1. A reticulocyte's cytoplasmic RNA may be visualized after staining with NMB stain or other vital stains. In cats, reticulocytes are grouped into two types (aggregate and punctate) based on the staining pattern of the RNA.
   2. A reticulocyte's cytoplasmic RNA may also be visualized after staining with Wright stains, in which case reticulocytes will appear as polychromatophilic erythrocytes. All polychromatophilic erythrocytes are reticulocytes, but not all reticulocytes have enough RNA to appear as polychromatophilic erythrocytes.
   3. *Reticulocytosis* (increased blood RC), like increased polychromasia, is an important indicator of accelerated erythropoiesis.

IV. Erythrocyte organisms
   A. Identifying features are listed in Table 3.5.
   B. Major aspects of the anemias or disorders caused by organisms are included in the Nonregenerative Anemia and the Hemolytic Anemias sections.

V. Inclusions other than organisms (Table 3.6)
   A. Basophilic stippling (punctate basophilia) (Plate 4G)
      1. *Basophilic stippling* is the presence of fine to coarse, blue to dark purple dots of aggregated ribosomes (RNA) dispersed within the erythrocyte cytoplasm. Basophilic

Table 3.5. Erythrocyte organisms: identifying features and associated pathogenic processes

Organism	Identifying features[a]	Associated pathogenic processes
Anaplasma marginale	Marginal body is a small, dark-staining coccus about 0.5 μm in diameter on the internal margin of erythrocytes; typically one organism per cell but may be multiple (Plate 3H)	Immune hemolysis, possibly others
Anaplasma centrale	Small dark-staining coccus about 0.5 μm in diameter within erythrocytes; typically one organism per cell but may be multiple (Plate 3I)	Immune hemolysis, possibly others
Babesia spp.	Intracellular oval to teardrop or pear-shaped (pyriform) trophozoites (piroplasms); sizes vary with species (see the text); typically pale blue with a darker outer membrane and a reddish purple eccentric nucleus (Plate 3J and K)	Several theories, including immune mechanisms, protease activity, decreased cell pliability, and oxidative damage
Cytauxzoon felis	Intracellular oval structures (0.1–2.0 μm) with outer thin rim and eccentric nucleus; may resemble signet ring or safety pin; one to several piroplasms per cell (Plate 3L)	Pathogenesis of the anemia may be multifaceted (anemia of inflammation, marrow damage, possibly hemolysis in some cases)
Distemper in dogs	Round or variably shaped, pale blue or pink homogeneous inclusions; variable sizes (< 0.3 to 3 μm); more apparent with Diff-Quik than with Wright staining; also in leukocytes (Plate 4A and B)	Indicates active distemper infection; rare finding wherever distemper is controlled by vaccination
Mycoplasma[b] spp. of cattle	Rings, rods, or cocci on surface of erythrocytes; 0.3–1.0 μm in diameter (Plate 4C)	Immune hemolysis
Mycoplasma haemocanis[c,d]	Typically thin chains of cocci on membrane that may form pleomorphic patterns (violin bow, figure 8, oval, cross); occasionally seen as individual cocci or rods (Plate 4D)	Immune hemolysis
Mycoplasma haemofelis[c]	Typically cocci (individual or in short chains) and small rings or doughnuts (< 1 μm) on erythrocyte surface; stain blue-grey to pale purple (Plate 4E)	Immune hemolysis
"*Candidatus* Mycoplasma haemominutum"[e]	Typically cocci (0.1–0.2 μm) (individual or in short chains)	Immune hemolysis (but has low virulence)
Theileria spp.	Highly pleomorphic piroplasms including cocci, rings, rods, pears, and Maltese crosses (Plate 4F)	Several theories, including immune mechanisms, protease activity, decreased cell pliability, and oxidative damage

[a] Appearance as seen on a Wright-stained blood film unless stated otherwise
[b] Basonym, *Eperythrozoon*
[c] Basonym, *Haemobartonella canis*
[d] A smaller organism ("*Candidatus* Mycoplasma haematoparvum") has also been found in dogs (see the text)
[e] Basonym, *Haemobartonella felis*

Table 3.6. Erythrocyte inclusions other than organisms: identifying features, clinical significance, and associated pathogenic processes

Inclusions	Identifying features[a]	Clinical significance	Associated pathogenic processes
*Basophilic stippling	Fine to coarse, blue to dark purple dots or specks that represent aggregated ribosomes dispersed in an erythrocyte's cytoplasm (Plate 4G)	Regenerative anemia (especially cattle), plumbism	Young cells—persistence of ribosomal RNA; plumbism—inhibition of pyrimidine 5'-nucleotidase
Heinz body	Slightly pale, rounded, protruding structure that creates a membrane defect; may occur as free body; stains blue with NMB stain (Plate 4H and I)	Exposure to oxidants	Oxidants overwhelm reductive capacity of erythrocyte; hemoglobin precipitates and may bind with erythrocyte membrane
Hemoglobin crystals	Intensely stained, crystallized hemoglobin that forms a pencil, parallelogram, cube, or other polyhedron within erythrocytes (Plate 4J)	None in domestic mammals; most frequent in cats (and camelids)	Occurs with hemoglobinopathies in people
*Howell-Jolly body	Usually a homogeneous, dark purple–staining, round structure in erythrocytes; not associated with membrane; can be ring forms (especially in cats) (Plate 4K and L)	Increased erythropoiesis, decreased splenic function	Nuclear remnant that remained free in the cytoplasm after mitosis; persists in erythrocyte if the spleen does not pit it
Siderotic granules	Loose aggregate of fine granular basophilic inclusions; stain blue with Fe stains (Prussian blue) (Plate 5B)	Excess Fe in body; plumbism in dogs; myeloproliferative disease, usually unknown	Fe accumulates in damaged mitochondria or in autophagocytic vacuoles

* A relatively common inclusion (Note: Basophilic stippling is more common in cattle than in dogs and cats, and it is not expected in horses.)

[a] Appearance as seen on a Wright-stained blood film unless stated otherwise

stippling must be differentiated from siderotic granules, which are usually located in clusters.

2. Basophilic stippling is seen with regenerative anemias, especially in cattle, but also in dogs and cats.

3. When seen without corresponding polychromasia or reticulocytosis, or in nonanemic animals, plumbism is a common cause, especially in dogs. Lead inhibits the pyrimidine 5′-nucleotidase that helps degrade nucleotides in RNA.

B. Heinz bodies (Plate 4H and I)

1. *Heinz bodies* are aggregates of denatured Hgb caused by oxidative damage.

2. Heinz bodies are visualized with NMB stain as pale blue, protruding, rounded structures associated with erythrocyte membranes. In Wright-stained films, Heinz bodies have nearly the same staining features as normal Hgb but appear as slightly pale structures that create membrane defects or protrude. Heinz bodies may detach from erythrocytes and occur as free bodies in a blood film.

3. Except in cats, the presence of Heinz bodies in an animal with a hemolytic anemia indicates Heinz body hemolysis. Small single Heinz bodies (diameter ≈ 0.5 μm; see the smallest forms in Plate 4I) can be found in the erythrocytes of cats without clinical anemia or hemolysis.

C. *Hgb crystals* (Plate 4J)

1. These are seen occasionally in domestic mammal erythrocytes (including dogs and cats), but their significance is unknown. Some may form in vitro because of sample storage conditions.

2. Hgb electrophoresis has failed to demonstrate abnormal Hgb molecules in domestic mammals that have had Hgb crystals.

D. Howell-Jolly bodies (Plate 4K and L)

1. A *Howell-Jolly body* is a nuclear remnant that has remained free in the cytoplasm after mitosis of an erythrocyte precursor. The Howell-Jolly body is nuclear material that was not incorporated into a new nucleus.

2. Howell-Jolly bodies can be found in healthy mammals, frequently in cats and occasionally in dogs and horses. The number of Howell-Jolly bodies in blood increases during accelerated erythropoiesis and also may increase in mammals with decreased splenic function (including after splenectomy).

E. Refractile artifacts (Plate 5A)

1. Erythrocyte refractile artifacts are frequently found in stained blood films. Objects are *refractile* when they change from dark to shiny as the focal plane is changed; refractile artifacts are recognized by focusing up and down and assessing for this property. They may appear as crescents or as small to large, irregular shapes within the erythrocytes. Erythrocyte refractile structures in blood films stained with Romanowsky-type stains are always artifacts. The defect that creates the refractile structure develops during the drying or staining of the erythrocytes.

2. When refractile artifacts are in a plane of focus that makes them resemble black structures, they can be confused with erythrocyte inclusions or parasites.

3. Refractile artifacts are different from erythrocyte refractile bodies as described by Schalm.[27] Erythrocyte refractile bodies are Heinz bodies seen on air-dried blood films by using a wet NMB stain under a cover glass. In these preparations, Heinz bodies appear as erythrocyte refractile bodies in erythrocytes; the bodies are dark foci in one focal plane but become refractile when slightly out of focus.

Heinz bodies are not refractile in films stained with a Romanowsky-type stain (e.g., Wright, Wright-Giemsa, or Wright-Leishman).

F. Siderotic granules (Pappenheimer bodies) (Plate 5B)

1. *Siderotic granules* in Wright-stained erythrocytes are basophilic granular structures that represent Fe-laden mitochondria. Siderotic granules may be difficult to differentiate from basophilic stippling on Wright-stained blood films. Siderotic granules tend to occur as loose basophilic aggregates that are often palely stained. Basophilic stippling tends to be dispersed throughout an erythrocyte's cytoplasm, and staining is often more prominent. Confirmation of siderotic granules requires identification of positive-blue staining of granules with a Prussian blue stain.

2. A *siderocyte* is a nonnucleated erythroid cell (reticulocyte or mature erythrocyte) that contains one or more siderotic granules. If the siderotic granules are in a nucleated erythrocyte, the cell is a *sideroblast*; if the granules encircle the nucleus, the cell is a *ringed sideroblast*.

3. A transient siderocytosis has been associated with chloramphenicol therapy in dogs. Siderocytosis and sideroblastosis may be related to Fe overload and also have been reported as features of sideroblastic anemias.[28] An association with hemolytic anemias has been suggested,[29] but, in many cases, siderocytes occur without a known cause.

VI. Abnormal erythrocyte volume

A. Erythrocytes appear two-dimensional on a Wright-stained blood film, and thus a cell's diameter is frequently considered to reflect its size. However, it is important to recognize that two cells with the same diameter, but with different thicknesses, have different volumes. An erythrocyte's thickness is reflected by the cell's staining intensity. A thin cell will be lightly stained (hypochromic), whereas a thick cell will be stained more intensely (hyperchromic).

B. *Anisocytosis* is variation in the volumes of erythrocytes

1. Anisocytosis can be caused by macrocytes, microcytes, or both. Because of their decreased diameters, spherocytes may produce apparent anisocytosis even if the spherocyte volumes are not decreased.

2. Its diagnostic significance depends on the cells that are creating the anisocytosis (see the next sections on macrocytes and microcytes). It is commonly associated with macrocytosis and thus regenerative anemias.

3. *RDW* (see Analytical Principles and Method, sect. II.E.6) is an automated measure of anisocytosis based on volumes, not on the microscopic assessment of cell diameters.

C. A *macrocyte* is an erythrocyte that has increased volume (Plate 5C).

1. *Macrocytosis* is an increased concentration of macrocytes in peripheral blood, which can be reflected by a shift in the erythrocyte cytogram or by an increased MCV. If normocytes or microcytes are also present, there will be anisocytosis and the RDW will be increased.

2. Macrocytosis is frequently seen with accelerated erythropoiesis, because immature erythrocytes are typically larger than mature erythrocytes. Macrocytes may result from a skipped mitosis in disorders of abnormal erythropoiesis.

3. Poodles with hereditary poodle marrow dyscrasia (see Other Nonneoplastic Leukocyte Disorders, sect. II, in Chapter 2) have uniform normochromic macrocytes (MCV: 85–95 fL).

D. A *microcyte* is an erythrocyte that has decreased volume (Plates 5D and E and 6B).

1. *Microcytosis* is an increased concentration of microcytes in peripheral blood, which can be reflected by a decreased MCV. If normocytes or macrocytes are also present, there will be anisocytosis and the RDW will be increased.

2. Causes of microcytosis include Fe deficiency (concurrent hypochromasia is usually seen), hepatic failure in dogs (especially caused by portosystemic shunts), and probably copper deficiency (see Anemia, sects. II.B.6 and 7).

3. As seen with Fe deficiency, microcytes are created by increased erythroid cell divisions that occur because the cellular Hgb concentration is not great enough to inhibit mitosis. A microcyte can have a normal diameter but increased central pallor because of its thinness (a *hypochromic microcyte* and leptocyte).

4. Dogs in some breeds (e.g., Akitas, Shibas, and possibly Jindos, chow-chows, and shar-peis) may have erythrocytes whose MCVs are 50–60 fL, though most breeds have MCVs of 60–77 fL.[30] Young horses (up to 6 mo of age) have lower MCVs than mature horses.[31] Young kittens have lower MCVs than mature cats.[32]

5. Spherocytes may microscopically appear microcytic because of decreased diameters, but their volumes are typically WRI, and MCVs for the sample may be WRI or increased because of a regenerative response.

6. Sideroblastic anemias occurring in association with other diseases in dogs may be microcytic (see Other Erythrocyte Disorders, sect. X).[28]

VII. Abnormal erythrocyte shape (Table 3.7)

A. A *poikilocyte* is any erythrocyte with an abnormal shape, including all the shapes named in this section, as well as shapes for which there are no accepted labels. *Poikilocytosis* is an increased concentration of poikilocytes in blood. The significance of poikilocytosis depends on the type of poikilocyte present, so specific terms should be used whenever possible. Poikilocytes can represent artifacts or pathologic cells.

1. Erythrocytes of neonatal calves (especially if anemic) can have spiculated erythrocytes with features of acanthocytes, echinocytes, or schizocytes. The pathogenesis of the changes is not established but may be related to the presence of a unique Hgb molecule or its interactions with erythrocyte membrane proteins.[33] Fe deficiency may also contribute to the anemia and poikilocytosis.[33,34]

2. Erythrocytes in some ill cats assume an irregular, elongated form that may have a broad appendage (Plate 5F). Although these poikilocytes have not been specifically described or named (often described as some combination of ovalocytes, elliptocytes, acanthocytes, burr cells, and keratocytes), and their pathogenesis(es) is (are) unknown, they have been noted repeatedly in cats that have hepatic disease.

3. There are substantial differences among veterinary laboratory professionals and clinical pathology resources regarding identification, naming, semiquantitation, and interpretation of poikilocytes. The poikilocytes are typically defined by their identifying microscopic features (see Table 3.7).

B. Acanthocyte (spur cell and burr cell) (Plates 5G and 6J)

1. Acanthocytes are most common in dogs. In dogs, acanthocytosis is associated with splenic and hepatic disorders, especially splenic hemangiosarcoma and other infiltrative splenic disorders. Why acanthocytes form in these disorders is not known.

2. Poikilocytes that have the microscopic features of acanthocytes (see Table 3.7) have been seen concurrently with keratocytes and schizocytes in cases of lymphoma,

Table 3.7. Poikilocytes: identifying features, clinical significance, and pathogeneses in domestic mammals

Poikilocyte	Other name	Identifying features	Clinical significance	Pathogenesis
Acanthocyte (*acantho* = "spur")	Spur cell, burr cell[a]	1–20 irregularly spaced, membrane projections of variable lengths; projections may be blunt spurs or clubs (Plate 5G and 6J)	Hemangiosarcoma; occasionally splenic, hepatic, and renal disorders	Unknown in domestic mammals; can form from changes in membrane lipids; possibly fragmentation
*Codocyte (*codo* = "hat")	Target cell, Mexican hat cell	Central focus of Hgb that is surrounded by a ring of pallor that separates it from peripheral Hgb; one form of leptocyte (Plate 5H)	Typical with regenerative anemias; also seen with hepatic, renal, and lipid disorders	Excess membrane relative to Hgb content; may occur with membrane lipid changes
Dacryocyte (*dacyro, dacry* = "tear")	—	Teardrop shaped (Plate 5I and J)	Marrow diseases such as myelofibrosis and neoplasia; also may be an artifact	Unknown except artifacts caused by stretching during film preparation
Eccentrocyte (*eccentro* = "eccentric")	Bite cell, cross-bonded cells, hemighost	Eccentric dense-staining Hgb and adjacent clear space or crescent (Plate 5K)	Overwhelming exposure to oxidants; also rare cases of G6PD or FAD deficiencies	Fusion of membranes damaged by oxidants
*Echinocyte (*echino* = "spiny")	Burr cell[a]	Vary from irregularly shaped cells (type I), to regularly spaced blunt projections (type II), to regularly spaced pointed projections (type III) (Plate 5L)	Hyponatremic dehydration, doxorubricin toxicosis, anionic drugs	Multiple causes (see the text)
	Crenated erythrocyte		Crenated cells are artifacts	Prolonged exposure to alkaline glass while drying

Cell Type	Synonym	Description	Associated Conditions	Pathogenesis
Elliptocyte	(See ovalocyte)	—	—	—
*Keratocyte (*kerato* = "horn")	Helmet cell	Notched, flattened margin between two membrane projections (horns); variant has one horn (Plate 6A)	Vasculitis, intravascular coagulation, hemangiosarcoma, caval syndrome, endocarditis	Unclear: trauma, oxidative injury, and vesiculation have all been proposed
Leptocyte (*lepto* = "thin")	—	Thin cell that appears as a hypochromic cell with increased central pallor (Plate 6B)	Fe deficiency	Incomplete hemoglobin synthesis
Ovalocyte (*ovalo* = "egg")	Elliptocyte	Elliptical or oval cell (Plate 6C)	Protein band 4.1 deficiency in dogs, mutant spectrin in a dog, myelofibrosis, idiopathic in cats, iron deficiency	Abnormal membrane proteins in hereditary form, otherwise unknown
Pincered cell	—	Button or knob joined to rest of cell by a pinched area (Plate 6D)	PK deficiency, intravascular trauma	Unknown
Pyknocyte (*pykno* = "condensed")	Irregularly contracted cell	Spheroid erythrocyte with condensed or contracted Hgb and perhaps small tags of fragmented membrane (Plate 6E and F)	Overwhelming exposure to oxidants; also rare cases of G6PD or FAD deficiencies	Unclear; may form from eccentrocytes

Continues

145

Table 3.7. *continued*

Poikilocyte	Other name	Identifying features	Clinical significance	Pathogenesis
Schizocyte (schizo = "cut")	RBC fragment, schistocyte	Triangular, comma-shaped, small round, or irregularly shaped piece of an erythrocyte (Plate 6G)	Intravascular coagulation, vasculitis, hemangiosarcoma, caval syndrome, endocarditis	Same as keratocyte
Selenocyte (*seleno* = "moon")	—	A damaged erythrocyte that is crescent-shaped and has a large clear space	Associated with hemolytic anemias, fragile erythrocytes	Artifact (See the text)
Spherocyte (sphero = "round")	—	Decreased central pallor, decreased cell diameter, increased Hgb staining intensity, and smooth margins (Plate 6I and J)	Immune hemolysis, fragmentation hemolysis, envenomations, clostridial infections, hereditary band 3 deficiency	Membrane loss due to action of macrophages or trauma or abnormal cytoskeleton
Stomatocyte (*stomato* = "mouth")	—	Elongated (slitlike or mouthlike) area of cytoplasmic pallor (Plate 6K)	Young erythrocytes or hereditary stomatocytosis of dogs	Folding of excess membrane
Torocyte (*toro* = "donut shaped")	—	Punched-out, central clear space that creates a donut-shaped cell (Plate 6L)	None; do not confuse with hypochromia	Artifact

* A relatively common poikilocyte

[a] Classifying cells as burr cells is not recommended because the name is used for acanthocytes and echinocytes.

hemangiosarcoma, cirrhosis, pancreatitis, intravascular coagulopathy, and glomerulo-nephritis. The concurrent finding of acanthocytes, keratocytes, and schizocytes suggests that the acanthocytes may represent another form of poikilocyte formed by intravascular trauma.[35]

3. In people, acanthocytic change is considered the result of abnormal lipid composition (high cholesterol to phospholipid ratio) acquired within an erythrocyte's membrane during circulation. Similar findings have not been described for domestic mammal acanthocytes.

4. Some acanthocytes may be difficult to distinguish from echinocytes.

C. Blister cell (see eccentrocyte and keratocyte in the following sects. H and K)

D. *Burr cell* is common name for many spiculated erythrocytes.
1. Echinocytes, acanthocytes, and other spiculated erythrocytes (those with membrane projections) are called burr cells by different people.
2. Because the term may refer to several types of poikilocytes, its use may lead to confusion and thus its clinical value is limited.

E. Codocyte (target cell or Mexican hat cell) (Plate 5H)
1. A codocyte's shape results from a central bulge in the cell caused by an increased ratio of cell membrane to Hgb content.
2. Codocytosis is commonly seen in regenerative anemias because young erythrocytes have excess membrane and a decreased cellular Hgb concentration. When not associated with a regenerative anemia, codocytosis is seen in hypochromic states (e.g., Fe deficiency) and when erythrocytes have excess membrane (e.g., hepatic, renal, and lipid metabolism disorders).

F. Crenated erythrocytes (see echinocyte in the following sect. I)

G. Dacryocyte (Plate 5I and J)
1. Dacryocytosis is occasionally seen in animals with marrow diseases such as myelofibrosis and neoplasia.
2. Artifactual dacryocytes may form because of erythrocyte stretching during blood film preparation. Artifactual dacryocytes tend to have sharp points, occur in streaks, and tend to point in the same direction because directional forces of the slide preparation create them.
3. Some people use the term dacryocyte for cells that others would call keratocytes (with one horn) or even just poikilocytes.

H. Eccentrocyte (bite cell, cross-bonded cell, or hemighost cell) (Plate 5K)
1. Eccentrocytes form when oxidation leads to a bonding of erythrocyte membranes and results in a collapsed, peripheral, crescent-shaped region of the cell (sometimes called a blister) and the cell's Hgb is displaced eccentrically.
2. The membranes are damaged by some of the same oxidants that cause Heinz body anemias.
3. Eccentrocytes may form when reducing pathways in erythrocytes are defective (e.g., in G6PD-deficient[36] or FAD-deficient[37] horses).
4. If enough erythrocytes in a blood sample are eccentrocytes, the sample's CHCM and MCHC may be increased.

I. Echinocyte (burr cell) (Plate 5L)
1. The number and shape of spicules classify echinocytes: type I (irregular or angular cells lacking distinct spicules), type II (multiple regularly spaced blunt spicules), and type III (multiple regularly spaced sharp projections).[38,39] This classification is similar to stage 1, stage 2, and stage 3 echinocytic changes seen with electron microscopy.[40]

2. Echinocytes are thought to form when the surface area of the outer lipid layer of the cell membrane increases relative to that of the inner lipid layer because of insertion of lipids or amphipathic drugs. They may also form secondary to increases in pH, erythrocyte ATP depletion, damage by phospholipases, and cellular dehydration.

3. Pathologic echinocytosis has been associated with several disorders.
   a. Erythrocyte dehydration (especially with hyponatremia and hypochloremia in horses)[38,41]
   b. Strenuous exercise (in racing horses)[39]
   c. Doxorubicin toxicosis[42]
   d. Reaction to anionic drugs such as phenothiazine[43]
   e. PK deficiency (echinocytes or spheroechinocytes seen in some canine cases)[44,45]
   f. Rattlesnake and coral snake envenomation[46,47]
   g. Hemolytic anemia caused by clostridial infection in a horse[48]

4. Artifactual echinocytes are called *crenated erythrocytes* and may have features of type I, II, or III echinocytes. Clinically, an echinocyte is often considered a crenated erythrocyte until proven otherwise. Crenation occurs after blood is collected and while the blood film is drying: The membrane changes are probably due to the alkalinity of glass.[49] Erythrocytes of some sick animals are more prone to crenation. Crenation may increase with storage (erythrocyte ATP depletion or increased plasma lysolecithin formation).[49]

5. Differentiation of artifactual and pathologic echinocytes can be difficult. These three methods might assist with the challenge:
   a. Make another blood film and use a hair drier or other means to dry the blood quickly.
   b. Examine blood films prepared on plastic slides or coverslips. Crenation is less likely to occur on plastic.
   c. Examine erythrocytes in a wet mount of blood on a slide. If echinocytes are not present, those seen in the stained film can be considered artifacts.

J. Elliptocyte (see ovalocyte in the following sect. M)
   1. Elliptocytosis (ovalocytosis) in domestic mammals can be caused by either acquired or congenital disorders.
   2. *Ovalocytosis* and *elliptocytosis* are typically considered synonyms. Some prefer one term over the other, using ovalocyte for plumper cells and elliptocyte for more elongated or elliptical cells.

K. Keratocyte (helmet cell) (Plate 6A)
   1. Keratocytosis may be caused by trauma to erythrocytes within the vascular system; the same processes may create schizocytes. Other mechanisms may also be involved. Keratocytes and schizocytes are both seen in Fe deficiency when the cells are more fragile and less deformable. Keratocytes have also been reported in feline liver disease,[50] doxorubicin toxicity in cats,[51] and canine myelodysplastic syndrome.[52] Keratocytosis is also described as an in vitro change that occurs in feline blood collected in EDTA, but the mechanism was not provided.[29]
   2. An intermediate form sometimes called a *prekeratocyte* (blister cell) has a cytoplasmic clear space (blister) that may represent a vacuole or a hole through the cell. Others suggest it represents fused membranes. Scanning electron microscopic assessment of these cells has revealed holes, not vacuoles or fused membranes (M.A.S. unpublished observations). The mechanisms by which these cells form are not certain.

3. Some forms of keratocytes, such as those with one horn, have also been classified as budding fragmentation, acanthocytes, or dacryocytes.

L. Leptocyte (Plate 6B)

1. Some codocytes and most hypochromic erythrocytes are leptocytes (see codocytes and hypochromic erythrocytes, in Morphologic Features of Erythrocytes, sects. III.C and VII.E).

2. Some people consider leptocyte a synonym for codocyte or a term for a hypochromic erythrocyte. Codocytes and hypochromic erythrocytes may be leptocytes, but not all leptocytes are codocytes or hypochromic erythrocytes. Also, immature erythrocytes may be hypochromic, based on the CHCM or MCHC (but not microscopically), or codocytic, without being leptocytes.

M. Ovalocyte (elliptocyte) (Plate 6C)

1. Acquired ovalocytosis is seen in dogs with myelofibrosis[53] and in animals with Fe-deficiency anemias (along with other abnormal erythrocyte features).

2. Ovalocytosis has been found in cats with hepatic lipidosis,[50] portosystemic shunts,[54] and doxorubicin toxicity.[51] Ovalocytosis is occasionally seen in blood films of cats with other disorders. Erythrocyte membrane analysis has failed to detect qualitative or quantitative defects (unpublished reports).

3. Two types of canine hereditary ovalocytosis (elliptocytosis) have been reported: one associated with a protein band 4.1 deficiency[55] and one with mutant membrane spectrin.[56] Clinical aspects of these disorders are presented in this chapter (Other Erythrocyte Disorders, sects. VI and VII).

4. Elliptocytes have been subclassified: Type I is nearly circular, type II is oval, and type III is more elongated.[149]

5. Healthy camelid, avian, reptilian, and amphibian species have ovalocytes as the expected erythrocytes. Round discocytes would be poikilocytes in these species.

N. Pincered cell (Plate 6D)

1. Pincered cells have been associated with erythrocyte trauma and PK deficiency in a Cairn terrier (unpublished case report) but is rarely reported.

2. In people, pincered cells have been associated with erythrocyte fragmentation, hereditary spherocytosis,[57] and erythroleukemia.[58]

O. Pyknocyte (irregularly contracted cell) (Plate 6E and F)

1. Pyknocytosis is seen concurrently with eccentrocytosis in dogs and horses and probably will be seen in other animals. Pyknocytes likely form from eccentrocytes, but oxidative damage might cause both directly.

2. Pyknocytes stain more intensely with NMB stain than do discocytes or spherocytes, at least in horses.

3. Via light microscopy, some pyknocytes look like spherocytes. However, these spheroid pyknocytes are usually accompanied by eccentrocytes and pyknocytes with membrane tags, so the pathologic changes can be recognized. Via electron microscopy, pyknocytes had membrane irregularities or tags and were not perfect spheres.[36]

P. Schizocyte (schistocyte or RBC fragment) (Plate 6G)

1. Schizocytosis occurs when rigid structures or rheologic forces traumatize erythrocytes.

2. Pathologic states associated with schizocytosis include intravascular coagulation, vasculitis including glomerulonephritis and hemolytic uremic syndrome, hemangiosarcoma, caval syndrome of dirofilariasis, endocarditis, liver disease, heart failure,

hemophagocytic histiocytic disorders, acquired dyserythropoiesis, and Fe deficiency.[29] Schizocytosis may become prominent after splenectomy.[29]

Q. Selenocyte (selenoid bodies) (Plate 6H)
   1. Selenocytes are not a commonly recognized poikilocyte in domestic mammals but have been found in anemic and nonanemic animals (M.A.S. and S.L.S. observations).
   2. Their formation is described as a two-step process: (1) a hole is formed in the erythrocyte membrane, and (2) the hole becomes much larger while the cell is spreading on the slide, and the remaining erythrocyte appears as a large lightly colored crescent.[49] Erythrocytes in lipemic blood may be more prone to selenocyte formation.[59]

R. Spherocyte (Plate 6I and J)
   1. For domestic mammals, spherocytes are most easily recognized in canine blood films because erythrocytes of most dogs have enough central pallor to contrast clearly with the spherocytes that lack central pallor. With careful evaluation, however, spherocytes can be recognized or suspected in other species. A moderate to marked spherocytosis is typically associated with IMHA.
   2. In IMHA, the spherical shape results from the loss of erythrocyte membrane without a corresponding loss in erythrocyte volume. These cells cannot flatten on a slide, so their diameters are decreased and they appear microcytic, but their volumes are typically not altered appreciably.
   3. Spherocytes are frequently seen in immune hemolytic anemias and may be seen with other fragmentation-induced poikilocytes in fragmentation anemias. Spherocytes created by fragmentation may have decreased volume (*microspherocytes*). They also are reported to occur in PK-deficient dogs,[60] in bee-sting anemias,[61,62] with some snake envenomations, in hereditary band 3 deficiency in Japanese black cattle,[63] and with dyserythropoiesis in English springer spaniels.[64]
   4. Spherocytosis may be falsely detected if one assesses cells too near the feathered edge of a smear where artifactual distortion of erythrocytes makes erythrocytes lack central pallor. Pyknocytes may be falsely considered spherocytes.
   5. Processes that produce spherocytes may also produce spheroid cells that are not perfect spheres and have small amounts of central pallor that cannot be definitively categorized as spherocytes. These may be called *stomatospherocytes*.

S. Stomatocyte (Plate 6K)
   1. Stomatocytes result from folding of excess membrane to form an elongated area of pallor (a slit or stoma) instead of a circular central pallor. Young erythrocytes (polychromatophilic erythrocytes or young macrocytes) frequently are stomatocytes, although this is typically not noted in CBC reports.
   2. Stomatocytosis also can be caused by a hereditary defect in the erythrocyte membrane: hereditary stomatocytosis of Alaskan malamutes with concurrent chondrodysplasia, Drentse patrijshonds with concurrent hypertrophic gastritis,[65] miniature schnauzers (asymptomatic),[66] standard schnauzers (asymptomatic),[67] and a Pomeranian[29] (see Other Erythrocyte Disorders, sect. IV).

T. Torocyte (Plate 6L)
   1. Represents an artifactual shape change
   2. Torocytes should not be confused with hypochromic cells that have marked central pallor. A torocyte has a sharply punched out center and a dense ring of Hgb staining

in its periphery, whereas a hypochromic cell has a paler ring of peripheral Hgb staining that fades into central pallor.

ANEMIA

I. General information
   A. *Anemia* is a decreased [RBC], a decreased blood [Hgb], or a decreased Hct.
   B. A blood's Hct, blood [Hgb], and [RBC] generally change proportionately because they are all assessments of the erythrocyte content of blood. However, they may not be uniformly decreased, because of variations in reference intervals or the presence of abnormal erythrocytes; that is, an abnormal erythrocyte volume or intracellular Hgb concentration.
   C. Anemia is a pathologic state or diagnostic problem rather than a disease. Its major significance is a reduced capacity of blood to transport O_2 to tissues. Anemia develops when there is one or more of the following:
      1. Increased erythrocyte loss due to blood loss
      2. Accelerated erythrocyte destruction (pathologic hemolysis)
      3. Decreased effective erythrocyte production
   D. Clinical signs caused by anemia reflect decreased O_2-carrying capacity and include decreased exercise tolerance, weakness, depression, and rapid respiration (tachypnea).
   E. The major physical examination finding is pale mucous membranes (gingival, conjunctival, or vulvar) due to anemic blood in capillaries. With a marked anemia, blood becomes less viscous and may cause a systolic heart murmur.

II. Classifications of anemias
   There are three common classification systems, each with its advantages and limitations in certain clinical situations.
   A. Classification by marrow responsiveness
      1. This classification system is primarily based on the presence or absence of reticulocytosis in blood, but other blood film and marrow findings may influence the classification.
         a. *Regenerative anemia* is anemia with a concurrent reticulocytosis. Marrow may be responsive prior to a reticulocytosis (preregenerative anemia). Until there is a reticulocytosis (or progressive Hct increases), one cannot be certain that erythropoiesis will be effective and the anemia will be regenerative.
         b. *Nonregenerative anemia* is anemia without a concurrent reticulocytosis.
      2. Reticulocytosis is typically established by finding an increased RC, increased CRP, or increased polychromasia (see Analytical Principles and Methods, sects. III.I and K, and Morphologic Features of Erythrocytes, sect. III.D).
         a. Documenting reticulocytosis is the most reliable, single routine method of establishing accelerated erythropoiesis (except in horses).
         b. In most species, reticulocytosis is expected about 3–4 d after Epo stimulates marrow. Peak production is expected about 7–10 d after stimulation. The reticulocyte response in cats is different.[12,14] In a study with five cats and after a single episode of blood loss, the aggregate reticulocytosis peaked 4 d later and then diminished to pre–blood loss concentration by day 9. The punctate

reticulocytosis peaked 9 d after blood loss and did not return to baseline until after day 21.[12]

c. Animals in each species vary in their ability to produce a reticulocytosis.
   (1) Dogs have a great ability. RC or CRP may increase sixfold to eightfold in response to severe anemia.
   (2) Cats have moderate ability (maybe threefold to fivefold).
   (3) Cattle have mild ability. Increased polychromasia is frequently accompanied by erythrocytes with basophilic stippling.
   (4) Horses very rarely release polychromatophilic erythrocytes from marrow, so attempting to establish peripheral blood reticulocytosis has not been valuable. However, horses with an erythropoietic stimulus may release reticulocytes that are detectable by automated analyzers (e.g., ADVIA 120): RCs were $5-10 \times 10^3/\mu L$ after phlebotomy induced anemia in horses,[10] and the RC was $57 \times 10^3/\mu L$ in a horse with a hemolytic anemia.[48] The presence of macrocytes in equine blood suggests, but does not prove, marrow responsiveness to Epo in most clinical situations. Bone marrow examination may provide evidence for marrow Epo responsiveness in horses. Similarly, early marrow responses may be noted in other species prior to reticulocytosis.

3. The following erythrocyte abnormalities would support a regenerative status, but each may also be found in nonregenerative anemias: macrocytic and/or hypochromic indices, anisocytosis, Howell-Jolly bodies, rubricytosis, codocytosis, or basophilic stippling.

4. Mild to moderate bone marrow erythroid hyperplasia without a reticulocytosis may reflect a pending regenerative anemia, particularly when the erythroid series is left-shifted. Marked erythroid hyperplasia with a moderate to severe anemia and without a reticulocytosis is usually caused by ineffective erythropoiesis. If there is a mild anemia, erythroid hyperplasia could represent the later stages of effective erythropoiesis when there is increased release of mature erythrocytes.

5. A progressively increasing Hct, even in the absence of a reticulocytosis, indicates a responsive marrow and a regenerative anemia. This may occur in horses or in other animals that have mild anemias or that are in the resolving stages of more severe anemias. Once an anemic animal has established erythroid hyperplasia and its anemia improves, the Epo stimulus is reduced; therefore, more erythrocytes will mature in the bone marrow before being released, and a reticulocytosis will diminish or disappear.

6. Regenerative anemia (responsive anemia)
   a. This occurs primarily in response to blood loss or hemolysis. It is rarely associated with erythroid neoplasia in cats. It may occur with resolution of some causes of nonregenerative anemia.
   b. Regenerative status indicates that a bone marrow is regenerating a replacement population of erythrocytes.
   c. Regeneration may be blunted by concurrent conditions associated with nonregenerative anemias

7. Nonregenerative anemia (nonresponsive anemia)
   a. This occurs diseases that directly or indirectly cause defective or reduced erythrocyte production. (During the first few days after hemolysis or blood loss, an anemia will be classified as nonregenerative because the marrow has not had time to produce a reticulocytosis.)

b. A persistent nonregenerative status indicates that bone marrow is not regenerating a replacement population of erythrocytes. A severe, nonregenerative anemia typically reflects severe and prolonged damage to erythroid cell precursors.

c. Findings in bone marrow examinations include erythroid hypoplasia, marrow aplasia, red cell aplasia, myelofibrosis, myelitis, myelophthisis, relatively normal erythroid series (hypoplasia may be too mild to detect), mild to moderate erythroid hyperplasia in early responsive anemias, or marked erythroid hyperplasia with or without maturation arrest in conditions of ineffective erythropoiesis.

d. Most nonregenerative anemias are normocytic normochromic anemias without poikilocytosis or other erythrocyte abnormalities. However, blood may contain the following erythrocyte abnormalities related to the underlying disease process: Howell-Jolly bodies, rubricytosis, codocytosis, basophilic stippling, macrocytes or microcytes, or hypochromic erythrocytes.

B. Classification by erythrocyte indices (morphologic classification)

1. This classification system is based on MCV and MCHC (or CHCM) (Table 3.8). Classification should be further characterized by examining erythrocytes on a Wright-stained blood film. In the original classification system, there was not a category for blood samples with increased MCHC values because such values were considered to be erroneous. However, an increased MCHC or CHCM may be valid and reflect a pathologic state; thus we have added them to the system. (Note: The MCV and MCHC or CHCM values are used mostly to characterize erythrocytes in anemic blood, but abnormal values can also be found when anemia is not present. In such samples, they are frequently related to dyserythropoiesis or in vitro artifacts.)

2. General concepts

a. The Hgb concentration within the cytoplasm of a developing erythrocyte provides negative feedback on both DNA and RNA synthesis. In physiologic conditions, once an optimal cytoplasmic Hgb concentration is reached (near 33–35 g/dL), negative feedback stops DNA synthesis (thus no more mitoses) and RNA synthesis (thus no more Hgb synthesis). However until that optimal concentration is reached, the immature erythroid cells may continue to divide (and thus produce microcytes) or may make more Hgb than usual (i.e., more Hgb is needed to reach the optimal concentration in larger erythrocytes).[3]

b. MCV and MCHC or CHCM suggest the type of erythrocyte that is being produced by the marrow, although postproduction processes can influence the values if severe enough.

(1) Normocytic: Erythroid cell maturation is not defective.

(2) Macrocytic: Young erythrocytes are present or erythrocyte maturation is defective.

(3) Microcytic: Mitoses during erythropoiesis may create smaller cells.

(4) Normochromic: Hgb synthesis is complete.

(5) Hypochromic: Hgb synthesis is incomplete (young erythrocytes or defective synthesis).

(6) Hyperchromic: Erythrocytes were not hyperchromic when produced. Either they lost volume (in vivo or in vitro) or there is an erroneous MCHC.

Table 3.8. Causes of anemias classified by erythrocyte indices (MCV and MCHC or CHCM)

Anemia classification	MCV	MCHC or CHCM	Disorders or conditions that cause the anemia
Normocytic normochromic	WRI	WRI	If persistent, then typically disorders that reduce erythropoiesis; most anemias begin as normocytic normochromic
Macrocytic hypochromic	↑	↓	Regenerative response after blood loss or hemolysis
Macrocytic normochromic	↑	WRI	Regenerative response after blood loss or hemolysis; occasionally due to defective erythropoiesis (FeLV induced, poodle macrocytosis); in vitro changes[a]
Microcytic hypochromic	↓	↓	Fe deficiency, pyridoxine deficiency
Microcytic normochromic	↓	WRI	Fe deficiency, hepatic failure including portosystemic shunts, in vitro changes[a]
Normocytic hypochromic	WRI	↓	Rarely seen, suspect error
Normocytic hyperchromic[b]	WRI	↑	MCHC or CHCM may be factitiously increased or a pathologic state may cause true increases (see the text for explanation)
Macrocytic hyperchromic[b]	↑	↑	
Microcytic hyperchromic[b]	↓	↑	

[a] See the text for the cause of in vitro changes that can produce higher or lower MCV values.

[b] The *hyperchromic* classification was not part of the original morphologic classification system because increased MCHC values were considered to be erroneous. However, the increased MCHC or CHCM rarely may represent a pathologic state (see the text) and thus we have added *hyperchromic* to the system.

Note: Erythrocyte concentrations in juvenile animals typically are lower than in mature animals.

    c. Because MCV and MCHC or CHCM are averages, erythrocyte cytograms or blood film examinations are typically more sensitive methods of detecting macrocytic, microcytic, or hypochromic cells. With either method, it is possible to have a normocytic normochromic anemia with detectable macrocytic, microcytic, or hypochromic populations.

3. Normocytic normochromic anemias

    a. Blood film findings: Erythrocytes are typically uniform but may occasionally have morphologic abnormalities.

    b. Most anemias begin as normocytic normochromic anemias. When marrow releases many larger or smaller erythrocytes with normal or decreased Hgb concentrations, then MCV or MCHC (and CHCM) will change. MCV or MCHC (and CHCM) must be outside of reference intervals before the morphologic classification changes.

    c. Persistent normocytic normochromic anemias are expected to be nonregenerative.

    d. Most anemias in horses are normocytic normochromic because their marrows release few reticulocytes. If sufficient macrocytes are released, the anemia will become macrocytic.

4. Macrocytic hypochromic anemias

    a. Blood film findings: One can expect polychromasia (except in horses), macrocytosis, and anisocytosis. Visual hypochromasia is not expected because reticulocytes are large and contain a normal mass of Hgb (MCH is not decreased); they do not spread thin enough to have an increased central pallor.

    b. Concurrent macrocytosis and hypochromasia support the presence of immature erythrocytes, and thus the anemia is probably due to blood loss or hemolysis.

    c. Dogs (e.g., schnauzers) with stomatocytosis may have macrocytic hypochromic cells.[67]

    d. In automated hematologic instruments, the MCHC is calculated from the measured blood [Hgb] and a Hct that is calculated from a measured MCV and [RBC]. If the [RBC] is accurate and the MCV is falsely increased (see the following sect. 5.c), then the calculated MCHC will be falsely decreased.

5. Macrocytic normochromic anemias

    a. Blood film findings: One can expect polychromasia, macrocytosis, and anisocytosis.

    b. Disorders or conditions

       (1) They are common in regenerative anemias because of blood loss or hemolysis.

       (2) They are sometimes associated with defective erythropoiesis.

          (a) FeLV-infected cats may have defective erythroid maturation that yields megaloblastic cells (Plate 9L) with defective DNA synthesis and thus decreased mitoses; megaloblastic cells mature to macrocytes.

          (b) Folic acid and cobalamin (vitamin B_{12}) deficiencies cause defective nucleic acid metabolism that could cause macrocytosis (possible, but rarely documented). Cattle that graze a cobalt-deficient pasture may have a normocytic or macrocytic anemia due to a cobalamin deficiency.[68] Cobalt is an essential component of cobalamin. Cobalamin deficiency depresses the activity of a methyltransferase that blocks folate metabolism by trapping a methyl group in 5-methyltetrahydrofolate. Thus, in the absence of cobalamin, a functional folate deficiency may exist even though the serum [folate] may be WRI. (5-Methyltetrahydrofolate is detected in folate assays; see the Folate Concentration in Dogs and Cats section in Chapter 15.)

          (c) Poodles with the poodle marrow dyscrasia (see Other Nonneoplastic Leukocyte Disorders, sect. II, in Chapter 2) will have a macrocytosis and may have an anemia due to another pathologic process. The pathogenesis of the macrocytosis is not established.

          (d) Erythroleukemia

          (e) Congenital dyserythropoiesis and progressive alopecia of polled Hereford calves[69]

   c. The MCV may be increased by certain sample or patient conditions.

     (1) Erythrocyte agglutination: An electronic cell counter may detect an aggregate (mostly doublets and triplets) of erythrocytes to be one large erythrocyte; agglutination could be immune-mediated or, in horses, induced by heparin. However, if the electronic cell counter is programmed to exclude particles that are unrealistically large, the agglutinated cells may be ignored.

     (2) Cell swelling during storage before testing: This occurs most frequently with mail-in samples. The MCHC (and CHCM) may be decreased.

     (3) In vivo hyperosmolar states (e.g., hypernatremia) can lead to increased intracellular osmolality. When the blood within the analyzer is diluted by fluid of lower osmolality (approximately isoosmotic with normal plasma), H_2O moves into the cells and causes acute swelling. The MCHC (and CHCM) may be decreased.[21]

     (4) Excess dipotassium-EDTA anticoagulant may cause erythrocyte swelling and decrease the MCHC (CHCM) with the Bayer Technicon instrument when the cells mix with analyzer diluent. Excess tripotassium-EDTA did not have the same effect.[70,71]

6. Microcytic hypochromic anemias

   a. Blood film findings: Expect microcytosis, leptocytosis, codocytosis, hypochromasia, and anisocytosis. Other poikilocytes may include ovalocytes, schizocytes, and folded erythrocytes. Polychromasia may be present but less than expected for the severity of the anemia.

   b. Microcytosis and hypochromasia may be due to defective Hgb synthesis caused by the following:

     (1) Fe deficiency (see Blood Loss Anemias, sect. II.B)

     (2) Copper deficiency in dogs may cause a microcytic hypochromic anemia.[72] However, an experimental Cu deficiency in dogs produced a normocytic normochromic anemia.[73]

     (3) Potentially, vitamin B_6 (pyridoxine) deficiency

   c. Hepatic failure (rarely; more likely microcytic normochromic)

   d. The MCV may be decreased by certain sample or patient conditions (see Table 3.3) and microcytic hyperchromic states (see the following sect. 11).

7. Microcytic normochromic anemias

   a. Blood film findings vary from those seen in microcytic hypochromic anemia to normocytic normochromic anemia.

   b. Causes of microcytosis

     (1) Fe deficiency (early or mild): Prior to causing a microcytic hypochromic anemia, Fe deficiency may produce a microcytic normochromic anemia, but the MCH is decreased.

     (2) Hepatic failure due to hepatic disease or portosystemic shunts: The cause of microcytosis is not known, but data suggest a defect in Fe transport to erythrocyte precursors. MCH is decreased, but the MCHC (CHCM) typically remains WRI.

     (3) Dyserythropoiesis in English springer spaniels[64]

     (4) Some healthy Akitas and Shibas have lower MCV values (in the 50–60 fL range) than do dogs of other breeds. The same may be true of some dogs belonging to other Asian breeds (e.g., Jindos, chow-chows, and shar-peis).

Also, foals and kittens have lower MCV values than do adult animals of the respective species.[31,32]

8. Normocytic hypochromic anemias
   a. These are uncommon. If found, one must consider that the data may be inaccurate or that the reference intervals may be inappropriate.
   b. They can be found when erythrocytes are hypochromic (because of immaturity or Fe deficiency) and the MCV has not changed enough to be outside of reference interval. Examination of blood film may reveal marked anisocytosis, but overall there were not enough macrocytes or microcytes to increase or decrease the MCV.

9. Macrocytic hyperchromic anemias: Typically, the MCHC is falsely increased (see the following sect. 12). Compare to the CHCM, if available.

10. Normocytic hyperchromic anemias: Typically, the MCHC is falsely increased (see the following sect. 12). Compare to the CHCM if it is available.

11. Microcytic hyperchromic anemias
    a. Falsely low MCV and high MCHC (CHCM) may be produced when erythrocytes are in hypoosmolal plasma.[21,74] Erythrocytes adjust in vivo to the hypoosmolal environment caused by hyponatremia and hypochloremia by having decreased cytoplasmic osmolality. When placed in a diluent prior to counting, osmosis results in H_2O leaving the erythrocytes and thus decreasing volume of erythrocytes.
    b. If the MCHC (or CHCM) is falsely increased for other reasons, then potential causes of a pathologic microcytosis should be considered.

12. Increased MCHC or CHCM
    a. In theory, it is not physiologically possible to produce hyperchromic erythrocytes because Hgb synthesis stops in an erythrocyte precursor when an optimal [Hgb] is reached within its cytoplasm.
    b. Most increased MCHCs are falsely increased, and the blood samples' MCH values also are falsely increased. CHCMs are more reliable but can also be falsely increased. Causes of falsely increased MCHC, CHCM, and MCH include the following:
       (1) Pathologic hemoglobinemia: Blood [Hgb] is used to calculate MCHC and MCH, and it would include Hgb from erythrocytes and the Hgb in plasma. The CHCM would not be affected. A more accurate MCHC could be calculated by correcting the blood [Hgb] by using a value for Hgb_{delta}.
       (2) Oxyglobin: The free Hgb from therapeutic use of Hgb-based O_2 carriers causes an overestimation of intracellular Hgb and falsely increases the MCHC. The CHCM is not affected. A more accurate MCHC could be calculated by correcting the blood [Hgb] by using a value for Hgb_{delta}.
       (3) In vitro hemolysis: Blood [Hgb] is used to calculate the MCHC, and it truly represents the blood [Hgb], but the Hct and [RBC] for the sample are falsely decreased and thus the MCHC and MCH are falsely increased.
       (4) Spectral interferences in the blood Hgb assay: Interferences that produce a falsely increased blood [Hgb] include lipid droplets in grossly lipemic samples, pigments in markedly icteric samples, nuclei or intact WBCs in samples with extreme leukocytosis, Heinz bodies (due to incomplete erythrocyte lysis), and precipitates of immunoglobulins (e.g., immuno-

globulin A).[75] This would yield a falsely increased MCHC. The CHCM may also be falsely increased when many Heinz bodies are present because Heinz bodies alter the light-scattering properties of affected erythrocytes.[17]

    (5) As discussed in the preceding section 11, the MCHC and CHCM may be falsely increased because of cell shrinkage related to in vivo hypoosmolal states (e.g., hyponatremia) followed by cell contact with a relatively hyperosmolal diluent in the analyzer.

  c. The ADVIA methods of evaluating erythrocytes can detect whether a MCHC is erroneous or reflects an uncommon hyperchromic state.

    (1) If the MCHC is increased and the CHCM is not, then the MCHC is probably falsely increased because of Hgb in plasma or because of a spectral interference in the blood [Hgb] assay.

    (2) If both the MCHC and CHCM are increased, then there may truly be a hyperchromic state.

  d. Pathologic conditions that can cause true increases in MCHC (and CHCM) are rare.

    (1) Blood with eccentrocytosis and pyknocytosis sometimes has an increased MCHC because oxidative condensation of Hgb and fusion of cell membranes cause a loss of cell volume without a proportionate loss of cell Hgb.[36,76] These cells may also be microcytic.

    (2) Spherocyte populations with increased MCHC and CHCM may potentially form in some spherocytic anemias if the spherocytic process causes loss of cell volume in excess of Hgb. These cells may also be microcytic. Generally, however, spherocytes in domestic species only appear to be hyperchromic and microscopically small because of their thickness, and their MCHCs, CHCMs, and MCVs are WRI.

C. Pathophysiologic classification

  1. It is based on the pathologic mechanism or process that produced the anemia. Multiple pathologic processes may contribute to an anemia.

    a. Blood loss anemias can be acute (hours to days) to chronic (weeks to months).

      (1) In *external blood loss anemias*, erythrocytes are lost from the body or lost into the alimentary or urinary tract.

      (2) In *internal blood loss anemias*, erythrocytes move from the intravascular to the extravascular space (typically into peritoneal or pleural cavities).

    b. Hemolytic anemias

      (1) In *extravascular hemolysis*, there is erythrocyte lysis outside of blood vessels (in macrophages). It does not include hemorrhage.

      (2) In *intravascular hemolysis*, there is erythrocyte lysis within the blood vascular system. It does not include phagocytosis by tissue macrophages while they pass through the sinuses of the spleen, liver, or bone marrow.

    c. Anemias caused by decreased erythrocyte production

      (1) Inflammatory diseases

      (2) Renal disease

      (3) Marrow hypoplasia or aplasia

      (4) Erythroid hypoplasia or ineffective erythropoiesis

  2. The pathophysiologic classification system is frequently used in one of these two ways:

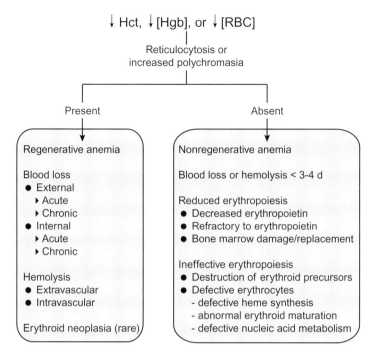

Fig. 3.7. An approach to problem-solving anemias: After anemia has been detected or confirmed, the presence or absence of a regenerative response is determined by assessing RC or CRP or detecting increased polychromasia (see Anemia, sect. II.A). If it is a regenerative anemia, then the anemia is probably due to either blood loss or hemolysis. If the anemia is nonregenerative and has been present for several days, then it is due to reduced or ineffective erythropoiesis.

a. It serves as a differential diagnosis list or to answer questions such as "What are the basic causes of anemias?" (Fig. 3.7)
b. It is used to group specific diseases based on the method or methods by which they cause anemia.

NONREGENERATIVE ANEMIAS

I. General concepts
  A. The major reason for a persistent nonregenerative anemia is decreased erythrocyte production; defective erythropoiesis can also contribute. Since erythrocyte life spans of domestic animals are generally 2–5 mo, an anemia will take several weeks to months to develop if it is caused only by decreased erythropoiesis. For example, a dog's erythrocyte life span is about 100 d. In health, half of its erythrocytes are > 50 d old and half are < 50 d old. If a disease stopped erythropoiesis completely and did not alter erythrocyte life span, it would take 25 d for the dog's Hct to drop from 40 % to 30 %, and about 50 d to drop from 40 % to 20 %. Because cat erythrocytes have shorter life spans (approximately 70 d), such anemias would develop quicker. Likewise, production-failure anemia would develop slower in horses and cattle because their erythrocytes have longer life spans (approximately 150 d).

B. Most diseases do not stop erythrocyte production completely but only decrease the rate of production. Therefore, nonregenerative anemias may take even longer to develop. However, many diseases that reduce erythropoiesis also shorten erythrocyte life span, and thus anemia may develop quicker than expected from reduced erythropoiesis alone.

C. Most animals with nonregenerative anemias have been anemic for several weeks before clinical signs are detected. Because the anemia is chronic, the disease or disorder causing the anemia is chronic. Severity of a nonregenerative anemia will depend on duration of the disease, degree of decreased erythropoiesis, and presence of other processes that shorten erythrocyte life span.

D. When a persistent nonregenerative anemia is detected, most erythrocytes in the animal's blood were produced when the animal had the disease that caused the anemia. Thus, characteristics of the circulating erythrocytes may help determine the cause of the persistent nonregenerative anemia (see Anemia, sect. II.B).

II. Disorders that cause nonregenerative anemias (Table 3.9)
  A. Inflammatory disease
    1. Inflammation causes AID (also called *anemia of chronic disease* and *anemia of chronic inflammation*). It is the most common nonregenerative anemia of domestic mammals and varies from mild to moderate severity. Typically, it is a normocytic normochromic anemia but, rarely, is microcytic.

Table 3.9. Disorders and conditions that cause nonregenerative anemias

Reduced erythropoiesis
  Inflammatory diseases (primarily chronic)
    *Infectious: bacterial, fungal, viral, protozoal, parasitic
    *Noninfectious
  *Renal disease (chronic)
  Diseases causing marrow hypoplasia or aplasia
    Infectious agents: bacterial, fungal, viral, protozoal
    Toxicosis: chemotherapeutic agents, estrogen, bracken fern, phenylbutazone
    Irradiation: whole body or environmental
    Marrow neoplasia or replacement: neoplasia, myelofibrosis, osteopetrosis
  Diseases causing selective erythroid hypoplasia or aplasia
    Pure red cell aplasia (including immune-mediated mechanisms)
    *FeLV-induced erythroid hypoplasia[a]
    *Endocrine: hypothyroidism, hypoadrenocorticism, hypoandrogenism
    *Liver disease or failure (including portosystemic shunts)
Ineffective erythropoiesis
  Nutritional: Fe, copper, cobalt, folate, or vitamin B_{12} deficiency
  Immune-mediated nonregenerative anemia (includes at least some pure red cell aplasias)
  FeLV-induced erythroid neoplasia[a]
  Dyserythropoiesis of English springer spaniels
  Congenital dyserythropoiesis of polled Hereford calves

  * A relatively common disease or condition
  [a] FeLV may cause hypoplasia or ineffective erythropoiesis.
  Note: Blood loss or hemolysis of less than 3–4 d duration must be differentiated from conditions causing nonregenerative anemias (see Fig. 3.7).

2. AID is of relatively little clinical significance after it is recognized. Most diagnostic efforts are directed toward the primary disease and not the secondary abnormalities caused by the inflammatory disease.

3. Almost any chronic disorder with an inflammatory component will initiate the processes that cause the anemia.
   a. Chronic infections: bacterial (including anaplasmal), fungal, viral, and protozoal
   b. Noninfectious disorders: immune, toxic, and neoplastic (usually a malignant neoplasm that causes necrosis and/or inflammation around or within the neoplasm)

4. Pathogenesis of the anemia involves these three concurrent mechanisms initiated by inflammation:[77]
   a. Shortened erythrocyte survival
      (1) Pathologic events are not understood entirely but are associated with increased [IL-1].
      (2) Oxidant damage to erythrocyte membranes and subsequent binding of immunoglobulin molecules may accelerate the removal of erythrocytes.[78]
   b. Impaired Fe mobilization or utilization
      (1) Hepcidin production by hepatocytes is stimulated by IL-6, and the binding of hepcidin to ferroportin in cell membranes internalizes ferroportin. Without membrane ferroportin, the macrophages cannot export Fe.[9]
      (2) Alterations in ferritin production and alterations in transferrin receptors increase Fe storage and therefore decrease the availability of Fe for Hgb synthesis.
      (3) Cytokines involved in altered Fe kinetics include IL-1, IL-6, interferon, and TNF.
   c. Impaired erythrocyte production
      (1) Erythroid cells become refractory (nonresponsive) to increased Epo because of the effects of inflammatory cytokines (IL-1, interferon, and TNF) on precursors.
      (2) Blunted Epo response to anemia (Epo production is increased but not as much as expected) is due to actions of IL-1, TNF, and tumor growth factor β.

5. These laboratory findings support the conclusion that an animal has AID:
   a. Mild to moderate normocytic normochromic anemia with little to no poikilocytosis
   b. Chronic inflammatory leukogram: mature neutrophilia, lymphocytosis, or monocytosis
   c. Hyperproteinemia due to increased concentrations of γ-globulins or positive acute-phase proteins
   d. Marrow that contains essentially normal to mildly reduced erythroid population, mild to moderate granulocytic hyperplasia, possibly plasmacytosis, and abundant hemosiderin (except in feline marrow, where it is not expected)
   e. Hypoferremia, serum [ferritin] WRI to increased, and adequate to increased stainable Fe in tissues (marrow except for cats, spleen, or liver)

B. Renal disease (chronic)
   1. Most patients with chronic renal disease are anemic. The anemias are slight to moderate in severity, and essentially all are normocytic normochromic.
   2. Pathogenesis of anemia

   a. Inadequate Epo production: Chronic renal disease damages the kidneys sufficiently so that Epo production decreases, and thus the stimulation of erythrocyte production is inadequate. (Epo therapy is effective.)

   b. Decreased erythrocyte life span (mild): Substances not cleared by the kidneys may decrease erythrocyte life span.

   c. Decreased marrow response to Epo

   d. Other factors: hemorrhage caused by uremic ulcers or vascular damage; poor nutritional status

 3. Laboratory findings

   a. Normocytic normochromic, nonregenerative anemia

   b. Evidence of chronic renal disease or dysfunction, such as azotemia, urine specific gravity in the isosthenuric range, and electrolyte disturbances

C. Diseases causing marrow hypoplasia or aplasia of multiple cell lineages

 1. Major concepts

   a. Damage can be to one or more of the components of the marrow's microenvironment: blood vessels and/or sinusoids, reticular adventitial cells, marrow stroma (fat cells or fibrocytes), or hematopoietic stem cells. The resulting marrow will be hypoplastic or aplastic.

   b. Damage may be irreversible or reversible and may cause aplastic anemia (hypoplastic pancytopenia).

 2. Disorders

   a. Marrow hypoplasia or aplasia in domestic animals often has an unproven disorder (idiopathic). In people, aplastic anemia is usually immune mediated.

   b. Infectious agents may suppress hematopoiesis through direct hemic cell infection, myelitis, or secondary effects such as immune reactions.

     (1) Suppression may occur with bacterial septicemias, ehrlichiosis, disseminated mycoses (e.g., histoplasmosis), viral infections (e.g., EIAV or FeLV infection), or protozoal infections (e.g., leishmaniasis or cytauxzoonosis)

     (2) Infections with *Cytauxzoon felis* are somewhat unique among these infectious agents because the agent has piroplasms in erythrocytes and schizonts in macrophages.[79] Clinically, cytauxzoonosis is often a rapid and highly fatal disease,[80] but a few cats do survive natural infections.[81]

       (a) When blood erythrocytes contain the piroplasms, cats may or may not be anemic. When present, anemias can range from mild to severe, are nonregenerative, and probably are caused by AID and damage to marrow, spleen, and liver.

       (b) Fever and icterus are common clinical findings. The moderate to marked hyperbilirubinemia and resultant bilirubinuria are primarily caused by hepatic damage and cholestasis. Erythrophages are found in many organs, but hemolysis usually is considered a minor contributor to the anemia.[79]

       (c) Other laboratory findings may include the following: thrombocytopenia, leukopenia (sometimes with toxic changes), large macrophages laden with schizonts in the blood films (rarely), and other hematologic and clinical chemistry abnormalities caused by hepatic, splenic, lymph node, and marrow damage associated with the schizont stage of the parasitic infection.

    c. Toxicoses involving compounds such as chemotherapeutic agents, estrogen,[82,83] phenylbutazone,[84,85] and chemicals in bracken fern (*Pteridium aquilinum*)

    d. Irradiation damage produced by whole body therapeutic or environmental exposure to X-rays, gamma irradiation, or beta irradiation

    e. Marrow replacement

        (1) Diseases may cause anemia and other cytopenias by replacing hematopoietic cells in the marrow. Such anemias are commonly called *myelophthisic anemias.*

        (2) Disorders that may cause myelophthisis (*myelo-* "marrow" plus *-phthisis* "wasting")

            (a) Myeloproliferative diseases: granulocytic, monocytic, erythroid, or megakaryocytic neoplasia

            (b) Lymphoproliferative neoplasia: lymphoid and plasma cell neoplasia

            (c) Metastatic neoplasia

                (i) Lymphoproliferative neoplasia (primary in lymph nodes, spleen, or other tissues)

                (ii) Mast cell neoplasia

                (iii) Carcinomas and nonhemic sarcomas can metastasize to marrow, but such lesions are not expected to cause sufficient marrow damage to produce anemia.

            (d) Nonneoplastic cell proliferation

                (i) Myelofibrosis is fibrous tissue proliferation, usually for unknown reasons. It may occur after inflammation and/or necrosis, with myeloproliferative disease, or with a chronic erythropoietic stimulus.

                (ii) Osteopetrosis: bone proliferation into medullary space

D. Diseases causing selective erythroid hypoplasia or ineffective erythropoiesis (without generalized marrow hypoplasia)

    1. Pure red cell aplasia

        a. *Pure red cell aplasia* is a descriptive term for disorders in which a nonregenerative anemia is caused by marked erythroid hypoplasia or aplasia, but other hematopoietic cell lines are not defective. It has been recognized in dogs,[86] cats, and people.

        b. Pathogenesis of the anemia

            (1) In people, there is often either a viral infection of erythroid cells or an antibody-mediated or T-lymphocyte–mediated destruction of erythroid precursors that has been associated with T-lymphocyte clonal disorders. Antibodies may even be directed against Epo.

            (2) Some dogs have had a demonstrable serum substance (probably antibody) that inhibits erythropoiesis in vitro, but other dogs do not.[87]

        c. The disorder may be responsive to immune-suppressive dosages of glucocorticoid compounds or other immunosuppressive therapy, but therapy may take 2 wk or longer before evidence of response (e.g., reticulocytosis). Some dogs require long-term therapy to prevent recurrence of an anemia.

        d. Laboratory findings

            (1) Typically, they include normocytic normochromic anemia and sometimes spherocytic anemia.

      (2) Nonregenerative anemia

      (3) A Coombs' test might yield a positive result.

      (4) Marrow examination reveals marked hypoplasia or aplasia (absence) of the erythroid cell lineage, with preservation of the other lineages.

2. Immune-mediated nonregenerative anemia[86]

    a. *Immune-mediated nonregenerative anemia* is similar to pure red cell aplasia with the exception that the erythroid series is present in marrow and characterized by either a left shift and maturation arrest or by persistent erythroid hyperplasia concurrent with anemia.

    b. The disorder may respond to immunosuppressive therapy

    c. Laboratory findings

      (1) Typically, they include normocytic normochromic anemia and sometimes spherocytic anemia.

      (2) Nonregenerative anemia, often severe

      (3) A Coombs' test might yield a positive result.

      (4) Marrow examination reveals variations from erythroid hypoplasia with an incomplete left-shifted series (maturation arrest) to erythroid hyperplasia, often with subtle but detectable phagocytosis of intact erythroid precursors at the latest stage of orderly development (Plate 9G). The production of other cell lines is effective.

3. FeLV-induced erythroid hypoplasia

    a. FeLV may selectively damage erythroid cells to cause erythroid hypoplasia or transform a cell into a neoplastic cell line.

    b. Pathogenesis of anemia

      (1) If erythroid precursors are selectively damaged, then erythroid hypoplasia or aplasia develops and thus erythrocyte production decreases.

      (2) If erythroid cells undergo neoplastic transformation, the proliferation of cells may be marked, but their function, cell metabolism, and maturation will be defective. Accordingly, the cells may not mature or they may die before maturing to erythrocytes, and thus anemia develops because of decreased effective erythropoiesis.

    c. Laboratory findings

      (1) There may be mild to severe, nonregenerative anemia; either normocytic normochromic or macrocytic normochromic.

      (2) The anemia may have inappropriate rubricytosis, especially in myelodysplastic syndrome with erythroid predominance (MDS-Er).

      (3) Marrow findings may vary from erythroid hypoplasia to neoplasia of any marrow cell lineage.

      (4) Megaloblastic erythroid cells may be found in blood or marrow (*megaloblastic anemia*) (Plate 9L). Megaloblastic cells have asynchronous maturation of nuclei and cytoplasms: Cytoplasms mature but nuclear maturation is incomplete. The defective maturation produces larger erythroid precursors with atypically large nuclei for the degree of cytoplasmic maturation.

4. Nutrient deficiencies

    a. Fe deficiency

      (1) This occurs because of chronic external blood loss (e.g., alimentary tract blood loss because of ulcers or parasites or cutaneous blood loss because of fleas or ticks) or inadequate dietary Fe intake (especially in neonates).

(2) When diagnosed, the anemia is classically microcytic hypochromic but may be microcytic normochromic (for its pathogenesis, see Blood Loss Anemias, sect. II.B).

b. Copper deficiency

(1) This is uncommon in domestic mammals but has been reported in pigs and in dogs. Erythrocyte abnormalities develop because of defective Fe transport.

(a) Ceruloplasmin (ferroxidase) and hephaestin are related Fe oxidases that contain copper and promote the conversion of Fe^{2+} to Fe^{3+} during Fe^{2+} transport out of macrophages and enterocytes, respectively.

(b) If an animal is deficient in copper, there is less ferric oxidase activity, less Fe^{2+} absorption from the intestine, less release from macrophages, less Fe^{2+} available for heme synthesis, and thus defective Hgb synthesis. Because of the copper deficiency, there is a functional Fe deficiency, and thus a microcytic hypochromic anemia can develop. Serum Fe concentrations should not be decreased.

(2) In an experimental study, copper-deficient dogs developed a normocytic normochromic anemia.[73] The pathogenesis of the anemia was not established.

(3) An iatrogenic copper deficiency was created when trientine hydrochloride was used to treat copper storage disease.[72] A microcytic hypochromic anemia persisted after treatment for an Fe deficiency. The anemia resolved and the erythrocyte indices improved when the therapy for copper storage disease ceased. Interpretation of the case data was complicated by evidence of hepatic dysfunction.

(4) Microcytic hypochromic anemias do develop in copper-deficient pigs.

c. Folate or cobalamin (vitamin B_{12}) deficiency

(1) Folate and cobalamin are required for DNA synthesis, and thus deficiencies might cause abnormal erythrocyte development. Folate and cobalamin deficiencies may cause a macrocytic anemia in people but rarely are such disorders found in domestic mammals.

(2) Cats with experimental folate deficiency had megaloblastic marrow erythroid cells but neither macrocytosis nor anemia.[88] A cat with a congenital cobalamin deficiency had normocytic erythrocytes.[89]

(3) Giant schnauzers with an inherited malabsorption of cobalamin had a cobalamin deficiency and a normocytic nonregenerative anemia. Marrow samples contained megaloblastic erythroid cells, and macrocytes and ovalocytes were found in blood films. Reportedly, an increased MCV was not present because of concurrent microcytosis; an explanation of the microcytosis was not provided.[90] Dysplastic changes in the myeloid cells included hypersegmented neutrophils and giant neutrophils. Methylmalonic aciduria was also present.

(4) A Border collie with inherited malabsorption of cobalamin had a normocytic normochromic anemia.[91]

(5) Cattle that develop a cobalamin deficiency from grazing on cobalt-deficient soil may develop a normocytic normochromic anemia.[92]

d. Pyridoxine (vitamin B_6) deficiency: A dietary pyridoxine deficiency in growing kittens resulted in anemia, but the features and pathogenesis of the anemia were not described.[93]

5. Endocrine disorders
   a. Hypothyroidism
      (1) Seen primarily in dogs, this causes a mild normocytic normochromic anemia.
      (2) Pathogenesis of the anemia: Decreased [total thyroxine] and [total triiodothyronine] result in a decreased metabolic rate and thus a decreased need for O_2 in peripheral tissues. The decreased need for O_2 leads to decreased Epo production and thus less erythrocyte production. A new homeostasis develops in which metabolic needs for O_2 are met by a lower blood [RBC].
      (3) Laboratory findings
         (a) Mild normocytic normochromic, nonregenerative anemia
         (b) Evidence of thyroid dysfunction, such as decreased [total thyroxine], decreased [free thyroxine], and increased [thyroid-stimulating hormone]
   b. Hypoadrenocorticism
      (1) Seen primarily in dogs, this may cause a mild to moderate normocytic normochromic anemia.
      (2) Pathogenesis of the anemia is not established, but glucocorticoids have been reported to stimulate erythropoiesis in vitro, so their absence may be relatively marrow suppressive. Gastrointestinal blood loss may enhance the anemia.
      (3) Laboratory findings
         (a) Mild normocytic normochromic anemia, which may be masked by hemoconcentration caused by hypovolemia
         (b) Evidence of adrenal dysfunction, such as hyponatremia, hyperkalemia, azotemia, hypocortisolemia, lymphocytosis, and eosinophilia
   c. Hyperestrogenism
      (1) Blood [estrogen] may be increased because of excessive production by a neoplasm (e.g., Sertoli cell tumor or granulosa cell tumor) or by the administration of estrogen compounds.
      (2) Besides developing clinical signs of feminization, manifestations of hyperestrogenism in mammals (especially dogs and ferrets) may include a severe nonregenerative anemia as part of the pancytopenia of estrogen toxicosis.
6. Liver disease or insufficiency (including portosystemic shunts)
   a. Mammals with chronic and usually progressive liver disease or portosystemic shunts frequently have mild to moderate anemia. Typically, the anemias are normocytic normochromic, but decreased MCHC values have been reported. When the disease causes hepatic insufficiency in dogs, some will have a microcytic normochromic anemia.
   b. Pathogenesis of anemia
      (1) The normocytic normochromic anemia could be an AID in some cases.
      (2) Other potential mechanisms include defective amino acid and protein synthesis and abnormal lipid metabolism, which affect erythrocyte lipid content and life span.
      (3) In dogs with hepatic insufficiency, the microcytosis is not caused by total body Fe deficiency. However, defective protein synthesis may create a functional Fe deficiency because of defective Fe transport.
   c. Laboratory findings
      (1) Mild to moderate normocytic or microcytic normochromic (or rarely hypochromic) anemia

   (2) Evidence of liver disease (e.g., increased serum hepatic enzyme activities) or hepatic dysfunction (e.g., decreased serum [urea], hypoproteinemia, hypoalbuminemia, increased serum [bile acids], hyperammonemia, or ammonium biurate crystalluria)
7. Dyserythropoiesis in English springer spaniels[64]
   a. This multisystemic disorder is characterized by dyserythropoiesis, polymyopathy with megaesophagus, and varying degrees of cardiomegaly. The clinical findings in the young dogs included regurgitation and decreased muscle mass.
   b. The pathogenesis of the familial disorder is unknown.
   c. Laboratory findings
      (1) Features of peripheral blood included microcytic (MCV near 50 fL) normochromic nonregenerative anemias with rubricytosis, spherocytosis, codocytosis, dacryocytosis, schizocytosis, and "vacuolated erythrocytes."
      (2) Marrow findings indicated ineffective erythropoiesis. The findings included hyperplasia of early erythroid cells, frequent binucleated and mitotic nuclei, and macrophages containing erythroid cells and abundant Fe.
8. Congenital dyserythropoiesis and progressive alopecia of polled Hereford calves[69]
   a. The two major aspects of this syndrome are macrocytic normochromic anemia and cutaneous lesions characterized by a hyperkeratotic dermatitis with dyskeratosis in stratum spinosum and follicular infundibuli.
   b. The pathogenesis of the disorder is unknown but appears to be related to impaired cytokinesis during terminal cells divisions.
   c. Laboratory findings
      (1) Features of peripheral blood included macrocytic (MCV near 54 fL in affected calves and MCV near 41 in unaffected calves) normochromic anemia (Hct near 16 %) and rubricytosis. A mild reticulocytosis was considered inappropriate for the severity of anemia. Hyperferremia was present with normal TIBC.
      (2) Marrow findings included erythroid hyperplasia, multinucleated erythroid cells, irregular chromatin patterns, and slight megalocytosis. There appeared to be a maturation arrest in the late rubricyte stage, but with cytoplasmic staining indicating nearly complete Hgb synthesis in the rubricytes. Nuclear buds were common in the rubricyte nuclei. Hemosiderin was abundant.

BLOOD LOSS ANEMIAS

I. Causes of blood loss
   A. Hemorrhage
      1. Blood vessels damaged by trauma, ulceration, neoplasia, or other means
      2. Acquired or congenital coagulation factor deficiencies or von Willebrand disease
      3. Thrombocytopenia (marked)
   B. Parasitism: hookworms and whipworms (dogs), haemonchosis and ostertagiasis (ruminants), coccidiosis, ticks, bloodsucking lice, and fleas (dogs, cats, and calves)[94]
   C. Removal of blood that is to be used for a transfusion

II. Classifications based on duration and location
   A. Acute blood loss anemia
      1. This occurs when blood is lost from the vessels in a few hours. Anemia results from the dilution of erythrocytes that remain in vessels (Fig. 3.8).

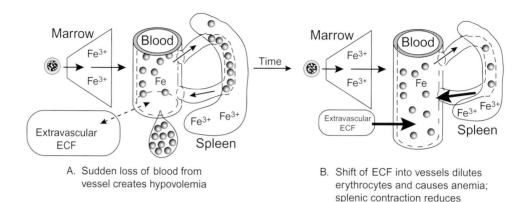

A. Sudden loss of blood from vessel creates hypovolemia

B. Shift of ECF into vessels dilutes erythrocytes and causes anemia; splenic contraction reduces severity of anemia

Fig. 3.8. Erythrocyte kinetics of acute blood loss.
A. Immediately after whole blood is lost, Hct and [total protein] should not change because erythrocytes and plasma are lost proportionately. However, blood volume is decreased.
B. Hypovolemia stimulates thirst to replenish ECF volume and induces movement of ECF from the extravascular space to the intravascular space, thus expanding blood volume. The fluid shift dilutes erythrocytes (and plasma proteins), and thus anemia (and hypoproteinemia) develops. The degree of anemia depends on the quantity and duration of hemorrhage and the time period from the onset of hemorrhage. Splenic contraction will diminish the severity of the anemia because splenic blood is rich in erythrocytes (especially in horses and dogs).

a. The severity of an anemia caused by hemothorax or hemoperitoneum may be diminished by resorption (autotransfusion) of about 65 % of erythrocytes within 2 d and 80 % within 1–2 wk.[95] Also, animals do not become Fe depleted, because erythrocytes are absorbed (autotransfusion) or destroyed and the Fe is reutilized.

b. Sudden anemia creates tissue hypoxia that stimulates Epo production. If marrow is responsive, reticulocytosis should be present 3–4 d after blood loss (except in horses).

2. Clinical data that support a conclusion that an anemia is caused by acute blood loss (major diagnostic features) include the following:

a. Blood loss was observed (historical or physical examination).

(1) Gross external hemorrhage is seen. If there is gastrointestinal hemorrhage, then the feces may be tarry (melena) or occult-blood positive (heme present). If there is urinary tract hemorrhage, there are erythrocytes in the urine sediment or a heme-positive reaction.

(2) Hemothorax or hemoperitoneum

b. Regenerative anemia, if sufficient time for response

c. Hypoproteinemia with a proportionate decrease in [albumin] and [globulin]: Hypoproteinemia caused by intracavitary hemorrhage tends not to be as severe as external hemorrhage because proteins may return to plasma via lymphatic vessels.

B. Chronic blood loss anemia that leads to Fe-deficiency anemia

1. Chronic blood loss occurs when blood is lost from the body (including into the gastrointestinal tract or urinary tract) over several weeks to months. Anemia results from a combination of factors but is primarily the result of Fe deficiency (Fig. 3.9).

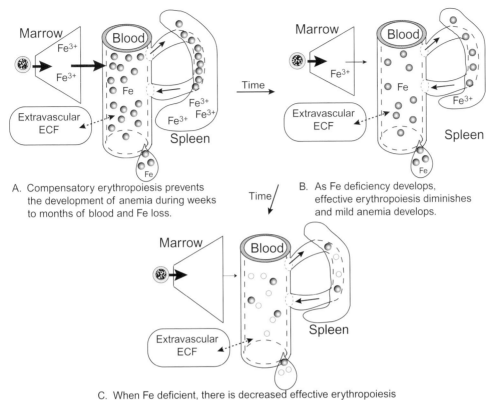

A. Compensatory erythropoiesis prevents
   the development of anemia during weeks
   to months of blood and Fe loss.

B. As Fe deficiency develops,
   effective erythropoiesis diminishes
   and mild anemia develops.

C. When Fe deficient, there is decreased effective erythropoiesis
   and marrow releases microcytic hypochromic erythrocytes.

Fig. 3.9. Erythrocyte kinetics of chronic blood loss that results in Fe deficiency.
A. Initially, there is a continual loss of small quantities of blood over weeks to months. Anemia does not
   develop as long as compensatory increased erythropoiesis (using stored Fe) replaces lost erythrocytes.
B. After prolonged blood loss, Fe deficiency develops (decreased total body Fe). When Fe deficiency is severe
   enough, effective erythropoiesis decreases sufficiently so that the compensation for blood loss is inadequate, and thus anemia ensues. Concurrently, the erythrocyte life span decreases because of increased
   erythrocyte membrane fragility. Fe deficiency affects many organs and is present before anemia occurs.
C. Microcytosis and hypochromasia result from the defective heme synthesis caused by Fe deficiency.
   Hypochromasia develops because the amount of Fe that is available is inadequate for incorporation into
   heme for Hgb formation. While attempting to reach optimal cytoplasmic Hgb concentration, erythroid
   precursors are thought to undergo additional mitoses, so microcytes are formed (microcytic normochromic anemia). With severe Fe depletion, precursors are eventually unable to reach optimal cytoplasmic
   Hgb concentration, and then hypochromic cells are formed (microcytic hypochromic anemia).

    a. Once Fe deficiency is present, maturation and release of erythrocytes are impaired
       such that those being lost cannot be replaced rapidly enough despite erythroid
       hyperplasia. The ongoing blood loss in the presence of Fe deficiency also
       contributes to the anemia, but the amount of blood loss itself typically is not the
       major factor.
    b. During Fe deficiency, the erythrocytes become more fragile and less deformable;[96]
       these changes decrease erythrocyte life span. The reduced deformability was

attributed to increased membrane rigidity, but the reason for the rigidity was not explained.[96] The presence of keratocytes and schizocytes in blood of an Fe-deficient animal is microscopic evidence of this pathologic process.

2. When Fe deficiency develops, reticulocytosis is usually present but less than expected for the degree of anemia (marrow is poorly responsive). Developing erythrocytes may become RNA depleted during the prolonged maturation.[97]

3. Clinical data supporting a conclusion that an anemia is due to chronic external blood loss include the following:

   a. One may find tarry feces (melena), urine or feces may be heme positive, and frank hemorrhage is not observed. If the anemia is caused by parasitism, one may find intestinal nematode ova, fleas, or other parasites.

   b. Poorly regenerative anemia or nonregenerative anemia

   c. Microcytic normochromic to microcytic hypochromic anemia

   d. Decreased CHr and MCVr[98]

   e. Erythroid hyperplasia in marrow but ineffective erythropoiesis because of the maturation defects

   f. Mild to moderate hypoproteinemia

   g. Hypoferremia, decreased total body Fe (depleted storage sites), and decreased serum [ferritin]

   h. A history of frequent blood donations

4. Young animals are more prone to develop Fe-deficiency anemias than are mature animals because young animals store relatively little Fe, consume less Fe while on a milk diet, and require a large amount of Fe during growth.

HEMOLYTIC ANEMIAS

I.   Concepts and classifications

   A. *Hemolysis (erythrolysis)* is erythrocyte necrosis and occurs at the end of every erythrocyte's life. When the rate of in vivo hemolysis increases, then it is a pathologic state. *Pathologic hemolysis* may be defined as an increased rate of erythrocyte destruction that decreases erythrocyte life span.

   B. Extravascular versus intravascular hemolysis

      1. Major differences

         a. Intravascular hemolysis

            (1) Erythrocyte destruction occurs in the blood within blood vessels or heart, not including phagocytosis by tissue macrophages while erythrocytes pass through sinuses of the spleen, liver, or bone marrow.

            (2) Intravascular hemolysis is clinically recognized when it causes hemoglobinemia and hemoglobinuria (or, if measured, decreased serum [haptoglobin]).

         b. Extravascular hemolysis

            (1) Erythrocyte destruction occurs outside of the arterial-capillary-venous system and is unrelated to hemorrhage. It has been called *intracellular hemolysis* because destruction occurs in macrophages near venular sinuses of the spleen, liver, and bone marrow. Splenic macrophages have greatest contact with erythrocytes in the red pulp (except in cats). Macrophages also can attach to erythrocytes within blood by reaching through noncontinuous capillary walls and then binding, engulfing, and lysing them.

            (2) Extravascular hemolysis does not cause hemoglobinemia or hemoglobinuria.

2. Why differentiate intravascular hemolysis from extravascular hemolysis?
   a. Establishing a major site of erythrocyte destruction may be a diagnostic clue; that is, certain diseases typically cause extravascular hemolysis, whereas others typically cause intravascular hemolysis (Table 3.10).
   b. Differentiation may be helpful in determining prognosis and treatment. Intravascular hemolysis usually occurs with life-threatening diseases, so its presence suggests a poorer prognosis, and immediate treatment and management of the case are indicated.

3. Problems with classification system
   a. "Diseases" don't read the book; that is, a disorder may be described as causing extravascular hemolysis, but your case may be the uncommon exception with intravascular hemolysis that was not mentioned.
   b. Diseases may cause anemia by both intravascular and extravascular hemolysis. Extravascular hemolysis typically accompanies intravascular hemolysis.
   c. Disorders may switch from one to another (i.e., an intravascular hemolytic crisis can develop in an animal that has a mild extravascular hemolytic disorder).

4. Major features of the hemolytic disorders are listed in Table 3.11.

C. Thorough examination of erythrocytes in a blood film is an essential diagnostic procedure for suspected or confirmed hemolytic anemias. A well-made and well-stained blood smear and a good microscope with a 100× oil objective are needed for such examinations. One may see organisms or definite clues of a hemolytic process.
   1. Organisms: *Mycoplasma*, *Anaplasma*, *Babesia*, and *Theileria*
   2. Clues of a hemolytic process: spherocytes, Heinz bodies, eccentrocytes, pyknocytes, schizocytes, keratocytes, and acanthocytes

D. Hemolytic icterus (jaundice) (Fig. 3.10)
   1. Pathologic hemolysis leads to increased Hgb degradation, thus increased bilirubin formation, and perhaps development of icterus. Icterus may develop in animals with either intravascular or extravascular hemolytic disorders. In both forms, Hgb degradation increases, but the sites of erythrocyte destruction differ. Icterus may develop in animals with intravascular hemolysis because of concurrent extravascular hemolysis.
   2. Hemolytic hyperbilirubinemia occurs when Bu travels through the blood from tissue macrophages to the liver. Except for uncommon situations, the capacity for Bu uptake greatly exceeds that of bilirubin excretion, so uptake is not rate limiting. If Bu formation exceeds an animal's ability to excrete it into the bile as Bc, hyperbilirubinemia will develop. If the capacity of the liver for Bu uptake, conjugation, and excretion (the rate-limiting step) are not exceeded, serum [bilirubin] may remain WRI even though pathologic hemolysis is present.
   3. The rate-limiting step in bilirubin excretion is the transport of Bc to the biliary system. Once the transport maximum is reached, Bc is "regurgitated" out of hepatocytes and into plasma.
   4. Bu and Bc compete for the same receptors on hepatocytes. Thus, once the excretion system becomes saturated, both forms increase in plasma. Generally, with icterus of hemolytic origin, [Bu] > [Bc]. In longer-standing hemolytic disorders (1 week or longer), the [Bc] may equal or exceed the [Bu], especially if there is liver damage (caused by hypoxia or other insults).

E. Bilirubinuria (bilirubin in urine)
   1. Bc is H_2O soluble and is not protein bound, so it easily passes through the glomerular filtration barrier and is not resorbed (it has a low renal threshold).

Table 3.10. Hemolytic disorders and conditions

Immune hemolytic disorders
  *Idiopathic[a] (includes autoimmune)
   Drug induced[a]
   Vaccine associated
   Alloimmune
     Neonatal isoerythrolysis[a]
     Blood transfusion reactions[a]
Hemolysis induced by bacterial and viral infections[a]
  *_Mycoplasma_ spp.
  *_Anaplasma_ spp.
   Leptospira spp.[b]
   Clostridium spp. causing erythrocyte membrane damage by phospholipases
     Bacillary hemoglobinuria (_Clostridium haemolyticum_ or _C. novyii_)[a]
     Yellow lamb disease (_Clostridium perfringens_, type A)
     Clostridial infections in horses
   EIAV[a,b]
   FeLV[b]
   Hemolysis associated with other infections (e.g., ehrlichial)[b]
Erythrocytic metabolic defects (acquired or inherited)
   Oxidative damage
     Heinz body hemolysis[a]
     Eccentrocytic hemolysis (acquired or inherited)[a]
   Defects in ATP generation
     Pyruvate kinase deficiency
     Phosphofructokinase deficiency[a]
     Hypophosphatemic hemolysis[b]
     L-sorbose intoxication
   Defects in heme synthesis that result in porphyria
     Bovine congenital erythropoietic porphyria
     Feline erythropoietic porphyria
Erythrocyte fragmentation in blood creating schizocytes, keratocytes, or acanthocytes
  *Intravascular coagulation (localized or disseminated)
  *Vasculitis
   Hemangiosarcoma
   Rheologic processes
     Caval syndrome of dirofilariasis
     Cardiac valvular disease
Hemolytic anemia of other or unknown pathogeneses
   Protozoal infections
     Babesia spp.[a,b]
     Theileria spp.[b]
     Trypanosoma spp.[b]
   Heparin-induced hemolysis
   Iatrogenic hypoosmolar hemolysis[a]
   Envenomation (snakes, spiders, insects)
   Hemophagocytic histiocytic sarcoma
   Idiopathic nonspherocytic hemolytic disorders with increased osmotic fragility
   Hereditary nonspherocytic hemolytic anemia of beagles
   Idiopathic hemolytic anemia of Abyssinian and Somali cats
   Hemolytic syndrome in horses with liver disease[a,b]

---

* A relatively common disease or condition

[a] Hemoglobinuria or hemoglobinemia may be present because of marked intravascular hemolysis.

[b] Other mechanisms may also contribute to anemia in these infections.

Table 3.11. Major features of intravascular and extravascular hemolytic disorders

Feature	Clinical intravascular hemolysis[a]	Predominantly extravascular hemolysis[b]
Site of hemolysis	Within blood vessels or heart	Macrophages near blood sinuses of spleen, liver, or marrow
Degree of RBC damage directly caused by the hemolytic agent or process	Marked	Mild to marked
Severity of anemia	Marked or rapidly falling	Mild to marked
Onset of illness	Hours to days	Days to weeks
Reticulocytosis	Usually after initial presentation	Usually at initial presentation
Hemoglobinemia	Yes, but may not be grossly visible	No
Hemoglobinuria	Yes	No
Hyperbilirubinemia	No or yes[c]	Usually at presentation; Bu > Bc
Bilirubinuria	No or yes[c]	Usually at presentation

[a] Clinical intravascular hemolysis is recognized by finding pathologic hemoglobinemia and pathologic hemoglobinuria. In most of these disorders, there will be concurrent extravascular hemolysis.

[b] During these disorders, intravascular hemolysis may be occurring but not severely enough to cause hemoglobinemia or hemoglobinuria.

[c] Soon after the onset of intravascular hemolysis, hyperbilirubinemia and bilirubinuria will probably not be present. With time, increased degradation of Hgb from intravascular hemolysis could contribute to the excess bilirubin formation and thus hyperbilirubinemia or bilirubinuria. Hyperbilirubinemia and bilirubinuria would be more expected when there is concurrent extravascular hemolysis of sufficient duration and severity.

2. Bu is H_2O insoluble and is bound with albumin in plasma, so very little Bu penetrates the glomerular filtration barrier in most animals (reflecting a high renal threshold).
3. Dogs have a very low renal threshold for bilirubin, and thus some bilirubin is present in the urine of healthy dogs. The bilirubin may be Bc because it freely passes through the glomerular filtration barrier. However, many apparently healthy dogs also have a mild albuminuria, and thus the bilirubin detected may be Bu bound to albumin.
4. Bilirubinuria usually occurs before clinical hyperbilirubinemia (icterus) because Bc is excreted in urine as soon as its concentration in blood starts to increase, and clinical icterus is usually not recognized until serum [bilirubin] reach 1.5–2.0 mg/dL. However, bilirubinuria may be missed because of false-negative urine bilirubin results.

F. Urobilinogenuria
1. Renal urobilinogen excretion increases in hemolytic anemias, but urobilinogenuria is not recognized frequently, perhaps because urobilinogen is unstable in urine.

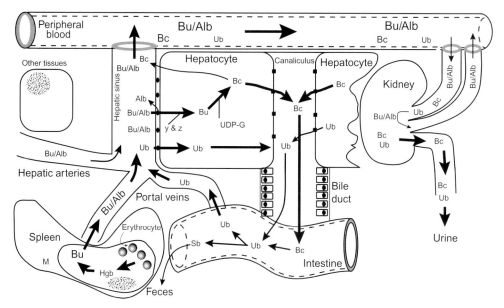

Fig. 3.10. Hemolytic icterus: Accelerated destruction of erythrocytes in macrophages of spleen (also liver and marrow) increases the production and delivery of Bu to the hepatocytes. If the rate of Bu formation exceeds the liver's ability to clear Bu from plasma, hyperbilirubinemia with increased [Bu] develops. Increased delivery of Bu to hepatocytes also increases Bc formation and biliary excretion. If Bc formation exceeds Bc transport to canaliculi, then excess hepatocellular Bc diffuses to sinusoidal plasma. The increased [Bc] in plasma will increase the Bc excretion in urine (bilirubinuria). If there is persistently increased plasma [Bc], there may be increased formation of Bδ (see the Bilirubin Concentration section in Chapter 13). Bu/Alb, Bu associated with albumin; Mφ, macrophage; Sb, stercobilinogen; Ub, urobilinogen; and UDP-G, uridine diphosphoglucoronide.

   2. Urinary urobilinogen excretion increases because all the pathways associated with the excretion of heme degradation products are enhanced.
G. Hemolytic hemoglobinemia and hemoglobinuria (Fig. 3.11)
   1. A key to recognizing intravascular hemolysis is differentiating the pathologic causes of red, brown, or black urine. These are primarily hemoglobinuria, hematuria, and myoglobinuria. These pigmenturias can typically be classified by criteria listed in Table 3.12. Other causes of pigmenturia are described in Physical Examination of Urine, Sect. I.C., in Chapter 8.
   2. Hgb nephropathy is a pathologic state seen in intravascular hemolytic disorders characterized by proximal tubular degeneration that may result in acute renal insufficiency. Hgb casts may be present in renal tubules and/or urine. Evidence suggests that the renal damage is primarily due to altered renal blood flow associated with the erythrocyte stroma and not with the Hgb; the altered renal blood flow might be due to release of vasoactive substances or consumptive coagulation initiated by the erythrocyte stroma.[99] However, a study in rats indicated that stroma-free Hgb could also be toxic to proximal tubular epithelial cells.[100]

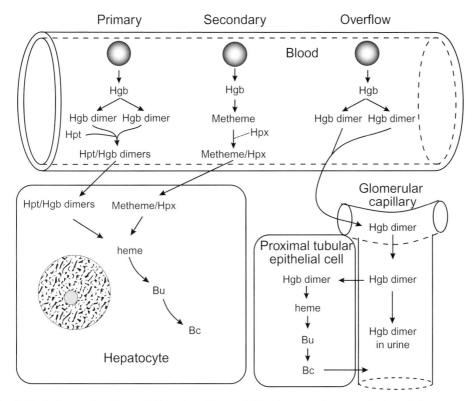

Fig. 3.11. Pathogenesis of hemoglobinemia and hemoglobinuria during intravascular hemolysis.

- The normal physiological processes that conserve Fe released during intravascular hemolysis can be divided into primary and secondary systems. These systems are not saturated during health, and thus hemoglobinemia is not seen in health. In pathologic states, saturation of the primary and secondary systems leads to hemoglobinemia and hemoglobinuria (loss of Hgb and Fe).
- The primary system of Fe conservation (the most important, which may become saturated or overwhelmed)
  - Intravascular erythrocyte damage or death causes release of Hgb to plasma. The unstable Hgb tetramer splits into dimers and immediately binds to Hpt (if available). The Hpt/Hgb dimer complexes are cleared from plasma primarily by hepatocytes,[251] which degrade Hgb dimers to Bu, Fe^{3+}, and amino acids.[252,253] There is evidence that macrophages have a receptor for the Hpt/Hgb complex and thus may also be involved in clearing the complexes from plasma.[254]
  - Plasma [Hgb] or [Hgb/Hpt] may be high enough to cause the plasma to be pink, and thus hemoglobinemia is recognized. Plasma will appear pink when plasma [Hgb] as low as 50 mg/dL.
- The secondary system of Fe conservation (becomes more important after plasma [Hpt] decreases)
  - Continued or more severe intravascular erythrocyte damage or death causes release of more Hgb to plasma. The plasma Hgb may oxidize to form methemoglobin, which dissociates and releases metheme and globin. Metheme binds to Hpx to form a metheme/Hpx complex.[251]
  - Metheme/Hpx complexes enter hepatocytes, where the complexes are degraded to Bu, amino acids, and Fe^{3+}.[251]
  - In people and nonhuman primates, metheme also binds to albumin, and the metheme/albumin complex enters hepatocytes so that Fe can be conserved. However, albumin molecules of dogs, cattle, horses, and other domestic mammals do not bind metheme, and thus this pathway is not functional in those animals.[255]
- Overflow (which occurs when Fe conservation systems are saturated and results in marked hemoglobinemia and concurrent hemoglobinuria)
  - If the rate of hemolysis exceeds the ability of Hgb-binding proteins to conserve Fe, free Hgb dimers accumulate in plasma (hemoglobinemia). The transport maximum of Hpt for Hgb dimers is near 150 mg/dL.
  - Hgb dimers pass through the glomerular filtration barrier and are excreted in the urine (hemoglobinuria). Proximal tubule epithelial cells have some ability to resorb Hgb dimers and degrade them to Bu for conjugation and urinary excretion.

Hpt, haptoglobin; and Hpx, hemopexin.

Table 3.12. Differential features of hematuria, hemoglobinuria, and myoglobinuria

	Hematuria	Hemoglobinuria	Myoglobinuria
Hct	WRI[a]	Decreased	WRI
Plasma color	Not pink to red[b]	Pink to red	Not pink to red
Urine color	Pink to red[c]	Pink to red[c]	Pink to red[c]
Urine heme reaction[c,d]	Positive	Positive	Positive
RBCs in urine sediment	Yes[e]	No[f]	No[f]
Information to support muscle damage[g]	No	No	Yes

[a] Unless there is an associated disorder that causes extensive hemorrhage

[b] Unless there is concurrent in vivo or in vitro hemolysis

[c] Heme typically is red but may become brown to black (with degradation or oxidation) because of metheme formation. Metheme will produce a positive urine heme reaction.

[d] The ammonium sulfate precipitation test does not reliably differentiate Hgb from myoglobin (see Chemical Examination of Urine, sect. VI.B.3, in Chapter 8).

[e] Erythrocytes may lyse after they enter urine (especially in dilute urine) and thus may not be seen in a urine sediment examination.

[f] There could be concurrent hematuria because of another pathologic process or to sample collection.

[g] Information may include historical or physical evidence of muscle damage (e.g., stiffness or trauma) or increased serum creatine kinase activity.

II.   Hemolytic disorders and diseases (Tables 3.10 and 3.13)
    A. Immune hemolytic anemias (not associated with infections)
        1. Concepts
            a. Immune hemolytic anemias occur when an animal's immune system produces antibodies that bind directly or indirectly to its own erythrocytes (ESAIg) and lead to erythrocyte destruction. The process may be initiated by a defective immune system, defective erythrocytes, or adsorbed antigens from drugs, infectious agents, or neoplasms. Factors that initiate the process are usually not known.
            b. Hemolysis may occur through three major processes as described in Fig. 3.12.
            c. Clinical evidence may suggest the presence of intravascular hemolysis, extravascular hemolysis, or both. ESAIg molecules of immune hemolysis may be IgG, IgM, or IgA.[101,102] Extravascular hemolysis occurs when erythrocytes coated with immunoglobulins are engulfed by macrophages. If the immunoglobulins fix complement, the membrane attack complex (C5b-9) may form and cause intravascular hemolysis. This complex consists of complement proteins C5b, C6, C7, C8, and multiple copies of C9, which form a ring in the membrane and enable free diffusion of molecules into and out of the cell. Variations in antibody involvement create variations in clinical manifestations.
            d. Direct antiglobulin tests (Coombs' test or flow cytometric methods) may be used to detect the presence of ESAIg or complement on a patient's erythrocytes (see the section on Methods for Detecting Erythrocyte Surface Antibody or Complement).
            e. To understand some of the clinical manifestations and laboratory findings in immune hemolytic anemias, the major features of warm and cold antibodies need to be understood.

Table 3.13. Recognized hemolytic anemias of dogs, cats, horses, and cattle

Type of anemia	Dogs	Cats	Horses	Cattle
Immune-mediated (not infectious)	IMHA Drug-induced NI Transfusion	IMHA NI Transfusion	IMHA Drug-induced NI Transfusion	IMHA Transfusion
Infectious	*Mycoplasma* *Babesia* *Ehrlichia*	*Mycoplasma* FeLV[a] *Ehrlichia*[a] *Cytauxzoon*[a,b]	*Babesia* *Leptospira*[a] Equine infectious anemia *Ehrlichia*[a] *Clostridium*	*Mycoplasma* *Anaplasma* *Babesia* *Theileria* *Leptospira* *Clostridium* *Trypanosoma*
Metabolic	Heinz body Eccentrocytic PK deficiency PFK deficiency Hypophosphatemia	Heinz body PK deficiency Erythropoietic porphyria	Heinz body Eccentrocytic	Heinz body Hypophosphatemia Congenital erythropoietic porphyria
Traumatic	Angiopathy	Angiopathy	Angiopathy	—
Other	Envenomation Hemophagocytic histiocytic sarcoma Hereditary nonspherocytic	Idiopathic ($\uparrow$ fragility)	Heparin-induced Liver disease	Hypoosmolar

[a] Firm evidence of hemolytic anemia was not found by the authors.

[b] Hemolysis may be a minor contributor to the anemia (see Nonregenerative Anemias, sect. II.C.2).

      (1) Warm antibodies (usually IgG)
        (a) Maximal binding activity at 37–39 °C
        (b) Warm antibodies are more common than cold antibodies. Warm antibodies may bind submaximally to erythrocytes at room temperatures and thus can cause autoagglutination in samples at routine handling temperatures.
      (2) Cold antibodies (usually IgM)
        (a) Maximal binding activity at 4–20 °C
        (b) Cold antibodies may be able to bind in vivo while passing through cool extremities, and thus they can activate complement and initiate immune hemolysis. They typically will cause autoagglutination as erythrocytes cool during or after collection. Not all cold antibodies are pathologic in vivo, even if they cause autoagglutination in vitro.
   2. Disorders
     a. IMHA (also called *idiopathic immune hemolytic anemia* or IIHA)
       (1) IMHA is the most common hemolytic anemia of dogs. It is also occasionally found in cats, horses, and cattle.

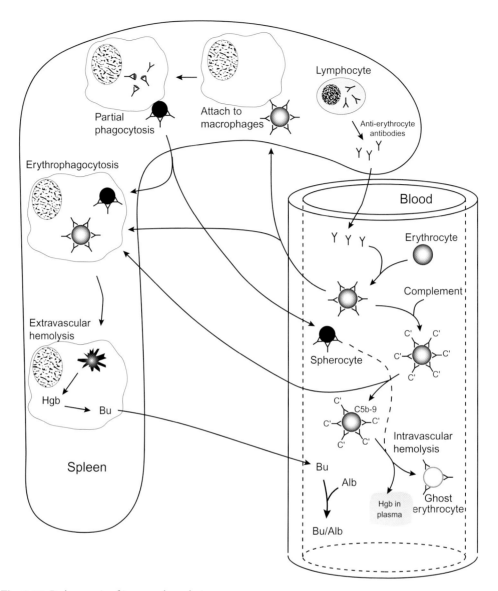

Fig. 3.12. Pathogenesis of immune hemolysis.
- Erythrocytes coated with ESAIg and/or C3 undergo extravascular hemolysis in macrophages.
- Erythrocytes coated with ESAIg and/or C3 are converted to spherocytes by macrophages removing the erythrocyte membrane. Spherocytes undergo either extravascular or intravascular hemolysis because of their rigidity and fragility, respectively.
- Some ESAIg may bind complement (especially IgM), which activates the complement cascade and leads to intravascular hemolysis via the membrane attack complex (C5b-9). Damaged cells will be removed from circulation by macrophages.

ESAIg, erythrocyte surface-associated immunoglobulin; C3, third component of complement; and C5b-9, complex of complement factors 5b through 9.

(2) IMHA is commonly referred to as *autoimmune hemolytic anemia* (AIHA), although the factors that initiated the immune hemolysis are unknown. Typically, it is assumed that the hemolysis is an autoimmune process because known causes of immune hemolysis are not found. However, conditions referred to as IMHA or AIHA have been associated with infections, neoplasia, and vaccinations and may not be autoimmune. Autoimmune cell destruction results from immune responses to normally occurring self epitopes. When the epitopes are from foreign antigens or alloantigens, the body's own cells are destroyed, but the process is not strictly speaking autoimmune in pathogenesis.

(3) Classic laboratory features of IMHA: regenerative anemia (mild to severe), icterus, possibly hemoglobinuria, spherocytosis (difficult to recognize in species other than dogs), positive Coombs' test, positive flow cytometric methods for ESAIg, inflammatory leukogram including neutrophilia with regenerative left shift and monocytosis, and absence of evidence of other immune hemolytic anemias

(4) Exceptions to classic features

  (a) Anemia may be nonregenerative if it lasts < 2–3 d, if antibodies also attack marrow erythrocyte precursors (e.g., pure red cell aplasia), or if another disease process interferes with erythropoiesis.

  (b) Evidence of extravascular hemolysis (icterus, bilirubinuria, etc.) may not be present if the rate of erythrocyte destruction is only slightly increased or if accelerated hemolysis is brief.

  (c) Spherocytosis may not be present because spherocytes may not accumulate in blood if their rate of formation is less than the rate of their removal.

  (d) The results of the Coombs' test may be negative due to a low density of ESAIg or technical problems, including prozone reaction, poor reagents, or poor sample.

(5) Other laboratory or diagnostic features of some IMHA cases: erythrocyte autoagglutination, ghost erythrocytes, thrombocytopenia, and splenomegaly

b. Drug-induced immune hemolytic anemias

(1) Drugs are thought to induce immune hemolysis through these three major mechanisms:[103]

  (a) Drug adsorption: A drug (e.g., penicillin) binds covalently to erythrocyte membranes and stimulates hapten-dependent antibodies. Such antibodies still bind to erythrocytes after the erythrocytes have been exposed to the drug and then washed.

  (b) Autoantibody induction: A drug (e.g., methyldopa and procainamide in people) induces formation of autoantibodies for erythrocyte membrane proteins. Antibodies bind to normal erythrocytes in the absence of drug.

  (c) Drug-dependent antibody induction: A drug (e.g., quinidine in people) induces antibodies that bind to erythrocytes only when soluble drug is present.

(2) Drugs reported to initiate IMHA in domestic mammals include penicillin in horses,[104,105] propylthiouracil in cats,[106] cephalosporins in dogs (supraphar-

macologic doses),[107] trimethoprim-sulfamethoxazole in horses,[108] levamisole in dogs,[109] and pirimicarb in dogs.[110] Many drugs are reported to cause IMHA in people.[111]

c. Vaccine-induced immune hemolytic anemia

(1) Some clinicians have associated the onset of immune-mediated anemia in dogs with recent vaccinations, but little data have been generated to support a cause-and-effect relationship. One retrospective study provided evidence to support the linkage.[112]

(2) An immune-mediated spherocytic anemia was found in a cow after it had been vaccinated with a polyvalent botulism vaccine.[113]

d. Alloimmune hemolysis

(1) NI (neonatal isoerythrolysis, also known as hemolytic disease of the newborn)

(a) In NI, ingested maternal colostral alloantibodies are absorbed by the intestine, enter blood, and then attach to the neonate's paternally derived erythrocyte surface antigens. The antibody-coated erythrocytes are then lysed by macrophages or complement.

(b) In cats, NI occurs when a queen with type B blood passes her anti-A alloantibodies to her type A or type AB kittens via colostrum. Type B erythrocytes are uncommon in American domestic shorthair cats (< 5 %), and the highest incidence is found in British shorthair (41 %), Devon rex (40 %), and Cornish rex (34 %) cats.[114] Anti-B alloantibodies of type A cats typically have weak activity and thus are not associated with NI. Type AB cats do not have alloantibodies.[115]

(c) In horses, NI may occur if a mare is negative for Aa or Qa antigens, she has acquired alloantibodies against such antigens during prior pregnancies or transfusions, and her foal is positive for the Aa or Qa alloantigen (paternally derived). Other alloantigens typically induce too weak an alloantibody response to cause isoerythrolysis,[116] although NI has been associated with several, including the Ab, Qb, Qc, Dg, and Pa alloantigens.[117] In one study involving 799 mares, anti-erythrocyte antibodies were detected via hemolytic or agglutination tests in 20 % of the Standardbred and 10 % of the Thoroughbred mares. However, most of the antibodies were anti-Ca; only 1 % of Thoroughbreds and 2 % of Standardbreds had either anti-Aa or anti-Qa antibodies.[118] Anti-Ca antibodies do not appear to mediate NI.

(d) Mules, from a donkey sire and a horse dam, are more likely than horses to have NI because all horses appear to lack an immunogenic donkey factor.

(e) In dogs, NI may occur if a DEA 1.1-negative bitch develops anti-(DEA 1.1) antibodies after being transfused with DEA 1.1-positive blood. Dogs are not known to have clinically significant naturally occurring alloantibodies to DEA 1.1, and other acquired alloantibodies probably do not cause hemolysis.[115]

(2) IMHA secondary to incompatible blood transfusions

(a) Transfused donor's erythrocytes are attacked by the recipient's (patient's) circulating anti-erythrocyte antibodies. Transfused erythrocytes are recognized as foreign because the donor and recipient have different antigens on their erythrocyte membranes. These are alloantigens causing alloimmune hemolytic anemia.

  (b) The alloantibodies that cause hemolysis are the same as those that cause NI. In dogs and horses, the alloantibodies are acquired antibodies that develop during pregnancy, parturition, or after whole blood transfusions. In cats, the antibodies are natural alloantibodies.

  (c) To reduce the possibility of a hemolytic transfusion reaction, blood typing or crossmatching may be used (see the Blood Typing and Crossmatching section).

  (3) Early attempts to develop a vaccine for bovine anaplasmosis resulted in production of anti-erythrocyte antibodies because of bovine erythrocyte stroma within the vaccine.[119] These antibodies were passed in colostrum and led to NI.[120] Purification of blood-derived vaccines reduced the stroma problem, but the vaccines became unavailable during the 1990s.[119]

  B. Infectious hemolytic anemias

    1. Hemotropic mycoplasma species

      a. Feline hemic *Mycoplasma* spp. (basonym, *Haemobartonella* spp.)[121–123] causing feline infectious anemia

        (1) *Mycoplasma haemofelis*: This organism was originally called the Ohio or Florida strain of *Haemobartonella felis* and is more pathogenic and larger than the other feline hemotropic *Mycoplasma* spp.

        (2) "*Candidatus* Mycoplasma haemominutum": This organism was called the smaller form or California species of *Haemobartonella felis*. It is less pathogenic than the *M. haemofelis*, and typically is considered an opportunist.

        (3) Another hemotropic *Mycoplasma* sp. that resembled the rodent hemotropic mycoplasmal organisms was identified in a cat in Switzerland.[124]

        (4) Parasitemia is usually present during hemolysis, but it may suddenly disappear (within hours). Also, organisms will fall off erythrocytes in vitro and thus it is advisable to examine blood films made from fresh blood.

      b. Canine hemic *Mycoplasma* spp.

        (1) *Mycoplasma haemocanis* (basonym, *Haemobartonella canis*)

          (a) Parasitemia is usually seen in splenectomized and in immunologically compromised dogs.

          (b) Like the feline hemotropic mycoplasmas, *M. haemocanis* may detach from erythrocytes as the sample ages and it is difficult to identify the organisms in plasma.

        (2) "*Candidatus* Mycoplasma haematoparvum"

          (a) This small organism was found in a splenectomized dog.[125]

          (b) Genetic analysis indicates the organism is more closely related to "*Candidatus* Mycoplasma haemominutum" than to *Mycoplasma haemocanis*.[126]

      c. Other hemic *Mycoplasma* spp. (all previously called *Eperythrozoon*)

        (1) *Mycoplasma haemosuis* and *M. parvum* in pigs

        (2) *Mycoplasma Wenyonii* in cattle

        (3) "*Candidatus* M. haemolamae" in llamas and alpacas

      d. Pathogeneses of these hemolytic anemias are thought to involve immune-mediated mechanisms. Antibodies bind to the parasitized erythrocytes either because of bound parasite antigens or antigens exposed on altered membranes.

    e. Major laboratory findings

       (1) These include *Mycoplasma* spp. on erythrocytes in films of fresh blood. Parasites are most numerous when Hct is falling. Organisms may detach from erythrocytes in vitro, so the best chance to detect and identify organisms is in blood films made immediately after blood collection.

       (2) Laboratory findings also include moderate to severe anemia, reticulocytosis and polychromasia, mild to moderate hyperbilirubinemia and bilirubinuria, positive direct Coombs' test, spherocytosis (dogs), autoagglutination, and PCR positivity for *Mycoplasma* spp. Findings may vary when associated with underlying disease.

2. *Anaplasma* spp. (erythrocytic species)

    a. *Anaplasma marginale* (cattle), *A. ovis* (sheep and goats), and *A. centrale* (cattle of South America, Africa, and the Middle East)

    b. *Anaplasma marginale* are most numerous when Hct is falling: 4–5 d later, it is difficult to find organisms. Via light microscopy, the marginal body may appear to protrude from the erythrocyte membrane, but the organism is an intracellular pathogen.

    c. Pathogenesis of anemia is mostly immune mediated. Antibodies bind to erythrocytes damaged by the anaplasmal infection and cause extravascular hemolysis.[127,128]

    d. Major laboratory findings

       (1) Organisms (marginal bodies) found early in disease

       (2) Moderate to severe anemia, reticulocytosis, increased polychromasia, basophilic stippling, mild to marked hyperbilirubinemia and bilirubinuria, and PCR positivity for *Anaplasma* spp.

3. *Leptospira* spp.

    a. *Leptospira interrogans* serovars *pomona* and *icterohemorrhagica* do not infect erythrocytes, but vasculitis and infection of kidneys or liver can lead to a hemolytic state.

    b. *Leptospira* spp. infect most domestic animals and many wild animals,[129] but the hemolytic state is seen primarily in calves, lambs, and pigs.[130,131] Toxins of *Leptospira* spp. are not known to be in vivo hemolysins in dogs and cats.

    c. Pathogenesis of the anemia is not established but may involve an immunologic response associated with an IgM cold agglutinin[132,133] or leptospiral phospholipase activity.[134–137]

    d. Major laboratory findings: moderate to severe anemia, hemoglobinemia and hemoglobinuria, hyperbilirubinemia and bilirubinuria, neutrophilia, leptospiral spirochetes detected in urine or other fluids by direct dark-field microscopic examination, at least a fourfold increase in convalescent titer to either *pomona* or *icterohemorrhagica* serotypes, PCR positivity for *Leptospira* spp., and *Leptospira* not found in blood films.

4. *Clostridium* spp.

    a. *Clostridium haemolyticum* and *C. novyii* type D

       (1) Disease: bacillary hemoglobinuria in cattle and sheep (red water disease and Nevada red water)

       (2) *Clostridium haemolyticum* and *C. novyii* type D are normal inhabitants of soil and may remain dormant in cattle until anaerobic conditions promote their growth. In the United States, bacillary hemoglobinuria is seen primar-

ily in poorly draining areas of Gulf Coast and Western states, and there is a reported association with liver flukes.

(3) Pathogenesis of anemia: Erythrocyte damage is caused primarily by a β-toxin (produced by either *C. haemolyticum* or *C. novyii* type D) that has phospholipase C or lecithinase activity. The β-toxin thus degrades membrane lecithin and causes lysis of erythrocytes. Other relatively minor hemolysins (lipase, proteinase, and another lecithinase) have also been reported as products of *C. haemolyticum*.[138]

(4) Major laboratory findings: acute severe anemia, hemoglobinemia, and hemoglobinuria

(5) Confirmatory diagnostic findings: postmortem lesions, Gram-positive bacilli in tissues (liver and spleen) or fluids (blood and peritoneal fluid), *C. haemolyticum* cultured from liver, and phospholipase C activity (β-toxin) detected in tissues

b. *Clostridium perfringens* type A (*C. welchii*) in ruminants

(1) Disease: yellow lamb disease in calves and lambs (also know as enterotoxemic jaundice or the yellows)

(2) *Clostridium perfringens* type A is part of normal intestinal flora in animals, but multiplication has been associated with highly proteinaceous diets, overfeeding, and starchy foods. In the United States, yellow lamb disease is a lethal disease that occurs in spring nursing lambs in northern California and in Oregon.[139] It also occurs in lambs and calves of other regions (e.g., Canada, Australia, New Zealand, and South Africa).

(3) Pathogenesis of anemia: An α-toxin that has phospholipase C activity and is produced by *C. perfringens* type A causes hydrolysis of membrane phospholipids and thus lysis of erythrocytes, leukocytes, platelets, endothelial cells, and myocytes.[140]

(4) Major laboratory findings

(a) Acute severe cases: anemia, hemoglobinemia, hemoglobinuria, and icterus

(b) Less severe forms: anemia, polychromasia, basophilic stippling, rubricytosis, and leukocytosis

c. *Clostridium perfringens* type A (*C. welchii*) in horses

(1) A horse with a clostridial abscess had a Coombs'-positive anemia with spheroechinocytes and autoagglutination. Retrospectively, other horses with clostridial myositis were also found to be anemic.[48]

(2) The exact relationship between the clostridial infection and the immune-mediated hemolysis has not been established but probably is related to erythrocyte membrane injury.

(3) Acute intravascular spherocytic anemia caused by a *C. perfringens* infection occurs in people.[141]

5. EIAV

a. *EIAV* is a retrovirus that infects cells of the mononuclear phagocytic systems of horses, ponies, donkeys, and mules. The disease is called *equine infectious anemia* (also know as swamp fever, equine malarial fever, mountain fever, and slow fever).

b. Persistent replication of EIAV in macrophages and a horse's response to the infection create the pathologic states that cause clinical disease.[142,143] The clinical disease may be an acute hemolytic state or a chronic debilitating disease caused by the recurrent episodes.

   c. Anemia pathogenesis: both decreased erythrocyte production and hemolysis

      (1) Production decreases because of TNF and other cytokines that inhibit erythroid precursors.

      (2) Hemolysis is due to immune complexes or complement fragments adhered to erythrocytes, which are then destroyed by macrophages.

   d. Major laboratory findings

      (1) Anemia may appear as an acute intravascular hemolytic anemia in acute stages. More commonly, it is a chronic extravascular hemolytic anemia or a chronic normocytic normochromic anemia.

      (2) Other findings: hemoglobinemia (acute), perhaps anisocytosis and macrocytosis, perhaps spherocytosis, thrombocytopenia, neutropenia or neutrophilia, Coombs' test positivity, and Coggins' test positivity

6. FeLV

   a. Most anemias associated with FeLV infections are caused by decreased erythrocyte production.[144] One study provided data suggestive of hemolytic anemia, but most data in the study could have represented ineffective erythropoiesis (erythroid hyperplasia) and dyserythropoiesis (macrocytosis and rubricytosis).[145]

   b. A FeLV infection may predispose a cat to certain infections (e.g., *Mycoplasma* spp.) or be associated with immune hemolytic processes.

7. *Babesia* spp.

   a. The expected number of piroplasms per infected erythrocyte is noted after each species and its host: *B. bigemina*, cattle (1 or 2); *B. caballi*, horse (2 or 4); *B. canis*, dog (1, 2, 4, or 8), *B. gibsoni*, dog (1 or 2). Another small canine *Babesia* has not been named.[146] *Babesia canis* has three recognized subspecies (*B. canis vogeli*, *B. canis canis*, and *B. canis rossi*), and the proposed name for another organism found in cats in Israel is *B. canis presentii*.[147] Other small babesial species also occur in cats (*B. felis* and *B. cati*).[148]

   b. Sizes: *Babesia gibsoni* and other small *Babesia* spp. are < 2 μm, whereas others are 2–4 μm long.

   c. Parasitemia: It may be difficult to find organisms in chronic forms of disease. They are more frequently found in capillary blood ear sticks, toenail clips, or in buffy coat preparations.[149] Babesial organisms can induce erythrocyte surface adhesion molecules that bind to endothelial cells. The binding may concentrate cells in capillary beds and also sequester them away from the animal's mononuclear phagocytic system.[150]

   d. Pathogenesis of anemia appears to involve nonhemolytic and hemolytic mechanisms.[151] Hemolysis may involve proteases produced by the invading parasite, an immune reaction to parasitized cells, and/or oxidative damage to erythrocytes.

   e. Major laboratory findings

      (1) Chronic form: few to rare organisms in blood, mild anemia, mild lymphocytosis (due to chronic antigenic stimulus), seropositivity to *Babesia* spp., and PCR positivity for *Babesia* spp.

      (2) In acute or subacute forms: many piroplasms in blood, moderate to severe anemia, reticulocytosis, increased polychromasia, macrocytosis, hyperbilirubinemia, bilirubinuria, possibly hemoglobinuria, sometimes spherocytosis, and occasionally eccentrocytosis

8. *Theileria* spp.
   a. Erythrocyte piroplasms are intracellular and highly pleomorphic, depending on species and stage of parasitemia. Many forms resemble *Cytauxzoon*, but others resemble small babesial piroplasms.
   b. *Theileria equi* (basonym, *Babesia equi*)[152] infects horses and is endemic in many tropical and subtropical areas. The infected horse may have a subclinical disease or may have pathologic states, including intravascular hemolytic anemia, icterus, hepatomegaly, and splenomegaly.[153]
   c. In the United States (Missouri, Texas, North Carolina, and Michigan), bovine cases of theileriosis have been caused by *T. buffeli*.[154–156] Numerous piroplasms were present in clinically ill cows; piroplasms were rare in subclinical cases. Pathogenesis of the anemia is not established and may include both decreased erythrocyte production and decreased erythrocyte life span (because of either immunologic or oxidative damage). Major laboratory findings are piroplasms in erythrocytes, macrocytosis, polychromasia, basophilic stippling, lymphocytosis, and hyperbilirubinemia and bilirubinuria.
   d. In other countries, many *Theileria* spp. are recognized as causing hemolytic anemias in cattle and other ungulates. Erythrocytic piroplasms are the major pathogenic forms in *T. mutans*, *T. orientalis*, and *T. sergenti*. The major pathogenic stage of *T. parva* is in the intralymphocytic schizont, whereas erythrocytic and lymphocytic forms are considered important for *T. annulata*.[157,158] A *Theileria* sp. was found in Swiss cattle that were concurrently infected with large *Babesia* sp., *Anaplasma marginale*, *Mycoplasma wenyonii*, and *A. phagocytophilum*.[159]
   e. In Spain, 21 dogs were reported to be infected with *B. microti*-like organisms, but analysis of ribosomal RNA from organisms in three dogs indicated that the organisms were *T. annae*.[160] The dogs were anemic and had evidence of a protein-losing glomerulopathy.
   f. PCR testing can be used to differentiate similar organisms.
9. *Trypanosoma* spp. (Plate 8K and L)
   a. These are flagellated protozoa that occur as free-living flagellated trypomastigotes in blood and as amastigotes in pseudocysts or macrophages in other tissues. The pathogenicity of the parasitic species varies, and the host specificity is minimal.[161]
   b. In the United States, *T. theileri* (basonym, *T. americanum*) is found in cattle and typically is not considered a pathogen. There are reports of finding it in Kansas, Wyoming, Oklahoma, Louisiana, Missouri, Illinois, Pennsylvania, and New York. It is also found in other countries.
   c. *Trypanosoma cruzi* infects dogs and cats in South and Central America and in the southern United States of America. Trypomastigotes are found in blood in the acute stages, but most lesions involve amastigotes in nonhemic tissues (heart, brain, and lymph node), and hemolytic anemia is not a feature of the disorder.[162] *Trypanosoma cruzi* causes Chagas disease in people.
   d. Major African trypanosomes of veterinary significance are *T. congolense*, *T. vivax*, *T. brucei*, and *T. simiae*. A subspecies of *T. brucei* causes African sleeping sickness in people.
      (1) In the acute stages of *T. vivax* infections in cattle, the animals may have an acute hemolytic anemia, leukopenia, and thrombocytopenia. Phagocytosis of

hemic precursors and platelets is a prominent finding in marrow, and thus ineffective hematopoiesis contributes to the pancytopenia.[163]

(2) *Trypanosoma congolense* infections in cattle and sheep have resulted in the coating of erythrocytes and leukocytes with trypanosomal antigen-antibody complexes.[164,165]

C. Erythrocytic metabolic defects (acquired or inherited)

   1. Oxidative damage

      a. Heinz body hemolytic anemia

         (1) *Heinz bodies* are foci of denatured Hgb, and their formation appears to involve the following sequence of events in erythrocytes:[166]

            (a) Erythrocytes are exposed to an oxidant that overwhelms the reductive pathways that keep Hgb in a reduced state (Fig. 3.5), and thus erythrocytic Hgb is converted to Hgb-Fe^{3+}.

            (b) Hgb-Fe^{3+} undergoes spontaneous conformational changes to form hemichromes (Hgb-Fe^{3+} with unique binding of Fe to nitrogenous bases of globins) or to form a heme-depleted Hgb.

            (c) Hemichromes or heme-depleted Hgb molecules precipitate and aggregate to form Heinz bodies. Oxidation of sulfhydryl groups and formation of disulfide bonds occur during the precipitation process. The Heinz bodies are frequently associated with the erythrocyte membrane through hydrophobic bonds.

         (2) Many oxidants or substances containing oxidants are reported to cause Heinz body formation in domestic mammals.

            (a) Dogs: acetaminophen, benzocaine, hydrogen peroxide, onions (sodium n-propylthiosulfate, n-propyl disulfide, and other sulfides),[167–169] vitamin K_1 (phytonadione), vitamin K_3 (menadione), naphthalene, phenylhydrazine, possibly zinc,[170] garlic (*Allium sativum*), Chinese chive (*Allium tuberosum*),[171] and possibly skunk spray[172]

            (b) Cats: acetaminophen, benzocaine, methionine, methylene blue (in old urinary antiseptics), onions (*Allium* spp.), phenazopyridine, propofol, and propylene glycol[173]

            (c) Horses: onions, phenothiazine, wilted or dry red maple (*Acer rubrum*) and red maple hybrid leaves (gallic acid and other oxidants),[174] possibly other maple leaves, and garlic (*Allium sativum*)[175]

            (d) Ruminants: *Brassica* spp. (kale and rape), copper, hydrogen peroxide (intravenous), onions, and ryegrass (red maple leaves in alpacas)

         (3) Cats are very susceptible to acetaminophen because they lack a glucuronyl transferase that is used by most animals to conjugate acetaminophen. Without the conjugation, acetaminophen is converted to reactive metabolites that deplete glutathione concentrations and therefore decrease protection from oxidative injury.

         (4) Pathogenesis of the anemia may involve multiple mechanisms[166]

            (a) Erythrocytes containing Heinz bodies are less deformable and are trapped and lysed in the spleen.

            (b) Structural damage caused by oxidation of membrane proteins or binding of Heinz body to erythrocyte membrane leads to fragile cells that may lyse within vessels or sinusoids.

            (c) Binding of hemichromes to band 3 proteins of the erythrocyte membrane causes a redistribution of band 3 proteins and formation of an antigen that is recognized by autologous antibodies. After antibody binding, the defective erythrocyte is removed by splenic or hepatic macrophages.

(5) Major laboratory features: mild to severe anemia, polychromasia and reticulocytosis, Heinz bodies in peripheral blood (NMB or an other vital stain may help confirm the presence of Heinz bodies), eccentrocytosis, hyperbilirubinemia and bilirubinuria, hemoglobinemia and hemoglobinuria in acute severe cases, and perhaps methemoglobinemia (dark or chocolate-colored blood)

(6) Feline Heinz bodies

(a) Clinically healthy, nonanemic cats and cats with nonhemolytic anemias frequently have circulating erythrocytes that contain single small Heinz bodies (diameter ≈ 0.5 μm) that are of little to no clinical significance. Typically, a minority of the erythrocytes contain Heinz bodies. Larger Heinz bodies or multiple Heinz bodies per cell in an anemic cat should alert one to the likelihood of a Heinz body hemolytic anemia.

(b) Feline Heinz bodies were described as erythrocyte refractile (ER) bodies by Schalm.[27] In the NMB-stained blood films (NMB applied to a dried blood film), Heinz bodies were dark-staining structures in one focal plane but became refractile when the focal plane was adjusted. (Do not confuse with refractile artifact on Wright-stained smears.)

(c) Theories that attempt to explain why healthy cats may have circulating Heinz bodies

(i) Feline erythrocytes containing Heinz bodies are probably not removed from the circulation as rapidly as in other species because the cat's spleen has a closed circulation. Therefore, erythrocytes do not flow through the red pulp in which pitting of Heinz bodies is thought to occur in other species.

(ii) Because feline Hgb has more sulfhydryl groups than other species, it may be prone to form more disulfide bridges and thus more denatured Hgb.

(iii) Feline erythrocytes may have less reductive capacity.

(d) Cats that eat semimoist food containing propylene glycol have more Heinz bodies, and their erythrocytes have shorter life spans, but clinically significant anemia is not expected.

(e) Cats with a variety of disorders (e.g., diabetes mellitus, hyperthyroidism, and lymphoma) may have increased percentages of erythrocytes containing Heinz bodies.

(f) Diagnosis of Heinz body hemolytic anemia in cats requires finding a regenerative anemia, evidence of hemolysis (usually hyperbilirubinemia or bilirubinuria), and demonstration of Heinz bodies in erythrocytes. Known exposure to an oxidant is very helpful.

b. Eccentrocytic hemolytic anemias (acquired or inherited)

(1) Pathogenesis of the anemia probably involves multiple mechanisms

(a) Eccentrocytes are more rigid and thus less able to pass through splenic sinusoids, where they are trapped and removed by macrophages.

(b) Eccentrocytes may be more fragile because of the damaged membrane or cytoskeleton and thus may spontaneously rupture in blood.

(2) Acquired states

(a) Oxidative damage to erythrocytes may cause formation of eccentrocytes, Heinz bodies, or both (for recognized oxidants, see Hemolytic Disorders and Diseases, sect. C.1.a).

(b) Factors that determine the outcome of oxidative damage are not understood. Oxidants reported to cause Heinz bodies in one animal may cause eccentrocytosis or methemoglobinemia in another.

(3) G6PD deficiency

(a) This X-linked defect is common in people and was found in one American saddlebred colt.[36] The nonsense mutation occurred in the colt's dam[176] and is not a breed problem because none of the colt's male siblings lived to produce progeny. One dog was reported to have erythrocytes with decreased G6PD activity (44 % of normal), but the dog did not have a clinical disorder related to the defect.[177]

(b) Pathogenesis of anemia: G6PD is the rate-controlling enzyme for the hexose monophosphate shunt from which NADPH is produced (Fig. 3.5). NADPH is a potent reducing agent that keeps GSH, and indirectly other substances, in a reduced state. With reduced G6PD activity, erythrocytes cannot repair damage caused by spontaneous oxidation; thus, the cells are prone to eccentrocyte and pyknocyte formation and reduced life spans.

(c) Major laboratory findings in horses: persistent macrocytic normochromic anemia (Hct near 20 %), eccentrocytosis and pyknocytosis, macrocytosis, and persistent icterus (primarily increased [Bu])

(d) Confirmatory diagnostic findings: greatly reduced erythrocyte G6PD activity, decreased erythrocyte [GSH] and [NADPH], and increased blood [$Hgb\text{-}Fe^{3+}$]

(4) Erythrocyte FAD deficiency

(a) A defective biochemical pathway in the erythrocytes of a Spanish mustang mare created a FAD deficiency.[37] The FAD deficiency led to deficient activity of Cb_5R and GR, enzymes that contain FAD (Fig. 3.5). Hereditary aspects of the defect were not determined.

(b) Major laboratory findings in horses: eccentrocytosis, pyknocytosis, Hgb crystals, and methemoglobinemia

2. Defects in ATP generation

a. PK deficiency

(1) *PK deficiency* is a hereditary disorder in people, several breeds of dogs (basenjis, beagles, cairn terriers, West Highland white terriers, American Eskimo dogs, and dachshunds)[60,178–180] and Abyssinian and Somali cats.[181–183] The clinical illness typically is seen in dogs in the first few weeks to months of age, but less severe deficiencies can be found in older dogs.

(2) Pathogenesis of anemia: Normal erythrocytes have R-type PK isoenzyme (R-PK) (R for RBC) that normally catalyzes the last ATP generation step of anaerobic glycolysis (Fig. 3.5). Without R-PK activity, erythrocytes become ATP deficient, erythrocyte membranes become defective, and hemolysis occurs. In this disorder, young erythrocytes have a little R-PK, the R-PK content decreases as the cell ages, and erythrocytes have a greatly decreased life span.

(3) Major laboratory findings include moderate anemia, moderate to extreme reticulocytosis (RP = 40–60 %), and mild to moderate icterus. Spheroechinocytes are reported to occur but are uncommon in canine cases. Pancytopenia may develop in later stages if myelofibrosis develops.

(4) Confirmatory diagnostic findings include decreased erythrocyte R-PK activity. Total erythrocyte PK activity may be increased because of increased heat-labile, M_2-type PK isoenzyme (M2-PK) (M for muscle). PCR testing can confirm some PK deficiencies.[184]

b. PFK deficiency

(1) This was first recognized in English springer spaniels with erythrocyte PFK activity near 10 % of healthy dogs.[185,186] Other cells in these dogs (e.g., muscle fibers) were also deficient in PFK. It was more recently recognized in American cocker spaniels[187] and mixed-breed dogs (which may have had spaniel parentage).

(2) Pathogenesis of anemia: PFK is a rate-controlling enzyme of glycolysis (Fig. 3.5). A deficiency in PFK results in less downstream formation of ATP and 2,3-DPG, the major impermeable anion in erythrocytes.

(a) Decreased ATP impairs erythrocyte functions and contributes to premature destruction. Studies of PFK-deficient human erythrocytes suggest they have a defective Ca^{2+} pump that needs ATP to function, and thus erythrocytes accumulate Ca^{2+} and become less deformable.[188] However, mechanisms that link the Ca^{2+}-transport defect with the alkaline-induced hemolysis and increased erythrocyte $[Cl^-]$ were not found.

(b) Decreased 2,3-DPG results in greater intracellular $[Cl^-]$, greater pH, and enhanced alkaline fragility (normal canine erythrocytes are generally sensitive to alkalinity). The low 2,3-DPG decreases O_2 delivery to tissues such that Epo production is increased. This results in a compensated regenerative state. When hyperventilation occurs because of excitement or exercise, blood P_aCO_2 decreases and alkalemia may lead to a hemolytic crisis.

(3) The major laboratory findings are anemia, hemoglobinemia, and hemoglobinuria after hyperventilation (producing respiratory alkalosis), and hemolytic icterus. When not in an active intravascular hemolytic state, dogs have mild regenerative anemias or reticulocytoses without anemias (compensated hemolysis).

(4) Confirmatory findings: PFK-deficient erythrocytes, decreased erythrocyte [2,3-DPG], and increased $[Cl^-]$. PCR testing can confirm PFK deficiencies.

c. Hypophosphatemic hemolysis

(1) Postparturient hemoglobinuria in cattle[189]

(a) Occurs 3–8 wk after calving

(b) Pathogenesis of anemia: Defective mobilization of phosphorus from bone and increased phosphorus loss via milk cause a pronounced hypophosphatemia. Without plasma phosphorus, the ATP production by erythrocytes is defective, which results in ATP deficiency, unstable erythrocyte membranes, and hemolysis.

(c) Major laboratory findings: hypophosphatemia, hemoglobinemia, hemoglobinuria, and moderate to marked anemia

(2) There are sporadic reports of concurrent hypophosphatemia and severe hemolysis in horses, dogs, and cats.[190,191] Severe hypophosphatemia may decrease erythrocyte ATP production and thus produce unstable erythrocyte membranes and hemolysis. In dogs, a low [2,3-DPG] may also play a role by making cells more susceptible to alkaline-associated hemolysis.[4]

(3) Bilirubin interference can cause artifactual hypophosphatemia with some assay methods, so one must be careful about interpreting the concurrent presence of hypophosphatemia and hemolytic anemia.

(4) Hyperinsulinism (primary or secondary to hyperglycemia) may cause hypophosphatemia by promoting movement of glucose and phosphate into cells other than erythrocytes. (Glucose transport into erythrocytes is not insulin dependent.) Persistent hypophosphatemia may deplete erythrocyte phosphate, decrease ATP production, and cause hemolysis.

d. L-sorbose intoxication[192,193]

(1) Dogs that have low-K^+ erythrocytes (most breeds) develop a hemolytic anemia after ingestion of L-sorbose, a sugar substitute. Dogs with high-K^+ erythrocytes (e.g., some Japanese Akitas and Japanese Shibas) and human erythrocytes are resistant to the effects of L-sorbose.

(2) Evidence indicates that the hemolysis is due to ATP depletion that results from the strong inhibition of hexokinase by sorbose-1-phosphate in dogs with low-K^+ erythrocytes. Sorbose-1-phosphate is also formed within high-K^+ erythrocytes but has less effect on their hexokinase.[193]

3. Defects in heme synthesis that cause porphyria

a. *Porphyrias* are a group of hereditary and acquired disorders in which porphyrins accumulate in cells and body fluids because of deficient enzyme activity in the heme synthetic pathway (Fig. 3.2). Collectively, porphobilinogen through protoporphyrin IX are called *porphyrins*. Some authors define porphyria as an inherited disorder and porphyrinuria as an acquired disorder.[194]

(1) Some forms of porphyria produce a hemolytic anemia, but others do not. The accumulation of certain porphyrins in erythrocytes reduces erythrocyte life span and thus causes a hemolytic anemia. The mechanism of erythrocyte destruction is not firmly established but may relate to porphyrin-induced damage of membrane lipids or photolysis when erythrocytes are near the skin surface.[195,196] When certain porphyrins absorb ultraviolet light, excitation of the molecule leads to oxidative damage to cells. Another common manifestation of oxidant damage is the dermatitis of photosensitivity.

(2) Congenital (hereditary) porphyrias can be classified as either erythropoietic or hepatic depending on the major expression of the enzymatic defect in heme synthesis.[195,196]

(3) The acquired (secondary) hepatic porphyrias are more common; for example, cattle and horses may develop porphyria and the resulting photosensitization when severe liver disease decreases excretion of phylloerythrin (a porphyrin derived from the breakdown of chlorophyll).

b. Congenital erythropoietic porphyria

(1) Bovine congenital erythropoietic porphyria

(a) The homozygous calves with this autosomal recessive disorder have reddish brown discoloration of teeth and bones, photosensitivity, and anemia of varying severity. The disorder is found primarily in Holsteins, but also in shorthorn and Jamaican cattle.[195]

   (b) The porphyria is caused by a hereditary deficiency of uroporphyrinogen III cosynthase, an enzyme that catalyzes one of the first porphyrin reactions shown in Fig. 3.2.

   (2) Feline erythropoietic porphyria

   (a) Erythropoietic porphyria was diagnosed in a female Siamese cat and two male offspring. The cats had photosensitivity, hemolytic anemia, and renal disease.[197]

   (b) The specific enzymatic defect was not established in the cats.

   c. Other hereditary erythropoietic porphyrias have been diagnosed in cattle, pigs, and cats; however, anemia was not reported as a feature of these forms.[195,198,199] Lead poisoning creates an acquired porphyria because lead inhibits enzymes in the heme synthetic pathway. Anemia may be present in plumbism but is not considered a hemolytic anemia caused by the porphyrin accumulation.

4. Hypoosmolar hemolysis

   a. Rapid infusion of hypotonic fluid intravenously (such as sterile H_2O) or the ingestion of large quantities of water by calves (water intoxication) can cause rapid intravascular hemolysis.

   b. Pathogenesis of the anemia: Infusion of a hypotonic solution or absorption of large quantities of water creates hypoosmolar plasma. Rapid movement of H_2O into erythrocytes via osmosis causes erythrocyte swelling and lysis.

   c. The major laboratory findings are anemia, hemoglobinemia, and hemoglobinuria, the severities of which depend on the severity of the hypoosmolar state.

D. Erythrocyte fragmentation in blood creating schizocytes, keratocytes, or acanthocytes

   1. Erythrocyte damage is thought to be due to trauma caused by relatively rigid structures (fibrin) or by rheologic forces (see Table 3.10 for disorders), but other factors may be involved.

   2. Pathogeneses of anemia: Because the erythrocyte trauma is a consequence of other pathologic states, processes that cause the anemia may be multifaceted.

   a. Erythrocyte trauma either directly causes lysis or creates poikilocytes that have a shortened life span. Acanthocytes may form in the circulation because of membrane lipid changes rather than mechanical or rheologic forces, but these forces may contribute to the accelerated fragmentation of acanthocytes (budding fragmentation).

   b. Primary diseases are frequently infectious or noninfectious inflammatory disorders, and thus the inflammatory state may be producing anemia (see Nonregenerative Anemias, sect. II.A).

   3. Major laboratory findings may include mild to moderate anemia with no reticulocytosis or moderate reticulocytosis and polychromasia, schizocytosis, keratocytosis, acanthocytosis, and thrombocytopenia. There may be other evidence of a consumptive coagulopathy. There may be evidence of renal failure with hemolytic uremic syndrome.

E. Hemolytic disorders of other or unknown pathogeneses

   1. Heparin-induced hemolysis

   a. Heparin anticoagulant therapy in some horses can cause erythrocyte agglutination, mild to moderate anemia, and increased biliary bilirubin excretion that reflects increased Hgb degradation.

(1) Pathogenesis of the decreased Hct is not established but probably involves hemolysis. In vivo erythrocyte agglutination appears to trap and destroy erythrocytes.[200]

(2) When determined by Coulter cell counters, in vitro erythrocyte agglutination can cause an erroneously low [RBC] and erroneously high MCV because a group of agglutinated cells is considered one large cell (a particle). Therefore, the falsely decreased measured [RBC] can produce a falsely low calculated Hct. The effects of heparin can be inhibited and reversed in vitro by trypsin administration.[201]

(3) When analyzed by the CELL-DYN, the group of agglutinated cells is also recognized as one "large cell" during impedance counting. However, volumes of the "large cells" that are outside the expected distribution curve are excluded from the data used for determination of the MCV. Thus, the derived MCV may be nearly correct but the [RBC] will be falsely decreased because many cells were not counted. Accordingly, the calculated Hct will be falsely decreased, and the MCHC and MCH will be falsely increased.

b. Major laboratory findings: In experimental studies, spun Hct (microhematocrit) decreased from near 30 % to near 20 % within 6–8 h after heparin treatment and then returned to baseline percentages by day 5. Bilirubin concentrations increased from near 0.6 mg/dL to 1.4 mg/dL within 24 h of heparin treatment.[200]

2. Envenomation

a. Venoms from some animals (e.g., snakes, spiders, and insects) cause hemolysis. Mechanisms include complement activation with subsequent destruction (e.g., cobra venom factor) and direct hemolysis from hemolysins (including phospholipase A_2 in rattlesnake venom).[46]

b. Spherocytic hemolytic anemias may occur after bee stings. The hemolysis may be due to hemolysins present in the venom: phospholipase A_2 and melittin. The spherocytosis may be related to altered membrane structure or antibody-mediated changes.[61,62]

3. Histiocytic neoplasia: When anemia accompanies hemophagocytic histiocytic sarcoma (*malignant histiocytosis*), extravascular hemolysis by neoplastic cells is one contributing factor to an animal's anemia.

4. Idiopathic nonspherocytic hemolytic disorders with increased osmotic fragility

a. Hereditary nonspherocytic hemolytic anemia in beagles

(1) Affected beagles had mild chronic anemia (Hct values of 30–39 %), persistent reticulocytosis, splenomegaly, erythroid hyperplasia in marrow samples, shortened erythrocyte life spans, and increased erythrocyte osmotic fragility.[202,203]

(2) Studies suggest that the defect is an autosomal recessive trait, but the specific defect has not been established.

b. Idiopathic hemolytic anemia in Abyssinian and Somali cats[204]

(1) A total of 18 cats (13 Abyssinian and 5 Somali, male and female) had macrocytic, regenerative anemias (Hct values of 5–25 %), splenomegaly, and increased erythrocyte osmotic fragility.

(2) Studies suggest that the defect is an autosomal recessive trait, but the specific defect has not been established.

5. Hemolytic syndrome in horses with liver disease[205]
   a. Nine horses with evidence of hepatic or hepatobiliary disease had intravascular hemolytic anemias. Five horses were considered to have pyrrolizidine alkaloid toxicity, but the causes in the other four were not determined.
   b. The cause of the hemolytic states was not determined.

ERYTHROCYTOSIS AND POLYCYTHEMIA

I. Terms and concepts
    A. *Erythrocytosis* is an increased [RBC] in peripheral blood. It is detected by finding an increased Hct, increased [RBC], or increased blood [Hgb].
    B. *Hemoconcentration* is an increased concentration of blood components (including erythrocytes) because of decreased plasma volume.
    C. *Polycythemia*
        1. *Polycythemia vera* (*polycythemia rubra vera*) is a clonal myeloproliferative disorder characterized by neoplastic proliferation of all marrow cell precursors that produces erythrocytosis, leukocytosis, and thrombocytosis. In this context, polycythemia means "many" (*poly-*) "cells" (*cyth-*) in the "blood" (*-emia*).
        2. In common use, polycythemia may refer to an erythrocytosis or increased total erythrocyte mass (i.e., an increased number of cells in the erythron because of either erythroid hyperplasia or erythroid neoplasia). However, there may or may not be a leukocytosis or thrombocytosis. Such use leads to confusion and misunderstandings. In this context, these are the two types of polycythemia:
            a. *Relative polycythemia*: Erythrocytosis occurs because of hemoconcentration or splenic contraction. It is also called *pseudo-polycythemia* or *spurious polycythemia* to emphasize that the state is really not an absolute increase in erythrocyte mass.
            b. *Absolute* or *true polycythemia*: Erythrocytosis occurs because of increased erythrocyte mass, and there is concurrent erythrocytosis. Polycythemia vera is one form of this type but also includes secondary erythrocytotic disorders.
        3. In this textbook, erythrocytosis and polycythemia are not considered synonyms. *Erythrocytosis* is an increased [RBC] in blood, just as a *leukocytosis* is an increased [WBC] in blood. Polycythemia will be used only in the context of the neoplastic state of polycythemia vera.
        4. Some people have combined terms and concepts to form another classification system.
            a. *Relative erythrocytosis*: The definition is the same as for *relative polycythemia*.
            b. *Absolute erythrocytosis*: Erythrocytosis associated with increased erythrocyte mass.
    D. Extreme erythrocytosis may cause sludging of blood and thus impaired blood flow and poor oxygenation of tissues. Related clinical signs may include purplish mucous membranes, congested retinal blood vessels, and seizures.

II. Erythrocytotic disorders and conditions (Table 3.14) (Fig. 3.13)
    A. Hemoconcentration
        1. Dehydration
            a. The most common cause of erythrocytosis in mammals, dehydration occurs as a mild to moderate erythrocytosis of no direct pathologic significance.
            b. Erythrocytosis is present, but it is not due to an increased mass of erythroid cells in the body.
            c. Pathogenesis of the erythrocytosis of hemoconcentration is shown in Fig. 3.14.

Table 3.14. Disorders and conditions that cause erythrocytosis

Hemoconcentration
    *Dehydration
    Endotoxic shock
*Splenic contraction
Secondary appropriate erythrocytotic disorders
    Right-to-left shunts, congenital or acquired
    Chronic pulmonary disease
    Hyperthyroidism
Secondary inappropriate erythrocytotic disorders
    Renal neoplasms, cysts, or diseases
    Other neoplasms (hepatoma)
Primary erythrocytotic disorders
    Primary erythrocytosis
    Polycythemia vera (polycythemia rubra vera)
Idiopathic erythrocytosis

*A relatively common disease or condition

Note: Animals that live at higher altitudes or perhaps those that have been physically trained (e.g., racing animals) have an increased need for Hgb to transport O_2 to tissues and may produce more erythrocytes. In addition, certain breeds of dogs and horses have greater Hct values than other animals of the same species (see list in Erythrocytosis and Polycythemia, sect. II.C.4).

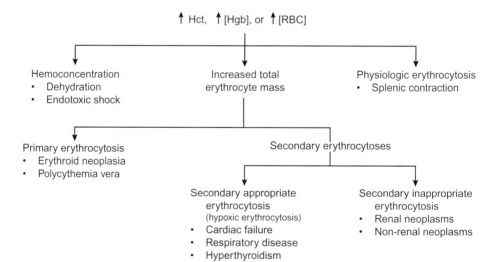

Fig. 3.13. An approach to problem-solving erythrocytoses: After erythrocytosis has been detected or confirmed, the animal is examined for evidence of the most common causes: hemoconcentration or splenic contraction. If they are not found and the erythrocytosis is persistent, then diagnostic plans are formulated to pursue identification of secondary or primary erythrocytotic disorders. However, the erythrocytosis may be idiopathic.

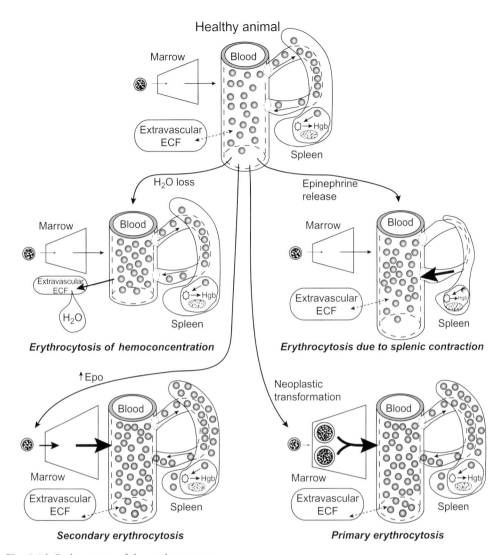

Fig. 3.14. Pathogeneses of the erythrocytoses.

- Erythrocytosis of hemoconcentration: Dehydration (decreased total body water) results in a decreased ECF volume and thus a decreased plasma volume. With a decreased plasma volume but no change in number of blood erythrocytes, the [RBC] is increased. Loss of plasma H_2O because of increased vascular permeability in endotoxic shock also causes an erythrocytosis via hemoconcentration.

- Erythrocytosis due to splenic contraction (physiologic erythrocytosis): The fight-or-flight response or exercise causes the release of epinephrine. Epinephrine administration causes the contraction of splenic smooth muscle and thus the release of splenic blood to peripheral blood vessels. Splenic blood with a high Hct (70–80 %) is mixed with peripheral blood (Hct = 40–50 %) and causes erythrocytosis.

- Secondary erythrocytosis: Increased Epo activity stimulates erythropoiesis to cause erythroid hyperplasia and erythrocytosis associated with an increase in total body erythrocyte mass. Increased Epo production may be appropriate (if stimulated by tissue hypoxia) or inappropriate (if not stimulated by tissue hypoxia). Several disease states can cause a secondary erythrocytosis (see Erythrocytosis and Polycythemia, sects. II.C and D).

- Primary erythrocytosis: There is a proliferation of erythroid cells in the absence of increased Epo production that causes an erythrocytosis and increases total body erythrocyte mass. This may be neoplastic or nonneoplastic. Nonneoplastic primary erythrocytosis caused by defective Epo receptors has been reported in people. If erythrocytosis is concurrent with a neoplastic proliferation of leukocytes and megakaryocytes, then polycythemia vera is present.

    d. Laboratory findings that support a conclusion that erythrocytosis is caused by dehydration
       (1) Hyperproteinemia with possibly a concurrent hyperalbuminemia
       (2) Hypernatremia and hyperchloremia if dehydration is hypertonic (loss of hypotonic fluid)
  2. Endotoxic shock
    a. The blood of some animals with endotoxemia may become hemoconcentrated because of the shift of H_2O from intravascular to extravascular space.
    b. Pathogenesis of the erythrocytosis: Endotoxins damage endothelial cells so that blood vessels become more permeable to proteins. The extravascular proteins reduce the oncotic pressure gradient, which promotes the shift of plasma H_2O from intravascular space to extravascular space, thus causing a decrease in plasma volume and an erythrocytosis.
    c. Laboratory findings that support endotoxic shock
       (1) Erythrocytosis is usually mild to moderate and of no direct pathologic significance.
       (2) Inflammatory leukogram (either neutropenia or neutrophilia)
       (3) Thrombocytopenia

B. Splenic contraction (physiologic erythrocytosis) (Fig. 3.14)
  1. This state is called *physiologic erythrocytosis* because it results from normal physiologic responses to excitement, fright, and exercise that cause epinephrine release from adrenal medullae.
  2. This erythrocytosis is more common in dogs and horses because of the large number and high concentration of erythrocytes in equine and canine splenic blood. After epinephrine injections in cats, Hct values were about 25 % greater than preinjection Hct values.[14]
  3. Erythrocytosis is not due to an increased mass of erythroid cells or erythrocytes in the body, but the erythrocyte number and concentration is increased in the peripheral blood.
  4. Laboratory findings
    a. Erythrocytosis is mild to moderate and of no direct pathologic significance.
    b. Erythrocytosis is transient. The Hct returns to WRI after the stimulus is removed.
    c. One may see a physiologic leukocytosis (mature neutrophilia and lymphocytosis).

C. Secondary appropriate erythrocytosis (sustained hypoxic erythrocytosis) (Fig. 3.14)
  1. This state is called *secondary* because erythroid cell proliferation is stimulated by Epo rather than being autonomous. It is called *appropriate* because Epo is increased by renal (usually systemic) hypoxia rather than being autonomous.
  2. Erythrocytosis and erythroid hyperplasia are due to increased production stimulated by Epo.
  3. Disorders that cause hypoxic erythrocytosis
    a. Cardiac disease that leads to persistent poor perfusion of the lungs (e.g., congenital right to left shunt)
    b. Pulmonary disorders that cause persistent poor oxygenation of blood
    c. Hyperthyroidism that increases the metabolic rate and thus increases the need for O_2 in tissues. In one study, about 45 % of 131 hyperthyroid cats had an erythrocytosis (Hct values from 38 % to 57 %).[206]

    d. In theory, a defective Hgb molecule that has decreased ability to transport or release O_2 could cause an erythrocytosis. Acquired disorders (such as cyanide poisoning, carbon monoxide poisoning, and nitrate poisoning) are typically acute and thus of insufficient duration to produce increased Hct. Hereditary Hgb disorders (*hemoglobinopathies*) are not documented in domestic animals.

   4. Physiologic processes

    a. Mammals that move to high altitudes may develop tissue hypoxia. The hypoxia stimulates Epo production and erythropoiesis, resulting in erythroid hyperplasia and erythrocytosis that resolve the tissue hypoxia. Mammals that live at high altitudes are expected to have greater Hct values than mammals that live at sea level, but without tissue hypoxia or pathologic consequence. Such animals really do not have erythrocytoses; rather, reference intervals for high altitudes are greater than those for low altitudes. However, one study involving dogs indicates that the erythrocytosis one expects does not always occur.[207]

    b. Prolonged exercise training in horses has produced differing results. In some studies the trained horses had greater Hct values but in other studies they did not. Increased O_2 demand during training might stimulate erythropoiesis, but other mechanisms may contribute.[208,209]

    c. Some breeds have greater erythrocyte concentrations than others.

      (1) Thoroughbreds, Standardbreds, and quarter horses have greater Hcts than draft horses.

      (2) Greyhounds, Afghan hounds, salukis, and whippets have greater Hcts than most other dogs. The Hcts of the former average in the high 50s to low 60s,[210] whereas most other dogs have average Hcts in the 40s in health. Poodles, German shepherds, boxers, beagles, dachshunds, and Chihuahuas are also mentioned as having Hcts greater than those of most dogs.[211]

   5. Pathogenesis: Hypoxemia or increased tissue O_2 consumption (hyperthyroidism) causes sustained tissue (renal) hypoxia, which leads to increased Epo production, increased erythropoiesis via erythroid hyperplasia, and, with time, erythrocytosis.

   6. Clinical data that would support secondary appropriate erythrocytosis

    a. Clinical history or evidence of a right to left shunt, chronic pulmonary disease, or hyperthyroidism

    b. Decreased P_aO_2 (strongly if < 70 mmHg[212] or < 60 mmHg[213])

    c. Hemoglobinopathy (rare)

D. Secondary inappropriate erythrocytosis (Fig. 3.14)

   1. This state is called *secondary* because erythroid cell proliferation is stimulated by Epo rather than being autonomous. It is called *inappropriate* because the increased Epo production is autonomous rather than being caused by systemic hypoxia.

   2. Disorders in this erythrocytotic group can cause mild to marked erythrocytosis and erythroid hyperplasia. Marked erythrocytosis may cause sluggish blood that leads to poor tissue perfusion.

   3. Pathologic causes (both rare or rarely recognized)

    a. Inappropriate Epo production by renal tissue because of renal cysts, renal neoplasms, and, rarely, other renal disease

    b. Inappropriate Epo production by other benign or malignant neoplasms (e.g., hepatoma, hepatoblastoma, schwannoma, or leiomyosarcoma)

   4. Clinical data that would support the conclusion that a persistent erythrocytosis is secondary and inappropriate

      a. Known associated pathologic disorders are found.

      b. Serum [total protein] and P_aO_2 are WRI.

E. Primary erythrocytosis (Fig. 3.14)

  1. This state is called *primary* because erythroid cell proliferation is autonomous rather than secondary to Epo.

  2. Disorders in this erythrocytotic group can cause mild to marked erythrocytosis that may cause sluggish blood, poor tissue perfusion, and therefore secondarily increased Epo production.

  3. Disorders

    a. *Primary erythrocytosis* is either a neoplastic or nonneoplastic condition in which the total number of mature erythrocytes in the body and blood is increased without increased production of Epo.

    b. *Polycythemia vera* is neoplasia of erythroid, myeloid, and megakaryocytic cell lines. Primary erythrocytosis may be a presenting form of polycythemia vera.

    c. In people, truncation of the Epo receptor can lead to sustained Epo stimulation and congenital nonneoplastic primary erythrocytosis. This has not been identified in domestic mammals but should be considered as a potential cause.

  4. Information that would support these disorders

    a. Absence of other causes of erythrocytosis

    b. With polycythemia vera, bone marrow with too many erythroid cell, myeloid cell, and megakaryocyte precursors

    c. Theoretically, blood [Epo] would not be increased with primary erythrocytosis but would be increased with secondary erythrocytosis. However, blood [Epo] may be increased because of hypoxia induced by primary erythrocytosis, and blood [Epo] may not be increased with secondary erythrocytosis if erythrocytosis has resolved tissue hypoxia such that here is little or no stimulus for increased Epo production at the time of testing.

F. *Idiopathic erythrocytosis* is the classification for patients whose erythrocytosis cannot be classified.

OTHER ERYTHROCYTE DISORDERS

I.   Methemoglobinemia

  A. *Methemoglobinemia* is the condition in which $Hgb\text{-}Fe^{3+}$ accumulates in erythrocytes. It may be hereditary or acquired.

    1. Hereditary

      a. Cb_5R deficiency in dogs (several breeds) and cats

      b. Associated with erythrocyte FAD deficiency in a horse (see Hemolytic Disorders and Diseases, sect. II.C.1.b)[37]

      c. GR deficiency in a horse[214]

    2. Acquired

      a. Nitrate poisoning

        (1) In ruminants, ingestion of feed with high nitrate content increases rumen formation and absorption of nitrites.

        (2) Nitrite (NO_2^-) binds to oxyhemoglobin and results in the release of O_2 and linked chain reactions that form $Hgb\text{-}Fe^{3+}$, hydrogen peroxide, nitrous dioxide radical, and more nitrite.

      b. Erythrocyte exposure to oxidants

(1) A variety of toxicants are oxidants that overwhelm the reductive capacity of erythrocyte pathways and thus can lead to conversion of Hgb to Hgb-Fe^{3+}.

(2) Many of these oxidants also damage the Hgb molecule and lead to the formation of Heinz bodies (see Hemolytic Disorders and Diseases, sect. C.1.a).

B. Diagnosis of methemoglobinemia

1. *Spot test*: A drop of blood is placed on white filter paper. Methemoglobinemic blood has a brown discoloration compared to blood containing primarily oxyhemoglobin.

2. *CO-oximeter*: This instrument uses polychromatic light to detect oxyhemoglobin, deoxyhemoglobin, carboxyhemoglobin, and Hgb-Fe^{3+} by means of their different absorption spectra. The results are expressed as a percentage of total Hgb; for example, 20 % Hgb-Fe^{3+} (see Analytical Concepts, sect. III, in Chapter 10).

3. *Pulse oximeter*: This device also uses the absorption spectra to measure percent Hgb saturation with Hgb (Spo_2). Unfortunately, the pulse oximeter cannot differentiate Hgb-Fe^{3+} from oxyhemoglobin, so the Spo_2 is falsely increased when methemoglobinemia is present. Methemoglobinemia should be considered if the Spo_2 is significantly greater than the So_2 (percentage of Hgb saturated with O_2) determined by blood gas analysis (see the Analytical Concepts section in Chapter 10).

II. Cytochrome-b_5 reductase (Cb_5R) (NADH-methemoglobin reductase) deficiency[215–220]

A. Cb_5R catalyzes the primary reaction involved in the conversion of Hgb-Fe^{3+} to Hgb. It uses FAD as a cofactor (Fig. 3.5). A Cb_5R deficiency allows Hgb-Fe^{3+} to accumulate in erythrocytes.

B. It is a hereditary disorder in people. The genetics are not known for dog and cats (reported in purebred and mongrel dogs).

C. Classic features

1. Young and old dogs with clinical signs of hypoxia because of poor O_2-carrying capacity of methemoglobin

2. Methemoglobinemia (dark to chocolate blood) and usually Heinz bodies present

3. No anemia or mild anemia; may be a compensatory reticulocytosis

III. Familial methemoglobinemia associated with GR deficiency in a horse[214]

A. GR catalyzes the conversion of glutathione disulfide to GSH. It uses FAD as a cofactor (Fig. 3.5). A deficiency in GR can lead to a decreased [GSH] in erythrocytes, thus making them more susceptible to oxidants.

B. A young mare and her dam both were exercise intolerant and had similar abnormalities.

C. Clinical features

1. Methemoglobinemia

2. Mild anemia (Hct near 25 %)

3. GR deficiency (about 30 % of activity of healthy horses)

4. Reduced [GSH] (about 50 % of healthy values)

5. Cb_5R activity and NADPH dehydrogenase activity were not decreased. (Note: Some methods give false values.)[37]

IV. Hereditary stomatocytosis

A. Hereditary stomatocytoses have been recognized in three canine breeds: Alaskan malamutes, Drentse patrijshonds, and schnauzers. The specific erythrocyte defects are not established; clinically, the dogs probably have different disorders.

B. In the Alaskan malamutes, there is a concurrent short-limb dwarfism.[221] The erythrocyte disorder is characterized by mild anemia, mild to moderate reticulocytosis, mild to moderate stomatocytosis, and shortened erythrocyte life span.

C. In the Drentse patrijshonds, the concurrent findings include hypertrophic gastritis, polycystic renal disease, and regenerative macrocytic hypochromic anemia due to hemolysis.[65] Studies of erythrocyte membranes and plasmas of affected dogs indicate that abnormal fatty acid composition in plasma phospholipids leads to abnormal phospholipid composition in erythrocyte membranes.[222]

D. Among the miniature and standard schnauzers, those with stomatocytosis were not anemic, but their erythrocytes were macrocytic and hypochromic.[66] The amount of stomatin (erythrocyte membrane protein 7.2b) in erythrocytes of standard schnauzers with stomatocytosis was variable but similar to the amount found in dogs without stomatocytosis.[223] The erythrocyte $[Na^+]$ and $[K^+]$ were increased; the stomatocytosis appeared to be due to erythrocyte overhydration caused by a defective cation exchange.[67]

V. Hereditary band 3 deficiency in Japanese black cattle[63]
  A. Homozygous cattle for this autosomal dominant disorder have a chronic hemolytic anemia, spherocytosis, and metabolic acidosis. They also suffer from retarded growth.
  B. *Erythrocyte band 3* is a membrane protein that has two major functions: (1) it serves as an ion-exchange protein for the rapid exchange of Cl^- and HCO_3^- to allow the transport of CO_2 from tissues to lungs, and (2) it contributes to the erythrocyte cytoskeleton.

VI. Hereditary elliptocytosis in dogs that is caused by protein band 4.1 deficiency[55,224]
  A. Elliptocytosis is caused by qualitative and quantitative defects of *erythrocyte membrane protein 4.1*, a protein that is needed to stabilize the cytoskeleton of the erythrocyte membrane by providing an anchor for the spectrin-ankyrin complex.
  B. Classic features of canine disorder
    1. Marked elliptocytosis is present.
    2. There is slight anemia but with moderate reticulocytosis (compensated anemia).
    3. In cases reported so far, the disorder was not a major problem for the dogs.

VII. Elliptocytosis in a mixed-breed dog with mutant spectrin[56]
  A. Elliptocytosis was caused by a mutation in the spectrin gene and was associated with an increased ratio of spectrin dimers compared to spectrin tetramers in erythrocyte membranes.
  B. *Spectrin*, a major protein of the erythrocyte cytoskeleton, is composed of heterodimers of two proteins: α-spectrin and β-spectrin. These proteins self-associate to form tetramers. Molecular defects in either α-spectrin or β-spectrin can reduce this association, and thus more dimers are present in the membrane. In people, the location of the mutation in either α-spectrin or β-spectrin produces elliptocytosis or spherocytosis.[225] Elliptocytosis occurs when there is a defective horizontal interaction of membrane proteins, whereas spherocytosis occurs when the vertical interaction of membrane proteins is defective.
  C. Clinical features of the canine disorder
    1. Elliptocytosis: Many erythrocytes are involved but to a varying degree. Typical findings are 40 % type I elliptocytes (nearly circular cells), 35 % type II elliptocytes (oval cells), and 25 % type III elliptocytes (elongated cells).

2. The dog was clinically healthy, not anemic, and thus its elliptocytosis was a subclinical disorder.

VIII. Spectrin deficiency in Dutch golden retrievers
   A. Spectrin is a membrane protein that is a major component of an erythrocyte's cytoskeleton. In people, a spectrin deficiency causes a disorder known as *hereditary spherocytosis*. Concurrently, these people have a hemolytic anemia and increased erythrocyte osmotic fragility.
   B. A partial spectrin deficiency was detected in a group of Dutch golden retrievers after they recovered from hemolytic anemias (three immune mediated and two of unknown mechanisms).[226] It was discovered because of the persistence of increased erythrocyte osmotic fragility. The erythrocyte [spectrin] in the affected dogs was 50–65 % of the concentrations found in golden retrievers without altered erythrocyte osmotic fragility. After recovery from the hemolytic anemias, the dogs with partial spectrin deficiency were not anemic. Spherocytes were detected only in dogs diagnosed with immune-mediated hemolytic anemia. A cause-and-effect association between spectrin deficiency and hemolytic anemia was not established in these dogs. Pedigree analysis indicated an autosomal dominant inheritance.

IX. Megaloblastic anemia
   A. A *megaloblastic anemia* has the concurrent findings of anemia and megaloblastic erythroid precursors in bone marrow or blood.
   B. Megaloblastic erythroid precursors form because of asynchronous maturation of nucleus and cytoplasm (Plate 9L). Nuclear maturation is arrested, so nuclei are large, with exaggerated euchromatin regions that persist to late rubricyte stages. Cytoplasmic maturation is relatively more complete, so Hgb is apparent in cells with relatively immature nuclei. The cells have relatively abundant cytoplasm and thus are larger than would be expected for the maturity of the nucleus.
   C. Causes
      1. The exact defect is rarely documented. It may be the result of neoplastic transformation of erythrocyte precursors, defective nucleic acid metabolism caused by folate or vitamin B_{12} deficiency, or defective metabolism.
      2. In cats, there is a high clinical association with FeLV infections (especially subtype C).
   D. Frequently, cats with this disorder have a nonregenerative, macrocytic normochromic anemia (mild to marked severity).
      1. Nonregenerative because of defective and reduced erythrocyte production
      2. Macrocytic because megaloblastic metarubricytes become macrocytes with erythrocyte diameters $1\frac{1}{2}$–2 times those of healthy cats
      3. Bone marrow findings in cats
         a. Erythroid cell numbers: variable, increased to decreased
         b. Erythroid cells: frequent megaloblastic rubricytes and/or megaloblastic metarubricytes
         c. Granulocytic cells: occasionally hypersegmented neutrophils
   E. Classification of megaloblastic disorders in cats that is based on exclusion of underlying diseases until cytogenetic markers of neoplastic transformation become available (see Bone Marrow Classifications, sect. IX.B, in Chapter 6)
      1. Acquired secondary dyshematopoiesis: Erythrocytes are dysplastic but are not neoplastic.

2. Erythroid neoplasia
   a. Acute myeloid leukemia: erythroleukemia or erythroleukemia with erythroid predominance
   b. Primary myelodysplastic syndromes: myelodysplastic syndrome or myelodysplastic syndrome with erythroid predominance

X. Sideroblastic anemia in dogs[28]
   A. A diagnosis of sideroblastic anemia was based on the concurrent presence of > 15 % sideroblasts in marrow and of ringed sideroblasts.
   B. Of the seven dogs, six had nonregenerative anemias, one had a regenerative anemia, five had hypochromic anemias, and two had microcytic anemias. Dysplastic features in marrow included dyserythropoiesis (asynchronous nuclear maturation, binucleation, and nuclear fragmentation or lobulation), asynchronous maturation in megakaryocytes, and dysmyelopoiesis (giant neutrophils and hypersegmentation).
   C. The anemias were not caused by Fe deficiency, because Fe stores in marrow were considered increased or normal. The siderocytes and sideroblasts indicated defective Fe metabolism and were associated with acute hepatitis, pancreatitis, glomerulonephritis, sepsis, and myelofibrosis.

XI. Distemper inclusions in dogs (Plate 4A and B)
   A. Erythrocyte distemper inclusions are generally rare findings. They may occur in the early viremic stage and before clinical illness in dogs. They may appear as pink or pale blue amorphous inclusions of varying shapes and sizes, are rarely observed in the United States, and are usually more easily detected with the quick-dip stains (e.g., Diff-Quik) than the Wright stains.
   B. Rarely, similar cytoplasmic inclusions are found in blood neutrophils and lymphocytes (see Plate 2D)

LABORATORY METHODS FOR ASSESSING IRON (Fe) STATUS[7]

Evaluation of an animal's Fe status may be helpful in confirming an Fe-deficient or an Fe-overload state, but serum [Fe] alone is an unreliable reflection of body Fe stores.

I. Serum [Fe]
   A. Analytical concepts
      1. Because nearly all Fe in nonhemolyzed serum is bound to transferrin, serum [Fe] typically represents the amount of Fe bound to transferrin. Fe in ferritin may contribute significantly to serum [Fe] if the hyperferritinemia is marked.
      2. Unit conversion: $\mu g/dL \times 0.01791\ \mu mol/\mu g \times 10\ dL/L = \mu mol/L$ (SI unit, nearest $1\ \mu mol/L$)[16]
      3. Sample
         a. Serum is preferred.
         b. Serum [Fe] is relatively stable if the sample is refrigerated, frozen, or kept at room temperatures for a few hours.
      4. Common principle of serum Fe assays: Fe^{3+} is liberated from transferrin in an acidic environment and then is reduced to Fe^{2+} by ascorbic acid. Fe^{2+} reacts with a dye or other compound to form a colored complex that is detected by photometric methods.

Table 3.15. Disorders and conditions that cause hyperferremia

Fe overload due to excess intake
   Iatrogenic: excess Fe injections or oral hematinics
   Genetic defect in regulation of Fe absorption
Release of Fe from tissues
   Hepatocyte damage
Increased glucocorticoid hormones: iatrogenic or endogenous (horses and dogs)

Note: Serum [Fe] can be falsely increased with hyperferritinemia or hemoglobinemia (in vitro or pathologic) as discussed in the text.

  B. Hyperferremia (increased [Fe] in blood) (Table 3.15)
    1. Excess Fe intake
      a. Iatrogenic
        (1) Excess ingestion of a hematinic in calves[227] and ingestion of a digestive inoculate (Primapaste) in foals[228] have produced Fe toxicosis.
        (2) Fe injections may be administered inappropriately to animals suspected of being Fe deficient, especially to racehorses.[229] If Fe cannot be excreted fast enough by urine and feces, hyperferremia will develop.
      b. Hereditary hemochromatosis was reported in cattle of the Salers breed.[230] In people, primary hemochromatosis occurs because intestinal absorption of Fe is not appropriately regulated.
    2. Increased glucocorticoid hormones: Hyperferremia occurs after administration of dexamethasone in horses (doubling within 2–3 d)[231] and in dogs,[7] but hypoferremia occurred in cattle. The reasons for changes in [Fe] are not known.
    3. Release of Fe from tissues
      a. Hepatocytes typically contain Fe-rich ferritin. When hepatocyte damage occurs, the Fe that is released may cause hyperferremia.
      b. Intravascular and extravascular hemolytic states are associated with increased serum [Fe]. Fe released from degraded Hgb is available to bind to transferrin so Fe^{3+} can be transported in plasma for either reutilization or storage.
    4. False increases
      a. The Fe in plasma Hgb (hemoglobinemia) has very little influence on serum [Fe] because Fe is not released from Hgb for detection by most clinical assay methods. However, the Hgb molecule may cause spectral interference to cause erroneous measurements (false increases in most assays).[232]
      b. Fe liberated from ferritin can cause hyperferremia when determined by some Fe assays. The amount of increase is minimal unless serum ferritin concentrations are greatly increased.[233]
    5. Neonatal foals had serum Fe concentrations > 400 µg/dL, but the [Fe] decreased to adult concentrations (about 125–130 µg/dL) by 3 d of age.[31]
  C. Hypoferremia (Table 3.16)
    1. Increased Fe loss caused by chronic external blood loss
      a. Because each mL of blood contains about 1 mg of Fe, blood loss results in a loss of Fe from the body. Hypoferremia may develop when Fe stores become depleted from chronic blood loss.
      b. Causes of blood loss that result in Fe deficiency include intestinal parasitism (hookworms and whipworms in dogs), fleas and ticks (in dogs, cats, and calves),

Table 3.16. Disorders and conditions that cause hypoferremia

Fe deficiency
  *Increased Fe loss: chronic external blood loss
  Decreased Fe intake or intestinal absorption
Shift of Fe to storage sites
  *Acute inflammation
  *Chronic inflammation
Other or unknown mechanisms
  Dexamethasone injections in cattle
  *Young animals (foals, kittens, calves)
  Dogs with congenital portosystemic shunts

  * A relatively common disease or condition

chronic gastrointestinal hemorrhage (caused by neoplasia, ulcers, or other lesions), and excessive donation of blood.

   c. Acute blood loss is not expected to cause hypoferremia, because Fe is mobilized from storage sites and carried in the plasma by transferrin.

2. Shift of Fe to storage sites

   a. In inflammatory diseases, serum [Fe] is decreased because of the sequestration of Fe in macrophages of liver, spleen, or marrow. IL-1 and IL-6 are involved in the altered Fe kinetics: IL-6 promotes the synthesis of hepcidin, and thus the amount of ferroportin available for the export of Fe from cells (including macrophages) is reduced.[9]

   b. The altered state of Fe kinetics in inflammation that causes hypoferremia has been called a *pseudo–Fe deficiency*.[234] In this condition, blood may be Fe deficient but the body is not.

3. Decreased Fe intake or intestinal absorption

   a. Veal calves are purposely fed an Fe-deficient diet that can produce Fe deficiency.

   b. Extensive intestinal mucosal disease that leads to impaired absorption of Fe will contribute to an Fe-deficient state.

4. Glucocorticoids in cattle caused a hypoferremia (from about 140 μg/dL to 50 μg/dL) within 1 d after dexamethasone (2 mg) was given intravenously.[235]

5. Portosystemic shunts in dogs

   a. Dogs with congenital portosystemic shunts may have a microcytic anemia, and some may have concurrent hypoferremia.[236] In experimental studies, the serum [Fe] did decrease in a group of 16 surgically induced portosystemic shunts (from a mean of 129 μg/dL to a mean of 92 μg/dL), but the individual serum [Fe] remained WRI.[237]

   b. The pathogenesis of the hypoferremia is not established, but data support the concept of defective transport of Fe because of decreased production of transferrin by hepatocytes.[236]

6. Young animals

   a. Of the 2- to 4-wk-old kittens in a specific-pathogen-free colony, 70 % had hypoferremia (relative to adult concentrations) that was associated with microcytosis.[32] This suggests a transient Fe-deficient state during early growth.

   b. In 18 dairy calves (< 3 d old), serum Fe concentrations were lower in calves with Hct values < 25 % than in those with Hct values > 25 %. Only the most severely anemic calf (Hct = 9 %) had clinical signs of anemia. The cause of the apparent congenital hypoferremia and Fe-deficient state was not determined.[34]

    c. Relative to adult MCV values, foals have a peak microcytosis between 3 mo and 5 mo of age.[31] However, their serum Fe concentrations were equal to or greater than concentrations found in healthy adult horses.[31] Stabled Dutch warmblood foals (1–3 mo of age) that were fed freshly cut grass had lower blood [Hgb], Hct, blood [Fe], and percentage transferrin saturation than similar foals raised on pasture. The data provided evidence of Fe deficiency in the stabled foals.[238]

7. Because plasma Fe is transported in transferrin, disorders that cause a loss of or decreased production of plasma proteins could cause hypoferremia. Renal disease, late pregnancy, and hypothyroidism have been listed as hypoferremic disorders,[239] but supportive data for domestic mammals were not found.

II.   TIBC and UIBC
    A. Analytical concepts
        1. Terms and units
            a. *TIBC*, a measure of plasma capacity to carry Fe, is the maximum concentration of Fe that can be bound by plasma or serum proteins. Because most plasma Fe is in *transferrin* (a complex of Fe and the protein apotransferrin), serum [Fe] depends on and correlates with the serum [transferrin].
            b. A transferrin molecule can contain two Fe^{3+} ions, but, in health, Fe^{3+} occupies only about a third of all plasma or serum transferrin Fe-binding sites. *UIBC*, a measure of the total unused (open) Fe-binding sites on transferrin, is the [Fe] that could be protein bound in the sample in addition to the [Fe] already present.
            c. Unit conversion: μg/dL × 0.01791 μmol/μg × 10 dL/L = μmol/L (SI unit, nearest 1 μmol/L)[16]
        2. Sample
            a. Serum is preferred.
            b. Serum [TIBC] is stable for a few days if the sample is refrigerated or kept at room temperatures, and it is stable for months if frozen.
        3. Principles of serum TIBC and UIBC assays
            a. Transferrin concentrations can be measured directly, but this rarely is done in veterinary medicine.
            b. Typical method
                (1) Excess Fe citrate is added to serum to saturate all Fe-binding sites, and then the bound-Fe and free-Fe fractions are separated by chemical methods. The Fe^{3+} in the saturated transferrin molecules reacts with a dye to determine the bound [Fe], which represents the TIBC.
                (2) The UIBC is calculated: UIBC = TIBC − serum [Fe].
            c. In some clinical assays, plasma Hgb (hemoglobinemia) may cause spectral interference in assays that measure [Fe] (see Laboratory Methods for Assessing Iron Status, sect. I.B.4) and thus could result in erroneous TIBC and UIBC results.
    B. Increased serum TIBC (Table 3.17)
        1. Fe deficiency
            a. People with Fe deficiency may have an increased TIBC because of the increased production of transferrin to carry available Fe to cells.
            b. Fe-deficient dogs typically do not have increased TIBC.[7]

Table 3.17. Disorders and conditions that cause increased TIBC

Increased apotransferrin production
  Fe deficiency: species variable
Other or unknown mechanisms
  Young animals (foals)

Table 3.18. Disorders and conditions that cause decreased TIBC

Decreased apotransferrin production
  *Inflammation
   Hepatic insufficiency
Increased transferrin loss (protein-losing nephropathies, potentially other protein-losing
     states)

* A relatively common disease or condition

2. Young foals, especially near 1 mo of age, have much greater TIBC (> 600 µg/dL) than neonates or adult horses. Colostrum is transferrin rich, but colostral intake does not explain the entire increase in TIBC during a foal's first month of life.
  C. Decreased serum TIBC (Table 3.18)
    1. Decreased transferrin production
       a. Inflammation: Apotransferrin is a negative acute-phase protein (i.e., its production is decreased by actions of inflammatory mediators such as IL-1), so inflammation may lead to hypotransferrinemia.
       b. Hepatic insufficiency: Because transferrin is a β-globulin produced by hepatocytes, liver disease that causes hypoproteinemia may cause hypotransferrinemia. Hypotransferrinemia may play a role in the microcytosis that develops in some animals with hepatic insufficiency.
    2. Increased transferrin loss
       a. Severe glomerular lesions that produce a protein-losing nephropathy may cause hypotransferrinemia. The relative molecular mass of transferrin is only slightly greater than albumin's.
       b. Potentially, other protein-losing states (e.g., severe protein-losing enteropathy and hemorrhage) could also cause the loss of plasma transferrin and thus decrease serum TIBC.

III. Percent transferrin saturation (% saturation)
  A. Analytical concepts
    1. *Percent transferrin saturation* is a calculated percentage that estimates the percentage of Fe-binding sites on apotransferrin molecules that are occupied by Fe.
    2. Percent transferrin saturation = (serum [Fe] × 100) ÷ TIBC
  B. Because the % transferrin saturation is a calculated percentage, changes depend on changes in the serum [Fe] and TIBC.
    1. Greater % transferrin saturation occurs when serum [Fe] is increased, TIBC is decreased, or both.
    2. Lower % transferrin saturation occurs when serum [Fe] is decreased, TIBC is increased, or both.

IV. Stainable Fe in macrophages of marrow, spleen, or liver
   A. In microscopic examinations of formalin-fixed tissue or air-dried cytologic preparations, hemosiderin is seen as a yellow to brown granular or globular pigment in macrophages.
   B. When attempting to quantify the amount of Fe in storage (especially for Fe deficiency), the use of an Fe-specific stain (such as Prussian blue) enables a more definitive assessment than does the use of routine stains. However, the process is subjective and requires knowledge of how much Fe is expected in tissues of healthy animals.
   C. The marrow of healthy cats does not contain stainable Fe, so feline marrow cannot be used to assess Fe stores. Fe stores may also be undetectable or minimal in young, growing animals without clinical Fe deficiency.

V. Serum Ferritin Concentrations
   A. Analytical concepts
      1. Unit conversion: ng/mL × 1000 mL/L × 1 µg/1000 ng = µg/L (SI unit, nearest 10 µg/L)[16]
      2. Sample: Serum is preferred. A [ferritin] is reported to be stable for 7 d at 2–8 °C and for 6 mo at −20 °C. Repeated thawing and refreezing is not recommended.
      3. Principles of serum ferritin assays: Species-specific immunoassays and other immunologic assays are used to measure ferritin in dogs, cats, and horses.[31,240] Plasma ferritin concentrations in horses increased with exercise. The exact mechanism for the increased [ferritin] is not established but appears to be release from tissues other than liver.[241] Samples for the assessment of Fe stores should be drawn at least 2 d after strenuous exercise.
   B. Hyperferritinemia (Table 3.19)
      1. Associated with increased total body Fe
         a. If neither inflammation nor hepatic disease is present, serum or plasma ferritin concentrations in people are correlated with Fe storage.[242] If Fe toxicity is present, the typical ferritin assay will measure tissue ferritin released from damaged cells, and thus the amount of Fe storage will be overestimated.
         b. In a group of 95 dogs, there was a weak but statistically significant correlation (r = 0.37) between serum [ferritin] and nonheme-Fe content of liver and spleen, but none of the dogs had increased Fe stores.[243] A similar correlation (r = 0.365) was present in 106 random-source cats.[240]

Table 3.19. Disorders and conditions that cause hyperferritinemia

Associated with increased total body Fe
    Iatrogenic: excess Fe injections or oral hematinics
    Genetic defect in regulation of Fe absorption
Increased apoferritin production
    *Inflammation
    Neoplasia: histiocytic sarcoma (malignant histiocytosis)
Shift of ferritin from tissue to plasma
    Liver disease
    Hemolysis
    Exercise in horses

  * A relatively common disease or condition

2. Increased ferritin production
   a. Inflammation: Because apoferritin is a positive acute-phase protein, cytokine (e.g., IL-1) stimulation of hepatocytes may cause hyperferritinemia. In people, the Fe saturation of ferritin decreases with inflammation.[244]
   b. Neoplasia: Hyperferritinemia has been considered a marker for several human neoplasms and may be caused by inflammation, accelerated erythrocyte turnover (hemolysis), or increased production by neoplastic cells. Hyperferritinemia has been associated with disseminated histiocytic sarcomas (malignant histiocytosis) in dogs.[245] It may also occur in reactive hemophagocytic syndrome.
3. Shift of ferritin from tissue to plasma
   a. Liver disease such as hepatitis and necrosis: Tissue ferritin is released from damaged hepatocytes and is measured by ferritin assays that do not selectively measure glycosylated (or plasma) ferritin.[242] Most clinical assays probably measure glycosylated and nonglycosylated ferritin.
   b. Hemolytic diseases: Hyperferritinemia may relate to underlying inflammation or to increased transport demands due to Fe recycling from lysed erythrocytes.
C. Hypoferritinemia
   1. Decreased Fe storage
      a. Serum or plasma ferritin concentrations decrease as Fe stores decrease.
      b. In people, ferritin concentrations decrease early in Fe deficiency and before decreased blood [Hgb], microcytosis, or decreased serum [Fe] is detected. Once Fe stores are depleted, the decreased plasma ferritin concentrations remain relatively constant while hematologic evidence of the deficiency (anemia or microcytosis) develops.
   2. Because serum ferritin concentrations may be the net result of opposing processes, an Fe-deficient animal with inflammatory disease may not be hypoferritinemic.

VI. Reticulocyte Hgb content (CHr) and volume (MCVr)
   A. The ADVIA 120 hematology analyzer directly measures individual reticulocyte Hgb concentration and volume by light scatter. From these measures, CHr (the average amount of Hgb in reticulocytes) and MCVr (average reticulocyte volume) are calculated.
   B. Decreased CHr and MCVr were associated with typical findings of Fe deficiency in dogs.[98] These values may prove useful as early detectors of Fe deficiency, when the circulating mature cells lack evidence of Fe deficiency (i.e., the MCV and CHCM or MCHC are WRI) but the forming cells have a decreased CHr and MCVr.

VII. Comparative Fe profile results
   A. Assessment of the Fe status of an animal is enhanced if the laboratory assays are grouped as a profile.
   B. As shown in Table 3.20, the two major causes of hypoferremia can be differentiated by the assessment of Fe stores (either by stainable marrow or serum ferritin concentrations). However, the other conditions or disorders that can alter serum [Fe], TIBC, and Fe stores need to be considered.

BLOOD TYPING AND CROSSMATCHING

I. Blood typing
   A. Blood groups are important for transfusion medicine and NI.
      1. If the transfused erythrocytes are recognized as having foreign surface antigens, these are the two major consequences:

Table 3.20. Comparative Fe profile results

	Serum [Fe]	Serum TIBC	Stainable Fe in marrow[a]	Serum [ferritin]
Fe deficiency	↓	WRI–↑	↓	↓
Inflammation	↓	↓	↑	↑
Overload of Fe due to excess intake (diet or iatrogenic)	↑	WRI–↑	↑	↑
Increased glucocorticoids (except cattle)	↑	?	?	?
Pathologic hemolysis (in vivo)	WRI[b]	WRI[b]	WRI–↑	↑
Young animals (compared to mature)	↓ (foals and kittens)	↑ (foals)	↓	↓
Hepatic insufficiency	?	↓	?	↓–↑[c]
Hepatocyte necrosis	?	?	?	↑
Protein-losing nephropathy	?	↓	?	?

[a] Marrow samples of healthy cats do not have stainable Fe.

[b] Plasma Hgb may cause erroneous values (see the text).

[c] [Ferritin] could be decreased because of decreased production or it could be increased because of hepatocyte damage.

> a. If there are circulating antibodies in the recipient, those antibodies can attach to the transfused cells, which then results in a transfusion reaction and/or hemolysis of the transfused cells.
> b. If there is not a circulating antibody in the recipient, the recipient's immune system will be triggered to produce one.
> 2. Anti-erythrocyte antibodies may be naturally occurring (i.e., present without previous exposure), or acquired if they develop after exposure to foreign erythrocyte antigens.
> 3. Knowledge of blood groups is needed to understand NI. In this hemolytic state of neonates, antibodies in the colostrum are absorbed and then bind to the neonate's erythrocytes and mediate their destruction.
> B. Blood typing involves methods to detect the erythrocyte blood-group factors on the surface of the erythrocytes. Most methods involve antibodies that are produced in laboratory animals by injecting the blood-group antigen. For many years, blood typing was limited to a few specialized research laboratories that produced or developed blood-typing reagents (either polyclonal or monoclonal). Blood typing in horses is still limited to a few laboratories.
> C. Blood-typing cards have been developed commercially for dog and cat blood. In these tests, a small drop of blood is added to a white card impregnated with an antibody (or other agglutinin). If there is a positive reaction, the erythrocytes agglutinate.
> 1. For dogs, the blood-typing card is used to determine whether the dog is DEA 1.1 positive or negative. The agglutinin is an antibody.

2. For cats, the blood-typing card is used to determine whether the cat is type A, B, or AB. Type A antigen is detected with an agglutinating antibody; type B antigen is detected with a wheat germ lectin.

II. Crossmatching
A. Crossmatching procedures are used to help determine whether an animal's blood can be safely transfused into another animal. Crossmatching is similar to blood typing in that the laboratory assays involve antibody reactions to erythrocyte antigens. However, they are different in that the antibody is present in a recipient's plasma (for major crossmatch) or in the donor's plasma (for minor crossmatch).
B. The basic aspects of the assay are as follows:
   1. Blood is drawn from a patient that needs a blood transfusion (the recipient) and from a donor. Plasma or serum is separated from the erythrocytes, and the erythrocytes are washed in saline several times to remove loosely bound proteins.
   2. Major crossmatch
      a. The procedure involves mixing and incubating a dilute suspension of potential donor's erythrocytes with the recipient's serum. Antibody binding is detected by agglutination, hemolysis, or a Coombs' test.
      b. A compatible major crossmatch indicates that alloantibodies against the donor's erythrocytes were not detected. An incompatible major crossmatch indicates that alloantibodies against the donor's erythrocytes were detected.
      c. There is not a standard crossmatching procedure in veterinary medicine, so results may vary. An incompatible crossmatch may occur when the alloantibody detected is not clinically significant. Conversely, some significant alloantibodies are not detected by agglutination and require complement reactions or Coombs' testing for detection.
   3. Minor crossmatch (not done as frequently as the major)
      a. The procedure involves mixing and incubating a dilute suspension of recipient's erythrocytes with potential donor's serum.
      b. An incompatible minor crossmatch is usually not a clinical concern because it is not expected to cause a major transfusion reaction.

III. Species variations
A. Natural antibodies against DEA 1.1 and DEA 1.2 have not been reported, and thus rejection of the first transfusion of blood of unknown type is not expected. However, if the donor dog is DEA 1.1 positive and the recipient is DEA 1.1 negative (about a 25 % chance), the recipient will develop acquired anti-(DEA 1.1) antibodies. The DEA 3 system does have natural antibodies that can attack transfused erythrocytes: About 6 % of US dogs are DEA 3 positive, and about 20 % of DEA 3-negative dogs have the natural antibody.[246]
B. Cats have natural isoantibodies against the antigen they are lacking; that is, type A cats have anti-B antibodies, type B cats have anti-A antibodies, and type AB cats do not have isoantibodies. If blood types are not known or if a cat has had a previous transfusion with untyped blood, crossmatching should be completed.[246,247]
C. Blood-type systems in horses are more complex, and crossmatching procedures are not as simple as those for dogs and cats. Some of the antibodies are agglutinins, but others are poor agglutinins and thus require complement as a reagent to detect antibody binding.[247]

1. Horses that lack an erythrocyte antigen may have natural isoantibodies.[248]
   a. Horses lacking erythrocyte antigen A (EEA) may have anti-Aa or anti-Ac antibodies.
   b. Horses lacking erythrocyte antigen C (EEC) will typically have a low titer of anti-C antibodies.
   c. Isoantibodies to other erythrocyte antigens D, K, P, and U are rare to infrequent.
2. Horses may be sensitized to erythrocyte antigens via blood transfusions or during pregnancy. The acquired antibodies that cause transfusion reactions or NI are primarily against EEA, EEQ, and EEC. The antibodies may cause an incompatible reaction in the major crossmatch.
D. Blood-type systems in cattle are extremely complex, and thus it is essentially impossible to give a compatible transfusion.

METHODS FOR DETECTING ERYTHROCYTE SURFACE ANTIBODY OR COMPLEMENT

I. Coombs' test (direct antiglobulin test)
   A. Purpose: To detect ESAIg or complement on a patient's erythrocytes, usually to help diagnose immune hemolytic anemia
   B. Method for the direct Coombs' test
      1. A patient's erythrocytes are washed three times with saline to remove nonbound proteins.
      2. Antiglobulin is added (species-specific anti-IgG, anti-IgM, and/or anticomplement). Sera that contain two or more types of antiglobulin are called *polyvalent antisera*. Antiglobulins will bind to any IgG, IgM, or complement on the washed erythrocytes.
      3. A source of fresh complement proteins is needed for a hemolytic reaction in the equine Coombs' test. The hemolytic reaction is needed because equine erythrocytes may not agglutinate in the direct Coombs' test.
      4. Positive reactions
         a. Agglutination indicates that a patient's erythrocytes are coated with hundreds of immunoglobulin or C3 molecules and that the binding of the antiserum's immunoglobulin was sufficient to cause agglutination (Fig. 3.15).
            (1) For agglutination to occur, there must be the appropriate ratio of antigen and antibodies. To reduce the possibility of false-negative results caused by the prozone response, Coombs' tests are frequently completed with multiple dilutions of antiglobulin sera.
            (2) If there is a prozone reaction, the Coombs' test might be negative with a low dilution but positive at higher dilutions; for example, negative at a 1:2 antiserum dilution, weakly positive at a 1:4 dilution, and strongly positive at a 1:8 dilution.
         b. Hemolysis suggests that immune complexes formed between the antiserum immunoglobulin and the ESAIg and that these immune complexes led to complement activation and erythrocyte lysis.
         c. Coombs' tests are not standardized and are often unnecessary, given other clinical and laboratory findings. Negative results are common in cases that present, progress, and respond like immune hemolytic anemias. Positive results do occur in samples from animals without clinically significant hemolysis.

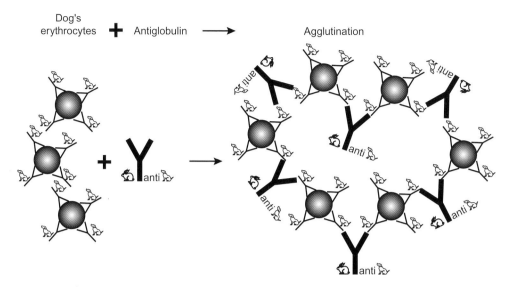

Fig. 3.15. Agglutination reaction of a positive canine Coombs' test. Washed canine erythrocytes are incubated with rabbit anti-(dog immunoglobulin). If the dog's washed erythrocytes are coated with dog immunoglobulin, the antiserum will cause agglutination of the dog's erythrocytes when the concentration of rabbit anti-(dog immunoglobulin) is appropriate. Tests may also detect erythrocyte-bound complement proteins by using anti-(dog complement) immunoglobulin.

II.   Flow cytometric detection of ESAIg
    A. Purpose: To detect ESAIg or complement on a patient's erythrocytes, usually to help diagnose immune hemolytic anemia.
    B. Analytic principles
        1. EDTA blood is the preferred sample and should be kept cool during transport. Erythrocytes are washed at least three times with saline or phosphate-buffered saline prior to a dilute erythrocyte suspension being made.
        2. Washed erythrocytes are incubated with fluorescein-labeled antibodies against IgG, IgM, or complement.
        3. If the patient's erythrocytes are coated with antibodies (or complement), the fluorescein-labeled antibodies will bind to them to make those erythrocytes fluorescent.
        4. Flow cytometry identifies those erythrocytes that are fluorescent and those that are not. A positive result has been identified by an increased percentage of fluorescent cells[249] or by an increased mean fluorescence intensity of the erythrocyte population.[250]
    C. Disorders with ESAIg
        1. Any of the immune-mediated hemolytic disorders can result in an accumulation of erythrocytes with increased ESAIg. These include idiopathic IMHA, drug-induced IMHA, vaccine-induced IMHA, NI, incompatible blood transfusion, and IMHA induced by bacterial and viral infections.
        2. Finding erythrocytes coated with increased ESAIg supports a conclusion of an IMHA but does not establish a diagnosis.

References

1. Koury ST, Bondurant MC, Semenza GL, Koury MJ. 1993. The use of in situ hybridization to study erythropoietin gene expression in murine kidney and liver. Microsc Res Tech 25:29–39.

2. Stockmann C, Fandrey J. 2006. Hypoxia-induced erythropoietin production: A paradigm for oxygen-regulated gene expression. Clin Exp Pharmacol Physiol 33:968–979.

3. Dessypris EN. 1999. Erythropoiesis. In: Lee GR, Foerster J, Lukens J, Paraskevas F, Greer JP, Rodgers GM, eds. *Wintrobe's Clinical Hematology*, 10th edition, 169–192. Philadelphia: Lippincott Williams & Wilkins.

4. Harvey JW. 1997. The erythrocyte: Physiology, metabolism, and biochemical disorders. In: Kaneko JJ, Harvey JW, Bruss ML, eds. *Clinical Biochemistry of Domestic Animals*, 5th edition, 157–203. San Diego: Academic.

5. Rettig MP, Low PS, Gimm JA, Mohandas N, Wang J, Christian JA. 1999. Evaluation of biochemical changes during in vivo erythrocyte senescence in the dog. Blood 93:376–384.

6. Kaneko JJ. 2000. Hemoglobin synthesis and destruction. In: Feldman BF, Zinkl JG, Jain NC, eds. *Schalm's Veterinary Hematology*, 5th edition, 135–139. Philadelphia: Lippincott Williams & Wilkins.

7. Smith JE. 1997. Iron metabolism and its disorders. In: Kaneko JJ, Harvey JW, Bruss ML, eds. *Clinical Biochemistry of Domestic Animals*, 5th edition, 223–239. San Diego: Academic.

8. Fry MM, Liggett JL, Baek SJ. 2004. Molecular cloning and expression of canine hepcidin. Vet Clin Pathol 33:223–227.

9. Ganz T. 2005. Hepcidin: A regulator of intestinal iron absorption and iron recycling by macrophages. Best Pract Res Clin Haematol 18:171–182.

10. Cooper C, Sears W, Bienzle D. 2005. Reticulocyte changes after experimental anemia and erythropoietin treatment of horses. J Appl Physiol 99:915–921.

11. Cramer DV, Lewis RM. 1972. Reticulocyte response in the cat. J Am Vet Med Assoc 160:61–67.

12. Alsaker RD, Laber J, Stevens J, Perman V. 1977. A comparison of polychromasia and reticulocyte counts in assessing erythrocytic regenerative response in the cat. J Am Vet Med Assoc 170:39–41.

13. Schalm OW, Jain NC, Carroll EJ. 1975. *Veterinary Hematology*, 3rd edition. Philadelphia: Lea & Febiger.

14. Fan LC, Dorner JL, Hoffmann WE. 1978. Reticulocyte response and maturation in experimental acute blood loss anemia in the cat. J Am Anim Hosp Assoc 14:219–224.

15. Schalm OW. 1980. Differential diagnosis of anemias in cattle. Part I: Massive blood loss by repeated phlebotomies. Bovine Pract 1:10–17.

16. Lundberg GD, Iverson C, Radulescu G. 1986. Now read this: The SI units are here. J Am Med Assoc 255:2329–2339.

17. Tvedten HW, Holan K. 1996. What is your diagnosis? Peripheral blood from a 13-year-old Abyssinian–mixed breed cat. Vet Clin Pathol 25:148–149 and 153–154.

18. Weiser MG. 1983. Comparison of two automated multi-channel blood cell counting systems for analysis of blood of common domestic animals. Vet Clin Pathol 12:25–32.

19. Weiser MG. 1987. Modification and evaluation of a multichannel blood cell counting system of blood analysis in veterinary hematology. J Am Vet Med Assoc 190:411–415.

20. Magona JW, Walubengo J, Anderson I, Olaho-Mukani W, Jonsson NN, Eisler MC. 2004. Portable haemoglobinometers and their potential for penside detection of anaemia in bovine disease diagnosis: A comparative evaluation. Vet J 168:343–348.

21. Boisvert AM, Tvedten HW, Scott MA. 1999. Artifactual effects of hypernatremia and hyponatremia on red cell analytes measured by the Bayer H*1 analyzer. Vet Clin Pathol 28:91–96.

22. McMahon DJ, Carpenter RL. 1990. A comparison of conductivity-based hematocrit determinations with conventional laboratory methods in autologous blood transfusions. Anesth Analg 71:541–544.

23. Green RA. 1999. Spurious platelet effects on erythrocyte indices using the CELL-DYN 3500 automated hematology system. Vet Clin Pathol 28:47–51.

24. Schisano T, Van Hove L. 2002. Abbott Cell-Dyn reticulocyte method comparison and reticulocyte normal reference range evaluation. Lab Hematol 8:85–90.

25. Cicha I, Suzuki Y, Tateishi N, Maeda N. 2001. Enhancement of red blood cell aggregation by plasma triglycerides. Clin Hemorheol Microcirc 24:247–255.

26. Canfield PJ, Watson ADJ. 1989. Investigations of bone marrow dyscrasia in a poodle with macrocytosis. J Comp Pathol 101:269–278.

27. Schalm OW, Smith R. 1963. Some unique aspects of feline hematology in disease. Small Anim Clin 3:311–318.

28. Weiss DJ. 2005. Sideroblastic anemia in 7 dogs (1996–2002). J Vet Intern Med 19:325–328.

29. Harvey JW. 2001. *Atlas of Veterinary Hematology: Blood and Bone Marrow of Domestic Animals*. Philadelphia: WB Saunders.

30. Gookin JL, Bunch SE, Rush LJ, Grindem CB. 1998. Evaluation of microcytosis in 18 Shibas. J Am Vet Med Assoc 212:1258–1259.

31. Harvey JW, Asquith RL, Sussman WA, Kivipelto J. 1987. Serum ferritin, serum iron, and erythrocyte values in foals. Am J Vet Res 48:1348–1352.

32. Weiser MG, Kociba GJ. 1983. Sequential changes in erythrocyte volume distribution and microcytosis associated with iron deficiency in kittens. Vet Pathol 20:1–12.

33. Okabe J, Tajima S, Yamato O, Inaba M, Hagiwara S, Maede Y. 1996. Hemoglobin types, erythrocyte membrane skeleton and plasma iron concentration in calves with poikilocytosis. J Vet Med Sci 58:629–634.

34. Tennant B, Harrold D, Reina-Guerra M, Kaneko JJ. 1975. Hematology of the neonatal calf. III. Frequency of congenital iron deficiency anemia. Cornell Vet 65:543–556.

35. Weiss DJ, Kristensen A, Papenfuss N. 1993. Qualitative evaluation of irregularly spiculated red blood cells in the dog. Vet Clin Pathol 22:117–121.

36. Stockham SL, Harvey JW, Kinden DA. 1994. Equine glucose-6-phosphate dehydrogenase deficiency. Vet Pathol 31:518–527.

37. Harvey JW, Stockham SL, Scott MA, Johnson PJ, Donald JJ, Chandler CJ. 2003. Methemoglobinemia and eccentrocytosis in equine erythrocyte flavin adenine dinucleotide deficiency. Vet Pathol 40:632–642.

38. Weiss DJ, Geor R, Smith CM II, McClay CB. 1992. Furosemide-induced electrolyte depletion associated with echinocytosis in horses. Am J Vet Res 53:1769–1772.

39. McClay CB, Weiss DJ, Smith CM II, Gordon B. 1992. Evaluation of hemorheologic variables as implications for exercise-induced pulmonary hemorrhage in racing thoroughbreds. Am J Vet Res 53:1380–1385.

40. Brecher G, Bessis M. 1972. Present status of spiculated red cells and their relationship to the discocyte-echinocyte transformation: A critical review. Blood 40:333–344.

41. Geor RJ, Lund EM, Weiss DJ. 1993. Echinocytosis in horses: 54 cases (1990). J Am Vet Med Assoc 202:976–980.

42. Badylak SF, Van Vleet JF, Herman EH, Ferrans VJ, Myers CE. 1985. Poikilocytosis in dogs with chronic doxorubicin toxicosis. Am J Vet Res 46:505–508.

43. Smith JE, Mohandas N, Shohet SB. 1982. Interaction of amphipathic drugs with erythrocytes from various species. Am J Vet Res 43:1041–1048.

44. Chandler FW Jr, Prasse KW, Callaway CS. 1975. Surface ultrastructure of pyruvate kinase–deficient erythrocytes in the basenji dog. Am J Vet Res 36:1477–1480.

45. Prasse KW, Crouser D, Beutler E, Walker M, Schall WD. 1975. Pyruvate kinase deficiency anemia with terminal myelofibrosis and osteosclerosis in a beagle. J Am Vet Med Assoc 166:1170–1175.

46. Walton RM, Brown DE, Hamar DW, Meador VP, Horn JW, Thrall MA. 1997. Mechanisms of echinocytosis induced by *Crotalus atrox* venom. Vet Pathol 34:442–449.

47. Marks S, Mannella C, Schaer M. 1990. Coral snake envenomation in the dog: Report of four cases and review of the literature. J Am Anim Hosp Assoc 26:629–634.

48. Weiss DJ, Moritz A. 2003. Equine immune-mediated hemolytic anemia associated with *Clostridium perfringens* infection. Vet Clin Pathol 32:22–26.

49. Bessis M. 1977. *Blood Smears Reinterpreted.* Berlin: Springer International.

50. Christopher MM, Lee SE. 1994. Red cell morphologic alterations in cats with hepatic disease. Vet Clin Pathol 23:7–12.

51. O'Keefe DA, Schaeffer DJ. 1992. Hematologic toxicosis associated with doxorubicin administration in cats. J Vet Intern Med 6:276–282.

52. Weiss DJ, Lulich J. 1999. Myelodysplastic syndrome with sideroblastic differentiation in a dog. Vet Clin Pathol 28:59–63.

53. Hoff B, Lumsden JH, Valli VEO. 1985. An appraisal of bone marrow biopsy in assessment of sick dogs. Can J Comp Med 49:34–42.

54. Scavelli TD, Hornbuckle WE, Roth L, Rendano VT Jr, de Lahunta A, Center SA, French TW, Zimmer JF. 1986. Portosystemic shunts in cats: Seven cases (1976–1984). J Am Vet Med Assoc 189:317–325.

55. Smith JE, Moore K, Arens M, Rinderknecht GA, Ledet A. 1983. Hereditary elliptocytosis with protein band 4.1 deficiency in the dog. Blood 61:373–377.

56. Di Terlizzi R, Mohandas N, Dolce K, Rowland K, Wilkerson MJ, Stockham SL. 2007. Canine elliptocytosis due to defective spectrin.

57. Cazzola M, Dacco M, Ascari E. 1981. Pincered red cells and hereditary spherocytosis. Haematologica 66:498–502.

58. Domingo-Claros A, Larriba I, Rozman M, Irriguible D, Vallespi T, Aventin A, Ayats R, Milla F, Sole F, Florensa L, Gallart M, Tuset E, Lopez C, Woessner S. 2002. Acute erythroid neoplastic proliferations: A biological study based on 62 patients. Haematologica 87:148–153.

59. Cuadra M. 1959. Mechanism of formation of selenoid bodies. Acta Haematol 22:103–111.

60. Chapman BL, Giger U. 1990. Inherited erythrocyte pyruvate kinase deficiency in the West Highland white terrier. J Small Anim Pract 31:610–616.

61. Wysoke JM, Van-den Berg PB, Marshall C. 1990. Bee sting–induced haemolysis, spherocytosis and neural dysfunction in three dogs. J S Afr Vet Assoc 61:29–32.

62. Noble SJ, Armstrong PJ. 1999. Bee sting envenomation resulting in secondary immune-mediated hemolytic anemia in two dogs. J Am Vet Med Assoc 214:1026–1027.

63. Inaba M, Yawata A, Koshino I, Sato K, Takeuchi M, Takakuwa Y, Manno S, Yawata Y, Kanzaki A, Sakai J, Ban A, Ono K, Maede Y. 1996. Defective anion transport and marked spherocytosis with membrane instability caused by hereditary total deficiency of red cell band 3 in cattle due to a nonsense mutation. J Clin Invest 97:1804–1817.

64. Holland CT, Canfield PJ, Watson ADJ, Allan GS. 1991. Dyserythropoiesis, polymyopathy, and cardiac disease in three related English springer spaniels. J Vet Intern Med 5:151–159.

65. Slappendel RJ, van der Gaag I, van Nes JJ, van den Ingh ThSGAM, Happæ RP. 1991. Familial stomatocytosis-hypertrophic gastritis (FSHG), a newly recognised disease in the dog (Drentse patrijshond). Vet Q 13:30–40.

66. Brown DE, Weiser MG, Thrall MA, Giger U, Just CA. 1994. Erythrocyte indices and volume distribution in a dog with stomatocytosis. Vet Pathol 31:247–250.

67. Bonfanti U, Comazzi S, Paltrinieri S, Bertazzolo W. 2004. Stomatocytosis in 7 related standard schnauzers. Vet Clin Pathol 33:234–239.

68. Smith SE, Loosli JK. 1957. Cobalt and vitamin B_{12} in ruminant nutrition: A review. J Dairy Sci 40:1215–1227.

69. Steffen DJ, Elliot GS, Leipold HW, Smith JE. 1992. Congenital dyserythropoiesis and progressive alopecia in polled Hereford calves: Hematologic, biochemical, bone marrow cytologic, electrophoretic, and flow cytometric findings. J Vet Diagn Invest 4:31–37.

70. Hinchliffe RF, Bellamy GJ, Lilleyman JS. 1992. Use of the Technicon H1 hypochromia flag in detecting spurious macrocytosis induced by excessive K_2-EDTA concentration. Clin Lab Haematol 14:268–269.

71. Goossens W, van Duppen V, Verwilghen RL. 1991. K_2- or K_3-EDTA: The anticoagulant of choice in routine hematology? Clin Lab Haematol 13:291–295.

72. Seguin MA, Bunch SE. 2001. Iatrogenic copper deficiency associated with long-term copper chelation for treatment of copper storage disease in a Bedlington terrier. J Am Vet Med Assoc 218:1593–1597.

73. van Wyk JJ, Baxter JH, Akeroyd JH, Motulsky AG. 1953. The anemia of copper deficiency in dogs compared with that produced by iron deficiency. Bull Johns Hopkins Hosp 93:41–49.

74. Bain BJ. 1995. Detecting erroneous blood counts. In: *Blood Cells: A Practice Guide*, 2nd edition, 132–146. Cambridge, MA: Blackwell Science.

75. Roberts WL, Fontenot JD, Lehman CM. 2000. Overestimation of hemoglobin in a patient with an IgA-kappa monoclonal gammopathy. Arch Pathol Lab Med 124:616–618.

76. Ham TH, Grauel JA, Dunn RF, Murphy JR, White JG, Kellermeyer RW. 1973. Physical properties of red cells as related to effects in vivo. IV. Oxidant drugs producing abnormal intracellular concentration of hemoglobin (eccentrocytes) with a rigid-red-cell hemolytic syndrome. J Lab Clin Med 82:898–910.

77. Means RT Jr. 1999. Advances in the anemia of chronic disease. Int J Hematol 70:7–12.

78. Weiss DJ, McClay CB. 1988. Studies on the pathogenesis of the erythrocyte destruction associated with the anemia of inflammatory disease. Vet Clin Pathol 17:90–93.

79. Meinkoth JH, Kocan AA. 2005. Feline cytauxzoonosis. Vet Clin North Am Small Anim Pract 35:89–101.

80. Hoover JP, Walker DB, Hedges JD. 1994. Cytauxzoonosis in cats: Eight cases (1985–1992). J Am Vet Med Assoc 205:455–460.

81. Meinkoth J, Kocan AA, Whitworth L, Murphy G, Fox JC, Woods JP. 2000. Cats surviving natural infection with *Cytauxzoon felis*: 18 cases (1997–1998). J Vet Intern Med 14:521–525.

82. Gaunt SD, Pierce KR. 1986. Effects of estradiol on hematopoietic and marrow adherent cells of dogs. Am J Vet Res 47:906–909.

83. Legendre AM. 1976. Estrogen-induced bone marrow hypoplasia in a dog. J Am Anim Hosp Assoc 12:525–527.

84. Watson ADJ, Wilson JT, Turner DM, Culvenor JA. 1980. Phenylbutazone-induced blood dyscrasias suspected in three dogs. Vet Rec 107:239–241.

85. Schalm OW. 1979. Phenylbutazone toxicity in two dogs. Canine Pract 6:47–51.

86. Stokol T, Blue JT, French TW. 2000. Idiopathic pure red cell aplasia and nonregenerative immune-mediated anemia in dogs: 43 cases (1988–1999). J Am Vet Med Assoc 216:1429–1436.

87. Weiss DJ. 1986. Antibody-mediated suppression of erythropoiesis in dogs with red blood cell aplasia. Am J Vet Res 47:2646–2648.

88. Thenen SW, Rasmussen KM. 1978. Megaloblastic erythropoiesis and tissue depletion of folic acid in the cat. Am J Vet Res 39:1205–1207.

89. Vaden SL, Wood PA, Ledley FD, Cornwell PE, Miller RT, Page R. 1992. Cobalamin deficiency associated with methylmalonic acidemia in a cat. J Am Vet Med Assoc 200:1101–1103.
90. Fyfe JC, Jezyk PF, Giger U, Patterson DF. 1989. Inherited selective malabsorption of vitamin B$_{12}$ in giant schnauzers. J Am Anim Hosp Assoc 25:533–539.
91. Battersby IA, Giger U, Hall EJ. 2005. Hyperammonaemic encephalopathy secondary to selective cobalamin deficiency in a juvenile Border collie. J Small Anim Pract 46:339–344.
92. Watson ADJ, Canfield PJ. 2000. Nutritional deficiency anemias. In: Feldman BF, Zinkl JG, Jain NC, eds. *Schalm's Veterinary Hematology*, 5th edition, 190–195. Philadelphia: Lippincott Williams & Wilkins.
93. Bai SC, Sampson DA, Morris JG, Rogers QR. 1989. Vitamin B-6 requirement of growing kittens. J Nutr 119:1020–1027.
94. Dryden MW, Broce AB, Moore WE. 1993. Severe flea infestation in dairy calves. J Am Vet Med Assoc 203:1448–1452.
95. Clark CH, Woodley CH. 1959. The absorption of red blood cells after parenteral injection at various sites. Am J Vet Res 20:1062–1066.
96. Anderson C, Aronson I, Jacobs P. 2000. Erythropoiesis: Erythrocyte deformability is reduced and fragility increased by iron deficiency. Hematology 4:457–460.
97. Burkhard MJ, Brown DE, McGrath JP, Meador VP, Mayle DA, Keaton MJ, Hoffman WP, Zimmermann JL, Abbott DL, Sun SC. 2001. Evaluation of the erythroid regenerative response in two different models of experimentally induced iron deficiency anemia. Vet Clin Pathol 30:76–85.
98. Steinberg JD, Olver CS. 2005. Hematologic and biochemical abnormalities indicating iron deficiency are associated with decreased reticulocyte hemoglobin content (CHr) and reticulocyte volume (rMCV) in dogs. Vet Clin Pathol 34:23–27.
99. Stone AM, Stein T, LaFortune J, Wise L. 1979. Renal vascular effects of stroma and stroma-free hemoglobin. Surg Gynecol Obstet 149:874–876.
100. Chan WL, Tang NLS, Yim CCW, Lai FM, Tam MSC. 2000. New features of renal lesion induced by stroma free hemoglobin. Toxicol Pathol 28:635–642.
101. Slappendel RJ. 1979. The diagnostic significance of the direct antiglobulin test (DAT) in anemic dogs. Vet Immunol Immunopathol 1:49–59.
102. Barker RN, Gruffydd-Jones TJ, Stokes CR, Elson CJ. 1992. Autoimmune haemolysis in the dog: Relationship between anaemia and the levels of red blood cell–bound immunoglobins and complement measured by an enzyme-linked antiglobulin test. Vet Immunol Immunopathol 34:1–20.
103. Petz LD, Mueller-Eckhardt C. 1992. Drug-induced immune hemolytic anemia. Transfusion 32:202–204.
104. McConnico RS, Roberts MC, Tompkins M. 1992. Penicillin-induced immune-mediated hemolytic anemia in a horse. J Am Vet Med Assoc 201:1402–1403.
105. Blue JT, Dinsmore RP, Anderson KL. 1987. Immune-mediated hemolytic anemia induced by penicillin in horses. Cornell Vet 77:263–276.
106. Aucoin DP, Peterson ME, Hurvitz AI, Drayer DE, Lahita RG, Quimby FW, Reidenberg MM. 1985. Propylthiouracil-induced immune-mediated disease in the cat. J Pharmacol Exp Ther 234:13–18.
107. Bloom JC, Thiem PA, Sellers TS, Deldar A, Lewis HB. 1988. Cephalosporin-induced immune cytopenia in the dog: Demonstration of erythrocyte-, neutrophil-, and platelet-associated IgG following treatment with cefazedone. Am J Hematol 28:71–78. [Erratum in Am J Hematol 1988;29:241.]
108. Thomas HL, Livesey MA. 1998. Immune-mediated hemolytic anemia associated with trimethoprim-sulphamethoxazole administration in a horse. Can Vet J 39:171–173.
109. Atwell RB, Johnstone I, Read R, Reilly J, Wilkins S. 1979. Haemolytic anaemia in two dogs suspected to have been induced by levamisole. Aust Vet J 55:292–294.
110. Jackson JA, Chart IS, Sanderson JH, Garner R. 1977. Pirimicarb induced immune haemolytic anaemia in dogs. Scand J Haematol 19:360–366.
111. Schwartz RS, Silberstein LE, Berkman EM. 1995. Autoimmune hemolytic anemias. In: Hoffman R, Benz EJ Jr, Shattil SJ, Furie B, Cohen HJ, Silberstein LE, eds. *Hematology: Basic Principles and Practice*, 2nd edition, 710–729. New York: Churchill Livingstone.
112. Duval D, Giger U. 1996. Vaccine-associated immune-mediated hemolytic anemia in the dog. J Vet Intern Med 10:290–295.
113. Yeruham I, Avidar Y, Harrus S, Fishman L, Aroch I. 2003. Immune-mediated thrombocytopenia and putative haemolytic anaemia associated with a polyvalent botulism vaccination in a cow. Vet Rec 153:502–504.
114. Oakley DA, Giger U. 1997. Just their type: Feline transfusions and blood donors. Vet Tech 18:747–752.
115. Giger U. 2000. Regenerative anemias caused by blood loss or hemolysis. In: Ettinger SJ, Feldman EC, eds. *Textbook of Veterinary Internal Medicine: Diseases of the Dog and Cat*, 5th edition, 1784–1804. Philadelphia: WB Saunders.

116. Morris DD. 1998. Disease of the hemolymphatic system. In: Reed SM, Bayly WM, eds. *Equine Internal Medicine*, 1st edition, 558–601. Philadelphia: WB Saunders.

117. Boyle AG, Magdesian KG, Ruby RE. 2005. Neonatal isoerythrolysis in horse foals and a mule foal: 18 cases (1988–2003). J Am Vet Med Assoc 227:1276–1283.

118. Bailey E. 1982. Prevalence of anti–red blood cell antibodies in the serum and colostrum of mares and its relationship to neonatal isoerythrolysis. Am J Vet Res 43:1917–1921.

119. Kocan KM, Blouin EF, Barbet AF. 2000. Anaplasmosis control: Past, present, and future. Ann NY Acad Sci 916:501–509.

120. Luther DG, Cox HU, Nelson WO. 1985. Screening for neonatal isohemolytic anemia in calves. Am J Vet Res 46:1078–1079.

121. Kewish KE, Appleyard GD, Myers SL, Kidney BA, Jackson ML. 2004. *Mycoplasma haemofelis* and *Mycoplasma haemominutum* detection by polymerase chain reaction in cats from Saskatchewan and Alberta. Can Vet J 45:749–752.

122. Tasker S, Braddock JA, Baral R, Helps CR, Day MJ, Gruffydd-Jones TJ, Malik R. 2004. Diagnosis of feline haemoplasma infection in Australian cats using a real-time PCR assay. J Feline Med Surg 6:345–354.

123. Sykes JE. 2003. Feline hemotropic mycoplasmosis (feline hemobartonellosis). Vet Clin North Am Small Anim Pract 33:773–789.

124. Willi B, Boretti FS, Cattori V, Tasker S, Meli ML, Reusch C, Lutz H, Hofmann-Lehmann R. 2005. Identification, molecular characterization, and experimental transmission of a new hemoplasma isolate from a cat with hemolytic anemia in Switzerland. J Clin Microbiol 43:2581–2585.

125. Sykes JE, Bailiff NL, Ball LM, Foreman O, George JW, Fry MM. 2004. Identification of a novel hemotropic mycoplasma in a splenectomized dog with hemic neoplasia. J Am Vet Med Assoc 224:1946–1951.

126. Sykes JE, Ball LM, Bailiff NL, Fry MM. 2005. "*Candidatus* Mycoplasma haematoparvum", a novel small haemotropic mycoplasma from a dog. Int J Syst Evol Microbiol 55:27–30.

127. Swenson C, Jacobs R. 1986. Spherocytosis associated with anaplasmosis in two cows. J Am Vet Med Assoc 188:1061–1064.

128. Giardina S, Aso PM, Bretana A. 1993. Antigen recognition on *Anaplasma marginale* and bovine erythrocytes: An electron microscopy study. Vet Immunol Immunopathol 38:183–191.

129. Hartskeerl RA, Terpstra WJ. 1996. Leptospirosis in wild animals. Vet Q 18(Suppl 3):S149–S150.

130. Carlson GP. 1996. Leptospirosis. In: Smith BP, ed. *Large Animal Internal Medicine*, 2nd edition, 1222–1223. St Louis: CV Mosby.

131. Timoney JF, Gillespie JH, Scott FW, Barlough JE. 1988. The spirochetes. In: Timoney JF, Gillespie JH, Scott FW, Barlough JE, eds. *Hagan and Bruner's Microbiology and Infectious Diseases of Domestic Animals*, 8th edition, 45–60. Ithaca, NY: Comstock.

132. Decker MJ, Freeman MJ, Morter RL. 1970. Evaluation of mechanisms of leptospiral hemolytic anemia. Am J Vet Res 31:873–878.

133. Bhasin JL, Freeman MJ, Morter RL. 1971. Properties of a cold hemagglutinin associated with leptospiral hemolytic anemia of sheep. Infect Immun 3:398–404.

134. Keenan KP, Alexander AD, Montgomery CA Jr. 1978. Pathogenesis of experimental *Leptospira interrogans*, serovar *bataviae*, infection in the dog: Microbiological, clinical, hematologic, and biochemical studies. Am J Vet Res 39:449–454.

135. Chorváth B, Bakoss P. 1972. Studies on leptospiral lipase. II. Lipase activity of virulent and avirulent leptospirae. J Hyg Epidemiol Microbiol Immunol 16:352–357.

136. Kasarov LB. 1970. Degradation of the erythrocyte phospholipids and haemolysis of the erythrocytes of different animal species by leptospirae. J Med Microbiol 3:29–37.

137. Trowbridge AA, Green JB III, Bonnett JD, Shohet SB, Ponnappa BD, McCombs WB III. 1981. Hemolytic anemia associated with leptospirosis: Morphologic and lipid studies. Am J Clin Pathol 76:493–498.

138. Lozano EA, Smith LDS. 1967. Electrophoretic fractionation of *Clostridium hemolyticum* toxic culture fluids. Am J Vet Res 28:1569–1576.

139. McGowan B, Moulton JE, Rood SE. 1958. Lamb losses associated with *Clostridium perfringens* type A. J Am Vet Med Assoc 113:219–221.

140. Songer JG. 1996. Clostridial enteric diseases of domestic animals. Clin Microbiol Rev 9:216–234.

141. Pun KC, Wehner JH. 1996. Abdominal pain and massive intravascular hemolysis in a 47-year-old man. Chest 110:1353–1355.

142. Ishii S. 1963. Equine infectious anemia or swamp fever. Adv Vet Sci 9:263–298.

143. McGuire TC, Henson JB, Quist SE. 1969. Viral-induced hemolysis in equine infectious anemia. Am J Vet Res 30:2091–2097.

144. Cotter SM. 1979. Anemia associated with feline leukemia virus infection. J Am Vet Med Assoc 175:1191–1194.

145. Mackey L, Jarrett W, Jarrett O, Laird H. 1975. Anemia associated with feline leukemia virus infection in cats. J Natl Cancer Inst 54:209–217.

146. Kjemtrup AM, Kocan AA, Whitworth L, Meinkoth J, Birkenheuer AJ, Cummings J, Boudreaux MK, Stockham SL, Irizarry-Rovira A, Conrad PA. 2000. There are at least three genetically distinct small piroplasms from dogs. Int J Parasitol 30:1501–1505.

147. Baneth G, Kenny MJ, Tasker S, Anug Y, Shkap V, Levy A, Shaw SE. 2004. Infection with a proposed new subspecies of *Babesia canis*, *Babesia canis* subsp. *presentii*, in domestic cats. J Clin Microbiol 42:99–105.

148. Penzhorn BL, Schoeman T, Jacobson LS. 2004. Feline babesiosis in South Africa: A review. Ann NY Acad Sci 1026:183–186.

149. Irwin PJ, Hutchinson GW. 1991. Clinical and pathological findings of *Babesia* infection in dogs. Aust Vet J 68:204–209.

150. O'Connor RM, Allred DR. 2000. Selection of *Babesia bovis*-infected erythrocytes for adhesion to endothelial cells coselects for altered variant erythrocyte surface antigen isoforms. J Immunol 164:2037–2045.

151. Furlanello T, Fiorio F, Caldin M, Lubas G, Solano-Gallego L. 2005. Clinicopathological findings in naturally occurring cases of babesiosis caused by large form *Babesia* from dogs of northeastern Italy. Vet Parasitol 134:77–85.

152. Mehlhorn H, Schein E. 1998. Redescription of *Babesia equi* Laveran, 1901 as *Theileria equi* Mehlhorn, Schein 1998. Parasitol Res 84:467–475.

153. Camacho AT, Guitian FJ, Pallas E, Gestal JJ, Olmeda AS, Habela MA, Telford SR III, Spielman A. 2005. *Theileria* (*Babesia*) *equi* and *Babesia caballi* infections in horses in Galicia, Spain. Trop Anim Health Prod 37:293–302.

154. Chae J, Lee J, Kwon O, Holman PJ, Waghela SD, Wagner GG. 1998. Nucleotide sequence heterogeneity in the small subunit ribosomal RNA gene variable (V4) region among and within geographic isolates of *Theileria* from cattle, elk and white-tailed deer. Vet Parasitol 75:41–52.

155. Stockham SL, Kjemtrup AM, Conrad PA, Schmidt DA, Scott MA, Robinson TW, Tyler JW, Johnson GC, Carson CA, Cuddihee P. 2000. Theileriosis in a Missouri beef herd caused by *Theileria buffeli*: Case report, herd investigation, ultrastructure, phylogenetic analysis, and experimental transmission. Vet Pathol 37:11–21.

156. Cossio-Bayugar R, Pillars R, Schlater J, Holman PJ. 2002. *Theileria buffeli* infection of a Michigan cow confirmed by small subunit ribosomal RNA gene analysis. Vet Parasitol 105:105–110.

157. Irvin AD. 1987. Characterization of species and strains of *Theileria*. Adv Parasitol 26:145–197.

158. Shimizu S, Yagi Y, Nakamura Y, Shimura K, Fujisaki K, Onodera T, Minami T, Ito S. 1990. Clinico-hematological observation of calves experimentally infected with *Theileria sergenti*. Jpn J Vet Sci 52:1337–1339.

159. Hofmann-Lehmann R, Meli ML, Dreher UM, Gonczi E, Deplazes P, Braun U, Engels M, Schupbach J, Jorger K, Thoma R, Griot C, Stark KD, Willi B, Schmidt J, Kocan KM, Lutz H. 2004. Concurrent infections with vector-borne pathogens associated with fatal hemolytic anemia in a cattle herd in Switzerland. J Clin Microbiol 42:3775–3780.

160. Camacho AT, Guitian EJ, Pallas E, Gestal JJ, Olmeda AS, Goethert HK, Telford SR III, Spielman A. 2004. Azotemia and mortality among *Babesia microti*-like infected dogs. J Vet Intern Med 18:141–146.

161. Radostits OM, Gay CC, Blood DC, Hinchcliff KW. 2000. Diseases caused by protozoa. In: Radostits OM, Gay CC, Blood DC, Hinchcliff KW, eds. *Veterinary Medicine*, 9th edition, 1289–1338. London: WB Saunders.

162. Barr SC. 2000. Trypanosomiasis: American trypanosomiasis. In: Greene CE, ed. *Infectious Diseases of the Dog and Cat*, 2nd edition, 445–448. Philadelphia: WB Saunders.

163. Anosa VO, Logan-Henfrey LL, Shaw MK. 1992. A light and electron microscopic study of changes in blood and bone marrow in acute hemorrhagic *Trypanosoma vivax* infection in calves. Vet Pathol 29:33–45.

164. Kobayashi A, Tizard IR, Woo PT. 1976. Studies on the anemia in experimental African trypanosomiasis. II. The pathogenesis of the anemia in calves infected with *Trypanosoma congolense*. Am J Trop Med Hyg 25:401–406.

165. Mackenzie PKI, Boyt WP, Nesham VW, Pirie E. 1978. The aetiology and significance of the phagocytosis of erythrocytes and leucocytes in sheep infected with *Trypanosoma congolense* (Broden, 1904). Res Vet Sci 24:4–7.

166. Winterbourn CC. 1990. Oxidative denaturation in congenital hemolytic anemias: The unstable hemoglobins. Semin Hematol 27:41–50.

167. Yamato O, Hayashi M, Yamasaki M, Maede Y. 1998. Induction of onion-induced haemolytic anaemia in dogs with sodium *n*-propylthiosulphate. Vet Rec 142:216–219.

168. Munday R, Munday JS. 2003. Comparative haemolytic activity of bis(phenylmethyl) disulphide, bis(phenylethyl) disulphide and bis(phenylpropyl) disulphide in rats. Food Chem Toxicol 41:1609–1615.

169. Munday R, Munday JS, Munday CM. 2003. Comparative effects of mono-, di-, tri-, and tetrasulfides derived from plants of the *Allium* family: Redox cycling in vitro and hemolytic activity and Phase 2 enzyme induction in vivo. Free Radic Biol Med 34:1200–1211.

170. Luttgen PJ, Whitney MS, Wolf AM, Scruggs DW. 1990. Heinz body hemolytic anemia associated with high plasma zinc concentration in a dog. J Am Vet Med Assoc 197:1347–1350.

171. Yamato O, Kasai E, Katsura T, Takahashi S, Shiota T, Tajima M, Yamasaki M, Maede Y. 2005. Heinz body hemolytic anemia with eccentrocytosis from ingestion of Chinese chive (*Allium tuberosum*) and garlic (*Allium sativum*) in a dog. J Am Anim Hosp Assoc 41:68–73.

172. Zaks KL, Tan EO, Thrall MA. 2005. Heinz body anemia in a dog that had been sprayed with skunk musk. J Am Vet Med Assoc 226:1516–1518.

173. DesNoyers M. 2000. Anemias associated with Heinz bodies. In: Feldman BF, Zinkl JG, Jain NC, eds. *Schalm's Veterinary Hematology*, 5th edition, 178–184. Philadelphia: Lippincott Williams & Wilkins.

174. Boyer JD, Breeden DC, Brown DL. 2002. Isolation, identification, and characterization of compounds from *Acer rubrum* capable of oxidizing equine erythrocytes. Am J Vet Res 63:604–610.

175. Pearson W, Boermans HJ, Bettger WJ, McBride BW, Lindinger MI. 2005. Association of maximum voluntary dietary intake of freeze-dried garlic with Heinz body anemia in horses. Am J Vet Res 66:457–465.

176. Nonneman D, Stockham SL, Shibuya H, Messer NT, Johnson GS. 1993. A missense mutation in the glucose-6-phosphate dehydrogenase gene is associated with hemolytic anemia in an American saddlebred horse. Blood 82(Suppl 1):466a (abstract).

177. Smith JE, Ryer K, Wallace L. 1976. Glucose-6-phosphate dehydrogenase deficiency in a dog. Enzyme 21:379–382.

178. Giger U, Mason GD, Wang P. 1991. Inherited erythrocyte pyruvate kinase deficiency in a beagle dog. Vet Clin Pathol 20:83–86.

179. Andresen E. 1977. Haemolytic anaemia in basenji dogs. 2. Partial deficiency of erythrocyte pyruvate kinase (PK; EC 2.7.1.40) in heterozygous carriers. Anim Blood Groups Biochem Genet 8:149–156.

180. Schaer M, Harvey JW, Calderwood-Mays M, Giger U. 1992. Pyruvate kinase deficiency causing hemolytic anemia with secondary hemochromatosis in a Cairn terrier. J Am Anim Hosp Assoc 28:233–239.

181. Harvey JW. 1996. Congenital erythrocyte enzyme deficiencies. Vet Clin North Am Small Anim Pract 26:1003–1011.

182. Ford S, Giger U, Duesberg C, Beutler E, Wang P. 1992. Inherited erythrocyte pyruvate kinase (PK) deficiency causing hemolytic anemia in an Abyssinian cat. J Vet Intern Med 6:123 (abstract).

183. Mansfield CS, Clark P. 2005. Pyruvate kinase deficiency in a Somali cat in Australia. Aust Vet J 83:483–485.

184. Whitney KM, Lothrop CD Jr. 1995. Genetic test for pyruvate kinase deficiency of basenjis. J Am Vet Med Assoc 207:918–921.

185. Giger U, Harvey JW, Yamaguchi RA, McNulty PK, Chiapella A, Beutler E. 1985. Inherited phosphofructokinase deficiency in dogs with hyperventilation-induced hemolysis: Increased in vitro and in vivo alkaline fragility of erythrocytes. Blood 65:345–351.

186. Giger U, Harvey JW. 1987. Hemolysis caused by phosphofructokinase deficiency in English springer spaniels: Seven cases (1983–1986). J Am Vet Med Assoc 191:453–459.

187. Giger U, Smith BF, Woods CB, Patterson DF, Stedman H. 1992. Inherited phosphofructokinase deficiency in an American cocker spaniel. J Am Vet Med Assoc 201:1569–1571.

188. Ronquist G, Rudolphi O, Engstrom I, Waldenstrom A. 2001. Familial phosphofructokinase deficiency is associated with a disturbed calcium homeostasis in erythrocytes. J Intern Med 249:85–95.

189. Stockdale CR, Moyes TE, Dyson R. 2005. Acute post-parturient haemoglobinuria in dairy cows and phosphorus status. Aust Vet J 83:362–366.

190. Adams LG, Hardy RM, Weiss DJ, Bartges JW. 1993. Hypophosphatemia and hemolytic anemia associated with diabetes mellitus and hepatic lipidosis in cats. J Vet Intern Med 7:266–271.

191. Justin RB, Hohenhaus AE. 1995. Hypophosphatemia associated with enteral alimentation in cats. J Vet Intern Med 9:228–233.

192. Goto I, Shimizu T, Maede Y. 1992. L-sorbose does not cause hemolysis in dog erythrocytes with inherited high Na, K-ATPase activity. Comp Biochem Physiol [C] 101:657–660.

193. Goto I, Inaba M, Shimizu T, Maede Y. 1994. Mechanism of hemolysis of canine erythrocytes induced by L-sorbose. Am J Vet Res 55:291–294.

194. Kaneko JJ. 1997. Porphyrins and the porphyrias. In: Kaneko JJ, Harvey JW, Bruss ML, eds. *Clinical Biochemistry of Domestic Animals*, 5th edition, 205–221. San Diego: Academic.

195. Kaneko JJ. 2000. The porphyrias and the porphyrinurias. In: Feldman BF, Zinkl JG, Jain NC, eds. *Schalm's Veterinary Hematology*, 5th edition, 1002–1007. Philadelphia: Lippincott Williams & Wilkins.

196. Sassa S. 2001. The hematologic aspects of porphyria. In: Beutler E, Lichtman MA, Coller BS, Kipps TJ, Seligsohn U, eds. *Williams Hematology*, 6th edition, 703–720. New York: McGraw-Hill.

197. Giddens WE Jr, Labbe RF, Swango LJ, Padgett GA. 1975. Feline congenital erythropoietic porphyria associated with severe anemia and renal disease: Clinical, morphologic, and biochemical studies. Am J Pathol 80:367–386.

198. Glenn BL, Glenn HG, Omtvedt IT. 1968. Congenital porphyria in the domestic cat (*Felis catus*): Preliminary investigations on inheritance pattern. Am J Vet Res 29:1653–1657.

199. With TK. 1980. Porphyrias in animals. Clin Haematol 9:345–370.

200. Engelking LR, Mariner JC. 1985. Enhanced biliary bilirubin excretion after heparin-induced erythrocyte mass depletion. Am J Vet Res 46:2175–2178.

201. Moore JN, Mahaffey EA, Zboran M. 1987. Heparin-induced agglutination of erythrocytes in horses. Am J Vet Res 48:68–71.

202. Maggio-Price L, Emerson CL, Hinds TR, Vincenzi FF, Hammond WR. 1988. Hereditary nonspherocytic hemolytic anemia in beagles. Am J Vet Res 49:1020–1025.

203. Pekow CA, Hinds TR, Maggio-Price L, Hammond WP, Vincenzi FF. 1992. Osmotic stress in red blood cells from beagles with hemolytic anemia. Am J Vet Res 53:1457–1461.

204. Kohn B, Goldschmidt MH, Hohenhaus AE, Giger U. 2000. Anemia, splenomegaly, and increased osmotic fragility of erythrocytes in Abyssinian and Somali cats. J Am Vet Med Assoc 217:1483–1491.

205. Tennant BC, Evans CD, Kaneko JJ, Schalm OW. 1972. Hepatic failure in the horse. Mod Vet Pract 53:40–42.

206. Peterson ME, Kintzer PP, Cavanagh PG, Fox PR, Ferguson DC, Johnson GF, Becker DV. 1983. Feline hyperthyroidism: Pretreatment clinical and laboratory evaluation of 131 cases. J Am Vet Med Assoc 183:103–110.

207. Glaus TM, Hassig M, Baumgartner C, Reusch CE. 2003. Pulmonary hypertension induced in dogs by hypoxia at different high-altitude levels. Vet Res Commun 27:661–670.

208. Rose RJ, Allen JR. 1985. Hematologic responses to exercise and training. Vet Clin North Am Equine Pract 1:461–476.

209. Lykkeboe G, Schougaard H, Johansen K. 1977. Training and exercise change respiratory properties of blood in race horses. Respir Physiol 29:315–325.

210. Hilppö M. 1986. Some haematological and clinical-chemical parameters of sight hounds (Afghan hound, saluki and whippet). Nord Vet Med 38:148–155.

211. Jain NC. 1986. *Schalm's Veterinary Hematology*, 4th edition. Philadelphia: Lea & Febiger.

212. Lumb WV, Johns EW. 1984. *Veterinary Anesthesia*, 2nd edition. Philadelphia: Lea & Febiger.

213. Nunn JF. 1987. *Applied Respiratory Physiology*, 3rd edition. Boston: Butterworth.

214. Dixon PM, McPherson EA. 1977. Familial methaemoglobinaemia and haemolytic anaemia in the horse associated with decreased erythrocytic glutathione reductase and glutathione. Equine Vet J 9:198–201.

215. Letchworth GJ, Bentinck-Smith J, Bolton GR, Wootton JF, Family L. 1977. Cyanosis and methemoglobinemia in two dogs due to a NADH methemoglobin reductase deficiency. J Am Anim Hosp Assoc 13:75–79.

216. Harvey JW, Ling GV, Kaneko JJ. 1974. Methemoglobin reductase deficiency in a dog. J Am Vet Med Assoc 164:1030–1033.

217. Atkins CE, Kaneko JJ, Congdon LL. 1981. Methemoglobin reductase deficiency and methemoglobinemia in a dog. J Am Anim Hosp Assoc 17:829–832.

218. Baker DC, Gaunt SD. 1985. Nicotinamide–adenine dinucleotide–methemoglobin reductase activity in erythrocytes from cats. Am J Vet Res 46:1354–1355.

219. Harvey JW. 2000. Hereditary methemoglobinemia. In: Feldman BF, Zinkl JG, Jain NC, eds. *Schalm's Veterinary Hematology*, 5th edition, 1008–1011. Philadelphia: Lippincott Williams & Wilkins.

220. Fine DM, Eyster GE, Anderson LK, Smitley A. 1999. Cyanosis and congenital methemoglobinemia in a puppy. J Am Anim Hosp Assoc 35:33–35.

221. Pinkerton PH, Fletch SM, Brueckner PJ, Miller DR. 1974. Hereditary stomatocytosis with hemolytic anemia in the dog. Blood 44:557–567.

222. Slappendel RJ, Renooij W, de Bruijne JJ. 1994. Normal cations and abnormal membrane lipids in the red blood cells of dogs with familial stomatocytosis-hypertrophic gastritis. Blood 84:904–909.

223. Paltrinieri S, Comazzi S, Ceciliani F, Prohaska R, Bonfanti U. 2007. Stomatocytosis of standard schnauzers is not associated with stomatin deficiency. Vet J 173:202–205.

224. Conboy JG, Shitamoto R, Parra M, Winardi R, Kabra A, Smith J, Mohandas N. 1991. Hereditary elliptocytosis due to both qualitative and quantitative defects in membrane skeletal protein 4.1. Blood 78:2438–2443.

225. Gallagher PG. 2005. Red cell membrane disorders. Hematology Am Soc Hematol Educ Program 13–18.

226. Slappendel RJ, van ZR, van LM, Schneijdenberg CT. 2005. Hereditary spectrin deficiency in golden retriever dogs. J Vet Intern Med 19:187–192.

227. Ruhr LP, Nicholson SS, Confer AW, Blakewood BW. 1983. Acute intoxication from a hematinic in calves. J Am Vet Med Assoc 182:616–618.

228. Mullaney TP, Brown CM. 1988. Iron toxicity in neonatal foals. Equine Vet J 20:119–124.

229. Lewis HB, Moyer WA. 1975. Iatrogenic iron overload in the horse. In: Kitchen H, Krehbiel JD, eds. *Proceedings of the First International Symposium on Equine Hematology*, 258–261. Golden, CO: American Association of Equine Practitioners.

230. House JK, Smith BP, Maas J, Lane VM, Anderson BC, Graham TW, Pino MV. 1994. Hemochromatosis in Salers cattle. J Vet Intern Med 8:105–111.

231. Smith JE, DeBowes RM, Cipriano JE. 1986. Exogenous corticosteroids increase serum iron concentrations in mature horses and ponies. J Am Vet Med Assoc 188:1296–1298.

232. Grafmeyer D, Bondon M, Manchon M, Levillain P. 1995. The influence of bilirubin, haemolysis and turbidity on 20 analytical tests performed on automatic analysers: Results of an interlaboratory study. Eur J Clin Chem Clin Biochem 33:31–52.

233. Yamanishi H, Iyama S, Fushimi R, Amino N. 1996. Interference of ferritin in measurement of serum iron concentrations: Comparison by five methods. Clin Chem 42:331–332.

234. Smith JE, Cipriano JE, DeBowes R, Moore K. 1986. Iron deficiency and pseudo–iron deficiency in hospitalized horses. J Am Vet Med Assoc 188:285–287.

235. Weeks BR, Smith JE, DeBowes RM, Smith JM. 1989. Decreased serum iron and zinc concentrations in cattle receiving intravenous dexamethasone. Vet Pathol 26:345–346.

236. Bunch SE, Jordan HL, Sellon RK, Cullen JM, Smith JE. 1995. Characterization of iron status in young dogs with portosystemic shunt. Am J Vet Res 56:853–858.

237. Laflamme DP, Mahaffey EA, Allen SW, Twedt DC, Prasse KW, Huber TL. 1994. Microcytosis and iron status in dogs with surgically induced portosystemic shunts. J Vet Intern Med 8:212–216.

238. Brommer H, van Oldruitenborgh-Oosterbaan MM. 2001. Iron deficiency in stabled Dutch warmblood foals. J Vet Intern Med 15:482–485.

239. Kaneko JJ. 1980. Iron metabolism. In: Kaneko JJ, ed. *Clinical Biochemistry of Domestic Animals*, 3rd edition, 649–669. San Diego: Academic.

240. Andrews GA, Chavey PS, Smith JE. 1994. Enzyme-linked immunosorbent assay to measure serum ferritin and the relationship between serum ferritin and nonheme iron stores in cats. Vet Pathol 31:674–678.

241. Hyyppa S, Hoyhtya M, Nevalainen M, Poso AR. 2002. Effect of exercise on plasma ferritin concentrations: Implications for the measurement of iron status. Equine Vet J Suppl 34:186–190.

242. Baynes RD. 1996. Assessment of iron status. Clin Biochem 29:209–215.

243. Weeks BR, Smith JE, Northrop JK. 1989. Relationship of serum ferritin and iron concentrations and serum total iron-binding capacity to nonheme iron stores in dogs. Am J Vet Res 50:198–200.

244. ten Kate J, Wolthuis A, Westerhuis B, van Deursen C. 1997. The iron content of serum ferritin: Physiological importance and diagnostic value. Eur J Clin Chem Clin Biochem 35:53–56.

245. Newlands CE, Houston DM, Vasconcelos DY. 1994. Hyperferritinemia associated with malignant histiocytosis in a dog. J Am Vet Med Assoc 205:849–851.

246. Andrews GA. 2000. Red blood cell antigens and blood groups in the dog and cat. In: Feldman BF, Zinkl JG, Jain NC, eds. *Schalm's Veterinary Hematology*, 5th edition, 767–773. Philadelphia: Lippincott Williams & Wilkins.

247. Wardrop KJ. 2000. Clinical blood typing and crossmatching. In: Feldman BF, Zinkl JG, Jain NC, eds. *Schalm's Veterinary Hematology*, 5th edition, 795–798. Philadelphia: Lippincott Williams & Wilkins.

248. Bowling AT. 2000. Red blood cell antigens and blood groups in the horse. In: Feldman BF, Zinkl JG, Jain NC, eds. *Schalm's Veterinary Hematology*, 5th edition, 774–777. Philadelphia: Lippincott Williams & Wilkins.

249. Wilkerson MJ, Davis E, Shuman W, Harkin K, Cox J, Rush B. 2000. Isotype-specific antibodies in horses and dogs with immune-mediated hemolytic anemia. J Vet Intern Med 14:190–196.

250. Kucinskiene G, Schuberth HJ, Leibold W, Pieskus J. 2005. Flow cytometric evaluation of bound IgG on erythrocytes of anaemic dogs. Vet J 169:303–307.

251. Bonkovsky HL. 1991. Iron and the liver. Am J Med Sci 301:32–43.

252. Zuwala-Jagiello J, Osada J. 1998. Internalization study using EDTA-prepared hepatocytes for receptor-mediated endocytosis of haemoglobin-haptoglobin complex. Int J Biochem Cell Biol 30:923–931.

253. Kino K, Mizumoto K, Watanabe J, Tsunoo H. 1987. Immunohistochemical studies on hemoglobin-haptoglobin and hemoglobin catabolism sites. J Histochem Cytochem 35:381–386.

254. Kristiansen M, Graversen JH, Jacobsen C, Sonne O, Hoffman HJ, Law SK, Moestrup SK. 2001. Identification of the haemoglobin scavenger receptor. Nature 409:198–201.

255. George JW. 1988. Methemalbumin: reality and myth. Vet Clin Pathol 17:43–46.

Chapter 4

PLATELETS

Physiologic Processes 224
Analytical Principles and Methods. 227
    I.   Complete Blood Count (CBC) 227
    II. Thrombogram 227
    III. Methods. 229
Microscopic Features of Platelets. 232
Thrombocytopenia 233
Thrombocytosis 244
Platelet Volume. 246
Reticulated Platelets. 247
Tests for Immune-mediated Thrombocytopenia (IMT) 249

Table 4.1. Abbreviations and symbols in this chapter

[x]	x concentration (x = analyte)
ATP	Adenosine triphosphate
DIC	Disseminated intravascular coagulation
DNA	Deoxyribonucleic acid
EDTA	Ethylenediaminetetraacetic acid
Fc	Fragment (crystallizable)
IL-6	Interleukin 6
IMHA	Immune-mediated hemolytic anemia
IMT	Immune-mediated thrombocytopenia
MPS	Mononuclear phagocyte system
MPV	Mean platelet volume
PDW	Platelet distribution width
PSAIg	Platelet surface–associated immunoglobulin
QBC	Quantitative buffy coat
RNA	Ribonucleic acid
SI	Système International d'Unités
SLE	Systemic lupus erythematosus
Tpo	Thrombopoietin
WRI	Within the reference interval

PHYSIOLOGIC PROCESSES

I. Platelets are small cytoplasmic fragments of megakaryocytes (*mega* = "large," *karyon* = "nucleus," and *cyte* = "cell") that are derived from pluripotent hematopoietic stem cells (see Fig. 2.1). Mammalian platelets share most of the following components, although with species variations:

   A. A phospholipid membrane containing glycoproteins important in cell-cell interactions and phospholipids important for coagulation

   B. An open canalicular system of membrane invaginations that serves as a conduit for substances moving between platelets and plasma (not developed in horses and cattle), and that contributes to a marked increase in external platelet surface area after activation

   C. A cytoskeleton, associated with a peripheral microtubular ring and abundant actin and myosin, that maintains discoid shape and allows for shape change and pseudopod formation with activation

   D. A dense tubular system of endoplasmic reticulum that stores Ca^{2+} for platelet activation and that is important in thromboxane synthesis

   E. α-Granules that store numerous proteins involved in hemostasis and vessel repair and whose contents are secreted with appropriate stimuli

   F. Dense granules containing Ca^{2+}, Mg^{2+}, adenosine diphosphate, ATP, and serotonin, all of which are secreted with appropriate stimuli

   G. Glycogen stores and mitochondria for energy

II. Platelet production: The process of generating circulating platelets from hematopoietic stem cells can be divided into megakaryopoiesis and thrombopoiesis. Adequate megakaryopoiesis is reflected by adequate numbers of megakaryocytes in the bone marrow but does not guarantee adequate thrombopoiesis.

A. *Megakaryopoiesis*, the proliferation and maturation of megakaryocytes, occurs in hematopoietic tissue, mostly bone marrow. Resident myeloid progenitor cells respond to cytokines, primarily Tpo, by undergoing proliferation and maturation.[1] Limited baseline megakaryocyte production occurs in the absence of Tpo.[2]

B. *Thrombopoiesis*, the formation of platelets from megakaryocytes and their delivery to the circulation, is also primarily mediated by Tpo,[1] but baseline platelet production can occur in the absence of Tpo.[2] Tpo is also important for maintaining adequate hematopoietic stem cell populations.

  1. Thrombopoiesis occurs in the bone marrow and at other sites of hematopoiesis (e.g., the spleen). It also occurs in the lungs, where megakaryocytes lodge after circulating from the bone marrow (see Plate 4A [for all plates, see the color section of this book]).[3]

  2. Platelets form from late-stage megakaryocytes. They appear to shed directly into the blood by cytoplasmic fragmentation or by the periodic constriction of megakaryocytic cytoplasmic pseudopodia that extend into vascular sinuses.

C. Tpo is produced primarily in hepatocytes, renal tubular epithelium, and stromal cells of the bone marrow.[1,4]

  1. In health, Tpo is produced constantly and is cleared by receptor-mediated uptake and destruction by platelets and megakaryocytes.[5,6] Therefore, platelet and megakaryocyte masses exert control over plasma [Tpo], and there is generally an inverse relationship between [platelet] and blood and bone marrow [Tpo].

    a. With decreased platelet mass, more Tpo remains unbound and is available to stimulate megakaryocytes. However, when megakaryocyte hyperplasia accompanies thrombocytopenia, more Tpo will become bound by megakaryocytes and the blood [Tpo] will be lower than expected based solely on the [platelet].

    b. As the [platelet] increases, more Tpo is bound and removed from the circulation, so there is less stimulation of megakaryocytes or other stem cells.

  2. Tpo production increases in certain pathologic states:[4]

    a. Inflammation causes increased IL-6, which induces hepatocytes to produce more Tpo, which in turn may cause thrombocytosis. Because of increased Tpo production, the plasma [Tpo] is greater with inflammatory thrombocytosis than expected, given the [platelet].

    b. Marrow stromal cells are induced to produce more Tpo in at least some thrombocytopenic states.

  3. Activated platelets may release intact Tpo in vivo, thus increasing blood concentrations during platelet consumptive states.[7]

D. Reticulated platelets: Just as the RNA content of circulating young erythrocytes (reticulocytes) is used to assess erythropoiesis, circulating reticulated platelets have been measured to assess thrombopoiesis in dogs and horses.[8,9] Reticulated platelets have increased cytoplasmic RNA and have been shown to be less than 24 h old in dogs.[10]

III. Platelet kinetics

A. The blood [platelet] is generally established by the relative rates of platelet production, consumption, and destruction, and by the shifting of platelets to and from the circulation (Fig. 4.1).

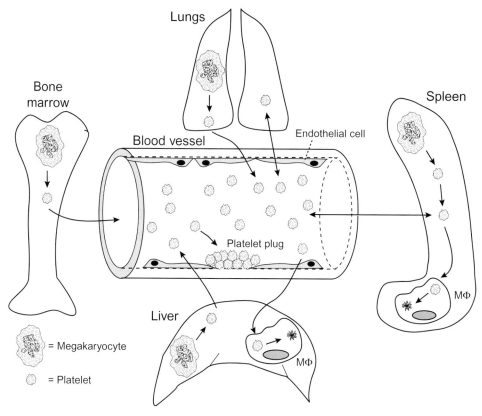

Fig. 4.1. Blood platelet concentrations are established mostly by the relative rates of platelet production, consumption, and destruction, and by the shifting of platelets to and from the circulation. In pathologic states, combinations of these factors often contribute to abnormal platelet concentrations.

- Production: Most megakaryopoiesis and thrombopoiesis occur in the bone marrow, and new platelets enter systemic circulation via marrow sinusoids. Some megakaryocytes appear to become lodged in the lungs after release from the bone marrow. These megakaryocytes release platelets into the blood, but the overall importance of this process is not known. Platelets produced by splenic hematopoietic tissue may contribute to the circulating platelet mass in health and disease. Hematopoietic foci may also arise in the liver and contribute to the circulating platelet mass.
- Consumption: Platelets may be removed from circulation during normal maintenance of vascular integrity or during accelerated consumptive states (e.g., thrombotic disease and vasculitis).
- Destruction: Macrophages (Mϕ), primarily in the spleen and liver, may destroy platelets that carry surface-associated antibodies or complement. Aged or damaged platelets may be similarly destroyed.
- Redistribution: Splenic platelet sequestration (reversible) may reduce the circulating platelet mass, and splenic contraction may increase it. Pulmonary sequestration of platelets has been associated with severe hypothermia and endotoxemia.
- Massive transfusion with blood products or other fluids may cause a dilutional decrease in platelet concentration.

B. Platelet production is affected mostly by the degree of cytokine stimulation and the number of responsive cells. In rodents and people, the total megakaryocyte maturation time ranges from about 2 d to 10 d.[11]

C. Platelet consumption is ongoing because of the continuous repair of minor vascular defects. Mean platelet life span appears to be decreased in any markedly thrombocytopenic state, even when thrombocytopenia is caused by decreased production. This can be explained by a fixed platelet requirement for maintenance of vascular integrity, so when marked thrombocytopenia is present, a substantially greater percentage of the circulating platelets is consumed during routine maintenance.[12]

D. Platelet life spans vary among species and are about 5–10 d in health.[13–15] Factors governing platelet life span are unclear, but the spleen is important in determining platelet life span in dogs. Splenectomized dogs had almost 50 % longer platelet life spans (8 d) than healthy nonsplenectomized dogs (about 5–6 d).[13]

E. Human and rabbit spleens have been shown to harbor about 33 % of blood platelets at any given moment.[11,16,17] Epinephrine and splenic contraction can mobilize these platelets to circulation, while splenic engorgement can trap more platelets there.[11,17] Splenic pooling and mobilization of platelets are expected in other species, too.[17]

IV. Platelet functions (see Chapter 5 for details regarding the roles of platelets in hemostasis)

A. The major function of platelets is to help repair vascular damage and prevent hemorrhage by participating in the formation of hemostatic plugs. Platelets are consumed in this ongoing process.

B. Energy for platelet functions is derived from ATP generated by aerobic glycolysis and oxidative phosphorylation. Glucose enters platelets by facilitated diffusion.

C. Nonhemostatic platelet functions: Platelets are important in inflammation and wound healing. They interact with leukocytes and release vasoactive amines, cytokines, mitogens, and growth factors.

ANALYTICAL PRINCIPLES AND METHODS

I. Complete blood count (CBC): Quantitative and qualitative data regarding blood platelets are routinely included in mammalian CBC results. Major concepts pertaining to the CBC are in Chapter 2.

II. Thrombogram: those portions of a CBC related to platelets (thrombocytes)

A. Blood film evaluation

1. Microscopic evaluation of platelets on a stained blood film is an important part of the thrombogram, especially in bleeding patients or when thrombocytopenia or extreme thrombocytosis is present.

2. It serves three major purposes:

a. It enables detection of platelet clumps, which may falsely decrease [platelet] values. Some analyzers detect the presence of platelet clumps and report their presence, but others do not.

b. It enables estimation of [platelet] for corroboration of automated values or when automated measures are unavailable or unreliable.

c. It enables evaluation of platelets for abnormal features.

  B. Platelet concentration

    1. The *platelet concentration* is the number of platelets per unit volume of blood (in clinical jargon, commonly referred to as *platelet count*).

    2. Unit conversion: $(\# \times 10^3/\mu L) \times 10^6 \, \mu L/L = \# \times 10^9/L$ (SI unit; suggest reporting to nearest $10 \times 10^9/L$)

  C. MPV

    1. *MPV* is the average apparent volume of all the particles in a blood sample that are counted as individual platelets

    2. Because MPV is an average, populations of large or small platelets may be present and detectable by microscopy when the MPV is WRI. Also, large platelets may be seen microscopically but excluded from analysis by the instrument.

    3. Unit: fL (μm^3)

  D. PDW

    1. *PDW* is an assessment of platelet anisocytosis calculated from the distribution of individual platelet volumes.

    2. There are several different methods of calculating PDW.

      a. For ADVIA instruments, it is the standard deviation of the distribution of platelet volumes recorded as a percentage of the MPV; that is, $100 \times$ (standard deviation of MPV)/MPV.

      b. For other analyzers, the calculation may exclude a certain proportion of the largest and smallest platelets.

    3. Units: %

  E. Thrombocrit: *thrombo-* ("platelet") plus *-crit* (from *krinein*, meaning "to separate"); also called *platelet crit*

    1. *Thrombocrit*, like hematocrit, is the percentage of blood volume filled by platelets (typically < 1 %). It is an assessment of circulating platelet mass.

    2. Unlike hematocrit, thrombocrit values have not been routinely reported but have become available with modern automated analyzers.

    3. Thrombocrit values are calculated from the MPV and [platelet], so abnormalities or errors with either of these measurements affect the thrombocrit value (see Eq. 4.1).

$$10 \text{ fL/platelet} \times 300{,}000 \text{ platelets}/\mu L = 3{,}000{,}000 \text{ fL}/\mu L = 0.003 \, \mu L/\mu L = 0.3 \, \% \qquad \textbf{(4.1)}$$

    4. Compared to the [platelet], thrombocrit may better represent the total platelet functional potential and the thrombopoietic stimulus.[18]

    5. Units: % or decimal form (L/L or unitless)

  F. Several other platelet values are generated by some analyzers and may be reported, although they are currently used mostly for investigative purposes.

    1. MPC: mean platelet component concentration

      a. The *MPC* is an approximation of the average platelet density based on two-angle light scatter of individual platelets (ADVIA)

      b. It is used to assess platelet activation, which leads to granule secretion and a decreased MPC.

      c. Values are affected by anticoagulant, sample age, sample storage temperature, and iatrogenic activation, so they must be interpreted cautiously.

      d. Unit: g/dL

    2. *PCDW*: mean platelet component concentration distribution width

      a. Variation in the MPC

      b. Unit: g/dL

3. Values for mean platelet mass (pg), variation in mean platelet mass, large platelets, and platelet clumps may also be reported by some analyzers.

III. Methods
A. Blood film evaluation of platelets
1. Scan the feathered edge and smear body for platelet clumps. If clumps are present, the following estimation of [platelet] will provide only a minimum value that may markedly underestimate the true [platelet].
2. One method of estimating the concentration of individualized platelets requires first finding the appropriate counting window, where leukocytes are flattened like fried eggs to expose nuclear and cytoplasmic detail.
   a. Appropriate counting windows contain fields of similar blood thickness and therefore similar volumes of blood per field. Differences in cell number per field will reflect differences in cell number per volume of blood (i.e., concentration).
   b. Smear thickness can be judged by the degree to which cells are flattened out (fried egg appearance) rather than by the proximity of cells to one another.
   c. If fields are chosen to normalize the density of erythrocytes, thicker areas of the smear (with more blood volume per field) will be evaluated in anemic animals and the [platelet] will be overestimated.
3. Using the 100× oil objective (1000× magnification), again assess for the presence of platelet clumps. If platelets are clumped, report "clumped platelets" and recognize that smear estimates and machine values for [platelet] in the sample may be falsely decreased.
4. If platelets are well distributed, estimate the average number of platelets per 1000× field in at least 5 (preferably 10) fields.
5. Convert the average number of platelets per field to an estimated [platelet] by using the following conversion factor: 1 platelet/1000× field = 15,000–20,000 platelets/µL.[19] For example, if the mean number per 1000× field was 4, then the estimated [platelet] would range from about $4 \times 15,000$ platelets/µL = 60,000 platelets/µL to about $4 \times 20,000$ platelets/µL = 80,000 platelets/µL.
   a. The area represented by a 1000× microscopic field varies with the optics of microscopes. The diameter of the field of view varies directly with the field number of the oculars, and field numbers vary considerably.
   b. Because of this, the appropriate conversion factor varies considerably. The 1:20,000 conversion may be more appropriate for regular oculars, and the 1:15,000 conversion may be more appropriate for wide-field oculars. Either should provide a useful estimate.
6. The estimated [platelet] should then be compared to species-specific reference intervals for interpretation. To exclude thrombocytopenia, dogs (most breeds), cats, and cattle should generally have at least 8–10 platelets per 1000× field, and horses should have at least 5 platelets per 1000× field.
7. Other methods may be used to estimate [platelet]:
   a. Some people advocate enumeration of platelets in 10 thick and thin areas of the film and use of a 1:8000 conversion factor to estimate [platelet] (the lower conversion factor reflects assessment of thicker areas with greater blood volume and more platelets per field).
   b. Others compare the ratio of platelets to either erythrocytes or leukocytes in several fields, and then use either the erythrocyte concentration or leukocyte

concentration to calculate the estimated [platelet] (e.g., for 5 platelets per leukocyte and a [leukocyte] of 20,000/μL, the estimated [platelet] = 5 × 20,000/μL = 100,000/μL). These methods require quantitative erythrocyte or leukocyte concentrations.

8. While estimating [platelet], platelets should be assessed for morphologic abnormalities (see the following section).

B. Platelet concentration

1. Sample

a. EDTA anticoagulation of venous blood is routine for CBCs (see Analytical Principles and Methods, sect. I.D, in Chapter 2), but citrated venous blood (1 part citrate to 9 parts blood) can be used (e.g., when EDTA-induced platelet clumping is suspected). Citrate dilution requires that the measured [platelet] be corrected (corrected platelet concentration = measured platelet concentration × 1.1).

b. Heparinized samples should not be used, because platelet clumping frequently occurs.

c. Platelets can be easily activated during blood collection, and activation causes clumping. Platelets can clump because they are hyperactive, because of slow or poor venipuncture technique, or because of delayed or inadequate mixing of blood and anticoagulant. Platelets of cats and cattle are very prone to clumping.

d. Blood collection tubes containing citrate, theophylline, dipyridamole, and adenosine (CTAD tubes) provide platelet inhibitory factors that help reduce in vitro platelet activation.[20] These may be particularly useful in cats.

e. There are various reported statements regarding the stability of platelet concentrations.[21,22] On average, concentrations appear reasonably stable for 8 h at room temperature and for 48 h at 4 °C. However, concentrations may increase or decrease considerably in individual samples, so prompt testing is recommended.

f. For all platelet quantitation methods, platelet clumping must be absent to be confident that a [platelet] is accurate. If platelet clumps are present, measured values should be considered minimum values.[23] If more accurate values are required (e.g., to confirm an apparent decrease), a new sample should be collected in such a way as to minimize platelet activation and therefore clumping (see Coagulation Sect. II.C, in Chapter 5).

2. Impedance cell counters (see Chapter 2 and Fig. 2.5 for basic principles and analyzers)

a. Typically, [platelet] is measured in the same path as erythrocyte parameters and is the concentration of particles that are within a defined particle volume interval (e.g., 2–30 fL) based on their electrical impedance.

b. For most samples, a properly adjusted and calibrated impedance cell counter provides reliable platelet concentrations for most dogs, horses, and cattle.

c. However, impedance cell counters cannot always accurately assess platelets; in some samples, they cannot differentiate small erythrocytes from platelets (e.g., in iron deficiency), or large platelets from erythrocytes (e.g., cats and Cavalier King Charles spaniels). Cats have a greater variation in platelet volume, with more large platelets than other species, so impedance methods are problematic for determining [platelet] accurately in cats.[24]

3. Optical or laser flow cell cytometers (see Chapter 2 and Fig. 2.5 for basic principles and analyzers)

      a. Assessment of low-angle (volume) and high-angle (refractive index) light scatter enables better differentiation of platelets from erythrocytes than does the use of electrical impedance.

      b. Platelets are defined as particles with certain light-scatter characteristics, and the number of these particles in a given volume of fluid is the [platelet].

      c. However, other particles, such as lipid droplets, can scatter light similarly and be counted as platelets.

  4. QBC (see Chapter 2 and Fig. 2.6 for basic principles)

      a. The QBC detects the thickness of the cell layer above the lymphocyte and monocyte layer that has characteristic fluorescence of RNA or lipoprotein.

      b. The thickness of this layer (essentially a thrombocrit) is converted to a [platelet] based on correlation studies with other analyzers.

      c. Because the value is affected by platelet size, it may not always match platelet concentrations based on other methods.

      d. The analytical method is less affected by small platelet clumps than are impedance methods.[23]

  5. Hemocytometer (see Chapter 2 and Fig. 2.4 for basic principles)

      a. Platelets are enumerated microscopically in defined grid regions after sample dilution and lysis of erythrocytes.

      b. This manual technique is relatively labor intensive and has much lower precision than automated methods, but it is adequate for most diagnostic uses and may be preferred when many giant platelets are present.

      c. It does not enable measurement of other platelet parameters.

      d. As with any method, platelet clumping prevents accurate measurement of [platelet].

C. MPV

  1. MPV values vary among analyzers and methods.[25] Electrical impedance methods may exclude large platelets from evaluation, and the diluting fluids used to sphere platelets in optical analyzers may falsely decrease the values.[26–28]

  2. MPV values also vary with the anticoagulant, the sample storage temperature, and the sample storage time, though not necessarily in the same manner with every analyzer.

      a. These variables usually have relatively minor effects (< 20 % differences), but the effects should be considered when values are interpreted, particularly for values near the upper or lower reference limits. Reference samples may have been handled differently from patient samples.

      b. With impedance measurements, EDTA was shown to induce artifactual and time-dependent increases in MPV that occurred within 5 min and could result in 3 h values that were 150 % of baseline for room temperature samples.[26,29] Artifactual increases also occur when EDTA samples are refrigerated (at 4 °C).[30]

      c. MPV increases over time in citrated samples stored at room temperature or 4 °C, but the increase is less than with EDTA samples.[26]

      d. When analyzed over time on the ADVIA, MPV values increased after an initial decrease, and the changes were slower at 4 °C. MPV was relatively stable when samples were anticoagulated by a mixture of EDTA and citrate, stored at 4 °C, and analyzed from 1 h through 3 h after blood collection.[31]

  3. Some impedance analyzers cannot generate reliable MPV values in severely thrombocytopenic patients, so the values may be unavailable when of interest.

4. Particulates such as lipid droplets or cell fragments may be detected as platelets, leading to false MPV values with either impedance or laser methods.

MICROSCOPIC FEATURES OF PLATELETS (see Plate 7 and 8)

I.   General
    A. In blood films, platelets are present individually or in small to large clumps (see Plate 7J–L).
    B. Clumps usually result from in vitro platelet activation, but anticoagulant-induced agglutination of nonhuman platelets has been reported.[32] Clumps are most frequent in feline and bovine samples. They may be found throughout a blood film but are best found at its feathered edge, sides, and base.

II. Features
    A. Shape
        1. Nonactivated platelets are discoid and appear mostly round, oval, or elongate in blood films made from non-anticoagulated blood (see Plate 7F).
        2. Platelets become spheroid with EDTA anticoagulation (also with citrate, but to a lesser degree) and more commonly appear round.
        3. Elongate platelets, which probably represent undivided megakaryocyte pseudopod segments (*proplatelets*), may be more numerous during stimulated thrombopoiesis (see Plate 7E).
        4. Activated platelets may have peripheral pseudopodia (see Plate 8A–C).
    B. Size
        1. In most healthy individuals, platelets are fairly uniform in size.
        2. The diameter of feline platelets, which is greater and more variable than in other common domestic mammals, may exceed that of feline erythrocytes.[33] This variability is reflected by a greater PDW in cats than in other domestic mammals.
        3. There is not a universal definition of a giant platelet (large platelet, shift platelet, stress platelet, megaplatelet, megathrombocyte, or macrothrombocyte) or how many must be seen to report them. However, platelets larger than normal erythrocytes are typically classified as *giant*, and when the number of such platelets appears increased to the microscopist, they may be reported.
        4. Because MPV is an average for all platelets, subpopulations of large platelets may be present without an increased MPV. Also, large platelets may not be included in MPV calculations if they are too large to be detected as platelets.
        5. On some blood films, many platelets appear larger than normal but not larger than erythrocytes. These platelets may not be reported as large, but the MPV may be increased.
        6. An increase in the number of giant platelets suggests accelerated thrombopoiesis within a few days of sample collection, usually because of a destructive or consumptive thrombocytopenia. It may be accompanied by an increased MPV (see Platelet Volume, sect. II.A). However, an increased number of giant platelets does not confirm adequate numbers of megakaryocytes and may occur with congenital platelet disorders, clonal hemic disorders, splenic contraction, and some acute feline leukemia virus infections.
    C. Inclusions
        1. Granules

a. With Wright staining, nonactivated platelets have clear to pale blue cytoplasms containing small pink to purple granules. These granules contain numerous substances that can be released to promote platelet functions, including hemostasis and repair.

b. With activation, the granules may be centralized (see Plate 8A and C) or absent (secreted) (see Plate 8B). Granules tend to be most prominent in feline and bovine platelets and least prominent in equine platelets.

c. Abnormalities in granule size, shape, and staining may be rarely seen with dysthrombopoiesis. More often, abnormalities are noted in megakaryocytes.

2. *Anaplasma platys* (basonym *Ehrlichia platys*) morulae may be present in platelets (see Plate 8E). They must be differentiated from stain precipitate and fragments of nuclear material (see Plate 8F). When they are suspected, specific analysis by polymerase chain reaction (PCR) may be used for confirmation.

THROMBOCYTOPENIA

I. General concepts

A. *Thrombocytopenia* is a pathologic state in which [platelet] is less than a valid lower reference limit (platelet clumps must be absent). Some healthy greyhounds[34–36] and perhaps Shiba Inus[37] have lower platelet concentrations than other dogs.

B. Thrombocytopenia reflects a pathologic process and is a diagnostic problem, not a disease. Its major significance is the potentiation of bleeding when platelet concentrations are markedly decreased. Also, its presence may suggest specific disorders or diseases.

C. Clinical signs: Petechiae and ecchymoses are the hallmarks of severe thrombocytopenia. Mucosal bleeding (epistaxis, hematochezia, or melena), hematuria, hyphema, and prolonged hemorrhage after accidental or intentional trauma (e.g., venipuncture) are common.

D. Thrombocytopenia can occur in many diseases,[38–41] but there are limited pathogenic mechanisms to be considered (see Fig. 4.1).

II. Diseases and conditions (Table 4.2)

A. *Pseudo-thrombocytopenia* is false thrombocytopenia that may occur when not all the platelets in a sample are counted. It can be suspected when automated analyzers indicate the presence of platelet clumps. It can also be recognized when microscopic examination reveals platelet clumps or yields an estimate of [platelet] that is substantially greater than the measured [platelet].

1. It often occurs because blood collection causes platelet activation and aggregation. Therefore, platelets are clumped and not counted individually.

2. It also occurs with automated analyzers, particularly impedance analyzers, when many large platelets are present (e.g., in cats and Cavalier King Charles spaniels) but not detected because they exceed the upper size limit of detection. For such samples, platelet concentrations should be determined by microscopic methods.

3. It can occur with cold agglutinins or anticoagulant-induced, antibody-mediated agglutination of platelets. Anticoagulants, especially EDTA, can unmask nonpathologic antigenic sites on platelet membranes so that immunoglobulins bind and bridge platelets together in vitro.[42] Although rarely reported in veterinary species,[32,43] it is quite common with human samples.

Table 4.2. Diseases and conditions that cause thrombocytopenia

Abnormal platelet distribution (sequestration): splenomegaly, severe hypothermia
Decreased platelet production (myelosuppression of one to all hemic cell lines)
    Acquired amegakaryocytic thrombocytopenia
    Drugs (toxicants)
  *Predictable: chemotherapeutic agents, estrogens in dogs (exogenous, endogenous), bracken
        fern poisoning (ruminants), trichothecene mycotoxins
    Idiosyncratic: phenylbutazone, meclofenamic acid, trimethoprim-sulfamethoxazole,
       griseofulvin
    Infectious (usually multifactorial; see the text)
    Irradiation (whole body or extensive): prior to autologous marrow transplantation
    Marrow replacement: bone marrow neoplasia (primary hemic or metastatic), myelofibrosis,
       osteopetrosis
    Megakaryocytic leukemia
    Myelonecrosis: infections, neoplasia, toxicants
Decreased platelet survival (accelerated platelet destruction and consumption)
    Immunologic
      *Primary (idiopathic) IMT
      Secondary IMT
        Drug induced: gold salts, sulfonamides
        Infectious (usually multifactorial; see the text)
        Neonatal alloimmune thrombocytopenia
        Neoplasia (usually multifactorial; see the text)
        Posttransfusion purpura
        Systemic immune-mediated disease: SLE, Evans' syndrome
    Nonimmunologic
        Blood loss, acute and severe: anticoagulant rodenticides
        Platelet activation with accelerated consumption or utilization
        Localized intravascular coagulation: hemangiosarcoma, hemorrhage, thrombosis
      *DIC: envenomation, hepatic disease, infections, massive necrosis, pancreatitis, neoplasia,
         overheating, septicemia
        Drugs: protamine sulfate
        Envenomation (without DIC)
      *Vasculitis/endocarditis: Rocky Mountain spotted fever, canine herpesvirus infection,
        hemolytic uremic syndrome, dirofilariasis, angiostrongylosis, bacterial endocarditis,
        hemolytic uremic syndrome (cutaneous and renal glomerular vasculopathy of
        greyhounds)
Hemodilution: massive infusion with colloids, crystalloids, platelet-poor blood products
Idiopathic mechanism or multifactorial (decreased production and decreased survival)
    Idiopathic thrombocytopenia of Cavalier King Charles spaniels
  *Infections: *Anaplasma platys, Anaplasma phagocytophilum, Babesia canis, Babesia gibsoni,* bovine
       viral diarrhea virus, canine distemper virus, canine parvovirus, *Cytauxzoon felis,*
       Ehrlichia spp., equine infectious anemia virus, feline leukemia virus, feline
       immunodeficiency virus, *Histoplasma capsulatum, Leishmania* spp., *Leptospira* spp.,
       Theileria spp.
    Endotoxemia
  *Neoplasia: carcinomas, hemangiosarcoma and other sarcomas, lymphoma, leukemias
    Drugs
    Hypophosphatemia associated with hyperalimentation
    Anaphylaxis

* A relatively common disease or condition
Note: Lists of specific disorders or conditions are not complete but are provided to give examples. Platelet concentrations in greyhounds and Shiba Inus may be lower than for other breeds of dogs. Pseudo-thrombocytopenia caused by platelet clumping or giant platelets should be considered before pursuing causes of true thrombocytopenia.

B. Abnormal platelet distribution (sequestration)
   1. Platelets may become reversibly redistributed into the vascular system of certain
       tissues (e.g., spleen), and therefore the concentration of freely circulating platelets is
       decreased. This thrombocytopenia occurs without decreased total body platelet mass
       and therefore does not stimulate thrombopoiesis.
   2. The term *sequestration* is often used for either reversible platelet redistribution or for
       irreversible trapping of platelets in organs because of destruction by the MPS.
       However, in this textbook, irreversible removal of platelets from circulation is
       regarded as decreased platelet survival, not sequestration.
   3. Abnormal platelet distribution may contribute to or (rarely) cause marked
       thrombocytopenia.
   4. Disorders
       a. Splenomegaly appears to cause splenic pooling of an exchangeable platelet fraction
           in some human conditions, though platelet survivals may also be decreased.[44]
           Similar effects of splenomegaly have been presumed to occur in other species.
       b. Severe hypothermia (e.g., a rectal temperature of 20 °C) may cause reversible
           platelet redistribution to liver and spleen in dogs.[45]
       c. Endotoxemia has been associated experimentally with transient pulmonary
           platelet pooling in dogs, but platelet consumption also occurs.[46,47]
C. Decreased platelet production
   1. Adequate platelet production requires a healthy megakaryocyte population; there
       must be enough megakaryocytes and they must be shedding platelets. Megakaryo-
       cytes can be unhealthy because of generalized bone marrow diseases or because of
       megakaryocyte-specific diseases that either diminish megakaryopoiesis or impair
       thrombopoiesis. Unexplained bicytopenia and pancytopenia suggest the possibility of
       generalized bone marrow disease.
   2. Idiopathic thrombocytopenia in Cavalier King Charles spaniels is likely caused by
       decreased platelet production rather than a compensated consumptive state, but it is
       included below (see Thrombocytopenia, sect. II.F.1) under idiopathic conditions
       until better characterized.
   3. Acquired amegakaryocytic thrombocytopenia is rarely reported in dogs and cats.[48–50]
       Some cases may be immune mediated, as in people.
       a. Bone marrow aspirate and core samples must be of excellent quality to conclude
           reliably that megakaryocytes are absent.
       b. In people, it may occur with antibody-mediated or cell-mediated[51] destruction of
           megakaryocytes or their precursors, or with antibody-mediated destruction of
           required cytokines.[52,53]
       c. Antimegakaryocyte antibodies may also impair thrombopoiesis[54,55] without
           megakaryocytic hypoplasia or aplasia. Dogs injected with rabbit anti-[canine
           platelet] antiserum developed marked thrombocytopenia with morphologic
           changes in megakaryocytes that suggested the possibility of impaired megakaryo-
           cyte function without megakaryocytic hypoplasia.[56] Plasma from some people
           with IMT inhibits megakaryopoiesis and thrombopoiesis in cell cultures.
   4. Drugs (toxicants)
       a. Drugs with predictable and dose-dependent myelosuppressive effects (examples)
           (1) Antineoplastic chemotherapeutic agents, including alkylating agents,
                antimetabolites, and antibiotics (e.g., doxorubicin), frequently induce
                thrombocytopenia 1–2 wk after drug administration.[57,58]

    (2) Estrogens from exogenous sources[59] or endogenous sources (e.g., testicular Sertoli cell neoplasm,[60] rare ovarian granulosa cell neoplasms,[61] and rare interstitial cell neoplasms[62] in dogs) can induce thrombocytopenia or aplastic pancytopenia. Suppressive doses cause thrombocytopenia after a week or more, and thrombocytopenia may persist for weeks. Myelosuppression may be mediated by an inhibitor produced by thymic stromal cells in response to estrogen.[63]

    (3) Bracken fern poisoning may induce aplastic anemia with thrombocytopenia in ruminants,[64] as may trichothecene mycotoxins.[65]

    (4) Albendazole has been implicated in a dog.[66]

  b. Drugs (toxicants) with idiosyncratic (i.e., sporadic and unpredictable) myelosuppressive effects (examples)

    (1) Idiosyncratic myelosuppression is suspected much more often than it is proven. Relapse of thrombocytopenia with rechallenge after initial recovery would support a cause-and-effect relationship, but such rechallenges are avoided. When suspected, potential offending drugs are withdrawn, but subsequent improvement may or may not be due to drug withdrawal.

    (2) Phenylbutazone and meclofenamic acid are nonsteroidal anti-inflammatory drugs that have been associated with bone marrow hypoplasia and bicytopenia or pancytopenia in dogs and probably in horses (only phenylbutazone).[67–69]

    (3) Trimethoprim-sulfadiazine and trimethoprim-sulfonamide have been associated with aplastic anemia in dogs and cats.[70–72] This occurrence is uncommon and unpredictable at doses commonly used. However, potentiated sulfonamides predictably inhibit sequential steps in folate pathways, thus suppressing DNA synthesis. This may contribute to aplastic anemia and thrombocytopenia in affected dogs. Thrombocytopenia caused by myelosuppression should be differentiated from immune-mediated platelet destruction caused by trimethoprim-sulfa–dependent antibodies.

    (4) Griseofulvin has caused marrow suppression in cats,[73,74] and an idiosyncratic reaction to albendazole has been implicated in a cat.[66]

5. Infections: The pathogenesis of thrombocytopenia associated with many infections is multifactorial (see Thrombocytopenia, sect. II.F.2) but often includes decreased platelet production. Several mechanisms of decreased production may be involved.

  a. Direct infection of megakaryocytes or other hematopoietic precursors may decrease megakaryopoiesis or thrombopoiesis. Examples are infections with bovine virus diarrhea virus (immunotolerant cattle persistently infected with bovine virus diarrhea virus do not have thrombocytopenia)[75] and canine distemper virus.[76]

  b. Myelosuppressive cytokines may be produced in response to infection (e.g., equine infectious anemia virus).[77,78]

  c. Some infections (e.g., chronic ehrlichiosis caused by *Ehrlichia canis* and canine parvoviral infection) are associated with generalized bone marrow hypoplasia and thrombocytopenia, but the mechanisms are not clear. Canine parvoviral infections may cause suppression thrombocytopenia by direct infection of hematopoietic precursor cells. However, viral antigen has minimally and inconsistently been found in the bone marrow of experimentally infected dogs and, when present, was not in recognizable cells of the megakaryocyte series.[79,80] Thrombocytopenia may also be caused by septicemia and/or endotoxemia associated with severe enteritis.

   d. Production failure may contribute to thrombocytopenia occurring in some cats with feline leukemia virus infections, but the effects may be indirect via secondary disorders, including hemic neoplasia.

6. Irradiation (whole body or extensive): This can cause generalized marrow suppression and thrombocytopenia through widespread cell death. Thrombocytopenia was prolonged (weeks to months) and severe in dogs receiving autologous bone marrow transplants after marrow-ablative total body irradiation.[81,82]

7. Marrow replacement (myelophthisis): Bone marrow neoplasia (primary hemic or metastatic), myelofibrosis, and osteopetrosis may each induce myelosuppression. Mechanisms may include physical replacement of normal cell populations, competition for nutrients, obstruction of blood supply, lysis of marrow cells, and secretion of inhibitors. Megakaryocytic leukemia may be associated with thrombocytopenia,[83–85] probably because of dysthrombopoiesis and decreased thrombopoiesis.

8. Myelonecrosis (with or without myelofibrosis): Infections, neoplasia, or toxicants may cause enough marrow necrosis to contribute to thrombocytopenia.[86,87]

D. Decreased platelet survival (accelerated platelet destruction or consumption)

1. If increased platelet production does not compensate for accelerated platelet destruction or consumption, thrombocytopenia will ensue.

   a. Platelet *consumption* usually refers to the use of platelets during hemostatic functions, whether physiologic or pathologic.

   b. Platelet *destruction* usually refers to the death of platelets by other means, usually immune-mediated destruction.

2. Immunologic causes of decreased platelet survival

   a. General concepts

      (1) IMT usually occurs when an animal's immune system produces antibodies that bind directly (e.g., autoantibody or alloantibody) or indirectly (e.g., adsorbed antigen) to its own platelets (PSAIg). This leads to accelerated platelet destruction by the MPS. Destruction is mediated by PSAIg, platelet surface–associated complement, or both. The process may be initiated by a defective immune system, defective platelets, or adsorbed antigens from drugs, infectious agents, or neoplasms. The cause is usually unknown.

      (2) Thrombocytopenia is often clinically classified as immune mediated based on clinical findings and response to immunosuppressive therapy. Detection of increased PSAIg by a validated direct assay, it available, would provide more support for the conclusion.

      (3) The abbreviation ITP is also used for IMT. It originally was used for "idiopathic thrombocytopenic purpura" in human patients, but it came to be used for "immune thrombocytopenic purpura" once an immunologic mechanism was demonstrated. However, purpura may not be present in patients with IMT, and idiopathic thrombocytopenia may not always be immune mediated.

      (4) IMT not associated with a detected disease or condition is *idiopathic IMT*, which is often called *primary IMT*. It may be autoimmune, but antibody specificity to normal self-epitopes is rarely documented in veterinary medicine.

(a) Destruction of one's own cells is an autoimmune phenomenon only if the body's immune system is directed against autoantigens.
(b) Alloantibodies from colostrum or transfusion are directed toward alloantigens and cause alloimmune thrombocytopenia.
(c) Antibodies to adsorbed antigens cause secondary IMT that is neither autoimmune nor alloimmune.

(5) IMT that is part of a more widespread disease (e.g., SLE) is also often called *secondary IMT* despite an autoimmune pathogenesis.

b. Idiopathic IMT (primary, often presumed to be autoimmune)

(1) Idiopathic IMT is well documented and relatively common only in dogs and people but appears to occur in other species, as well.[88–94] Immunoblotting and immunoprecipitation studies have confirmed a role for platelet membrane antigen targets in at least some cases of canine idiopathic IMT.[95] Antibodies may also target megakaryocytes. Diagnosis is primarily by exclusion, but increased PSAIg or positive megakaryocyte immunofluorescence results may support an immune pathogenesis (see the Tests for Immune-Mediated Thrombocytopenia section).

(2) Common laboratory features[96] are thrombocytopenia (usually $< 50 \times 10^3/\mu$L and often $< 10 \times 10^3/\mu$L); MPV increased, decreased, or WRI; anemia (in about 50 % of cases); and megakaryocytic hyperplasia (megakaryocytic hypoplasia can occur).

c. Drug-induced IMT

(1) Exposure to certain drugs may lead to increased PSAIg and therefore accelerated platelet destruction because of the production of drug-dependent or drug-independent antibodies.
(a) *Drug-independent antibodies* do not require the drug for binding; they may bind to a platelet epitope that is cross-reactive with the drug or a metabolite.
(b) *Drug-dependent antibodies*, which are more common in people than in domestic mammals,[97] can theoretically bind to any of the following: a drug or a metabolite adsorbed to the platelet surface, a platelet surface antigen exposed by the presence of the drug or a metabolite, or a combined drug-platelet neoantigen on the platelet membrane.

(2) Drug-induced IMT is suspected when otherwise unexplained thrombocytopenia, usually severe, develops a few days after drug exposure, and when the thrombocytopenia resolves rapidly after drug withdrawal.

(3) Strict criteria to be met for confirmation of drug-induced IMT by drug-dependent antibodies are the following:
(a) Increased PSAIg in a patient that developed thrombocytopenia at least a few days after drug exposure
(b) Patient plasma antibodies that bind in vitro to platelets or platelet antigens in the presence, but not in the absence, of drug or a metabolite
(c) Resolution of both thrombocytopenia and increased PSAIg after drug withdrawal
(d) Relapse after reexposure to the drug (not recommended)

(4) Numerous drugs have been suspected to cause IMT in dogs. Gold salts (auranofin, gold sodium thiomalate, and possibly aurothioglucose)[98] and sulfonamides (with or without trimethoprim)[99,100] have been strongly

implicated in dogs. Platelet antibody assay results have been supportive of drug-induced IMT.

    (5) Methimazole and propylthiouracil have been incriminated in cats,[101,102] and penicillin and trimethoprim-sulfadoxine may have led to IMT in horses.[103]

    (6) Heparin, a common cause of immune complex–induced IMT in people, has not been reported to produce an analogous condition in veterinary species. The pathogenesis of heparin-induced IMT involves platelet Fc receptors for immunoglobulin G (IgG) but not all species express them.[104]

d. IMT associated with infection (usually multifactorial; see Thrombocytopenia, sect. II.F.2)

    (1) Pathogeneses of thrombocytopenias associated with infection are usually multifactorial or unknown, but many bacterial, viral, fungal, and protozoal diseases have been associated with IMT in people. Similar associations are likely in domestic mammals.

    (2) Infection-associated IMT may be caused by cross-reactive antibodies, bacteria-induced production of autoantibodies, exposure of otherwise hidden platelet membrane antigens by the organism, binding of antiorganism antibodies to the infectious agent attached to the platelet membrane, or the induction of immune complexes that adhere to the platelet membrane.

    (3) Infection-associated IMT may occur with acute canine ehrlichiosis[105] and, by extension, infections with related organisms of the genera *Ehrlichia* and *Anaplasma*. Other infectious diseases with a likely immune component to the thrombocytopenia are Rocky Mountain spotted fever,[106] histoplasmosis,[107] leishmaniasis,[108,109] distemper or modified live virus distemper vaccination,[76] equine infectious anemia,[110] and babesiosis.[111]

    (4) Some people have considered vaccination a precipitating event in clinical canine IMT, but supporting data are lacking.

e. Neonatal alloimmune thrombocytopenia

    (1) Thrombocytopenia occurs when passively acquired (mainly via colostrum) maternal alloantibodies to paternal epitopes on a neonate's platelets circulate in the neonate's blood and mediate platelet destruction. The maternal alloantibodies are produced when the dam is sufficiently exposed to fetal platelets possessing paternally derived antigenic determinants that are recognized as foreign. It has been described in horses, mule foals, and pigs.[112–114]

    (2) It must be differentiated from other causes of thrombocytopenia in neonates, especially sepsis. Confirmation entails detection of increased PSAIg in the neonate but not in the dam, and demonstration of the presence of antibodies in the dam's blood that react with paternal and neonatal, but not maternal, platelets. Validated tests may be unavailable.

    (3) Thrombocytopenia concurrent with neutropenia and ulcerative dermatitis has been described in neonatal foals and may have an alloimmune pathogenesis.[115]

f. Neoplasia (usually multifactorial; see Thrombocytopenia, sect. II.F.3)

    (1) Thrombocytopenia occurs commonly in animals with neoplasia. The cause is often multifactorial but may include immunologic mechanisms.

    (2) Antibodies, possibly in the form of immune complexes, have been indirectly implicated in mediating thrombocytopenia in some dogs with a variety of

hemic and nonhemic neoplasms.[116] IMT has been associated with lymphoma in dogs and horses.[92,117]

  g. Posttransfusion purpura

    (1) In human transfusion recipients, this condition occurs about 1 wk after transfusion. It is associated with severe thrombocytopenia and high titers of platelet-reactive alloantibodies that mediate the destruction of transfused, as well as the patient's own platelets.

    (2) Rarely, posttransfusion thrombocytopenia has been reported in dogs, but the pathogeneses have not been established.[118]

  h. Systemic immune-mediated diseases such as SLE are caused by general B-lymphocyte activation and the production of autoantibodies directed against multiple targets, one of which may be platelets.

    (1) In dogs with SLE, there is evidence, though rarely documented, of increased PSAIg.[96] Primary IMT and SLE may be different disorders within a spectrum of autoimmune diseases.

    (2) Evans' syndrome

      (a) This was first described in people as idiopathic immune hemolytic anemia and concurrent thrombocytopenia or neutropenia,[119] but the term is now used to refer to concurrent IMT and IMHA.

      (b) In at least some human patients, the antibodies mediating the two cytopenias are distinct.[120] Information is unavailable for animals.

      (c) IMHA with concurrent presumed IMT occurs in dogs (first reported in 1965[121]). An immune pathogenesis has been implicated in some cases by indirect assays for platelet-reactive or megakaryocyte-reactive antibodies in patient plasma.[96]

      (d) Dogs with IMHA are often prothrombotic, so thrombocytopenia in some of them may reflect platelet consumption instead of, or in addition to, immunologic destruction.[122]

 3. Nonimmunologic causes of decreased platelet survival

  a. Blood loss, acute and severe

    (1) When bleeding accompanies severe thrombocytopenia, hemorrhage is probably secondary to the thrombocytopenia rather than severe thrombocytopenia being caused by the bleeding. However, platelet loss and consumption at sites of hemorrhage may cause or contribute to thrombocytopenia.

    (2) In dogs, experimental acute, severe blood loss via phlebotomy caused mild to moderate thrombocytopenia (up to 50 % reduction in [platelet]).[123–125]

    (3) Thrombocytopenia is sometimes present in bleeding dogs that have anticoagulant rodenticide toxicosis.[126] Platelets are probably consumed at an accelerated rate by use at sites of hemorrhage throughout the body. With extensive hemorrhage, platelet loss contributes to thrombocytopenia, and thrombocytopenia may become more severe during routine treatment with fluids, transfusions, and vitamin K_1.

  b. Platelet activation with accelerated consumption or use: Any disorder associated with increased platelet activation may accelerate platelet consumption and lead to thrombocytopenia if platelet production does not compensate.

    (1) Localized (controlled) intravascular coagulation (e.g., with hemangiosarcoma, thrombosis, or hemorrhage) may be associated with platelet consumption at the site(s) where coagulation occurs.

(a) Activation of the coagulation cascade leads to the generation of thrombin (factor IIa), a potent platelet activator.

(b) Thrombin activates platelets, and activated platelets release platelet-activating substances that recruit and consume more platelets. Thrombocytopenia may ensue.[127]

(2) DIC: Widespread, uncontrolled activation of the coagulation cascade may produce thrombocytopenia in the same way as localized coagulation, but the likelihood of thrombocytopenia is greater. DIC may be caused by envenomation, hepatic disease, infections, massive necrosis, pancreatitis, neoplasia, overheating, or septicemia.

(3) Drugs and foreign materials: Some drugs cause or contribute to thrombocytopenia by directly activating platelets.

(a) Protamine sulfate, used to reverse the effects of heparin, can induce severe thrombocytopenia in heparinized and nonheparinized dogs, apparently through a direct proaggregatory effect.[128]

(b) Foreign materials used within the vascular system (e.g., tubing and catheters) are tested and chosen to minimize platelet activation, but accelerated consumption may occur.

(4) Envenomation (without DIC): The numerous types of venoms from numerous animal species differ in their effects. Venom from some snakes may contain platelet-activating factors that induce thrombocytopenia in the absence of DIC.[129] Other venoms induce DIC.[130]

(5) Vasculitis or endocarditis: Inflammation of blood vessels or endocardium can alter endothelial cells or lead to exposure of subendothelium, each of which can lead to a prothrombotic state and platelet adhesion, aggregation, and secretion. Vasculitis has infectious, immune-mediated, and chemical causes.

(a) Infectious causes of vasculitis include Rocky Mountain spotted fever, canine herpesvirus infection, dirofilariasis, angiostrongylosis, infectious canine hepatitis, and equine viral arteritis.

(b) Thrombocytopenia is commonly associated with bacterial endocarditis and may have a multifactorial pathogenesis.

(c) Endothelial cell damage and necrosis lead to thrombocytopenia without DIC in dogs with hemolytic uremic syndrome (e.g., cutaneous and renal glomerular vasculopathy of greyhounds associated with ingestion of Shiga toxin produced by *Escherichia coli*).[131-135] When evaluating greyhounds, it is important to recognize that their platelet concentrations in health are often lower than commonly reported canine reference intervals.

E. Hemodilution: Massive dilution of blood with platelet-poor fluids (e.g., crystalloids, colloids, plasma, or packed erythrocytes) may cause mild to moderate decreases in blood [platelet].[136-138]

F. Idiopathic or multifactorial mechanisms

1. Idiopathic thrombocytopenia in Cavalier King Charles spaniels (inherited giant platelet disorder in Cavalier King Charles spaniels)[139,140]

   a. A congenital disorder reported to have an autosomal recessive inheritance pattern[141]

   b. The disorder is common in the breed. It is associated with large platelets (*macrothrombocytes*), particularly when platelet concentrations are < 100,000/μL. It may be referred to as a *macrothrombocytopenia*.

(1) The relationship between thrombocytopenia and macrothrombocytosis is unclear because investigators have used varied definitions of thrombocytopenia and macrothrombocytosis.

(2) These definitions also cloud the differentiation of affected from unaffected dogs.

c. Platelet concentrations of $50–100 \times 10^3/\mu L$ are common, and they may be < 25,000/μL in some dogs. However, thrombocrit may not be decreased when platelet volumes are increased in thrombocytopenic dogs.

d. Affected dogs have no clinical bleeding problem.

e. This breed also has a high incidence of mitral valve disease, but there is no clear relationship between the conditions.

f. Recognition of this condition is important to prevent unnecessary therapy and to employ appropriate methods for accurate platelet concentrations.

(1) Microscopic hemocytometer counts or estimates from blood smears are useful.

(2) Automated methods, particularly impedance methods, are unreliable when a substantial number of platelets are larger than the analyzer's upper threshold (which varies with the analyzer). Although the QBC VetAutoread may provide falsely increased platelet concentrations when platelets are large, the reported values will reflect the thrombocrit and functional platelet mass.

2. Infections

a. Thrombocytopenia is commonly associated with endotoxemia[142,143] and infections.[38,39,41,144,145]

(1) Etiologic agents frequently associated with thrombocytopenia include certain bacteria (*Ehrlichia* spp. and *Anaplasma* spp.), fungi (e.g., *Histoplasma* spp.), viruses (e.g., equine infectious anemia virus), and protozoa (e.g., *Leishmania* spp., *Babesia* spp., and *Theileria* spp.).

(2) Thrombocytopenia occurs somewhat less frequently, but not unexpectedly, with other organisms (e.g., *Leptospira* spp. and feline immunodeficiency virus).[146,147]

b. Infectious thrombocytopenias may be caused by various combinations of suppressed platelet production (e.g., direct infection, immune suppression, or local effects of inflammation within the bone marrow), altered platelet distribution, increased platelet consumption, and immune-mediated or nonimmune platelet destruction.

c. *Anaplasma platys* (formerly *Ehrlichia platys*) organisms are rickettsial bacteria that infect platelets and cause canine infectious cyclic thrombocytopenia.

(1) Infection may be subclinical or have clinical manifestations.[148]

(2) Parasitemias may be marked but are often mild, so organisms in blood films may be difficult to identify definitively.

(3) Molecular diagnostic techniques have been developed.[149,150]

3. Neoplasms[151]

a. Many types of neoplasia are associated with thrombocytopenia, including carcinomas, sarcomas, lymphomas, and leukemias. In one study, approximately 10 % of dogs with neoplasia were thrombocytopenic, though sometimes because of concurrent infections or therapy.[152]

b. Thrombocytopenia may result from many mechanisms, alone or combined. In specific cases, causes are usually speculative. Potential mechanisms include the following:

(1) Decreased production

   (a) Myelophthisis is a presumed contributor to thrombocytopenia in dogs with multiple myeloma, acute leukemia, or chronic lymphocytic leukemia. Other cytopenias are sometimes present.

   (b) Myelodysplasia

   (c) Estrogen secretion by the neoplasm

   (d) Chemotherapy

(2) Decreased platelet survival

   (a) DIC occurs in some cancer patients and may contribute to thrombocytopenia seen in dogs that have mast cell neoplasia or hepatic metastases.[152,153] However, most evaluated dogs with neoplasia and decreased platelet survival (kinetic studies) had hyperfibrinogenemia, and fibrinogen half-lives were not decreased.[154,155] This does not support DIC.

   (b) Vasculitis or thrombosis within a neoplasm (e.g., hemangiosarcoma, a malignancy of endothelial cells) may accelerate platelet consumption.

   (c) Secondary IMT may also occur and has been incriminated in dogs with certain types of neoplasia (e.g., lymphoma) by use of indirect platelet and megakaryocyte assays.[96]

   (d) Other contributors may include hemorrhage secondary to a neoplasm, sepsis secondary to immunosuppression, and destruction (phagocytosis) by neoplastic macrophages (e.g., malignant histiocytic neoplasia).

(3) Abnormal platelet distribution: Splenomegaly or hepatomegaly induced by neoplastic infiltration (e.g., hemangiosarcoma) or secondary organ congestion may be associated with platelet sequestration.

4. Drugs: As already noted (Thrombocytopenia, sects. II.C.4, D.2.c, and D.3.b), the thrombocytopenia associated with drugs may be caused by myelosuppression, accelerated platelet destruction (immune or nonimmune), or multiple mechanisms. In some cases, the pathogenesis of drug-induced thrombocytopenia is not clear.[156]

5. Hypophosphatemia caused by hyperalimentation in starved dogs decreased platelet survival and caused thrombocytopenia.[157]

   a. Thrombocytopenia was associated with decreased platelet ATP concentrations, probably because of an associated decrease in glycolysis. The specific mechanism of accelerated platelet clearance was not determined.

   b. Cats receiving total parenteral nutrition also developed thrombocytopenia, but they were not hypophosphatemic and the cause was not apparent.[158]

6. Anaphylaxis (type I hypersensitivity)

   a. This is an immune-mediated reaction, but the mechanism of thrombocytopenia is incompletely characterized. Nonimmune factors appear to be important in causing thrombocytopenia for at least some hypersensitivity reactions.

   b. Anaphylactic thrombocytopenia may be caused by inflammatory mediators, DIC, or immune-complex interactions with platelets. Membrane receptors for immunoglobulin E (IgE) exist on a subpopulation of human platelets and mediate inflammatory platelet reactions in some species.[159]

THROMBOCYTOSIS

I.   General concepts
     A. *Thrombocytosis* is a [platelet] greater than a valid upper reference limit.
     B. It may result from redistribution or increased production of platelets. Increased
        production may be associated with hemic neoplasia involving megakaryocytes, or it may
        occur as a secondary reaction to other conditions. Familial thrombocytoses including
        those caused by mutations of the Tpo receptor occur in people but have not been
        reported in animals.
     C. Appropriate reference intervals for [platelet] may be shifted upward for individuals at
        high altitudes.[160]
     D. Serum [K+] may become increased in vitro (a type of *pseudo-hyperkalemia*) by the
        increased amount of platelet K+ released during clotting.

II. Diseases and conditions (Table 4.3)
     A. Hemic neoplasia (clonal thrombocytosis)
        1. Primary (essential) thrombocythemia: a rare chronic myeloproliferative disease that
           has been reported in a few dogs and cats (see Plate 7I).[161–163]
           a. Platelet concentrations have been markedly increased (1000–5000 × 10^3/µL).
           b. Large, pleomorphic, or hypogranular platelets may be present and similar to
              those seen with some megakaryocytic leukemias (see Plate 8G).
           c. Increased numbers of mature megakaryocytes are in the bone marrow, and
              myeloid hyperplasia and erythroid hypoplasia have been reported. Megakaryo-
              cytes may have atypical features.
           d. Though not proven in dogs and cats, the human condition involves a clonal
              proliferation of pluripotent stem cells.[164] Diagnosis in animals is currently by
              exclusion of other causes of persistent thrombocytosis.

Table 4.3. Diseases and conditions that cause thrombocytosis

Hemic neoplasia (clonal thrombocytosis)
   Primary (essential) thrombocythemia and other chronic myeloproliferative diseases
   Acute megakaryoblastic leukemia
Reactive thrombocytosis (secondary, nonclonal)
   Redistribution
      Exercise
      Epinephrine
   Increased production
      *Inflammation: infection, immune mediated, surgery, trauma
      Nonhemic neoplasia
      *Iron deficiency
      Vinca alkaloids (vincristine, vinblastine)
      *Recovery from thrombocytopenia (rebound): withdrawal of myelosuppression, recovery
         from IMT
      Splenectomy (post)
      Blood loss

* A relatively common disease or condition

e. Data are lacking regarding the prevalence of thrombotic or hemorrhagic tendencies in animals with clonal thrombocytosis.
   2. Other chronic myeloproliferative diseases: polycythemia vera, primary erythrocytosis, and chronic myeloid leukemia
   3. Acute megakaryoblastic leukemia (M7 subtype of acute myeloid leukemia) has been reported rarely in dogs and cats (see Plate 8G–I).
      a. In contrast to essential thrombocythemia, ≥ 30 % of nucleated cells in the marrow are megakaryoblasts, marrow fibrosis may be present, and neoplastic megakaryoblasts may be present in blood and other organs.[83,84,165–168]
      b. Thrombocytosis or thrombocytopenia may be present.
   4. Myelodysplastic syndrome is sometimes associated with thrombocytosis.
B. Reactive thrombocytosis (secondary, nonclonal): Reactive thrombocytosis occurs secondary to other conditions and does not involve neoplasia of the megakaryocyte cell line. In most cases, thrombocytosis is mild to moderate and poses no threat to the patient. It is a nonspecific indicator of certain underlying abnormalities.
   1. Redistribution: Mild and transient physiologic thrombocytosis, even when corrected for hemoconcentration, may occur in some species (e.g., dogs, cats, and people) with strenuous exercise or epinephrine release.[16,169–172] In people, the thrombocytosis appears to result primarily from release of platelets from the spleen, but exercise may induce thrombocytosis in asplenic patients.[173] There is evidence for platelet redistribution from lungs.[173,174]
   2. Increased production
      a. Inflammation: Inflammatory cytokines, including IL-6, stimulate Tpo production and, therefore, increased thrombopoiesis in a wide variety of infectious and noninfectious inflammatory conditions, including surgical and nonsurgical trauma in people.[175,176] Thrombocytosis is frequently associated with inflammatory conditions in domestic mammals.[177,178]
      b. Nonhemic malignant neoplasia: Thrombocytosis may result from accompanying inflammation or from production of thrombopoietic cytokines (e.g., IL-6) by neoplastic cells.[179–181]
      c. Iron deficiency: Thrombocytosis is a common but inconsistent finding in canine and human patients with iron deficiency. The specific cause is not known, but blood concentrations of measured thrombopoietic cytokines (e.g., Tpo and IL-6) have not been increased in human patients with iron deficiency and thrombocytosis.[182] Cross-reactivity of Epo with Tpo receptors is also apparently not the cause.[183]
      d. *Vinca* alkaloids: Vincristine and vinblastine stimulate thrombopoiesis that can lead to thrombocytosis without increased MPV.[184,185] In patients with IMT, these drugs may lead to increased platelet concentrations by other mechanisms, including inhibition of the MPS and therefore decreased platelet destruction.
      e. Recovery from thrombocytopenia (rebound thrombocytosis): Thrombocytopenia may stimulate enough thrombopoiesis that production exceeds consumption/destruction and blood concentrations transiently overshoot the upper reference limit during recovery. This can occur after withdrawal of myelosuppression, with recovery from IMT, or after blood loss.[123,186–188]
      f. Postsplenectomy: Splenectomy causes thrombocytosis, sometimes marked, associated with increased thrombopoiesis and increased blood concentrations of Tpo.[189–191] Thrombocytosis is transient but may persist for weeks. Other

mechanisms that may contribute to the thrombocytosis include decreased platelet destruction or decreased sequestration.[192]

g. Blood loss, especially chronic, has been associated with thrombocytosis in several species, but iron deficiency, inflammation, rebound thrombocytosis, or neoplasia may cause or contribute to thrombocytosis in many of these cases. Thrombocytosis associated with blood loss may require the presence of a spleen; it occurred with repeated phlebotomy (chronic blood loss) in nonsplenectomized rabbits that were supplemented with iron, but did not occur in iron-supplemented, splenectomized rabbits.[193]

h. Hypercortisolemia: Hyperadrenocorticism and exogenous glucocorticoids have been associated with thrombocytosis in dogs,[177] but a cause-and-effect relationship is not clear. Thrombocytosis may relate to underlying or concurrent conditions. Prednisone administration to healthy dogs resulted in no increase[184] or a questionable increase[194] in platelet concentrations.

PLATELET VOLUME

I.   Interpretation of MPV values is limited by inaccuracies and inconsistencies of routine MPV measurement and limited knowledge of factors influencing platelet size,[26,195] especially in domestic species.

A. Values should be interpreted relative to reference intervals generated from samples handled in the same manner as the patient samples.

B. Anticoagulant, storage time, storage temperature, and analyzer all affect the results.

II. Among individuals, populations, and species, platelet volume is generally inversely related to the [platelet],[18] and MPV values tend to be greater with thrombocytopenia and lower with thrombocytosis.[196] A similar relationship was found in healthy cats.[197]

A. Increased MPV

1. This usually suggests accelerated thrombopoiesis caused by an increased stimulus for platelet production.[26]

   a. In people, MPV tends to be greater in patients with thrombocytopenia caused by shortened platelet survival (e.g., IMT) than with thrombocytopenia caused by bone marrow disease (e.g., aplastic anemia). A sufficiently increased MPV may have useful negative predictive value for excluding bone marrow disease.[198]

   b. Accelerated thrombopoiesis is usually associated with increased megakaryopoiesis.

   c. Although there are reports to suggest postproduction size modification of platelets,[188] platelet size is generally thought to be established primarily during production and not dramatically altered in the circulation.[26,199] Therefore, increased MPV may reflect accelerated thrombopoiesis occurring any time within 5–10 d (platelet life span in health) before testing. Increased MPV may precede increases in [platelet] in patients recovering from thrombocytopenia.[26]

2. Increased production of abnormal platelets in essential thrombocythemia and other clonal disorders may lead to an increased MPV or an unexpectedly high MPV for the degree of thrombocytosis.[25,26]

3. Abnormally large platelets are produced in certain congenital platelet disorders, so MPV may be increased. Large platelets were reported in the first dogs described with otterhound thrombopathia,[200] and they are present in many Cavalier King Charles spaniels (see Plate 8C).[139,140,201,202]

    4. MPV may increase with physiologic thrombocytosis, possibly because of mobiliza-tion of the splenic platelet pool, which is thought to be overrepresented by large platelets in some species.[26]

    5. Increased MPV is associated with hyperthyroxinemia in people and mice.[26]

    6. Acute infection with the Kawakami-Theilen strain of feline leukemia virus induced production of macrothrombocytes.[203] This was associated with decrements in [platelet] but no significant change in platelet mass.

  B. Decreased MPV

    1. Dogs with IMT may have decreased MPV values more often than dogs with thrombocytopenia for other reasons, but values may also be increased or WRI.[204] Increased numbers of platelet microparticles are detected by flow cytometry in blood of dogs with IMT.

    2. With severe thrombocytopenia ($< 5 \times 10^3/\mu L$), MPV may be affected by nonplatelet debris in the sample or instrument if special precautions are not taken. This debris is insignificant except at very low platelet concentrations when it can affect values from light scatter or impedance methods.

    3. Bone marrow failure and chemotherapeutic myelosuppression have been associated with decreased MPV in people.[25,198] However, MPV was WRI for seven of nine dogs with primary bone marrow disease, and increased in two of nine. The latter two dogs did not have megakaryocytic hypoplasia.[204]

III. An increased PDW indicates an increased population of large platelets, an increased population of small platelets, or both.

IV. Platelet volume is also subjectively assessed by microscopic inspection of blood films (see Microscopic Features of Platelets, sect. II.B). Populations of large platelets can be detected even when automated analyzers miss them. Interpretation is similar to that for increased MPV.

RETICULATED PLATELETS

I. Reticulated platelets: young platelets containing increased RNA; analogous to reticulocytes

  A. Assessment is primarily a research tool at this time, but testing may be available in specialized laboratories.

  B. Reticulated platelet percentage

    1. Percentage of platelets that have increased RNA

    2. Unit: %

  C. Reticulated [platelet]

    1. Concentration of reticulated platelets in blood calculated as the product of [platelet] and platelet reticulocyte percentage (in decimal form)

    2. Units: $(\# \times 10^3/\mu L) \times 10^6 \ \mu L/L = \# \times 10^9/L$ (SI unit)

II. Method

  A. Platelets are typically incubated with thiazole orange, which binds to platelet RNA and granule nucleotides and emits a fluorescence that is detected by flow cytometry. The percentage of platelets with increased fluorescence is determined, and a reticulated [platelet] can be calculated.

B. An increase in fluorescence may relate to an increase in platelet size or to an increase in RNA concentration within the platelets, depending on how the threshold limit for increased fluorescence is defined and the method used (e.g., thiazole orange concentration, incubation time, or fresh versus fixed).[9,205–207] Variations in methods complicate interpretation of reported findings.

C. With some methods, reticulated platelet percentages increase with sample fixation and with sample storage for 18 h at either 4 °C or 21 °C.[9]

III. Interpretation
   A. In theory, increases in reticulated platelets suggest increased thrombopoiesis and may therefore help with the following:
      1. Differentiating consumptive or destructive thrombocytopenias from at least some production-failure thrombocytopenias
      2. Differentiating reactive thrombocytosis from primary thrombocythemia
      3. Identifying when a patient is recovering from bone marrow suppression (e.g., after chemotherapy)
   B. The few studies reported to date generally support the aforementioned theory.
      1. Increased reticulated platelet percentages have been present, when evaluated, in most dogs and horses with thrombocytopenias caused by decreased platelet survival.[8,111,208]
      2. Erythropoietin administration to dogs was associated with increased numbers of reticulated platelets and platelet hyperreactivity.[209]
      3. In one study, four dogs with decreased [platelet] after carboplatin-induced myelosuppression did not have increased reticulated platelet percentages. However, the magnitude of the decrement in [platelet] was not reported.
      4. In people, reticulated platelet percentages are sometimes increased with marrow aplasia, but minimally compared to increases associated with thrombocytopenic disorders caused by platelet destruction or consumption.[210] Human patients recovering from myelosuppressive chemotherapy also had increases in reticulated platelets.[211]
      5. Non-thrombocytopenic dogs with a variety of illnesses had reticulated platelet percentages and concentrations similar to those in healthy dogs.[9] This suggests that abnormal reticulated platelet results may have some specificity for platelet disorders. However, samples with increased reticulated platelets were not reported in this study to confirm that an increase in reticulated platelets could be detected.
   C. Reticulated platelet values have usually been reported and interpreted as percentages rather than as concentrations.
      1. Analogous to interpretation of immature erythrocytes (reticulocytes), one must consider the possibility that reticulated platelet percentage increases may be relative and not truly indicative of increased platelet production.
      2. However, even with accelerated thrombopoiesis, reticulated platelet percentages may be increased in severe thrombocytopenias without increases in reticulated platelet concentrations because there may simply be too few platelets for even a high reticulated platelet percentage to yield an increased reticulated [platelet].[111,208]
         a. Reticulated platelet concentrations may also be suppressed by the markedly reduced platelet life spans in severe thrombocytopenias. The relatively few platelets must be consumed at an accelerated rate to maintain normal vascular integrity.[12,212]

      b. Also, the pathologic process consuming or destroying platelets may target young and old platelets alike.

D. The clinical utility of reticulated platelet assessment in domestic mammals is unclear and awaits further study in a variety of disorders.

TESTS FOR IMMUNE-MEDIATED THROMBOCYTOPENIA (IMT)

I. A variety of specialized assays have been developed to aid in the diagnosis of canine IMT, but the diagnosis remains primarily one of exclusion. Even in human medicine, where assays have been extensively evaluated, testing for antiplatelet antibodies is not considered a necessary part of the recommended diagnostic procedure for suspected primary IMT.[213]

II. Sample conditions (e.g., anticoagulant, storage time, and storage temperature) may affect results. For example, a few hours exposure of citrated blood samples to room temperature or refrigeration led to variable but sometimes marked increases in PSAIg in canine samples.[214] Storage-related increases in PSAIg also occur with EDTA anticoagulation,[215] but the relative contribution of anticoagulant, storage temperature, and other factors to these increases is not known.

III. Platelet assays
    A. Direct platelet assays that test for antibodies on the surface of a patient's platelets (PSAIg) are recommended.
        1. Most current assays are flow cytometric; PSAIg is detected by fluorescence-tagged, species-specific, anti-immunoglobulin antibodies.[94,103,105,106,111,216–218]
        2. Positive results generated from properly processed samples by using reliable assays support antibody-mediated platelet destruction but do not differentiate primary IMT from secondary IMT.
        3. Negative results suggest the need to search for a nonimmune pathogenesis for the thrombocytopenia.
    B. Indirect assays testing for antibodies in a patient's plasma or serum that can bind to "normal" platelets from healthy animals have been used but are not recommended. They have less diagnostic sensitivity and specificity for IMT than direct assays. Indirect assays do not differentiate autoantibodies from immune complexes, immunoglobulin aggregates that can form in frozen sera, or acquired and naturally occurring alloantibodies to platelet antigens.

IV. Direct megakaryocyte immunofluorescence assays have been used to detect the presence of megakaryocyte-associated immunoglobulins on a patient's megakaryocytes, usually on smears of a bone marrow aspirate.[116,219]
    A. Testing requires good bone marrow aspirates with ample megakaryocytes, so samples are not always adequate.
    B. If antibodies directed against platelets also bind shared epitopes on megakaryocytes, results may be positive.[220]
    C. False-positive results may occur if megakaryocytes are damaged and cytoplasmic immunoglobulin rather than surface immunoglobulin is detected.
    D. The cumulative reported diagnostic sensitivity for clinical diagnoses of canine IMT is about 50 %, which is too low to recommend.[96]

References

1. Alexander WS. 1999. Thrombopoietin. Growth Factors 17:13–24.
2. Gainsford T, Nandurkar H, Metcalf D, Robb L, Begley CG, Alexander WS. 2000. The residual megakaryocyte and platelet production in c-Mpl–deficient mice is not dependent on the actions of interleukin-6, interleukin-11, or leukemia inhibitory factor. Blood 95:528–534.
3. Zucker-Franklin D, Philipp CS. 2000. Platelet production in the pulmonary capillary bed: New ultrastructural evidence for an old concept. Am J Pathol 157:69–74.
4. Kaushansky K. 2005. The molecular mechanisms that control thrombopoiesis. J Clin Invest 115:3339–3347.
5. Yang C, Li YC, Kuter DJ. 1999. The physiological response of thrombopoietin (c-Mpl ligand) to thrombocytopenia in the rat. Br J Haematol 105:478–485.
6. Zent CS, Ratajczak J, Ratajczak MZ, Anastasi J, Hoffman PC, Gewirtz AM. 1999. Relationship between megakaryocyte mass and serum thrombopoietin levels as revealed by a case of cyclic amegakaryocytic thrombocytopenic purpura. Br J Haematol 105:452–458.
7. Folman CC, Linthorst GE, van Mourik J, van Willigen G, de Jonge E, Levi M, de Haas M, dem Borne AEGK. 2000. Platelets release thrombopoietin (Tpo) upon activation: Another regulatory loop in thrombocytopoiesis? Thromb Haemost 83:923–930.
8. Russell KE, Perkins PC, Grindem CB, Walker KM, Sellon DC. 1997. Flow cytometric method for detecting thiazole orange–positive (reticulated) platelets in thrombocytopenic horses. Am J Vet Res 58:1092–1096.
9. Smith R III, Thomas JS. 2002. Quantitation of reticulated platelets in healthy dogs and in nonthrombocytopenic dogs with clinical disease. Vet Clin Pathol 31:26–32.
10. Dale GL, Friese P, Hynes LA, Burstein SA. 1995. Demonstration that thiazole-orange–positive platelets in the dog are less than 24 hours old. Blood 85:1822–1825.
11. Stenberg PE, Hill RJ. 1999. Platelets and megakaryocytes. In: Lee GR, Foerster J, Lukens J, Wintrobe MM, eds. *Wintrobe's Clinical Hematology*, 10th edition, 615–660. Philadelphia: Lippincott Williams & Wilkins.
12. Hanson SR, Slichter SJ. 1985. Platelet kinetics in patients with bone marrow hypoplasia: Evidence for a fixed platelet requirement. Blood 66:1105–1109.
13. Dale GL, Wolf RF, Hynes LA, Friese P, Burstein SA. 1996. Quantitation of platelet life span in splenectomized dogs. Exp Hematol 24:518–523.
14. Zoghbi SS, Thakur ML, Sostman HD, Greenspan RH, Gottschalk A. 1988. Indium-111–oxinate labeled swine platelets and their survival in vivo. Lab Anim Sci 38:444–447.
15. Baker LC, Kameneva MV, Watach MJ, Litwak P, Wagner WR. 1998. Assessment of bovine platelet life span with biotinylation and flow cytometry. Artif Organs 22:799–803.
16. Aster RH. 1966. Pooling of platelets in the spleen: Role in the pathogenesis of "hypersplenic" thrombocytopenia. J Clin Invest 45:645–657.
17. Freedman ML, Karpatkin S. 1975. Heterogeneity of rabbit platelets. V. Preferential splenic sequestration of megathrombocytes. Br J Haematol 31:255–262.
18. Kuter DJ. 1996. The physiology of platelet production. Stem Cells 14(Suppl 1):88–101.
19. Tvedten H, Grabski S, Frame L. 1988. Estimating platelets and leukocytes on canine blood smears. Vet Clin Pathol 17:4–6.
20. Norman EJ, Barron RC, Nash AS, Clampitt RB. 2001. Evaluation of a citrate-based anticoagulant with platelet inhibitory activity for feline blood cell counts. Vet Clin Pathol 30:124–132.
21. Tietz NW. 1995. *Clinical Guide to Laboratory Tests*, 3rd edition. Philadelphia: WB Saunders.
22. Tvedten H, Kociba G. 1999. Hemostatic abnormalities. In: Willard MD, Tvedten H, Turnwald GH, eds. *Small Animal Clinical Diagnosis by Laboratory Methods*, 3rd edition, 75–89. Philadelphia: WB Saunders.
23. Koplitz SL, Scott MA, Cohn LA. 2001. Effects of platelet clumping on platelet concentrations measured by use of impedance or buffy coat analysis in dogs. J Am Vet Med Assoc 219:1552–1556.
24. Zelmanovic D, Hetherington EJ. 1998. Automated analysis of feline platelets in whole blood, including platelet count, mean platelet volume, and activation state. Vet Clin Pathol 27:2–9.
25. Jackson SR, Carter JM. 1993. Platelet volume: Laboratory measurement and clinical application. Blood Rev 7:104–113.
26. Threatte GA. 1993. Usefulness of the mean platelet volume. Clin Lab Med 13:937–950.
27. Reardon DM, Hutchinson D, Preston FE, Trowbridge EA. 1985. The routine measurement of platelet volume: A comparison of aperture-impedance and flow cytometric systems. Clin Lab Haematol 7:251–257.
28. Ross DW, Bentley SA. 1986. Evaluation of an automated hematology system (Technicon H-1). Arch Pathol Lab Med 110:803–808.

29. Macey MG, Carty E, Webb L, Chapman ES, Zelmanovic D, Okrongly D, Rampton DS, Newland AC. 1999. Use of mean platelet component to measure platelet activation on the ADVIA 120 haematology system. Cytometry 38:250–255.

30. Handagama P, Feldman B, Kono C, Farver T. 1986. Mean platelet volume artifacts: The effect of anticoagulants and temperature on canine platelets. Vet Clin Pathol 15:13–17.

31. Macey M, Azam U, McCarthy D, Webb L, Chapman ES, Okrongly D, Zelmanovic D, Newland A. 2002. Evaluation of the anticoagulants EDTA and citrate, theophylline, adenosine, and dipyridamole (CTAD) for assessing platelet activation on the ADVIA 120 hematology system. Clin Chem 48:891–899.

32. Hinchcliff KW, Kociba GJ, Mitten LA. 1993. Diagnosis of EDTA-dependent pseudothrombocytopenia in a horse. J Am Vet Med Assoc 203:1715–1716.

33. Norman EJ, Barron RC, Nash AS, Clampitt RB. 2001. Prevalence of low automated platelet counts in cats: Comparison with prevalence of thrombocytopenia based on blood smear estimation. Vet Clin Pathol 30:137–140.

34. Sullivan PS, Evans HL, McDonald TP. 1994. Platelet concentration and hemoglobin function in greyhounds. J Am Vet Med Assoc 205:838–841.

35. Clark P, Parry BW. 1997. Some haematological values of Irish wolfhounds in Australia. Aust Vet J 75:523–524.

36. Couto CG, Lara A, Iazbik MC, Brooks MB. 2006. Evaluation of platelet aggregation using a point-of-care instrument in retired racing Greyhounds. J Vet Intern Med 20:365–370.

37. Gookin JL, Bunch SE, Rush LJ, Grindem CB. 1998. Evaluation of microcytosis in 18 Shibas. J Am Vet Med Assoc 212:1258–1259.

38. Jordan HL, Grindem CB, Breitschwerdt EB. 1993. Thrombocytopenia in cats: A retrospective study of 41 cases. J Vet Intern Med 7:261–265.

39. Sellon DC, Levine J, Millikin E, Palmer K, Grindem C, Covington P. 1996. Thrombocytopenia in horses: 35 cases (1989–1994). J Vet Intern Med 10:127–132.

40. Russell KE, Grindem CB. 2000. Secondary thrombocytopenia. In: Feldman BF, Zinkl JG, Jain NC, eds. *Schalm's Veterinary Hematology*, 5th edition, 487–495. Philadelphia: Lippincott Williams & Wilkins.

41. Grindem CB, Breitschwerdt EB, Corbett WT, Jans HE. 1991. Epidemiologic survey of thrombocytopenia in dogs: A report on 987 cases. Vet Clin Pathol 20:38–43.

42. Schrezenmeier H, Muller H, Gunsilius E, Heimpel H, Seifried E. 1995. Anticoagulant-induced pseudothrombocytopenia and pseudoleucocytosis. Thromb Haemost 73:506–513.

43. Kubo Y, Amejima S, Miyagi A. 1993. Artifacts: Case A-5—EDTA dependent pseudothrombocytopenia. In: Tvedten HW, ed. *Multi-species Hematology Atlas: Technicon H·1E System*, 134–135. Tarrytown, NY: Miles.

44. Warkentin TE, Trimble MS, Kelton JG. 1995. Thrombocytopenia due to platelet destruction and hypersplenism. In: Hoffman R, Benz EJ Jr, Shattil SJ, Furie B, Cohen HJ, Silberstein LE, eds. *Hematology: Basic Principles and Practice*, 2nd edition, 1889–1909. New York: Churchill Livingstone.

45. Pina-Cabral JM, Ribeiro-da-Silva A, Almeida-Dias A. 1985. Platelet sequestration during hypothermia in dogs treated with sulphinpyrazone and ticlopidine: Reversibility accelerated after intra-abdominal rewarming. Thromb Haemost 54:838–841.

46. Gutmann FD, Murthy VS, Wojciechowski MT, Wurm RM, Edzards RA. 1987. Transient pulmonary platelet sequestration during endotoxemia in dogs. Circ Shock 21:185–195.

47. Sostman HD, Zoghbi SS, Smith GJ, Carbo P, Neumann RD, Gottschalk A, Greenspan RH. 1983. Platelet kinetics and biodistribution in canine endotoxemia. Invest Radiol 18:425–435.

48. Murtaugh RJ, Jacobs RM. 1985. Suspected immune-mediated megakaryocytic hypoplasia or aplasia in a dog. J Am Vet Med Assoc 186:1313–1315.

49. Gaschen FP, Smith Meyer B, Harvey JW. 1992. Amegakaryocytic thrombocytopenia and immune-mediated haemolytic anemia in a cat. Comp Haematol Int 2:175–178.

50. Lachowicz JL, Post GS, Moroff SD, Mooney SC. 2004. Acquired amegakaryocytic thrombocytopenia: Four cases and a literature review. J Small Anim Pract 45:507–514.

51. Gewirtz AM, Sacchetti MK, Bien R, Barry WE. 1986. Cell-mediated suppression of megakaryocytopoiesis in acquired amegakaryocytic thrombocytopenic purpura. Blood 68:619–626.

52 Hoffman R, Zaknoen S, Yang HH, Bruno E, LoBuglio AF, Arrowsmith JB, Prchal JT. 1985. An antibody cytotoxic to megakaryocyte progenitor cells in a patient with immune thrombocytopenic purpura. N Engl J Med 312:1170–1174.

53. Hoffman R, Briddell RA, van Besien K, Srour EF, Guscar T, Hudson NW, Ganser A. 1989. Acquired cyclic amegakaryocytic thrombocytopenia associated with an immunoglobulin blocking the action of granulocyte-macrophage colony–stimulating factor. N Engl J Med 321:97–102.

54. Ballem PJ, Segal GM, Stratton JR, Gernsheimer T, Adamson JW, Slichter SJ. 1987. Mechanisms of thrombocytopenia in chronic autoimmune thrombocytopenic purpura: Evidence of both impaired platelet production and increased platelet clearance. J Clin Invest 80:33–40.

55. McMillan R, Nugent D. 2005. The effect of antiplatelet autoantibodies on megakaryocytopoiesis. Int J Hematol 81:94–99.

56. Joshi BC, Jain NC. 1977. Experimental immunologic thrombocytopenia in dogs: A study of thrombocytopenia and megakaryocytopoiesis. Res Vet Sci 22:11–17.

57. Kisseberth NC, MacEwen EG. 2001. Complications of cancer and its treatment. In: Withrow SJ, MacEwen EG, eds. *Small Animal Clinical Oncology*, 3rd edition, 198–232. Philadelphia: WB Saunders.

58. Anderson KC. 2001. Hematologic complications and blood bank support. In: Holland JF, Bast RC Jr, Morton DL, Frei EI, Kufe DW, Weichselbaum RR, eds. *Cancer Medicine*, 4th edition, 3155–3177. Baltimore: Williams & Williams.

59. Aranda E, Pizarro M, Pereira J, Mezzano D. 1994. Accumulation of 5-hydroxytryptamine by aging platelets: Studies in a model of suppressed thrombopoiesis in dogs. Thromb Haemost 71:488–492.

60. Sherding RG, Wilson GP III, Kociba GJ. 1981. Bone marrow hypoplasia in eight dogs with Sertoli cell tumor. J Am Vet Med Assoc 178:497–501.

61. McCandlish IA, Munro CD, Breeze RG, Nash AS. 1979. Hormone-producing ovarian tumours in the dog. Vet Rec 105:9–11.

62. Suess RP, Barr SC, Sacre BJ, French TW. 1992. Bone marrow hypoplasia in a feminized dog with an interstitial cell tumor. J Am Vet Med Assoc 200:1346–1348.

63. Farris GM, Benjamin SA. 1993. Inhibition of myelopoiesis by conditioned medium from cultured canine thymic cells exposed to estrogen. Am J Vet Res 54:1366–1373.

64. Dalton RG. 1964. The effects of batyl alcohol on the haematology of cattle poisoned with bracken. Vet Rec 76:411–416.

65. Parent-Massin D. 2004. Haematotoxicity of trichothecenes. Toxicol Lett 153:75–81.

66. Stokol T, Randolph JF, Nachbar S, Rodi C, Barr SC. 1997. Development of bone marrow toxicosis after albendazole administration in a dog and cat. J Am Vet Med Assoc 210:1753–1756.

67. Watson ADJ, Wilson JT, Turner DM, Culvenor JA. 1980. Phenylbutazone-induced blood dyscrasias suspected in three dogs. Vet Rec 107:239–241.

68. Schalm OW. 1979. Phenylbutazone toxicity in two dogs. Canine Pract 6:47–51.

69. Weiss DJ, Klausner JS. 1990. Drug-associated aplastic anemia in dogs: Eight cases (1984–1988). J Am Vet Med Assoc 196:472–475.

70. McEwan NA. 1992. Presumptive trimethoprim-sulphamethoxazole associated thrombocytopenia and anaemia in a dog. J Small Anim Pract 33:27–29.

71. Weiss DJ, Adams LG. 1987. Aplastic anemia associated with trimethoprim-sulfadiazine and fenbendazole administration in a dog. J Am Vet Med Assoc 191:1119–1120.

72. Fox LE, Ford S, Alleman AR, Homer BL, Harvey JW. 1993. Aplastic anemia associated with prolonged high-dose trimethoprim-sulfadiazine administration in two dogs. Vet Clin Pathol 22:89–92.

73. Rottman JB, English RV, Breitschwerdt EB, Duncan DE. 1991. Bone marrow hypoplasia in a cat treated with griseofulvin. J Am Vet Med Assoc 198:429–431.

74. Kunkle GA, Meyer DJ. 1987. Toxicity of high doses of griseofulvin in cats. J Am Vet Med Assoc 191:322–323.

75. Walz PH, Bell TG, Steficek BA, Kaiser L, Maes RK, Baker JC. 1999. Experimental model of type II bovine viral diarrhea virus–induced thrombocytopenia in neonatal calves. J Vet Diagn Invest 11:505–514.

76. Axthelm MK, Krakowka S. 1987. Canine distemper virus–induced thrombocytopenia. Am J Vet Res 48:1269–1275.

77. Crawford TB, Wardrop KJ, Tornquist SJ, Reilich E, Meyers KM, McGuire TC. 1996. A primary production deficit in the thrombocytopenia of equine infectious anemia. J Virol 70:7842–7850.

78. Tornquist SJ, Oaks JL, Crawford TB. 1997. Elevation of cytokines associated with the thrombocytopenia of equine infectious anemia. J Gen Virol 78:2541–2548.

79. Macartney L, McCandlish IA, Thompson H, Cornwell HJ. 1984. Canine parvovirus enteritis 1: Clinical, haematological and pathological features of experimental infection. Vet Rec 115:201–210.

80. Macartney L, McCandlish IA, Thompson H, Cornwell HJ. 1984. Canine parvovirus enteritis 2: Pathogenesis. Vet Rec 115:453–460.

81. Abrams-Ogg AC, Kruth SA, Carter RF, Valli VE, Kamel-Reid S, Dube ID. 1993. Preparation and transfusion of canine platelet concentrates. Am J Vet Res 54:635–642.

82. Abrams-Ogg AC, Kruth SA, Carter RF, Dick JE, Valli VE, Kamel-Reid S, Dube ID. 1993. Clinical and pathological findings in dogs following supralethal total body irradiation with and without infusion of autologous long-term marrow culture cells. Can J Vet Res 57:79–88.

83. Colbatzky F, Hermanns W. 1993. Acute megakaryoblastic leukemia in one cat and two dogs. Vet Pathol 30:186–194.

84. Pucheu-Haston CM, Camus A, Taboada J, Gaunt SD, Snider TG, Lopez MK. 1995. Megakaryoblastic leukemia in a dog. J Am Vet Med Assoc 207:194–196.

85. Ledieu D, Palazzi X, Marchal T, Fournel-Fleury C. 2005. Acute megakaryoblastic leukemia with erythrophagocytosis and thrombosis in a dog. Vet Clin Pathol 34:52–56.

86. Janssens AM, Offner FC, Van Hove WZ. 2000. Bone marrow necrosis. Cancer 88:1769–1780.

87. Weiss DJ. 2005. Bone marrow necrosis in dogs: 34 cases (1996–2004). J Am Vet Med Assoc 227:263–267.

88. Garon CL, Scott MA, Selting KA, Cohn LA. 1999. Idiopathic thrombocytopenic purpura in a cat. J Am Anim Hosp Assoc 35:464–470.

89. Tasker S, Mackin AJ, Day MJ. 1999. Primary immune-mediated thrombocytopenia in a cat. J Small Anim Pract 40:127–131.

90. Humber KA, Beech J, Cudd TA, Palmer JE, Gardner SY, Sommer MM. 1991. Azathioprine for treatment of immune-mediated thrombocytopenia in two horses. J Am Vet Med Assoc 199:591–594.

91. Sockett DC, Traub-Dargatz J, Weiser MG. 1987. Immune–mediated hemolytic anemia and thrombocytopenia in a foal. J Am Vet Med Assoc 190:308–310.

92. Reef VB, Dyson SS, Beech J. 1984. Lymphosarcoma and associated immune-mediated hemolytic anemia and thrombocytopenia in horses. J Am Vet Med Assoc 184:313–317.

93. Yasuda J, Okada K, Sato J, Sato R, Tachibana Y, Takashima K, Naito Y. 2002. Idiopathic thrombocytopenia in Japanese black cattle. J Vet Med Sci 64:87–89.

94. Kohn B, Linden T, Leibold W. 2006. Platelet-bound antibodies detected by a flow cytometric assay in cats with thrombocytopenia. J Feline Med Surg 8:254–260.

95. Lewis DC, Meyers KM. 1996. Studies of platelet-bound and serum platelet-bindable immunoglobulins in dogs with idiopathic thrombocytopenic purpura. Exp Hematol 24:696–701.

96. Scott MA. 2000. Immune-mediated thrombocytopenia. In: Feldman BF, Zinkl JG, Jain NC, eds. *Schalm's Veterinary Hematology*, 5th edition, 478–486. Philadelphia: Lippincott Williams & Wilkins.

97. Rizvi MA, Shah SR, Raskob GE, George JN. 1999. Drug-induced thrombocytopenia. Curr Opin Hematol 6:349–353.

98. Bloom JC, Blackmer SA, Bugelski PJ, Sowinski JM, Saunders LZ. 1985. Gold-induced immune thrombocytopenia in the dog. Vet Pathol 22:492–499.

99. Lewis DC, Meyers KM, Callan MB, Bücheler J, Giger U. 1995. Detection of platelet-bound and serum platelet-bindable antibodies for diagnosis of idiopathic thrombocytopenic purpura in dogs. J Am Vet Med Assoc 206:47–52.

100. Sullivan PS, Arrington K, West R, McDonald TP. 1992. Thrombocytopenia associated with administration of trimethoprim/sulfadiazine in a dog. J Am Vet Med Assoc 201:1741–1744.

101. Peterson ME, Kintzer PP, Hurvitz AI. 1988. Methimazole treatment of 262 cats with hyperthyroidism. J Vet Intern Med 2:150–157.

102. Peterson ME, Hurvitz AI, Leib MS, Cavanagh PG, Dutton RE. 1984. Propylthiouracil-associated hemolytic anemia, thrombocytopenia, and antinuclear antibodies in cats with hyperthyroidism. J Am Vet Med Assoc 184:806–808.

103. McGurrin MKJ, Arroyo LG, Bienzle D. 2004. Flow cytometric detection of platelet-bound antibody in three horses with immune-mediated thrombocytopenia. J Am Vet Med Assoc 224:83–87.

104. Sinha RK, Santos AV, Smith JW, Horsewood P, Andrew M, Kelton JG. 1992. Rabbit platelets do not express Fc receptors for IgG. Platelets 2:35–39.

105. Waner T, Leykin I, Shinitsky M, Sharabani E, Buch H, Keysary A, Bark H, Harrus S. 2000. Detection of platelet-bound antibodies in beagle dogs after artificial infection with *Ehrlichia canis*. Vet Immunol Immunopathol 77:145–150.

106. Grindem CB, Breitschwerdt EB, Perkins PC, Cullins LD, Thomas TJ, Hegarty BC. 1999. Platelet-associated immunoglobulin (antiplatelet antibody) in canine Rocky Mountain spotted fever and ehrlichiosis. J Am Anim Hosp Assoc 35:56–61.

107. Kucera JC, Davis RB. 1983. Thrombocytopenia associated with histoplasmosis and an elevated platelet associated IgG. Am J Clin Pathol 79:644–646.

108. Slappendel RJ. 1988. Canine leishmaniasis: A review based on 95 cases in the Netherlands. Vet Q 10:1–16.

109. Terrazzano G, Cortese L, Piantedosi D, Zappacosta S, Di LA, Santoro D, Ruggiero G, Ciaramella P. 2006. Presence of anti-platelet IgM and IgG antibodies in dogs naturally infected by *Leishmania infantum*. Vet Immunol Immunopathol 110:331–337.

110. Clabough DL, Gebhard D, Flaherty MT, Whetter LE, Perry ST, Coggins L, Fuller FJ. 1991. Immune-mediated thrombocytopenia in horses infected with equine infectious anemia virus. J Virol 65:6242–6251.

111. Wilkerson MJ, Shuman W, Swist S, Harkin K, Meinkoth J, Kocan AA. 2001. Platelet size, platelet surface-associated IgG, and reticulated platelets in dogs with immune-mediated thrombocytopenia. Vet Clin Pathol 30:141–149.

112. Buechner-Maxwell V, Scott MA, Godber L, Kristensen A. 1997. Neonatal alloimmune thrombocytopenia in a quarter horse foal. J Vet Intern Med 11:304–308.

113. Stormorken H, Svenkerud R, Slagsvold P, Lie H. 1963. Thrombocytopenic bleedings in young pigs due to maternal isoimmunization. Nature 198:1116–1117.

114. Ramirez S, Gaunt SD, McClure JJ, Oliver J. 1999. Detection and effects on platelet function of anti-platelet antibody in mule foals with experimentally induced neonatal alloimmune thrombocytopenia. J Vet Intern Med 13:534–539.

115. Perkins GA, Miller WH, Divers TJ, Clark CK, Belgrave RL, Sellon DC. 2005. Ulcerative dermatitis, thrombocytopenia, and neutropenia in neonatal foals. J Vet Intern Med 19:211–216.

116. Kristensen AT, Weiss DJ, Klausner JS, Laber J, Christie DJ. 1994. Detection of antiplatelet antibody with a platelet immunofluorescence assay. J Vet Intern Med 8:36–39.

117. Keller ET. 1992. Immune-mediated disease as a risk factor for canine lymphoma. Cancer 70:2334–2337.

118. Wardrop KJ, Lewis D, Marks S, Buss M. 1997. Posttransfusion purpura in a dog with hemophilia A. J Vet Intern Med 11:261–263.

119. Evans RS, Duane RT. 1949. Acquired hemolytic anemia. I. The relation of erythrocyte antibody production to activity of the disease. II. The significance of thrombocytopenia and leukopenia. Blood 4:1196–1213.

120. Pegels JG, Helmerhorst FM, van Leeuwen EF, van de Plas-van Dalen, Engelfriet CP, dem Borne AE. 1982. The Evans syndrome: Characterization of the responsible autoantibodies. Br J Haematol 51:445–450.

121. Lewis RM, Schwartz RS, Gilmore CE. 1965. Autoimmune diseases in domestic animals. Ann NY Acad Sci 124:178–200.

122. Carr AP, Panciera DL, Kidd L. 2002. Prognostic factors for mortality and thromboembolism in canine immune-mediated hemolytic anemia: A retrospective study of 72 dogs. J Vet Intern Med 16:504–509.

123. Ingram M, Coopersmith A. 1969. Reticulated platelets following acute blood loss. Br J Haematol 17:225–229.

124. Ljungqvist U. 1971. The platelet response to haemorrhage in splenectomised dogs. Acta Chir Scand 137:97–102.

125. Minter FM, Ingram M. 1971. Platelet volume: Density relationships in normal and acutely bled dogs. Br J Haematol 20:55–68.

126. Lewis DC, Bruyette DS, Kellerman DL, Smith SA. 1997. Thrombocytopenia in dogs with anticoagulant rodenticide-induced hemorrhage: Eight cases (1990–1995). J Am Anim Hosp Assoc 33:417–422.

127. Marder VJ, Feinstein DI, Francis CW, Colman RW. 1994. Consumptive thrombohemorrhagic disorders. In: Colman RW, Hirsch J, Marder VJ, Salzman EW, eds. *Hemostasis and Thrombosis: Basic Principles and Clinical Practice*, 3rd edition, 1023–1063. Philadelphia: JB Lippincott.

128. Kresowik TF, Wakefield TW, Fessler RD, Stanley JC. 1988. Anticoagulant effects of protamine sulfate in a canine model. J Surg Res 45:8–14.

129. Budzynski AZ, Pandya BV, Rubin RN, Brizuela BS, Soszka T, Stewart GJ. 1984. Fibrinogenolytic afibrinogenemia after envenomation by western diamondback rattlesnake (*Crotalus atrox*). Blood 63:1–14.

130. Schaeffer RC Jr, Briston C, Chilton SM, Carlson RW. 1986. Disseminated intravascular coagulation following *Echis carinatus* venom in dogs: Effects of a synthetic thrombin inhibitor. J Lab Clin Med 107:488–497.

131. Cowan LA, Hertzke DM, Fenwick BW, Andreasen CB. 1997. Clinical and clinicopathologic abnormalities in greyhounds with cutaneous and renal glomerular vasculopathy: 18 cases (1992–1994). J Am Vet Med Assoc 210:789–793.

132. Hertzke DM, Cowan LA, Schoning P, Fenwick BW. 1995. Glomerular ultrastructural lesions of idiopathic cutaneous and renal glomerular vasculopathy of greyhounds. Vet Pathol 32:451–459.

133. Holloway S, Senior D, Roth L, Tisher CC. 1993. Hemolytic uremic syndrome in dogs. J Vet Intern Med 7:220–227.

134. Raife T, Friedman KD, Fenwick B. 2004. Lepirudin prevents lethal effects of Shiga toxin in a canine model. Thromb Haemost 92:387–393.

135. Dell'Orco M, Bertazzolo W, Pagliaro L, Roccabianca P, Comazzi S. 2005. Hemolytic-uremic syndrome in a dog. Vet Clin Pathol 34:264–269.

136. Jones PA, Tomasic M, Gentry PA. 1997. Oncotic, hemodilutional, and hemostatic effects of isotonic saline and hydroxyethyl starch solutions in clinically normal ponies. Am J Vet Res 58:541–548.

137. Jutkowitz LA, Rozanski EA, Moreau JA, Rush JE. 2002. Massive transfusion in dogs: 15 cases (1997–2001). J Am Vet Med Assoc 220:1664–1669.

138. Glowaski MM, Moon-Massat PF, Erb HN, Barr SC. 2003. Effects of oxypolygelatin and dextran 70 on hemostatic variables in dogs. Vet Anaesth Analg 30:202–210.

139. Singh MK, Lamb WA. 2005. Idiopathic thrombocytopenia in Cavalier King Charles spaniels. Aust Vet J 83:700–703.

140. Cowan SM, Bartges JW, Gompf RE, Hayes JR, Moyers TD, Snider CC, Gerard DA, Craft RM, Muenchen RA, Carroll RC. 2004. Giant platelet disorder in the Cavalier King Charles spaniel. Exp Hematol 32:344–350.

141. Pedersen HD, Haggstrom J, Olsen LH, Christensen K, Selin A, Burmeister ML, Larsen H. 2002. Idiopathic asymptomatic thrombocytopenia in Cavalier King Charles spaniels is an autosomal recessive trait. J Vet Intern Med 16:169–173.

142. Tsuchiya R, Kyotani K, Scott MA, Nishizono K, Ashida Y, Mochizuki T, Kitao S, Yamada T, Kobayashi K. 1999. Role of platelet activating factor in development of thrombocytopenia and neutropenia in dogs with endotoxemia. Am J Vet Res 60:216–221.

143. Yilmaz Z, Ilcol YO, Torun S, Ulus IH. 2006. Intravenous administration of choline or cdp-choline improves platelet count and platelet closure times in endotoxin-treated dogs. Shock 25:73–79.

144. Kettner F, Reyers F, Miller D. 2003. Thrombocytopaenia in canine babesiosis and its clinical usefulness. J S Afr Vet Assoc 74:63–68.

145. Garcia ATC. 2006. Piroplasma infection in dogs in northern Spain. Vet Parasitol 138:97–102.

146. Shelton GH, Linenberger ML, Grant CK, Abkowitz JL. 1990. Hematologic manifestations of feline immunodeficiency virus infection. Blood 76:1104–1109.

147. Goldstein RE, Lin RC, Langston CE, Scrivani PV, Erb HN, Barr SC. 2006. Influence of infecting serogroup on clinical features of leptospirosis in dogs. J Vet Intern Med 20:489–494.

148. Harrus S, Aroch I, Lavy E, Bark H. 1997. Clinical manifestations of infectious canine cyclic thrombocytopenia. Vet Rec 141:247–250.

149. Martin AR, Brown GK, Dunstan RH, Roberts TK. 2005. *Anaplasma platys*: An improved PCR for its detection in dogs. Exp Parasitol 109:176–180.

150. Sirigireddy KR, Ganta RR. 2005. Multiplex detection of *Ehrlichia* and *Anaplasma* species pathogens in peripheral blood by real-time reverse transcriptase–polymerase chain reaction. J Mol Diagn 7:308–316.

151. Chisholm-Chait A. 2000. Mechanisms of thrombocytopenia in dogs with cancer. Compend Contin Educ Pract Vet 22:1006–1018.

152. Grindem CB, Breitschwerdt EB, Corbett WT, Page RL, Jans HE. 1994. Thrombocytopenia associated with neoplasia in dogs. J Vet Intern Med 8:400–405.

153. O'Keefe DA, Couto CG, Burke-Schwartz C, Jacobs RM. 1987. Systemic mastocytosis in 16 dogs. J Vet Intern Med 1:75–80.

154. O'Donnell MR, Slichter SJ, Weiden PL, Storb R. 1981. Platelet and fibrinogen kinetics in canine tumors. Cancer Res 41:1379–1383.

155. Slichter SJ, Weiden PL, O'Donnell MR, Storb R. 1982. Interruption of tumor-associated platelet consumption with platelet enzyme inhibitors. Blood 59:1252–1258.

156. Bloom JC, Lewis HB, Sellers TS, Deldar A, Morgan DG. 1987. The hematopathology of cefonicid- and cefazedone-induced blood dyscrasias in the dog. Toxicol Appl Pharmacol 90:143–155.

157. Yawata Y, Hebbel RP, Silvis S, Howe R, Jacob H. 1974. Blood cell abnormalities complicating the hypophosphatemia of hyperalimentation: Erythrocyte and platelet ATP deficiency associated with hemolytic anemia and bleeding in hyperalimented dogs. J Lab Clin Med 84:643–653.

158. Lippert AC, Faulkner JE, Evans AT, Mullaney TP. 1989. Total parenteral nutrition in clinically normal cats. J Am Vet Med Assoc 194:669–676.

159. Hasegawa S, Pawankar R, Suzuki K, Nakahata T, Furukawa S, Okumura K, Ra C. 1999. Functional expression of the high affinity receptor for IgE (FcεRI) in human platelets and its' [*sic*] intracellular expression in human megakaryocytes. Blood 93:2543–2551.

160. Hudson JG, Bowen AL, Navia P, Rios-Dalenz J, Pollard AJ, Williams D, Heath D. 1999. The effect of high altitude on platelet counts, thrombopoietin and erythropoietin levels in young Bolivian airmen visiting the Andes. Int J Biometeorol 43:85–90.

161. Bass MC, Schultze AE. 1998. Essential thrombocythemia in a dog: Case report and literature review. J Am Anim Hosp Assoc 34:197–203.

162. Hopper PE, Mandell CP, Turrel JM, Jain NC, Tablin F, Zinkl JG. 1989. Probable essential thrombocythemia in a dog. J Vet Intern Med 3:79–85.

163. Hammer AS, Couto CG, Getzy D, Bailey MQ. 1990. Essential thrombocythemia in a cat. J Vet Intern Med 4:87–91.

164. Fialkow PJ, Faguet GB, Jacobson RJ, Vaidya K, Murphy S. 1981. Evidence that essential thrombocythemia is a clonal disorder with origin in a multipotent stem cell. Blood 58:916–919.

165. Messick J, Carothers M, Wellman M. 1990. Identification and characterization of megakaryoblasts in acute megakaryoblastic leukemia in a dog. Vet Pathol 27:212–214.

166. Cain GR, Kawakami TG, Jain NC. 1985. Radiation-induced megakaryoblastic leukemia in a dog. Vet Pathol 22:641–643.

167. Hamilton TA, Morrison WB, DeNicola DB. 1991. Cytosine arabinoside chemotherapy for acute megakaryocytic leukemia in a cat. J Am Vet Med Assoc 199:359–361.

168. Park HM, Doster AR, Tashbaeva RE, Lee YM, Lyoo YS, Lee SJ, Kim HJ, Sur JH. 2006. Clinical, histopathological and immunohistochemical findings in a case of megakaryoblastic leukemia in a dog. J Vet Diagn Invest 18:287–291.

169. Field ME. 1930. The effect of emotion on the blood platelet count. Am J Physiol 93:245–248.

170. Chamberlain KG, Tong M, Penington DG. 1990. Properties of the exchangeable splenic platelets released into the circulation during exercise-induced thrombocytosis. Am J Hematol 34:161–168.

171. Freedman M, Altszuler N, Karpatkin S. 1977. Presence of a nonsplenic platelet pool. Blood 50:419–425.

172. Lepherd EE. 1977. Effect of exercise on platelet size and number in ponies. Vet Rec 101:488.

173. Dawson AA, Ogston D. 1969. Exercise-induced thrombocytosis. Acta Haematol 42:241–246.

174. Schmidt KG, Rasmussen JW. 1984. Exercise-induced changes in the in vivo distribution of ^{111}In-labelled platelets. Scand J Haematol 32:159–166.

175. Margiotta MS, Kasabian AK, Karp NS, Ting V, Dublin BK, Sagiroglu J, Dublin BA. 1998. Humorally mediated thrombocytosis in major lower extremity trauma. Ann Plast Surg 40:463–468.

176. Folman CC, Ooms M, Kuenen BB, de Jong SM, Vet RJ, de Haas M, dem Borne AE. 2001. The role of thrombopoietin in post-operative thrombocytosis. Br J Haematol 114:126–133.

177. Hammer AS. 1991. Thrombocytosis in dogs and cats: A retrospective study. Comp Haematol Int 1:181–186.

178. Sellon DC, Levine JF, Palmer K, Millikin E, Grindem C, Covington P. 1997. Thrombocytosis in 24 horses (1989–1994). J Vet Intern Med 11:24–29.

179. Gastl G, Plante M, Finstad CL, Wong GY, Federici MG, Bander NH, Rubin SC. 1993. High IL-6 levels in ascitic fluid correlate with reactive thrombocytosis in patients with epithelial ovarian cancer. Br J Haematol 83:433–441.

180. Hogan DF, Dhaliwal RS, Sisson DD, Kitchell BE. 1999. Paraneoplastic thrombocytosis–induced systemic thromboembolism in a cat. J Am Anim Hosp Assoc 35:483–486.

181. Levine SP. 1999. Thrombocytosis. In: Lee GR, Foerster J, Lukens J, Wintrobe MM, eds. *Wintrobe's Clinical Hematology*, 10th edition, 1648–1660. Philadelphia: Lippincott Williams & Wilkins.

182. Akan H, Guven N, Aydogdu I, Arat M, Beksac M, Dalva K. 2000. Thrombopoietic cytokines in patients with iron deficiency anemia with or without thrombocytosis. Acta Haematol 103:152–156.

183. Geddis AE, Kaushansky K. 2003. Cross-reactivity between erythropoietin and thrombopoietin at the level of Mpl does not account for the thrombocytosis seen in iron deficiency. J Pediatr Hematol Oncol 25:919–920.

184. Mackin AJ, Allen DG, Johnstone IB. 1995. Effects of vincristine and prednisone on platelet numbers and function in clinically normal dogs. Am J Vet Res 56:100–108.

185. Mandel EM, Bessler H, Djaldetti M. 1977. Effect of a low dose of vincristine on platelet production in mice. Exp Hematol 5:499–504.

186. Corash L, Mok Y, Levin J, Baker G. 1990. Regulation of platelet heterogeneity: Effects of thrombocytopenia on platelet volume and density. Exp Hematol 18:205–212.

187. Hunt P, Zsebo KM, Hokom MM, Hornkohl A, Birkett NC, del Castillo JC, Martin F. 1992. Evidence that stem cell factor is involved in the rebound thrombocytosis that follows 5-fluorouracil treatment. Blood 80:904–911.

188. Kraytman M. 1973. Platelet size in thrombocytopenias and thrombocytosis of various origin. Blood 41:587–598.

189. Ichikawa N, Kitano K, Shimodaira S, Ishida F, Ito T, Kajikawa S, Tahara T, Kato T, Kiyosawa K. 1998. Changes in serum thrombopoietin levels after splenectomy. Acta Haematol 100:137–141.

190. Jain NC. 1986. Qualitative and quantitative disorders of platelets. In: Jain NC, ed. *Schalm's Veterinary Hematology*, 4th edition, 466–486. Philadelphia: Lea & Febiger.

191. Bessler H, Notti I, Djaldetti M. 1981. The effect of partial splenectomy on platelet production in mice. Thromb Haemost 46:602–603.

192. Tanum G, Sønstevold A, Jakobsen E. 1984. The effect of splenectomy on platelet formation and megakaryocyte DNA content in rats. Blood 63:593–597.

193. Weintraub AH, Khan I, Karptkin S. 1976. Evidence for a splenic release factor of platelets in chronic blood loss plasma of rabbits. Br J Haematol 34:421–426.

194. Moore GE, Mahaffey EA, Hoenig M. 1992. Hematologic and serum biochemical effects of long-term administration of anti-inflammatory doses of prednisone in dogs. Am J Vet Res 53:1033–1037.

195. Corash L. 1989. The relationship between megakaryocyte ploidy and platelet volume. Blood Cells 15:81–107.

196. Levin J, Bessman JD. 1983. The inverse relation between platelet volume and platelet number: Abnormalities in hematologic disease and evidence that platelet size does not correlate with platelet age. J Lab Clin Med 101:295–307.

197. Weiser MG, Kociba GJ. 1984. Platelet concentration and platelet volume distribution in healthy cats. Am J Vet Res 45:518–522.

198. Bowles KM, Cooke LJ, Richards EM, Baglin TP. 2005. Platelet size has diagnostic predictive value in patients with thrombocytopenia. Clin Lab Haematol 27:370–373.

199. Thompson CB, Love DG, Quinn PG, Valeri CR. 1983. Platelet size does not correlate with platelet age. Blood 62:487–494.

200. Catalfamo JL, Dodds WJ. 2000. Thrombopathies. In: Feldman BF, Zinkl JG, Jain NC, eds. *Schalm's Veterinary Hematology*, 5th edition, 1042–1050. Philadelphia: Lippincott Williams & Wilkins.

201. Brown SJ, Simpson KW, Baker S, Spagnoletti MA, Elwood CM. 1994. Macrothrombocytosis in Cavalier King Charles spaniels. Vet Rec 135:281–283.

202. Smedile LE, Houston DM, Taylor SM, Post K, Searcy GP. 1997. Idiopathic, asymptomatic thrombocytopenia in Cavalier King Charles spaniels: 11 cases (1983–1993). J Am Anim Hosp Assoc 33:411–415.

203. Boyce JT, Kociba GJ, Jacobs RM, Weiser MG. 1986. Feline leukemia virus–induced thrombocytopenia and macrothrombocytosis in cats. Vet Pathol 23:16–20.

204. Northern J Jr, Tvedten HW. 1992. Diagnosis of microthrombocytosis and immune-mediated thrombocytopenia in dogs with thrombocytopenia: 68 cases (1987–1989). J Am Vet Med Assoc 200:368–372.

205. Balduini CL, Noris P, Spedini P, Belletti S, Zambelli A, Da Prada GA. 1999. Relationship between size and thiazole orange fluorescence of platelets in patients undergoing high-dose chemotherapy. Br J Haematol 106:202–207.

206. Joutsi-Korhonen L, Sainio S, Riikonen S, Javela K, Teramo K, Kekomaki R. 2000. Detection of reticulated platelets: Estimating the degree of fluorescence of platelets stained with thiazole orange. Eur J Haematol 65:66–71.

207. Robinson M, Machin S, Mackie I, Harrison P. 2000. In vivo biotinylation studies: Specificity of labelling of reticulated platelets by thiazole orange and mepacrine. Br J Haematol 108:859–864.

208. Weiss DJ, Townsend E. 1998. Evaluation of reticulated platelets in dogs. Comp Haematol Int 8:166–170.

209. Wolf RF, Peng J, Friese P, Gilmore LS, Burstein SA, Dale GL. 1997. Erythropoietin administration increases production and reactivity of platelets in dogs. Thromb Haemost 78:1505–1509.

210. Abe Y, Wada H, Sakakura M, Nishioka J, Tomatsu H, Hamaguchi Y, Oguni S, Shiku H, Nobori T. 2005. Usefulness of fully automated measurement of reticulated platelets using whole blood. Clin Appl Thromb Hemost 11:263–270.

211. Salvagno GL, Montagnana M, Degan M, Marradi PL, Ricetti MM, Riolfi P, Poli G, Minuz P, Santonastaso CL, Guidi GC. 2006. Evaluation of platelet turnover by flow cytometry. Platelets 17:170–177.

212. Ault KA, Rinder HM, Mitchell J, Carmody MB, Vary CP, Hillman RS. 1992. The significance of platelets with increased RNA content (reticulated platelets): A measure of the rate of thrombopoiesis. Am J Clin Pathol 98:637–646.

213. British Committee for Standards in Haematology General Haematology Task Force. 2003. Guidelines for the investigation and management of idiopathic thrombocytopenic purpura in adults, children and in pregnancy. Br J Haematol 120:574–596.

214. Scott MA, Kaiser L, Davis JM, Schwartz KA. 2002. Development of a sensitive immunoradiometric assay for detection of platelet surface-associated immunoglobulins in thrombocytopenic dogs. Am J Vet Res 63:124–129.

215. Wilkerson MJ, Shuman W. 2001. Alterations in normal canine platelets during storage in EDTA anticoagulated blood. Vet Clin Pathol 30:107–113.

216. Kristensen AT, Weiss DJ, Klausner JS, Laber J, Christie DJ. 1994. Comparison of microscopic and flow cytometric detection of platelet antibody in dogs suspected of having immune-mediated thrombocytopenia. Am J Vet Res 55:1111–1114.

217. Lewis DC, McVey DS, Shuman WS, Muller WB. 1995. Development and characterization of a flow cytometric assay for detection of platelet-bound immunoglobulin G in dogs. Am J Vet Res 56:1555–1558.

218. Nunez R, Gomes-Keller MA, Schwarzwald C, Feige K. 2001. Assessment of equine autoimmune thrombocytopenia (EAT) by flow cytometry. BMC Blood Disord 1:1.

219. Joshi BC, Jain NC. 1976. Detection of antiplatelet antibody in serum and on megakaryocytes of dogs with autoimmune thrombocytopenia. Am J Vet Res 37:681–685.

220. Hyde P, Zucker-Franklin D. 1987. Antigenic differences between human platelets and megakaryocytes. Am J Pathol 127:349–357.

Chapter 5

HEMOSTASIS

Hemostasis 261
Platelets (Thrombocytes) 262
    I.   Physiologic Processes 262
    II.   Platelet Concentration 262
    III.   Platelet Function Tests 263
von Willebrand Factor (vWF) 265
    I.   Physiologic Processes 265
    II.   von Willebrand Disease (vWD) 265
    III.   Analytical Concepts 266
    IV.   Decreased von Willebrand Factor to Antigen (vWF : Ag) Ratio 267
    V.   Interpretive Considerations 268
    VI.   Genetic Tests 268
Coagulation 268
    I.   Physiologic Processes 268
    II.   Analytical Concepts 274
    III.   Whole Blood Clotting Times 279
        A. Lee-White Method 279
        B. Activated Coagulation (Clotting) Time (ACT) 279
        C. Synbiotics SCA2000 Veterinary Coagulation Analyzer 280
    IV.   Activated Partial Thromboplastin Time (PTT, APTT, or aPTT) 280
    V.   Prothrombin Time (PT) 282
    VI.   Thrombin Time (TT) 284
    VII. Fibrinogen 285
    VIII. Other Specific Coagulation Factor Activities (II, VII, VIII, IX, X, XI, XII,
         PK, and HMWK) 286
    IX.   Proteins Induced by Vitamin K Antagonism or Absence (PIVKA) 287
    X.   Russell's Viper Venom Time (RVVT) 288
    XI.   Endogenous Anticoagulants 288
        A. Antithrombin (AT) 288
        B. Protein C 291
        C. Protein Z 291
    XII. Coagulation Factor Antibodies (Inhibitors) 292
    XIII. Anti-(phospholipid-protein) Antibodies 292
Fibrinolysis 293
    I.   Physiologic Processes 293
    II.   Fibrin or Fibrinogen Degradation Products (FDPs) 293
    III.   Fibrin Fragment D-Dimer 299
    IV.   Other Assays 300
Blood Vessels (Endothelial Cells) 300
Major Bleeding Disorders: Findings and Pathogeneses 300
    I.   Diagnosis 300
    II.   Pathogenesis 304
Thrombosis 310

Table 5.1. Abbreviations and symbols in this chapter

[x]	x concentration (x = analyte)
ACT	Activated coagulation (clotting) time
ADP	Adenosine diphosphate
APC	Activated protein C
AT	Antithrombin (antithrombin III)
ATP	Adenosine triphosphate
BMBT	Buccal mucosal bleeding time
Ca^{2+}	Calcium
DDAVP	1-deamino-8-D-arginine vasopressin
DIC	Disseminated intravascular coagulation
DNA	Deoxyribonucleic acid
EDTA	Ethylenediaminetetraacetic acid
ELISA	Enzyme-linked immunosorbent assay
fCa^{2+}	Free ionized calcium
FDPs	Fibrin or fibrinogen degradation products; fibrin fragments + fibrinogen fragments
GPIb	Glycoprotein Ib
Hct	Hematocrit
HMWK	High molecular weight kininogen
INR	International normalized ratio
ISI	International Sensitivity Index
I–XIII	Inactive coagulation factors one through thirteen; terminal "a" denotes that the factor has been activated (e.g., IIa)
LMWH	Low molecular weight heparin
MPS	Mononuclear phagocyte system
M_r	Relative molecular mass
PAI	Plasminogen activator inhibitor
PIVKA	Proteins induced by vitamin K antagonism, absence, or deficiency
PK	Prokallikrein or prekallikrein (synonyms)
PT	Prothrombin time
PTT	Activated partial thromboplastin time
PZI	Protein Z–dependent protease inhibitor
RMSF	Rocky mountain spotted fever
RVVT	Russell's viper venom time
SI	Système International d'Unités
TAFI	Thrombin-activatable fibrinolysis inhibitor
TAT	Thrombin-antithrombin complexes
TF	Tissue factor, tissue thromboplastin factor
TFPI	Tissue factor pathway coagulation inhibitor
t-PA	Plasminogen activator, tissue type
TT	Thrombin time
TT_{Clauss}	Modified TT for [fibrinogen] by using the method of von Clauss
u-PA	Plasminogen activator, urokinase type
vWD	Von Willebrand disease
vWF	Von Willebrand factor
vWF:Ag	Von Willebrand factor as detected antigenically
vWF:CBA	Von Willebrand factor collagen-binding activity
WRI	Within the reference interval

HEMOSTASIS

I.   *Hemostasis* is the arrest of bleeding or the interruption of blood flow through a vessel. The term is also used more generally to refer to the intricate and balanced physiologic processes that maintain blood in a freely flowing state but allow the rapid formation of localized solid plugs to seal injured vessels. Normal hemostasis depends on the complex interactions of its major components: platelets, coagulation factors, fibrinolytic factors, and blood vessels (Fig. 5.1).

II.   Abnormal hemostasis causes hemorrhage or thrombosis. Laboratory testing of the individual components of the hemostatic system may be used to discover, explain, monitor, or prognosticate these pathologic states.

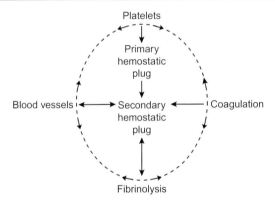

Fig. 5.1. Hemostasis in health. Normal hemostasis is maintained by the numerous and complex interactions of blood vessels, platelets, coagulation pathways, and the fibrinolytic system that lead to the formation and resolution of a secondary hemostatic plug after vascular injury. The following events occur with blood vessel damage:
- Vasoconstriction reduces blood loss, and activated endothelial cells express both prothrombotic functions to limit bleeding and antithrombotic functions to limit clotting.
- Platelets adhere to exposed subendothelium, spread to patch the defect, release products that activate other platelets, and aggregate to form a primary hemostatic plug. Their secretory products also help maintain vasoconstriction and promote coagulation, and their membranes are an important source of phospholipid to accelerate coagulation.
- The surface-induced and TF coagulation pathways are activated, leading to the production of thrombin and subsequent conversion of fibrinogen to fibrin within the primary hemostatic plug. This forms a stable secondary hemostatic plug that controls bleeding. Thrombin also activates platelets, endothelial cells, and TAFI.
- When coagulation pathways are activated, fibrinolysis is also. Fibrinolysis helps control the extent of coagulation by breaking down fibrin, thus contributing to the formation of an appropriate secondary hemostatic plug and promoting eventual removal of the plug to maintain normal blood flow.

Abnormalities of any component of this system can upset the balance and lead to either hemorrhage or thrombosis.

PLATELETS (THROMBOCYTES)

I. Physiologic processes
  A. See Chapter 4 for platelet structure, production, kinetics, and nonhemostatic functions.
  B. Hemostatic functions
    1. Platelets are required for formation of primary hemostatic plugs to repair small vascular defects. They amplify minute stimuli into explosive production of fibrin to form more secure secondary hemostatic plugs.
    2. Platelet hemostatic functions can be divided into five major categories:
      a. Adhesion: Platelets adhere to and spread over (patch) perturbed endothelium or exposed subendothelium, mostly via vWF that binds to platelet GPIb and collagen in the vessel wall.
      b. Aggregation: When adherence or platelet agonists (e.g., ADP, collagen, platelet-activating factor, or thrombin) activate receptors for platelet membrane glycoprotein $\alpha_{IIb}\beta_3$, platelets aggregate via fibrinogen or vWF bridges that bind to $\alpha_{IIb}\beta_3$ on neighboring platelets.
      c. Release (secretion): Activated platelets can release preformed granular contents (e.g., fibrinogen, factor V, ADP, ATP, and plasminogen) and newly formed mediators such as thromboxane A_2 and arachidonic acid. These products help mediate the hemostatic process.
      d. Facilitation of coagulation: When platelets are stimulated, anionic membrane phospholipids that support coagulation move from the inner membrane to the outer membrane, where they are available for use as cofactors in the coagulation pathways. These phospholipids include phosphatidylserine and are referred to as *platelet factor 3*.[1,2] Platelets provide specific high-affinity binding sites for coagulation enzymes, cofactors, and zymogens. Platelets also release platelet agonists that activate other platelets.
      e. Clot (coagulum) retraction: Platelets within a thrombus facilitate wound closure and vessel patency by a contractile process involving activated platelets, inter-platelet bridging via the fibrinogen receptor $\alpha_{IIb}\beta_3$, and platelet actin and myosin.[3]
    3. Mediators released from platelets during the hemostatic process contribute to local tissue repair.

II. Platelet concentration (often called platelet count in clinical jargon)
  A. See Chapter 4 for analytical concepts and disorders associated with thrombocytopenia and thrombocytosis.
  B. Thrombocytopenia may cause mucocutaneous hemorrhage when severe. Hemorrhage from thrombocytopenia alone is not expected with a [platelet] above about $30 \times 10^3/\mu L$ and may not occur with a [platelet] $< 5 \times 10^3/\mu L$.
    1. Thrombocrit may be a better reflection of platelet hemostatic potential than is [platelet], because large platelets may have greater hemostatic potential.
    2. Hemorrhage may occur at greater [platelet] if there are concurrent platelet functional deficits or increased vascular trauma.
  C. Thrombocytosis has been associated with thrombosis or hemorrhage in people. Similar reports are rare in domestic mammals.
    1. Thrombosis is not expected with reactive thrombocytosis.

2. Thrombosis associated with human clonal thrombocythemic disorders may relate to altered function of platelets, endothelial cells, or leukocytes. It is not predictable based solely on the [platelet].[4]

3. Hemorrhage in clonal thrombocythemic disorders of people may relate to altered platelet function or acquired vWD.[4]

III. Platelet function tests

A. BMBT is a standardized in vivo test of primary hemostasis used in dogs and cats. Mucosal membranes or skin sites[5] have been used in large animals. The skin bleeding time is less repeatable,[6] and cuticle bleeding times assess secondary hemostasis in addition to primary hemostasis.

1. Analytical concepts

a. Units are not standardized. Results are sometimes reported in seconds (e.g., 202 s), minutes and seconds (e.g., 3 min 22 s), or minutes (e.g., 3, 3.4, or 3.37 min). Interobserver and intraobserver imprecision[7] suggests it would be most appropriate to report to the nearest minute. The BMBT of healthy dogs has been reported to range from 1 to 5 min, but it usually is less than 4 min.[6,7]

b. Procedure: The upper lip is rolled out and usually secured with a gauze strip around the maxilla. Timing begins when a standardized cut (or duplicate cuts) is made in the mucosal surface of the upper lip by using a spring-loaded device (e.g., Surgicutt devices). The cut is small enough (5 mm × 1 mm) for primary hemostasis alone to resolve the bleeding; coagulation and generation of fibrin are not necessary. Filter paper is used to blot away excess blood without touching or disturbing the incision itself. The end point is when bleeding ceases and a crescent of blood no longer forms on the filter paper.

2. Prolonged BMBT: The BMBT test is relatively insensitive, but BMBT will be prolonged (> 4–5 min in dogs) with moderate to marked defects of primary hemostasis.

a. Thrombocytopenia (Table 4.2): Marked thrombocytopenia is a contraindication to BMBT because it is already known that BMBT will be prolonged. The degree of thrombocytopenia required to prolong the BMBT is not clear, but it is commonly stated that BMBT prolongations may occur with platelet concentrations of < 70–100 × 10^3/μL. This decision threshold varies with other factors, such as mean platelet volume, vWF : Ag, and Hct.

b. Thrombopathia (platelet dysfunction) (Table 5.2)

(1) Terms used to describe a disorder of abnormal platelet function include *thrombopathia*, *thrombopathy*, *thrombocytopathy*, and *thrombocytopathia*. The precise definition and usage of each term vary. *Thrombopathia* is used herein as a general term to indicate any disorder of platelet function.

(2) Thrombopathia should be suspected if BMBT is prolonged, but platelet concentrations, Hct, and vWF : Ag values are WRI.

(a) Hereditary thrombopathias are uncommon. Additional reading is available.[8]

(b) Acquired thrombopathia occurs concurrently with diseases or conditions that are usually diagnosed by other findings. The thrombopathia may be subclinical or it may contribute obviously to morbidity.

c. vWD: BMBT can be used as a screening test for vWD in breeds predisposed to the disease (e.g., Doberman pinschers). BMBT should be prolonged when vWF : Ag < 20 % and may be prolonged with greater values.

Table 5.2. Diseases and conditions that cause thrombopathias

Hereditary: Ca^{2+} diacylglycerol guanine nucleotide exchange factor I mutations (basset hound thrombopathia, Simmental hereditary thrombopathia, Spitz thrombopathia), Chédiak Higashi syndrome (Persian cats; Hereford, Brangus, and Japanese black cattle), cyclic hematopoiesis (grey collie), dense-granule storage pool disease of American cocker spaniels, Glanzmann's thrombasthenia (great Pyrenees, otterhounds, horses), idiopathic thrombopathia in a Thoroughbred, platelet procoagulant defect of German shepherds, thrombasthenic thrombopathia (otterhounds—original variant)

Acquired
*Drug exposure: anesthetics (barbiturates), anti-inflammatories (nonsteroidal anti-inflammatory drugs), membrane-active drugs (local anesthetics, β-adrenergic blockers, antihistamines), antibiotics (penicillins and cephalosporins), antiplatelets (ticlopidine), dietary factors (garlic, ethanol, caffeine)

Envenomation (certain venoms)

*Increased FDPs (increased fibrinolysis, DIC)

Hepatic disease

Hyperglobulinemia (multiple myeloma, ehrlichiosis)

Immune-mediated thrombocytopenia (some antiplatelet antibodies)

Infections: bovine virus diarrhea virus, feline leukemia virus

Neoplasia involving megakaryocytes: myeloproliferative diseases, acute megakaryoblastic leukemia

*Renal failure (uremia)

Synthetic colloids (dextran, hetastarch)

* A relatively common disease or condition

Note: Thrombopathia (decreased platelet function) should be considered when (1) petechiae, ecchymoses, or mucosal hemorrhages occur without marked thrombocytopenia, or (2) bleeding time or clot retraction is prolonged in the absence of thrombocytopenia (also consider vWD).

    d. Anemia: This may prolong BMBT. Proposed mechanisms include (1) the lower erythrocyte concentration enables more platelets to circulate centrally and forces fewer platelets to circulate near the vessel wall where they can readily interact with it, and (2) fewer erythrocytes result in decreased erythrocyte ADP, a platelet agonist.[9,10]

    e. Vascular disease: BMBT rarely may be prolonged with certain vascular diseases.

    f. Antiplatelet drugs: Aspirin increased forelimb cutaneous bleeding times in horses[5] and also increased canine BMBT values, although the latter were still WRI. Other antiplatelet drugs often do not prolong the BMBT.[11–13]

    g. Afibrinogenemia: BMBT may be prolonged in patients with afibrinogenemia, presumably because of the lack of fibrinogen for interplatelet bridging.[14–16]

  3. Defects restricted to secondary hemostasis and the formation of fibrin (e.g., hemophilia, but not afribinogenemia) should not prolong BMBT unless a larger vessel is cut.[17]

  4. Bleeding time has not been useful as a screening test for predicting the occurrence of excessive surgical bleeding in human patients.[12]

B. Clot (coagulum) retraction is mediated by platelets, so some thrombopathias (e.g., Glanzmann's thrombasthenia) (Table 5.2) or marked thrombocytopenia (Table 4.2) prolong clot retraction. This may be noted by a decreased yield of serum after

60–90 min of clotting but is more reliably determined by standardized tests of clot retraction:[18]

1. Blood (0.5 mL) is collected into cold saline (4.5 mL) and maintained at 4 °C until being transferred to a glass tube and mixed with thrombin (10 U/mL final).
2. The tubes are then placed in a 37 °C water bath. At 1 h, 2 h, and 4 h, clot retraction is graded 1+ (the least retraction) through 4+ (the most retraction) based on the size of the clot and the volume of surrounding serum.
3. Testing should not be done if the patient has thrombocytopenia or has recently received aspirin or other cyclooxygenase inhibitors, because poor clot retraction is expected.
4. Clot retraction is not impaired in vWD.

C. Other specialized tests are used to assess platelet responses in vitro.[8] These tests are available in labs with specialized expertise and equipment including flow cytometers, aggregometers, and the PFA-100 analyzer (Dade Behring, Miami, FL). In addition to detecting and characterizing decreased platelet function, these tests can also detect hyperactive platelets as may occur with infections (e.g., feline infectious peritonitis or heartworm disease), malignancies, the nephrotic syndrome, and other disorders.[19–22] A suspected specific thrombopathia may be demonstrable by specific testing; for example, basset hound thrombopathy by platelet aggregation and secretion studies or by molecular genetic detection of the mutation.

VON WILLEBRAND FACTOR (vWF)

I. Physiologic processes
   A. *vWF* is a large multimeric plasma glycoprotein ($M_r \approx 500,000–20,000,000$) important in platelet adhesion and aggregation.
      1. Adhesion: vWF bridges platelets to injured vessel walls via platelet GPIb and exposed subendothelial proteins such as collagen.
      2. Aggregation: vWF contributes to platelet-platelet bridging via GPIb and the platelet integrin $\alpha_{IIb}\beta_3$.
      3. The largest multimers of vWF are the most functional.[23]
   B. Most vWF is produced by endothelial cells[24,25] and secreted constitutively or stored and secreted later upon endothelial cell activation. Megakaryocytes also synthesize vWF. Megakaryocytes and platelets contain a substantial percentage of total circulating vWF in most species (e.g., cats and people), but canine platelets contain very little.[26,27]
   C. Secreted vWF forms noncovalent complexes with coagulation factor VIII and serves as a stabilizing and protective carrier molecule for factor VIII.[28]

II. von Willebrand disease (vWD)
   A. *vWD*, which is a disorder of primary hemostasis caused by a deficiency in functional vWF, is the most common hereditary bleeding disorder in dogs but is rare in cattle,[29] cats,[30] and horses.[31–33]
   B. vWD is usually an inherited disorder, but acquired vWD occurs rarely in people.[34,35] Acquired vWD has not been clearly documented in veterinary species.
      1. One of the diseases associated with human acquired vWD is hypothyroidism, and treatment of these people for hypothyroidism has resolved the concurrent vWF deficiencies.[36]

2. An association between hypothyroidism and vWD has also been suggested in dogs, particularly in Doberman pinschers.[37] However, studies have produced conflicting results, and the concurrence of common diseases does not prove a cause-and-effect relationship.[23] The finding of vWF : Ag values that were WRI for hypothyroid dogs before treatment with levothyroxine and significantly decreased (not increased) after treatment indicates that there is not a predictable association between hypothyroidism and vWD in dogs.[38]

C. Three general types of vWD have been defined (though subtypes exist):[39]

1. Type 1: All vWF multimers are present but at decreased concentrations. The severity of type 1 vWD varies. It is the most common form and occurs in many dog breeds, including Doberman pinschers.[40]

2. Type 2: This severe, uncommon form is a deficiency of vWF with a disproportionate decrease in large multimers. It occurs in German shorthaired pointers and German wirehaired pointers[41] and has been reported in horses.[31,33]

3. Type 3: This severe form, which involves an absence of all vWF multimers, occurs particularly in Chesapeake Bay retrievers, Dutch kooikers, Scottish terriers, and Shetland sheepdogs.[42–45]

D. Clinical and laboratory signs of vWD

1. Mild to severe mucosal hemorrhage (epistaxis, gastrointestinal hemorrhage, or prolonged estral bleeding), cutaneous bruising, and prolonged hemorrhage from nonsurgical or surgical trauma (e.g., tail docking, dewclaw removal in puppies, or tooth extraction); hemarthrosis and hematomas in horses

2. Absence of petechiae may help differentiate vWD from platelet disorders.

3. Prolonged BMBT without thrombocytopenia and without prolonged coagulation times

4. PTT may be mildly prolonged because decreased factor VIII coagulation activity (which may be denoted FVIII : C) occurs secondary to reductions in circulating vWF, a carrier molecule for factor VIII. However, in contrast to human patients with vWD, FVIII : C in dogs with vWD is usually > 30 % of the activity in reference plasma, so PTT is usually WRI, even in dogs with type 3 vWD and therefore no vWF.[23,42,46] PTT may be prolonged in horses with vWD.[33]

III. Analytical concepts

A. Sample

1. Plasma from blood drawn into sodium citrate or EDTA; citrate tubes should be filled to give a 1 : 9 volume ratio of citrate to blood. The vWF : Ag may be markedly decreased in samples with clots or in vitro hemolysis, but lipemia has no significant effect.[47]

2. The vWF : Ag is reportedly stable for at least 8 h in canine plasma or whole blood stored at room temperature.[47] However, values are significantly increased at 24 h after collection when whole blood samples are stored at room temperature, and values are increased at 48 h (but not 24 h) after collection when plasma is stored at room temperature.[48] These increases did not occur when samples were refrigerated. It is generally recommended that plasma be collected promptly after blood collection, frozen, and shipped overnight with ice.

B. Units: %, U/dL, or U/mL relative to 100 %, 100 U/dL, or 100 U/mL, respectively, of vWF : Ag in pooled plasma from healthy individuals of the same species. Units may be written to indicate the species of the patient and reference samples (e.g., CU/dL for canine (C) samples). Variations in the composition of pooled plasma from the reference animals can affect results.

   C. vWF : Ag assays[23,49–52]

     1. ELISA: vWF is usually measured by a quantitative ELISA with species-specific antibodies to vWF (i.e., vWF : Ag). Values < 50 % are usually considered decreased. ELISA testing has largely replaced electroimmunoassay methods involving electrophoresis of plasma vWF in agarose gels containing antibodies to vWF.

     2. Multimeric analysis (immunoelectrophoresis)

       a. vWF multimers are separated by agarose electrophoresis so that the relative amounts of different sized multimers can be determined.

       b. Differentiates type 1 vWD (high molecular weight multimers present) from type 2 vWD (high molecular weight multimers absent)

     3. Functional assays

       a. Botrocetin cofactor assay: Platelets agglutinate in the presence of botrocetin and vWF. The rate of this vWF-dependent platelet agglutination correlates well with the amount of plasma vWF : Ag except with type 2 vWD. In type 2 vWD, botrocetin cofactor activity may be markedly reduced while the amount of plasma vWF : Ag may be WRI or mildly decreased. This is because the more functional large multimers are deficient.

       b. vWF collagen-binding activity (vWF : CBA) may be measured in canine plasma by an ELISA that detects only the vWF that can bind to collagen. The assay therefore measures the quantity of functional vWF and preferentially detects the more functional large multimers. The ratio of vWF : Ag to vWF : CBA may be increased in type 2 vWD because of a decrease in large multimers and therefore a greater decrease in functional vWF than in vWF antigen.

IV. Decreased von Willebrand factor to antigen (vWF : Ag) ratio (Table 5.3)

   A. Decreased plasma vWF : Ag is indicative of the vWD trait or a carrier state for it, depending on the degree of the decrease. Clinical signs of impaired hemostasis may not be present. The following are common guidelines for ELISA vWF : Ag results in dogs:[53]

     1. Dogs with vWF : Ag values < 50 % are considered carriers of the vWD trait. They are at risk for clinical disease and are likely to transmit the trait to offspring. The risk of clinical vWD is greater at lower vWF : Ag values.

     2. Dogs with borderline vWF : Ag values of 50–69 % are at little or no risk for clinical disease but may be carriers that can transmit the trait to offspring. Repeated testing may clarify if affected (value < 50 %) or not (value > 69 %).

Table 5.3. Diseases and conditions that cause decreased vWF : Ag

vWD: vWF : Ag usually < 35 %
*Type I: all vWF multimers present but proportionately deficient
Type II: deficiency of vWF multimers with high M_r
Type III: absence of all vWF multimers, vWF : Ag ≈ 0 %
*vWD carrier (rarely symptomatic): vWF : Ag usually 30–70 %

  * A relatively common disease or condition

  Note: Hemolysis or clotted samples may cause marked false decreases in vWF : Ag values. vWF : Ag units: % of result for plasma pooled from healthy dogs.

    3. Dogs with type 3 vWD have essentially no vWF : Ag.

    4. Most dogs that bleed because of vWD have vWF : Ag values < 35 %.

  B. Dogs with at least 70 % plasma vWF : Ag are considered free from the vWD trait. They are not at risk for clinical disease and have a very low risk for transmitting the trait to offspring.

  C. Multimer analysis is necessary to document type 2 vWD. Functional testing may be suggestive.

V. Interpretive considerations

  A. See the foregoing section (Analytical concepts, sect. III, A) for effects of improper sample processing.

  B. Intraindividual biological variation: The amount of plasma vWF : Ag has been shown to vary considerably from day to day when healthy or diseased (vWD) dogs are sampled serially.[47]

  C. Exercise: Amounts of the plasma vWF : Ag in dogs may be increased after very strenuous exercise.[54,55] The vWF : Ag in horses increased as much as 100 % within minutes after strenuous exercise.[56]

  D. Pregnancy: Substantial increases occurred in bitches at parturition, with lesser increases in the last trimester of pregnancy and for the first 1–2 wk after parturition.[57]

  E. DDAVP (1-deamino-8-D-arginine vasopressin):[54]

    1. DDAVP increases the plasma vWF : Ag in dogs with type 1 vWD or in dogs without vWD by releasing vWF from stores, probably in endothelial cells.[58] Improved hemostasis after DDAVP may not be due to preferential release of larger multimers as in people. In one study, the vWF : CBA increased proportionally to the vWF : Ag after DDAVP administration to dogs, without a disproportionate increase in large multimers.[52]

    2. DDAVP can be used effectively to increase the amount of vWF in blood donor animals when administered 30–90 min prior to blood collection.[59]

  F. vWF : Ag values may also be increased by epinephrine,[54] endotoxin,[60] azotemia,[61] liver disease,[62] and other illnesses.

VI. Genetic tests have been developed that can detect some vWF gene mutations in several breeds of dogs and may be useful in detecting carriers in specific breeds.[45,63,64]

COAGULATION

I. Physiologic processes[65,66]

  A. Coagulation is not synonymous with hemostasis. It is only one component of hemostasis and although intimately associated with endothelial cells, platelets, the fibrinolytic system, and other blood cells, it is distinct from these components and can be evaluated independently in vitro.

  B. Coagulation involves an interconnected series of enzyme-activating steps that form thrombin (factor IIa) and convert soluble fibrinogen (factor I) into an insoluble fibrin plug called the *secondary hemostatic plug*.

  C. Most steps involve an enzyme, a substrate (fibrinogen, fibrin, or proenzyme forms of coagulation enzymes), and a cofactor (e.g., factor Va or VIIIa) assembled and localized on a phospholipid surface (e.g., platelet, leukocyte, or endothelial cell membranes) in the presence of fCa^{2+}.

  D. The coagulation cascade or web can be divided into three pathways that can be assessed separately in vitro but that have considerable cross talk in vivo (Fig. 5.2).

1. TF (extrinsic) pathway
   a. This pathway is initiated by TF expressed on vascular smooth muscle cells, activated monocytes, or other extravascular cells. Endothelial cells do not normally express TF, and it is not certain whether they do when stimulated.
   b. It activates factor X at the start of the common pathway.
   c. It is inhibited by TFPI.
   d. It is important in initiating thrombin generation.
2. Surface-induced (intrinsic) pathway
   a. This pathway is initiated when the contact coagulation factors HMWK, PK, and factor XII contact negatively charged surfaces (e.g., collagen).
   b. It activates factor X at the start of the common pathway.
   c. It is inhibited by AT, protein C, protein S, and protein Z.
   d. It is also activated secondary to TF and common pathway activation.
      (1) TF-VIIa activates factor IX.
      (2) Thrombin activates factors XI and VIII.
   e. It is important in propagating and amplifying thrombin generation initiated by the TF pathway.
3. Common pathway (common continuation of surface-induced and TF pathways)
   a. This pathway is initiated by activation of factor X to factor Xa by either the surface-induced pathway or the TF pathway.
   b. It leads to the formation of thrombin from prothrombin by the prothrombinase complex.
   c. Thrombin acts on fibrinogen to generate fibrin monomers and then multimers, which are cross-linked via factor XIIIa.
   d. The pathway is inhibited by AT, protein C, protein S, and protein Z.
   e. Thrombin activation of factor V amplifies the common pathway.
E. Coagulation factors (Table 5.4)
   1. Enzymatic coagulation factors circulate as inactive proenzymes (zymogens) until they are activated.
      a. They are produced primarily in hepatocytes. The production of factors II, VII, IX, and X is vitamin K dependent (Fig. 5.3). The "K" in vitamin K is derived from the German *Koagulations Vitamin* (i.e., "coagulation vitamin").[65]
      b. Factor IX is sex linked. Its gene is on the X chromosome.[67,68]
      c. Half-lives of proenzymes in health: In people, half-lives range from a few hours (factor VII) to several days (factors II and XIII), with most ranging about 1–2 d.[69] Half-lives of coagulation factors in domestic animals are presumed to be similar. The half-life of factor VII was < 5 h in factor VII–deficient beagles transfused with plasma from healthy dogs.[69]
      d. Most enzymatic factors are not directly destroyed during coagulation (they are present in serum). The activated factors are complexed by inhibitors, and the complexes are cleared by hepatocytes or the MPS. Enzymatic degradation of some enzymatic factors (e.g., factor XIII by plasmin) does occur. Some thrombin bound to thrombomodulin is internalized and destroyed by endothelial cells.
   2. Nonenzymatic coagulation factors include TF, fibrinogen, protein pro-cofactors (factors V and VIII), fCa^{2+}, and phospholipid.
      a. *TF* is the transmembrane cellular receptor and cofactor for factors VII and VIIa, and the major activator of coagulation in vivo. It can mediate cell signaling and

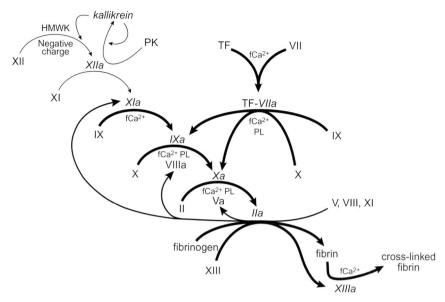

Fig. 5.2. Coagulation cascade. The coagulation cascade begins with activation of the TF (extrinsic) or surface-induced (intrinsic) pathways, and results in the formation of cross-linked fibrin by the common pathway (beginning with factor X). *Bold arrows* represent major coagulation pathways in vivo.

- TF pathway: It was originally thought to require extravascular activation and was therefore named *extrinsic*. This pathway is initiated by TF released from, or exposed on, damaged tissue or activated monocytes, macrophages, and possibly endothelial cells. These cells can be activated by endotoxin and certain inflammatory cytokines. Cell membrane TF binds to factor VII (and VIIa) in the presence of fCa^{2+}, and the resulting activated TF-VIIa complex rapidly activates factor X (common pathway) and factor IX (surface-induced pathway) in the presence of fCa^{2+} and phospholipid (PL). TFPI rapidly inactivates TF-VIIa, but not until thrombin is generated through the common pathway. Thrombin activates factor XI and the amplification pro-cofactors V and VIII for sustained production of factor Xa via the surface-induced pathway.

- Surface-induced pathway: It was originally considered the pathway activated by intravascular (intrinsic) factors. This pathway is initiated by so-called contact activation, which is the activation of factor XII by contact with a negatively charged surface. In vivo, this could be subendothelial collagen exposed at the site of vascular injury. In vitro, kaolin, silica, celite, diatomaceous earth, or glass surfaces may be involved.

  ◆ Once formed, surface-bound factor XIIa facilitates the binding of HMWK to the activating surface, probably by enzymatic cleavage of HMWK. Because HMWK circulates in association with PK and factor XI, factor XI and the three contact activation factors (PK, HMWK, and factor XIIa) become closely associated.

  ◆ Factor XIIa activates PK to kallikrein, which enzymatically produces more kallikrein and more factor XIIa in a potent amplification pathway.

  ◆ Factor XIIa cleaves factor XI, yielding factor XIa, which cleaves factor IX in the presence of fCa^{2+} to form factor IXa. Factor IXa then binds to the PL surface (in the presence of fCa^{2+}) to form the "tenase" or "Xase" complex with factor VIIIa (activated mostly by thrombin), which cleaves factor X to form factor Xa.

  ◆ In vivo, the TF pathway is thought to initiate thrombin generation through activation of factors IX and X, and the surface-induced pathway is thought to propagate coagulation via thrombin feedback on factors XI, V and VIII. Surface activation plays a minor role in activating coagulation in vivo; patients with single contact factor deficiencies (e.g., factor XII, HMWK, or PK) do not have clinical bleeding disorders.

appears to participate in several nonhemostatic processes (e.g., angiogenesis and metastasis).

   b. *Fibrinogen* is a positive acute-phase protein produced by hepatocytes. It has a half-life of 2–3 d in healthy dogs[70] and is consumed during coagulation as it is converted to fibrin by thrombin.

   c. Factors V and VIII markedly accelerate coagulation by facilitating surface attachment and localization of coagulation factors.

   (1) Factor V may be produced in hepatocytes, megakaryocytes, lymphocytes, and vascular smooth muscle cells.[71] It has a half-life of about 0.5–1.5 d and is consumed by APC during coagulation.

   (2) Factor VIII may be produced in multiple cell types, but hepatocytes appear to be most important.

   (a) It is sex linked. Its gene is on the X chromosome.[72]

   (b) It circulates in a noncovalent complex with vWF but is distinct from vWF.

   (c) The half-life of human factor VIII is about 0.5 d, but it is less in the absence of vWF, its carrier protein.

   (d) It is consumed by APC during coagulation.

   (e) It is a positive acute-phase protein, increasing in plasma with exercise and inflammation.[73,74]

   (3) Factors V and VIII are consumed during clotting and are not present in serum.

   d. EDTA, oxalate, and citrate function as in vitro anticoagulants by binding fCa^{2+} and preventing it from interacting with coagulation proteins. In vivo, there is always enough fCa^{2+} for coagulation even with hypocalcemia.

 F. Physiologic inhibitors of coagulation help prevent excessive coagulation. Deficiencies of these anticoagulants are associated with thromboembolic disease. Some of the inhibitors can be measured.

Fig. 5.2. *continued*

• Common pathway: This is the common continuation of the TF and surface-induced pathways, beginning with activation of factor X. Factor Xa complexes with factor Va (activated mostly by thrombin) and fCa^{2+} on a phospholipid surface to form the active *prothrombinase complex*, which results in the enzymatic conversion of prothrombin (factor II) to thrombin (factor IIa). Thrombin then activates platelets and cleaves its many substrates (not all shown), which include the following:

   • Fibrinogen: Fibrinopeptides A and B are cleaved from fibrinogen to form fibrin monomers, which polymerize into fibrin polymers (see Fig. 5.6).

   • Factor XIII: Proteolytic cleavage of factor XIII leads to activation. Factor XIIIa, in the presence of fCa^{2+}, cross-links fibrin and reinforces the secondary hemostatic plug.

   • Protein pro-cofactors (factors V and VIII): Proteolytic cleavage leads to cofactor activation and accelerated coagulation.

   • Factor XI: Thrombin activation provides positive feedback on the surface-induced and common pathways through factor XIa.

   • Protein C: APC inactivates factors Va and VIIIa, and promotes fibrinolysis via t-PA.

   • TAFI: TAFIa formed via thrombin and thrombomodulin inhibits fibrinolysis by cleaving plasminogen-binding sites from fibrin.

Table 5.4. Coagulation factors, abbreviations, and roles

Factor	Name	Pathway	Function
I	Fibrinogen	Common	Substrate for thrombin—converted to fibrin
II	Prothrombin	Common	Proenzyme: IIa (thrombin) cleaves fibrinogen and activates V, VIII, XI, XIII, protein C, and platelets
(III)[a]	Tissue factor (TF), tissue thromboplastin factor	TF	Cofactor: TF binds and activates VII, and the TF/VIIa complex activates IX and X
(IV)	Free ionized calcium	All	Cofactor for IIa, VIIa, IXa, Xa, and XIIIa
V	Proaccelerin	Common	Pro-cofactor for Xa; cofactor after activation to Va
VII	Proconvertin, stable factor	TF	Proenzyme: VIIa activates IX and X
VIII	Antihemophilic factor	Surface	Pro-cofactor for IXa; cofactor after activation to VIIIa
IX	Christmas factor	Surface	Proenzyme: IXa activates X
X	Stuart factor, Stuart-Prower factor	Common	Proenzyme: Xa activates II
XI	Plasma thromboplastin antecedent	Surface	Proenzyme: XIa activates IX
XII	Hageman factor	Surface	Proenzyme: XIIa activates XI, PK, HMWK, and plasminogen
XIII	Fibrin-stabilizing factor, fibrinase	Common	Proenzyme: XIIIa cross-links fibrin and protects it from plasmin degradation
HMWK	Fitzgerald factor	Surface	Cofactor for activation of XII and XI
PF3	Platelet factor 3, mostly phosphatidylserine	Surface, common	Negatively charged platelet membrane lipoproteins important for in vivo activation of X and II
PK	Fletcher factor	Surface	Proenzyme: kallikrein activates XII and PK, generates bradykinin from HMWK, and leads to plasmin generation

[a] Parentheses indicate that the Roman numeral is rarely used.

Note: Roman numeral VI is unassigned; a proposed factor VI was later identified as factor Va.

The TF pathway is also called the extrinsic pathway, and the surface-induced pathway is also called the contact pathway or the intrinsic pathway.

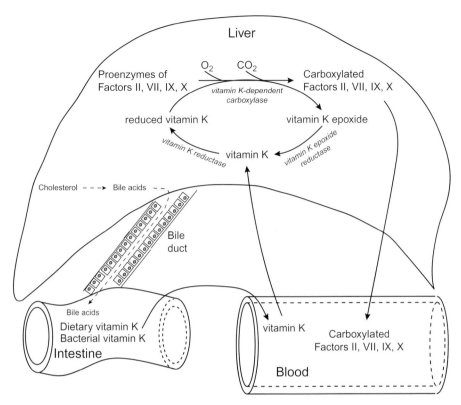

Fig. 5.3. Synthesis of vitamin K–dependent factors. Coagulation factors II (prothrombin), VII, IX, and X are synthesized primarily in hepatocytes. Vitamin K is required for these factors to be functional; that is, they are vitamin K dependent (as are the anticoagulants protein C, protein S, and protein Z).
- Vitamin K is ingested and also produced by intestinal bacteria. As a fat-soluble vitamin, it is absorbed with lipid that is digested by lipase and emulsified by the action of bile acids.
- In hepatocytes, vitamin K becomes reduced to its active form (reduced vitamin K). Reduced vitamin K is a cofactor for vitamin K–dependent carboxylase, the enzyme responsible for posttranslational gamma-carboxylation of glutamic acid residues in these coagulation factors. Carboxylation is needed so that the factors can bind fCa^{2+}, which induces conformational changes and enables binding to phospholipid membranes.
- Reduced vitamin K becomes oxidized to vitamin K epoxide during carboxylation, requiring enzymatic reduction before it can again function as a cofactor for vitamin K–dependent carboxylase.
- Carboxylated factors II, VII, IX, and X enter the blood, where they can be activated to participate in enzymatic reactions of the coagulation system.

Vitamin K reductase is also known as NAD(P)H dehydrogenase (quinone).

---

1. *AT* (short for *ATIII*) is the major inhibitor of coagulation enzymes. (Note: The inhibitory activity of fibrin on thrombin is sometimes referred to as *antithrombin I activity*.)
   a. It is a protein ($M_r \approx 58,000$) produced primarily by hepatocytes.
   b. It binds, inactivates, and removes most coagulation enzymes from the circulation, most importantly thrombin (factor IIa), factor IXa, and factor Xa.
   c. AT-enzyme complexes are rapidly cleared via receptors on hepatocytes.[75]

    d. AT activity is markedly enhanced by heparin (exogenous, or endogenous from mast cells) and heparan sulfate on endothelial cells (Fig. 5.4).

  2. *Protein C* is a vitamin K–dependent proenzyme anticoagulant and profibrinolytic agent ($M_r \approx 62,000$). The *C* stands for the third (a, b, and c) fraction eluted from a column.[76]

    a. It is produced in hepatocytes and circulates in plasma with a half-life of 8–10 h in people.

    b. It can be activated by thrombin, primarily when thrombin is bound to thrombomodulin, a thrombin receptor present on most endothelial cell membranes.

    c. APC then inactivates factors Va and VIIIa by proteolytic cleavage in the presence of factor V[77] and membrane-bound protein S (the *S* stands for "Seattle," where the protein was first described).[76]

    d. *Protein S* is a vitamin K–dependent, nonenzymatic cofactor produced by endothelial cells, hepatocytes, and megakaryocytes.

    e. Additional anticoagulation occurs by this pathway because thrombin bound to thrombomodulin cannot cleave fibrinogen, and the complex is internalized and degraded by endothelial cells.

    f. APC also promotes fibrinolysis by inhibition of PAI.

  3. *TFPI* ($M_r \approx 40,000$) is produced by endothelial cells, monocytes, macrophages, and hepatocytes. It also circulates in platelets and in plasma, mostly bound to lipoproteins. In the presence of fCa^{2+}, TFPI inhibits TF-VIIa by forming a stable quaternary complex: TF-VIIa–factor Xa–TFPI.[78] This inhibits further generation of factors IXa and Xa via TF-VIIa.

  4. Other circulating inhibitors of coagulation include PZI, heparin cofactor II, α_2-macroglobulin, and α_1-proteinase.

II. Analytical concepts

  A. Assay optimization for one species (e.g., humans) does not necessarily optimize for other species.[79–82] Veterinary assays for routine coagulation testing are not standardized, and many are not optimized for the species being tested. This compromises their sensitivity in detecting impaired coagulation.

  B. Proper sampling and sample handling are critical for accurate results from most coagulation assays.

  C. Sample collection

    1. For most tests, use a citrate vacuum tube or plastic syringe containing the right amount of citrate for the volume of blood to be drawn. Drawing into a syringe without anticoagulant and then transferring the sample to a citrate tube is not recommended, because coagulation may begin during venipuncture and progress far enough to alter hemostasis test results prior to mixing with the citrate.

    2. Sampling through nonheparinized catheters may be done, if necessary, after flushing the catheter with 5 mL saline and discarding at least the first 5 mL of blood removed (at least six times the catheter dead space).[83,84]

    3. Sampling through heparinized catheters should be avoided, though a similar flush-and-discard approach produced results for *healthy* dogs that did not differ significantly from direct venipuncture results.[85]

    4. Care should be taken to minimize activation of platelets and the coagulation and fibrinolytic systems.

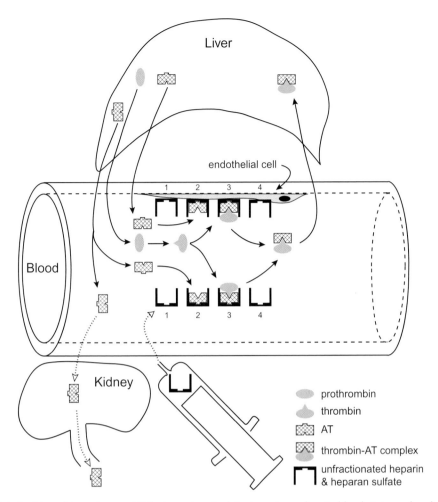

Fig. 5.4. Antithrombin pathways. AT is the major physiologic anticoagulant in blood. It is produced primarily by hepatocytes and circulates in the blood, where it can inactivate thrombin (shown here) and the other coagulation enzymes. As shown schematically, AT activity is markedly enhanced in the presence of circulating unfractionated heparin or heparan sulfate on endothelial cells (1). Heparin or heparan sulfate bind to lysine sites of AT (2), inducing a conformational change in AT (note the larger triangular notches) that increases its affinity for thrombin. Thrombin, generated from the activation of prothrombin, then binds to the heparin-AT complex, forming a covalent 1:1 complex with AT (3). The thrombin-AT complexes (TAT) dissociate from the heparin or heparan sulfate and are cleared from circulation by hepatocytes. The heparin and heparan sulfate act as catalysts and are available (4) for forming more complexes. Anticoagulation by AT and heparin limits excessive clotting, but AT and heparin do not inhibit coagulation enzymes bound to fibrin or platelets. Therefore, localized and controlled coagulation can proceed where needed. LMWH molecules also induce conformational changes in AT that enable it to bind to and inhibit factor Xa, but not thrombin.

- Decreased plasma AT activity and concentration occur via consumption when intravascular coagulation is increased or after injection of exogenous heparin. Decreased concentrations may also occur from decreased hepatic production or from excessive loss due to protein-losing nephropathy or enteropathy. Decreased AT produces a prothrombotic state that heparin cannot counter well because heparin requires AT for most of its function.
- Increased plasma AT activity and concentration may occur with increased hepatic production of AT. This may occur secondary to the production of inflammatory cytokines.

Note: Nonphysiologic pathways are represented by *dotted arrows*.

    a. Traumatic venipuncture exposes blood to TF, thus initiating coagulation that can produce clotted samples or cause platelet activation and clumping.

    b. Freely flowing blood should be collected by "clean" venipuncture on the first attempt. Probing with the needle, sampling through a hematoma, or exiting and reentering the vein will expose the blood to TF and activate the pathways to be tested.

    c. If collection is difficult, a new vein should be selected.

    d. An excessive vacuum may cause turbulence and platelet activation.

    e. The first few drops or a complete tube of blood may be discarded to decrease TF in the test sample, but this is not necessary with "clean sticks."

  5. The blood and anticoagulant should be mixed immediately and thoroughly, but gently.

D. Sample

  1. Most coagulation tests: citrated plasma

  2. Point-of-care instruments: citrated whole blood or citrated plasma

  3. ACT: whole blood in special ACT tubes containing diatomaceous earth

  4. Lee-White clotting time: non-anticoagulated whole blood tested immediately

  5. Citrated samples

    a. Siliconized glass tubes have been used routinely for hemostasis testing, but the use of plastic tubes is becoming common. Although statistically significant differences in test results have been documented in comparisons of plastic and glass tubes with human samples, differences have been small and rarely of clinical significance.[86]

    b. Plasma or whole blood should be anticoagulated with trisodium citrate at a 1:9 (anticoagulant to blood) ratio by using 3.2 % or 3.8 % citrate tubes (check with the laboratory for a preference).

    c. The citrate concentration significantly affects the results of coagulation tests on human samples (3.2 % is usually recommended),[84,87,88] and it can have significant effects on some results with canine samples.[89] The magnitude of the effect is not known for most conditions or most species, but a standard citrate concentration with reference intervals generated by using that citrate concentration, instrument, and method is recommended.

    d. Similarly, it is important to maintain the 1:9 citrate to blood volume ratio because overcitrated samples (too little blood) may have reduced coagulation activity (prolonged times) and undercitrated samples (too much blood) may be hypercoagulable (reduced times). Problems associated with suboptimal filling of human samples appear to be greater with 3.8 % citrate tubes than with 3.2 % citrate tubes.[90]

    e. Even with the correct blood volume, Hct may affect the appropriate amount of citrate to use.[91]

      (1) With anemia, plasma may be undercitrated because there is more plasma with the same amount of citrate. This may result in falsely shortened coagulation times, but the degree of the effect was of questionable clinical significance when PT and PTT results for unadjusted samples from anemic human patients were compared to PT and PTT results from paired samples adjusted to 3.8 % citrate.[92]

      (2) With erythrocytosis, plasma may be overcitrated because there is less plasma with the same amount of citrate. This may prolong coagulation times

because the excess citrate binds too much of the Ca^{2+} added to the assay system.

(3) Decreased citrate to blood ratios are recommended when Hct > 55 % in people.[84,93] Increased ratios may be indicated for Hct < 25 %, but the need has not been clearly shown.[92]

(4) The following formula (Eq. 5.1) may be used to calculate the citrate volume required for anticoagulating a volume of blood with a given Hct > 55 %:

$$C = 0.002 \times (100 - Hct) \times V \hspace{4cm} \textbf{(5.1.)}$$

C: citrate volume (mL)
Hct: blood hematocrit (%)
V: collected blood volume (mL)

E. Sample processing and stability[84]
   1. Time and temperature before processing[94]
      a. Except for whole blood clotting assays, studies of human blood indicate that whole blood samples may be refrigerated or kept at room temperature for up to 8–12 h (PTT assay for nonheparinized patients, TT assay, and coagulation factor analyses) or up to 24 h (PT assay) before processing.[95,96]
      b. However, a good general recommendation is to centrifuge and remove plasma within 1 h (room temperature storage) and test within 4 h of sample collection, because this time frame is necessary for certain tests and certain samples.[95,97]
   2. Centrifugation and plasma harvest
      a. After confirming the absence of clots in the sample, blood should be centrifuged for 10–15 min at high g-force (e.g., 15 min at 1500× g), and the platelet-poor plasma should be removed by plastic pipette.
      b. Plasma that cannot be tested within 4 h should be frozen.
      c. Excessive platelets (10–200 × 10^3/μL) remaining in the plasma because of inadequate centrifugation forces will not interfere with PT and PTT assays for routine diagnostic work but will interfere with heparin monitoring (via PTT assay) and tests for other inhibitors of coagulation.[98,99]
   3. Plasma storage time and temperature
      a. Plasma should not be placed in a serum tube containing a clot activator. This will promote coagulation.
      b. Frozen samples
         (1) Human plasma may be stored for 3 mo at −24 °C or for 18 mo at −74 °C before testing, but the use of frost-free freezers should be avoided.[100]
         (2) The results of stability studies of common hemostatic analytes in canine plasma suggest a similar stability at −70 °C for all plasma tests but PTT.[101]
      c. Room temperature plasma storage
         (1) Plasma from *healthy* dogs yielded stable hemostasis results (PT, PTT, TT, AT, specific coagulation factors, and D-dimers) for 48 h when stored at 24 °C, except for mild decreases in [fibrinogen] at 48 h (it appeared to start dropping by 24 h).[94]
         (2) However, similar storage of human plasma resulted in stable [fibrinogen] for 7 d, and TT, PTT, and factor VIII activity were decreased by 8 h in samples from *heparinized* patients.[97]

  d. Refrigerated plasma storage
    (1) Plasma from *healthy* dogs had less stability at 4 °C than at room temperature. Values for factors VIII and IX were decreased by 48 h (they appeared to be dropping by 24 h), and PTT was prolonged by 72 h (it appeared to be dropping by 48 h).[94]
    (2) In a similar study of human plasma, PT was stable for only 24 h at 6 °C, and factor VIII activity was decreasing by 8 h. Samples from *heparinized* patients were stable for 8 h, although activities of factors V and VIII were dropping by 8 h.[97]
  e. Stability of values in samples from sick or heparinized dogs has not been reported and may differ from stability in samples from healthy dogs.[94] Effects of heparin may be decreased with release of platelet factor 4 from platelets during storage.[97]
  f. When mailing samples for testing, frozen plasma should be packed in ice and mailed to arrive frozen within 24 h.
    (1) Samples should be tested promptly after thawing, and thawing should be rapid to minimize cryoprecipitate formation and therefore loss of hemostatic factors.
    (2) Concurrently collecting, processing, and mailing a sample from a healthy patient of the same species can be used as evidence that sample handling did not induce abnormal results.
  4. Hemolysis: Samples hemolyzed by in vitro factors should not be tested because coagulation and platelets may have been activated by the same factors responsible for hemolysis.
F. Instruments: A variety of automated coagulation analyzers, including point-of-care instruments, are replacing manual and fibrometer methods of measuring coagulation times for human and veterinary samples. Specific methods and sample requirements vary with the analyzer. End-point detection of a fibrin clot varies with the type of analyzer.
  1. Electromechanical methods
    a. Electrical conductance: Increased electrical conductance is detected between a stationary electrode and a moving electrode as fibrin forms (fibrometers).
    b. Electromagnetic viscosity: Analyzers detect decreased movement of a small metal ball suspended in the sample as it oscillates in an electromagnetic field.
  2. Photooptical methods detect changes in light transmission or light scatter as fibrin forms.
  3. Optical methods may function better with a low [fibrinogen] but may generate inaccurate results when optical interferents are present (e.g., lipemia, Oxyglobin, hemolysis, or icterus).
  4. Synbiotics SCA2000 Veterinary Coagulation Analyzer: The clotting end point is based on optical detection of decreased movement of a small volume of blood as it is pumped back and forth within a channel in the test cartridge.
G. General analytical approach: In vitro analysis enables independent testing of different parts of the coagulation web (simplified to a "Y") so that defects may be localized within the surface-induced (intrinsic), TF (extrinsic), or common pathways (Fig. 5.5). Testing generally begins with common screening tests, with more specialized tests used when indicated.
H. Severe hypothermia may contribute to hemorrhage, in part because coagulation is a temperature sensitive enzymatic pathway. However, coagulation testing is routinely

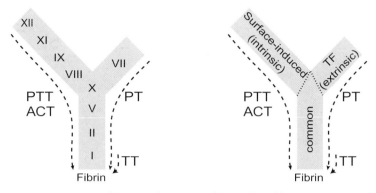

Fig. 5.5. Schematic representation of the coagulation cascade as evaluated by in vitro screening coagulation tests. Fibrin formation is the end point for each test. PTT and ACT evaluate coagulation factors in the surface-induced pathway (factors XII, XI, IX, and VIII) and in the common pathway (factors X, V, II, and I). PT evaluates the short TF pathway (factor VII) and the common pathway. TT (and TT_{Clauss}) assesses only the conversion of fibrinogen (factor I) to fibrin with the addition of thrombin. Factor XIII is not assessed.

done at or near normal body temperature, so routine assays may not identify hypothermia-induced coagulation abnormalities.

III. Whole blood clotting times
    A. Lee-White method[102,103]
        1. This is a standardized, but rarely used, insensitive method of screening for defects in the surface-induced and common pathways that uses non-anticoagulated whole blood immediately after collection. Activation of coagulation is initiated by the glass tube.
        2. Protocols require multiple analyses, standardization of blood volume, clean glass test tubes of a standard size, and a water bath (25–37 °C). Several modifications of the method have been used.[104] Variations in protocol, including venipuncture technique, blood volume, glass tubes size and coating, temperature, and sample Hct, influence the results.
        3. Reported reference values are 4–15 min for horses and cattle, 3–13 min for dogs, and about 8 min for cats.[102] Longer times (8–21 min) were found in a group of nine healthy dogs.[105]
        4. When confounding variables are controlled, prolonged times indicate severe defects in the surface-induced and/or common pathways, including those caused by coagulation inhibitors (see Coagulation, sect. IV).
    B. Activated coagulation (clotting) time (ACT)
        1. Point-of-care whole blood screening coagulation test of the surface-induced and common pathways
        2. Several ACT methods are used in human medicine, largely for monitoring heparinization. Negatively charged particulate materials such as kaolin, celite, or diatomaceous earth are used to activate the contact factors.
        3. Principle and method (conventional visual method)

a. Surface-induced activation: Blood (2 mL) is drawn by atraumatic jugular venipuncture into a prewarmed (37 °C) ACT vacuum tube containing silaceous (diatomaceous) earth, which activates the surface-induced (intrinsic) pathway.

b. The blood is mixed by five inversions, and the tube is incubated (37 °C) for 60 s. The tube is then checked (visually while tipping it) every 5 or 10 s for the first definite evidence of a clot.

c. The time from contact of blood with silaceous earth to the initial definite signs of a clot is the *ACT*.

d. Units: seconds (nearest 5 or 10 s, depending on the frequency of inspection)

4. Interpretive considerations

a. Interpretation is similar to that for PTT (see Coagulation, sect. IV), but the test has less diagnostic sensitivity and may require > 90–95 % deficiency of a single factor for a prolonged result.

b. Severe thrombocytopenia (< 10×10^3 platelets/μL) is commonly stated to prolong ACT, because of decreased phospholipid availability. However, ACT values may be WRI with severe thrombocytopenia, and moderate thrombocytopenia has no effect.[106,107]

c. A standard protocol should be followed because modifications of the protocol may affect expected values. Variations have related to syringe versus vacuum collection, incubation temperature (various axillary temperatures versus a heating block), length of initial incubation period, and frequency of inspection for clots.

5. A prolonged ACT indicates decreased in vitro function of the surface-induced or common pathways (see Table 5.5).

6. ACT may be used to monitor heparin therapy.

7. Automated point-of-care instruments are available, and manufacturer recommendations should be followed.

C. Synbiotics SCA2000 Veterinary Coagulation Analyzer

1. This is a point-of-care analyzer that measures PT, PTT, and ACT in whole blood or plasma.

2. Manufacturer recommendations should be followed.

3. Reference intervals may be markedly different from those of other methods.

IV. Activated partial thromboplastin time (PTT, APTT, or aPTT)[108]

A. A screening coagulation test of the surface-induced and common pathways

B. Principle and method

1. Surface-induced activation: Citrated test plasma is incubated (37 °C) with an excess of procoagulant phospholipids (partial thromboplastin) and a surface activator (e.g., kaolin, silicates, or ellagic acid) to activate the contact factors. The chelation of fCa^{2+} by citrate in the sample limits activation beyond factor XIa.

a. The partial thromboplastin reagent consists of procoagulant phospholipids devoid of TF, and therefore the reagent is unable to activate the TF pathway (factor VII).

b. In the original PTT assay, the glass tube (rather than added particulates) was the surface activator.[109] To differentiate tests with and without added particulates, the current test is referred to as the *activated partial thromboplastin time* (APTT or aPTT). However, PTT is used as the abbreviation in this text for simplicity. The original test without added particulates is no longer used, so there should be no confusion.

Table 5.5. Diseases or conditions that may cause prolonged PTT

Deficiencies of functional surface-induced or common pathway coagulation factors
  Acquired (usually multiple defects)
    Decreased production
      *Hepatic disease (necrosis, cirrhosis, portosystemic shunt)
      Vitamin K antagonism or absence
        *Decreased vitamin K recycling in hepatocytes: anticoagulant rodenticide
          ingestion, coumadin overdose, moldy sweet clover ingestion (*Melilotus* spp.),
          phenoprocoumon toxicity
        Decreased vitamin K absorption: biliary obstruction, infiltrative bowel disease,
          chronic oral antimicrobials, exocrine pancreatic insufficiency
    Increased coagulation factor inactivation and consumption
      *Disseminated intravascular coagulation or coagulopathy
      Localized consumptive coagulation or coagulopathy
    Dilution of coagulation factors: acute, massive blood loss treated with massive
      transfusion of plasma-poor fluids; e.g., packed RBCs and crystalloid or colloid
      fluids, including Oxyglobin solution
  Hereditary (usually single defect, but may be multiple)
  Intrinsic pathway: PK, XII, XI, IX, VIII
  Common pathway: X, V, II, I
*Inhibition of surface-induced or common pathway coagulation factors: heparin, FDPs,
    anti-(phospholipid-protein) antibodies, antibodies to coagulation factors

  * A relatively common disease or condition
  Note: ACT may also be prolonged in most of these conditions, but ACT prolongation requires
greater deficits in factor activities.

   2. After a defined incubation time, a measured amount of prewarmed (37 °C) calcium
      chloride is added to counteract the effects of citrate and enable the cascade of
      coagulation to proceed to the formation of fibrin monomers, which polymerize to
      form an insoluble fibrin clot that is detected optically or electromechanically,
      depending on the instrument. *The time from addition of calcium chloride to clot
      detection is the* PTT.
   3. Units: seconds (usually reported to nearest 0.1 s, though reporting to the nearest
      half-second or second may be more appropriate for some methods)
 C. Interpretive considerations
   1. Values greater than a valid upper reference limit should be considered prolonged.
      Values are sometimes interpreted by comparing them to values from a concurrently
      tested healthy animal of the same species, but this is not recommended. Neither is
      requiring a 25 % increase over the URL to conclude that the PTT is abnormal.
   2. Laboratory-specific and species-specific reference intervals must be used because
      results vary substantially with variations in species, analyzers, reagents, and
      protocols.
   3. As equine data indicate, values in healthy newborns (< 24 h old) may be greater
      than reference intervals established for adults.[110,111]
   4. The test is relatively insensitive, but, for optimized assays, results should be
      prolonged when there is about a 70 % decrease in the activity of a single

coagulation factor (30 % of expected activity). In one study of various PT reagents and methods, the factor VII activity needed to keep PT WRI varied from 16 % to 39 %.[112]

5. Milder reductions in individual factor activities may be detected when multiple factors are affected.

6. PTT assayed at 37 °C may overestimate in vivo coagulation in markedly hypothermic patients because enzyme activities are temperature dependent.[113,114]

7. Lipemia, hemolysis, Oxyglobin solution, and icterus interfere with PTT assays that detect clot formation optically.

8. Excessive citrate or improper handling (delayed processing, an old sample, or an inappropriate temperature) may prolong PTT.

D. A prolonged PTT indicates decreased in vitro function of the surface-induced or common pathways (see Table 5.5)

1. Pure deficiencies of either factor XII or PK are typically not associated with clinical hemorrhage, but they are associated with prolonged PTT results in most assay systems.[81] A prolonged PTT caused by PK deficiency may be corrected by increasing the incubation time of plasma with the particulate surface activator or by using ellagic acid for surface activation.[115]

2. Carriers of hemophilia cannot be detected by PTT because they have only a moderate decrease in factor activity (approximately 50 % of normal).

3. Unexplained prolongations in PTT, without other evidence of impaired hemostasis, have been reported in cats.[116]

E. Shortened PTT is not reliable for detecting hypercoagulability, though increases in fibrinogen, factor V, or factor VIII with inflammation may shorten the PTT.[117]

F. PTT has been used to monitor unfractionated heparin therapy, but targets of prolongation used for people (e.g., 1.5–2.5 times baseline) do not appear to reflect appropriate anticoagulation in animals. Target prolongations vary with the PTT assay and reagents, in part because partial thromboplastin reagents have different sensitivities to heparin.[118,119] PTT was less prolonged in dogs than in people for a given plasma heparin activity, possibly because of greater factor V and VIII activity.[120] LMWH has minimal effect on PTT because of reduced anti–factor IIa activity.[121]

V. Prothrombin time (PT), also called one-stage prothrombin time (OSPT)

A. A screening coagulation test of the TF and common pathways

B. Principle and method

1. Test plasma and a Ca^{2+}-thromboplastin reagent (containing phospholipid and excess TF) are separately prewarmed (37 °C).

2. A measured amount of the prewarmed Ca^{2+}-thromboplastin reagent is forcibly added to a measured amount of the prewarmed plasma so that TF will activate factor VII in the TF pathway. Activation should proceed along the common pathway so as to form fibrin monomers, which polymerize to form an insoluble fibrin clot that can be detected optically or electromechanically, depending on the instrument. *The time from plasma-thromboplastin mixing to clot detection is the* PT.

3. A heparin inactivator is generally included in PT assays.

4. Different thromboplastin reagents produce different results.[122,123] Some appear to be affected by PIVKA, which interfere with the generation of thrombin and inhibit coagulation in vitro.

Table 5.6. Diseases or conditions that may cause prolonged PT

Deficiencies of functional coagulation factors in the TF or common pathway
    *Acquired (usually multiple defects); see Table 5.5
    Hereditary (usually single defect)
       TF pathway: VII
       Common pathway: X, V, II, I
*Inhibition of coagulation factors in the TF or common pathway: FDPs, anti-(phospholipid-
       protein) antibodies, antibodies to coagulation factors, sometimes heparin

  * A relatively common disease or condition

5. Reagents and plasma may be diluted to prolong PT and increase the analytical sensitivity for detecting abnormalities. Fibrinogen may be added to diluted samples to ensure adequate fibrinogen concentration.

6. Point-of-care instruments are available, and manufacturer recommendations should be followed.

7. Units
   a. Seconds (usually reported to nearest 0.1 s, though reporting to the nearest half-second may be more appropriate for some methods)
   b. PT may be reported as a unitless INR for monitoring warfarin therapy (see Coagulation, sect. V.G)

C. Interpretive considerations are the same as previously described for PTT. Unless used to monitor warfarin therapy, PT values are best interpreted relative to a valid reference interval.

D. Prolonged PT indicates decreased in vitro function of the TF or common pathways (see Table 5.6). PT is typically not sensitive to heparin because of the presence of heparin inactivators in most thromboplastin reagents, but it may be prolonged with certain thromboplastin reagents when blood contains therapeutic heparin concentrations.[124]

E. Shortened PT is not reliable for detecting hypercoagulability but may occur with increased [fibrinogen] or factor V.[117]

F. PT is used to monitor warfarin therapy (target PT ≈ 1.5–2.0 times baseline).

G. *INR* is a unitless ratio (Eq. 5.2) used widely in human medicine to help standardize the reporting of PT values to help correct for differences in thromboplastin reagents among laboratories.[125] In Eq. 5.2, reference PT is the mean of a valid reference interval for the species in question, not a random control sample value. The *ISI* (International Sensitivity Index) is a number determined and provided by the thromboplastin reagent manufacturer for each lot of reagent by using a particular PT method. The ISI, which reflects the relative sensitivity of the reagent to factor deficiencies, is determined by calibration against an international reference preparation. Thromboplastins with higher ISI values are less sensitive than are thromboplastins with lower ISI values.

$$INR = \left(\frac{\text{Patient PT}}{\text{Reference PT}} \right)^{ISI} \tag{5.2.}$$

1. The INR was developed and used for monitoring oral anticoagulant therapy (warfarin) in people.

2. It may enable more meaningful comparisons of PT results among laboratories but does not eliminate significant interlaboratory differences.[126]
3. A reliable reference mean for the species in question is required for valid use of the INR.
   a. If a local human hospital is used for coagulation tests of veterinary patients, INR results may be reported by using a human reference mean. Such values are not valid for nonhuman samples.
   b. Substituting a control sample value for the reference mean is not acceptable.
4. Examples using the INR
   a. Different patients and different thromboplastin reagents but the same PT value
      (1) Patient 1, ISI = 1.5: PT = 12.0 s; reference mean = 8.0 s (Eq. 5.3a)
      (2) Patient 2, ISI = 2.3: PT = 12.0 s; reference mean = 8.0 s (Eq. 5.3b)
      (3) Patients 1 and 2 had the same PT (12.0 s) when patient 2 was tested with a less sensitive thromboplastin reagent (which had a greater ISI). The amount of anticoagulation was actually greater for patient 2, despite the same PT value. This is reflected by a greater INR.
   b. Different thromboplastin reagents but the same patient sample
      (1) Patient 1, ISI = 1.5: PT = 12.0 s; reference mean = 8.0 s (Eq. 5.3a)
      (2) Patient 1, ISI = 2.3: PT = 10.3 s; reference mean = 8.0 s (Eq. 5.3c)
      (3) When patient 1 was tested with the less sensitive reagent (which had a greater ISI), the PT was only 10.3 s, but the INR, and therefore degree of anticoagulation, was unchanged.

$$\text{Patient \#1 INR} = \left(\frac{12.0}{8.0}\right)^{1.5} = 1.8 \tag{5.3a.}$$

$$\text{Patient \#2 INR} = \left(\frac{12.0}{8.0}\right)^{2.3} = 2.5 \tag{5.3b.}$$

$$\text{Patient \#1 INR} = \left(\frac{10.3}{8.0}\right)^{2.3} = 1.8 \tag{5.3c.}$$

VI. Thrombin time (TT), also called thrombin clotting time (TCT)
   A. This assesses the thrombin-induced conversion of fibrinogen to an insoluble fibrin clot without being affected by thrombin generation. It differentiates hypofibrinogenemia, dysfibrinogenemia, and effects of heparin, FDPs, and paraproteins from other causes of prolonged PT and PTT.
   B. Principle and method
      1. Thrombin is added to prewarmed test plasma (37 °C). Thrombin cleaves fibrinogen to form monomers, which polymerize into an insoluble fibrin clot that can be detected optically or electromechanically, depending on the instrument. *The time from thrombin addition to detection of a fibrin clot is the* TT.
      2. Units: seconds (usually reported to nearest 0.1 s)
   C. Interpretive considerations
      1. TT should be differentiated from TT_{Clauss} (see Coagulation, sect. VII), which uses diluted plasma and high thrombin concentrations to better measure functional [fibrinogen] with less interference by heparin and FDPs.[127]

2. Lab-specific reference intervals should be used for interpretation because of method variations.[120]

D. Prolonged TT[128]

1. Hypofibrinogenemia or afibrinogenemia: There is an inadequate amount of fibrinogen to form a normal fibrin clot.[16,129–132]

   a. Increased consumption from localized coagulation or DIC

   b. Congenital or hereditary deficiency (rare)

   c. Possibly because of hepatic failure and decreased fibrinogen production

2. Dysfibrinogenemia: Polymerization of fibrin is impaired because of abnormal fibrinogen molecules.[130–132]

   a. Hereditary or acquired production of abnormal fibrinogen (rare)

   b. Acquired form that may occur with a variety of liver diseases

3. Heparinized patient or sample: Unfractionated heparin interferes with thrombin activity via AT, so TT can be used to monitor unfractionated heparinization.[120] TT prolongation by heparin can be normalized with heparin neutralization. TT is affected relatively little by LMWH.[121]

4. Increased [FDPs]: This interferes with fibrin polymerization and thrombin's action on fibrinogen.[133] Fibrinolytic therapy can be monitored with the TT.

5. Paraproteinemia: Abnormal immunoglobulins from multiple myelomas may interfere with fibrin polymerization.[134]

6. Systemic amyloidosis (reported in people): Plasma from affected patients may contain an inhibitor of fibrin polymerization.[135]

7. Hyperfibrinogenemia: Rarely, in people, hyperfibrinogenemia has prolonged the TT, but the cause is not clear.[136,137]

8. TT is unaffected by decreased activity of any coagulation factor (including factor XIII) other than fibrinogen.

E. Shortened TT: This may occur with increased or activated clotting factors, or with soluble fibrin in the sample, but it is not a reliable measure of hypercoagulability.

VII. Fibrinogen

A. [Fibrinogen] measured as fibrinogen activity[127,128,138]

1. Calculated from TT_{Clauss}, a modification of the TT

   a. Plasma is diluted so that fibrinogen is rate limiting.

   b. Greater concentrations of thrombin are used to override much of the inhibition caused by heparin and FDPs.

   c. TT_{Clauss} values of samples with a known [fibrinogen] and therefore activity are used to construct a reference (standard) curve from which a test plasma [fibrinogen] can be estimated.

2. TT_{Clauss} is inversely proportional to [fibrinogen] when high concentrations of inhibitors and dysfibrinogenemia are absent.

3. TT_{Clauss} is measured in seconds, but values for [fibrinogen] are read from the reference (standard) curve and reported in units of mg/dL or μmol/L.

4. Unit conversion: mg/dL × 0.0294 = μmol/L (SI unit)

5. Heparin will not interfere at clinically therapeutic concentrations in human samples, but it will interfere at high concentrations occurring after a bolus injection, with inappropriate blood collection from a heparinized catheter, or with blood collected into a heparinized tube.

      6. FDPs have a minimal effect on TT_{Clauss} in human samples unless present at high concentrations concurrently with hypofibrinogenemia.
- B. [Fibrinogen] may be measured by detection of fibrinogen antigen
  1. Anti-fibrinogen antibodies are used to detect fibrinogen antigen by immunoassay.
  2. Prolonged TT and TT_{Clauss} with decreased fibrinogen antigen indicate hypofibrinogenemia.
  3. Prolonged TT and TT_{Clauss} without decreased fibrinogen antigen support the presence of a dysfibrinogenemia (rare).
- C. [Fibrinogen] by heat precipitation is not precise or accurate enough technique for use in hemostasis testing.
- D. Interpretive considerations
  1. Plasma [fibrinogen] reflects the balance between production and consumption, not production or consumption alone.
  2. Accelerated consumption of fibrinogen during hypercoagulable states may be masked by increased production associated with inflammation or pregnancy.[70,139]
  3. As equine data indicate, values in healthy newborns (<24 h old) may be lower than reference intervals established for adults.[110,111]

VIII. Other specific coagulation factor activities (II, VII, VIII, IX, X, XI, XII, PK, and HMWK)
- A. Other specific coagulation factor assays may be used in specialized veterinary laboratories if screening tests and clinical findings suggest factor deficiencies. The assays may be used to characterize acquired deficiencies but usually are done to identify hereditary deficiencies (Table 5.7).[130,140,141]

Table 5.7. Hereditary or congenital coagulation factor deficiencies reported in animals

Pathway Factor	Condition	Species	Expected Test Results		
			PTT	PT	TT
Tissue factor					
VII	Factor VII deficiency	Dogs	WRI	↑	WRI
Surface-induced					
PK	PK deficiency	Dogs, horses	↑	WRI	WRI
XII	Hageman trait	Dogs, cats	↑	WRI	WRI
XI	Factor XI deficiency	Dogs, cats, cattle	↑	WRI	WRI
IXa	Hemophilia B[a]	Dogs, cats	↑	WRI	WRI
VIIIa	Hemophilia A[a]	Dogs, cats, cattle, horses	↑	WRI	WRI
Common					
X	Factor X deficiency	Dogs	↑	↑	WRI
II	Hypoprothrombinemia	Dogs	↑	↑	WRI
I	Hypo- or afibrinogenemia	Dogs, goats	↑	↑	↑
Combined					
II, VII, IX, X	Vitamin K–dependent multifactor deficiency	Cats (Devon rex), possibly dogs	↑	↑	WRI

[a] These conditions have an X-linked recessive transmission and rarely occur in females.

Note: Hemorrhage is not associated with isolated PK or factor XII deficiency. Factor XI deficiency is also called hemophilia C. Multiple hereditary or congenital factor deficiencies also occur.

B. Factor deficiencies are indicated if a 1:1 dilution of test plasma with normal plasma corrects prolonged PT or PTT (provides the missing factor or factors), whereas failure to correct coagulation times supports the presence of an inhibitor (see sects. XII and XIII).

C. Clotting assays for specific factors assess the ability of the patient plasma to correct the PT or PTT of specific factor-deficient plasmas.[142]
   1. PTT is used for evaluating surface-induced and common pathway factor deficiencies.
   2. PT is used for evaluating TF or common pathway factor deficiencies.
   3. Prolonged PTT or PT of the known factor-deficient plasma usually corrects with a 1:1 dilution of patient plasma if the patient plasma contains the missing factor. However, the PTT or PT will not correct if the patient plasma has the same factor deficiency.
   4. To determine the amount of factor activity in the test plasma, a reference curve (coagulation time versus reference plasma dilution) is generated from mixtures of known factor-deficient plasma and serial dilutions of species-specific pooled plasma considered to have 100 % factor activity prior to dilution.
      a. By using the reference curve, observed clotting times for dilutions of the test plasma are converted to % activity relative to the reference plasma pool.
      b. Units of U/dL or U/mL relative to the plasma pool that is considered to have activity of 100 U/dL or 100 U/mL, respectively, are also used.

D. Chromogenic assays assess the capability of a factor or cofactor to lead to enzymatic cleavage of a chromogenic substrate, thus producing a detectable color change that is proportional to the amount of factor or cofactor present.[143]
   1. Prothrombin activity can be assessed this way by using citrated plasma or EDTA-anticoagulated plasma.[144]
   2. Factor Xa activity can be used to assess the activity of unfractionated heparin or LMWH in a sample.[119] In this chromogenic assay, increased heparin activity is associated with increased inhibition of factor Xa and therefore decreased formation of a chromogen from a substrate for factor Xa.

IX. Proteins induced by vitamin K antagonism or absence (PIVKA)
   A. PIVKA are the incompletely gamma-carboxylated vitamin K–dependent coagulation factors (e.g., des-γ-carboxy prothrombin, often referred to as PIVKA-II because pro-thrombin is coagulation factor II) that are produced by hepatocytes during periods of vitamin K antagonism, absence, or deficiency (see Major Bleeding Disorders, sect. II.B).[65]
   B. In these conditions, plasma concentrations of normally carboxylated coagulation factors are decreased, and PIVKA are secreted and circulate in the blood at increased concentrations. The potential of PIVKA to become activated to functional coagulation enzymes is severely limited.
   C. Human assays
      1. Clinical immunoassays are used in human medicine to specifically and directly measure plasma [PIVKA], but they are not used in veterinary medicine. They can detect abnormalities in the vitamin K–dependent factors that PIVKA-sensitive coagulation tests cannot.[145]
      2. Charge differences between PIVKA and their carboxylated forms also enable detection by high-performance liquid chromatography.[146]

3. Increased plasma [PIVKA] may occur with vitamin K deficiency, vitamin K antagonism, or as a result of production by malignant hepatocytes in human patients with hepatocellular carcinomas.[147]

D. The Thrombotest PT, a modification of the PT assay that is PIVKA sensitive, has been referred to as a PIVKA test, but it is not specific for PIVKA and does not directly measure [PIVKA].[148,149]

1. It is a PT test that detects decreased activities of coagulation factors II, VII, and X from any cause. Factor V and fibrinogen are not assessed because they are provided in the assay.

2. If PIVKA are present in the sample, the Thrombotest PT will be further prolonged because PIVKA appear to act as competitive substrates that delay the generation of thrombin. PIVKA do not appear to interfere with functional factors in vivo.[150]

3. Causes of a prolonged Thrombotest PT

a. Vitamin K antagonism or deficiency: The Thrombotest PT may have greater sensitivity (than the regular PT) to detect mild vitamin K antagonism or deficiency, and it may help differentiate these conditions from other coagulopathies when appropriately high decision thresholds are used. However, when the investigators' recommended decision thresholds were used, diagnostic sensitivity and specificity for vitamin K antagonism or deficiency were similar for the Thrombotest PT (78.6 % and 99.7 %, respectively) and a traditional PT (83.3 % and 97.2 %, respectively).[151,152]

b. Other acquired and hereditary coagulopathies as for PT, excluding factor V and factor I deficiencies (see Table 5.6)[122,153,154]

c. Cats with a variety of hepatic, biliary, or inflammatory bowel diseases had prolonged Thrombotest PT values, often without clinical evidence of a bleeding tendency.[148]

(1) In a subset of these cats treated with vitamin K_1, Thrombotest PT values were WRI 3–5 d after treatment was instituted, indicating that prolonged Thrombotest PT values were at least transiently vitamin K responsive.

(2) Although the assay appears sensitive in cats, its diagnostic specificity for clinically significant bleeding tendencies is unknown.

d. Endogenous or exogenous heparin[151]

X. Russell's viper venom time (RVVT): The test is not widely offered. Direct activation of factor X by venom of the Russell's viper leads to a clot. Prolonged clotting times indicate an abnormality of the common pathway (factor X, V, II, or I).

XI. Endogenous anticoagulants

A. Antithrombin (AT), also known as antithrombin III (ATIII), is assayed to provide information about a patient's anticoagulant status

1. Plasma AT is usually measured by chromogenic (functional) assays rather than immunoassays that detect AT antigen but not function.[127]

2. Principle and method

a. Test plasma is added to a reagent containing heparin, excess thrombin or factor Xa (depending on the assay), and the corresponding chromogen-labeled substrate for thrombin or factor Xa.

b. Increased AT in the test plasma causes less activity of thrombin or factor Xa and therefore less color change (measured spectrophotometrically).

Table 5.8. Diseases or conditions that cause decreased antithrombin (AT) activity

Decreased production
    Hereditary (not reported in animals)
    Acquired
        Hepatic disease
        Inflammation (possibly, in some species)
        Hyperestrogenism
Loss
   *Protein-losing nephropathy
   Protein-losing enteropathy
   Severe hemorrhage
Consumption: increased hepatic clearance of AT-enzyme complexes
    Localized coagulation (e.g., hemorrhagic trauma) or thrombosis
   *DIC
   *Sepsis
   *Heparin administration

* A relatively common disease or condition
Note: Neonates may have lower AT values than adults.

3. Units
   a. Units are % activity compared to either a species-specific or human plasma pool considered to have 100 % activity. Because of species differences in AT activity, reference and reported values vary with the species used for the reference pool.[155–157]
   b. AT also has been reported in U/mL or U/dL, where 1 U/mL or 100 U/dL, respectively, is arbitrarily assigned as the mean value of the reference sample pool.
4. Stability: AT appears to be stable in citrated plasma for 6 mo at −70 °C and for 6 wk in whole blood stored at 4 °C.[157]
5. Interpretive considerations
   a. Foals and human neonates have been shown to have plasma AT activities that are substantially lower than adult values.[110,158] This must be considered when interpreting AT values in young patients, especially in the absence of age-matched reference intervals.
   b. AT activity may be overestimated when measured by some thrombin chromogenic assays because heparin cofactor II activity may be detected in addition to AT activity.[157,159]
6. Decreased AT activity[155,157,160] (Fig. 5.4 and Table 5.8)
   a. Decreased AT activity may be either a cause or an effect of hypercoagulable (prothrombotic) states. Other clinical and laboratory findings should be used to help determine its pathogenesis.
   b. Decreased production
      (1) Inherited deficiencies have not been reported in animals but occur in people as type I (decreased antigen and activity, a quantitative disorder) and type II (decreased activity but normal amounts of antigen, a qualitative disorder).[161]
      (2) Liver disease (including portosystemic shunts)[162] may cause or contribute to AT deficiency in several ways, including decreased AT production related to decreased hepatocellular mass.

(3) Inflammation may decrease AT production in some species. AT was shown to be a negative acute-phase protein in human liver cells and in baboons,[163] but increased AT activity has been suggested to reflect a positive acute-phase response in rabbits[164] and cats.[162,165,166]

(4) Estrogens may contribute to AT deficiency by causing a mild to moderate decrease in AT synthesis[158,167]

c. AT loss
  (1) Like albumin, AT may be lost from the body in animals with protein-losing nephropathy and with protein-losing enteropathy.[168]
  (2) Urinary loss of AT without concurrent impairment of coagulation contributes to severe thrombotic disease in nephrotic syndrome patients, though other factors are involved.[169]
  (3) Severe hemorrhage may contribute to AT loss.

d. AT consumption: increased hepatic clearance of AT-enzyme complexes
  (1) Localized coagulation or disseminated consumptive coagulation states (see Thrombosis, sect. II) may cause decreased plasma AT activities when hepatic clearance of AT-enzyme complexes exceeds AT production.[127,157,162,170]
  (2) Sepsis has been associated with a prothrombotic condition and decreased AT activity.[111,171]
  (3) Heparin therapy (unfractionated and LMWH) accelerates the use and, therefore, hepatic clearance of AT, leading to decreased plasma activity.[172,173] Because AT is required for heparin's full anticoagulant effects, patients with subnormal AT activities are expected to have diminished responses to heparin and may be heparin resistant.[174]

7. Increased AT activity
  a. This is of unknown diagnostic utility and not considered a problem.
  b. Exogenous cortisol administration to dogs was associated with mildly to moderately increased AT synthesis,[167] but dogs with hyperadrenocorticism had decreased AT activity (evidence for a hypercoagulable state).[175]
  c. Inflammation may increase AT synthesis as part of the positive acute-phase response in some species, including cats.[162,164–166]
  d. Cats that were made taurine deficient had greater plasma AT activities than they had prior to being fed a taurine-deficient diet,[165] and cats with cardiac disease and hyperthyroidism had increased AT activities.[166] A role for thyroid hormones in increasing plasma AT activities in cats has not been reported but could be considered.[176–179]

8. Thrombin-antithrombin complexes (TAT)
  a. These form whenever thrombin is generated in the presence of AT.
  b. The [TAT] is measured to assess for activation of coagulation, especially latent coagulation that is not otherwise apparent.
  c. Increased plasma [TAT] indicates an increase in local or systemic thrombin generation, which is associated with thromboembolic disease or hypercoagulable states.[180–182]
  d. Decreased hepatic clearance of TAT could theoretically contribute to increased plasma [TAT].
  e. Increased [TAT] may occur without appreciable decreases in AT activity.
  f. Equine and canine plasma TAT have been measured with a human ELISA, primarily for research purposes.[175,183–185]

      g. Units: µg/L or ng/mL

      h. TAT may readily form in vitro if collection techniques are poor and coagulation occurs.[186]

B. Protein C

  1. This is infrequently assayed in veterinary medicine but provides information about a patient's anticoagulant and fibrinolytic status. Low plasma concentrations or activities predispose individuals to thrombosis because of decreased inactivation of factors Va and VIIIa and because of decreased fibrinolysis.

  2. Antigen concentration can be measured immunologically (by ELISA, radioimmunoassay, or Laurell rocket electroimmunoassay),[187] or activity can be measured by clot-based or amidolytic-based functional assays.[188]

      a. Antigenic assessment does not detect functional deficiencies, including those induced by vitamin K antagonism or deficiency (protein C is vitamin K dependent).

      b. Results of functional assays vary with the method, and species-specific modifications may be required.[189,190] Amidolytic assays do not assess all functional aspects of the molecule and do not directly measure its capability of inactivating factors Va and VIIIa. However, these assays are less sensitive than clot-based assays to coagulation inhibitors such as heparin. Some human patients have had abnormal clot-based results but normal antigen and amidolytic test results.

  3. Results are reported as % activity or antigen relative to a reference plasma pool considered to have 100 % activity or antigen.

  4. Decreased protein C activity

      a. Decreased production

         (1) Hereditary deficiencies (type I, antigenic; or type II, functional): A functional deficiency was identified in a colt.[191]

         (2) Vitamin K antagonism or deficiency (protein C is vitamin K dependent)

         (3) Decreased protein S (cofactor of protein C, which also is vitamin K dependent)

         (4) Liver disease with decreased functional hepatic mass

      b. Decreased survival: consumptive coagulation and its predisposing causes (see Thrombosis, sect. II);[192] sepsis[171]

      c. Inhibition: Anti-(phospholipid-protein) antibodies may inhibit the function of protein S, protein C, or factor V.[161,190,193]

      d. As equine data indicate, protein C activity (not antigen) values in healthy neonates (< 24 h old) may be greater than reference intervals established for adults.[110,111]

C. Protein Z

  1. *Protein Z* is a vitamin K–dependent protein that serves as a cofactor for PZI. *PZI*, first isolated from bovine plasma,[194] forms a complex with protein Z on membrane phospholipids and degrades factor Xa. PZI also degrades factor XIa but independently of protein Z.

  2. Roles for PZI and protein Z in health and disease are not clear, but mutations of the PZI gene and deficiencies of protein Z or PZI have been associated with abnormal hemostasis, usually thromboembolic disease, in people.[195]

  3. Protein Z is similar to albumin in molecular mass, and plasma concentrations have correlated positively with AT and negatively with proteinuria in people with

nephrotic syndrome. Urinary loss of protein Z may contribute to the prothrombotic state seen in some patients with protein-losing nephropathy.

4. Protein Z and PZI have not been assessed in veterinary patients.

XII. Coagulation factor antibodies (inhibitors)

A. Antibodies to coagulation factors are commonly referred to as *inhibitors*. These inhibitors must be differentiated from endogenous physiologic anticoagulants, exogenous anticoagulants, and anti-(phospholipid-protein) antibodies.

B. Conditions associated with coagulation factor antibodies

1. Antibodies may form spontaneously as part of an autoimmune disorder.
2. Antibodies may result from repeated transfusions to hemophiliacs who develop antibodies to the deficient factor.

C. Coagulation factor antibodies may predispose patients to hemorrhage.

D. Approach to detecting coagulation factor antibodies

1. Coagulation factor antibodies prolong whichever coagulation times are dependent on the target factor, usually PTT, so unexplained prolongations of PTT, PT, or both should prompt consideration of relevant deficiencies and inhibitors.
2. When PTT is prolonged but PT is not, unfractionated heparin should be considered a potential cause. Resampling, analysis with a heparin inactivator, or evaluation of TT (prolonged with heparin) could be considered.
3. If heparin cannot be incriminated, the coagulation times should be determined by use of mixing studies that assess the effects of diluting the sample 1:1 with platelet-free normal plasma. Coagulation times should be assessed immediately and after a 1–2 h incubation at 37 °C because some antibodies are time and/or temperature dependent.

    a. Immediate correction of the coagulation time, with no prolongation upon further incubation, supports a factor deficiency (including those caused by vitamin K antagonism) rather than a coagulation factor antibody. Factor analysis can be done to identify the deficient factor(s).
    b. Failure to correct the coagulation time supports the presence of a coagulation factor antibody or an anti-(phospholipid-protein) antibody (or heparin, if not already excluded).
    c. Immediate correction, but with inhibition after incubation, supports a coagulation factor antibody.

4. If mixing studies suggest an antibody, specialized tests can be done to assess for the presence of anti-(phospholipid-protein) antibodies. Specific coagulation factor antibodies can be assessed by combining mixing studies with specific factor assays.

XIII. Anti-(phospholipid-protein) antibodies

A. Rarely reported in veterinary medicine,[196] these antibodies are immunoglobulin G (IgG), IgM, or IgA associated with phospholipids (e.g., cardiolipin, phosphatidylcholine, phosphatidylserine, and phosphatidylethanolamine), but they appear to react with specific proteins that bind to the phospholipids (e.g., prothrombin, HMWK, factor XI, protein C, and protein S).

B. Lupus anticoagulants are a subset of anti-(phospholipid-protein) antibodies that inhibit phospholipid-dependent coagulation tests (e.g., PT and PTT), thus prolonging times if the test plasma is sufficiently devoid of platelets (and therefore phospholipid). Despite the name, they are not restricted to patients with lupus erythematosus.

    C. Although inhibitors of in vitro coagulation, clinical manifestations are thrombosis or thromboembolism, not hemorrhage.[99]

    D. A series of specialized tests may be required to identify and characterize anti-(phospho-lipid-protein) antibodies, but the following support their presence:

       1. Prolongation of a phospholipid-dependent coagulation assay

       2. Failure of normal, species-specific, pooled, platelet-poor plasma to correct the prolonged coagulation times when mixed with patient plasma[197]

       3. Neutralization of the inhibitor by increased phospholipid in the test system

       4. Exclusion of other coagulopathies

FIBRINOLYSIS

I.   Physiologic processes

    A. *Fibrinolysis* is the enzymatic degradation of fibrin. It counteracts coagulation and helps restore normal vessel architecture and patency after hemorrhage has been controlled with a secondary hemostatic plug.

    B. The fibrinolytic system, like the coagulation system, is a complex network of zymogens, enzymes, activators, and inhibitors (see Table 5.9).

    C. Fibrinolysis is initiated simultaneously with coagulation and is normally localized to the hemostatic plug.

       1. When coagulation occurs, plasminogen (inactive zymogen) binds to fibrin.

       2. t-PA released from stimulated endothelial cells binds to the fibrin-plasminogen complex and proteolytically cleaves plasminogen to form plasmin. u-PA from circulating cells or damaged tissue may play a similar role.

       3. Plasmin enzymatically degrades fibrin, fibrinogen, factors Va and VIIIa, vWF, HMWK, and other prothrombotic factors.

       4. Plasmin released into circulation is rapidly inhibited, primarily by plasmin inhibitor (α_2-antiplasmin), and cleared by the liver.

    D. The activation of plasmin is promoted by APC and inhibited by PAI, which APC inactivates.

    E. Plasmin degradation of fibrin and fibrinogen produces FDPs (Fig. 5.6), which can be measured to assess fibrinolysis.

    F. FDPs appear to be cleared from circulation by the liver (hepatocytes and macrophages) and kidneys (via catabolism or excretion).[198–201] Nonhepatic parts of the MPS may also be involved.[202,203]

II.   Fibrin or fibrinogen degradation products (FDPs) (fibrin fragments + fibrinogen fragments)

    A. Purpose: The measurement of FDPs is primarily used to detect increased fibrinolysis associated with excessive coagulation. It also may be used to detect increased fibrinogenolysis.

    B. Sample: serum or plasma

       1. Serum assays: Blood is collected into special tubes containing thrombin or *Botrox atrox* venom (reptilase), either of which can be used to consume fibrinogen via coagulation. Soybean trypsin inhibitor or aprotinin are present to inhibit plasmin and therefore in vitro FDP formation.

       2. Plasma assays: Blood is collected as for screening coagulation tests (see Coagulation, sect. II); citrated plasma is used.

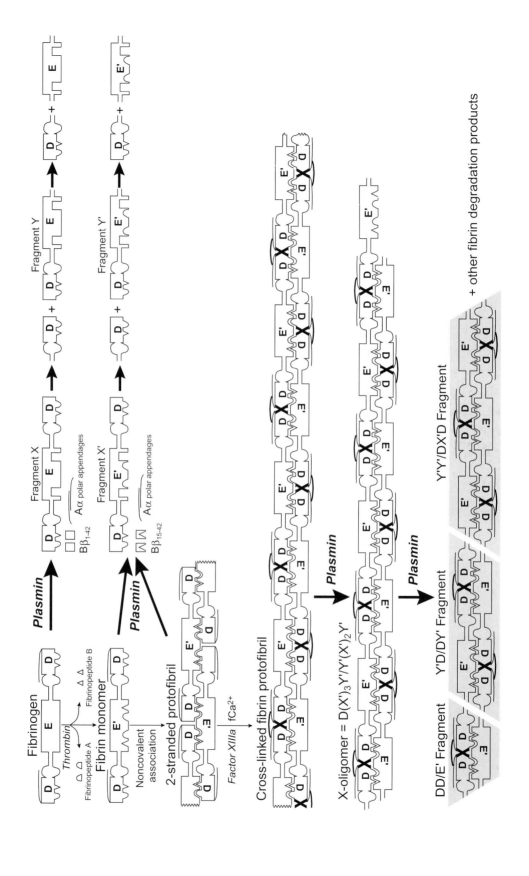

Fig. 5.6. Schematic representation of the formation of cross-linked fibrin from fibrinogen (*thin arrows*) and of the plasmin-mediated degradation of fibrinogen and fibrin to form FDPs (*thick arrows*).

- Fibrin formation: Fibrin is formed from fibrinogen, an elongated molecule that has a central E region and peripheral D regions (named for presence in the D and E fractions of FDPs eluted from an ion-exchange column). When thrombin is generated, it cleaves fibrinopeptides A and B from the E region of fibrinogen to form fibrin monomers. Unlike fibrinogen, fibrin monomers can polymerize (noncovalently) to form protofibrils of two or more strands (two are shown here). Thrombin also activates factor XIII to factor XIIIa, which cross-links adjacent D regions of different fibrin monomers to form stable cross-linked fibrin protofibrils. These can associate to form larger fibrin fibers (not shown) and a stable clot or thrombus.

- FDP formation: Plasmin cleaves fibrin and fibrinogen at specific sites to form fibrin fragments + fibrinogen fragments, collectively referred to as fibrin and fibrinogen degradation products (FDPs).

  - Fibrinogen: This is cleaved to form fragment X, and smaller fragments referred to as $B\beta_{1-42}$ and $A\alpha$ polar appendages. Fragment X is further degraded to fragments D and Y, and fragment Y is degraded to fragments D and E.

  - Non-cross-linked fibrin: Note that the degradation of non-cross-linked fibrin is similar, differing only because of the removal of fibrinopeptides A and B from fibrinogen during the formation of fibrin. Fibrin monomers and non-cross-linked protofibrils are degraded to form fragment X′ and smaller fragments $B\beta_{15-42}$ and $A\alpha$ polar appendages. Fragment X′ is further degraded to fragments D and Y′, and fragment Y′ is degraded to fragments D and E′.

  - Cross-linked fibrin: Plasmin-mediated degradation of cross-linked fibrin produces a different set of FDPs because of the covalent bonds formed by factor XIIIa between adjacent D regions. Initial degradation of cross-linked fibrin yields X-oligomers, high molecular weight compounds containing series of end-to-end X′ segments. These may be further degraded to other FDPs, including fragments DD/E′ (the major terminal breakdown product), Y′D/DY′, and Y′Y′/DX′D.[220]

  - Antigenic similarities of FDPs produced from fibrinogen and fibrin make the current FDP assay nonspecific for fibrinogenolysis or fibrinolysis (with or without cross-linking). However, D-dimer assays detect a variety of cross-linked fibrin compounds that occur only with coagulation and fibrinolysis.

Table 5.9. Fibrinolytic factors and their major functions

Factor[a]	Function
α_2-Macroglobulin	Binds, inhibits, and clears plasmin from circulation
Fibrin	Major protein in a stable thrombus; source of FDPs
Fibrin fragment D-dimer	FDP that contain D-dimer moieties generated by factor XIIIa–mediated cross-linking of fibrin; includes high and low molecular weight products
Fibrin fragments + fibrinogen fragments (FDPs)	Fragments of fibrinogen or fibrin produced from enzymatic degradation (fibrinolysis or fibrinogenolysis); inhibit platelets, thrombin, and fibrin polymerization
Fibrinogen (factor I)	Required for coagulation to progress to fibrin; converted to fibrin via thrombin (factor IIa)
Plasmin	Major enzyme that breaks down fibrin; also may degrade fibrinogen and other proteins
Plasmin inhibitor (PI, α_2-antiplasmin)	Binds, inhibits, and clears plasmin from circulation
Plasminogen	Inactive plasma protein precursor of plasmin; becomes localized to thrombi by binding to fibrin and fibrinogen
Plasminogen activator inhibitor 1 (PAI-1)	Inhibitor of fibrinolysis produced by endothelial cells; inactivates t-PA and u-PA
Plasminogen activator, tissue type (t-PA)	Converts plasminogen to plasmin; important in fibrinolysis within the vasculature
Plasminogen activator, urokinase type (u-PA)	Converts plasminogen to plasmin; important in tissue remodeling
Thrombin-activatable fibrinolysis inhibitor (TAFI)	Zymogen activated by thrombin and thrombomodulin; TAFIa cleaves plasminogen-binding sites from fibrin, thus inhibiting fibrinolysis

[a] The nomenclature follows recommendations made jointly by the Scientific and Standardization Committee of the International Society on Thrombosis and Haemostasis and the Committee (Commission) on Quantities and Units (in Clinical Chemistry) of the International Federation of Clinical Chemistry (IFCC) and the International Union of Pure and Applied Chemistry (IUPAC).[273]

    3. As with other tests of hemostasis, care must be taken to prevent or minimize coagulation during collection and processing. When plasma is the test sample, clotted samples should be discarded.

    4. Stability: It is often recommended to test plasma within 24 h when it is stored at 4 °C and within 20 d when it is frozen at −20 °C.

  C. Analytical concepts

    1. Latex agglutination immunoassays are used.[204] Dilutions of test serum or plasma are incubated with latex beads coated with antibodies to human FDPs. Agglutination of the beads indicates increased [FDPs].

    2. Antibody specificity

      a. The specific reactivity of assay antibodies with different FDP fragments from veterinary species is not known, but cross-reactivity of some polyclonal reagents with canine FDPs has been shown.[205] Clinical correlations with disease also support that there is at least partial cross-reactivity in dogs.

      b. Two FDP assays, one serum and one plasma, did not appear to have clinical utility in identifying fibrinolysis in horses with colic because there were positive results in healthy horses and few increased values in horses suspected of having DIC.[206]

      c. The plasma assay uses a monoclonal antibody to FDPs that does not react with fibrinogen, thus allowing the use of plasma (which contains fibrinogen) as the test sample.

      d. The serum assay uses a polyclonal antibody to FDPs that also binds fibrinogen, thus necessitating the in vitro removal of fibrinogen by means of reptilase or thrombin.

  3. Unit: usually μg/mL (may also be reported in ng/mL or μg/L)

  4. Reported semiquantitatively as the following:

      a. Less than a low decision threshold (e.g., < 5 μg/mL with plasma tests and <10 μg/mL with serum tests), below which values are considered normal)

      b. Increased (5–20 μg/mL with plasma tests and 10–40 μg/mL with serum tests)

      c. Increased more (> 20 μg/mL with plasma tests and > 40 μg/mL with serum tests)

  5. Interpretive considerations

      a. Prozone: With a high [FDPs], agglutination may occur at the greater dilution but not at the lesser dilution.

      b. False results

        (1) Serum assay results may be falsely decreased by FDP incorporation into the clot as it forms.[207]

        (2) Serum assays may be falsely increased by incomplete removal of fibrinogen from the sample due to the presence of dysfibrinogenemia (rare) or heparin (if thrombin rather than reptilase is used to activate clotting).[208]

        (3) Generation of FDPs during blood collection can cause false increases with plasma or serum assays.

        (4) Results may be false if antibodies do not bind to target FDPs or if they bind to other proteins.

      c. As equine data indicate, values in apparently healthy neonates may be greater than reference intervals established for adults.[110,111]

      d. Values in apparently healthy elderly people are often increased, probably related to changes in clearance rates or to an increased incidence of occult disease.[209]

D. Increased [FDPs] occurs in numerous diseases and conditions in which at least one of the following is present (see Table 5.10):[210]

  1. Increased fibrinolysis

      a. Localized intravascular coagulation (e.g., isolated thrombosis or thromboembolism, following surgery)

      b. Disseminated intravascular coagulation

      c. Sepsis[171] and probably many inflammatory conditions:[211] The prothrombotic state may progress to consumptive coagulation, but clinically recognizable thrombi or associated signs are often absent when inflammation is associated with an increased [FDPs].

      d. Hemorrhage: Bloody fluid collected from body cavities after hemorrhage contains high concentrations of FDPs, and an increased blood [FDPs] has been measured in such affected patients.[212] Increased [FDPs] and [D-dimer] have been detected in the serum or plasma of dogs with hemorrhage, but values were usually not as great as those in dogs classified as having thromboembolic disease or DIC.[213,214]

Table 5.10. Diseases or conditions that cause increased concentrations of FDPs[a]

Increased fibrinolysis
Localized intravascular coagulation
*Disseminated intravascular coagulation
*Sepsis and other inflammatory conditions
Internal hemorrhage
Increased fibrinogenolysis
Envenomations
Administration of plasminogen activators
Excessive release of t-PA (hypotensive shock, surgical trauma, heatstroke)
Decreased FDP clearance
Liver disease
Renal failure

* A relatively common disease or condition
[a] FDPs include D-dimers, but increased fibrinogenolysis alone will not increase [D-dimer].

However, an increased serum [FDPs] was not detected in dogs when hemorrhage into tissue was experimentally mimicked by pumping blood from the jugular vein to the peritoneal cavity or to muscle.[215]

  2. Increased fibrinogenolysis from hyperplasminemia or high local concentrations of plasmin
    a. Certain envenomations[216]
    b. Administration of plasminogen activators (e.g., t-PA or streptokinase)[217]
    c. Excessive endothelial release of t-PA, for which causes are not clearly defined but may include hypotensive shock, surgical trauma, and heatstroke[218]
    d. It may accompany fibrinolysis associated with thrombotic disease,[219] but some consider this very unlikely.[220]
  3. Decreased FDP clearance
    a. Decreased hepatic clearance may contribute to the increased [FDPs] in some patients with liver disease.[201]
    b. Decreased renal function may contribute to increased [FDPs] in some patients with renal failure.[198]
    c. Theoretically, decreased MPS activity could contribute to increased [FDPs].
E. Effects of increased [FDPs] on other hemostatic functions and tests
  1. Prolongs values for tests with clot end points (PT, PTT, TT, ACT, and Lee-White clotting time)
  2. Impairs platelet function
  3. Mechanisms of anticoagulation and antiplatelet effects
    a. FDPs compete with fibrinogen for the active site of thrombin and thus may inhibit the conversion of fibrinogen to fibrin.[221,222]
    b. FDPs compete with fibrinogen for platelet-binding sites and thus may inhibit platelet aggregation.[223]
    c. FDPs associate with fibrin monomers and may disrupt normal polymerization.[133,224]
  4. An increased concentration of FDPs promotes an antithrombotic and prohemorrhagic state.

III. Fibrin fragment D-dimer
   A. Theory: It can be used to assess increased fibrinolysis associated with coagulation. It should not detect fibrinogenolysis because antibodies should react only with fibrin cross-linked by the action of factor XIIIa (Fig. 5.6)
   B. Sample
      1. The sample is usually citrated plasma collected and handled as described for FDP analysis and coagulation assays. As with the FDP assay, when serum samples are used, in vitro D-dimer formation must be prevented and D-dimer fragments may be lost into the clot.
      2. Stability: It is recommended to test plasma within 24 h when stored at 4 °C and within 20 d when frozen at −20 °C.[225]
   C. Analytical concepts
      1. Although a canine assay was developed,[213] it is no longer available, and routine assays used to detect fibrin fragment D-dimer were developed for human D-dimer measurement. These assays are immunoassays.
         a. Results vary among assays because the assays vary in method, sample, and antibody used, and have lacked standardized and universal calibrators.
         b. The diagnostic utility of the assays in animals is being explored and varies with the assay and species.[206,225,226]
         c. Immunoturbidimetric, ELISA, card immunofiltration, and latex agglutination tests (semiquantitative) have been evaluated or used in animals.[206,225,227] Latex agglutination is most widely used and can be run as a point-of-care test.
      2. Antibody specificity: Most kits use monoclonal antibodies to human D-dimers that do not react with human fibrinogen, fibrinogen fragment D, or other FDPs lacking D-dimer domains.[228]
         a. Although the assay name suggests that only terminal D-dimer fragments are measured, assays detect D-dimer domains on a spectrum of human fibrin compounds.[228]
            (1) Compounds include high molecular weight cross-linked fibrin complexes, fibrin X-oligomers, and fibrin fragment DD/E' (Fig. 5.6).
            (2) Antibodies vary in reactivity, some preferentially reacting with high molecular weight fibrin oligomers, and others preferentially binding to low molecular weight D-dimer compounds.
            (3) D-dimer assays are specific for fibrin formation, but antibodies in some kits bind human D-dimer domains without plasmin-induced degradation.[229]
            (4) Some antibodies detect D-dimer moieties produced by cathepsin or elastase activities.
         b. The target molecules detected by D-dimer test antibodies in veterinary samples are uncharacterized, and the specificity of the test antibodies for D-dimer domains of veterinary species has not been proven. However, certain assays appear useful.
            (1) Clinical correlations with disease suggest at least partial reactivity, although these studies usually assess for positive results in animals suspected of having DIC based on imperfect criteria.
            (2) A point-of-care immunochromatographic assay with a monoclonal antibody for canine D-dimer (not currently available) compared well to ELISA and latex agglutination assays with anti-(human D-dimer) antibodies.[213]

    3. Unit: μg/mL, ng/mL, or μg/L, reported variably as D-dimer units (D-DU) or as fibrinogen equivalent units (FEU); 1 ng/mL D-DU = 2 ng/mL FEU.

  D. Increased plasma [D-dimer]: Interpretation is similar to that for increased [FDPs], except that values should reflect only increased cross-linked fibrin formation and fibrinolysis (not fibrinogenolysis) or decreased clearance of fibrin degradation products (not fibrinogen degradation products) by the liver or MPS.[230,231]

    1. In human medicine, D-dimer assays have been most useful in excluding clinically significant thrombotic disease; such conditions are rare when [D-dimer] is not increased. However, latex agglutination assays may not detect mild increases detectable with other assays and therefore cannot be used to exclude thrombotic disease in people.

    2. As for increases in the [FDPs], a variety of conditions cause increases in [D-dimer] without overt DIC or thrombotic disease; for example, with inflammation, with hemorrhage, and after surgery.[214]

      a. Testing serial sample dilutions of up to 1:8 and using increased decision thresholds increase the diagnostic specificity of results for clinically significant thrombotic or thromboembolic disease.[214]

      b. Diagnostic specificity for thromboembolic disease was 94 % in one canine study using a decision threshold of 1000 ng/mL and including postsurgery dogs and dogs with hepatic disease, renal disease, cardiac disease, and neoplasia. Diagnostic sensitivity was still 80 % with this decision threshold.

    3. Unlike in dogs and people, healthy horses have a detectable [D-dimer] when current assays are used. Detectable concentrations are therefore abnormal only when exceeding a defined decision threshold (e.g., > 1000 ng/mL).[206]

IV.   Other assays may be used to measure fibrinolytic components (e.g., plasminogen, plasmin inhibitor, t-PA, and PAI-1) (see Table 5.9) or fibrinolytic activity (euglobulin lysis time test), but they are not widely used in clinical settings. Thromboelastography and resonance thrombography are more global in vitro tests of hemostasis that assess the functional contributions of platelets, coagulation, and fibrinolysis to the hemostatic process. Further reading about these specialized techniques is available.[232–235]

BLOOD VESSELS (ENDOTHELIAL CELLS)

Although blood vessels (especially the endothelial cells) are very important in maintaining normal hemostasis via prothrombotic and antithrombotic properties,[236] their assessment in the clinical pathology laboratory is limited primarily to tissue biopsy and histologic evaluation (e.g., for vasculitis or thrombosis). Vascular lesions are usually obvious when hemorrhage is the result of surgical or accidental vascular trauma. Diseases involving small vessels, such as RMSF and equine purpura hemorrhagica, may be associated with petechiae and ecchymoses caused by combinations of direct vascular damage, thrombocytopenia, and thrombopathia. Hemostasis testing may help exclude other disorders but will not provide a specific diagnosis.

MAJOR BLEEDING DISORDERS: FINDINGS AND PATHOGENESES

I.   Diagnosis: The diagnosis of bleeding disorders requires knowledge of the general types of bleeding disorders, consideration of clinical findings, accurate interpretation of hemostasis test results, and recognition of hemostasis test patterns.

A. Types of bleeding disorders
   1. Blood vessel disorders are typically identified by nonhemostatic tests (e.g., gross examination, imaging, serology, and biopsy), but hemostatic tests are useful for excluding primary blood disorders and may provide diagnostic clues because of secondary changes in blood constituents (e.g., thrombocytopenia with vasculitis).
      a. Large vessels: surgical or nonsurgical trauma, invasion, aneurysms, and anomalies
      b. Small vessels: vasculitides (infectious, immune mediated, and chemical) and vasculopathies (rare)
   2. Blood disorders: typically identified by hemostatic tests
      a. Impaired primary hemostasis: thrombocytopenia, thrombopathia, and vWD
      b. Impaired secondary hemostasis: hereditary or acquired defects in coagulation
      c. Excessive fibrinolysis: DIC and some envenomations
B. Clinical findings are essential for establishing a final diagnosis, but the bleeding pattern, breed, age, and gender may be of particular value in directing diagnostic plans.
   1. Bleeding pattern
      a. Petechiae and ecchymoses should prompt consideration of severe thrombocytopenia or thrombopathia, though concurrent defects in secondary hemostasis may also be present. Vascular diseases may cause similar hemorrhages.
      b. Subcutaneous hematomas and hemorrhage into body cavities suggest defects in secondary hemostasis, especially when petechiae and ecchymoses are absent. However, hematomas may form with platelet defects.
      c. Hemorrhage through mucosal surfaces (e.g., epistaxis, gastrointestinal hemorrhage, or prolonged estral bleeding) may occur with thrombocytopenia, thrombopathia, vWD, or defects in coagulation. Prolonged hemorrhage secondary to venipuncture or surgical or nonsurgical trauma is also not specific.
   2. Breed and age
      a. Breed predispositions for inherited diseases may help in selection of appropriate diagnostic tests.[237]
      b. Hemorrhage in a young animal should prompt consideration of an inherited defect of platelets (Table 5.2), vWD, or coagulation factor deficiency (Table 5.7) if another cause is not apparent. Molecular genetic testing may be available for some characterized mutations in some affected and carrier animals (e.g., vWD).[238]
   3. Gender
      a. Hemophilia A (factor VIII deficiency) and hemophilia B (factor IX deficiency) are sex-linked (X chromosome), recessively inherited disorders.
         (1) Males are either affected or not. They are not carriers.
         (2) Females may be free of the defect, carriers (heterozygous), or, rarely, affected (homozygous).
         (3) About 50 % of the offspring of carrier females mated to unaffected males will inherit a defective X chromosome, so 50 % of male offspring will be affected and 50 % of female offspring will be carriers.
         (4) All female offspring of a clear female and an affected male are asymptomatic carriers.
         (5) Female offspring from a carrier female and an affected male can be affected.
      b. Therefore, these disorders almost always occur in males. Hemorrhage in females is unlikely to be caused by one of these disorders.

Table 5.11. Possible causes of abnormal results for the major tests of hemostasis

Test or analyte	Result	Possible causes
ACT	↑ Time	Defect in surface-induced and/or common pathways
AT	↓ Activity[a]	Renal or intestinal loss, consumptive coagulation, heparin administration, or decreased production
BMBT	↑ Time	Thrombocytopenia, thrombopathia, vWF deficiency, anemia
Clot retraction	↓ Extent	Thrombocytopenia, thrombopathia
Coagulation factors	↓ Activity	Hereditary or acquired factor deficiencies (hypocoagulable state)
D-dimers	↑ Concentration	Coagulation and fibrinolysis, decreased clearance
FDPs	↑ Concentration	Increased fibrin(ogen)olysis, decreased clearance
Fibrinogen[b]	↓ Concentration	Decreased hepatic production, increased consumption (may be hypocoagulable)
	↑ Concentration	Inflammation, hypovolemia (dehydration)
Protein C	↓ Activity[c]	Decreased hepatic production, abnormal production (vitamin K antagonism or absence), loss, consumption (may be hypercoagulable)
PT	↑ Time	Defect in TF and/or common pathways
PTT	↑ Time	Defect in surface-induced and/or common pathways
RVVT	↑ Time	Defect in common pathway
TT	↑ Time	Hypofibrinogenemia, dysfibrinogenemia, heparinized patient or sample, increased FDPs
vWF:Ag	↓ Concentration	vWD or vWD carrier
	↑ Concentration	Exercise, excitement, pregnancy, vasopressin

[a] Chromogenic assays assess activity, but there are immunologic assays that assess concentration. Proteins may be present but not functional.

[b] For assessment of hemostasis, fibrinogen concentrations are usually determined from TT_{Clauss} values, which are inversely correlated with fibrinogen concentrations unless prolonged by high concentrations of heparin or high concentrations of FDPs when fibrinogen concentrations are low.

[c] Chromogenic assays assess activity, but immunologic assays assess concentration. Concentration may be WRI while activity is decreased if there is abnormal production of protein C (e.g., vitamin K antagonism or absence).

C. Hemostasis tests: A summary of available screening and specialized hemostasis tests is presented in Table 5.11 to aide in selection and interpretation of specific tests.

D. Major patterns of hemostasis test results: Hemostasis in bleeding patients is best evaluated by multiple tests (hemostasis profiles). Examples of the major patterns of common hemostatic test results in bleeding patients are listed in Table 5.12.

1. Pattern 1: Prolonged BMBT without thrombocytopenia or severe anemia suggests vWD or a thrombopathia. vWF analysis or platelet function studies may be indicated. Specifically defining thrombopathias may be difficult. PTT may occasionally be prolonged with canine vWD if factor VIII is concurrently deficient enough, and it may be prolonged in horses with vWD.

2. Pattern 2: Prolonged BMBT associated with moderate to severe thrombocytopenia can be explained by the thrombocytopenia, though concurrent defects in platelet

Table 5.12. Interpretation of the major patterns of common hemostasis test results

Pattern	PT	PTT[a]	FDPs[b]	Fibrinogen[c]	Platelets	BMBT	Interpretation[d]
1	WRI	WRI	WRI	WRI	WRI	↑	Thrombopathia, vWD[e]
2	WRI	WRI	WRI	WRI	↓	↑	Thrombocytopenia
3	WRI	↑	WRI	WRI	WRI	WRI	Intrinsic pathway defect[f]
4	↑	WRI	WRI	WRI	WRI	WRI	Factor VII deficiency[f]
5	↑	↑	WRI	WRI	WRI	WRI	Common pathway defect or multiple defects
6	↑	↑	WRI	↓	WRI	WRI–↑	Dys- or afibrinogenemia
7	↑	↑	↑	↓	↓	↑	Fulminant DIC[g]

[a] ACT would mirror PTT results in most diseases, but has less diagnostic sensitivity and therefore may be WRI.

[b] Plasma [FDPs], including [D-dimer], may increase with hemorrhage (see the text).

[c] For assessment of hemostasis, fibrinogen concentrations are usually determined from TT_{Clauss} values, which are inversely correlated with fibrinogen concentrations unless prolonged by high concentrations of heparin or high concentrations of FDPs.

[d] See the text (Major Bleeding Disorders, sect. I.D) for expanded interpretive comments.

[e] PTT may be prolonged in horses and occasionally in dogs with vWD if factor VIII is concurrently deficient.

[f] This pattern may also occur with early stages of hepatic disease or vitamin K antagonism or absence.

[g] This pattern applies only to the severe, fulminant form of DIC.

function or vWF cannot be excluded. BMBT testing is not indicated in patients with moderate to severe thrombocytopenia because prolongations of BMBT are expected and thus will not add new information.

3. Pattern 3: Isolated prolongation of the PTT indicates a surface-induced pathway defect, though insensitivity of the PT assay may mask other abnormalities.
    a. Acquired PTT prolongations: This may be caused by hepatic disease, heparin contamination of the sample (e.g., inappropriate collection from a heparinized catheter), or heparin therapy, and rarely is caused by vitamin K antagonism. Rare surface-induced pathway coagulation factor or anti-(phospholipid-protein) antibodies should be considered.
    b. Inherited or congenital PTT prolongations (Table 5.7)
        (1) Hemophilia A and B caused by deficiencies of factor VIII and factor IX, respectively, are the most common inherited causes and may be associated with severe hemorrhage. They are extremely rare in females because they are X-linked recessive traits.
        (2) Deficiencies in factor XII and PK are not associated with hemorrhage when either occurs alone.
        (3) Deficiency of factor XI is associated with mild hemorrhage, usually in response to trauma. Hemorrhage may be delayed.
        (4) Deficiencies may be multiple (e.g., factor XII plus factor IX deficiency).
4. Pattern 4: Isolated prolongation of PT indicates a TF pathway (factor VII) defect.
    a. Acquired PT prolongations: Hepatic or hepatobiliary disease and vitamin K antagonism or deficiency should be considered. Factor VII has the shortest half-life of the vitamin K–dependent factors, and three of the five factors in the combined TF and common pathways are vitamin K dependent. Therefore, the

PT may be affected by vitamin K antagonism or absence before the PTT, especially when a PIVKA-sensitive PT method is used.

    b. Inherited or congenital PT prolongations (Table 5.7): Factor VII deficiencies are rare and associated with mild hemorrhage, usually in response to surgical or nonsurgical trauma.

5. Pattern 5: Prolonged PT and PTT without other screening abnormalities suggest multiple factor deficiencies or a common pathway defect (excluding afibrinogenemia or dysfibrinogenemia, which would be recognized by a low [fibrinogen]).

    a. Acquired disorders: Combined deficiencies of vitamin K–dependent factors (II, VII, IX, and X) caused by vitamin K antagonism or deficiency may lead to severe hemorrhage. Thrombocytopenia may also develop. Increases in [fibrinogen] and decreases in [FDPs] have been reported in people receiving warfarin and may occur in other species. Hepatic disease should also be considered, especially if [fibrinogen] or activity is low-normal. Variations of this pattern seen with hepatic disease include combinations of increased [FDPs], decreased [fibrinogen], thrombocytopenia, and prolonged BMBT.

    b. Inherited or congenital disorders (Table 5.7): Rare inherited factor X or factor II deficiency could be considered and may be associated with severe hemorrhagic tendencies. A similar clinical and laboratory pattern could be caused by rare hereditary defects in vitamin K–dependent carboxylase (so-called vitamin K–dependent multifactor deficiency, reported in Devon rex cats and possibly found in a Labrador retriever).[239,240]

6. Pattern 6: Prolonged PT and PTT with hypofibrinogenemia and possibly prolonged BMBT

    a. Acquired disorders: Hepatic disease is a consideration for this pattern (see the discussion of pattern 5). Consumptive coagulation (e.g., DIC) could also be considered, but thrombocytopenia and increased [FDPs] and/or [D-dimer] are usually expected with DIC.

    b. Inherited or congenital disorders: A marked decrease in [fibrinogen] along with prolonged PT and PTT should prompt consideration of rare inherited dysfibrinogenemia or afibrinogenemia.[16] Severe hemorrhagic tendencies are expected, and BMBT may be prolonged.

7. Pattern 7: Prolonged PT and PTT with increased [FDPs], hypofibrinogenemia, and thrombocytopenia are typical of fulminant DIC, whatever the cause. Such a patient would appear very ill, likely with evidence of multiple organ damage. Findings with hepatic failure could be similar.

II. Pathogenesis: The pathogeneses of hemorrhagic defects in primary hemostasis relate to specific abnormalities or deficiencies in platelets, vWF, or the vessel wall. Inherited disorders of secondary hemostasis are caused by various genetic alterations that result in decreased, absent, or abnormal hemostatic factors. Acquired bleeding disorders often have a more complex pathogeneses. The pathogeneses of hemostatic abnormalities are discussed for the following selected acquired bleeding disorders:

    A. Hepatic disease[116]

        1. Liver disease can cause defects in the production and clearance of procoagulants, anticoagulants, profibrinolytics, and antifibrinolytics. The net result is often clinically silent despite abnormalities in hemostatic laboratory tests.

2. Bleeding is uncommon but may occur if hepatic failure is severe or associated with DIC. Other laboratory evidence of hepatic failure would be expected in a patient bleeding because of the hepatic failure.

3. Potential abnormal hemostatic test results and their causes

   a. Prolonged PT, PTT, ACT, or TT
      (1) Decreased hepatic production of coagulation factors because of decreased functional hepatic mass (including portosystemic shunts[241])
      (2) Abnormal production of vitamin K–dependent coagulation factors because of decreased vitamin K absorption secondary to cholestasis or, possibly, decreased food intake

   b. Increased [FDPs] and/or [D-dimer]
      (1) Decreased hepatic clearance of FDPs and plasminogen activators
      (2) Increased FDP production (fibrinolysis) because of accompanying intravascular coagulation, which is sometimes disseminated

   c. Thrombocytopenia
      (1) Increased splenic sequestration caused by portal hypertension, splenomegaly, and possibly decreased thrombopoietin production
      (2) Consumption secondary to accompanying intravascular coagulation

   d. Prolonged BMBT
      (1) Thrombocytopenia
      (2) Acquired thrombopathia

   e. Decreased [fibrinogen]
      (1) Decreased hepatic production
      (2) Consumption secondary to accompanying intravascular coagulation

   f. Decreased AT activity
      (1) Decreased hepatic production
      (2) Consumption secondary to accompanying intravascular coagulation

   g. Thrombopathia: increased [FDPs] or unknown causes

4. Laboratory findings may mimic consumptive coagulation and/or consumptive coagulopathy.

5. Results of routine hemostatic tests are not good predictors of surgical hemorrhage in human patients with hepatic disease[242] or of hemorrhage induced by collecting liver biopsy samples.[131] This is likely because the net balance of all antithrombotic and prothrombotic processes is not altered as much as the function of the isolated processes that are tested. Similarly, bleeding secondary to biopsy procedures in dogs and cats does not appear to be predictable from PT and PTT results, although, in cats, there was an association between major complications and PTT prolongation of at least 1.5× the mean of the reference interval.[243] Bleeding complications in dogs and cats are more strongly associated with thrombocytopenia than with prolonged PT and PTT.

B. Vitamin K antagonism or deficiency

1. Vitamin K antagonism: Bleeding is common and may be external and obvious or internal and occult. It usually occurs 3–7 d after exposure.

   a. Vitamin K antagonists may be ingested in several forms:
      (1) Hydroxycoumarins or indanediones in anticoagulant rodenticide products; for example, warfarin, bromadiolone, brodifacoum, and diphacinone (specifically detectable by high-performance liquid chromatography).

(2) Sweet clover or sweet vernal grass containing bishydroxycoumarin, a metabolite produced from the actions of certain molds[244,245]

(3) Therapeutic coumadins: From an overdose, because of displacement from plasma proteins by additional protein-binding drugs (e.g., phenylbutazone), or by ingestion of medication intended for human patients (includes warfarin and phenoprocoumon)[246]

(4) Excess sulfaquinoxaline, a coccidiostat with vitamin K antagonistic effects[247–249]

b. Once absorbed, these compounds inhibit the enzymatic recycling of oxidized vitamin K back to its reduced and functional form in hepatocytes, thus leading to production of coagulation factors with decreased functional potential (Fig. 5.7).[65] When normal coagulation factors in the circulation ($t_{1/2} = 6$–40 h) decrease enough, coagulation times become prolonged (within 24 h)[250] and hemorrhage may occur.

2. Vitamin K deficiency (hypovitaminosis K) is rarely deficient enough to cause hemorrhage.

a. Vitamin K is absorbed in the intestine after ingestion or production by intestinal bacteria.

b. Causes of clinically significant vitamin K deficiency have not been clarified in most species, but the following should be considered:

(1) Prolonged anorexia or ingestion of an abnormal diet may cause or contribute to vitamin K deficiency. In contrast, normal diets contain excess vitamin K.[251,252]

(2) Gut sterilization by antimicrobials may cause or contribute to vitamin K deficiency.[251,253]

(3) Malabsorption of vitamin K (a fat-soluble vitamin)[148]

(a) Intrahepatic or extrahepatic cholestasis (decreased fat digestion and absorption, and therefore decreased vitamin K absorption)

(b) Intestinal malabsorption diseases (e.g., infiltrative bowel disease)

(c) Exocrine pancreatic insufficiency (decreased fat digestion and absorption, and therefore decreased vitamin K absorption)

c. Diminished, but not absent, vitamin K may lead to a subclinical mixture of normal coagulation factors and PIVKA. Vitamin K supplementation was associated with a correction of prolonged PIVKA-sensitive PT values in cats with intestinal or hepatic diseases.[148]

3. Causes of abnormal hemostatic test results

a. Prolonged PT, PTT, or ACT

(1) Decreased amounts of functional vitamin K–dependent coagulation factors participating in the surface-induced (factor IX), TF (factor VII), and common (factors X and II) pathways

(2) Although PT is expected to be prolonged before PTT, there may be prolongation of PTT alone, PT alone, or both values, depending on the optimization of the assays and, perhaps, the species involved.[254]

b. Thrombocytopenia

(1) If present, thrombocytopenia probably results mostly from consumption at multiple sites of hemorrhage.

(2) When moderate or marked, BMBT prolongation would be expected, especially if the patient is anemic.

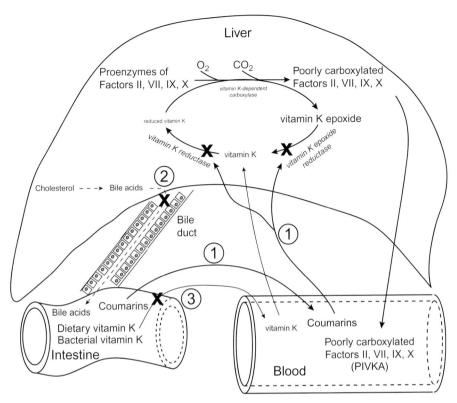

Fig. 5.7. Effects of vitamin K antagonism or deficiency on hepatocyte production of vitamin K–dependent coagulation factors (II, VII, IX, and X). *Circled numbers* in the figure denote the three following processes that result in production of defective factors II, VII, IX, and X:

1. Antagonism: Ingested anticoagulant rodenticides or other coumarins are absorbed in the intestine. In hepatocytes, they inhibit the enzymatic reduction of vitamin K epoxide back to reduced vitamin K, which is the form of vitamin K required for the vitamin K–dependent carboxylase enzyme to carboxylate the coagulation proteins. Failure to recycle vitamin K leads to decreased amounts of reduced vitamin K and increased amounts of vitamin K epoxide. Factors II, VII, IX, and X are still produced, however. They enter the blood and circulate in a permanently hypofunctional or nonfunctional state. These poorly carboxylated or noncarboxylated coagulation factors are known as PIVKA (proteins induced by vitamin K antagonism) and in people can be measured with specific antibodies. Plasma vitamin K epoxide concentrations increase (not shown). Vitamin K_1 administration overrides competitive inhibition of vitamin K reductase and enables functional factors to be produced.

2. Absence because of cholestasis (intrahepatic or posthepatic): Impaired bile flow reduces fat absorption because not enough bile acids are reaching the intestine to emulsify ingested fats properly. Consequently, fewer fat-soluble vitamins, including vitamin K, are absorbed, and a vitamin K deficiency may develop. The deficiency causes impaired carboxylation of vitamin K–dependent coagulation factors despite normal activity of reducing enzymes. Noncarboxylated factors are produced and enter the blood, where they are known as PIVKA (proteins induced by vitamin K absence). Amounts of vitamin K epoxide would not increase in this case.

3. Absence because of other causes: Anorexia (decreased dietary intake of vitamin K), decreased vitamin K production by intestinal bacteria (e.g., after antibiotics), intestinal malabsorptive disease, or exocrine pancreatic insufficiency can contribute to, or rarely cause, vitamin K deficiency.

       c. Factor analysis is typically not necessary, but deficiencies in vitamin K–dependent factors would be noted.

       d. Other abnormalities have not been widely described, but decreased [FDPs], including D-dimer, and increased [fibrinogen] may result from decreased coagulation and consequently decreased fibrinolysis. Prolonged TT reported in people correlated with increases in [fibrinogen].[137]

    4. Rare hereditary defects in vitamin K–dependent carboxylase (vitamin K–dependent multifactor deficiency) produce similar hemostatic abnormalities, but vitamin K is neither deficient nor antagonized in this disorder.[239,240]

C. Consumptive coagulopathy

    1. *Consumptive coagulation* is the process of accelerated or unbalanced coagulation that may cause a disorder of deficient coagulation referred to as *consumptive coagulopathy*.

    2. *Consumptive coagulopathy* results from local or disseminated consumptive coagulation when procoagulant blood components are destroyed or removed from circulation (consumed) and FDPs are generated.

    3. It may arise from DIC, in which case bleeding is common.

       a. *DIC* is a syndrome of consumptive coagulation occurring throughout the vasculature (disseminated and intravascular).

       b. It is always secondary to a condition that causes unbalanced or excessive coagulation.

         (1) Causes include severe tissue necrosis, angiostrongylosis, heatstroke, disseminated neoplasia, endotoxemia, sepsis, pancreatitis, hepatic disease, or some envenomations.

         (2) Coagulation is often initiated by TF release from damaged tissues, neoplastic cells, or endotoxin-stimulated cells or by surface-induced activation caused by massive endothelial cell damage or activation. Many snake venoms initiate the process by activating the common pathway directly.[131,255,256]

       c. It may be acute or chronic, compensated or uncompensated.

       d. When production of procoagulant factors does not keep up with consumption, excessive coagulation can lead to defective coagulation (i.e., consumptive coagulopathy).

    4. Consumptive coagulopathy may arise from localized consumptive coagulation, in which case bleeding is rare.[257]

       a. Excessive coagulation in a localized area or organ can produce laboratory signs of consumptive coagulation and, rarely, clinical bleeding. Correction of the localized problem may be curative.

       b. Human examples include aortic aneurysm and large hemangiomas. With these conditions, disseminated intravascular coagulation does not occur, but localized hemostatic abnormalities may lead to a coagulopathy. Large cutaneous and splenic hemangiomas and hemangiosarcomas may be examples of localized consumptive coagulation in dogs. However, the changes have usually been interpreted as DIC.

    5. Clinical signs vary from subclinical to serious hemorrhage, shock, or signs of multiple organ failures caused by thromboembolism or hemorrhage. Signs of the underlying disease may also be present.

    6. Consumptive coagulopathy can be recognized when the typical laboratory and clinical signs accompany a condition known to trigger the process. Typical findings are thrombocytopenia, prolonged PT and PTT, increased [D-dimer] and [FDPs],

decreased AT activity, or trends toward these abnormalities with serial measure-ments. However, combinations of these abnormalities can occur without consump-tive coagulation/coagulopathy, and the patterns of laboratory abnormalities vary considerably and depend on severity, duration, and underlying or concurrent disorders.

7. Causes of abnormal hemostatic test results
   a. Hypofibrinogenemia: Fibrinogen is consumed as it is transformed into fibrin during excessive coagulation. Because fibrinogen is a positive acute-phase protein, increased hepatic production may occur in inflammatory states and mask the hypofibrinogenemia typical of consumptive coagulation.
   b. Thrombocytopenia: Platelets are consumed as they patch exposed vascular defects, become incorporated into thrombi, or become activated secondary to thrombin and other platelet agonists formed in the blood.
   c. Prolonged PT, PTT, and ACT: Hypofibrinogenemia, increased [FDPs], and decreased functional coagulation factors may all contribute.
      (1) Once the nonenzymatic coagulation cofactors V and VIII become activated to factors Va and VIIIa, they are inactivated by APC. Decreased factor V and VIII concentrations will develop if activation and inactivation occur at a greater rate than production and secretion.
      (2) Coagulation enzymes in the surface-induced and common pathways are bound by AT or other antiproteases and removed from circulation by hepatocytes. Thrombin also binds thrombomodulin on endothelial cell membranes, and the complex is internalized and degraded. If the rate of enzyme inactivation and removal remains greater than the rate of production and release of new proenzymes, plasma activity of these coagulation factors decreases.
      (3) FDPs from fibrinolysis interfere with fibrin formation.
   d. Decreased AT activity: After AT binds to activated coagulation enzymes, the complexes are removed from the circulation by hepatocytes. If the rate of removal remains greater than the rate of production and release of new AT, plasma AT activity decreases.
   e. Increased [FDPs] and [D-dimer]: With activation of coagulation pathways, cross-linked fibrin forms, with concurrent activation of fibrinolysis and plasmin-mediated degradation of fibrin and possibly fibrinogen. This leads to the increased formation of FDPs and D-dimers.
   f. Prolonged TT and TT$_{Clauss}$: This can be caused by hypofibrinogenemia and increased [FDPs].
   g. Prolonged BMBT: This can be caused by thrombocytopenia and increased [FDPs]. FDPs interfere with platelet function.
   h. Erythrocyte fragmentation: This occurs from intravascular trauma (microangio-pathic fragmentation). Schizocytes, keratocytes, and low numbers of spherocytes may be found in blood films.

D. Dilutional coagulopathy: Infusion of large volumes of colloid fluids, crystalloid fluids, plasma-poor packed erythrocytes, or Oxyglobin solution (a hemoglobin-based oxygen carrier) to treat massive, acute blood loss expands blood volume and transiently dilutes blood components, including coagulation factors, platelets, vWF, and fibrinogen.[258] This may result in prolonged coagulation times and contribute to hemorrhage, but it alone is not expected to cause hemorrhage.[259–261] Compared to saline, high molecular weight colloids (dextrans, oxypolygelatin, and hetastarch) may have additional effects on hemostasis, such as causing greater decrements in the amount of plasma fibrinogen and vWF:Ag. The effects depend on the fluid infused, the rate of infusion, and the recipient species.[262]

E. Afibrinogenemia/dysfibrinogenemia (rare):[16,129–132] Without adequate functional fibrinogen, fibrin clots cannot form, thus prolonging PT, PTT, ACT, and TT. Because fibrinogen is the major interplatelet bridge during aggregation, BMBT may be prolonged.

F. Inhibition of functional coagulation factors[263]
1. Heparinization
   a. Heparin administration or release from neoplastic mast cells may prolong coagulation times and predispose patients to hemorrhage (see Fig. 5.4 for the mechanism of action).
   b. Unfractionated heparin prolongs PTT and ACT values but typically not PT values. PT assays generally contain a heparin inactivator.
   c. LMWH decreases factor Xa activity and may or may not prolong PTT.
   d. AT activity decreases after heparin administration.
2. FDPs: They contribute to hemorrhage, prolong coagulation times (PT, PTT, ACT, and TT), and decrease platelet function.
3. Antibodies to coagulation factors:[264]
   a. As with human hemophiliac patients receiving multiple transfusions, dogs transfused for hemophilia A and hemophilia B have also produced antibodies to the factor they lack.[265,266]
   b. Antibodies may also form as an autoimmune phenomenon, and they may have reactivity to coagulation factors other than factors VIII and IX.
   c. Antibodies can prolong coagulation times of the affected pathway or pathways because of antibody-mediated inhibition of the target protein.
   d. Normal pooled plasma does not correct the prolonged coagulation times when mixed with patient plasma; prolonged coagulation times reflect an increased propensity to bleed.

THROMBOSIS

I. *Thrombosis* is the formation of thrombi within the vascular system. Thrombi are in vivo "clots" but adherent to the vessel or heart wall and composed of varying amounts of fibrin and blood cells. Thrombi that form under high-flow conditions (arterial) contain more platelets. Thrombi that form under low-flow conditions (venous) contain more erythrocytes and fewer platelets.

II. Thrombi form when the normal balance between prothrombotic factors and antithrombotic factors shifts to favor thrombosis (i.e., thrombophilia). The specific reasons for this shift are not completely understood for many conditions.
A. The shift may occur with disorders involving one or more of the following mechanisms:
1. Endothelial cell activation or damage
2. Platelet activation
3. Activation of coagulation
4. Blood stasis

   5. Inhibition of fibrinolysis
   6. Deficiencies or abnormalities in anticoagulant proteins (e.g., AT, protein C, protein S, factor V, and possibly protein Z or PZI) or abnormalities in coagulant proteins (e.g., prothrombin)[267]
   B. Acquired conditions associated with thrombosis include the following:
       1. Vasculitis, endocarditis, intravascular catheterization, and injection of chemical irritants
       2. Congestive heart failure, feline cardiomyopathy, and vascular defects
       3. Surgical or nonsurgical trauma
       4. Malignant neoplasia
       5. Sepsis, endotoxemia, and equine colic and colitis
       6. Immune-mediated hemolytic anemia in dogs
       7. Hypothyroidism and hyperadrenocorticism
       8. AT deficiency from protein-losing nephropathy, enteropathy, blood loss, or liver failure
       9. Protein C deficiency
       10. Anti-(phospholipid-protein) antibodies (antiphospholipid antibodies)[99]

III. Thrombi may cause clinical signs by obstructing blood flow and causing ischemia, by forming emboli (fragments) that travel to distant sites and cause ischemia, or by consuming platelets and other hemostatic factors, which may lead to hemorrhage. Thrombi may occur in a single area because of local disturbances (e.g., chemical irritants injected into the jugular vein) or at multiple sites because of more systemic abnormalities (e.g., DIC).

IV. Clinical signs are variable and depend on the underlying disease and location and severity of the lesion(s). Dyspnea may occur with pulmonary thromboembolism, hematuria with renal infarction, edema of the head with cranial vena cava thrombosis, and distal aortic thrombosis may cause rear-limb weakness and pain, decreased femoral pulse pressure and quality, and cool extremities.[268–272]

V. Potential hemostatic abnormalities
   A. Increased [D-dimer] is evidence of cross-linked fibrin formation and degradation and therefore intravascular coagulation.
   B. Increased [FDPs] can be evidence of fibrin degradation, but it could be the result of fibrinogenolysis without intravascular coagulation.
   C. Decreased AT activity can be evidence of consumption caused by intravascular coagulation, but it may result from AT loss or decreased production and may contribute to intravascular coagulation.
   D. Increased [TAT] is evidence of increased thrombin generation and therefore intravascular coagulation.
   E. Decreased protein C activity can be evidence of consumption caused by intravascular coagulation, but it may also result from other causes, such as vitamin K antagonism or hereditary deficiency, in which case it may contribute to intravascular coagulation.
   F. Thrombocytopenia can be evidence of consumption caused by intravascular coagulation, but there are many other causes.
   G. Decreased [fibrinogen] can be evidence of consumption caused by intravascular coagulation, but increased production associated with inflammation may mask shortened fibrinogen survival.

References

1. Dachary-Prigent J, Toti F, Satta N, Pasquet JM, Uzan A, Freyssinet JM. 1996. Physiopathological significance of catalytic phospholipids in the generation of thrombin. Semin Thromb Hemost 22:157–164.

2. Solum NO. 1999. Procoagulant expression in platelets and defects leading to clinical disorders. Arterioscler Thromb Vasc Biol 19:2841–2846.

3. Osdoit S, Rosa JP. 2001. Fibrin clot retraction by human platelets correlates with alpha(IIb)beta(3) integrin–dependent protein tyrosine dephosphorylation. J Biol Chem 276:6703–6710.

4. Elliott MA, Tefferi A. 2005. Thrombosis and haemorrhage in polycythaemia vera and essential thrombocythaemia. Br J Haematol 128:275–290.

5. Kopp KJ, Moore JN, Byars TD, Brooks P. 1985. Template bleeding time and thromboxane generation in the horse: Effects of three non-steroidal anti-inflammatory drugs. Equine Vet J 17:322–324.

6. Forsythe LT, Willis SE. 1989. Evaluating oral mucosal bleeding time in healthy dogs using a spring-loaded device. Can Vet J 30:344–345.

7. Sato I, Anderson GA, Parry BW. 2000. An interobserver and intraobserver study of buccal mucosal bleeding time in greyhounds. Res Vet Sci 68:41–45.

8. Catalfamo JL, Dodds WJ. 2000. Thrombopathies. In: Feldman BF, Zinkl JG, Jain NC, eds. *Schalm's Veterinary Hematology*, 5th edition, 1042–1050. Philadelphia: Lippincott Williams & Wilkins.

9. Blajchman MA, Bordin JO, Bardossy L, Heddle NM. 1994. The contribution of the haematocrit to thrombocytopenic bleeding in experimental animals. Br J Haematol 86:347–350.

10. Valeri CR, Cassidy G, Pivacek LE, Ragno G, Lieberthal W, Crowley JP, Khuri SF, Loscalzo J. 2001. Anemia-induced increase in the bleeding time: Implications for treatment of nonsurgical blood loss. Transfusion 41:977–983.

11. Jergens AE, Turrentine MA, Kraus KH, Johnson GS. 1987. Buccal mucosa bleeding times of healthy dogs and of dogs in various pathologic states, including thrombocytopenia, uremia, and von Willebrand's disease. Am J Vet Res 48:1337–1342.

12. Lind SE. 1991. The bleeding time does not predict surgical bleeding. Blood 77:2547–2552.

13. Forsyth SF, Guilford WG, Lawoko CR. 1996. Endoscopic evaluation of the gastroduodenal mucosa following non-steroidal anti-inflammatory drug administration in the dog. NZ Vet J 44:179–181.

14. Gugler E, Lüscher EF. 1965. Platelet function in congenital afibrinogenemia. Thromb Diath Haemorrh 14:361–373.

15. Rodgers GM, Greenberg CS. 1999. Inherited coagulation disorders. In: Lee GR, Foerster J, Lukens J, Wintrobe MM, eds. *Wintrobe's Clinical Hematology*, 10th edition, 1682–1732. Philadelphia: Lippincott Williams & Wilkins.

16. Wilkerson MJ, Johnson GS, Stockham S, Riley L. 2005. Afibrinogenemia and a circulating antibody against fibrinogen in a bichon frise dog. Vet Clin Pathol 34:148–155.

17. Brooks M, Catalfamo J. 1993. Buccal mucosa bleeding time is prolonged in canine models of primary hemostatic disorders. Thromb Haemost 70:777–780.

18. Boudreaux MK, Catalfamo JL. 2001. Molecular and genetic basis for thrombasthenic thrombopathia in otterhounds. Am J Vet Res 62:1797–1804.

19. Boudreaux MK, Dillon AR, Spano JS. 1989. Enhanced platelet reactivity in heartworm-infected dogs. Am J Vet Res 50:1544–1547.

20. Green RA, Russo EA, Greene RT, Kabel AL. 1985. Hypoalbuminemia-related platelet hypersensitivity in two dogs with nephrotic syndrome. J Am Vet Med Assoc 186:485–488.

21. Boudreaux MK, Weiss RC, Toivio-Kinnucan M, Cox N, Spano JS. 1990. Enhanced platelet reactivity in cats experimentally infected with feline infectious peritonitis virus. Vet Pathol 27:269–273.

22. Thomas JS, Rogers KS. 1999. Platelet aggregation and adenosine triphosphate secretion in dogs with untreated multicentric lymphoma. J Vet Intern Med 13:319–322.

23. Thomas JS. 1996. von Willebrand's disease in the dog and cat. Vet Clin North Am Small Anim Pract 26:1089–1110.

24. Meinkoth JH, Meyers KM. 1995. Measurement of von Willebrand factor–specific mRNA and release and storage of von Willebrand factor from endothelial cells of dogs with type-I von Willebrand's disease. Am J Vet Res 56:1577–1585.

25. Smith JM, Meinkoth JH, Hochstatter T, Meyers KM. 1996. Differential distribution of von Willebrand factor in canine vascular endothelium. Am J Vet Res 57:750–755.

26. McCarroll DR, Waters DC, Steidley KR, Clift R, McDonald TP. 1988. Canine platelet von Willebrand factor: Quantification and multimeric analysis. Exp Hematol 16:929–937.

27. Parker MT, Turrentine MA, Johnson GS. 1991. Von Willebrand factor in lysates of washed canine platelets. Am J Vet Res 52:119–125.

28. Benson RE, Johnson GS, Dodds WJ. 1981. Binding of low-molecular-weight canine factor VIII coagulant from von Willebrand plasma to canine factor VIII–related antigen. Br J Haematol 49:541–550.

29. Sullivan PS, Grubbs ST, Olchowy TWJ, Andrews FM, White JG, Catalfamo JL, Dodd PA, McDonald TP. 1994. Bleeding diathesis associated with variant von Willebrand factor in a Simmental calf. J Am Vet Med Assoc 205:1763–1766.

30. French TW, Fox LE, Randolph JF, Dodds WJ. 1987. A bleeding disorder (von Willebrand's disease) in a Himalayan cat. J Am Vet Med Assoc 190:437–439.

31. Brooks M, Leith GS, Allen AK, Woods PR, Benson RE, Dodds WJ. 1991. Bleeding disorder (von Willebrand disease) in a quarter horse. J Am Vet Med Assoc 198:114–116.

32. Laan TT, Goehring LS, van Oldruitenborgh-Oosterbaan MM. 2005. Von Willebrand's disease in an eight-day-old quarter horse foal. Vet Rec 157:322–324.

33. Rathgeber RA, Brooks MB, Bain FT, Byars TD. 2001. Clinical vignette: Von Willebrand disease in a thoroughbred mare and foal. J Vet Intern Med 15:63–66.

34. Hennessy BJ, White B, Byrne M, Smith OP. 1998. Acquired von Willebrand's disease. Ir J Med Sci 167:81–85.

35. Rinder MR, Richard RE, Rinder HM. 1997. Acquired von Willebrand's disease: A concise review. Am J Hematol 54:139–145.

36. Michiels JJ, Schroyens W, Berneman Z, van der Planken M. 2001. Acquired von Willebrand syndrome type 1 in hypothyroidism: Reversal after treatment with thyroxine. Clin Appl Thromb Hemost 7:113–115.

37. Avgeris S, Lothrop CD Jr, McDonald TP. 1990. Plasma von Willebrand factor concentration and thyroid function in dogs. J Am Vet Med Assoc 196:921–924.

38. Panciera DL, Johnson GS. 1994. Plasma von Willebrand factor antigen concentration in dogs with hypothyroidism. J Am Vet Med Assoc 205:1550–1553.

39. Sadler JE, for the Subcommittee on von Willebrand Factor of the Scientific and Standardization Committee of the International Society on Thrombosis and Haemostasis. 1994. A revised classification of von Willebrand disease. Thromb Haemost 71:520–525.

40. Brooks MB, Erb HN, Foureman PA, Ray K. 2001. Von Willebrand disease phenotype and von Willebrand factor marker genotype in Doberman pinschers. Am J Vet Res 62:364–369.

41. Brooks M, Raymond S, Catalfamo J. 1996. Severe, recessive von Willebrand's disease in German wirehaired pointers. J Am Vet Med Assoc 209:926–929.

42. Slappendel RJ, Beijer EGM, van Leeuwen M. 1998. Type III von Willebrands [sic] disease in Dutch kooiker dogs. Vet Q 20:93–97.

43. Johnson GS, Lees GE, Benson RE, Rosborough TK, Dodds WJ. 1980. A bleeding disease (von Willebrand's disease) in a Chesapeake Bay retriever. J Am Vet Med Assoc 176:1261–1263.

44. Raymond SL, Jones DW, Brooks MB, Dodd WJ. 1990. Clinical and laboratory features of a severe form of von Willebrand disease in Shetland sheepdogs. J Am Vet Med Assoc 197:1342–1346.

45. Venta PJ, Li J, Yuzbasiyan-Gurkan V, Brewer GJ, Schall WD. 2000. Mutation causing von Willebrand's disease in Scottish terriers. J Vet Intern Med 14:10–19.

46. Stokol T, Parry BW, Mansell PD. 1995. Factor VIII activity in canine von Willebrand disease. Vet Clin Pathol 24:81–90.

47. Moser J, Meyers KM, Meinkoth JH, Brassard JA. 1996. Temporal variation and factors affecting measurement of canine von Willebrand factor. Am J Vet Res 57:1288–1293.

48. Mansell PD, Parry BW. 1991. Stability of canine factor VIII activity and von Willebrand factor antigen concentration in vitro. Res Vet Sci 51:313–316.

49. Johnson GS, Turrentine MA, Kraus KH. 1988. Canine von Willebrand's disease: A heterogeneous group of bleeding disorders. Vet Clin North Am Small Anim Pract 18:195–229.

50. Johnstone IB. 1999. Plasma von Willebrand factor–collagen binding activity in normal dogs and in dogs with von Willebrand's disease. J Vet Diagn Invest 11:308–313.

51. Johnstone IB. 1997. Multimeric analysis of von Willebrand factor in animal plasmas using sodium dodecyl sulfate agarose gel electrophoresis, semidry electrotransfer, and immunoperoxidase detection. J Vet Diagn Invest 9:314–317.

52. Callan MB, Giger U, Catalfamo JL. 2005. Effect of desmopressin on von Willebrand factor multimers in Doberman Pinschers with type 1 von Willebrand disease. Am J Vet Res 66:861–867.

53. Brooks M. 1992. Management of canine von Willebrand's disease. Probl Vet Med 4:636–646.

54. Meyers KM, Wardrop KJ, Dodds WJ, Brassard J. 1990. Effect of exercise, DDAVP, and epinephrine on the factor VIII:C/von Willebrand factor complex in normal dogs and von Willebrand factor deficient Doberman pinscher dogs. Thromb Res 57:97–108.

55. Turrentine MA, Hahn AW, Johnson GS. 1986. Factor VIII complex in canine plasma after submaximal treadmill exercise. Am J Vet Res 47:39–42.

56. Smith JM, Meyers KM, Barbee DD, Schott H, Bayly WM. 1997. Plasma von Willebrand factor in thoroughbreds in response to high-intensity treadmill exercise. Am J Vet Res 58:71–76.

57. Moser J, Meyers KM, Russon RH, Reeves JJ. 1998. Plasma von Willebrand factor changes during various reproductive cycle stages in mixed-breed dogs with normal von Willebrand factor and in Doberman pinschers with type I von Willebrand's disease. Am J Vet Res 59:111–118.

58. Johnstone IB. 1999. Desmopressin enhances the binding of plasma von Willebrand factor to collagen in plasmas from normal dogs and dogs with type I von Willebrand's disease. Can Vet J 40:645–648.

59. Sato I, Parry BW. 1998. Effect of desmopressin on plasma factor VIII and von Willebrand factor concentrations in greyhounds. Aust Vet J 76:809–812.

60. Novotny MJ, Turrentine MA, Johnson GS, Adams HR. 1987. Experimental endotoxemia increases plasma von Willebrand factor antigen concentrations in dogs with and without free-radical scavenger therapy. Circ Shock 23:205–213.

61. Brassard JA, Meyers KM. 1994. Von Willebrand factor is not altered in azotemic dogs with prolonged bleeding time. J Lab Clin Med 124:55–62.

62. Badylak SF, Dodds WJ, Van Vleet JF. 1983. Plasma coagulation factor abnormalities in dogs with naturally occurring hepatic disease. Am J Vet Res 44:2336–2340.

63. Brooks M. 2000. Von Willebrand disease. In: Feldman BF, Zinkl JG, Jain NC, eds. *Schalm's Veterinary Hematology*, 5th edition, 509–515. Philadelphia: Lippincott Williams & Wilkins.

64. van Oost BA, Versteeg SA, Slappendel RJ. 2004. DNA testing for type III von Willebrand disease in Dutch Kooiker dogs. J Vet Intern Med 18:282–288.

65. Greenberg CS, Orthner CL. 1999. Blood coagulation and fibrinolysis. In: Lee GR, Foerster J, Lukens J, Wintrobe MM, eds. *Wintrobe's Clinical Hematology*, 10th edition, 684–764. Philadelphia: Lippincott Williams & Wilkins.

66. Gentry PA. 2004. Comparative aspects of blood coagulation. Vet J 168:238–251.

67. Maggio-Price L, Dodds WJ. 1993. Factor IX deficiency (hemophilia B) in a family of British shorthair cats. J Am Vet Med Assoc 203:1702–1704.

68. Feldman DG, Brooks MB, Dodds J. 1995. Hemophilia B (factor IX deficiency) in a family of German shepherd dogs. J Am Vet Med Assoc 206:1901–1905.

69. Dodds WJ, Packham MA, Rowsell HC, Mustard JF. 1967. Factor VII survival and turnover in dogs. Am J Physiol 213:36–42.

70. O'Donnell MR, Slichter SJ, Weiden PL, Storb R. 1981. Platelet and fibrinogen kinetics in canine tumors. Cancer Res 41:1379–1383.

71. Rodgers GM. 1988. Vascular smooth muscle cells synthesize, secrete and express coagulation factor V. Biochim Biophys Acta 968:17–23.

72. Clark P, Parry BW. 1997. Cytogenetic analysis of German shepherd dogs with haemophilia A. Aust Vet J 75:521–522.

73. Stirling D, Hannant WA, Ludlam CA. 1998. Transcriptional activation of the factor VIII gene in liver cell lines by interleukin-6. Thromb Haemost 79:74–78.

74. Topper MJ, Prasse K. 1998. Analysis of coagulation proteins as acute-phase reactants in horses with colic. Am J Vet Res 59:542–545.

75. Wells MJ, Sheffield WP, Blajchman MA. 1999. The clearance of thrombin-antithrombin and related serpin-enzyme complexes from the circulation: Role of various hepatocyte receptors. Thromb Haemost 81:325–337.

76. Griffin JH. 2001. Control of coagulation reactions. In: Beutler E, Lichtman MA, Coller BS, Kipps TJ, Seligsohn U, eds. *Williams Hematology*, 6th edition, 1435–1449. New York: McGraw-Hill.

77. Shen L, He X, Dahlbäck B. 1997. Synergistic cofactor function of factor V and protein S to activated protein C in the inactivation of the factor VIIIa–factor IXa complex: Species specific interactions of components of the protein C anticoagulant system. Thromb Haemost 78:1030–1036.

78. McVey JH. 1999. Tissue factor pathway. Bailliere's Clin Haematol 12:361–372.

79. Gentry PA, Feldman BF, O'Neill SL. 1992. An evaluation of the effect of reagent modification on routine laboratory coagulation tests. Equine Vet J 24:30–32.

80. Mischke R, Nolte I. 1997. Optimization of prothrombin time measurements in canine plasma. Am J Vet Res 58:236–241.

81. Lisciandro GR, Brooks M, Catalfamo JL. 2000. Contact factor deficiency in a German shorthaired pointer without clinical evidence of coagulopathy. J Vet Intern Med 14:308–310.

82. Mischke R. 2001. Optimization of coagulometric tests that incorporate human plasma for determination of coagulation factor activities in canine plasma. Am J Vet Res 62:625–629.

83. Mayo DJ, Dimond EP, Kramer W, Horne MK III. 1996. Discard volumes necessary for clinically useful coagulation studies from heparinized Hickman catheters. Oncol Nurs Forum 23:671–675.

84. Arkin CF, Bowie EJW, Carroll JJ, Day HJ, Joist JH, Lenahan JG, Marlar RA, Triplett DA. 1998. Collection, transport, and processing of blood specimens for coagulation testing and general performance of coagulation assays: Approved guideline. National Committee for Clinical Laboratory Standards, 18:1–24.

85. Millis DL, Hawkins E, Jager M, Boyle CR. 1995. Comparison of coagulation test results for blood samples obtained by means of direct venipuncture and through a jugular vein catheter in clinically normal dogs. J Am Vet Med Assoc 207:1311–1314.

86. Kratz A, Stanganelli N, Van Cott EM. 2006. A comparison of glass and plastic blood collection tubes for routine and specialized coagulation assays: A comprehensive study. Arch Pathol Lab Med 130:39–44.

87. Adcock DM, Kressin DC, Marlar RA. 1997. Effect of 3.2% vs 3.8% sodium citrate concentration on routine coagulation testing. Am J Clin Pathol 107:105–110.

88. von Pape KW, Aland E, Bohner J. 2000. Platelet function analysis with PFA-100 in patients medicated with acetylsalicylic acid strongly depends on concentration of sodium citrate used for anticoagulation of blood sample. Thromb Res 98:295–299.

89. Stokol T, Brooks MB, Erb HN. 2000. Effect of citrate concentration on coagulation test results in dogs. J Am Vet Med Assoc 217:1672–1677.

90. Adcock DM, Kressin DC, Marlar RA. 1998. Minimum specimen volume requirements for routine coagulation testing: Dependence on citrate concentration. Am J Clin Pathol 109:595–599.

91. O'Brien SR, Sellers TS, Meyer DJ. 1995. Artifactual prolongation of the activated partial thromboplastin time associated with hemoconcentration in dogs. J Vet Intern Med 9:169–170.

92. Siegel JE, Swami VK, Glenn P, Peterson P. 1998. Effect (or lack of it) of severe anemia on PT and APTT results. Am J Clin Pathol 110:106–110.

93. Marlar RA, Potts RM, Marlar AA. 2006. Effect on routine and special coagulation testing values of citrate anticoagulant adjustment in patients with high hematocrit values. Am J Clin Pathol 126:400–405.

94. Furlanello T, Caldin M, Stocco A, Tudone E, Tranquillo V, Lubas G, Solano-Gallego L. 2006. Stability of stored canine plasma for hemostasis testing. Vet Clin Pathol 35:204–207.

95. Adcock D, Kressin D, Marlar RA. 1998. The effect of time and temperature variables on routine coagulation tests. Blood Coagul Fibrinolysis 9:463–470.

96. Rao LV, Okorodudu AO, Petersen JR, Elghetany MT. 2000. Stability of prothrombin time and activated partial thromboplastin time tests under different storage conditions. Clin Chim Acta 300:13–21.

97. Heil W, Grunewald R, Amend M, Heins M. 1998. Influence of time and temperature on coagulation analytes in stored plasma. Clin Chem Lab Med 36:459–462.

98. Carroll WE, Wollitzer AO, Harris L, Ling MCC, Whitaker WL, Jackson RD. 2001. The significance of platelet counts in coagulation studies. J Med 32:83–96.

99. Triplett DA. 1997. Lupus anticoagulants: Diagnostic dilemma and clinical challenge. Clin Lab Sci 10:223–228.

100. Woodhams B, Girardot O, Blanco MJ, Colesse G, Gourmelin Y. 2001. Stability of coagulation proteins in frozen plasma. Blood Coagul Fibrinolysis 12:229–236.

101. Bateman SW, Mathews KA, Abrams-Ogg ACG, Lumsden JH, Johnstone IB. 1999. Evaluation of the effect of storage at −70 degrees C for six months on hemostatic function testing in dogs. Can J Vet Res 63:216–220.

102. Schalm OW, Jain NC, Carroll EJ. 1975. Blood coagulation and fibrinolysis. In: Schalm OW, Jain NC, Carroll EJ, eds. Veterinary Hematology, 3rd edition, 284–300. Philadelphia: Lea & Febiger.

103. Johnstone IB. 1988. Clinical and laboratory diagnosis of bleeding disorders. Vet Clin North Am Small Anim Pract 18:21–33.

104. Sirridge MS. 1964. Pitfalls in the performance and interpretation of laboratory studies for hemorrhagic disorders. Am J Med Technol 30:399–410.

105. Byars TD, Ling GV, Ferris NA, Keeton KS. 1976. Activated coagulation time (ACT) of whole blood in normal dogs. Am J Vet Res 37:1359–1361.

106. Rodgers GM, Bithell TC. 1999. The diagnostic approach to the bleeding disorders. In: Lee GR, Foerster J, Lukens J, Wintrobe MM, eds. Wintrobe's Clinical Hematology, 10th edition, 1557–1578. Philadelphia: Lippincott Williams & Wilkins.

107. Ammar T, Fisher CF, Sarier K, Coller BS. 1996. The effects of thrombocytopenia on the activated coagulation time. Anesth Analg 83:1185–1188.

108. Arkin CF, Bowie EJW, Carroll JJ, Day HJ, Joist JH, Lenahan JG, Marlar RA, Triplett DA. 1996. One-stage prothrombin time (PT) test and activated partial thromboplastin time (APTT) test: Approved guideline. National Committee for Clinical Laboratory Standards, 16:1–17.

109. Proctor RR, Rapaport SI. 1961. The partial thromboplastin time with kaolin. Am J Clin Pathol 36:212–219.

110. Barton MH, Morris DD, Crowe N, Collatos C, Prasse KW. 1995. Hemostatic indices in healthy foals from birth to one month of age. J Vet Diagn Invest 7:380–385.

111. Barton MH, Morris DD, Norton N, Prasse KW. 1998. Hemostatic and fibrinolytic indices in neonatal foals with presumed septicemia. J Vet Intern Med 12:26–35.

112. Mischke R, Diedrich M, Nolte I. 2003. Sensitivity of different prothrombin time assays to factor VII deficiency in canine plasma. Vet J 166:79–85.

113. Reed RL II, Bracey AW Jr, Hudson JD, Miller TA, Fischer RP. 1990. Hypothermia and blood coagulation: Dissociation between enzyme activity and clotting factor levels. Circ Shock 32:141–152.

114. Felfernig M, Blaicher A, Kettner SC, Felfernig D, Acimovic S, Kozek-Langenecker SA. 2001. Effects of temperature on partial thromboplastin time in heparinized plasma in vitro. Eur J Anaesthesiol 18:467–470.

115. Geor RJ, Jackson ML, Lewis KD, Fretz PB. 1990. Prekallikrein deficiency in a family of Belgian horses. J Am Vet Med Assoc 197:741–745.

116. Lisciandro SC, Hohenhaus A, Brooks M. 1998. Coagulation abnormalities in 22 cats with naturally occurring liver disease. J Vet Intern Med 12:71–75.

117. Kurata M, Sasayama Y, Yamasaki N, Kitazawa I, Hamada Y, Horii I. 2003. Mechanism for shortening PT and APTT in dogs and rats: Effect of fibrinogen on PT and APTT. J Toxicol Sci 28:439–443.

118. Mischke R. 2003. Heparin in vitro sensitivity of the activated partial thromboplastin time in canine plasma depends on reagent. J Vet Diagn Invest 15:588–591.

119. Brooks MB. 2004. Evaluation of a chromogenic assay to measure the factor Xa inhibitory activity of unfractionated heparin in canine plasma. Vet Clin Pathol 33:208–214.

120. Mischke R, Jacobs C. 2001. The monitoring of heparin administration by screening tests in experimental dogs. Res Vet Sci 70:101–108.

121. Mischke R, Grebe S, Jacobs C, Kietzmann M. 2001. Amidolytic heparin activity and values for several hemostatic variables after repeated subcutaneous administration of high doses of a low molecular weight heparin in healthy dogs. Am J Vet Res 62:595–598.

122. Hall DE. 1970. Sensitivity of different thromboplastin reagents to factor VII deficiency in the blood of beagle dogs. Lab Anim 4:55–59.

123. Mischke R, Junker J, Deegen E. 2006. Sensitivity of commercial prothrombin time reagents to detect coagulation factor deficiencies in equine plasma. Vet J 171:114–119.

124. Leech BF, Carter CJ. 1998. Falsely elevated INR results due to the sensitivity of a thromboplastin reagent to heparin. Am J Clin Pathol 109:764–768.

125. Riley RS, Rowe D, Fisher LM. 2000. Clinical utilization of the international normalized ratio (INR). J Clin Lab Anal 14:101–114.

126. Adcock DM, Duff S. 2000. Enhanced standardization of the International Normalized Ratio through the use of plasma calibrants: A concise review. Blood Coagul Fibrinolysis 11:583–590.

127. Bateman SW, Mathews KA, Abrams-Ogg ACG, Lumsden JH, Johnstone IB, Hillers TK, Foster RA. 1999. Diagnosis of disseminated intravascular coagulation in dogs admitted to an intensive care unit. J Am Vet Med Assoc 215:798–804.

128. Santaro SA, Eby CS. 1995. Laboratory evaluation of hemostatic disorders. In: Hoffman R, Benz EJ Jr, Shattil SJ, Furie B, Cohen HJ, Silberstein LE, eds. *Hematology: Basic Principles and Practice*, 2nd edition, 1622–1632. New York: Churchill Livingstone.

129. Fecteau G, Zinkl JG, Smith BP, O'Neil S, Smith S, Klopfer S. 1997. Dysfibrinogenemia or afibrinogenemia in a Border Leicester lamb. Can Vet J 38:443–444.

130. Dodds WJ. 2000. Other hereditary coagulopathies. In: Feldman BF, Zinkl JG, Jain NC, eds. *Schalm's Veterinary Hematology*, 5th edition, 1030–1036. Philadelphia: Lippincott Williams & Wilkins.

131. Grosset ABM, Rodgers GM. 1999. Acquired coagulation disorders. In: Lee GR, Foerster J, Lukens J, Wintrobe MM, eds. *Wintrobe's Clinical Hematology*, 10th edition, 1733–1780. Philadelphia: Lippincott Williams & Wilkins.

132. Martinez J. 1995. Quantitative and qualitative disorders of fibrinogen. In: Hoffman R, Benz EJ Jr, Shattil SJ, Furie B, Cohen HJ, Silberstein LE, eds. *Hematology: Basic Principles and Practice*, 2nd edition, 1703–1717. New York: Churchill Livingstone.

133. Williams JE, Hantgan RR, Hermans J, McDonagh J. 1981. Characterization of the inhibition of fibrin assembly by fibrinogen fragment D. Biochem J 197:661–668.

134. O'Kane MJ, Wisdom GB, Desai ZR, Archbold GPR. 1994. Inhibition of fibrin monomer polymerisation by myeloma immunoglobulin. J Clin Pathol 47:266–268.

135. Gastineau DA, Gertz MA, Daniels TM, Kyle RA, Bowie EJW. 1991. Inhibitor of the thrombin time in systemic amyloidosis: A common coagulation abnormality. Blood 77:2637–2640.

136. Carr ME Jr, Gabriel DA. 1986. Hyperfibrinogenemia as a cause of prolonged thrombin clotting time. South Med J 79:563–570.

137. Fricke WA, McDonagh J. 1983. Thrombin clotting time and fibrinogen concentration in patients treated with coumadin. Thromb Res 31:23–28.

138. Day HJ, Arkin CF, Bovill EG, Bowie EJW, Carroll JJ, Joist JH, Lenahan JG, Marlar RA, Triplett DA. 1994. Procedure for the determination of fibrinogen in plasma: Approved guideline. National Committee for Clinical Laboratory Standards, 14:1–13.

139. Concannon PW, Gimpel T, Newton L, Castracane VD. 1996. Postimplantation increase in plasma fibrinogen concentration with increase in relaxin concentration in pregnant dogs. Am J Vet Res 57:1382–1385.

140. Mansell P. 2000. Hemophilia A and B. In: Feldman BF, Zinkl JG, Jain NC, eds. *Schalm's Veterinary Hematology*, 5th edition, 1026–1029. Philadelphia: Lippincott Williams & Wilkins.

141. Gentry PA. 2000. Factor XI deficiency. In: Feldman BF, Zinkl JG, Jain NC, eds. *Schalm's Veterinary Hematology*, 5th edition, 1037–1041. Philadelphia: Lippincott Williams & Wilkins.

142. Arkin CF, Bowie EJW, Carroll JJ, Day HJ, Joist JH, Lenahan JG, Marlar RA, Triplett DA. 1997. Determination of factor coagulant activities: Approved guideline. National Committee for Clinical Laboratory Standards, 17:1–21.

143. Topper MJ, Prasse KW. 1998. Chromogenic assays for equine coagulation factors VII, VIII:C, IX, and X, and C1-esterase inhibitor. Am J Vet Res 59:538–541.

144. Gentry PA, Christopher MM. 2001. Determination of prothrombin in feline plasma. Vet Clin Pathol 30:53–56.

145. Widdershoven J, Kolleæ L, van Munster P, Bosman AM, Monnens L. 1986. Biochemical vitamin K deficiency in early infancy: Diagnostic limitation of conventional coagulation tests. Helv Paediatr Acta 41:195–201.

146. Soute BAM, de Boer-vd Berg MA, Vermeer C. 1984. The separation of bovine prothrombin and descarboxyprothrombin by high-performance liquid chromatography. Anal Biochem 137:227–229.

147. Huisse MG, Leclercq M, Belghiti J, Flejou JF, Suttie JW, Bezeaud A, Stafford DW, Guillin MC. 1994. Mechanism of the abnormal vitamin K–dependent gamma-carboxylation process in human hepatocellular carcinomas. Cancer 74:1533–1541.

148. Center SA, Warner K, Corbett J, Randolph JF, Erb HN. 2000. Proteins invoked by vitamin K absence and clotting times in clinically ill cats. J Vet Intern Med 14:292–297.

149. Hemker HC, Veltkamp JJ, Hensen A, Loeliger EA. 1963. Nature of prothrombin biosynthesis: Preprothrombinemia in vitamin K-deficiency. Nature 200:589–590.

150. Arnesen H, Smith P. 1991. The predictability of bleeding by prothrombin times sensitive or insensitive to PIVKA during intensive oral anticoagulation. Thromb Res 61:311–314.

151. Mount ME, Kim BU, Kass PH. 2003. Use of a test for proteins induced by vitamin K absence or antagonism in diagnosis of anticoagulant poisoning in dogs: 325 cases (1987–1997). J Am Vet Med Assoc 222:194–198.

152. Giger U. 2003. Differing opinions on value of PIVKA test. J Am Vet Med Assoc 222:1070–1071.

153. Mount ME. 1986. Proteins induced by vitamin K absence or antagonists ("PIVKA"). In: Kirk RW, ed. *Current Veterinary Therapy IX: Small Animal Practice*, 513–515. Philadelphia: WB Saunders.

154. Rozanski EA, Drobatz KJ, Hughes D, Scotti M, Giger U. 2001. Thrombotest (PIVKA) test results in 25 dogs with acquired and hereditary coagulopathies. J Emerg Crit Care 9:73–78.

155. Pusterla N, Braun U, Forrer R, Lutz H. 1997. Antithrombin-III activity in plasma of healthy and sick cattle. Vet Rec 140:17–18.

156. Mischke R, Nolte IJA. 2000. Hemostasis: Introduction, overview, laboratory techniques. In: Feldman BF, Zinkl JG, Jain NC, eds. *Schalm's Veterinary Hematology*, 5th edition, 519–525. Philadelphia: Lippincott Williams & Wilkins.

157. Green RA. 1988. Pathophysiology of antithrombin III deficiency. Vet Clin North Am Small Anim Pract 18:95–104.

158. Johnstone IB, Physick-Sheard P, Crane S. 1989. Breed, age, and gender differences in plasma antithrombin III activity in clinically normal young horses. Am J Vet Res 50:1751–1753.

159. Demers C, Henderson P, Blajchman MA, Wells MJ, Mitchell L, Johnston M, Ofosu FA, Fernandez-Rachubinski F, Andrew M, Hirsh J, Ginsberg JS. 1993. An antithrombin III assay based on factor Xa inhibition provides a more reliable test to identify congenital antithrombin III deficiency than an assay based on thrombin inhibition. Thromb Haemost 69:231–235.

160. Vinazzer H. 1999. Hereditary and acquired antithrombin deficiency. Semin Thromb Hemost 25:257–263.

161. Rodgers GM. 1999. Thrombosis and antithrombotic therapy. In: Lee GR, Foerster J, Lukens J, Wintrobe MM, eds. *Wintrobe's Clinical Hematology*, 10th edition, 1781–1818. Philadelphia: Lippincott Williams & Wilkins.

162. Thomas JS, Green RA. 1998. Clotting times and antithrombin III activity in cats with naturally developing diseases: 85 cases (1984–1994). J Am Vet Med Assoc 213:1290–1295.

163. Niessen RWLM, Lamping RJ, Jansen PM, Prins MH, Peters M, Taylor FB Jr, de Vijlder JJ, ten Cate JW, Hack CE, Sturk A. 1997. Antithrombin acts as a negative acute phase protein as established with studies on HepG2 cells and in baboons. Thromb Haemost 78:1088–1092.

164. Plesca LA, Bodizs G, Cucuianu M, Colhon D. 1995. Hemostatic balance during the acute inflammatory reaction; with special reference to antithrombin III. Rom J Physiol 32:71–76.

165. Welles EG, Boudreaux MK, Tyler JW. 1993. Platelet, antithrombin, and fibrinolytic activities in taurine-deficient and taurine-replete cats. Am J Vet Res 54:1235–1243.

166. Welles EG, Boudreaux MK, Crager CS, Tyler JW. 1994. Platelet function and antithrombin, plasminogen, and fibrinolytic activities in cats with heart disease. Am J Vet Res 55:619–627.

167. Kobayashi N, Takeda Y. 1977. Studies of the effects of estradiol, progesterone, cortisol, thrombophlebitis, and typhoid vaccine on synthesis and catabolism of antithrombin III in the dog. Thromb Haemost 37:111–122.

168. Clare AC, Kraje BJ. 1998. Use of recombinant tissue-plasminogen activator for aortic thrombolysis in a hypoproteinemic dog. J Am Vet Med Assoc 212:539–543.

169. Joist JH, Remuzzi G, Mannucci PM. 1994. Abnormal bleeding and thrombosis in renal disease. In: Colman RW, Hirsch J, Marder VJ, Salzman EW, eds. *Hemostasis and Thrombosis: Basic Principles and Clinical Practice*, 3rd edition, 921–935. Philadelphia: JB Lippincott.

170. Welch RD, Watkins JP, Taylor TS, Cohen ND, Carter GK. 1992. Disseminated intravascular coagulation associated with colic in 23 horses (1984–1989). J Vet Intern Med 6:29–35.

171. de Laforcade AM, Freeman LM, Shaw SP, Brooks MB, Rozanski EA, Rush JE. 2003. Hemostatic changes in dogs with naturally occurring sepsis. J Vet Intern Med 17:674–679.

172. Hellebrekers LJ, Slappendel RJ, van den Brom WE. 1985. Effect of sodium heparin and antithrombin III concentration on activated partial thromboplastin time in the dog. Am J Vet Res 46:1460–1462.

173. Marciniak E, Gockerman JP. 1977. Heparin-induced decrease in circulating antithrombin-III. Lancet 2:581–584.

174. Levy JH, Montes F, Szlam F, Hillyer CD. 2000. The in vitro effects of antithrombin III on the activated coagulation time in patients on heparin therapy. Anesth Analg 90:1076–1079.

175. Jacoby RC, Owings JT, Ortega T, Gosselin R, Feldman EC. 2001. Biochemical basis for the hypercoagulable state seen in Cushing syndrome. Arch Surg 136:1003–1006.

176. Chapital AD, Hendrick SR, Lloyd L, Pieper D. 2001. The effects of triiodothyronine augmentation on antithrombin III levels in sepsis. Am Surg 67:253–255.

177. Niessen RW, Pfaffendorf BA, Sturk A, Lamping RJ, Schaap MC, Hack CE, Peters M. 1995. The influence of insulin, beta-estradiol, dexamethasone and thyroid hormone on the secretion of coagulant and anticoagulant proteins by HepG2 cells. Thromb Haemost 74:686–692.

178. Rennie JA, Bewsher PD, Murchison LE, Ogston D. 1978. Coagulation and fibrinolysis in thyroid disease. Acta Haematol 59:171–177.

179. Erem C, Ersoz HO, Karti SS, Ukinc K, Hacihasanoglu A, Deger O, Telatar M. 2002. Blood coagulation and fibrinolysis in patients with hyperthyroidism. J Endocrinol Invest 25:345–350.

180. Hoek JA, Sturk A, ten Cate JW, Lamping RJ, Berends F, Borm JJJ. 1988. Laboratory and clinical evaluation of an assay of thrombin–antithrombin III complexes in plasma. Clin Chem 34:2058–2062.

181. Pelzer H, Schwarz A, Heimburger N. 1988. Determination of human thrombin–antithrombin III complex in plasma with an enzyme-linked immunosorbent assay. Thromb Haemost 59:101–106.

182. Hoek JA, Nurmohamed MT, ten Cate JW, Büller HR, Knipscheer HC, Hamelynck KJ, Marti RK, Sturk A. 1989. Thrombin–antithrombin III complexes in the prediction of deep vein thrombosis following total hip replacement. Thromb Haemost 62:1050–1052.

183. Topper MJ, Prasse KW, Morris MJ, Duncan A, Crowe NA. 1996. Enzyme-linked immunosorbent assay for thrombin–antithrombin III complexes in horses. Am J Vet Res 57:427–431.

184. Topper MJ, Prasse KW. 1996. Use of enzyme-linked immunosorbent assay to measure thrombin–antithrombin III complexes in horses with colic. Am J Vet Res 57:456–462.

185. Maruyama H, Watari T, Miura T, Sakai M, Takahashi T, Koie H, Yamaya Y, Asano K, Edamura K, Sato T, Tanaka S, Hasegawa A, Tokuriki M. 2005. Plasma thrombin-antithrombin complex concentrations in dogs with malignant tumours. Vet Rec 156:839–840.

186. Bartels PC, Schoorl M, van Bodegraven AA. 2001. Reduction of preanalytical errors due to in vitro activation of coagulation. Clin Lab 47:449–452.

187. Welles EG, Prasse KW, Duncan A, Morris MJ. 1990. Antigenic assay for protein C determination in horses. Am J Vet Res 51:1075–1079.

188. Welles EG, Prasse KW, Moore JN. 1991. Use of newly developed assays for protein C and plasminogen in horses with signs of colic. Am J Vet Res 52:345–351.

189. Johnstone IB, Martin CA. 2000. Comparative effects of the human protein C activator, Protac, on the activated partial thromboplastin clotting times of plasmas, with special reference to the dog. Can J Vet Res 64:117–122.

190. Johnstone IB. 2000. Coagulation inhibitors. In: Feldman BF, Zinkl JG, Jain NC, eds. *Schalm's Veterinary Hematology*, 5th edition, 538–543. Philadelphia: Lippincott Williams & Wilkins.

191. Edens LM, Morris DD, Prasse KW, Anver MR. 1993. Hypercoagulable state associated with a deficiency of protein C in a thoroughbred colt. J Vet Intern Med 7:190–193.

192. Madden RM, Ward M, Marlar RA. 1989. Protein C activity levels in endotoxin-induced disseminated intravascular coagulation in a dog model. Thromb Res 55:297–307.

193. Esmon NL, Safa O, Smirnov MD, Esmon CT. 2000. Antiphospholipid antibodies and the protein C pathway. J Autoimmun 15:221–225.

194. Prowse CV, Esnouf MP. 1977. The isolation of a new warfarin-sensitive protein from bovine plasma. Biochem Soc Trans 5:255–256.

195. Van de Water N, Tan T, Ashton F, O'Grady A, Day T, Browett P, Ockelford P, Harper P. 2004. Mutations within the protein Z–dependent protease inhibitor gene are associated with venous thromboembolic disease: A new form of thrombophilia. Br J Haematol 127:190–194.

196. Stone MS, Johnstone IB, Brooks M, Bollinger TK, Cotter SM. 1994. Lupus-type "anticoagulant" in a dog with hemolysis and thrombosis. J Vet Intern Med 8:57–61.

197. Clyne LP. 1986. Species specificity of lupus-like anticoagulants. Blut 53:287–292.

198. Iio A, Rutherford WE, Wochner RD, Spilberg I, Sherman LA. 1976. The roles of renal catabolism and uremia in modifying the clearance of fibrinogen and its degradative fragments D and E. J Lab Clin Med 87:934–946.

199. Pasqua JJ, Pizzo SV. 1983. The clearance of human fibrinogen fragments X and Y in mice: A process mediated by the fragment D receptor. Thromb Haemost 49:78–80.

200. Pizzo SV, Pasqua JJ. 1982. The clearance of human fibrinogen fragments D_1, D_2, D_3 and fibrin fragment D_1 dimer in mice. Biochim Biophys Acta 718:177–184.

201. Ardaillou N, Yvart J, Le Bras P, Larrieu MJ. 1980. Catabolism of human fibrinogen fragment D in normal subjects and patients with liver cirrhosis. Thromb Haemost 44:146–149.

202. Rajagopalan S, Pizzo SV. 1986. Characterization of murine peritoneal macrophage receptors for fibrin(ogen) degradation products. Blood 67:1224–1228.

203. Ahlgren T, Berghem L, Lagergren H, Lahnborg G, Schildt B. 1976. Phagocytic and catabolic function of the reticuloendothelial system in dogs subjected to defibrinogenation. Thromb Res 8:819–828.

204. Stokol T, Brooks M, Erb H, Mauldin GE. 1999. Evaluation of kits for the detection of fibrin(ogen) degradation products in dogs. J Vet Intern Med 13:478–484.

205. Slappendel RJ, van Arkel C, Mieog WH, Bouma BN. 1972. Response to heparin of spontaneous disseminated intravascular coagulation in the dog. Zentralbl Veterinarmed [A] 19:502–513.

206. Stokol T, Erb HN, De Wilde L, Tornquist SJ, Brooks M. 2005. Evaluation of latex agglutination kits for detection of fibrin(ogen) degradation products and D-dimer in healthy horses and horses with severe colic. Vet Clin Pathol 34:375–382.

207. Gaffney PJ, Perry MJ. 1985. Unreliability of current serum fibrin degradation product (FDP) assays. Thromb Haemost 53:301–302.

208. Connaghan DG, Francis CW, Ryan DH, Marder VJ. 1986. Prevalence and clinical implications of heparin-associated false positive tests for serum fibrin(ogen) degradation products. Am J Clin Pathol 86:304–310.

209. Hager K, Platt D. 1995. Fibrin degeneration product concentrations (D-dimers) in the course of ageing. Gerontology 41:159–165.

210. Raimondi P, Bongard O, de Moerloose P, Reber G, Waldvogel F, Bounameaux H. 1993. D-dimer plasma concentration in various clinical conditions: Implication for the use of this test in the diagnostic approach of venous thromboembolism. Thromb Res 69:125–130.

211. Shorr AF, Thomas SJ, Alkins SA, Fitzpatrick TM, Ling GS. 2002. D-dimer correlates with proinflammatory cytokine levels and outcomes in critically ill patients. Chest 121:1262–1268.

212. Broadie TA, Glover JL, Bang N, Bendick PJ, Lowe DK, Yaw PB, Kafoure D. 1981. Clotting competence of intracavitary blood in trauma victims. Ann Emerg Med 10:127–130.

213. Griffin A, Callan MB, Shofer FS, Giger U. 2003. Evaluation of a canine D-dimer point-of-care test kit for use in samples obtained from dogs with disseminated intravascular coagulation, thromboembolic disease, and hemorrhage. Am J Vet Res 64:1562–1569.

214. Nelson OL, Andreasen C. 2003. The utility of plasma D-dimer to identify thromboembolic disease in dogs. J Vet Intern Med 17:830–834.

215. McCaw DL, Jergens AE, Turrentine MA, Johnson GS. 1986. Effect of internal hemorrhage on fibrin(ogen) degradation products in canine blood. Am J Vet Res 47:1620–1621.

216. Budzynski AZ, Pandya BV, Rubin RN, Brizuela BS, Soszka T, Stewart GJ. 1984. Fibrinogenolytic afibrinogenemia after envenomation by western diamondback rattlesnake (*Crotalus atrox*). Blood 63:1–14.

217. Weitz JI, Leslie B, Ginsberg J. 1991. Soluble fibrin degradation products potentiate tissue plasminogen activator–induced fibrinogen proteolysis. J Clin Invest 87:1082–1090.

218. Francis CW, Marder VJ. 1994. Physiologic regulation and pathologic disorders of fibrinolysis. In: Colman RW, Hirsch J, Marder VJ, Salzman EW, eds. *Hemostasis and Thrombosis: Basic Principles and Clinical Practice*, 3rd edition, 1076–1103. Philadelphia: JB Lippincott.

219. Takahashi H, Wada K, Hanano M, Niwano H, Takizawa S, Yazawa Y, Shibata A. 1992. Fibrinolysis and fibrinogenolysis in patients with thrombotic disease. Blood Coagul Fibrinolysis 3:193–196.

220. Gaffney PJ. 2001. Fibrin degradation products: A review of structures found in vitro and in vivo. Ann NY Acad Sci 936:594–610.

221. Bouton MC, Jandrot-Perrus M, Bezeaud A, Guillin MC. 1993. Late-fibrin(ogen) fragment E modulates human α-thrombin specificity. Eur J Biochem 215:143–149.

222. Mischke R, Wolling H. 2000. Influence of fibrinogen degradation products on thrombin time, activated partial thromboplastin time and prothrombin time of canine plasma. Haemostasis 30:123–130.

223. Gouin I, Lecompte T, Morel MC, Lebrazi J, Modderman PW, Kaplan C, Samama MM. 1992. In vitro effect of plasmin on human platelet function in plasma: Inhibition of aggregation caused by fibrinogenolysis. Circulation 85:935–941.

224. Khavkina LS, Rozenfeld MA, Leonova VB. 1995. Mechanism of inhibition of fibrinolysis and fibrinogenolysis by the end fibrinogen degradation products. Thromb Res 78:173–187.

225. Caldin M, Furlanello T, Lubas G. 2000. Validation of an immunoturbidimetric D-dimer assay in canine citrated plasma. Vet Clin Pathol 29:51–54.

226. Welles EG. 1996. Antithrombotic and fibrinolytic factors: A review. Vet Clin North Am Small Anim Pract 26:1111–1127.

227. Stokol T, Brooks MB, Erb HN, Mauldin GE. 2000. D-dimer concentrations in healthy dogs and dogs with disseminated intravascular coagulation. Am J Vet Res 61:393–398.

228. Dempfle CE, Zips S, Ergül H, Heene DL, for the FACT Study Group. 2001. The Fibrin Assay Comparison Trial (FACT): Evaluation of 23 quantitative D-dimer assays as basis for the development of D-dimer calibrators. Thromb Haemost 85:671–678.

229. Dempfle CE. 2005. Validation, calibration, and specificity of quantitative D-dimer assays. Semin Vasc Med 5:315–320.

230. Sato N, Takahashi H, Shibata A. 1995. Fibrinogen/fibrin degradation products and D-dimer in clinical practice: Interpretation of discrepant results. Am J Hematol 48:168–174.

231. Gordge MP, Faint RW, Rylance PB, Ireland H, Lane DA, Neild GH. 1989. Plasma D dimer: A useful marker of fibrin breakdown in renal failure. Thromb Haemost 61:522–525.

232. Mischke R. 2003. Alterations of the global haemostatic function test "resonance thrombography" in spontaneously traumatised dogs. Pathophysiol Haemost Thromb 33:214–220.

233. Mischke R, Wohlsein P, Schoon HA. 2005. Detection of fibrin generation alterations in dogs with haemangiosarcoma using resonance thrombography. Thromb Res 115:229–238.

234. Wiinberg B, Jensen AL, Rojkjaer R, Johansson P, Kjelgaard-Hansen M, Kristensen AT. 2005. Validation of human recombinant tissue factor–activated thromboelastography on citrated whole blood from clinically healthy dogs. Vet Clin Pathol 34:389–393.

235. Mischke R, Schulze U. 2004. Studies on platelet aggregation using the Born method in normal and uraemic dogs. Vet J 168:270–275.

236. Michiels C. 2003. Endothelial cell functions. J Cell Physiol 196:430–443.

237. Giger U. 2000. Hereditary blood diseases. In: Feldman BF, Zinkl JG, Jain NC, eds. *Schalm's Veterinary Hematology*, 5th edition, 955–959. Philadelphia: Lippincott Williams & Wilkins.

238. Mostoskey UV, Padgett GA, Stinson AW, Brewer GJ, Duffendack JC. 2000. Canine molecular genetic diseases. Compend Contin Educ Pract Vet 22:480–489.

239. Soute BA, Ulrich MM, Watson AD, Maddison JE, Ebberink RH, Vermeer C. 1992. Congenital deficiency of all vitamin K–dependent blood coagulation factors due to a defective vitamin K–dependent carboxylase in Devon rex cats. Thromb Haemost 68:521–525.

240. Mason DJ, Abrams-Ogg A, Allen D, Gentry PA, Gadd KR. 2002. Vitamin K–dependent coagulopathy in a black Labrador Retriever. J Vet Intern Med 16:485–488.

241. Niles JD, Williams JM, Cripps PJ. 2001. Hemostatic profiles in 39 dogs with congenital portosystemic shunts. Vet Surg 30:97–104.

242. Gerlach H, Slama KJ, Bechstein WO, Lohmann R, Hintz G, Abraham K, Neuhaus P, Falke K. 1993. Retrospective statistical analysis of coagulation parameters after 250 liver transplantations. Semin Thromb Hemost 19:223–232.

243. Bigge LA, Brown DJ, Penninck DG. 2001. Correlation between coagulation profile findings and bleeding complications after ultrasound-guided biopsies: 434 cases (1993–1996). J Am Anim Hosp Assoc 37:228–233.

244. Bartol JM, Thompson LJ, Minnier SM, Divers TJ. 2000. Hemorrhagic diathesis, mesenteric hematoma, and colic associated with ingestion of sweet vernal grass in a cow. J Am Vet Med Assoc 216:1605–1608.

245. Puschner B, Galey FD, Holstege DM, Palazoglu M. 1998. Sweet clover poisoning in dairy cattle in California. J Am Vet Med Assoc 212:857–859.

246. Lutze G, Romhild W, Elwert J, Leppelt J, Kutschmann K. 2003. Case report: Phenprocoumon (Marcumar, Falithrom) as an unusual reason for coumarin poisoning in a dog [in German]. Dtsch Tierarztl Wochenschr 110:31–33.

247. Neer TM, Savant RL. 1992. Hypoprothrombinemia secondary to administration of sulfaquinoxaline to dogs in a kennel setting. J Am Vet Med Assoc 200:1344–1345.

248. Patterson JM, Grenn HH. 1975. Hemorrhage and death in dogs following the administration of sulfaquinoxaline. Can Vet J 16:265–268.

249. Green RA, Roudebush P, Barton CL. 1979. Laboratory evaluation of coagulopathies due to vitamin K antagonism in the dog: Three case reports. J Am Anim Hosp Assoc 15:691–697.

250. Woody BJ, Murphy MJ, Ray AC, Green RA. 1992. Coagulopathic effects and therapy of brodifacoum toxicosis in dogs. J Vet Intern Med 6:23–28.

251. Lipsky JJ. 1994. Nutritional sources of vitamin K. Mayo Clin Proc 69:462–466.

252. Strieker MJ, Morris JG, Feldman BF, Rogers QR. 1996. Vitamin K deficiency in cats fed commercial fish-based diets. J Small Anim Pract 37:322–326.

253. Conly J, Stein K. 1994. Reduction of vitamin K_2 concentrations in human liver associated with the use of broad spectrum antimicrobials. Clin Invest Med 17:531–539.

254. Boermans HJ, Johnstone I, Black WD, Murphy M. 1991. Clinical signs, laboratory changes and toxicokinetics of brodifacoum in the horse. Can J Vet Res 55:21–27.

255. Schaeffer RC Jr, Briston C, Chilton SM, Carlson RW. 1986. Disseminated intravascular coagulation following *Echis carinatus* venom in dogs: Effects of a synthetic thrombin inhibitor. J Lab Clin Med 107:488–497.

256. Mammen EF. 2000. Disseminated intravascular coagulation (DIC). Clin Lab Sci 13:239–245.

257. Marder VJ, Feinstein DI, Francis CW, Colman RW. 1994. Consumptive thrombohemorrhagic disorders. In: Colman RW, Hirsch J, Marder VJ, Salzman EW, eds. *Hemostasis and Thrombosis: Basic Principles and Clinical Practice*, 3rd edition, 1023–1063. Philadelphia: JB Lippincott.

258. Jutkowitz LA, Rozanski EA, Moreau JA, Rush JE. 2002. Massive transfusion in dogs: 15 cases (1997–2001). J Am Vet Med Assoc 220:1664–1669.

259. Jones PA, Tomasic M, Gentry PA. 1997. Oncotic, hemodilutional, and hemostatic effects of isotonic saline and hydroxyethyl starch solutions in clinically normal ponies. Am J Vet Res 58:541–548.

260. Concannon KT, Haskins SC, Feldman BF. 1992. Hemostatic defects associated with two infusion rates of dextran 70 in dogs. Am J Vet Res 53:1369–1375.

261. Brooks M. 2000. Coagulopathies and thrombosis. In: Ettinger SJ, Feldman EC, eds. *Textbook of Veterinary Internal Medicine: Diseases of the Dog and Cat*, 5th edition, 1829–1841. Philadelphia: WB Saunders.

262. Glowaski MM, Moon-Massat PF, Erb HN, Barr SC. 2003. Effects of oxypolygelatin and dextran 70 on hemostatic variables in dogs. Vet Anaesth Analg 30:202–210.

263. de Gopegui RR. 2000. Acquired coagulopathy IV: Acquired inhibitors. In: Feldman BF, Zinkl JG, Jain NC, eds. *Schalm's Veterinary Hematology*, 5th edition, 571–573. Philadelphia: Lippincott Williams & Wilkins.

264. Sahud MA. 2000. Laboratory diagnosis of inhibitors. Semin Thromb Hemost 26:195–203.

265. Tinlin S, Webster S, Giles AR. 1993. The development of homologous (canine/anti-canine) antibodies in dogs with haemophilia A (factor VIII deficiency): A ten-year longitudinal study. Thromb Haemost 69:21–24.

266. Brooks MB, Gu W, Ray K. 1997. Complete deletion of factor IX gene and inhibition of factor IX activity in a Labrador retriever with hemophilia B. J Am Vet Med Assoc 211:1418–1421.

267. Federman DG, Kirsner RS. 2001. An update on hypercoagulable disorders. Arch Intern Med 161:1051–1056.

268. Morley PS, Allen AL, Woolums AR. 1996. Aortic and iliac artery thrombosis in calves: Nine cases (1974–1993). J Am Vet Med Assoc 209:130–136.

269. Laste NJ, Harpster NK. 1995. A retrospective study of 100 cases of feline distal aortic thromboembolism: 1977–1993. J Am Anim Hosp Assoc 31:492–500.

270. Boswood A, Lamb CR, White RN. 2000. Aortic and iliac thrombosis in six dogs. J Small Anim Pract 41:109–114.

271. Brianceau P, Divers TJ. 2001. Acute thrombosis of limb arteries in horses with sepsis: Five cases (1988–1998). Equine Vet J 33:105–109.

272. Norris CR, Griffey SM, Samii VF. 1999. Pulmonary thromboembolism in cats: 29 cases (1987–1997). J Am Vet Med Assoc 215:1650–1654.

273. Blombäck M, Dybkaer R, Jorgensen K, Olesen H, Thorsen S. 1997. Properties and units in the clinical laboratory sciences. V. Properties and units in thrombosis and haemostasis. Pure Appl Chem 69:1043–1079.

Chapter 6

BONE MARROW AND LYMPH NODE

Bone Marrow: Major Concepts and Terms 324
Bone Marrow Classifications. 334
    I.   Bone Marrow Hyperplasia. 334
    II.   Bone Marrow Hypoplasia 338
    III. Bone Marrow Lymphocytosis 340
    IV. Bone Marrow Mastocytosis. 340
    V.   Myelofibrosis. 341
    VI. Myelitis 341
    VII. Bone Marrow Necrosis 341
    VIII. Myelophthisis 342
    IX. Bone Marrow Hemic Cell Neoplasia. 342
Interpreting Results of Bone Marrow Examinations 357
Lymph Node: Major Concepts and Terms. 358
Lymph Node Classifications 363
    I.   Hyperplastic Lymph Node. 363
    II.   Reactive Lymph Node 363
    III. Lymphadenitis. 363
    IV. Lymphoid Neoplasia (Lymphoma and Lymphosarcoma) 363
    V.   Nonlymphoid Neoplasia (Typically Metastatic). 365
    VI. Other Findings 365

Table 6.1. Abbreviations and symbols in this chapter

ALSG	Animal Leukemia Study Group
AML	Acute myeloid leukemia
CBC	Complete blood count
CD	Cluster of differentiation
CMMoL	Chronic myelomonocytic leukemia
DNA	Deoxyribonucleic acid
Epo	Erythropoietin
Fe	Iron
FeLV	Feline leukemia virus
G:E	Granulocytic to erythroid
G-CSF	Granulocyte colony–stimulating factor
GM-CSF	Granulocyte/macrophage colony–stimulating factor
M:E	Myeloid to erythroid
M6-Er	Acute erythroleukemia with erythroid predominance
MDS	Myelodysplastic syndrome
MDS-EB	Myelodysplastic syndrome–excess blasts
MDS-Er	Myelodysplastic syndrome–erythroid predominance
MDS-RC	Myelodysplastic syndrome–refractory cytopenia
MPD	Myeloproliferative disease
MPO	Myeloperoxidase
NK	Natural killer
TCR$\alpha\beta$	$\alpha\beta$-Antigen–binding hetcrodimer of the T-lymphocyte receptor (T-cell receptor)
TCR$\gamma\delta$	$\gamma\delta$-Antigen–binding heterodimer of the T-lymphocyte receptor (T-cell receptor)
WHO	World Health Organization

BONE MARROW: MAJOR CONCEPTS AND TERMS

I.   Composition of bone marrow (medulla ossea)
     A. *Bone marrow* is the tissue enclosed by cortical and cancellous bone, and it consists
        mostly of hematopoietic cells, adipose tissue, and supportive tissue. When hematopoi-
        etic cells predominate, as in young animals, the marrow appears red. When adipose
        tissue predominates, as in the diaphyseal regions of long bones in healthy adults, the
        marrow appears yellow because of its high fat content. The extent of red marrow (active
        hematopoiesis) diminishes as neonates grow to adult size, but red marrow remains
        within bones of the axial (ilium, ribs, sternebrae, and vertebrae) and proximal appen-
        dicular (humeri and femurs) skeleton. Yellow marrow can convert to red marrow during
        pathologic states that stimulate hematopoiesis.
     B. Nutrients are delivered by vessels branching from one or more nutrient (medullary)
        arteries that enter through the cortical bone. New hemic cells enter blood through the
        walls of medullary sinuses.
     C. Hematopoietic cells develop in a supportive extravascular microenvironment controlled
        by a myriad of local and systemic cytokines.

II. *Hematopoietic cells* are precursors to hemic cells found in the blood or tissue. Microscopi-
     cally recognizable hematopoietic cells include cells in the proliferation pools and the
     maturation pools of the megakaryocyte, erythrocyte, and leukocyte lineages.

Table 6.2. Nomenclature of the erythroid series

Rubricyte system[a]	Erythroblast system[b]	Normoblast system[b]
Rubriblast	Proerythroblast	Pronormoblast
Prorubricyte	Basophilic proerythroblast	Basophilic normoblast
Basophilic rubricyte	Basophilic erythroblast	Basophilic normoblast
Polychromatophilic rubricyte	Polychromatophilic erythroblast	Polychromatophilic normoblast
Normochromic rubricyte	Early orthochromatic erythroblast	Early orthochromatic normoblast
Metarubricyte	Late orthochromatic erythroblast	Late orthochromatic normoblast

[a] The usual nomenclature in veterinary medicine
[b] Nomenclature used primarily in human medicine

A. Megakaryocyte lineage
  1. *Megakaryocytes* account for < 1 % of hematopoietic cells, but they are very large polyploid cells, each with the capability of producing many platelets.
  2. Thrombopoietin and other cytokines (see Chapter 4) stimulate the formation of mature megakaryocytes from megakaryoblasts through *endomitosis*: the nucleus divides repeatedly without cytokinesis to form cells of progressively greater ploidy (most about 16N).
    a. *Megakaryoblasts*, which are the first microscopically recognizable cells of the series, are similar in size to rubriblasts, myeloblasts, and monoblasts, and have single nuclei and deeply basophilic cytoplasms that may form blebs.
    b. *Promegakaryocytes* develop from megakaryoblasts and have what appear to be two or four nuclei and scant amounts of basophilic cytoplasm that may form blebs (Plate 9A [for all plates, see the color section of this book]).
    c. Megakaryocytes vary in size and ploidy. As they develop from promegakaryocytes, they become larger, have more nuclear lobulations, and have more abundant, paler cytoplasms that break up into anucleate platelets. Mature forms predominate (Plate 9B).
B. Erythrocyte lineage (Table 6.2)
  1. In veterinary medicine, the nucleated erythroid precursors are usually named using a *rubri-* prefix. The cells within the series are the rubriblast, prorubricyte, basophilic rubricyte, polychromatophilic rubricyte, normochromic rubricyte, and metarubricyte, although there is a continuum of development making cell subclassification difficult at times. Metarubricytes give rise to reticulocytes and mature erythrocytes.
  2. As cells proliferate and mature (see Fig. 3.1) from the first recognizable stage, the rubriblast, they decrease in size and cytoplasmic basophilia while increasing hemoglobin content and associated eosinophilic staining (Plate 9C).
  3. In human medicine, and sometimes in veterinary medicine, the nucleated erythroid precursors are named by using either erythroblast or normoblast terms (Table 6.2).
  4. Accordingly, an increased concentration of nucleated erythroid precursors in the blood may be called rubricytosis in veterinary medicine, but it is sometimes called either erythroblastosis or normoblastosis as in human medicine.

C. Nonlymphoid leukocyte (myeloid) lineages
1. Nonlymphoid leukocyte precursors are often collectively labeled myeloid cells. However, there are different meanings of *myeloid* and the prefix *myelo-*. Thus, a word beginning with *myelo-* must be interpreted in context.
    a. *Myel-* or *myelo-* meanings:
        (1) Combining form denoting the relationship to bone marrow
        (2) Referring to the nonlymphoid hemic cells of the megakaryocyte, leukocyte, and erythroid series (as in myeloproliferative disease)
        (3) Referring to granulocytes, as in myelomonocytic leukemia
        (4) Often used in specific reference to spinal cord
    b. *Myeloid* meanings:
        (1) Pertaining to or derived from bone marrow
        (2) Pertaining to all nonlymphoid leukocyte precursors, as in the myeloid to erythroid ratio
        (3) Pertaining to nonlymphoid hemic cells of the megakaryocyte, leukocyte, and erythroid series, as in acute myeloid leukemia (which includes pure erythroleukemia)
        (4) Having the appearance of the myelocyte
        (5) Pertaining to spinal cord
    c. *Myelocyte* meanings:
        (1) Intermediate precursor cell of the granulocyte series
        (2) Any cell of the grey matter of the nervous system
    d. *Myelitis* meanings:
        (1) Inflammation of bone marrow
        (2) Inflammation of spinal cord
    e. *Myelogenous* meanings:
        (1) Produced in bone marrow
        (2) Pertaining to nonlymphoid hemic cells of the megakaryocyte, leukocyte, and erythroid series, as in acute myelogenous (myeloid) leukemia
2. Nonlymphoid leukocytes: monocytes, granulocytes (neutrophils, eosinophils, and basophils), and mast cells (see Chapter 2 and Fig. 2.1).
    a. Neutrophils predominate. The mature neutrophils in the bone marrow are collectively referred to as the *neutrophil storage pool*.
    b. Granulocytes are derived from myeloblasts and promyelocytes, acquiring specific secondary granules at the myelocyte stage (neutrophil myelocyte, eosinophil myelocyte, and basophil myelocyte) (Plate 9D).
    c. Monocytes develop from monoblasts and promonocytes, populations that are inconspicuous in bone marrow from healthy animals. Macrophages, derived from monocytes, are present in low numbers.
    d. Mast cell precursors are not detectable in the bone marrow, but low numbers of resident mast cells derived from hemic stem cells may be present.
D. Lymphocyte lineage
1. Lymphocytes and plasma cells are present in relatively low numbers.
2. All lymphoid cells are derived from a common bone marrow precursor cell (Fig. 2.1).
3. Cells destined to be B-lymphocytes mature in the bone marrow or in some other tissues, whereas cells destined to be T-lymphocytes migrate to the thymus and mature there.

E. Dendritic cells

1. Dendritic cells are specialized for uptake, transport, processing, and presenting antigens to T-lymphocytes. There are several subtypes, including Langerhans cells, interstitial dendritic cells, and plasmacytoid dendritic cells.[1]

2. All dendritic cells are bone marrow derived, but their origins are not completely understood and their precursors are not recognized microscopically.

3. Dendritic cells are believed to originate from both myeloid and lymphoid precursors.[2,3]

F. Bone marrow nucleated cell differential count in health

1. The expected ratio of nonlymphoid leukocytes to erythroid precursors (myeloid to erythroid ratio) varies with the species and the individual. Average ratios in healthy dogs, cats, horses, and cattle are reported to be 1.25, 1.63, 0.93, and 0.71, respectively.[4]

2. In health, cells of the neutrophil and erythroid series predominate, and the majority of cells in each lineage are the more mature cells.[4]

   a. Myeloblasts and promyelocytes account for < 4 % of the nucleated cells.

   b. Segmented and band neutrophils are the predominant leukocytes.

   c. Cells of the eosinophil series usually account for < 5 % of the nucleated cells, whereas cells of the basophil series are rare.

   d. Rubriblasts and prorubricytes account for < 4 % of the nucleated cells.

   e. Metarubricytes and late-stage rubricytes are the predominant nucleated erythrocytes. Polychromatophilic erythrocytes are present.

   f. Lymphocytes usually account for < 5 % of the nucleated cells except in cats. Up to about 20 % lymphocytes have been reported in healthy cats.

   g. Cells of the monocyte series constitute < 2 % of nucleated cells.

III. Indications for bone marrow examinations

A. Whenever the following are unexplained and persistent:

1. Decreased cell concentrations

   a. Nonregenerative anemia

   b. Neutropenia

   c. Thrombocytopenia

   d. Pancytopenia

2. Increased cell concentrations

   a. Lymphocytosis, especially if atypical lymphocytes are seen in blood films or there is other evidence of lymphoid neoplasia

   b. Thrombocytosis, especially extreme

   c. Erythrocytosis, especially if there is no evidence of hemoconcentration, splenic contraction, or cardiopulmonary disease

   d. Granulocytosis or monocytosis if chronic leukemia is suspected

   e. Mastocytemia

3. Atypical or immature cells in blood films

4. Hyperproteinemia, especially if there is no evidence of hemoconcentration or dehydration

5. Hypercalcemia

B. To search for the following:

1. Evidence of metastatic neoplasia, especially of lymphocytes and mast cells

2. Evidence of Fe storage, especially when considering Fe deficiency

      3. Evidence of specific diseases: histoplasmosis, leishmaniasis, plasma cell myeloma, or lysosomal storage diseases

IV. Methods
   A. Complete descriptions of a bone marrow biopsy (collection, fixation, staining, and examination of bone marrow from a living animal) are beyond the scope of this text. Procedures of a bone marrow biopsy are described in several sources.[4–11]
   B. Bone marrow collection and processing
      1. Typically, bone marrow samples are collected from sites that are expected to have active hematopoietic tissue.
         a. In dogs and cats, such tissue is expected in the iliac crest or in the medullary cavities of proximal femurs or humeri.
         b. In horses, such tissue is most accessible in the sternebrae. In cattle, medullary cavities of proximal ribs can be sampled.
      2. The two major methods of collecting bone marrow samples are aspiration and core collection.
         a. *Aspiration*: A Rosenthal or Illinois biopsy needle is inserted into a bone marrow site, the stylet is removed, and bone marrow is aspirated into the needle and perhaps syringe by negative pressure. Excessive hemodilution is limited by terminating aspiration as soon as blood is seen entering the syringe. The Rosenthal and Illinois needles are straight shafted with a beveled end. Nondisposable forms require sterilization and sharpening. Disposable forms are available.
         b. *Core cutting*: A Jamshidi biopsy needle is inserted into the cortical bone adjacent to bone marrow, the stylet is removed, the needle is advanced 1 inch or more into the bone marrow with a forceful twisting motion, the needle is rotated 360 ° several times, and then the needle is withdrawn. After the needle is withdrawn, the stylet is used to push the core sample out the top of the needle (not the tip end that is narrower than most of a Jamshidi needle's bore); this promotes retrieval of a cylindrical core of tissue.
      3. Processing bone marrow aspirate samples
         a. To reduce clot formation and autolytic changes, it is critical that such samples be processed (sample distributed and fixed onto glass slides) within seconds of collection. A variety of smear, "squash", roll, and imprint methods may be used to produce slides that have monolayers of intact cells and foci of bone marrow particles that may be stained and examined.
            (1) After aspiration, drops may be placed on a series of glass slides and quickly spread by either a wedge blood smear technique or a horizontal "squash" technique. The latter better spreads cells that are present within particles. However, drops may be large, resulting in smears that are too long or too thick. Therefore, one should consider lifting parts of each drop up with the end of a spreader slide and then using the spreader slide to make squash preparations with this smaller amount of sample. Repeating this process can yield many good smears.
            (2) Other techniques can be used to decrease hemodilution of the final smears and maximize cellularity and marrow particle density.
               (a) Aspirated fluid can be expressed at the top of inclined slides so that the blood flows downward, leaving more particles and less blood at the application point. The short edge of a spreader slide can then be used to

lift particle-rich material repeatedly from the top of the slide and make horizontal squash preparations.

  (b) Alternatively, collected material can be placed in a watch glass or Petri dish with anticoagulant, and the particles can be extracted and spread onto slides without the concern of clotting. Anticoagulants may induce artifacts.

 b. Aspiration may yield a "dry tap" containing essentially no material, in which case additional aspiration attempts or core biopsy samples are required. "Dry taps" do not indicate that the marrow is hypocellular; they may occur with bone marrow hypercellularity in a variety of disorders.

 c. For routine microscopic examinations, the air-dried samples are stained with a stain that is used for blood films (a Romanowsky stain such as a Wright stain or Diff-Quik). A Prussian blue stain may be applied to assess the amount of stainable Fe in a sample.

 d. Processing requirements for cytochemical or immunocytologic procedures should be obtained from the relevant laboratory.

4. Processing core biopsy samples

 a. After making imprints by touching or rolling the core on a glass slide, the core sample is placed in a fixative. B5 or Zenker's fixative is preferable, but routine buffered formalin is adequate. (Note: keep the air-dried samples far away from the fixative because formalin fumes can severely alter the staining properties of cells). The fixation procedures vary with the type of fixative fluid that is used.

 b. The fixed core sample is submitted to a hematology or histology laboratory that can process and stain the sample for microscopic examination. Core samples require decalcification before the sample can be sectioned and prepared for staining. A variety of stains, including immunohistochemical stains, may be applied to demonstrate the types of cells or other contents of the sample.

C. Bone marrow examination

1. Gross examination

 a. Aspirated bone marrow samples will contain peripheral blood cells, but the best samples have very little contaminant blood. A representative sample typically contains small pieces of tissue known as bone marrow fragments, bone marrow units, bone marrow grains, bone marrow particles, or bone marrow spicules. The bone marrow fragments that contain adipose tissue will glisten. Bone marrow fragments should not be confused with clotted blood or platelet clumps.

 b. The appearance of bone marrow core samples will vary from hypercellular red tissue to hypocellular fatty tissue to cortical bone or blood clots.

2. Microscopic examination: A complete microscopic examination of bone marrow samples involves the characterization of the bone marrow tissue architecture, differentiation and enumeration of cells, and evaluation of individual cell structure. Such examinations are best completed on quality stained histologic and cytologic samples with a quality microscope by a person who is trained for such examinations. A complete examination with differential cell counts and special stains can be time-consuming. Frequently, just as much clinically useful information can be learned from a subjective assessment of cell populations by an experienced hematologist. The following bone marrow features are assessed:

 a. *Hematopoietic cellularity* is the percentage of the marrow cavity occupied by hematopoietic cells rather than by adipose tissue or stroma (assessed at low magnification)

(1) The hematopoietic cellularity of bone marrow fragments reflects the hematopoietic cellularity of the bone marrow, and the more fragments there are to examine, the better is the assessment. However, hematopoietic cellularity of bone marrow is best assessed in a core sample, especially when there is bone marrow hypocellularity and it is unclear whether fragments of fat are from the bone marrow or from extramedullary adipose tissue.

(2) Cellularity of the preparation is not the same as the hematopoietic cellularity of the bone marrow. If bone marrow fragments, on average, are < 25 % adipose tissue, the bone marrow is hypercellular (Plate 9E). If bone marrow fragments, on average, are > 75 % adipose tissue, the bone marrow is hypocellular (Plate 9F). If bone marrow fragments are not present and the preparation is very cellular, the bone marrow is likely hypercellular and unlikely hypocellular. If bone marrow fragments are not present and the preparation is not very cellular, the bone marrow may be hypocellular or the sample may be poorly representative of bone marrow tissue.

b. Hematopoietic populations (see Figs. 2.1 and 6.1)

(1) Number and structure of megakaryocytes

(a) The expected number of mature megakaryocytes in a sample varies among species and is highly dependent on the quality of the sample, especially the number of bone marrow fragments in aspirates. In health, there is usually at least one megakaryocyte per marrow fragment. If more megakaryocytes are found than are expected, then megakaryocytic hyperplasia is present. If fewer are present, then megakaryocytic hypoplasia is probably present.

(b) An increased number of immature forms of the megakaryocytic series (i.e., megakaryoblasts or promegakaryocytes) usually indicates increased megakaryopoiesis and megakaryocytic hyperplasia but may occur as an early response before there is clear-cut hyperplasia. It may also occur with dysplastic diseases and megakaryocytic neoplasia.

(2) G:E ratio (M:E ratio)

(a) A G:E or (M:E) ratio is often estimated but may be calculated using cytologic samples by differentiating 500–1000 consecutive granulocytic (or myeloid) and nucleated erythroid precursors and then dividing the number of granulocytic (or myeloid) cells by the number of erythroid cells. For example, if out of 500 counted cells there were 300 cells of the granulocyte series and 200 nucleated erythrocytes, the G:E ratio would be 300/200 = 1.5.

(b) Most authors seem to use G:E and M:E as synonyms. However, a M:E ratio may include monocyte precursors or megakaryocytes in the myeloid category, and a G:E ratio may exclude these cells even though it may be difficult or impossible to definitively differentiate monoblasts and promonocytes from granulocyte precursors. The difference between these ratios would usually be insignificant because there are usually few recognizable cells of the monocyte series and relatively few megakaryocytes.

(c) Other cells (e.g., lymphocytes, macrophages, mast cells, and stromal cells) are not included in the G:E or M:E ratios.

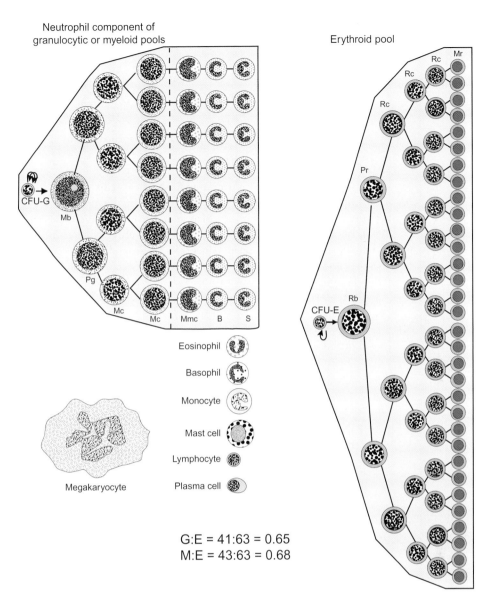

Fig. 6.1. Schematic representation of the hemic cells that may be found in bone marrow of healthy mammals. The two major pools are cells of the neutrophil series in the granulocytic pool and cells of the erythroid pool. Eosinophils and basophils and their precursors are also components of the granulocytic pool. Monocytes are part of the myeloid pool but not the granulocytic pool. Megakaryocytes may be considered part of the myeloid pool or may be evaluated as a separate cell line and not included in the M:E ratio. Mast cells are terminally differentiated tissue cells rather than hematopoietic cells and are not included in the M:E ratio. Lymphocytes and plasma cells belong to the nonmyeloid lymphoid pool.

B, band neutrophil; CFU-E, colony-forming unit–erythroid; CFU-G, colony-forming unit–granulocyte; Mb, myeloblast; Mc, myelocyte; Mmc, metamyelocyte; Mr, metarubricyte; Pg, progranulocyte; Pr, prorubricyte; Rb, rubriblast; Rc, rubricyte; and S, segmented neutrophil.

(d) A G:E or M:E ratio is estimated in histologic samples, but it is subjective and based mostly on the more mature granulocytic and erythroid cells. Immature cells are difficult to differentiate definitively into the appropriate cell lines.

(e) The G:E or M:E ratio (Plate 9D) may be increased because of granulocytic or myeloid hyperplasia, erythroid hypoplasia, or both. If the marrow hematopoietic cellularity is increased, granulocytic or myeloid hyperplasia is contributing to the increased G:E or M:E ratio. If hematopoietic cellularity is decreased, erythroid hypoplasia is contributing to an increased G:E or M:E ratio. If the hematopoietic cellularity is not clearly increased or decreased, CBC results may help with interpretation. For example, concurrent neutrophilia supports granulocytic hyperplasia, whereas concurrent nonregenerative anemia supports erythroid hypoplasia.

(f) The G:E or M:E ratio (Plate 9C) may be decreased because of granulocytic (myeloid) hypoplasia, erythroid hyperplasia, or both. If the marrow hematopoietic cellularity is increased, erythroid hyperplasia is contributing to the decreased G:E or M:E ratio. If hematopoietic cellularity is decreased, granulocytic (myeloid) hypoplasia is contributing to the decreased G:E or M:E ratio. If the hematopoietic cellularity is not clearly increased or decreased, CBC results may help with interpretation. For example, concurrent neutropenia supports granulocytic hypoplasia, whereas concurrent regenerative anemia supports erythroid hyperplasia.

(3) Maturation progression
  (a) Because nearly all cells of the erythroid series can undergo mitosis, there should be many more of the late stages than the early stages (a pyramidal distribution; see Figs. 2.1 and 6.1). There also should be an orderly and synchronous maturation between nuclei and cytoplasms. As nuclei become smaller and chromatin denser, the cell size decreases, the cytoplasmic basophilia decreases, and the eosinophilic staining of hemoglobin increases.
  (b) The granulocytic precursors are divided into two pools (see Figs. 2.2 and 6.1). The early pool (proliferation pool) contains cells capable of mitosis, and thus more myelocytes are expected than myeloblasts or progranulocytes. Most of the granulocytes are segmented neutrophils in the maturation pool (including the storage pool). There should be an orderly and synchronous maturation between nuclei and cytoplasms throughout the series.

(4) Lymphocytes: Most of the lymphocytes in bone marrow of healthy animals are small, but occasional larger forms and plasma cells can be found. Hematopoietic stem cells have the appearance of small lymphocytes but are expected to be present in very low numbers.

c. Other cells: Mast cells, macrophages, fibroblasts, osteoclasts, osteoblasts, and other stromal cells are usually present in very low numbers. Their numbers may be subjectively categorized as normal or increased. Increased numbers can indicate or suggest certain pathologic processes.

    d. Fe
       (1) In aspirate and core samples, the Fe pigment in hemosiderin will range from yellow to yellow-green to yellow-brown (Plate 9E). A more complete assessment of Fe storage can be determined if the samples are stained with an Fe stain such as Prussian blue.
       (2) The amount of Fe pigment in the sample is estimated and reported by using a variety of terms:
          (a) Absent or decreased
          (b) Adequate, within normal limits, or moderate
          (c) Increased or abundant
       (3) Healthy cats lack detectable marrow Fe stores, but Fe may be present because of hemolytic disorders, after a transfusion, and in myeloproliferative disorders.[12,13] Stores may be absent in healthy young animals of any species.
  3. Comparison of histologic and cytologic examinations
    a. Histologic examination of core samples
       (1) Advantages
          (a) Tissue architecture (how cells are arranged), necrosis, infiltrative patterns, focal lesions, and myelofibrosis can be better assessed.
          (b) Bone marrow cellularity can be better assessed.
          (c) Megakaryocyte number can be better assessed.
          (d) Abnormalities of bone and vessels can be better assessed.
          (e) Further tissue sections can be cut for special stains.
       (2) Disadvantages
          (a) It is more expensive, with greater turnaround time.
          (b) Cell differentiation is more difficult, especially if sections are not cut thin enough (target $\approx 3\ \mu m$).
          (c) Phagocytosis of hematopoietic cells is difficult to detect.
          (d) Many dysplastic features are difficult to detect.
       (3) Potential problems with core samples include short samples of uncertain representation, samples consisting mostly of cortical and subcortical bone, sample damage related to prior aspiration, crush artifact from traumatic collection, improper fixation, and thick sections or damage induced during sectioning.
    b. Cytologic examination of aspirate samples
       (1) Advantages
          (a) Individual cells and cell populations can be critically differentiated and evaluated, enabling better assessment of the G:E (M:E) ratio and the maturation progression.
          (b) Phagocytosis of hematopoietic cells or organisms can be better detected.
          (c) Dysplastic or neoplastic cell features can be better detected.
          (d) The processing cost is relatively little; most of the technique expense is in the collection procedure.
          (e) The technique can be used for cytochemical staining and immunocyto-chemistry, including use of antibodies that do not work on fixed tissues.
       (2) Disadvantages
          (a) Tissue architecture can be minimally assessed.
          (b) Necrosis or myelofibrosis are difficult to detect.

           (c) Interpretations are limited if marrow particles are not obtained.

           (d) It may be difficult to determine whether a sample is representative (i.e., to differentiate a poor sample from hypocellular bone marrow).

      (3) Potential problems with cytologic preparations include collection of extramedullary samples, "dry taps," excessive hemodilution, clotted samples, thick smears, lysed cells, and poor staining.

    c. Combining examinations of core and aspirate marrow samples provides the most complete information.

      (1) Cytologic evaluation of aspirates is almost always indicated.

      (2) Histologic examination is useful when marrow architecture is required to reach a diagnosis, myelofibrosis is suspected (connective tissue exfoliates poorly), or hypoplastic states are suspected (e.g., when pancytopenia is present) and therefore an aspirate may yield few cells and a pattern that may not be distinct from poor sampling.

      (3) When both samples are collected, care should be taken to avoid the first collection procedure from diminishing the quality of the second sample. A core can be artifactually altered when collected after an aspirate in the same area, and an aspirate may be more hemodiluted if collected after a core sample at the same site.

  4. Postmortem bone marrow samples

    a. Hematopoietic cells undergo autolysis rapidly because the insides of bones stay warm much longer than most tissues, and precursors of leukocytes contain many proteolytic and lipolytic enzymes that enable the digestion of cells.

    b. Samples should be collected as soon as possible after an animal's death so the they will be adequate for evaluation (guideline: $< \frac{1}{2}$ h for cytologic assessment).

    c. Samples should be collected from cancellous bone in the proximal humerus or femur, or from the axial skeleton (e.g., ilium, rib, or sternum). Although it is easier to collect samples from the diaphysis of long bones, these regions are not reliably representative of hematopoietic activity.

  5. Flow cytometry has been used to assess bone marrow aspirates and provide partial differentials[14] but is not routinely used for clinical cases and cannot replace microscopic evaluation.

BONE MARROW CLASSIFICATIONS

I.   *Bone marrow hyperplasia* is a term that indicates an increased number of nonneoplastic hematopoietic cells in bone marrow because of a stimulus that causes one or more cell lines to proliferate. The stimulus usually results from an increased need for cells but may occur secondary to aberrant production of stimulating cytokines (Table 6.3).

  A. Erythroid hyperplasia (erythroblastic or normoblastic hyperplasia)

    1. *Effective erythropoiesis*: Epo stimulation of precursor cells leads to a proliferation of erythroid cells, erythroid hyperplasia, and increased release of reticulocytes, nucleated erythrocytes, or erythrocytes into blood.

      a. It is usually secondary to hemolytic (Table 3.10) or blood loss disorders (see Fig. 3.8). The mechanisms that lead to erythroid hyperplasia begin immediately after the onset of anemia, but the resultant erythroid hyperplasia may not be present until a few days later. The degree of erythroid hyperplasia should correspond to the duration and severity of the anemia.

Table 6.3. Disorders and conditions that cause erythroid, granulocytic, or megakaryocytic hyperplasia in marrow

Erythroid hyperplasia
  Effective erythropoiesis
    *Secondary to hemolytic or blood loss disorders
    Secondary appropriate erythrocytotic disorders
        Right-to-left shunts, congenital or acquired
        Chronic pulmonary disease
        Hyperthyroidism
    Secondary inappropriate erythrocytotic disorders
        Renal neoplasms, cysts, or diseases
        Other neoplasms (hepatoma)
  Ineffective erythropoiesis
    *Immune-mediated nonregenerative anemia
    *Nutritional: Fe, copper, folate, or vitamin B_{12} deficiency
  Cyclic hematopoiesis of grey collies and FeLV-infected cats
Granulocytic hyperplasia
  Effective granulopoiesis
    Inflammatory
        *Infections: bacterial, fungal, viral, protozoal
        *Immune-mediated hemolytic anemia
        *Necrosis: hemolysis, hemorrhage, infarcts, burns, neoplasia, sterile inflammation
        Sterile foreign body
    Others or unknown mechanisms
        Paraneoplastic neutrophilia
        Neutrophilia of leukocyte adhesion deficiency
        G-CSF administration
        Estrogen toxicosis (early)
        Cyclic hematopoiesis of grey collies and in FeLV-infected cats
  Ineffective granulopoiesis
    Immune-mediated neutropenia
    Diphenylhydantoin and phenylbutazone toxicosis (suspected in animals)
    Chronic idiopathic neutropenia (G-CSF deficiency)
Megakaryocytic hyperplasia
  *Recovery from thrombocytopenia: withdrawal of myelosuppression or in response to a
        disorder that causes decreased platelet survival
  Inflammation: infection, immune-mediated, surgery, trauma

* A relatively common disease or condition
Note: Information about eosinophilic, basophilic, mononuclear-phagocytic, lymphoid, mast cell, and generalized marrow hyperplasia is provided in the text. Lists of specific disorders or conditions are not complete but are provided to give examples.

b. *Secondary appropriate erythrocytotic disorders*: Persistent hypoxia or increased tissue demand for O_2 promotes Epo release, which causes erythroid hyperplasia and erythrocytosis (see Chapter 3 for disorders).

c. *Secondary inappropriate erythrocytotic disorders*: Inappropriate Epo production in the absence of hypoxia causes erythroid hyperplasia and erythrocytosis (see Chapter 3 for disorders).

2. *Ineffective erythropoiesis*: Erythroid hyperplasia occurs concurrently with a nonregenerative or poorly regenerative anemia.

    a. Immune-mediated destruction of nucleated erythroid cells

        (1) These disorders are typically considered immune mediated based on the apparent response to immunosuppressive therapy and/or the presence of phagocytized erythroid precursors. In some cases, the results of a concurrent Coombs' test are positive.

        (2) In bone marrow samples, the erythroid series can have the appearance of maturation arrest with erythroid stages prior to the target cell stage being numerous.[15] Macrophages containing mid- to late-stage nucleated erythrocytes may be found on cytologic and rarely histologic preparations (Plate 9G). When earlier stage cells are targeted, generally too few erythroid cells are present to yield erythroid hyperplasia despite expansion of stages preceding the target stage. If erythroid stem cells are the target of an immune-mediated attack, there may be pure red cell aplasia (see Bone Marrow Classifications, sect. II.B).

    b. Nutritional deficiencies

        (1) Fe-deficiency anemia: In the Fe-deficient state, anemia develops despite erythroid hyperplasia. Erythropoiesis is defective, late-stage erythroid precursors do not mature properly, and erythrocytes are not released adequately into the blood. Reticulocytosis may be present, but the release of reticulocytes is not enough to meet the need. As the deficiency progresses, the rubricytes may appear smaller and have less hemoglobin in their cytoplasms.

        (2) Rare cases of copper, folate, and cobalamin deficiencies:[4,16] Cobalamin deficiency, which may occur secondary to abnormal intestinal cobalamin receptors, has been reported in giant schnauzers, beagles, Border collies, and Australian shepherds.[17] Dysplastic changes may be present.

B. *Granulocytic hyperplasia*: Unless stated otherwise, granulocytic hyperplasia (also called *myeloid hyperplasia*) typically is characterized by an increased number of neutrophil precursors. An orderly and complete proliferation and maturation series is expected with hyperplasia, but granulocytic hyperplasia may occur with a depleted storage pool and a left shift. Other forms of granulocytic hyperplasia are identified as eosinophilic granulocytic hyperplasia and basophilic granulocytic hyperplasia (rare). Because early stages of neutrophil and monocyte precursors are not easily differentiated, monocytic hyperplasia may or may not be recognized when there is neutrophilic granulocytic hyperplasia.

1. *Effective granulopoiesis*: Continual stimulation of neutrophil precursors by G-CSF, GM-CSF, or certain interleukins leads to granulocytic hyperplasia, increased release of neutrophils to blood, and typically a neutrophilia (with or without a left shift) (see Chapter 2).

    a. Inflammatory: The granulocytic hyperplasia is typically caused by an inflammatory process that results from any of a wide variety of infectious and noninfectious diseases.

    b. Other or unknown mechanisms of granulocytic hyperplasia are listed in Table 6.3 and Chapter 2.[18]

2. *Ineffective granulopoiesis*: This form of hyperplasia is recognized when there is a neutropenia and concurrent granulocytic hyperplasia. There may be a left shift with too few of the latest stages to complete the pyramidal maturation sequence.

a. Immune-mediated neutropenia:[19–21] Granulocytic hyperplasia results from persistent differentiation and proliferation of neutrophil precursors in an attempt to replace neutrophils being destroyed before or soon after release from bone marrow. There may or may not be a left shift, depending on the targeted neutrophil stage. Phagocytosis of neutrophils may be detected in bone marrow, liver, or spleen. Factors that lead to the generation of antineutrophil antibodies typically are not known but might be drug induced in some cases.

b. Drug-induced neutropenia: There have been rare reports of ineffective granulopoiesis associated with anticonvulsant (phenobarbital or primidone) treatments. The mechanism of the neutrophil destruction has not been established but might be immune mediated.[22]

c. Chronic idiopathic neutropenia caused by G-CSF deficiency: The bone marrow in the rottweiler with this disorder had numerous myeloblasts and progranulocytes, but myelocytes and later neutrophil stages were rare. The defect in maturation resulted from G-CSF deficiency, and G-CSF is needed for terminal neutrophil differentiation.[23]

C. *Megakaryocytic hyperplasia*, a nonneoplastic increase in megakaryocytes, occurs when megakaryopoiesis is persistently stimulated. Thrombopoiesis is concurrently stimulated. Platelet concentrations may be decreased, increased, or within the reference interval.

1. Recovery from thrombocytopenia

a. In response to thrombocytopenia, stimuli (stem cell factor, thrombopoietin, interleukin 3, and GM-CSF) promote the proliferation of megakaryocytes to replace the missing platelets.

b. The thrombocytopenia frequently is caused by disorders that decrease platelet survival. When thrombocytopenia is caused by a myelosuppressive agent or process, there may be a rebound megakaryocytic hyperplasia after removal of the suppression.

2. Mild megakaryocytic hyperplasia may be found concurrently with one of the several forms of reactive or secondary thrombocytosis, including inflammation and nonhemic neoplasia (see Chapter 4).

D. *Eosinophilic granulocytic hyperplasia* is characterized by increased numbers of eosinophils and eosinophil precursors in bone marrow.

1. Specific mediators, including interleukin 5 (eosinophil differentiation factor) and GM-CSF from mast cells, macrophages, and lymphocytes, stimulate eosinopoiesis.

2. Eosinophilic hyperplasia may or may not be recognized in animals with eosinophilia (see Table 2.12).

3. Cats with MDS may have eosinophilic granulocytic hyperplasia with or without peripheral blood eosinophilia.[24,25]

E. *Basophilic granulocytic hyperplasia* is characterized by increased numbers of basophils and basophil precursors in bone marrow. This type of hyperplasia is rarely recognized but might be found in animals with basophilias (see Table 2.14).

F. *Monocytic hyperplasia* is a hyperplastic state that is present when monocytic precursors are increased in the bone marrow. It typically is not seen as a primary bone marrow finding but may be found concurrently with granulocytic hyperplasia, particularly when there is a macrophagic or granulomatous component to the inflammatory process.

G. *Generalized bone marrow hyperplasia* is present when there is concurrent granulocytic, erythroid, and megakaryocytic hyperplasia. It is seen in some cases of immune-mediated hemolytic anemia in which thrombocytopenia and inflammatory neutrophilia

Table 6.4. Disorders and conditions that cause hypoplastic states in marrow

Generalized marrow hypoplasia
  *Infection in bone marrow: bacterial, fungal, viral, protozoal
  Toxicosis: bracken fern, cephalosporins, chemotherapeutic agents, estrogen, griseofulvin,
    mycotoxins, phenylbutazone, trichloroethylene, trimethoprim-sulfadiazine
  Irradiation: whole body or environmental
  *Marrow necrosis caused by ischemia, infections, or other states
  *Marrow replacement: neoplasia, myelofibrosis, osteopetrosis
Selective erythroid hypoplasia
  *Pure red cell aplasia: immune mediated, after recombinant Epo treatment, possibly
    parvovirus infection
  *FeLV-induced erythroid hypoplasia
  Endocrine: hypothyroidism, hypoadrenocorticism, hypoandrogenism
  Drug induced: chloramphenicol
Selective granulocytic hypoplasia
  Infectious: parvovirus (dogs, cats), FeLV, *Toxoplasma, Ehrlichia* (chronic)
  Toxic: bracken fern, chemotherapeutic drugs, chloramphenicol (cats), estrogen,
    griseofulvin, phenylbutazone, diphenylhydantoin
  Immune-mediated neutropenia
Selective megakaryocytic hypoplasia
  Toxic: bracken fern poisoning (ruminants), chemotherapeutic agents, estrogens in dogs
    (exogenous, endogenous), griseofulvin, meclofenamic acid, phenylbutazone,
    trimethoprim-sulfamethoxazole
  Immune-mediated: amegakaryocytic thrombocytopenia

* A relatively common disease or condition
Note: Lists of specific disorders or conditions are not complete but are provided to give examples.

are concurrent. It can be seen whenever there is a need for a proliferation of neutrophils, erythrocytes, and platelets. It should not be confused with polycythemia vera, a neoplastic state that involves the same cell lines and concurrent erythrocytosis, leukocytosis, and thrombocytosis.

II. *Bone marrow hypoplasia* is a nonspecific term that indicates a decreased number of hematopoietic cells in the bone marrow. Hypoplastic disorders may be caused by absence of stimulating agents, presence of inhibitors, direct damage to the marrow, or direct damage to individual cell lines (Table 6.4).

   A. Generalized marrow hypoplasia

      1. *Aplastic anemia (aplastic pancytopenia)* is the pathologic state in which severe generalized marrow hypoplasia causes nonregenerative anemia, neutropenia, and thrombocytopenia.

      2. Generalized marrow hypoplasia is most reliably identified with a good core bone marrow biopsy sample that consists of what should be active marrow spaces. Tangential cores sometimes yield mostly subcortical marrow that may not be representative of the hematopoietic state.

      3. Many disorders or conditions cause generalized bone marrow hypoplasia, and other disorders have been associated with it,[26,27] but identifying and proving the cause of

the disorder is frequently difficult. The insult to the bone marrow may have occurred weeks before the animal became clinically ill.

B. *Selective erythroid hypoplasia* is a pathologic state in which the number of erythroid precursors is decreased but the granulocytic and megakaryocytic cell lines are not.

1. *Pure red cell aplasia* is a pathologic state in which there is selective erythroid aplasia or severe hypoplasia. It causes development of normocytic, normochromic, nonregenerative anemia.[28]

   a. *Primary pure red cell aplasia* is considered an immune-mediated disorder and may be seen concurrently with immune spherocytic hemolytic anemia. The sera of affected dogs can suppress erythropoiesis. Bone marrow examinations reveal marked erythroid hypoplasia. There have been many reported cases in dogs[15,29] and rare reports in cats.[12]

   b. *Secondary pure red cell aplasia* has occurred secondary to treatment with recombinant human Epo in dogs,[30,31] horses,[32,33] and cats. The selective erythroid hypoplasia that occurs in some FeLV-infected cats and possibly in parvovirus-infected or parvovirus-vaccinated dogs is also considered a form of secondary pure red cell aplasia.[28]

2. Immune-mediated destruction of nucleated erythroid cells: When anemia is caused by destruction of early erythroid precursors (e.g., prorubricytes), an erythropoietic stimulus expands the rubriblast compartment, but erythroid hypoplasia will be present because cell destruction prevents the accumulation of many later stage erythroid cells. The series will be left-shifted and have the appearance of a maturation arrest beginning at the targeted stage.

3. FeLV-induced erythroid hypoplasia

   a. The Kawakami-Theilen strain of FeLV (A, B, and C subgroups present) causes severe erythroid hypoplasia in neonatal kittens but not in weanling or adult cats.[34]

   b. Weanling cats and older cats infected with another strain of FeLV (A and C subgroups present) also can develop erythroid hypoplasia and nonregenerative anemia.[35]

4. Anemia of inflammatory disease (see Chapter 3): Decreased erythropoiesis is part of the pathogenesis of this nonregenerative anemia. Erythroid hypoplasia may not be recognized because it is mild or because concurrent granulocytic hyperplasia may make it difficult to determine whether there is an absolute or a relative decrease in erythroid precursors. However, the presence of nonregenerative anemia in the absence of erythroid hyperplasia supports suppressed erythropoiesis even when erythroid hypoplasia is not apparent.

5. Selective erythroid hypoplasia caused by endocrine disorders: The nonregenerative anemias of hypothyroidism, hypoadrenocorticism, and hypoandrogenism are caused by erythroid hypoplasia, but the degree of hypoplasia in bone marrow samples can be very mild and not recognized in routine bone marrow examinations. The presence of nonregenerative anemia in the absence of erythroid hyperplasia supports suppressed erythropoiesis.

6. Drugs: Chloramphenicol can induce a transient erythroid hypoplasia in dogs[36] and cats.[37] There may be concurrent myeloid and megakaryocytic hypoplasia in cats.

C. *Selective granulocytic hypoplasia* (*agranulocytosis*) is a pathologic state in which the number of granulocyte (neutrophil) precursors is decreased, but the erythroid and megakaryocytic cell lines are not. There are not enough eosinophil and basophil precursors in health for a decrease in these lines to cause granulocytic hypoplasia.

1. Several infections and drugs have been reported to cause selective granulocytic hypoplasia (Table 6.4). However, since many of them have also been associated with hypoplasia of other cell lines, there may be the appearance of selective granulocytic hypoplasia, but damage to other cell lines might not be detected in the same marrow sample. In parvovirus infections, the granulocytic hypoplasia could be caused by damage to cells with mitotic potential, depletion of neutrophil pools because of excessive tissue demand, or endotoxin-induced damage to marrow cells.[38,39] In canine monocytic ehrlichiosis (*Ehrlichia canis*), hypoplasia (typically generalized) may be seen in chronic infections, whereas hyperplasia is seen in acute infections.

2. Animals with immune-mediated neutropenias can have either selective granulocytic hypoplasia accompanied by a left shift (early-stage to midstage destruction) or by ineffective granulopoiesis with granulocytic hyperplasia (late-stage destruction).

D. *Selective megakaryocytic hypoplasia* is a pathologic state in which the number of mega-karyocytes is decreased, but the erythroid and granulocytic cell lines are not.

1. Several infections and drugs have been reported to cause selective megakaryocytic hypoplasia (Table 6.4).

2. Rare cases of apparent immune-mediated amegakaryocytic thrombocytopenia have been reported in dogs.[40] Ineffective thrombopoiesis or megakaryocytic hypoplasia may contribute to thrombocytopenia secondary to immune-mediated damage to megakaryocytes.

III. *Bone marrow lymphocytosis* is a neoplastic (see Bone Marrow Classifications, sect. IX.C) or nonneoplastic accumulation of lymphocytes in the bone marrow. Nonneoplastic lymphocy-tosis may occur from infiltration or local hyperplasia. In tissue sections of bone marrow, the lymphoid cells may occur in nodules, in germinal centers, or as a diffuse population.

A. Because bone marrow is a lymphoid tissue, an inflammatory disease may cause lym-phoid hyperplasia in bone marrow samples, as well as lymph nodes and spleen. The hyperplastic lymphocytes are typically small lymphocytes, but larger forms and plasma cells may be prominent.

B. Small lymphocytes may be up to about 20 % of the nucleated cells in bone marrow samples from healthy cats, but the mean value is about 5–10 %.[41] In contrast, < 5 % (usually < 1 %) are expected in dogs, cattle, and horses.

C. A variety of disorders that involve stimulation of the immune system may cause bone marrow lymphocytosis. Examples include canine ehrlichiosis,[6] systemic lupus erythematosus,[42] and griseofulvin toxicosis.[43] When bone marrow lymphocytosis in cats was defined as > 16 % lymphocytes with > 50 % hematopoietic cellularity, it was associated most commonly with immune-mediated anemia and pure red cell aplasia.[41] Lymphocytes were mostly B-lymphocytes and were often present in aggregates, as opposed to diffusely distributed T-lymphocytes in cases of feline chronic lymphocytic leukemia.

D. When there is granulocytic and erythroid hypoplasia, the lymphocyte population may appear more prominent but be relatively increased rather than absolutely increased.

IV. *Bone marrow mastocytosis* is a neoplastic (see Bone Marrow Classifications, sect. IX.B.5) or nonneoplastic accumulation of mast cells in the bone marrow. Nonneoplastic accumulations may be called mast cell hyperplasia, but mast cells may accumulate by homing of mast cell progenitor cells rather than by increased production of mast cells through cell divisions.

A. Undifferentiated mast cell precursors originate in bone marrow but are not recognized as a separate cell population in routine bone marrow examinations. Occasional mast cells are found in the bone marrow of healthy dogs, cats, and horses and probably represent a resident population.

B. Bone marrow mastocytosis has been reported in dogs with aplastic anemia,[44] regenerative anemia, Fe-deficiency anemia, hypoplasia secondary to a Sertoli cell tumor, and lymphoma.[45]

C. Bone marrow mastocytosis probably represents a reactive state associated with an inflammatory process. Concurrent plasmacytosis is common.

V.   Myelofibrosis
A. *Myelofibrosis* is a pathologic state of increased fibrous connective tissue and collagen in the bone marrow (Plate 9H).

B. In dogs, myelofibrosis is often accompanied by a moderate to severe nonregenerative or poorly regenerative anemia without other cytopenias. However, with extensive myelofibrosis, there is a deficiency in all hematopoietic tissue, and an aplastic anemia (pancytopenia) may develop.

C. The cause of myelofibrosis is usually unknown in domestic mammals. It may be secondary to focal or widespread bone marrow damage, or it may be secondary to a clonal disorder of hemic cells (e.g., MDS), in which mediators from the hemic cells stimulate fibrocytic hyperplasia.[46]

VI. Myelitis
A. *Myelitis*, in the context of hemic disorders, is bone marrow inflammation. Some people use the word *osteomyelitis* to differentiate bone marrow myelitis from spinal cord myelitis, whereas others use the word to indicate concurrent bone inflammation and bone marrow inflammation.

B. There are several agents that can cause myelitis; the inflammatory populations vary with the agent.
   1. Fungal myelitis (histoplasmosis and blastomycosis)
   2. Protozoal myelitis (leishmaniasis) (Plate 9I)
   3. Bacterial myelitis, usually caused by bacteremia or a penetrating wound

VII. Bone marrow necrosis
A. Criteria for establishing the presence of bone marrow necrosis vary, as does the extent and relative significance of necrosis when it is reported. The term bone marrow necrosis may be restricted to bone marrow samples in which necrosis is the primary and predominant abnormality, or it may be applied when necrosis is not the major pathologic process.

B. Bone marrow necrosis must be differentiated from collection and processing artifacts, both cytologically and histologically.
   1. Cytologically, staining and preservation artifacts can mimic cell death, as can cell trauma and lysis during smearing.
   2. Crush artifact and plasma pools have been interpreted as evidence of necrosis in sections of bone marrow cores.

    C. Bone marrow necrosis has been reported in association with many disorders, including toxicants, bacterial sepsis, monocytic ehrlichiosis, canine parvovirus infection, feline panleukopenia, systemic lupus erythematosus, lymphoma, disseminated intravascular coagulation, and hypoxia.[47] However, the extent of the necrosis has not always been reported, cause-and-effect relationships are generally unproven, and the clinical significance of the finding is often unknown.

    D. Bone marrow necrosis has been considered idiopathic when unassociated with an underlying disease or with drug exposure,[47] though association with a disorder does not make it a cause-and-effect relationship, so it is usually idiopathic in those cases, as well. Eight of nine dogs classified as having idiopathic bone marrow necrosis had evidence of individual cell death rather than coagulation necrosis; the extent of cell death was not reported. These dogs also had marked anemia (sometimes with neutropenia or thrombocytopenia), mild to marked myelofibrosis, and sometimes a prominent macrophage population. The significance of cell death in these cases and its contribution to the hematologic abnormalities are not clear.

    E. Myelofibrosis may be the "healing" stage or chronic stage of some bone marrow necrosis disorders.

VIII. Myelophthisis

    A. Strictly speaking, *myelophthisis* means "marrow wasting" (*myelo-* plus *-phthisis*) or wasting of the spinal cord.

    B. The term is commonly used to indicate failure of the bone marrow to produce cells because of replacement or displacement of bone marrow by abnormal tissue. Causes of myelophthisis include neoplastic cell proliferation, myelofibrosis, and osteopetrosis. If the disease process has affected most bone marrow sites, animals will develop anemia, neutropenia, and thrombocytopenia (aplastic anemia; also known as aplastic pancytopenia).

IX. Bone marrow hemic cell neoplasia

    A. General concepts and terms

        1. Neoplasia of bone marrow hemic cells is not as common as many other forms of neoplasia in domestic mammals. The general diagnosis of hemic cell neoplasia is not difficult when there are numerous poorly differentiated cells in a blood or bone marrow sample, but establishing the cell of origin can be difficult. It can also be difficult to differentiate neoplasia of well-differentiated hemic cells from inflammatory conditions. Specific diagnoses may be reached by a combination of exclusionary tests, immunophenotyping and possibly cytochemical staining of blood or bone marrow by means of panels of antibodies and stains, bone marrow examination, and molecular genetic testing (Fig. 6.2).

        2. Characterization and classification of hemic neoplasms in domestic mammals[24,48,49] (see Table 6.5) has generally followed developments in understanding and classification of similar human neoplasms, many of which are now defined by specific genetic mutations.[50] The human model has provided useful insights into the forms of hemic neoplasia that may occur in domestic animals, but substantial investigation is needed in veterinary medicine to reach a similar degree of characterization.

        3. Bone marrow hemic cell neoplasia may arise in the bone marrow (e.g., acute myeloid leukemias) or spread to the bone marrow (e.g., lymphoma).

Table 6.5. Classifications of hemic cell neoplasia involving blood or marrow

Classification	Cell type
Lymphoproliferative neoplasia	Lymphocyte
*Acute lymphocytic leukemia	B-, T-, or NK-lymphocyte
Chronic lymphocytic leukemia	B-, T-, or NK-lymphocyte
*Lymphoma	B-, T-, or NK-lymphocyte
Plasma cell myeloma	B-lymphocyte
Myeloid neoplasia	Nonlymphoid hemic cell
Acute myeloid leukemias[a]	Nonlymphoid hemic cell
Acute myeloblastic with minimal differentiation (M0)[b]	Granulocyte
Acute myeloblastic without maturation (M1)	Granulocyte
Acute myeloblastic with maturation (M2)	Granulocyte
Acute promyelocytic leukemia (M3)[c]	Granulocyte
*Acute myelomonocytic leukemia (M4)	Granulocyte and monocyte
Acute monocytic leukemia (M5)[d]	Monocyte
Acute erythroleukemia (M6)	Erythrocyte, nonlymphoid leukocyte, megakaryocyte
Acute erythroleukemia with erythroid predominance (M6-Er)[e]	Erythrocyte, nonlymphoid leukocyte, megakaryocyte[e]
Megakaryoblastic leukemia (M7)	Megakaryocyte
Acute leukemia of ambiguous lineage	Unknown, mixed, or multiple (see the text)
Chronic myeloproliferative disorders	Nonlymphoid hemic cell
Chronic myeloid leukemia	Neutrophil
Eosinophilic leukemia	Eosinophil
Basophilic leukemia	Basophil
Primary erythrocytosis	Erythrocyte
Polycythemia vera	Erythrocyte, neutrophil, and megakaryocyte
Thrombocythemia	Megakaryocyte
Myelodysplastic/myeloproliferative disease	Nonlymphoid hemic cell
Chronic myelomonocytic leukemia[f]	Neutrophil and monocyte
Myelodysplastic syndrome[g]	Leukocyte, erythroid cell, and/or megakaryocyte
Mast cell neoplasia[h]	Mast cell
*Metastatic mast cell neoplasms (cutaneous or visceral)	Mast cell
Mast cell leukemia	Mast cell

* A relatively common disease or condition

[a] Modified from the classification system recommended by an Animal Leukemia Study Group of the American Society for Veterinary Clinical Pathology.[24] These leukemias fall into the WHO category of *acute myeloid leukemia not otherwise categorized.*[50]

[b] The "M" abbreviation system is used in the French-American-British classification and was used by the ALSG but is not used in the current WHO nomenclature. The ALSG classification omitted acute myeloblastic leukemia with minimal differentiation, a diagnosis requiring immunophenotyping and ultrastructural evaluation that were not available to the study group.

[c] Human acute promyelocytic leukemia is typically associated with defined mutations and is therefore categorized as *AML with recurrent genetic abnormalities* rather than as an otherwise uncategorized leukemia.

[d] The ALSG did not separate M5 into acute monoblastic leukemia (M5a) and acute monocytic leukemia (M5b) because of difficulties in differentiating monoblasts from promonocytes, but others have made the distinction in animals as is done in human classification schemes.

[e] The current human WHO system includes a pure erythroid leukemia.

[f] CMMoL is classified here according to the WHO system, which recognizes that this condition has features of a myeloproliferative disease and a MDS.

[g] See the text for proposed MDS classifications.

[h] Because mast cells originate from a myeloid stem cell (see Chapter 2), mast cell neoplasia is considered myeloid neoplasia.

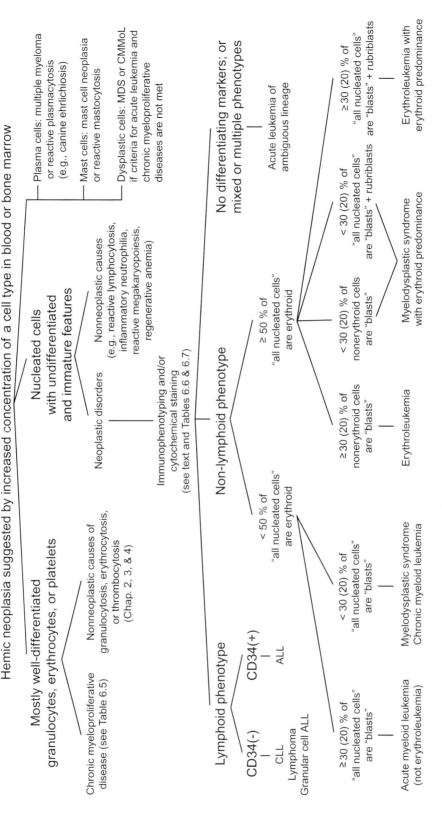

Fig. 6.2. The algorithm to use when hemic neoplasia is suspected because of an increased concentration of well-differentiated or atypical cells in blood or bone marrow:

- An increased concentration of well-differentiated erythrocytes, platelets, lymphocytes, monocytes, neutrophils, eosinophils, or basophils could be neoplastic or nonneoplastic.
    - ◆ Nonneoplastic disorders or conditions include appropriate or secondary inappropriate erythrocytosis, reactive thrombocytosis, or various types of inflammation.
    - ◆ Exclusion of nonneoplastic disorders or conditions incriminates one of the chronic myeloproliferative diseases (see Table 6.5), but confirmatory cytogenetic tests are currently unavailable.
- An increased population of nucleated cells with undifferentiated and immature features may be neoplastic or nonneoplastic. Neoplasia may or may not be obvious, depending mostly on the size of the population.
    - ◆ Nonneoplastic immature populations in blood or bone marrow may increase with reactive lymphocytosis, proliferation of immature granulocytes in a severe inflammatory reaction, reactive megakaryocytic hyperplasia, or markedly stimulated erythropoiesis in a severe regenerative anemia.
    - ◆ If findings do not support nonneoplastic disorders or conditions, hemic neoplasia should be characterized by immunophenotyping and possibly cytochemical staining of blood or bone marrow by means of panels of antibodies and stains.
        - ■ If cells have a lymphoid phenotype, CD34 positivity supports ALL, whereas a CD34-negative population of lymphocytes may be chronic lymphocytic leukemia, lymphoma involving bone marrow and/or blood, or ALL of granular lymphocytes.
        - ■ If atypical cells do not express identifying markers, that is evidence for an acute undifferentiated leukemia. Other rare acute leukemias of ambiguous origin include those consisting of more than one distinct atypical population (e.g., lymphoid blasts and myeloid blasts) or of one population of atypical cells expressing multiple phenotypes (e.g., lymphoid and myeloid markers).
        - ■ If cells have a nonlymphoid phenotype, they may be identified as megakaryoblasts, rubriblasts, monoblasts, myeloblasts, or myelomonoblasts. Bone marrow analysis is needed to classify these proliferations.
- If erythroid cells are the minority of "all nucleated cells" and at least 30 % (or 20 % using the current human guideline) of "all nucleated cells" are "blasts," then the patient has an acute myeloid leukemia other than erythroleukemia.
- If the erythroid cells are the minority of "all nucleated cells" and less than 30 % (20 %) of "all nucleated cells" are "blasts," one should consider MDS or a chronic myeloid leukemia. Prominent dysplasia and ineffective hematopoiesis support MDS. A left-shifted granulocyte series with effective granulopoiesis would support chronic myeloid leukemia.
- When erythroid cells are at least half of "all nucleated cells," either the percentage of nonerythroid cells that are "blasts" or the percentage of "all nucleated cells" that are "blasts" plus rubriblasts is used to determine whether there is erythroleukemia, erythroleukemia with erythroid predominance, or MDS with erythroid predominance.
- If the atypical cells are clearly plasma cells, reactive plasmacytosis must be differentiated from a plasma cell myeloma.
- If the cells are clearly mast cells, reactive mastocytosis must be differentiated from metastatic mast cell neoplasia and mast cell leukemia.
- If dysplasia is prominent and the cells do not fulfill criteria for acute myeloid leukemia or one of the chronic myeloproliferative diseases, then a MDS or myelodysplastic/myeloproliferative disease (e.g., CMMoL) should be considered.

All nucleated cells includes granulocytic, erythroid, and megakaryocytic cells, and excludes lymphocytes, plasma cells, monocytes, macrophages, and mast cells. *Nonerythroid cells* means "all nucleated cells" that are not nucleated erythroid cells, and *blasts* means myeloblasts, megakaryoblasts, monoblasts ± promonocytes, and atypical promyelocytes but not rubriblasts and lymphoblasts. ALL, acute lymphocytic leukemia; CLL, chronic lymphocytic leukemia; MDS, myelodysplastic syndrome; and CMMoL, chronic myelomonocytic leukemia, classified by the WHO system for hemic neoplasia as a myelodysplastic/myeloproliferative disease rather than MDS or one of the chronic myeloproliferative diseases.

4. The term *leukemia* is from the Greek *leukos* ("white") + *haima* ("blood") = "white blood" and refers to an increased buffy coat layer. It is the presence of neoplastic hemic cells in either blood or bone marrow because of a neoplastic proliferation originating in the bone marrow or, sometimes, the spleen. Not all hemic neoplasia originating in the bone marrow is considered leukemia; for example, myelodysplastic syndrome, plasma cell myeloma, and some chronic myeloproliferative diseases such as essential thrombocythemia are not leukemias.

5. *Acute leukemia* is a relatively more rapid proliferation of less differentiated hemic cells. It typically consists of many blast cells, and the illness is brief (unless treated). The microscopic criteria used for considering cells to be blasts are neither clear nor uniform, but CD34 expression supports classification as an acute leukemia.

6. A *blast cell* is an immature cell with replicative potential. Blasts typically have smooth or finely stippled chromatin and lack features of well-differentiated cells.
   a. The term is often used for certain relatively large cells with basophilic cytoplasms and visible nucleoli (e.g., myeloblasts, monoblasts, rubriblasts, megakaryoblasts, and some lymphoblasts).
   b. However, the term also refers to cells of small to intermediate size that lack increased cytoplasmic basophilia and prominent nucleoli (e.g., pluripotent stem cells).
   c. Commonly, lymphoblasts are defined as large lymphocytes with basophilic cytoplasms, finely stippled chromatin patterns, and prominent nucleoli. However, in the context of lymphoproliferative neoplasia, lymphoblasts are defined as small lymphocytes with finely stippled chromatin patterns and inconspicuous or absent nucleoli. Therefore, the term *lymphoblast* may be used to refer to cells with different microscopic appearances.
   d. CD34 expression supports the blastic nature of a hemic cell.
   e. Note that the term *erythroblast* refers to any nucleated erythrocyte in human medicine.

7. *Chronic leukemia* is a slower proliferation or accumulation (decreased apoptosis) of relatively well-differentiated hemic cells that are similar in appearance to the mature cells (e.g., neutrophils or lymphocytes). An animal may live for months after diagnosis, even without treatment. The microscopic criteria used for considering cells to be well-differentiated are neither clear nor uniform.

8. The term *myeloproliferative disease* is used specifically in a restricted context referring to those clonal conditions classified as *chronic myeloproliferative disease* (see Bone marrow hemic cell neoplasia in the following sect. B.4). However, it is often used more generally to refer to any proliferative neoplastic disorder of nonlymphoid hemic cells, including neutrophils, eosinophils, basophils, monocytes, erythrocytes, megakaryocytes, and perhaps mast cells.

9. *Lymphoproliferative disease* refers to a proliferation of lymphocytes, usually implying a neoplastic proliferation. *Lymphoproliferative neoplasia* (lymphoid neoplasia) clarifies that the proliferation is not reactive inflammation and includes any neoplastic proliferation of any type of lymphoid cell, including plasma cells. In some conditions, the major reason for increased lymphocyte numbers may actually be decreased cell death rather than increased cell proliferation.

B. Myeloid neoplasia: Classification of myeloid neoplasms in dogs and cats was described in 1991 by the ALSG, a multi-institutional group of veterinary clinical pathologists using human classification systems that have since been modified.[24,50] It is also addressed in a publication of the Armed Forces Institute of Pathology (AFIP) and the WHO (AFIP/WHO classification) as part of a series on histologic classification of tumors of domestic animals.[49] However, as noted in a recent review, further investigations are needed to define appropriate classifications and diagnostic criteria for myeloid neoplasia in domestic animals.[48] Until that occurs, the ALSG, AFIP/WHO, and human classifications are useful guidelines to understand the types of myeloid neoplasms that may affect veterinary patients. These guidelines were used to construct the algorithm presented in Fig. 6.2.

1. *AMLs* are acute leukemias involving nonlymphoid leukocyte, erythroid, megakaryocyte, or undifferentiated precursors. *Differentiation* refers to commitment to a particular lineage.
   a. In the human classification scheme, except in cases of erythroid leukemias or when a specific genetic mutation is identified that defines a human leukemia as AML, blasts or so-called blast equivalents (myeloblasts, megakaryoblasts, monoblasts ± promonocytes, and atypical promyelocytes) must account for > 20 % of all nucleated cells in the bone marrow (excluding plasma cells, lymphocytes, macrophages, and mast cells).
      (1) The blast percentage decision threshold used to be 30 %, and that is what was adopted by the ALSG for animals. However, human conditions with 20–29 % blasts (previously MDS rather than AML) appear to behave clinically like those with 30 % or more blasts (AML) (Fig. 6.2).
      (2) In erythroid leukemias, when > 50 % of the nucleated cells in the marrow are erythroid, there may be too few blasts or blast equivalents to meet criteria for AML. Different criteria are used in these cases (Fig. 6.2):
         (a) Blasts (myeloblasts, megakaryoblasts, monoblasts ± promonocytes, and atypical promyelocytes) are enumerated relative to the number of nonerythroid cells rather than all nucleated cells. When at least 20 % (30 % previously and according to the ALSG) of the nonerythroid cells are blasts, acute erythroid leukemia can be diagnosed.
         (b) In cases of rare erythroid leukemia with little or no myeloblastic component, criteria for pure erythroid leukemia (also referred to as DiGuglielmo disease, acute erythremic myelosis, or "true erythroleukemia") have been established in people and criteria for erythroid leukemia with erythroid predominance (M6-Er) have been defined for dogs and cats (usually cats). According to the ALSG, criteria for M6-Er are fulfilled in cats when blasts (myeloblasts, megakaryoblasts, monoblasts ± promonocytes, and atypical promyelocytes) are < 30 % of nonerythroid cells, but these blasts plus rubriblasts are at least 30 % of all nucleated cells.
   b. Five general categories of AML have been described in human medicine.[50] They are provided here as a basis for understanding categories that may be defined in domestic mammals.
      (1) *AML with recurrent genetic abnormalities*: This classification requires identification of specific recognized clonal genetic abnormalities (translocations or inversions) that define the neoplastic population.
      (2) *AML with multilineage dysplasia*: These leukemias either arise following MDS or MDS/MPD, or they have dysplasia in at least 50 % of the cells in two or more myeloid lineages.

(3) Therapy-related AML and MDS: These clonal proliferation arise months to years after therapies including alkylating agents, radiation, and topoisomerase inhibitors.

(4) *AML not otherwise categorized*: This category is used for AMLs that do not fit into one of the other categories, including when genetic information is lacking, and is where most veterinary AMLs fall. Classification is similar to the French-American-British system and is based mostly on lineage(s) and the degree of maturation, where *maturation* refers to microscopic structural changes associated with development of cell functions. The current WHO classification is similar to the ALSG classification, but with several differences (Table 6.5).

    (a) The WHO now uses only names and not M numbers (i.e., M1 to M7) to classify AMLs.

    (b) The WHO does not include the acute promyelocytic leukemia category.

    (c) The WHO also includes the following: acute myeloid leukemia, minimally differentiated; acute monoblastic leukemia; pure erythroleukemia; acute basophilic leukemia; acute panmyelosis with myelofibrosis; and myeloid sarcoma.

(5) Acute leukemias of ambiguous lineage: Blast cells lack identifying characteristics and can appear lymphoid. This category includes bilineal leukemias consisting of two distinct blast populations, combined myeloid and lymphoid leukemias, undifferentiated acute leukemias lacking lymphoid or myeloid markers, and biphenotypic acute leukemias with lymphoid and myeloid markers.

2. *Myelodysplastic syndromes* (MDSs) are a group of clonal disorders in which there is typically ineffective hematopoiesis (marrow proliferation of a cell line concurrent with cytopenia of the same cell line) and microscopic evidence in blood or bone marrow of abnormal maturation of hemic cells (i.e., dyshematopoiesis such as dysmyelopoiesis).[51] Involvement of multiple cell lines appears to stem from neoplastic transformation of multipotential hematopoietic stem cells.

    a. To be classified as MDS, blasts (defined as myeloblasts, megakaryoblasts, monoblasts ± promonocytes, and atypical promyelocytes) can account for only up to 20 % (30 % according to the ALSG) of all marrow nucleated cells (excluding plasma cells, lymphocytes, macrophages, and mast cells) when < 50 % of all marrow nucleated cells are erythroid; with ≥ 20 % (or ≥ 30 %) blasts, the diagnosis would be AML. When erythroid cells account for > 50 % of all marrow nucleated cells, MDS-Er is defined by blasts (myeloblasts, megakaryoblasts, monoblasts ± promonocytes, and atypical promyelocytes) being < 20 % (30 %) of nonerythroid cells, and rubriblasts plus blasts (as just defined) being < 20 % (30 %) of all nucleated cells (Fig. 6.2).

    b. The dysplastic changes that may be observed in MDS include the following:[24,52]

        (1) *Dysmyelopoiesis* (Plate 9K): giant cell size, abundance of azurophilic granules, hypogranular cytoplasms, polyploidy or hypersegmented neutrophil nuclei, or Pelger-Huët cell features (hyposegmentation)

        (2) *Dyserythropoiesis* (Plate 9L): multiple nuclei, nuclear fragmentation, megaloblastic appearance, excessive cytoplasm relative to the nucleus, abnormal distribution of siderosomes, macrocytosis, or unequal nuclear division

(3) *Dysmegakaryopoiesis* (Plate 9M) and *dysthrombopoiesis*: nonlobed large nucleus, multiple small nuclei, dwarf megakaryocytes (micro-megakaryocytes), megaplatelets, or abnormal cytoplasmic granularity or vacuolation of platelets

c. Microscopic detection of dysplastic changes is subjective, and the degree of concordance among clinical pathologists for recognizing dyshematopoieis in veterinary medicine is unknown. It is the authors' experience that there is a great deal of variation in the stringency of individual clinical pathologist's criteria for labeling changes as dysplastic as opposed to within the normal spectrum of variation.

d. Classifications

(1) A basic veterinary MDS classification proposed by the ALSG divided MDS into three groups: MDS, MDS-Er, and CMMoL.[24] This system was modified by Raskin by dividing MDS into two groups (MDS-RC and MDS-EB), thus generating four classifications of MDS in mammals: MDS-RC, MDS-EB, MDS-Er, and CMMoL.[52] Three categories of MDS are described in the *Histological Classification of Hematopoietic Tumors of Domestic Animals*:[49] idiopathic myelofibrosis/myeloid metaplasia (categorized as a chronic myeloproliferative disease), CMMoL, and refractory anemia with excess blasts (RAEB). Other categories have been proposed.[48,53,54] CMMoL has most recently been categorized as a myelodysplastic/myeloproliferative neoplasia in people (see the following sect. 3 and Table 6.5), not a MDS.

(2) The WHO classifications of human MDS are provided here because there is no clear consensus on the classification categories or criteria for MDS in domestic animals.

(a) *Refractory anemia (RA)*: bone marrow with < 5 % blasts, < 15 % ringed sideroblasts (nucleated erythrocytes with a ring of stainable Fe around the nucleus), and erythrodysplasia

(b) *Refractory anemia with ringed sideroblasts (RARS)*: similar to RA but with at least 15 % ringed sideroblasts

(c) *Refractory cytopenia with multilineage dysplasia (RCMD)*: cytopenias with < 1000 monocytes/μL; and bone marrow with < 5 % blasts, < 15 % ringed sideroblasts, and bilineage or trilineage dysplasia

(d) *Refractory cytopenia with multilineage dysplasia and ringed sideroblasts (RCMD-RS)*: similar to RCMD but with at least 15 % ringed sideroblasts

(e) *Refractory anemia with excess blasts 1 (RAEB-1)*: cytopenias with < 1000 monocytes/μL and < 5 % blasts in blood, one or more dysplastic cell lines, and 5–9 % bone marrow blasts

(f) *Refractory anemia with excess blasts 2 (RAEB-2)*: like RAEB-1 but with < 19 % blasts in blood and 10–19 % bone marrow blasts

(g) *Myelodysplastic syndrome, unclassified (MDS-U)*: cytopenias with granulocytic or megakaryocytic dysplasia and < 5 % blasts in bone marrow

(h) *MDS associated with isolated del(5q)*: anemia with < 5 % blasts in blood and normal to increased platelet concentration; also with normal to increased numbers of megakaryocytes with hypolobulated nuclei in bone marrow, < 5 % blasts, and isolated del(5q)

   e. Domestic mammals and people with a MDS may develop AML, and thus MDS has been considered a preleukemic disorder.

   f. MDS must be differentiated from nonneoplastic congenital dyshematopoiesis disorders:

      (1) Hereditary poodle marrow dyscrasia (poodle macrocytosis)

      (2) Malabsorption of cobalamin (vitamin B_{12}) in giant schnauzers, Border collies, Australian shepherd dogs, and beagles

      (3) Dyserythropoiesis in English springer spaniels

      (4) Congenital dyserythropoiesis and progressive alopecia of polled Hereford calves

      (5) Possibly idiopathic thrombocytopenia in Cavalier King Charles spaniels.[55]

   g. MDS must also be differentiated from *acquired secondary dyshematopoiesis* disorders in which dysplastic changes are neither congenital nor clonal.[56] Dysplastic features should resolve with alleviation of the underlying condition. Dyshematopoiesis had been reported in association with the following acquired conditions in dogs and cats:[53–55]

      (1) Toxicants: lead toxicity, chemotherapeutic drugs, estrogen, cephalosporins, chloramphenicol, phenobarbital, and colchicine

      (2) Nutritional deficiency: Fe deficiency

      (3) Immune-mediated disease: immune-mediated hemolytic anemia and immune-mediated thrombocytopenia (dysmegakaryopoiesis)

      (4) Inflammation (sideroblastic anemias): septicemia, pyometra, pancreatitis, hepatitis, glomerulonephritis, and feline infectious peritonitis

      (5) Neoplasia: lymphoma, multiple myeloma, and polycythemia vera (primary erythrocytosis by the criteria of this textbook)

      (6) Myelofibrosis, although dyshematopoiesis associated with myelofibrosis may prove to be neoplastic in some cases

3. Myelodysplastic/myeloproliferative diseases (Table 6.5) include conditions that may have myelodysplastic and/or myeloproliferative features.

   a. *Chronic myelomonocytic leukemia* fulfills the criteria and occurs in dogs. There is typically leukopenia and nonregenerative anemia with a hypercellular bone marrow and atypical hypersegmented monocytoid cells in blood, bone marrow, and often lymph nodes. Fewer than 10 % of the nucleated cells are blasts, and the disorder has a chronic course.

   b. Other conditions described in human patients have not been recognized in animals: atypical chronic myeloid leukemia, juvenile myelomonocytic leukemia, and unclassifiable myelodysplastic/myeloproliferative disease.

4. *Chronic myeloproliferative diseases*: This group, which includes several specific chronic clonal disorders of pluripotential stem cells, is characterized by excessive proliferation or accumulation of differentiated neoplastic cells that have few or no microscopic or functional abnormalities (Table 6.5). Tools to detect clonality and prove neoplasia are generally unavailable for these conditions in domestic animals. Diagnosis is often based on exclusion of other conditions, but differentiation from nonneoplastic conditions is difficult because the cells are well differentiated (Fig. 6.2).

   a. *Chronic myelogenous leukemia* (also known as chronic granulocytic leukemia or chronic myeloid leukemia) is characterized by a neutrophilia and typically a left shift. Chronic eosinophilic leukemia (and possibly hypereosinophilic syndrome) and chronic basophilic leukemia are variants.

   b. *Polycythemia vera* and *primary erythrocytosis* must be differentiated from other causes of erythrocytosis (see Chapter 3).

   c. *Megakaryocyte myelosis* or *essential thrombocythemia* must be differentiated from marked megakaryocyte hyperplasia and reactive thrombocytosis.

   d. *Chronic idiopathic myelofibrosis with extramedullary hematopoiesis* must be differentiated from secondary myelofibrosis. Proof that idiopathic myelofibrosis is a neoplastic entity in domestic animals is currently lacking.

5. *Mast cell disease* (*mastocytosis*): Mastocytemia may be reactive (nonneoplastic) or neoplastic. When neoplastic, it is usually associated with solid tissue mast cell tumors and rarely caused by mast cell leukemia. *Mast cell leukemia* is characterized by a bone marrow and blood distribution of mast cells with secondary infiltrates in other organs, particularly liver and spleen. Cells may be atypical, and myelophthisis may be severe.

C. *Lymphoid neoplasia* (Fig. 6.2) is neoplasia of undifferentiated or differentiated lymphoid cells, including plasma cells. *Lymphocytic neoplasia*, neoplasia of lymphocytes, has been classically divided into *lymphomas* (solid tissue origin) and *leukemias* (primarily bone marrow and blood origin and distribution). Lymphomas may enter a leukemic phase with bone marrow and blood involvement, but a predominant tissue distribution and late development of blood involvement signal lymphoma.

1. Lymphoid leukemias may be divided by cell type into B-lymphocyte, T-lymphocyte, or NK-lymphocyte leukemias (see Table 6.5). Immunophenotyping is required to identify the cell type (see the following sect. E.4 and Table 6.7). They may be acute or chronic.

   a. Granular lymphocyte leukemias consist of lymphocytes with cytoplasmic granules. The cells are either T-lymphocytes or NK-lymphocytes, and the leukemias may be acute or chronic.

   b. Clinical studies incorporating immunophenotyping and assessment of involved organs supports that chronic lymphocytic leukemia of B-lymphocytes in dogs is a primary bone marrow disease, but acute and chronic lymphocytic leukemias of granular T-lymphocytes appear to originate in the spleen with later marrow involvement.[57]

2. Lymphoma originating in any tissue may eventually involve the bone marrow (see the Lymph Node: Major Concepts and Terms section).

3. *Plasma cell myeloma* is a clonal proliferation of differentiated B-lymphocytes within the bone marrow, typically at multiple sites (*multiple myeloma*). Circulating plasma cells are rarely seen (Plate 9N).

   a. Although the cells are differentiated, they may have varying degrees of maturation and may not have a mature plasma cell appearance.

   b. These neoplasms are often associated with osteolysis and monoclonal gammopathies due to excessive production of immunoglobulin A (IgA), IgG, or IgM.

   c. Other laboratory abnormalities may include Bence Jones proteinuria, hypercalcemia, hypoalbuminemia, azotemia, and hyperviscosity

   d. A cutaneous or noncutaneous proliferation of neoplastic plasma cells outside of the bone marrow is an *extramedullary plasmacytoma*.

D. *Histiocytic neoplasia*: Histiocytic malignancies consist of cells that are derived from monocytes. Dendritic cells are specialized for antigen presentation, and macrophages are more specialized for phagocytosis. The functions of these two cell types are reflected by their immunophenotypes.

1. In dogs, *hemophagocytic histiocytic sarcoma* is a proliferation of splenic red pulp and bone marrow macrophages that express, among other markers, CD11d and, inconsistently, CD1c and CD11c.[58]
   a. Neoplastic cells in the bone marrow cells may appear relatively well differentiated or atypical. Neoplastic cells are consistently present in the spleen, where they may have more atypia. Other tissues may be involved (e.g., liver and lung).
   b. Most dogs have a regenerative anemia, thrombocytopenia, hypoalbuminemia, and hypocholesterolemia.

2. *Malignant histiocytic sarcoma* (*malignant histiocytosis*) of dendritic cell origin is a malignant proliferation of interstitial dendritic cells which express, among other markers, CD1c and CD11c, but not CD11d.[59]
   a. Pleomorphic populations of neoplastic cells are present in bone marrow and spleen, lungs, liver, or lymph nodes. Phagocytosis may be present.
   b. Other findings are variable and nonspecific, including anorexia, lethargy, weakness, and weight loss.

3. These malignancies must be differentiated from (1) systemic histiocytosis, (2) nonneoplastic hemophagocytic syndromes occurring in association with infections and other malignancies, (3) immune-mediated destruction of hematopoietic cells, and (4) macrophagic inflammation.
   a. Malignant histiocytic proliferations typically have atypia, though it may be more apparent in other tissues (Plate 9O). The number of cells in the bone marrow is typically greater than in other conditions, and cells are more likely to be in clusters.
   b. Phagocytic activity appears nonselective in hemophagocytic histiocytic sarcoma and hemophagocytic syndrome (authors' experience) (Plate 9O), but is typically selective for a particular lineage and maturation stage in marrow-directed immune-mediated anemia (Plate 9G) and neutropenia.
   c. With inflammation, other inflammatory cells may be present along with organisms or necrotic cells.
   d. Attempts have been made using flow cytometry to differentiate malignant and benign histiocytic bone marrow proliferations.[60]

E. Methods of classifying hemic cell neoplasia (Fig 6.2)
   1. The major goal of classification schemes is to determine and communicate the cell of origin with hopes that it can be used to reliably provide prognostic information and therapeutic recommendations. Two major problems with current classifications schemes are (1) the most simple and inexpensive method, microscopic appearance on a Wright-stained sample, has major limitations and can be inaccurate, and (2) other methods are not widely available and are expensive.
   2. Microscopic evaluation of Wright-stained blood films or bone marrow preparations
      a. The primary value of these evaluations is to detect the presence of neoplastic hemic cells. This may be obvious when there is a large population of atypical cells, but it may be difficult when there are fewer cells or when neoplastic cells have mature features compatible with an inflammatory population.
      b. Finding cells that have nuclear or cytoplasmic features that are unique or more common in certain differentiated cell lines is the first step in characterizing the neoplasia. When the cells are immature or lack differentiation, it can be very difficult to classify the cells reliably by their light microscopic appearance; that is, blast cells could be of one of several cell types.

Table 6.6. Expected cytochemical staining reactions of normal or neoplastic hemic cells in dogs and cats

Cell	Cytochemical stains[a]				
	PO	SBB	CAE	LAP	NBE
Neutrophil	+	+	+	+ (immature)	−
Lymphocyte	−	−	−	−[b]	−/focal +
Monocyte	±	±	−	−[b]	+ (diffuse)
Eosinophil	+ in dog − in cat	+ in dog − in cat	−	±	−
Basophil	−	−	+	±	−
Megakaryocyte	−	−	±	−	±

[a] PO, peroxidase; SBB, Sudan black B; CAE, chloracetate esterase; LAP, leukocyte alkaline phosphatase; and NBE, α-naphthyl butyrate esterase

[b] Positive results have been reported.

Note: Negative staining does not exclude cell lines; positive staining supports certain cell lines; ± indicates that weak or sporadic staining may occur in normal or neoplastic cells.

    c. The neoplasia is classified most accurately by other methods after first being identified by visual inspection.

  3. Cytochemical stains[48,61]

    a. These are helpful for differentiating the lineage(s) of leukemic cells.

    b. The basic premise behind the use of cytochemical stains is that leukemic cells may contain enzymes or compounds that are common or unique to certain cell lines. For example, neutrophils and monocytes contain peroxidase, whereas lymphocytes, erythrocyte precursors, and megakaryocytes do not. However, poorly differentiated myeloid precursors may not contain enough analyte for a positive reaction, or staining may be equivocal.

    c. Staining may be more prominent in immature cells than in mature cells. For example, alkaline phosphatase activity is present in canine myeloblasts but not mature neutrophils.

    d. The use of cytochemical stains for differentiation of leukemias is limited to a few special hematology laboratories and is of most value when a panel of stains is used (Table 6.6) and when assessed in conjunction with other findings.

    e. Positive staining of acute leukemia cells for peroxidase, phospholipid, chloracetate esterase, leukocyte alkaline phosphatase, or α-naphthyl butyrate esterase (diffuse) supports a nonlymphoid lineage. Staining with α-naphthyl butyrate esterase (diffuse) and chloracetate esterase supports a myelomonocytic population. Cells that appear lymphoid in Wright-stained marrow or blood often prove to be myeloid/monocytic when cytochemical stains are applied.

    f. Some cytochemical stains can be used on appropriately fixed plastic-embedded tissues.[48]

  4. *Immunophenotyping*[62,63] is the use of antibodies to detect cellular epitopes that help to classify cell types. It is typically used to characterize neoplasia, not to confirm it.

    a. The use of monoclonal antibodies has enabled the identification of surface antigens on a variety of cell types. If a group or cluster of monoclonal antibodies recognizes the same antigen, that antigen is assigned a CD number (Table 6.7).

Table 6.7. Selected immunophenotyping targets useful in immunodiagnostics of hemic cells in dogs

Cell marker	Function	Cells detected	Comments
CD1 (a–c)	Antigen-presenting molecules	Cortical thymocytes, dendritic cells; CD1c is expressed on some monocytes and B-lymphocytes	Useful to detect dendritic antigen presenting cells; not expressed by mature T-lymphocytes
CD3 (CD3ε)[a]	Part of the TCR complex	Mature T-lymphocytes, activated NK-lymphocytes (cytoplasm)	Useful to identify T-lymphocyte leukemia/lymphoma; αβ- and γδ-T-lymphocytes not differentiated
CD4	Protein that associates with TCR	MHC[b] class II–restricted T-helper cells, neutrophils	Monocytes, macrophages, dendritic cells can express when activated
CD8	Dimeric protein associated with TCR	MHC class I–restricted cytotoxic T-lymphocytes (usually CD8αβ heterodimer)	A subset of NK-lymphocytes may express (CD8αα homodimer)
CD11[a]	α-Subunit of the leukocyte adhesion molecule family of β2-integrins	CD11a: All leukocytes CD11b: Granulocytes, monocytes, some macrophages CD11c: Granulocytes, monocytes, dendritic antigen-presenting cells CD11d: Macrophages and T-lymphocytes in splenic red pulp, granular lymphocytes including NK-lymphocytes	Useful as a panleukocyte marker Useful as a marker of nonlymphoid leukocytes Useful to recognize histiocytic neoplasms of antigen-presenting cells Useful to recognize hemophagocytic histiocytic sarcoma
CD18[a]	β2-Subunit of the leukocyte adhesion molecule family of β2-integrins	All leukocytes but less expression in lymphocytes	Useful to confirm the hemic cell origin of round cells in tissue; deficient in Irish setters with leukocyte adhesion deficiency

Marker	Description	Cell expression	Comments
CD21 and CD21-like[a]	Complement receptor (CR2) associated with the BCR[b] complex	Mature B-lymphocytes, follicular dendritic cells of germinal centers	Useful to identify B-cell lymphoma and B-cell leukemia
CD34	Surface glycoprotein that binds selectins	Lympho-hematopoietic stem cells and progenitor cells	Helps differentiate ALL[b] from lymphoma; CLL[b], lymphoma, myeloma cells are negative
CD41	α_2-Integrin (GPIIb)[b] of the fibrinogen receptor	Megakaryocytes (and platelets)	By flow cytometry, cells may appear positive because of adherent platelets
CD45[a]	Membrane tyrosine phosphatase	All hemic cells but erythroid cells; cells express different isoforms	CD45RA isoform detected in fixed tissues but not expressed on all leukocytes (some T-lymphocytes)
CD61	β_3-Integrin (GPIIIa) of the fibrinogen receptor	Megakaryocytes, platelets; other cells include endothelial cells	By flow cytometry, cells may appear positive because of adherent platelets
CD79a[a]	Part of the BCR complex	B-lymphocytes, plasma cells; megakaryocytes also positive	Useful for B-cell leukemia and B-cell lymphoma
Calprotectin (MAC387)[a]	Cytoplasmic calcium-binding protein	Neutrophils, monocytes, and macrophages	Also expressed by some nonhemic cells (epithelial)
MPO	Myeloperoxidase	Granulocytic and monocytic cells	Helpful for identifying AML (nonlymphoid leukocytes)
vWf[a]	von Willebrand factor	Megakaryocytes, platelets	Intracytoplasmic location; relatively low levels in dogs

[a] The following can be detected in formalin-fixed tissues with appropriate antigen retrieval: CD3ε, CD11d, CD18, CD21-like, CD45, CD45RA, CD79a, calprotectin, and vWf.

[b] ALL, acute lymphocytic leukemia; BCR, B-cell receptor; CLL, chronic lymphocytic leukemia; GP, glycoprotein; and MHC, major histocompatability complex

Note: Not all targets are currently detectable by all methods (flow cytometry, immunocytochemistry, immunohistochemistry on fixed tissues). Reactivities and antibody availability vary with species.

b. The CD antigens are best characterized on human and mouse cells, but many of the same CD antigens are found on cells of domestic mammals.

c. Cells from blood, bone marrow, or other tissues may be immunophenotyped by flow cytometry, immunocytochemical staining of air-dried preparations, or immunohistochemical staining of fixed or frozen histologic sections. Some antibodies can be used on unfixed tissue but not on fixed tissue, and some antibodies are not available with fluorochromes for flow cytometry.

d. Immunophenotyping should be done with panels of antibodies to detect constellations of antigen expression that reflect the cell lineage and stage of maturation. Patterns are more likely to predict outcome than individual antigen reactivity. Individual antigen reactivity may be misleading because most immunophenotyping antibodies react with cells of multiple lineages, and neoplastic cells may have aberrant antigen expression.

e. The following panel has been recommended as a minimal immunophenotyping panel for animal leukemias:[48] CD79a for B-lymphocytes, CD3 for T-lymphocytes, CD11b for myeloid cells, MPO for myeloid cells, CD41 for megakaryoblastic cells, CD1c for dendritic cells, and CD34 for acute leukemia (hemic blast cells).

f. Immunophenotyping results should be interpreted in light of all historical, clinical, microscopic, cytochemical, cytogenetic, and molecular genetic findings that are available.

g. Canine chronic lymphocytic leukemias: Immunophenotyping indicates that most are T-lymphocyte neoplasms, including many granular lymphocyte leukemias. They do not express CD34.[57,64]

   (1) Nongranular T-lymphocyte leukemias are typically proliferations of TCR$\alpha\beta$ cells that lack a consistent pattern of CD4 and CD8 expression. Granular cell leukemias are typically CD8+ and CD11d+, and express TCR$\alpha\beta$ about twice as often as TCR$\gamma\delta$.

   (2) B-lymphocyte leukemias express CD21 (without T-lymphocyte markers) or CD79a and usually CD1c.

h. Canine acute leukemias, whether lymphoid or nonlymphoid, usually express CD34 (except for granular lymphocytes).

   (1) Nongranular acute lymphocytic leukemia is usually of B-lymphocyte (CD79a+) origin.

   (2) Granular lymphocyte leukemias may consist of either T-lymphocytes (CD3+, TCR$\alpha\beta$+, CD8$\alpha\beta$+, and CD11d+) or, probably, NK-lymphocytes (CD3−, CD11d+, and CD8α+).

   (3) MPO expression supports an acute myeloid leukemia other than pure erythroleukemia. MPO expression has not been detected in some leukemias of megakaryocyte or monocyte lineage.[63]

i. B-lymphocytes and T-lymphocytes of lymphomas are CD34−, so this marker is helpful in differentiating primary acute lymphocytic leukemias of agranular lymphocytes (CD34+) from leukemic phases of lymphoma.

j. Aberrant expression of CD18 and CD45 has been evaluated for recognizing and classifying atypical cell populations.[65,66]

5. Electron microscopy may be useful in some leukemias to provide evidence of a particular cell line; for example, the ultrastructure of leukemic cell cytoplasmic granules may be distinctive for basophil, eosinophil, or mast cell granules. Rarely, immunogold staining may be used to detect lineage-selective markers.

6. Molecular and cytogenetic studies may be employed to detect genetic abnormalities that may predict behavior and outcome of some neoplasms. Chromosomal abnormalities in canine leukemia cells have been detected by karyotyping but have offered little prognostic value to date. Chromosomal banding studies and molecular genetic techniques are being evaluated. These include fluorescent in situ hybridization, comparative genomic hybridization, and microarrays. Currently, the most used genetic technique is the polymerase chain reaction (PCR) for assessment of clonality:[57,67]

   a. With only rare exceptions, neoplasia of lymphoid cells is an uncontrolled proliferation or accumulation of one clone of lymphocytes.

   b. Antigen-binding regions of B- and T-lymphocyte receptors are encoded by the CDR3 region of the immunoglobulin and TCR genes. The CDR3 region is produced by various recombinations of several genes, generating numerous genetic combinations. Primers are used to amplify conserved regions of these genes, and the products are separated by size. If there is a clonal expansion of cells with one particular CDR3 region detectable with the test primers, separation will yield a dominant band.

   c. Polymerase chain reaction assays for B- and T-lymphocyte antigen receptor gene rearrangements are useful to help differentiate lymphoid neoplasia from inflammatory conditions.

      (1) The presence of gene rearrangements supports neoplasia. B-lymphocyte and T-lymphocyte gene rearrangements usually occur in neoplasms of the respective cell types.

      (2) The absence of a detected gene rearrangement does not exclude lymphoid neoplasia.

      (3) Clonal rearrangements of the TCR gene have been detected in dogs with *Ehrlichia canis* infections, and lymphocyte receptor gene rearrangements sometimes occur in nonlymphoid leukemias.[67]

      (4) The assay sensitivity varies with the tissue and proportion of lymphocytes that are neoplastic, but clonality can be detected when as little as 0.1–10.0 % of sample DNA is from neoplastic cells. Therefore, it can be used to detect residual disease after treatment or otherwise undetectably small amounts of neoplasia during staging.

      (5) Small samples may yield discrete bands that appear to be clones; these are called pseudoclones. Duplicate testing with separate DNA extractions can be done to decrease the likelihood of misinterpreting pseudoclones as real clones. Detection of clones should be repeatable.

INTERPRETING RESULTS OF BONE MARROW EXAMINATIONS

I.   Interpretation of the results of bone marrow examinations is easier if one uses the bone marrow examination to answer specific questions:
   A. Why does an animal have a nonregenerative anemia?
   B. Why does an animal have a persistent neutropenia?
   C. Why does an animal have a thrombocytopenia?
   D. Is there a neoplastic process in the bone marrow?

II. Complete interpretation of most bone marrow samples is only possible when there are CBC results for the day the bone marrow was collected.

A. Hyperplastic and hypoplastic conditions can usually be recognized independently of CBC findings, but the CBC findings help explain the disorder. For example, a hypercellular bone marrow with an increased G : E (M : E) ratio indicates there is myeloid hyperplasia (rarely neoplasia) no matter what the CBC findings are. However, the CBC may indicate there is ineffective neutropoiesis (granulocytic hyperplasia with severe neutropenia) or effective neutropoiesis (granulocytic hyperplasia with a marked neutrophilia). The former case suggests immune-mediated neutropenia, whereas the latter case supports an inflammatory process.

B. When marrow cellularity is neither clearly increased nor clearly decreased and there is an abnormal G : E (M : E) ratio, the CBC provides clues as to the cause of the abnormal ratio.

   1. If the G : E (M : E) ratio is increased, it may be due to erythroid hypoplasia, granulocytic (myeloid) hyperplasia, or both. A nonregenerative anemia would support erythroid hypoplasia, whereas a neutrophilia and hematocrit within the reference interval would support granulocytic (myeloid) hyperplasia.

   2. If the G : E (M : E) ratio is decreased, it may be due to erythroid hyperplasia, granulocytic (myeloid) hypoplasia, or both. A regenerative anemia or erythrocytosis would support erythroid hyperplasia, whereas a leukopenia would support granulocytic (myeloid) hypoplasia.

C. Unless a condition is clearly chronic and stable, it is important that CBC results are collected the same day as the bone marrow sample.

   1. An animal may have a nonregenerative anemia one day but a regenerative anemia the next day (or the reverse).

   2. An animal may have a neutropenia one day but a normal to increased neutrophil concentration the next day (or the reverse).

   3. An animal may have a thrombocytopenia one day but a normal to increased platelet concentration the next day (or the reverse).

D. Examples of the correlation of CBC and bone marrow results for five dogs are shown in Fig. 6.3. Findings must also be interpreted in light of other clinical findings.

LYMPH NODE: MAJOR CONCEPTS AND TERMS

I. Terms and conditions

   A. *Lymphadenopathy* is a pathologic state involving a lymph node. In clinical diseases, the lymphadenopathies typically cause enlarged lymph nodes (i.e., *lymphadenomegaly*). Frequently, but inaccurately, lymphadenopathy and enlarged lymph node are considered synonyms.

   B. The primary reason for a lymph node biopsy is to determine the pathologic process that is causing lymphadenomegaly. Pathologic processes may be present in lymph nodes that are not enlarged, but not as frequently. The following are major disorders or conditions that cause enlarged lymph nodes:

      1. Hyperplasia of lymphoid cells
      2. Inflammation involving lymph nodes
      3. Neoplasia of lymphoid cells
      4. Neoplasia of nonlymphoid cells (typically metastatic neoplasia)

II. Methods

   A. Complete descriptions of a lymph node biopsy (collection, fixation, staining, and examination of lymph node tissue from a living animal) are beyond the scope of this text. Procedures of a lymph node biopsy are described in several sources.[8,68–70]

B. Major features of a lymph node biopsy
   1. Sample collection and processing
      a. Typically, lymph node samples are collected from enlarged peripheral lymph nodes: mandibular, prescapular, axillary, popliteal, inguinal and, occasionally, facial. Internal lymph nodes are also sampled, usually by ultrasound-guided aspiration or during a celiotomy or thoracotomy. When multiple lymph nodes are enlarged, it is wise to sample multiple nodes.
      b. Samples may be collected from the lymph node by fine needles, Tru-cut needles, wedge incision, or lymph node excision. After the sample is collected, it may be prepared for microscopic analysis, tissue sectioning, culturing, or other procedures.
      c. Fine-needle collection is a relatively simple procedure for obtaining cytologic samples, but many errors can be made that result in inadequate or suboptimal samples. The following steps may be used as a guide for collecting cytologic samples from lymph nodes or other superficial masses:
         (1) Slides should be made ready.
         (2) Select a 22 gauge needle and a 5–12 mL syringe.
         (3) Prepare the skin as for a venipuncture.
         (4) Isolate and stabilize the lymph node with one hand.
         (5) Insert the needle into the skin and lymph node. (A syringe is not necessary at this time, but if using a needle attached to a syringe, moderate suction can be applied after the needle is in the lymph node to help hold cores of tissue in the needle. Forceful aspiration should be avoided, particularly while leaving the needle in one place, because this can cause significant hemodilution.)
         (6) Cut a core of tissue with a sharp forward cutting motion followed by an optional rotation of the needle to help free the core, withdraw the needle without leaving the node, and repeat up to three times in different directions to obtain a representative sample.
         (7) Withdraw and attach syringe (relieve suction before withdrawing if using a needle and syringe).
         (8) Place the needle against a slide, bevel down, and express the sample in a pool. Do not spray small droplets onto the slide.
         (9) Spread the material by one of several techniques to obtain areas on one or more slides that contain monolayers of intact cells.
             (a) A wedge blood smear technique may be used for thin (more fluid) samples.
             (b) Horizontal or vertical "squash" techniques can be used for thicker samples. A wavy spreading motion can be used with a horizontal technique in order to obtain thin zones of cells.
             (c) Lymph node samples are often very cellular and thick, sometimes too thick for evaluation, so care should be taken to spread material well. If the drop is moderate to large, instead of spreading it all into one thick smear, some of the material can be picked up on the edge of another slide and spread by a horizontal spread technique onto one or more other slides.
         (10) The air-dried slides should not be fixed (with heat or other fixative) prior to staining or submission, and they should not be exposed to formalin fumes

CBC results	Dog 1	Dog 2	Dog 3	Dog 4	Dog 5	Ref. Int.
Hct (%)	10	10	10	15	10	37-55
Reticulocytes (#/µL)	10,000	200,000	10,000	200,000	10,000	0-80,000
Neutrophils (#/µL)	8,000	8,000	500	30,000	1,000	3,000-12,000
Platelets (#/µL)	300,000	300,000	20,000	20,000	20,000	155,000-393,000
Atypical cells (#/µL)	0	0	0	0	100,000	none
Bone marrow biopsy results						
Hematopoietic cellularity (%)	20	80	10	85	90	25-75
G:E	2.4	0.5	1.0	0.7	3.5	0.9-1.8
Megakaryocyte pool						
Granulocytic pool						
Erythroid pool						

Fig. 6.3. Schematic examples of the interpretation of CBC and bone marrow biopsy results. Reference intervals and other expected results for healthy dogs are provided in the *right column*. The number of marrow megakaryocytes is represented by the number and size of schematic megakaryocytes. Granulocytic and erythroid pools are represented by pool diagrams that are miniatures of those shown in Chapters 2 and 3. G:E ratios were calculated from the number of cells illustrated in the granulocytic and erythroid pools:

- Dog 1: Decreased fragment hematopoietic cellularity and an increased G:E ratio indicate erythroid hypoplasia. CBC results of a nonregenerative anemia without abnormal platelet or neutrophil concentrations support that it is selective erythroid hypoplasia.
- Dog 2: Increased fragment hematopoietic cellularity and a decreased G:E ratio indicate erythroid hyperplasia. CBC data indicate it is associated with a regenerative anemia; therefore, it is probably caused by blood loss or hemolysis. If CBC data indicated a persistent nonregenerative anemia, one would have to consider causes of ineffective erythropoiesis (see the text).
- Dog 3: Decreased fragment hematopoietic cellularity, a G:E ratio within the reference interval, and decreased megakaryocytes indicate generalized marrow hypoplasia. CBC data support the presence of an aplastic anemia (aplastic pancytopenia).
- Dog 4: Increased fragment hematopoietic cellularity with a decreased G:E ratio indicates erythroid hyperplasia. Increased density of megakaryocytes indicates megakaryocytic hyperplasia. CBC data further indicate effective erythropoiesis (reticulocytosis) and a stimulus for megakaryocytic hyperplasia (thrombocytopenia). Neutrophilia is evidence for myeloid hyperplasia despite a decreased G:E ratio; the granulocytic series is expanded, but the erythroid series is expanded more. The regenerative anemia is probably caused by blood loss or hemolysis, the neutrophilia is caused by an inflammatory process, and the thrombocytopenia is caused by decreased platelet survival. This dog's inflammatory neutrophilia could be associated with an immune-mediated anemia and immune-mediated thrombocytopenia.
- Dog 5: Increased fragment hematopoietic cellularity and an increased G:E ratio with a predominance of atypical immature granulocytic cells indicates granulocytic neoplasia. A paucity of megakaryocytes and erythroid cells suggests the possibility of myelophthisic megakaryocytic and erythroid hypoplasia. CBC findings of thrombocytopenia and nonregenerative anemia further support this interpretation. Neutropenia is caused by defective neutropoiesis (neoplasia).

Hct, hematocrit.

because the gas can severely alter the staining properties of the cells. Keep them clean, covered, and at ambient temperature.

    d. To process samples for histologic evaluation, thin slices of excised samples should be placed in fixative for paraffin-embedded sectioning. Formalin is used most often, but B5 fixation improves cell detail.

2. Cytologic examination of lymph node aspirates and imprints

    a. This involves the differentiation and characterization of nucleated cells and the identification of organisms or other noncellular structures (e.g., hemosiderin).

        (1) The types of lymphocytes are determined by their nuclear diameters, chromatin patterns, the presence of enlarged nucleoli, and cytoplasmic features. In health, most lymphocytes should be small lymphocytes with clumped chromatin patterns, scant cytoplasms, and inapparent nucleoli.

        (2) Other cells are identified by their unique features. Nonlymphoid cells include neutrophils, macrophages, eosinophils, mast cells, metastatic neoplastic cells, and hematopoietic precursors.

    b. Examinations are best completed on a quality stained sample with a quality microscope by a person who is trained for such examinations.

3. Methods involved in the histologic examination of lymph node sections are beyond the scope of this textbook. Such examinations should be performed by veterinary pathologists.

E. Cells in lymph nodes of healthy mammals

1. Lymph nodes from healthy mammals are not commonly evaluated. However, microscopists should have a clear image of what should be seen in normal lymph nodes so that abnormal cell populations or other significant findings will be recognized (Plate 10A).

2. The expected cell populations in lymph nodes vary with the location of the lymph node. Mandibular and mesenteric lymph nodes in healthy mammals typically have greater percentages of resident macrophages, plasma cells, neutrophils, and large lymphocytes than do other lymph nodes.

3. Lymph nodes from healthy animals consist of a heterogeneous population of cells. Small to intermediate lymphocytes account for the vast majority of the cells, and there are low percentages of plasma cells, large lymphocytes, neutrophils, eosinophils, and macrophages.

4. The size of lymphocytes should be judged where cells are well spread (diameters are maximized). They can be measured with a micrometer or compared to "cellular micrometers" to estimate sizes: canine erythrocyte diameter is about 7 μm; canine neutrophil diameter is 12–14 μm; and mature plasma cell nuclei have diameters similar to erythrocytes.

    a. One system classifies canine lymphocytes by nuclear diameter relative to canine erythrocyte diameter, but there are gaps between categories:[71]

        (1) Small: 1–1.5 times the diameter of erythrocytes (≈ 7–10 μm)

        (2) Intermediate: 2–2.5 times the diameter of erythrocytes (≈ 14–18 μm)

        (3) Large: > three times the diameter of erythrocytes (> 21 μm)

        (4) Erythrocytes from other species are smaller, so the classification scale must be modified accordingly.

    b. Others have used different numeric diameters for classification:[72]

        (1) Small: < 10 μm

        (2) Intermediate: 10–15 μm

        (3) Large: > 15 μm

5. Large lymphocytes with basophilic cytoplasms, finely stippled chromatin, and nucleoli are often referred to as *lymphoblasts* as is consistent with the terms myeloblast, monoblast, and rubriblast. However, others reserve this term for the relatively small lymphocyte without conspicuous nucleoli that proliferates in lymphoblastic leukemia/lymphoma.

LYMPH NODE CLASSIFICATIONS

I. Hyperplastic lymph node
   A. *Lymph node hyperplasia* is characterized by increased numbers of B-lymphocytes, T-lymphocytes, or both. The proportions of different types of lymphocytes may appear normal, in which case hyperplasia is suggested by normal cell populations in association with lymphadenomegaly. There may be increases in large lymphocytes and/or plasma cells, in which case the terms *reactive* or *reactive hyperplasia* are often used in place of hyperplasia, though the nodes are enlarged because of hyperplasia.
   B. A variety of infectious and noninfectious diseases, including bacterial, viral, fungal, and neoplastic disorders, can lead to the stimulation and proliferation of lymphocytes. If there is generalized lymph node hyperplasia, a systemic illness should be considered. If only one node is hyperplastic, a disease within the drainage field of that node should be considered.
   C. There may or may not be a concurrent inflammatory lymphocytosis in mammals with hyperplastic lymph nodes.

II. Reactive lymph node
   A. A node classified as *reactive* typically has increased numbers of plasma cells and/or large lymphocytes (Plate 10B). The percentage of large lymphocytes is expected to be < 50 % in a reactive node and is usually < 10 %. An increase in plasma cells indicates B-lymphocyte stimulation.
   B. The causes of a reactive lymph node are essentially the same as those for lymph node hyperplasia.

III. Lymphadenitis
   A. *Lymphadenitis* is characterized by an increased number of nonlymphoid inflammatory cells in a lymph node. One inflammatory cell type might dominate (e.g., neutrophils), or there can be a mixture of inflammatory cells (e.g., neutrophils, macrophages, and eosinophils) (Plate 10C and D).
   B. The cause of the inflammatory state may be within the lymph node or, more commonly, in the node's drainage field. For example, an allergic dermatitis may lead to an eosinophilic lymphadenitis, or a lymph node draining a necrotic hemorrhagic lesion may have many macrophages containing cell debris and Fe pigments.
   C. There may or may not be a concurrent inflammatory leukocytosis.
   D. Organisms such as pyogenic bacteria, *Mycobacterium* sp. (Plate 10E), *Histoplasma* sp. (Plate 10F), *Blastomyces* sp. (Plate 10G), *Leishmania* sp. (Plate 10H), *Prototheca* sp., and *Neorickettsia* sp. may be present.
   E. Lymphadenitis is often associated with reactive (proplastic) changes, and the term *reactive lymphadenitis* is sometimes used to reflect both changes.

IV. Lymphoid neoplasia (lymphoma and lymphosarcoma)
   A. Anatomic classification, histologic classification, and staging of lymphomas are beyond the scope of this book.

B. Cytologically, lymphoma can be diagnosed when there is nearly a single population of atypical lymphocytes rather than the heterogeneous mixture of typical cell types present in normal, reactive, or inflamed lymph nodes. However, depending on the appearance of the cells, lymphoma can be an easy or difficult diagnosis cytologically.

1. When cytologic preparations consist of single populations of large lymphocytes with prominent nucleoli, the diagnosis of lymphoma is clear (Plate 10I and J).

2. The diagnosis is more difficult when the cells are small to intermediate in size or when substantial numbers of nonneoplastic cells are intermixed with neoplastic cells because of a nondiffuse form or a recent onset (Plate 10K). In these cases, histologic examination may be necessary for a diagnosis.

3. A lymph node is unlikely to be reactive and likely to be lymphomatous if > 50 % of the lymphoid cells are large lymphocytes.

C. Over the past 30 yr, several classification systems for lymphomas have been based on tissue patterns, cell sizes, nuclear shapes, nucleolar sizes, and cytoplasmic granulation. Most classifications were formulated for the classification of human lymphomas, and their application to other mammalian lymphomas has been inconsistent. Ideally, a classification system would differentiate neoplasms of differing clinical behavior and prognosis such that they could receive the most appropriate management.

1. The Rappaport classification is based primarily on sizes of the lymphocytes and patterns of cell growth (nodular and diffuse).

2. The Kiel classification is based on lymphocyte sizes and nuclear and cytoplasmic features, and separates lymphomas into B-lymphocyte and T-lymphocyte neoplasms.

3. The Lukes-Collins classification is based on the sizes and shapes of the nuclei (e.g., small, large, cleaved, noncleaved, and convoluted) and on cellular features (small, immunoblastic, plasmacytoid, and histiocytic), and separates lymphomas into B-lymphocyte and T-lymphocyte neoplasms.

4. The Working Formulation system uses growth patterns (follicular and diffuse), nuclear outline (cleaved, noncleaved, and convoluted), and cell sizes to classify the lymphomas into three grades (low, intermediate, and high).

5. The revised European/American Lymphoma (REAL) system divides lymphomas into B-lymphocyte or T-lymphocyte lymphomas on the basis of immunophenotyping, cell structure, genetic features, and clinical features. A group of specialists organized by the WHO modified the REAL system by incorporating aspects of the prior classifications (B-lymphocyte, T-lymphocyte, and NK-lymphocyte).[73] A similar veterinary histologic classification of lymphoid neoplasia in domestic animals has been published by the AFIP in cooperation with the American Registry of Pathology and the WHO Collaborating Center for Worldwide Reference on Comparative Oncology.[49]

D. Lymphomas can be evaluated by using methods described previously (Bone Marrow Classifications, sect. IX.E) for other hemic neoplasia, although cytochemical staining would be useful only to exclude a nonlymphoid cell lineage.

1. Microscopic evaluation of stained cells is the easiest method of evaluation and has the most clinical application, but classification of lymphoma is limited without further information. Microscopic appearance does not consistently differentiate B-lymphocytes and T-lymphocytes or predict genetic abnormalities, but it does provide information important for classification.

2. Immunophenotyping is used primarily to differentiate B-lymphocyte lymphomas from T-lymphocyte lymphomas, but it may also help differentiate acute lymphoblas-

tic leukemias (CD34+) from lymphoma with bone marrow and blood involvement
(CD34−). However, CD34+ B-lymphocyte lymphomas have been reported.[74]
  a. At a minimum, a B-lymphocyte marker and a T-lymphocyte marker should be
      assessed (often CD79a and/or CD21 for B-lymphocytes and CD3 for T-
      lymphocytes). T-lymphocyte lymphomas have a poorer prognosis.[74]
  b. Direct cytologic smears may be used for immunocytochemistry. Alternatively,
      cells can be collected into fluid for evaluation by a number of techniques:
      (1) immunocytochemistry on concentrated preparations of the cell suspensions,
      (2) immunohistochemistry on cell blocks made from cell suspensions by pelleting
      and fixing cells, or (3) flow cytometry. Immunohistochemistry may also be used
      on frozen or fixed tissue sections.
  c. Coexpression of CD3 and CD21 or CD79a has been reported,[74] and cells have
      had either TCR or immunoglobulin receptor gene rearrangements. This aberrant
      expression may be a useful diagnostic marker for malignancy.
  d. Lymphomas may also be assessed for p53 tumor-suppressor protein, which has
      been significantly increased in high-grade lymphomas.[75]
 3. Polymerase chain reaction analysis for rearrangements of the immunoglobulin and
    TCR genes can aid in detection of lymphoma (see immunophenotyping of hemic
    neoplasia in Bone Marrow Classifications, sect. IX.E.4). It is likely that cytogenetic
    and molecular techniques will be of diagnostic and prognostic value.

V. Nonlymphoid neoplasia (typically metastatic)
  A. Lymph nodes can be enlarged because of the growth of nonlymphoid neoplastic cells in
      the node. Metastatic cells can also be found during biopsies of lymph nodes that do not
      appear enlarged.
  B. Many neoplasms have the potential to spread to regional lymph nodes. Those seen
      more frequently in the peripheral lymph nodes include squamous cell carcinoma,
      mammary carcinoma or adenocarcinoma, melanoma, mast cell neoplasia, and some
      hemic neoplasms (Plate 10L–N).

VI. Other findings
  A. Edema may be suggested in aspirates by the loose arrangement of cells that suggests
      dispersion of cells by fluid.
  B. The presence of nonlymphoid hemic precursors (rubricytes, megakaryocytes, and
      granulocytes) indicates extramedullary hematopoiesis or, rarely, nonlymphoid hemic
      neoplasia involving the lymph node. Lymph node hematopoiesis may occur when bone
      marrow damage is extensive and stimuli promote proliferation of hemic precursors in
      extramedullary sites.
  C. The presence of erythrocytes in the sample indicates hemorrhage. If only erythrocytes
      are found, it may be difficult to differentiate pathologic hemorrhage from hemorrhage
      caused by sampling. The presence of erythrophages and siderophages supports the
      conclusion of pathologic hemorrhage either within the lymph node or its drainage
      field.
  D. A diagnosis of metastatic melanoma should be considered any time melanin pigment is
      found. However, melanin pigment can be found in macrophages (melanophages) when
      the lymph node's drainage field contains a melanoma, necrosis, or inflammation of
      pigmented tissue.
  E. Various combinations of multiple abnormalities may be present.

References

1. Zenke M, Hieronymus T. 2006. Towards an understanding of the transcription factor network of dendritic cell development. Trends Immunol 27:140–145.

2. Wu L, Dakic A. 2004. Development of dendritic cell system. Cell Mol Immunol 1:112–118.

3. Adolfsson J, Månsson R, Buza-Vidas N, Hultquist A, Liuba K, Jensen CT, Bryder D, Yang L, Borge OJ, Thoren LA, Anderson K, Sitnicka E, Sasaki Y, Sigvardsson M, Jacobsen SE. 2005. Identification of Flt3+ lympho-myeloid stem cells lacking erythro-megakaryocytic potential a revised road map for adult blood lineage commitment. Cell 121:295–306.

4. Harvey JW. 2001. *Atlas of Veterinary Hematology: Blood and Bone Marrow of Domestic Animals*. Philadelphia: WB Saunders.

5. Tyler RD, Cowell RL, Meinkoth JH. 2001. Bone marrow. In: Cowell RL, Tyler RD, Meinkoth JH, eds. *Diagnostic Cytology and Hematology of the Dog and Cat*, 2nd edition, 284–304. St Louis: CV Mosby.

6. Wellman ML, Radin MJ. 1999. *Bone Marrow Evaluation in Dogs and Cats*. St Louis: Gloyd.

7. Jain NC. 1993. *Essentials of Veterinary Hematology*, 1st edition. Philadelphia: Lea & Febiger.

8. Cowell RL, Tyler RD. 1992. *Cytology and Hematology of the Horse*, Goleta, CA: American Veterinary.

9. Grindem CB. 1989. Bone marrow biopsy and evaluation. Vet Clin North Am Small Anim Pract 19:669–696.

10. Jain NC. 1986. *Schalm's Veterinary Hematology*, 4th edition. Philadelphia: Lea & Febiger.

11. Grindem CB, Neel JA, Juopperi TA. 2002. Cytology of bone marrow. Vet Clin North Am Small Anim Pract 32:1313–1374.

12. Stokol T, Blue JT. 1999. Pure red cell aplasia in cats: 9 cases (1989–1997). J Am Vet Med Assoc 214:75–79.

13. Harvey JW. 1981. Myeloproliferative disorders in dogs and cats. Vet Clin North Am Small Anim Pract 11:349–381.

14. Weiss DJ. 2004. Flow cytometric evaluation of canine bone marrow based on intracytoplasmic complexity and CD45 expression. Vet Clin Pathol 33:96–101.

15. Stokol T, Blue JT, French TW. 2000. Idiopathic pure red cell aplasia and nonregenerative immune-mediated anemia in dogs: 43 cases (1988–1999). J Am Vet Med Assoc 216:1429–1436.

16. Watson ADJ, Canfield PJ. 2000. Nutritional deficiency anemias. In: Feldman BF, Zinkl JG, Jain NC, eds. *Schalm's Veterinary Hematology*, 5th edition, 190–195. Philadelphia: Lippincott Williams & Wilkins.

17. Battersby IA, Giger U, Hall EJ. 2005. Hyperammonaemic encephalopathy secondary to selective cobalamin deficiency in a juvenile Border collie. J Small Anim Pract 46:339–344.

18. Dole RS, MacPhail CM, Lappin MR. 2004. Paraneoplastic leukocytosis with mature neutrophilia in a cat with pulmonary squamous cell carcinoma. J Feline Med Surg 6:391–395.

19. Brown CD, Parnell NK, Schulman RL, Brown CG, Glickman NW, Glickman L. 2006. Evaluation of clinicopathologic features, response to treatment, and risk factors associated with idiopathic neutropenia in dogs: 11 cases (1990–2002). J Am Vet Med Assoc 229:87–91.

20. Perkins MC, Canfield P, Churcher RK, Malik R. 2004. Immune-mediated neutropenia suspected in five dogs. Aust Vet J 82:52–57.

21. McManus PM, Litwin C, Barber L. 1999. Immune-mediated neutropenia in 2 dogs. J Vet Intern Med 13:372–374.

22. Jacobs G, Calvert C, Kaufman A. 1998. Neutropenia and thrombocytopenia in three dogs treated with anticonvulsants. J Am Vet Med Assoc 212:681–684.

23. Lanevschi A, Daminet S, Niemeyer GP, Lothrop CD Jr. 1999. Granulocyte colony–stimulating factor deficiency in a rottweiler with chronic idiopathic neutropenia. J Vet Intern Med 13:72–75.

24. Jain NC, Blue JT, Grindem CB, Harvey JW, Kociba GJ, Krehbiel JD, Latimer KS, Raskin RE, Thrall MA, Zinkl JG. 1991. Proposed criteria for classification of acute myeloid leukemia in dogs and cats. Vet Clin Pathol 20:63–82.

25. Jain NC. 1993. Classification of myeloproliferative disorders in cats using criteria proposed by the animal leukaemia study group: A retrospective study of 181 cases (1969–1992). Comp Haematol Int 3:125–134.

26. Weiss DJ. 2006. Aplastic anemia in cats: Clinicopathological features and associated disease conditions 1996–2004. J Feline Med Surg 8:203–206.

27. Brazzell JL, Weiss DJ. 2006. A retrospective study of aplastic pancytopenia in the dog: 9 cases (1996–2003). Vet Clin Pathol 35:413–417.

28. Weiss DJ. 2000. Pure red cell aplasia. In: Feldman BF, Zinkl JG, Jain NC, eds. *Schalm's Veterinary Hematology*, 5th edition, 210–211. Philadelphia: Lippincott Williams & Wilkins.

29. Weiss DJ, Stockham SL, Willard MD, Schirmer RG. 1982. Transient erythroid hypoplasia in the dog: Report of five cases. J Am Anim Hosp Assoc 18:353–359.

30. Randolph JF, Stokol T, Scarlett JM, MacLeod JN. 1999. Comparison of biological activity and safety of recombinant canine erythropoietin with that of recombinant human erythropoietin in clinically normal dogs. Am J Vet Res 60:636–642.

31. Stokol T, Randolph J, MacLeod J. 1997. Pure red cell aplasia after recombinant human erythropoietin treatment in normal beagle dogs. Vet Pathol 34:474 (abstract).
32. Piercy RJ, Swardson CJ, Hinchcliff KW. 1998. Erythroid hypoplasia and anemia following administration of recombinant human erythropoietin to two horses. J Am Vet Med Assoc 212:244–247.
33. Woods PR, Campbell G, Cowell RL. 1997. Nonregenerative anaemia associated with administration of recombinant human erythropoietin to a thoroughbred racehorse. Equine Vet J 29:326–328.
34. Rojko JL, Olsen RG. 1984. The immunobiology of the feline leukemia virus. Vet Immunol Immunopathol 6:107–165.
35. Jarrett O, Golder MC, Toth S, Onions DE, Stewart MF. 1984. Interaction between feline leukaemia virus subgroups in the pathogenesis of erythroid hypoplasia. Int J Cancer 34:283–288.
36. Watson AD. 1977. Chloramphenicol toxicity in dogs. Res Vet Sci 23:66–69.
37. Watson ADJ, Middleton DJ. 1978. Chloramphenicol toxicosis in cats. Am J Vet Res 39:1199–1203.
38. Smith GS. 2000. Neutrophils. In: Feldman BF, Zinkl JG, Jain NC, eds. *Schalm's Veterinary Hematology*, 5th edition, 281–296. Philadelphia: Lippincott Williams & Wilkins.
39. Weiss DJ. 2000. Aplastic anemia. In: Feldman BF, Zinkl JG, Jain NC, eds. *Schalm's Veterinary Hematology*, 5th edition, 212–215. Philadelphia: Lippincott Williams & Wilkins.
40. Lachowicz JL, Post GS, Moroff SD, Mooney SC. 2004. Acquired amegakaryocytic thrombocytopenia: Four cases and a literature review. J Small Anim Pract 45:507–514.
41. Weiss DJ. 2005. Differentiating benign and malignant causes of lymphocytosis in feline bone marrow. J Vet Intern Med 19:855–859.
42. Felchle LM, McPhee LA, Kerr ME, Houston DM. 1996. Systemic lupus erythematosus and bone marrow necrosis in a dog. Can Vet J 37:742–744.
43. Rottman JB, English RV, Breitschwerdt EB, Duncan DE. 1991. Bone marrow hypoplasia in a cat treated with griseofulvin. J Am Vet Med Assoc 198:429–431.
44. Walker D, Cowell RL, Clinkenbeard KD, Feder B, Meinkoth JH. 1997. Bone marrow mast cell hyperplasia in dogs with aplastic anemia. Vet Clin Pathol 26:106–111.
45. McManus P. 1997. Canine mastocytemia and marrow mastocytosis: Disease associations, incidence and severity. Vet Pathol 34:474 (abstract).
46. Lichtman MA. 2001. Idiopathic myelofibrosis (agnogenic myeloid metaplasia). In: Beutler E, Lichtman MA, Coller BS, Kipps TJ, Seligsohn U, eds. *Williams Hematology*, 6th edition, 1125–1136. New York: McGraw-Hill.
47. Weiss DJ. 2005. Bone marrow necrosis in dogs: 34 cases (1996–2004). J Am Vet Med Assoc 227:263–267.
48. McManus PM. 2005. Classification of myeloid neoplasms: A comparative review. Vet Clin Pathol 34:189–212.
49. Valli VE, Jacobs RM, Parodi AL, Vernau W, Moore PF. 2002. *Histological Classification of Hematopoietic Tumors of Domestic Animals*. Washington DC: Armed Forces Institute of Pathology.
50. Vardiman JW, Harris NL, Brunning RD. 2002. The World Health Organization (WHO) classification of the myeloid neoplasms. Blood 100:2292–2302.
51. Blue JT. 2000. Myelodysplastic syndromes and myelofibrosis. In: Feldman BF, Zinkl JG, Jain NC, eds. *Schalm's Veterinary Hematology*, 5th edition, 682–688. Philadelphia: Lippincott Williams & Wilkins.
52. Raskin RE. 1996. Myelopoiesis and myeloproliferative disorders. Vet Clin North Am Small Anim Pract 26:1023–1042.
53. Weiss DJ. 2005. Recognition and classification of dysmyelopoiesis in the dog: A review. J Vet Intern Med 19:147–154.
54. Weiss DJ. 2006. Evaluation of dysmyelopoiesis in cats: 34 cases (1996–2005). J Am Vet Med Assoc 228:893–897.
55. Weiss DJ, Aird B. 2001. Cytologic evaluation of primary and secondary myelodysplastic syndromes in the dog. Vet Clin Pathol 30:67–75.
56. Blue JT. 2003. Myelodysplasia: Differentiating neoplastic from nonneoplastic syndromes of ineffective hematopoiesis in dogs. Toxicol Pathol 31(Suppl):44–48.
57. Vernau W, Moore PF. 1999. An immunophenotypic study of canine leukemias and preliminary assessment of clonality by polymerase chain reaction. Vet Immunol Immunopathol 69:145–164.
58. Moore PF, Affolter VK, Vernau W. 2006. Canine hemophagocytic histiocytic sarcoma: A proliferative disorder of CD11d+ macrophages. Vet Pathol 43:632–645.
59. Affolter VK, Moore PF. 2002. Localized and disseminated histiocytic sarcoma of dendritic cell origin in dogs. Vet Pathol 39:74–83.
60. Weiss DJ. 2002. Flow cytometric evaluation of hemophagocytic disorders in canine bone marrow. Vet Clin Pathol 31:36–41.
61. Raskin RE, Valenciano A. 2000. Cytochemical tests for diagnosis of leukemia. In: Feldman BF, Zinkl JG, Jain NC, eds. *Schalm's Veterinary Hematology*, 5th edition, 755–763. Philadelphia: Lippincott Williams & Wilkins.

62. Dean GA. 2000. CD antigens and immunophenotyping. In: Feldman BF, Zinkl JG, Jain NC, eds. *Schalm's Veterinary Hematology*, 5th edition, 689–695. Philadelphia: Lippincott Williams & Wilkins.

63. Vernau W. 2004. Flow cytometric assessment of hematopoietic neoplasia in the dog. In: 55th Annual Meeting of the American College of Veterinary Pathologists (ACVP) and 39th Annual Meeting of the American Society for Veterinary Clinical Pathology (ASVCP), Orlando, FL, 24–28.

64. Workman HC, Vernau W. 2003. Chronic lymphocytic leukemia in dogs and cats: The veterinary perspective. Vet Clin North Am Small Anim Pract 33:1379–1399.

65. Comazzi S, Gelain ME, Riondato F, Paltrinieri S. 2006. Flow cytometric expression of common antigens CD18/CD45 in blood from dogs with lymphoid malignancies: A semi-quantitative study. Vet Immunol Immunopathol 112:243–252.

66. Comazzi S, Gelain ME, Spagnolo V, Riondato F, Guglielmino R, Sartorelli P. 2006. Flow cytometric patterns in blood from dogs with non-neoplastic and neoplastic hematologic diseases using double labeling for CD18 and CD45. Vet Clin Pathol 35:47–54.

67. Burnett RC, Vernau W, Modiano JF, Olver CS, Moore PF, Avery AC. 2003. Diagnosis of canine lymphoid neoplasia using clonal rearrangements of antigen receptor genes. Vet Pathol 40:32–41.

68. Baker R, Lumsden JH. 2000. The lymphatic system. In: *Color Atlas of Cytology of the Dog and Cat*, 71–94. St Louis: CV Mosby.

69. Mills JN. 1989. Lymph node cytology. Vet Clin North Am Small Anim Pract 19:697–717.

70. Duncan JR. 1999. The lymph nodes. In: Cowell RL, Tyler RD, Meinkoth JH, eds. *Diagnostic Cytology and Hematology of the Dog and Cat*, 2nd edition, 97–103. St Louis: CV Mosby.

71. Raskin RE, Meyer DJ. 2001. *Atlas of Canine and Feline Cytology.* Philadelphia: WB Saunders.

72. Cowell RL, Dorsey KE, Meinkoth JH. 2003. Lymph node cytology. Vet Clin North Am Small Anim Pract 33:47–67.

73. Harris NL, Jaffe ES, Diebold J, Flandrin G, Muller-Hermelink HK, Vardiman J. 2000. Lymphoma classification—From controversy to consensus: The R.E.A.L. and WHO classification of lymphoid neoplasms. Ann Oncol 11(Suppl 1):S3–S10.

74. Wilkerson MJ, Dolce K, Koopman T, Shuman W, Chun R, Garrett L, Barber L, Avery A. 2005. Lineage differentiation of canine lymphoma/leukemias and aberrant expression of CD molecules. Vet Immunol Immunopathol 106:179–196.

75. Sueiro FA, Alessi AC, Vassallo J. 2004. Canine lymphomas: A morphological and immunohistochemical study of 55 cases, with observations on p53 immunoexpression. J Comp Pathol 131:207–213.

Chapter 7

PROTEINS

General Concepts for Total Protein, Albumin, and Globulins. 370
Analytical Principles for Total Protein, Albumin, and Globulins. 372
Hyperproteinemia. 379
Hypoproteinemia 385
Hyperalbuminemia. 390
Hypoalbuminemia 391
Hyperglobulinemia. 392
Hypoglobulinemia 392
Positive Acute-Phase Proteins. 392
    I.   General Concepts 392
    II. Fibrinogen 393
    III. Other Acute-Phase Proteins. 396
Immunoglobulins 398
Colloidal Osmotic Pressure (COP) (Oncotic Pressure) 405

Table 7.1. Abbreviations and symbols in this chapter

(TP:Fib)$_p$	Total protein to fibrinogen in plasma
[x]	x concentration (x = analyte)
ADH	Antidiuretic hormone
AL	Amyloid light chain
Alb	Albumin
APP	Acute-phase protein
BCG	Bromcresol green
BCP	Bromcresol purple
C3	Complement factor 3
COP	Colloidal osmotic pressure
CRP	C-reactive protein
DIC	Disseminated intravascular coagulation
ECF	Extracellular fluid
EDTA	Ethylenediaminetetraacetic acid
Fc	Crystallizable fragment
FPT	Failure of passive transfer
Hgb	Hemoglobin
IgA	Immunoglobulin A
IgE	Immunoglobulin E
IgG	Immunoglobulin G
IgG(T)	Immunoglobulin G, subtype T (T is for tetanus)
IgM	Immunoglobulin M
M_r	Relative molecular mass
Na_2SO_3	Sodium sulfite
NH_4^+	Ammonium
PLE	Protein-losing enteropathy
PLN	Protein-losing nephropathy
PP:F	Plasma protein to fibrinogen
pTP$_{ref}$	Plasma total protein by refractometry
RID	Radial immunodiffusion
SAA	Serum amyloid A
SI	Système International d'Unités
SIADH	Syndrome of inappropriate ADH secretion
SPE	Serum protein electrophoresis
sTP$_{ref}$	Serum total protein by refractometry
TP$_{ref}$	Total protein by refractometry
TP	Total protein
WRI	Within reference interval
$ZnSO_4$	Zinc sulfate

GENERAL CONCEPTS FOR TOTAL PROTEIN, ALBUMIN, AND GLOBULINS

I. Physiologic processes
   A. Proteins are polypeptide chains of amino acids. Over 1000 individual proteins have been characterized in serum. Most are not biochemically pure proteins; they are proteins combined with other substances. For example, lipoproteins are composed of

proteins, triglyceride, and cholesterol, whereas glycoproteins contain proteins and polysaccharides (sugar).
B. Plasma contains albumin and globulins, including fibrinogen and other clotting factors. A major difference between serum and plasma is that serum does not contain fibrinogen.
C. Most plasma proteins (albumin and globulins) are synthesized by hepatocytes. The major exceptions are the immunoglobulins that are produced by B-lymphocytes and plasma cells. The plasma half-life of albumin varies among species and generally increases with body size; reported values include 8.2 d in dogs,[1] 2–3 wk in cattle,[1,2] and an average of 19.4 d (n = 5) in horses.[3] There is a large variation in the half-life of the various proteins in the globulin fraction, and there are very few publications regarding half-lives for the plasma globulins in domestic mammals. The average γ-globulin half-life in horses (n = 5) was 11.0 d in one study,[3] whereas the half-life of IgG in foals was 26 d.[4]
D. In addition to a wide variety of specific functions, proteins also contribute to COP, which helps maintain intravasular fluid volume.

II. Protein disorders
A. *Protein dyscrasia* is a condition where there is an abnormal protein (abnormal structure).
B. *Dysproteinemia* is the presence of normal protein at abnormal concentration or abnormal protein (dyscrasia) in blood.
1. Selective or nonselective dysproteinemias
a. *Nonselective hyperproteinemia*: All protein concentrations are increased (*panhyperproteinemia*). It results from hemoconcentration.
b. *Selective hyperproteinemia*: The [total protein] is increased, and some protein concentrations are increased more than others. Typically, it results from inflammation or B-lymphocyte neoplasia.
c. *Nonselective hypoproteinemia*: The [total protein] is decreased, and all protein concentrations are decreased (*panhypoproteinemia*). Its cause is a proportional loss of proteins or proportional decrease in synthesis.
d. *Selective hypoproteinemia*: The [total protein] is decreased, and some protein concentrations are decreased more than others. Its cause is selective loss (typically small proteins selectively lost) or selectively decreased synthesis of one or more proteins.
2. To determine whether the dysproteinemia is selective or nonselective, serum protein electrophoresis may be needed to evaluate the relative concentrations of protein groups, especially in the globulin regions. An animal with hypoproteinemia, hypoalbuminemia, and hypoglobulinemia may or may not have a nonselective hypoproteinemia.
a. If hypoalbuminemia and hypoglobulinemia are present and electrophoresis results indicate that all protein fractions are decreased proportionately, then there is a nonselective hypoproteinemia.
b. If hypoalbuminemia and hypoglobulinemia are present and electrophoresis results indicate that protein fractions are not decreased proportionately, then there is a selective hypoproteinemia.
c. The same concepts apply to hyperproteinemia evaluations.
C. Other than the hyperproteinemia of dehydration, the most frequent dysproteinemias are caused by alterations in protein concentrations during inflammatory diseases. There

are three major groups of proteins whose plasma concentrations change because of inflammation.

1. *Positive APPs* are those proteins that have increased plasma or serum concentrations because of an inflammatory process. SAA and CRP concentrations may increase in < 1 d.[5,6] Concentrations of other APPs may be increased within 2 d after the onset of inflammation.[7] Their concentrations increase because of increased production by hepatocytes after stimulation by cytokines such as interleukin 6 and interleukin 1. The major positive APPs and some of their physiologic functions follow.

    a. *Fibrinogen*, the precursor of fibrin, is used to form secondary hemostatic plugs at sites of vascular injury. It is absent in serum.

    b. *C-reactive protein* promotes binding of complement to bacteria and induces cytokine production.

    c. *Serum amyloid A* promotes recruitment of inflammatory cells to inflammatory site.

    d. *Haptoglobin* binds Hgb dimers so that iron is not available to organisms.

    e. *α_1-Acid glycoprotein* has several anti-inflammatory activities.

    f. *Ceruloplasmin* is an enzyme that transports copper and has oxidase activity. It also helps convert ferrous iron into ferric iron for transport in the plasma in association with transferrin.

    g. *Ferritin* serves as a storage form of Fe (in Fe^{3+} form). Most ferritin is in tissues, but small amounts leave cells and enter plasma.[8,9]

2. *Negative APPs* are those proteins that have decreased plasma or serum concentrations because of an inflammatory process. Their concentrations decrease because of decreased production by hepatocytes due to the actions of cytokines such as interleukin 6 and interleukin 1. The major negative APPs and some of their physiologic functions follow.

    a. *Albumin* is the major contributor to plasma COP, serves as a source of amino acids, and transports many cationic substances (e.g., Ca^{2+}, Mg^{2+}, and drugs).

    b. *Transferrin* is the major transport protein for iron.

3. *Delayed response proteins* are proteins for which plasma or serum concentrations increase 1–3 wk after onset of inflammation. The two major delayed response proteins are immunoglobulins and complement.

    a. *Immunoglobulins* are produced by B-lymphocytes or plasma cells and are classified by their heavy chains as IgG, IgM, IgA, or IgE. Subclassifications also exist.

    b. *Complement proteins* (primarily C3), part of the innate immune system, accumulate in plasma in some inflammatory conditions.

ANALYTICAL PRINCIPLES FOR TOTAL PROTEIN, ALBUMIN, AND GLOBULINS

I. [Total protein]

    A. Refractometry for measuring [total protein] (plasma or serum)

        1. Principle: The degree of light refraction in an aqueous solution is proportional to the quantity of solids in solution. Because most solids in plasma are proteins, the degree of light refraction is highly dependent on protein concentration.

        2. The refractometer's total protein scale is calibrated with the assumption that changes in refractive index reflect changes in protein concentration alone. A temperature-compensated refractometer is recommended over a non–temperature-compensated refractometer for two reasons:

    a. It does not require daily adjustments based on ambient temperatures.

    b. It will probably be more accurate. If compensated and noncompensated refractometers are calibrated to agree at 68 °F, they will disagree by about 0.3 g/dL at 75 °F and by about 0.7 g/dL at 85 °C (Leica TS400 Total Solids Refractometer literature).

3. Interferences

    a. Because the refractive index of a solution depends on the concentration of solids in the sample, high concentrations of a variety of substances (e.g., glucose, urea, Na^+, and Cl^-) could increase the refractive index and thus the total protein reading. The total protein reading is reported to be falsely increased by 0.6 g/dL if the plasma glucose concentration is approximately 700 mg/dL (or 0.7 g/dL) or the urea nitrogen concentration is approximately 300 mg/dL.[10]

    b. Gross lipemia will increase the refractive index and thus falsely increase the total protein reading.

    c. Hemolysis causing a plasma [Hgb] of 0.5 g/dL did not interfere with refractive index values but made reading of the dividing line in the refractometer more difficult.[11]

    d. Bilirubin concentrations at 0.4 mg/dL did not interfere with refractive index values.[11] However, icterus is commonly listed as a cause of falsely increased values in clinical chemistry textbooks. Perhaps interference occurs at higher concentrations.

4. Unit conversion: g/dL × 10 = g/L (SI unit, nearest 1 g/L)[12]

5. Comments

    a. The [TP$_{ref}$] is also referred to as the *plasma total solids concentration* because the value is affected by solutes other than protein. However, most refractometer scales are calibrated for protein concentration, not total solids, and thus other substances (e.g., urea or glucose) are interferents rather than the targets of measurement.

    b. Determination of the [TP$_{ref}$] is part of a complete blood count (CBC) in many veterinary laboratories because it is a simple, quick, and inexpensive method for detection of hyperproteinemia and hypoproteinemia.

    c. Most refractometers are calibrated for the normal proteins in human plasma. The calibration scale will vary among species because of the different composition of plasma proteins,[11] but the difference is typically considered clinically insignificant.

    d. The [total protein] in serum may also be estimated with a refractometer. The serum concentration will be lower than the plasma [total protein] because of the absence of fibrinogen in serum. However, there are other factors that cause differences between plasma and serum [total protein] even if measured by the same method.[13]

        (1) H_2O diffuses from erythrocytes during clotting and thus lowers serum [total protein]. As this change is rarely described, it may cause only minor changes.

        (2) Some anticoagulants (e.g., citrate, oxalate, and fluoride) cause H_2O to diffuse from erythrocytes, but heparin (if used in appropriate amounts) does not. The solutes of the anticoagulant will add to the refractive index.

    e. As light refraction is a physical property, the [total protein] determined via refractometry may not be the same as determined by biuret reaction. In fact, it is frequently mildly different (≤ 0.3 g/dL) but occasionally different by as much as 2.0 g/dL in samples that are not hemolyzed, icteric, or lipemic (authors' observations).

B. Biuret reaction for measuring [total protein] (serum)
   1. Principle: Copper binding to peptide bonds creates a violet complex; the number of peptide bonds, and therefore amount of color change, is proportional to [total protein]. However, not all individual proteins react in the same way, and not all proteins are pure polypeptides that contain the same amount of nitrogen by weight. Therefore, [total protein] determinations are not completely accurate.
   2. Interferences: In some assays, hemolysis may cause a positive interference (e.g., Hgb at 400 mg/dL will produce a 12 % bias). Dextran (polysaccharide used as a plasma expander) may also cause a positive interference. Small peptides may react but contribute very little to total color change. NH_4^+ may interfere with the biuret reaction but not at concentrations found in plasma or serum.[14]
   3. Unit conversion: g/dL × 10 = g/L (SI unit, nearest 1 g/L)[12]
   4. Comment: The biuret or modified biuret reaction is the most common spectrophotometric method of measuring serum [total protein].

II. Albumin concentration
   A. BCG dye-binding reaction (serum)
      1. Principle: BCG preferentially binds to albumin and produces a color complex. The quantity of BCG-albumin complex is proportional to the [albumin], though binding varies among species; for example, the binding of BCG to bovine albumin is much stronger than to canine and feline albumin.[15]
      2. Interferences
         a. The binding of BCG to globulins will result in a falsely elevated [albumin]. The nonalbumin binding may lead to significant errors when the true serum [albumin] is very low (< 1 g/dL) compared to the concentration of interfering globulin (e.g., α_2-macroglobulin).
         b. In some assays, Hgb at 0.4 g/dL will cause a positive 24 % bias, whereas triglycerides at 0.8 g/dL will yield a negative interference of about 0.2 g/dL.
         c. Some BCG methods, but not others, are affected by the presence of anticoagulants. Measuring [Albumin] in heparinized plasma resulted in greater albumin values compared to serum with a standard BCG assay (median difference, 0.2 g/dL; −0.6 g/dL to 1.2 g/dL), but lower values (median difference, −0.1 g/dL; −0.9 g/dL to 0.1 g/dL) with a modified assay.[16] About 50 % of the difference in the standard assay was due to the presence of fibrinogen.
         d. Unit conversion: g/dL × 10 = g/L (SI unit, nearest 1 g/L)[12]
      3. Comment: BCG dye binding is the most common spectrophotometric method of measuring serum [albumin].
   B. BCP dye-binding reaction (serum): BCP binding is used in some human medical laboratories, but BCP does not reliably bind with all mammalian albumin molecules. BCP assays may give falsely low (sometimes markedly low) results in some domestic species (e.g., dogs).
   C. HABA (2-[4'-hydroxyazobenzene]-benzoic acid) dye-binding reactions (serum): unreliable in domestic mammal serum,[17] but the reagents are still available
   D. Protein electrophoresis can be used to determine [albumin], but is used more for quantitating globulin fractions.

III. Total [globulin]
   A. This is typically determined by subtraction (serum).
      1. Principle: All proteins in serum other than albumin are globulins.
      2. [Globulins] = [total protein] − [albumin].
   B. Protein electrophoresis (see the next section)
   C. Unit conversion: g/dL × 10 = g/L (SI unit, nearest 1 g/L)[12]
   D. Comments
      1. [Globulin] will be only as accurate as the measured [total protein] and [albumin].
      2. [Globulin] represents the total concentration of all serum proteins other than albumin (> 1000 proteins; e.g., haptoglobin, transferrin, α_2-macroglobulin, lipoproteins, and immunoglobulins).

IV. Serum protein electrophoresis (SPE) for determining protein fractions
   A. Principles
      1. Serum proteins separate into 4–6 major groups of one or more bands based on their ability to migrate through cellulose acetate or agarose in an electrical field. The degree of migration toward the anode (positively charged terminal) is based on electrical charge and a protein's mass and shape. In domestic mammal sera, albumin migrates the farthest because it is small and very anionic. Smaller proteins may not migrate as far because they lack the marked negative charge. Other globulins (e.g., α_2-macroglobulin) are very large, but negative charges cause an anodal migration. Some immunoglobulins are large and cationic and thus migrate toward the cathode (negatively charged terminal) or do not migrate. The pH of the electrophoresis medium affects the charge and migration of proteins.
      2. Major variations
         a. The same protein groups in each animal species have slight to moderate differences in migrations.
         b. Electrophoresis using cellulose acetate separates the proteins into 5–9 protein bands, whereas using agarose separates the proteins into 10–15 protein bands. A protein band may represent one protein or several proteins that have migrated the same distance.
         c. Protein bands that represent globulin proteins are grouped into electrophoretic regions. Via routine cellulose acetate methods, the common groups for domestic animals are as follows (note: a protein concentration > 0.1 g/dL is needed before it can be detected by this method):
            (1) In most dog, cat, and horse sera, five globulin regions can be seen: α_1, α_2, β_1, β_2, and γ.
            (2) In most cattle sera, only three globulin regions are seen: α, β, and γ.
   B. Calculating concentrations of the protein fractions
      1. The protein concentration of an electrophoretic group is the product of the [total protein] (preferably from a biuret reaction) and the percentage of total protein occupied by a region. When a stained cellulose acetate strip is scanned with a densitometer, stained proteins cause less light to be transmitted through the strip to a detector. The decreased transmittance is recorded as a deflection on a densitometer scan or tracing. After the cellulose acetate strip is scanned, the resulting curve represents the relative quantities of proteins (Fig. 7.1). The area under the curve represents the total quantity of stained protein.

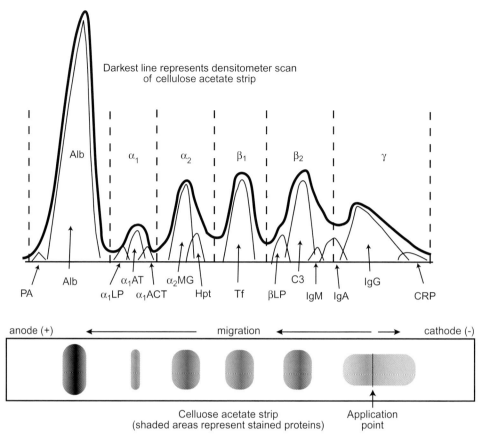

Fig. 7.1. Schematic representation of SPE results (cellulose acetate strip and densitometer tracing). Proteins are separated during electrophoresis in an alkaline medium on cellulose acetate. Albumin migrates the farthest toward the anode, and globulin fractions separate into bands or fractions (e.g., α_1-globulins, α_2-globulins, β_1-globulins, β_2-globulins, and γ-globulins). After electrophoresis, the strip is stained with a protein stain (e.g., Ponceau S). Bands that contain the most protein stain the darkest. When scanned with a densitometer, the tracer pen draws a line that corresponds with the intensity of protein staining. The darkest band causes the highest peak on the tracing, and other peaks are relatively lower depending on the relative staining intensities of the corresponding bands. One peak may represent the staining of one protein (e.g., albumin) or may represent the sum of multiple proteins (e.g., the α_2-globulin region contains Hpt and α_2-macroglobulin). α_1ACT, α_1-antichymotrypsin; α_1AT, α_1-antitrypsin; α_1LP, α_1-lipoprotein; α_2MG, α_2-macroglobulin; βLP, β-lipoprotein; and PA, prealbumin.

2. Older densitometers are calibrated so that complete transmittance through the acetate strip does not deflect the needle (zero response). In addition, densitometers may be calibrated so that the most blockage of light caused by the darkest protein band deflects the needle nearly 100 % (maximum response). The darkest band (or the maximal response) is normally the albumin band but can be found in the globulin fractions. Newer systems use flat-bed scanners to obtain digital data that are transformed into relative percentages (e.g., Helena QuickScan 2000).

3. The percentage of the total area under the curve for each region is calculated to determine the percentage of [total protein] represented by each electrophoretic region. Then, the percentages are multiplied by the [total protein] to determine the approximate protein concentrations in each electrophoretic region. For example, if the [total protein] is 6.0 g/dL and electrophoresis results indicate that 50 % of the stained protein is in the albumin band, then the [albumin] is calculated to be 3.0 g/dL.

4. The concentrations of the protein fractions determined by electrophoresis will vary because of several factors: variable affinities of stains for certain proteins, accuracy of the measured [total protein], accuracy of densitometry, and the sometimes substantial differences in marking of protein fractions. Coomassie brilliant blue and amido black stains have greater capabilities of detecting small amounts of protein than do Ponceau S stain and thus tend to be used in high-resolution electrophoretic systems.

C. Proteins that are the major contributors to the electrophoretic pattern are shown in Fig. 7.1 and listed in Table 7.2. Migration regions are for human proteins; there is evidence of similar migration in domestic mammals. When using agarose gel electrophoresis for canine sera, the protein migrations were similar to those listed in Table 7.2 except C3 was a β_1-globulin and transferrin was a β_2-globulin.[18] For some sera (e.g., bovine), only three or four globulin fractions will be detected.

D. Comments

1. SPE has limited diagnostic value. It may be helpful in differentiating the causes of hyperproteinemia, characterizing hypoproteinemias into selective or nonselective categories, screening for a monoclonal gammopathy in normoproteinemic and hyperproteinemic sera, and providing a more accurate estimation of [albumin] when globulins interfere with the BCG assay. Analysis of serum proteins by SPE is not common in clinical medicine, but understanding SPE results aids in understanding routine serum concentrations of total protein, albumin, and globulins.

2. The protein bands on the cellulose acetate or ararose should be examined in addition to the densitometric findings, because the tracings do not always demonstrate the abnormalities in the protein fractions.

3. The calculated concentrations of the electrophoretic fractions are at best estimates. The true value is usually within 0.3 g/dL of the calculated value (assuming proper marking of fractions). The calculated concentrations are frequently not needed to classify or interpret dysproteinemia patterns.

V. Immunoelectrophoresis

A. This is a method of identifying the presence of specific proteins or protein components. It can be used to identify the presence of immunoglobulin classes or subclasses, heavy chains, or light chains.

B. The serum proteins are first separated by electrophoresis. Appropriate antibodies are added to long troughs cut parallel to the electrophoretic separation. The antibody and the electrophoretically separated serum proteins diffuse toward each other and form precipitant arcs if there is a reactive antigen (e.g., heavy chain of IgG) for the antibody.

VI. Sia euglobulin test

A. A *euglobulin* is a protein that does not dissolve in pure water. The *Sia euglobulin test* is simply adding 1 drop of serum to demineralized H_2O; formation of a precipitate or flocculates is a positive test. When first described by Sia in 1921, the euglobulin test

Table 7.2. Serum proteins that contribute to electrophoretic regions

Region	Proteins	M_r (in thousands)	Function and other information
Pre-albumin	—	—	Not recognized in routine SPE of animal sera; includes thyroxine-binding albumin and retinol-binding protein
Albumin	Albumin[a]	69	Major contributor to oncotic pressure; transports Ca^{2+}, Mg^{2+}, unconjugated bilirubin, fatty acids, thyroxine, and many other substances
α_1	α_1-Lipoprotein	180–350	Transports lipids (especially cholesterol); also called HDL; relatively very low concentrations in domestic mammals when compared to people
	α_1-Antitrypsin[b]	54	Inactivates proteases, including trypsin, and thus is an anti-inflammatory protein
	α_1-Antichymotrypsin[b]	68	Inactivates proteases, including chymotrypsin, and thus is an anti-inflammatory protein
α_2	α_2-Macroglobulin[b]	820	Inactivates proteases and thus is an anti-inflammatory protein
	Haptoglobins[b]	80–160	Bind and transport free hemoglobin
β_1	Transferrin[a]	76	Binds and transports iron; measured as total iron-binding capacity in chemical assays
β_2	β-Lipoprotein	2400	Transports lipids (cholesterol and triglyceride); also called LDL
	Complement (C3a)[b]	180	Promotes inflammation; chemotactic substance
	IgM and IgA	IgA: 160 IgM: 900	Bind to specific antigens; concentrations are too low in health to be seen via routine SPE
γ	IgG	150	Binds to specific antigens; many different isotypes and idiotypes of IgG give a broad and usually indistinct gamma region
	C-reactive protein[b]	110	Positive acute-phase protein; rarely seen in mammalian sera via routine SPE

[a] Negative acute-phase protein
[b] Positive acute-phase protein

Note: Most information is based on human plasma proteins. Proteins in domestic mammal plasma are assumed to migrate in similar regions. There are hundreds of other plasma proteins of clinical significance, but their concentrations are too low in physiologic and pathologic states to alter the electrophoretic pattern in cellulose acetate electrophoresis. If plasma is electrophoresed, fibrinogen (M_r: 341,000, a positive acute-phase protein) should migrate in the cathodal end of the β_2-region.

Source: Ritzmann and Daniels[106]

was a screening test for macroglobulins. However, analyses of human sera indicate that the positive test may result from a variety of monoclonal and polyclonal gammopathies and thus is not diagnostically useful.[19] A modified Sia test (using weak electrolyte solutions) for macroglobulins resulted in fewer false positives but more false negatives.

B. Recognizing the precipitant property of immunoglobulins is important in two situations. First, this property can be used to separate immunoglobulins from other serum proteins; the precipitated immunoglobulins can then be dissolved in saline. Second, the precipitates can interfere with the analysis of sera or blood samples; for example, falsely increased serum phosphorus concentrations (Chapter 11), falsely increased blood [Hgb] (Chapter 3), and falsely increased serum bilirubin concentration (Chapter 13).

HYPERPROTEINEMIA (INCREASED TOTAL PROTEIN CONCENTRATION IN SERUM OR PLASMA)

The diseases and conditions that cause hyperproteinemia are listed in Table 7.3.

I.   Hemoconcentration is a common cause of hyperproteinemia.
    A. Pathogenesis: Hyperproteinemia results from the concentration of plasma proteins caused by the loss of plasma H_2O. The plasma H_2O loss and resultant decreased ECF volume may be due to vomiting, diarrhea, impaired renal concentrating ability, sweating, insensible loss via respiration, increased vascular permeability, or decreased H_2O intake combined with normal losses.
    B. If proteins were the only solids in plasma, then plasma would contain about 93 % H_2O and 7 % proteins and the [total protein] would be about 7.0 g/dL in health. If dehydration led to a 10 % decrease in plasma volume, the [total protein] would increase to about 7.8 g/dL (7.0/0.9 = 7.78).
    C. All proteins are concentrated by loss of plasma H_2O; therefore, hemoconcentration results in a nonselective hyperproteinemia. Concentrations of albumin, globulins, and fibrinogen are proportionately increased if dehydration is the only cause of the dysproteinemia (Plate 12B).
    D. Other expected laboratory findings
       1. Erythrocytosis
       2. Prerenal azotemia
       3. Hypersthenuria, if renal concentrating mechanisms are functional

Table 7.3. Diseases and conditions that cause hyperproteinemia

*Hemoconcentration
Increased protein synthesis
  Inflammatory diseases
    *Infection: bacterial, viral, fungal, protozoal
    *Noninfectious disease: necrosis, neoplasia, immune-mediated disease
  B-lymphocyte neoplasia
    Plasma cell: multiple myeloma, plasmacytoma
    Lymphocyte: lymphoma, lymphocytic leukemia

  * A relatively common disease or condition
  Note: All of these diseases or conditions may cause hyperglobulinemia, but only hemoconcentration will cause concurrent hyperalbuminemia.

II.   Increased protein synthesis
  A. Inflammation is a common cause of hyperproteinemia but does not necessarily cause hyperproteinemia.
    1. Pathogenesis: Inflammation (caused by infections or other processes) stimulates the synthesis of certain globulins by hepatocytes and perhaps immunoglobulins by B-lymphocytes. Several cytokines, especially interleukin 6, alter protein synthesis in, or protein release from, hepatocytes.[20] Cytokines primarily regulate transcription (either up-regulate or down-regulate) to alter protein production to produce these changes.
      a. Increased concentrations of the positive APPs (see General Concepts for Total Protein, Albumin, and Globulins, sect. II.C)
        (1) Production of these proteins may increase within hours and may persist as long as an inflammatory process is present. Increased plasma or serum concentrations may be seen by 2 d after the onset of inflammation.
        (2) Individually, fibrinogen and haptoglobin concentrations can increase enough to increase [total protein] (e.g., [fibrinogen] may increase from 0.3 g/dL to > 1.0 g/dL, and [haptoglobin] may increase from 0.3 g/dL to 0.9 g/dL). The concentrations of other APPs are relatively much less in health, and thus a marked increased in an individual protein concentration adds little to the [total protein] (e.g., [C-reactive protein] may increase from 1 mg/dL to 50 mg/dL, and [serum amyloid A] may increase from 0.2 mg/dL to 100 mg/dL).[6]
      b. Decreased concentrations of the negative APPs
        (1) Negative APPs are proteins whose plasma or serum concentrations decrease because of decreased production by hepatocytes during inflammation. This group includes albumin and transferrin.
        (2) Due to the plasma half-life of albumin in various animals (e.g., ≈ 8 d in dogs and ≈ 19 d in horses) and the variable degrees of reduced production, an inflammatory hypoalbuminemia may not be seen until inflammation has persisted for at least several days in dogs and at least 2 wk in horses. The magnitude of decrease is typically mild (i.e., a decrease by < 30 %; e.g., from 3.0 g/dL to 2.4 g/dL) if inflammation is the only reason for the hypoalbuminemia.
        (3) The plasma half-lives of transferrin are not firmly established in domestic species. However, decreased total iron binding capacity (as a measure of transferrin concentration) may not be seen until inflammation has persisted for at least a week.
      c. Delayed-response proteins
        (1) These are proteins whose plasma or serum concentrations increase 1–3 wk after the onset of inflammation; the increase is caused by increased production.
        (2) This group includes all immunoglobulins (IgG mostly) and complement (C3). Increased synthesis of a variety of immunoglobulins by many clones of B-lymphocytes produces a *polyclonal gammopathy*.
        (3) The magnitude of increases in [C3] (as detected by β-globulin increase) is typically < 1.0 g/dL. The magnitude of increases in [immunoglobulin] can be mild (< 1.0 g/dL) to marked (> 4.0 g/dL)
    2. Expected dysproteinemia patterns

a. Acute-phase response: hyperproteinemia caused by acute inflammation lasting 2–7 d
   (1) Mild hyperproteinemia caused by hyperglobulinemia (increased α_1- and/or α_2-globulins and hyperfibrinogenemia)
   (2) Possibly mild hypoalbuminemia or low-normal serum albumin concentration
b. Delayed response: hyperproteinemia caused by inflammation lasting more than 7 d
   (1) Hyperproteinemia (mild to marked) is caused by hyperglobulinemia (increased positive acute-phase and/or delayed response proteins). A polyclonal gammopathy may or may not be detected by SPE (Plate 12C–F).
   (2) Mild to moderate hypoalbuminemia may be present.
   (3) The net change in protein concentrations may produce a dysproteinemia with a lower [albumin] and greater concentrations of some globulin fractions.
   (4) A polyclonal gammopathy with a restricted migration has been called an *oligoclonal gammopathy* (Plate 12D). In human medicine, it is not considered a monoclonal gammopathy because its proteins do not meet the criteria for monoclonal proteins (i.e., increases in κ- or λ-light chains, not both). The "monoclonal" gammopathies that some authors have described in animals with infectious diseases (e.g., ehrlichiosis and leishmaniasis) may have been oligoclonal gammopathies or compact polyclonal gammopathies.[21–26] They were considered monoclonal gammopathies because of the narrow spike in an electrophoretic pattern, and the authors established that the gammopathy was primarily caused by one class of immunoglobulin (i.e., IgG) via immunoelectrophoresis or radial immunodiffusion. However, the gammopathy could include more than one immunoglobulin subclass and thus not be monoclonal, and light-chain analyses were not done to support clonality.
   (5) A biclonal pattern (electrophoretic α_2- and β_1-spikes) caused by an increased [IgG_3] was found in a horse. The gammopathy disappeared after the horse was treated for a strongyle infection.[26] IgG_3 is also referred to as IgG(T).
c. A monoclonal expansion of T-lymphocytes has been found in dogs infected with *Ehrlichia canis* that concurrently had gammopathies with narrow electrophoretic spikes. We are not aware of cases in which a clonal expansion of B-lymphocytes could be producing a true monoclonal gammopathy.
3. Other laboratory data associated with inflammatory hyperproteinemias
   a. Anemia of inflammatory disease may develop if inflammation persists.
   b. Inflammatory neutrophilia or neutropenia may develop.
   c. Inflammatory lymphocytosis or lymphopenia may develop.
   d. Inflammatory monocytosis may develop.
4. Concurrent pathologic processes may complicate interpretation of the protein data. For example, there can be a concurrent increased fibrinogen production because of inflammation and increased fibrinogen consumption because of intravascular coagulation. Or, there can be concurrent inflammation and hemoconcentration or inflammation and protein-losing states.
B. B-lymphocyte neoplasia
1. Pathogenesis: Neoplastic B-lymphocytes may produce large quantities of an immunoglobulin; typically, there is one neoplastic cell line or one clone of neoplastic

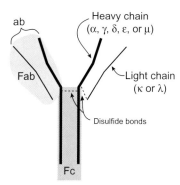

Fig. 7.2. Schematic structure of an immunoglobulin. Immunoglobulin consists of two heavy chains of the same class (α for IgA, γ for IgG, δ for IgD, ε for IgE, and μ for IgM) and two light chains (either κ or λ but not both). The combination of a light chain and the slanted segment of a heavy chain is a fragment (F) that contains an antigen-binding site (ab) (F + ab = Fab). The tail of the Y (vertical segments of two heavy chains) is called the crystallizable (c) fragment (F + c = Fc).

lymphocytes. The single clone of lymphocytes produces an electrophoretically, structurally, and antigenically homogeneous immunoglobulin or a comparably homogeneous immunoglobulin subunit. The resulting dysproteinemia is called a *monoclonal gammopathy*.

2. Proteins produced by B-lymphocyte neoplasia are sometimes called *M proteins* (for monoclonal proteins). *M protein* has also been used as an abbreviation for myeloma proteins or macroglobulin, and thus one must interpret "M protein" in context. An intact monoclonal immunoglobulin consists of two heavy chains of the same class (e.g., IgM) and subclass (e.g., IgG$_1$ or IgG$_2$) and two light chains of the same type (either κ or λ but not both) (Fig. 7.2).[27] The neoplastic cells may produce intact immunoglobulins, free light chains, only heavy chains, or abnormal fragments.[28] The proteins that are produced by neoplastic B-lymphocytes and accumulate in plasma, urine, or tissues are *paraproteins*.

3. Types of B-lymphocyte neoplasia that may cause a gammopathy
   a. Plasma cell neoplasia: multiple myeloma (most frequent cause) or extramedullary plasmacytoma
   b. Lymphocyte neoplasia: lymphoma or lymphocytic leukemia

4. Expected dysproteinemia pattern
   a. Mild to marked hyperproteinemia produced by hyperglobulinemia that contains a monoclonal gammopathy. The monoclonal protein may migrate in β- or γ-globulin fractions.
      (1) IgG typically migrates in the γ-globulin fraction, whereas IgM and IgA typically migrate at the β-γ junction or in the β-globulin fraction (Plate 12G).[29] In a horse with a plasma cell myeloma, a monoclonal spike was found in the α$_2$-globulin fraction and single radial immunodiffusion indicated the paraprotein was IgG$_3$. IgG$_3$ is also referred to as IgG(T).[30]
      (2) Atypical electrophoretic migrations may be caused by protein degradation, immunoglobulin binding to other proteins, formation of immunoglobulin complexes, or production of incomplete immunoglobulins (e.g., light chains,

heavy chains, or abnormal fragments).[27] Two electrophoretic peaks were detected in a dog's serum that had an IgA-producing myeloma; the two peaks were determined to be complexes of IgA (dimers, trimers, or tetramers).[31] Similar biclonal peaks were found in a cat with IgA-producing myeloma, but only one peak (thus suggesting a monoclonal peak) was present after the sera were exposed to a reducing agent.[32] In another case, the authors concluded that their data indicated that two clones of IgA-producing plasma cells were present.[33]

    (3) Concentrations of immunoglobulins other than the monoclonal protein frequently are decreased.

  b. Mild to moderate hypoalbuminemia may be caused by decreased albumin synthesis due to inflammatory cytokines, or by a negative feedback mechanism involving an oncotic pressure receptor on hepatocytes. Increased concentration of γ-globulins (either by infusion or endogenous production) does decrease albumin synthesis, but the mechanism has not been established.[34]

5. The presence of a monoclonal gammopathy in domestic mammals is rarely confirmed.

  a. Serum protein electrophoresis

    (1) An increased concentration of an immunoglobulin is called a gammopathy regardless of where the immunoglobulin migrates with SPE. It could be in the α-, β-, or γ-globulin regions.

    (2) The presence of a narrow protein band or the resulting narrow spike in a densitometer scan (i.e., resembling an albumin band or albumin peak) in either β-globulin or γ-globulin regions after serum electrophoresis is frequently stated to represent a monoclonal gammopathy.[21,35–37] However, such findings can be due to either one immunoglobulin or a group of proteins that are migrating in the same region. Serum electrophoresis is useful to screen for potential monoclonal gammopathies but frequently lacks sufficient specificity to reliably differentiate a monoclonal gammopathy from a restricted or compact polyclonal or oligoclonal gammopathy.

      (a) A narrow globulin spike in the γ-globulin fraction could be a monoclonal gammopathy (caused by B-lymphocyte neoplasia) or an oligoclonal (or restricted polyclonal) gammopathy (caused by an immune response).[38]

      (b) A narrow globulin spike that is not in the γ-globulin fraction is probably a monoclonal gammopathy since such bands are usually due to either IgA or IgM and not to IgG. High concentrations of IgA or IgM are not expected in a nonneoplastic immune response.

    (3) Compared to cellulose acetate methods, agarose electrophoresis or high-resolution electrophoretic methods will improve detection of protein bands; that is, what appears to be one band on cellulose acetate may be seen as two bands on agarose. However, the presence of a single band on agarose does not confirm the presence of a monoclonal gammopathy.[28]

  b. Immunoelectrophoresis

    (1) If a monoclonal gammopathy is suspected, then immunoelectrophoresis with species-specific anti-IgG (including subclasses), anti-IgM, anti-IgA, anti-(κ-chain), or anti-(λ-chain) antibodies is needed to differentiate monoclonal and polyclonal gammopathies by protein analysis.[27]

    (2) If immunoelectrophoresis results indicate that nearly all of the gammopathy is due to IgM or IgA, then the gammopathy very likely is monoclonal. If nearly all of the gammopathy is due to IgG, then it could be either monoclonal or polyclonal with multiple classes of IgG; such a polyclonal state was found in a dog with canine ehrlichiosis.[39] If the gammopathy is due to only one IgG subclass, then it is probably monoclonal.

    (3) If there is a monoclonal gammopathy, then the increased concentration of one heavy-chain class (or subclass) will be associated with either κ- or λ-chains because a lymphocyte clone produces either κ- or λ-chains, not both.[27]

    (4) A potential monoclonal gammopathy associated with canine ehrlichiosis was investigated by analysis of urinary light chains. Finding both κ- and λ-light chains (in a 2:1 ratio) in the dog's urine suggested that the gammopathy was polyclonal and not monoclonal. The light-chain concentrations were measured by an immunoprecipitation assay designed for human light chains.[40] These findings suggest there is cross-immunoreactivity for human and canine light chains, but the degree of cross-immunoreactivity is not known.

  c. Immunofixation is reported to have greater analytical sensitivity than immunoelectrophoresis and, like immunoelectrophoresis, requires monospecific (and possibly species specific) antisera to IgG, IgM, IgA, and free and bound κ- or λ-chains.[28]

  d. RID

    (1) RID assays for [IgM] and [IgA] may be used to support a monoclonal gammopathy conclusion because high concentrations of IgM or IgA are not expected in inflammatory states.

    (2) However, like immunoelectrophoresis, RID assays for total [IgG] cannot be used to differentiate an IgG polyclonal gammopathy from an IgG monoclonal gammopathy because the IgG gammopathy may contain more than one subclass of IgG.

6. Identification of light chains

  a. Immunohistochemical assays using anti-(human λ-light chain) antibodies and anti-(human κ-light chain) antibodies have been used to characterize neoplastic plasma cells in dogs and cats. Out of 117 canine plasmacytomas, 114 were λ positive and three were κ positive.[41] In several feline cases, nearly all were λ positive.[42] Establishing significance of these reactions is complicated by the distribution of λ-light chains and κ-light chains in domestic mammals. Results of studies using anti-(human λ-light chain) and anti-(human κ-light chain) antibodies for immunohistochemical analysis of plasma cells in lymphoid organs of healthy dogs, horses, cats, and cattle indicated the λ to κ ratios were about 9:1.[43] Therefore, a dominance of λ-light chains (when antibodies to human light chain are used) in tissue or serum could potentially be either a polyclonal or monoclonal proliferation in dogs, cats, horses, and cattle.

  b. Considering the need for species-specific antisera for the analysis of many proteins and polypeptides, the results of the aforementioned studies would be strengthened by establishing the degree of cross-reactivity of the anti-(human light chain) antibodies with domestic mammal light chains, especially with κ-light chains.

7. Associated laboratory or clinical problems
   a. Bence Jones proteinuria (BJ proteins = light chains of immunoglobulins) (see Chapter 8) (Plate 12J.2)
   b. Hyperviscosity syndrome
      (1) High immunoglobulin concentrations may cause the plasma to become viscous. Hyperviscosity syndrome is seen with high concentrations of IgA, IgG, or IgM.
      (2) Viscous plasma leads to sluggish blood flow in capillaries and causes poor perfusion and thus tissue hypoxia (stagnant hypoxia). Major tissues affected include brain, eyes, and kidneys.
      (3) The high plasma [total protein] may also cause abnormal platelet function that may lead to clinical bleeding.
   c. Hypercalcemia may be found in some lymphoproliferative disorders (see Chapter 11).
   d. Animals can develop systemic AL amyloidosis. AL-type amyloid is composed of immunoglobulin light chains. A horse with multiple myeloma was found to have systemic AL amyloidosis with an amyloid that reacted with anti-(human λ-chain) antibodies.[44] The horse had hypoglobulinemia, which suggests that the neoplastic plasma cells were producing λ-chains and not intact immunoglobulins. AL amyloidosis was also diagnosed in a cat that had an extramedullary plasmacytoma.[45] Peptides within the amyloid had amino acid sequences very similar to sequences of human λ-chains.
8. Amplification of variable regions of immunoglobulin genes by polymerase chain reaction is being used to characterize the clonality of B-lymphocyte neoplasia.[46] However, analysis of small biopsy samples from reactive lymphoid tissue may yield what appears to be a monoclonal proliferation because of clonal expansion within a germinal center or because of random amplification of small amounts of DNA.[47,48] Pseudoclonality is present if amplification produces one or more distinct bands, but the results are not reproducible.

HYPOPROTEINEMIA (DECREASED [TOTAL PROTEIN] IN SERUM OR PLASMA)

The diseases and conditions that cause hypoproteinemia are listed in Table 7.4.

I. Increased protein loss from vascular space
   A. Blood loss (primarily external hemorrhage; acute or chronic)
      1. Pathogenesis: Hypoproteinemia occurs when the remaining plasma proteins are diluted by movement of extracellular fluid from extravascular space to intravascular space (see Fig. 3.8). Hypoproteinemia will persist as long as the rate of protein loss exceeds the rate of protein production.
      2. Major laboratory findings
         a. *Panhypoproteinemia*, which is a decreased [total protein] with decreased concentrations of albumin and globulins, is a nonselective hypoproteinemia.
         b. Anemia: The type of anemia depends on duration and magnitude of blood loss (see Chapter 3).
   B. PLN
      1. Pathogenesis: Renal glomerular damage (e.g., by immune complex or amyloid deposition) causes either a retraction of podocytes or loss of the selective permeability

Table 7.4. Diseases and conditions that cause hypoproteinemia

Increased protein loss from vascular space
  *Blood loss
  *Protein-losing nephropathy: glomerulonephritis, amyloidosis
  *Protein-losing enteropathy: small intestinal mucosal disease, lymphangiectasia, intestinal
    blood loss
  Protein-losing dermatopathy: burns, generalized exudative skin disease
  Plasma loss: peritonitis, pleuritis, vasculitis
Decreased protein synthesis and/or increased protein catabolism
  *Hepatic insufficiency
  *Malabsorption or maldigestion: intestinal mucosal disease, exocrine pancreatic
    insufficiency
  *Cachectic states: chronic diseases, neoplasia, malnutrition, starvation
  Lymphoid hypoplasia or aplasia
Failure of passive transfer (FPT)
Hemodilution
  Excess administration of intravenous fluid
  Edematous disorders: congestive heart failure, cirrhosis, nephrotic syndrome
  Excess ADH secretion: SIADH

* A relatively common disease or condition
Note: Total protein concentrations in healthy pups, kittens, calves, and foals may be 1.0–2.0 g/dL
less than those found in mature animals.

of the glomerular basement membrane. Either or both lesions allow larger and more negatively charged proteins through the glomerular filtration barrier. When proteins enter the filtrate at a rate greater than proximal tubules can resorb, then proteinuria occurs. When the rate of protein loss exceeds protein production, hypoproteinemia occurs. The largest proteins (e.g., α_2-macroglobulin and β-lipoprotein) typically are not lost through glomeruli, and thus a selective hypoproteinemia occurs. Because dogs and cats normally have very little β-lipoprotein, the β_2-globulin fraction typically is not relatively increased as it is in people with a PLN.

2. Diseases
   a. Animals with a PLN (as defined in this section) have a glomerulopathy. Glomerulonephritis or renal amyloidosis may be apparent histologically.
   b. Soft-coated Wheaten terriers have an increased incidence of PLN and PLE.[49]
3. Major laboratory findings
   a. Mild to marked hypoproteinemia with hypoalbuminemia and normoglobulinemia (occasionally hypoglobulinemia)
   b. SPE results: There is a selective hypoproteinemia pattern with α_2-globulins WRI or only mildly decreased (but appear relatively increased). Other protein fractions are typically definitely decreased (Plate 12I.1). The degree of decrease of the γ-globulin fraction will depend on the porosity of the glomeruli.
   c. Moderate to marked proteinuria dominated by albuminuria (Plate 12I.2)
   d. Perhaps evidence of renal insufficiency (azotemia or isosthenuria) if the disease has destroyed enough nephrons

       e. Hypercholesterolemia and peritoneal transudate if nephrotic syndrome has developed

C. PLE

  1. Pathogenesis

    a. Intestinal secretions, which are relatively protein rich, typically are digested and absorbed in the small intestine, and then transported to the portal system and lymphatic vessels. When generalized small intestinal mucosal diseases or lymphatic diseases prohibit the absorption or transport of the proteins, the proteins are lost in feces. When the rate of protein loss exceeds the capability of the liver and lymphocytes to produce proteins, hypoproteinemia occurs.

    b. In some disorders, inflammatory exudation and decreased protein intake contribute to the hypoproteinemia.

    c. Intestinal blood loss because of parasitism is one form of PLE.

  2. Diseases

    a. Generalized small intestinal mucosal diseases: lymphoma, histoplasmosis, and lymphocytic/plasmacytic/eosinophilic enteritis

    b. Horses with acute enteritis

    c. Lymphatic disease: lymphangiectasia or lymphoma

    d. Intestinal blood loss: hookworms, whipworms, or neoplasia

  3. Major laboratory findings

    a. Mild to marked hypoproteinemia with hypoalbuminemia and hypoglobulinemia (or normoglobulinemia)

    b. SPE results: The pattern is usually nonselective but may be selective.

    c. Other findings may indicate or suggest the inciting pathologic state (e.g., *Histoplasma* organisms or neoplastic lymphocytes in biopsy samples, or melena or other evidence of blood loss).

D. Protein-losing dermatopathy

  1. Pathogenesis

    a. Thermal or chemical burns allow plasma proteins to exude from cutaneous lesions at a rate greater than the rate of protein production. If the animal is not seen soon after the injury, the dysproteinemia will reflect a mixture of cutaneous protein loss and an acute-phase inflammatory response.[50]

    b. Generalized exudative skin disease can cause a hypoproteinemic state, but the dysproteinemia probably reflects a mixture of protein loss and an inflammatory dysproteinemia.

  2. Major laboratory findings

    a. Early: nonselective hypoproteinemia

    b. Later: nonselective hypoproteinemia masked by either an acute or chronic inflammatory dysproteinemia

E. Plasma loss caused by peritonitis, pleuritis, or vasculitis

  1. Pathogenesis

    a. Pleuritis and peritonitis: Acute inflammation of pleura or peritoneum allows for extravasation of protein-rich fluid into the pleural and peritoneal cavities, respectively. Such protein loss is sometimes referred to as *third-space loss*. Subsequent hemodilution causes hypoproteinemia.

    b. Vasculitis: A similar loss of protein-rich fluid can occur with vasculitis; the fluid enters the interstitial fluid adjacent to the inflamed vessels.

    2. Major laboratory findings
      a. Early: nonselective hypoproteinemia
      b. Later: nonselective hypoproteinemia masked by either an acute or chronic inflammatory dysproteinemia

II. Decreased protein synthesis and/or increased protein catabolism
  A. Hepatic insufficiency (or hepatic failure)
    1. Pathogenesis: A marked reduction in functional hepatic mass (< 20 % remaining) decreases the synthesis of nearly all plasma proteins except immunoglobulins. Normal protein catabolism combined with decreased protein synthesis produces the hypoproteinemia.
    2. Disorders
      a. Cirrhosis
      b. Hepatic necrosis or inflammation (not acute)
      c. Hepatic atrophy secondary to portosystemic shunts
      d. Neoplasms that damage the liver extensively
    3. Major laboratory findings
      a. Hypoproteinemia, hypoalbuminemia, and normoglobulinemia or hypoglobulinemia
      b. SPE results: The pattern is frequently nonselective, but there may be a relative excess in β_2- or γ-globulins because of one of two theories:
        (1) There may be a compensatory increased synthesis of immunoglobulins to attempt to maintain a colloidal osmotic (oncotic) pressure in the vascular system.
        (2) The liver removes antigenic material and IgA from the portal blood. With hepatic insufficiency, the antigenic material gains entrance to peripheral blood and induces a systemic immune response (increased IgM, IgA, or IgG). Because IgM and IgA migrate in the β_2-globulin fraction and IgG in the γ-globulin fraction, there may not be a clear distinction between β_2- and γ-globulin fractions (called a *beta-gamma bridge*).
    4. Other chemical findings of hepatic disease or dysfunction: increased hepatic enzyme activities, decreased urea concentration, or increased bile acid or ammonium concentrations
  B. Malabsorption or maldigestion
    1. Pathogenesis: A malabsorptive or maldigestive state results in a deficient intake of basic body fuels (carbohydrates, proteins, or lipids) to replace fuels used by metabolic pathways for daily energy. Once depleted, protein catabolism and the use of amino acids for gluconeogenesis lead to a deficiency in energy and amino acids for hepatocellular and lymphocytic protein synthesis. When catabolism exceeds production, hypoproteinemia occurs.
    2. Disorders
      a. Malabsorption: Small intestinal diseases with generalized mucosal involvement may cause malabsorption of digested proteins, carbohydrates, and lipids.
      b. Maldigestion: Exocrine pancreatic insufficiency (because of chronic pancreatitis or pancreatic atrophy) creates deficiencies in proteases, lipase, and amylase and thus maldigestion of proteins, lipids (fat), or carbohydrates (starches).
    3. Major laboratory findings
      a. Hypoproteinemia, hypoalbuminemia, and normoglobulinemia or hypoglobulinemia

b. SPE results: The pattern typically is nonselective (Plate 12H).
c. Other findings dependent on the primary pathologic state (e.g., decreased trypsin-like immunoreactivity with exocrine pancreatic insufficiency, or poor xylose absorption with malabsorptive states [see Chapter 15])

C. Cachectic states
1. Pathogenesis: When the rate of protein catabolism exceeds protein production, the negative protein status causes hypoproteinemia. Before hypoproteinemia develops, glucose and most serum protein concentrations (especially albumin) are maintained at the expense of other tissues. Therefore, this hypoproteinemia is expected when body weight has been lost due to decreased fat and muscle mass.
2. Disorders
   a. Chronic diseases such as chronic infections and malignant neoplasia (Plate 12J.1)
   b. Marked malnutrition or starvation
3. Major laboratory findings
   a. Hypoproteinemia, hypoalbuminemia, and normoglobulinemia or hypoglobulinemia
   b. SPE results: The pattern typically is nonselective.
   c. Other findings dependent on the primary pathologic state

D. Lymphoid hypoplasia or aplasia
1. B-lymphocytes produce immunoglobulins and not other major plasma proteins. A mild hypoproteinemia potentially can be created by lymphoid hypoplasia if concentrations of other proteins are WRI.
2. Expected dysproteinemia
   a. The [total protein] is WRI to slightly decreased. The [albumin] is WRI, and the [globulin] is WRI or slightly decreased.
   b. SPE results: The [γ-globulin] is decreased.
3. Disorders
   a. Combined immunodeficiency occurs in horses (Arabian and Appaloosa) and dogs (basset hounds, Cardigan Welsh corgis, and Jack Russell terriers). Quantitative immunoglobulin techniques are needed to confirm decreases or deficiencies of immunoglobulins (see the Immunoglobulin section).
   b. Chemotherapy or infections may cause lymphoid hypoplasia.[51]

III. FPT
A. Neonates who fail to ingest or absorb colostral antibodies will have lower serum or plasma [total protein] because of lower [IgG]. However, inflammation or dehydration can increase the [total protein] in such animals and thus mask the FPT.
B. This relationship between [IgG] and [total protein] has been explored and resulted in the following findings in sera from 1- to 8-d-old calves when compared to an [IgG] decision value of 1000 mg/dL.[52]
   1. With a [sTP$_{ref}$] of 5.0 g/dL as a decision limit, 83 % were correctly classified regarding passive transfer status.
   2. With a [sTP$_{ref}$] of 5.5 g/dL as a decision limit, 82 % were correctly classified regarding passive transfer status.

IV. Hemodilution: increased ECF volume
A. By itself, increased ECF is a very uncommon cause of hypoproteinemia, but it may lower protein concentrations that were already decreased because of another problem.

  B. Disorders or conditions
     1. Excess administration of intravenous fluid (too fast or too much)
     2. Edematous disorders (congestive heart failure, cirrhosis, and nephrotic syndrome)
     3. Excess ADH secretion (SIADH)
     4. Use of plasma expanders, when extravascular fluid is pulled into plasma soon after administration (may not result in increased ECF volume but does dilute the plasma protein concentration)

HYPERALBUMINEMIA

The diseases and conditions that cause hyperalbuminemia are listed in Table 7.5.

I.   Hemoconcentration (dehydration): decreased ECF volume
      A. Decreased plasma H_2O leads to greater concentrations of those substances (including albumin) that have circulating life spans longer than the time it took to become dehydrated.
      B. Hemoconcentration is the most common reason for hyperalbuminemia. Concurrent hyperproteinemia and perhaps erythrocytosis are expected.

II.   Induced synthesis by glucocorticoid therapy
      A. Glucocorticoid therapy might cause mild hyperalbuminemia in dogs[53,54] and in cats (unpublished S.L.S. data). In dogs given prednisone (0.55 mg/kg, q12h) for 4 wk, the [albumin] and [total protein] increased more in the prednisone-treated dogs than in a control group.[54] In another study with dogs receiving prednisone (0.55 mg/kg, q12h) for 4 wk, [albumin] and [total protein] increased along with a concurrent increase in [haptoglobin]; the changes in [albumin] were not significantly different from the changes in the control dogs.[53] The [albumin] may be increased because of increased production[55] or possibly increased albumin life span.
      B. One study reported a large increase in [albumin] (about 2 g/dL) after 4–5 d of treatment with methylprednisolone (4 mg/kg IM q24h). However, the [albumin] was measured by a biuret method after Na_2SO_3 precipitation, so the increase may have included proteins other than albumin (e.g., haptoglobin). The [total protein] increased concurrently, but the [globulin] (calculated by subtraction) did not.[56]

III. Falsely increased concentration determined by the BCG dye method
      A. BCG dye preferentially binds to albumin. However, it also binds to some α-globulins and β-globulins, and thus a measured albumin concentration represents the dye binding to albumin and some globulins.[57] The binding of BCG to globulins is reduced if the assay's incubation time is reduced.[58] Falsely increased [albumin] is also found in heparinized plasma because of the binding of BCG with fibrinogen.[16]

Table 7.5. Diseases and conditions that cause hyperalbuminemia

*Hemoconcentration
Increased albumin synthesis induced by glucocorticoid drugs or hormones

* A relatively common disease or condition
Note: If [albumin] is determined by the BCG method, the BCG dye may bind to proteins other than albumin and thus yield a pseudo-hyperalbuminemia.

B. The anomalous [albumin] may not be recognized in hypoalbuminemic samples; that is, the hypoalbuminemia is more severe than indicated by the measured concentration. For example, in sera of dogs with PLN, the [albumin] from SPE may be considerably less than the BCG value.

HYPOALBUMINEMIA

I. This commonly occurs with hyperproteinemia and hypoproteinemia but also can be seen when there is normoproteinemia.

II. The diseases and conditions that cause hypoalbuminemia are listed in Table 7.6. Pathogeneses of the hypoalbuminemic states are described in the appropriate dysproteinemia sections (see the Hyperproteinemia and Hypoproteinemia sections).
   A. Hypoalbuminemia may be found in hyperproteinemic states not related to hemoconcentration.
      1. Inflammatory hypoalbuminemia occurs because albumin is a negative APP. The following two major concepts are related to inflammatory hypoalbuminemia:
         a. The hypoalbuminemia does not develop until the inflammation has persisted for days to weeks, especially in horses because equine albumin has a plasma half-life of nearly 3 wk.
         b. If inflammation is the only cause of the hypoalbuminemic state, hypoalbuminemia is expected to be mild.
      2. The pathogeneses of hypoalbuminemias seen concurrently with B-lymphocyte neoplasia vary and may relate to inflammatory cytokines, response to increased colloidal osmotic (oncotic) pressure caused by hyperglobulinemia, or damaged tissues such as liver, intestines, or kidneys.

Table 7.6. Diseases and conditions that cause hypoalbuminemia

Decreased albumin synthesis
  *Inflammation
  *Hepatic insufficiency
  *Malabsorption and maldigestion
  *Cachectic states
   Hypergammaglobulinemia
Increased albumin loss
  *Blood loss
  *Protein-losing nephropathy: glomerulonephritis, amyloidosis
  *Protein-losing enteropathy: small intestinal mucosal disease, lymphangiectasia, intestinal blood loss
   Protein-losing dermatopathy: burns, generalized exudative skin disease
Hemodilution
   Excess administration of intravenous fluid
   Edematous disorders: congestive heart failure, cirrhosis, nephrotic syndrome
   Excess ADH secretion: SIADH

* A relatively common disease or condition
Note: [Albumin] in healthy pups, kittens, calves, and foals may be 0.5–1.0 g/dL less than those found in mature animals.

B. Hypoalbuminemia is commonly found concurrently with hypoproteinemia. As described in the Hypoproteinemia section, hypoalbuminemias are usually caused by decreased production of albumin, increased loss of plasma albumin, or both.

HYPERGLOBULINEMIA (see the Hyperproteinemia section)

I.   Hyperglobulinemia is typically present concurrently with hyperproteinemia. In fact, the reason for the hyperproteinemia is typically the hyperglobulinemia. However, it is not uncommon to find hyperglobulinemia with normoproteinemia because of concurrent hypoalbuminemia.

II. There are four major concepts to consider:
A. The major causes of hyperglobulinemia are hemoconcentration, inflammation (especially chronic), and B-lymphocyte neoplasia.
B. By way of routine clinical chemistry methods, the globulin concentration is determined by subtraction; that is, [total protein] minus [albumin]. Thus, errors in those values can result in erroneous globulin concentrations.
C. Because the routine [globulin] represents the sum of the concentrations of all proteins other than albumin, hyperglobulinemia may result from the increased concentration of one or more different globulins.
D. SPE results typically will differentiate the hyperproteinemias of hemoconcentration from hyperglobulinemias of inflammation and lymphoid neoplasia, but they may not be able to differentiate inflammatory from lymphoid neoplastic hyperglobulinemias.

HYPOGLOBULINEMIA (see the Hypoproteinemia section)

I.   For animals other than neonates, hypoglobulinemia commonly occurs concurrently with hypoproteinemia and might be seen with normoproteinemia, whereas it is not expected with hyperproteinemia if reference intervals are appropriate.

II. As with the hypoproteinemic disorders, the major causes of hypoglobulinemia fall into two categories:
A. Globulin production is decreased. Remember that most globulins other than γ-globulins are produced by hepatocytes.
B. Plasma globulin loss is increased because of blood loss or loss via damaged glomeruli, intestinal mucosa, or skin.

POSITIVE ACUTE-PHASE PROTEINS (APPs)

I.   General concepts
A. Major aspects of the stimulated production of positive APPs are described in earlier sections of this chapter (see General Concepts for Total Protein, Albumin, and Globulins, Sect. II.C). Physiologic aspects of positive APPs and clinical application of positive APP assays in domestic mammals have been reviewed.[6,7]
B. Essentially any injury that produces an acute inflammatory reaction can increase concentrations of the positive APPs. These injuries can be due to infections (e.g., bacterial, viral, fungal, or protozoal) or noninfectious conditions (e.g., physical trauma, burns, or necrosis). As a group of proteins, the increased concentration of positive APPs

can increase [total protein] and [globulin]. Individually, the magnitude of increase varies considerably.

C. Positive APP results typically are valuable for two reasons:

1. Other methods of detecting inflammation (i.e., pyrexia or neutrophilia) may be too insensitive or nonspecific for the pathologic state of interest.

2. They provide another method of monitoring an inflammatory process either for therapeutic decisions or for prognostic classification.

D. Other factors need to be considered when interpreting concentrations of positive APPs:

1. If chronic inflammation is considered to be the persistence of acute inflammation, then it is easy to understand that concentrations of positive APPs can be increased in animals with chronic inflammatory disorders.

2. Concurrent with the pathologic state that is increasing the concentration of the positive APP, there may be processes that are decreasing the concentrations.

   a. Disorders that cause the loss of plasma proteins (e.g., blood loss or glomerular disease) can lower positive APP concentrations.

   b. Disorders that activate plasmin or thrombin can lower [fibrinogen] by fibrinogenolysis and coagulation.

   c. Intravascular hemolysis will lower [haptoglobin].

II. Fibrinogen

A. Physiologic process

1. Fibrinogen is a plasma protein that is produced by hepatocytes.

2. When enzymatic processes in plasma convert prothrombin to thrombin, thrombin then promotes the conversion of soluble fibrinogen to insoluble fibrin. Interactions of fibrin, platelets, and endothelial cells help prevent blood loss from blood vessels. Fibrin formation is limited by plasmin-induced fibrinolysis.

3. Because fibrinogen is a positive APP, plasma [fibrinogen] is expected to increase during inflammatory states. However, when inflammation is concurrent with coagulation and fibrinolysis, increased fibrinogen consumption may mask increased fibrinogen production and vice versa.

B. Analytical concepts

1. Heat-precipitant method

   a. Principle: The difference in the [TP_{ref}] in a sample before and after removal of fibrinogen via heat precipitation (56–58 °C) and centrifugation estimates the [fibrinogen].

   b. Unit conversion: mg/dL × 0.01 = g/L (SI unit, nearest 0.1 g/L)[12]

   c. Comments

      (1) It is a semiquantitative technique used to screen plasma for hyperfibrinogenemia. It is usually applied to bovine and equine samples because inflammation is less reliably detected by inflammatory leukograms in these species compared to dogs and cats. (Note: Reporting heat-precipitant fibrinogen results in mg/dL units [e.g., 300 mg/dL instead of 0.3 g/dL] implies much greater precision than the assay can deliver.)

      (2) The method's analytical sensitivity (i.e., capability of detecting small changes) is inadequate to document hypofibrinogenemia. As each refractometric reading is at best only accurate to the nearest 0.1 g/dL, the calculated fibrinogen value should be considered to be at best within 0.2 g/dL of the

true value. In most species, the lower reference limit is either 0.1 g/dL or 0.2 g/dL.

   d. Outline of the heat-precipitant method
      (1) Fill two microhematocrit tubes (at least three-quarters full) with EDTA-anticoagulated blood. Spin tubes in a microhematocrit centrifuge (as for hematocrit) for 5 min.
         (a) First tube: Determine the $[pTP_{ref}]$ to the nearest 0.1 g/dL.
         (b) Second tube: Place it in a 56–58 °C H_2O bath for 3 min, spin it in a microhematocrit centrifuge (for at least 1 min) to pack the precipitated fibrinogen, and then determine the [total protein] via refractometer to the nearest 0.1 g/dL.
      (2) Calculate the [fibrinogen].
         (a) The estimated [fibrinogen] = $[pTP_{ref}]$ of the first tube – $[TP_{ref}]$ of the second tube.
         (b) Example: 7.0 g/dL – 6.7 g/dL = 0.3 g/dL
2. Thrombin time, von Clauss modification
   a. Principle: A [fibrinogen] can be determined from the time required for fibrin formation after the addition of a high concentration of thrombin to diluted citrated plasma. This time primarily depends on the [fibrinogen]: the lower the [fibrinogen] is, the longer will be the time until clot formation.
   b. See Chapter 5 for details pertaining to measurement of fibrinogen concentration.
3. Some people have attempted to calculate a [fibrinogen] by determining the difference between the $[pTP_{ref}]$ of EDTA-plasma and the $[sTP_{ref}]$ from a serum sample. Such a method is not recommended because solutes other than fibrinogen alter the refractive index and thus cause differences between plasma and serum [total protein] (see the section on Analytical Principles for Total Protein, Albumin, and Globulins). Errors can arise when two different samples are collected and compared.
C. Hyperfibrinogenemia (plasma) (Table 7.7)
   1. Two major causes:
      a. Hemoconcentration: decreased plasma H_2O
      b. Inflammation: increased fibrinogen production by the liver
   2. The [total protein] is usually also increased with these disorders but may be WRI. Unless fibrinogen consumption is increased enough, the [fibrinogen] increases relatively more than the [total protein] in inflammation. With dehydration, the increases in the [total protein] and [fibrinogen] should be relatively the same; for example, they both increase by 5 %. These concepts led to the development of the PP : F ratio (Eq. 7.1a).[59] The ratio was simplified a few years later by not subtracting the [fibrinogen] from the $[TP_{ref}]$ (Eq. 7.1b).[60]

Table 7.7. Diseases and conditions that cause hyperfibrinogenemia

Increased fibrinogen production
   *Inflammation
   *Hemoconcentration

* A relatively common disease or condition

$$\text{PP:F ratio} = \frac{[\text{plasma TP}] - [\text{fibrinogen}]}{[\text{fibrinogen}]} \qquad\qquad \textbf{(7.1a.)}$$

$$(\text{TP:Fib})_p \text{ ratio} = \frac{[\text{plasma TP}]}{[\text{fibrinogen}]} \qquad\qquad \textbf{(7.1b.)}$$

Example: [pTP] = 8.8 g/dL & [fibrinogen] = 0.8 g/dL

$$\text{PP:F ratio} = \frac{8.8 \text{ g/dL} - 0.8 \text{ g/dL}}{0.8 \text{ g/dL}} = \frac{8.0 \text{ g/dL}}{0.8 \text{ g/dL}} = 10$$

$$(\text{TP:Fib})_p \text{ ratio} = \frac{8.8 \text{ g/dL}}{0.8 \text{ g/dL}} = 11$$

3. PP:F ratio or (TP:Fib)$_p$ ratio
   a. These ratios help in differentiating hyperfibrinogenemias of inflammation and dehydration.
   b. The original interpretive guides and reference intervals were established with the PP:F ratio.[59,61] The PP:F ratios in healthy mammals varied among species and by age group, mostly because of different total protein concentrations.[62]
      (1) Cattle: If the ratio is > 15, hyperfibrinogenemia is probably caused by dehydration. If the ratio is < 10, hyperfibrinogenemia is probably caused by inflammation.
      (2) Horses: If the ratio is > 20, hyperfibrinogenemia is probably caused by dehydration. If the ratio is < 15, hyperfibrinogenemia is probably caused by inflammation.
      (3) If the simpler calculation, (TP:Fib)$_p$ ratio, is used, a "1" should be added to guideline values to be consistent with guidelines determined by using the PP:F ratio (e.g., > 16 in cattle is probably dehydration).
   c. Guidelines are based on the assumptions that a healthy animal's [total protein] and [fibrinogen] are WRI, and then one of two things happens: the animal becomes dehydrated or develops an inflammatory disease.
      (1) Dehydration will increase concentrations of all proteins to the same degree, and thus the PP:F and (TP:Fib)$_p$ ratios do not change.
      (2) Inflammation will increase concentrations of fibrinogen and some proteins but also decrease concentrations of other proteins. Thus, the PP:F and (TP:Fib)$_p$ ratios will decrease because the denominator will increase relatively more than the numerator.
   d. Additional factors to be considered
      (1) Concurrent dehydration and inflammation will make interpretation of the ratios more difficult. Increased fibrinogen consumption in the pathologic state will also cloud the issue.
      (2) Dehydration by itself will cause only minor increases in [fibrinogen].
      (3) The aforementioned ratio guidelines are not appropriate for calves and foals because the ratio reference intervals are for mature animal values. They also are not appropriate for cattle and horses that have a concurrent pathologic state that causes hypoproteinemia.

Table 7.8. Diseases and conditions that cause hypofibrinogenemia

Increased fibrinogen consumption
*Intravascular coagulation (localized or disseminated)
Increased fibrinogenolysis
Decreased synthesis of fibrinogen
Hepatic insufficiency
Afibrinogenemia (congenital or inherited)

    * A relatively common disease or condition

        (4)   The accuracy of refractometric values is at best ± 0.1 g/dL. Thus, the accuracy of the calculated ratio is probably better with a higher [fibrinogen]. Even then, however, they should be considered estimates.

   D. Hypofibrinogenemia (plasma) (Table 7.8)

      1. Heat-precipitation techniques lack sufficient analytical sensitivity and precision to be used for detection or confirmation of hypofibrinogenemia. Quantitative assays are needed for documentation of hypofibrinogenemia. The common assay for detecting hypofibrinogenemia is the von Clauss modification of the thrombin time (see Chapter 5).

      2. Causes of hypofibrinogenemia (more information in Chapter 5)

         a. Increased consumption of fibrinogen

           (1) Intravascular coagulation: local or disseminated

           (2) Increased fibrinogenolysis: uncommon but may occur with fibrinolytic therapy, DIC, or certain envenomations

         b. Decreased synthesis of fibrinogen

           (1) Hepatic insufficiency: reduction in hepatic function must be marked before hypofibrinogenemia occurs

           (2) Inherited or congenital disorders: afibrinogenemia, hypofibrinogenemia, and dysfibrinogenemia

              (a) Afibrinogenemia was found in a bichon frise that developed antibodies to fibrinogen after transfusions.[63] Afibrinogenemia also has been described in goats and people.

              (b) Congenital hypofibrinogenemia was reported in a Bernese mountain dog (Berner sennenhund) (note: sometimes translated as Saint Bernard).[64]

              (c) Hypofibrinogenemia or dysfibrinogenemia has also been mentioned as occurring in Lhasa apsos, vizslas, collies, and borzois (W.J. Dodds, unpublished), but the laboratory data to characterize these states have not been published.

III.   Other acute-phase proteins

   A. Analytical concepts[6]

      1. Like most plasma proteins, the positive APPs are relatively stable analytes when stored frozen. Except for fibrinogen, serum is the preferred sample for most APPs. Anticoagulants (EDTA, heparin, and citrate) have been reported to cause a variety of effects on APP results. The effects of Hgb, bilirubin, or lipemia on the assays vary with the analyte and the assays used. As would be expected for a haptoglobin assay based on Hgb binding, the use of hemolyzed samples must be avoided.

2. A variety of analytical methods are used to measure increased concentrations of specific positive APPs. Some of the immunologic methods are species specific. In health, the concentrations of some positive APPs are near the detection limits of the assays, so detecting decreased concentrations is difficult or impossible.

    a. Serum C-reactive protein is usually measured by immunologic methods: immunoturbidimetry, enzyme-linked immunosorbent assay (ELISA), or latex agglutination.

    b. Haptoglobin assays typically are based on haptoglobin's binding to Hgb. The binding is detected either via spectral differences of bound versus unbound Hgb or by diminished peroxidase activity. Because of the species differences in haptoglobin's amino acid compositions, immunoassays designed for human haptoglobin may or may not detect a domestic mammal's haptoglobin.

    c. Serum amyloid A is measured with immunologic assays: immunoturbidimetric assays or enzyme-linked immunosorbent assays. Assays using anti-(canine SAA) or anti-(feline SAA) antibodies have been developed, but there is sufficient homology in the canine and feline proteins to cross-react with some anti-(human SAA) antibodies.

    d. α_1-Acid glycoprotein is measured with species-specific immunoassays: single radial immunodiffusion assays and immunoturbidimetric assays.

    e. Ceruloplasmin assays are typically spectrophotometric assays based on the oxidation of specific substrates.

    f. Ferritin: Generally, species-specific immunoassays are needed to measure serum or plasma [ferritin]. Assays have been developed for canine,[65] feline,[66] and equine[67] ferritin specifically. Occasionally, the cross-reactivity is sufficient to measure ferritin concentrations of species other than the one for which the assay was developed; for example, the equine ferritin assay can be used to measure concentrations of rhinoceros, tapir, and lemur ferritin. When possible, the ferritin used in calibrating (standard) solutions should be isolated from the species of interest; for example, the use of lemur ferritin to calibrate an assay for lemur ferritin that uses an anti-(equine ferritin) antibody.

B. Increased concentrations of positive APPs other than fibrinogen

    1. Examples of potential increases are provided in Table 7.9. It should be noted that the increase in [haptoglobin] may be sufficient to produce a recognizable increase in the serum [total protein] by itself, whereas increased concentrations of the other APPs typically are not.

    2. Conditions other than inflammation can cause increased positive APP concentrations.

        a. Pregnancy in bitches will increase [C-reactive protein].[68]

        b. In dogs, glucocorticoid therapy can cause increased [haptoglobin] similar to haptoglobin concentrations seen during inflammation.[53,69] Also, certain anthelmintic compounds (potassium melarsonyl, levamisole hydrochloride, and milbemycin oxime) can increase [haptoglobin].[70]

        c. Phenobarbital therapy in dogs can increase [α_1-acid glycoprotein].[71]

        d. [C-reactive protein] increases in cattle during lactation. The highest values were during the first 4 mo of lactation.[72]

        e. If an animal does not have an inflammatory disease, a plasma [ferritin] tends to reflect iron storage in the animal. Thus, if iron storage is increased (e.g.,

Table 7.9. Examples of changes in acute-phase protein concentrations

Acute-phase Protein	Concentration in healthy dog (mg/dL)	Magnitude of response (× baseline)	First detection of increase (h)	Time to peak concentration (d)
Fibrinogen	< 300	3 ×	—	—
C-reactive protein	< 1	95 ×	4	1
Serum amyloid A	< 0.4	800 ×	2	—
Haptoglobin	< 300	3 ×	24	3–4
α_1-Acid glycoprotein	< 60	3 ×	—	3
Ceruloplasmin	< 5	3 ×	24	4

Note: More information (except for fibrinogen) is available in a review article that was the source of the data. Note that units were converted from "/L" to "/dL" so they could be more easily compared to other protein concentrations (reported as g/dL) in this chapter.

Source: Ceron et al.[6]

hemochromatosis, hemosiderosis, or chronic hemolysis), then the plasma [ferritin] might be increased.

    f. Serum [ferritin] may increase after exercise in horses, so samples for ferritin analysis should be collected at least 2 d after strenuous exercise.[73] The exact mechanism for the increase is not established but appears to be release from tissues other than liver.

IMMUNOGLOBULINS

The most common reason for measuring [IgG] is to determine whether there has been successful passive transfer of IgG from a mother (mare or cow) to her foal or calf via colostrum. Accordingly, passive transfer is the focus of this section. Immunoglobulin concentrations may also be measured when evaluating congenital and acquired immunodeficiency states or when assessing potential monoclonal gammopathies.

I.   Failure of passive transfer (FPT)
    A. Physiologic concepts
       1. Placentation in horses and cattle prevents in utero transfer of immunoglobulins to the fetus, so neonatal horses and ruminants must ingest colostrum soon after birth (before "gut closure") to obtain maternal immunoglobulins, especially IgG. After ingestion and absorption, the half-life of maternal IgG is about 20–30 d in foals[74] and 20 d in calves.[75] Inadequate immunoglobulin transfer for a particular environment increases the risk of infectious diseases and decreases the rate of weight gain.
       2. Neonatal foals, prior to ingestion of colostrum, have essentially no IgG in their plasma, and calves have very low concentrations. Once exposed to antigens, neonatal foals are stimulated to produce IgG and protective immunity in about 10–14 d.[74] Synthesis of IgG by calves can be detected by 8–16 d.[76]
       3. Fetal foals and calves have limited ability to produce IgM, so neonatal foals and calves should have low concentrations of IgM.
       4. Intestinal absorption of colostrum rapidly increases plasma [total protein]. Most of the increase is due to increased [IgG], but colostrum also contains positive acute-

phase proteins such as amyloid A that is produced by mammary gland epithelial cells.[77]

5. Immunoglobulin uptake is mediated by the neonatal Fc receptor on epithelial cells.

B. Causes of FPT

1. Lack of colostrum ingestion (the neonate is too weak or because of other factors)

2. Inadequate IgG in the colostrum (a decreased concentration or inadequate volume of colostrum)

3. Failure to absorb enough ingested IgG could occur if the colostrum is ingested after "gut closure" and has been associated with certain haplotypes of the neonatal Fc receptor in calves.[78]

C. Establishing the presence or absence of passive transfer

1. Appropriate decision thresholds to define FPT vary with the assay because of assay biases (inaccuracies). Despite these biases, general recommendations have been made. Laboratory-specific decision thresholds should be used when available.

2. Foal guidelines: Blood samples are collected between 18 and 48 h after birth, when antibody absorption should be essentially complete.

   a. For several years, [IgG] > 400 mg/dL was considered evidence of passive transfer. However, [IgG] > 800 mg/dL may be a better criterion for adequate passive transfer and is currently recommended,[74,79] although adequacy may vary with different management and environmental factors.

   b. [IgG] < 200 mg/dL is considered evidence of complete FPT.

   c. [IgG] between 200 mg/dL and 800 mg/dL is considered evidence of partial FPT. Such concentrations may not provide adequate humoral protection, especially for foals with higher risk factors.

3. Calf guidelines are not firmly established; two published guidelines follow. For each, blood samples are collected between 1 and 8 d after birth.

   a. One recommendation[52,80]

   (1) [IgG] > 1000 mg/dL is considered evidence of passive transfer.

   (2) [IgG] < 500 mg/dL is considered evidence of complete FPT.

   b. Another recommendation[81,82]

   (1) [IgG] > 1600 mg/dL is considered evidence of passive transfer.

   (2) [IgG] = 800–1600 mg/dL is considered partial passive transfer.

   (3) [IgG] < 800 mg/dL is considered FPT.

   c. When refractometry was used to estimate serum [total protein], decision thresholds of 5.0 g/dL and 5.5 g/dL correctly classified the passive transfer status in 83 % and 82 % of the calves, respectively.[52]

4. Results for blood samples collected from older foals or calves, especially if ill, will be more difficult to interpret because the half-life of maternal IgG and a neonate's response to antigens after birth must be considered.

D. Analytical concepts for methods of measuring or estimating [IgG] in foals and calves: Because of the lack of standardization of assay methods and reference standard sera, there may be marked variations in [IgG] measured by different IgG assays. The evaluation of various analytical methods is frequently compared to [IgG] determined by RID. However, a RID assay might be inaccurate.[83] Thus, the interpretive guidelines will vary.

1. RID test for foal or calf serum

   a. Principle: IgG diffuses in a gel containing anti-(equine IgG) antibodies or anti-(bovine IgG) antibodies for 18–24 h. The diameter of a precipitant ring is proportional to the [IgG] in serum.

  b. Results: RID is considered to be a quantitative assay for measuring [IgG]. Assays for measuring bovine [IgG$_1$] are also available.

  c. Comments

   (1) Usually RID is considered too time consuming (24 h diffusion time) and expensive for routine clinical use.

   (2) RID has been considered the gold standard method in veterinary laboratories. However, some commercial RID assays overestimate [IgG], especially at [IgG] > 2000 mg/dL.[84] In one study, a commercial RID assay for bovine IgG had a positive proportional bias, thus indicating the provided standard solutions had lower IgG concentrations than labeled.[83]

 2. Glutaraldehyde coagulation test for foal or calf serum

  a. Principle: Glutaraldehyde (10 %) promotes the formation of molecular cross-linkages to coagulate basic proteins such as immunoglobulins and fibrinogen. Because fibrinogen is absent in serum and very little IgM is present in neonatal foal serum, the amount of coagulated protein is primarily dependent on [IgG].

  b. Results

   (1) For estimation of equine [IgG][85,86]

    (a) Reported semiquantitative values (gelling times may vary with newer assays)

     • [IgG] ≥ 800 mg/dL if serum forms gel ≤ 10 min.

     • [IgG] > 400 mg/dL if serum forms gel ≤ 60 min.

     • [IgG] ≤ 400 mg/dL if serum did not gel by 60 min.

    (b) Excellent agreement with the RID assay when [IgG] < 400 mg/dL and very good agreement with the RID assay when [IgG] > 800 mg/dL[85]

   (2) For estimation of bovine [IgG]

    (a) Semiquantitative values[82]

     • [IgG] > 600 mg/dL if the serum forms a firm opaque clot by 60 min.

     • [IgG] ≈ 400–600 mg/dL if the serum forms a semisolid gel by 60 min.

     • [IgG] < 400 mg/dL if the serum did not gel by 60 min.

    (b) Comments

     • To determine the [IgG] at the decision thresholds for FPT (either > 1000 mg/dL or > 1600 mg/dL), the serum would need to be diluted prior to analysis.

     • The results of the glutaraldehyde coagulation test (Gamma-Check-B) were unreliable when whole blood was used.[87]

  c. The test is very inexpensive and simple because it just requires glutaraldehyde, reaction tubes, and pipettes. It does require that serum be harvested from blood.

 3. Latex agglutination (Foalcheck) for foal serum

  a. Principle: Latex beads coated with anti-(equine IgG) antibodies will agglutinate in the presence of equine IgG.

  b. Results: It is a semiquantitative assay that generally agrees with the RID assay results but is not as good as the glutaraldehyde coagulation test.[85]

  c. Comments: The test is moderately expensive but takes only about 10 min to complete after the serum is collected.

 4. ZnSO$_4$ turbidity test for foal or calf serum

  a. Principle: Sulfates selectively precipitate cationic proteins such as immunoglobulins; other proteins are neutral or negatively charged. At a constant [ZnSO$_4$], a greater turbidity corresponds to a higher [immunoglobulin]. Since there is very little IgA or IgM in foal or calf sera, the amount of turbidity reflects the [IgG] in a sample.

b. The results can be assessed visually or turbidimetrically. Turbidimetric assessment requires a spectrophotometer and standard solutions to establish a standard curve.

(1) In foals, visual turbidity occurs when the [IgG] is near 400–500 mg/dL, which does not match with the current decision thresholds for FPT.[88]

(2) In calves:

(a) With a $ZnSO_4$ solution of 208 mg/L, sufficient turbidity to obscure newsprint occurs when [IgG] > 1600 mg/dL.[82] In this study, the $ZnSO_4$ turbidity test provided a good estimate of the [IgG] but was not considered to be as useful as the Na_2SO_3-precipitant test.

(b) In another study, the results with a $ZnSO_4$ solution (208 mg/L) were compared with RID assay results.[52] Inadequate turbidity was found in samples with $[IgG_1]$ values that ranged from 0 to 2825 mg/dL (mean, 955 mg/dL). Adequate turbidity (newsprint not legible) was found in samples with $[IgG_1]$ values that ranged from 1085 to 4305 mg/dL (mean, 2219 mg/dL). The marked variations in the results suggest that the assays were too inaccurate to enable confident decisions regarding passive transfer in calves.

(c) With higher concentrations of $ZnSO_4$ (250–400 mg/L), lower [IgG] produces the same degree of turbidity as higher [IgG] when 200 mg/L $ZnSO_4$ is used.[89]

c. Comments

(1) $ZnSO_4$ reagents may be made from scratch or purchased in kits. Stock solutions need to be sealed to prevent carbon dioxide absorption.

(2) For foals, turbidity tests have essentially been replaced by more accurate and convenient assays. The $ZnSO_4$ turbidity test tends to underestimate [IgG] when > 400 mg/dL.[90]

(3) The presence of Hgb from hemolysis will falsely increase the measured [IgG] if turbidity is assessed by spectrophotometry (at 660 nm): Hgb-induced increments are about 200 mg/dL at 1 % hemolysis and 1300 mg/dL at 5 % hemolysis.[84]

5. Na_2SO_3 precipitant test for calf serum

a. Principle: Sulfites selectively precipitate cationic proteins such as immunoglobulins; other proteins are neutral or negatively charged. Higher concentrations of sulfites have greater capability of precipitating IgG at lower concentrations. Since there is very little IgA or IgM in calf sera, the amount of turbidity reflects the quantity of IgG in the sample.

b. Guidelines for the interpretation of results with 14 %, 16 %, and 18 % Na_2SO_3 solutions.[82] (Note: Estimated concentrations do not match some recommended decision thresholds and thus would be difficult to interpret.[81])

(1) If [IgG] > 1500 mg/dL, precipitates are seen in 14 %, 16 %, and 18 % solutions.

(2) If [IgG] ≈ 500–1500 mg/dL, precipitates are seen in 16 % and 18 % solutions.

(3) If [IgG] < 500 mg/dL, precipitate is seen in the 18 % solution.

  c. In another study, results were compared with the [IgG] from a RID assay.[52] (Note: The marked variation in these results highlights the potentially poor accuracy or lack of precision of such assays.)

  (1) [IgG] ranged from 0 to 2400 mg/dL with no precipitate.

  (2) [IgG] ranged from 645 to 2450 mg/dL with precipitate in the 18 % solution.

  (3) [IgG] ranged from 1025 to 4305 mg/dL with precipitate in 16 % and 18 % solutions.

  (4) [IgG] ranged from 2380 to 3625 mg/dL with precipitate in 14 %, 16 %, and 18 % solutions.

  d. Comments

  (1) The Na_2SO_3-precipitant test is relatively inexpensive and quick. The major advantage over $ZnSO_4$ is the capability of estimating the [IgG] in a broad range.

  (2) Compared to the RID assay results, the precipitant test is at best a semi-quantitative assay.

  (3) The assay does not work well for foal serum.

6. Changes in γ-globulin concentration that are determined by protein electrophoresis: The difference between γ-globulin concentration in precolostral serum and postcolostral serum (1 d after colostrum ingestion) should reflect the increase in [IgG]. However, this method of measuring [IgG] is not applicable to clinical decisions because of the associated time and expense.

7. Changes in serum [total protein] determined by refractometry

  a. Calves

  (1) When measured by refractometry, the changes in total protein concentrations in precolostral and postcolostral samples (1 d after ingestion) reflected the changes in γ-globulin concentrations in calves.[83]

  (2) Because a precolostral sample is typically not available, guidelines for classifying the passive transfer status in calves have been proposed. If the decision threshold for serum [total protein] is 5.0 g/dL, there is a 83 % chance of correctly classifying the calf's status.[52]

  b. Foals

  (1) When a decision threshold of 6.0 g/dL was used to detect FPT, the refractometric serum [total protein] had a diagnostic sensitivity of 95 % and diagnostic specificity of 21 %.[91]

  (2) The study used two radial immunodiffusion tests as the reference methods. There was not good agreement between the results of the two methods.

E. Each of the methods of measuring or estimating [IgG] in foal or calf sera has its advantages and disadvantages. Factors that should be considered when selecting a procedure include associated expenses (reagents, equipment, and personnel), time required to obtain results, convenience, and the potential reasons for incorrect results. The most accurate test may not be clinically applicable, whereas the most convenient test may be prone to unreliable results.

II. Immunoglobulin deficiencies

  A. Other than directly or indirectly assessing [IgG] for the purpose of detecting FPT (see Immunoglobulins, sect. I), an immunoglobulin concentrations are measured to detect or confirm the presence of congenital immunodeficiencies.

1. Horses[92,93]
   a. Severe combined immunodeficiency in Arabian and Appaloosa foals: Affected foals do not produce functional T- or B-lymphocytes, and thus they succumb to infections shortly after maternal antibodies obtained by the colostrum are degraded ($\approx$ 6 d for IgM, and $\approx$ 2–3 wk for IgG). Other than the absence of IgM in presuckle serum, other diagnostic features include persistent lymphopenia and marked lymphoid hypoplasia in lymphoid organs.
   b. Primary agammaglobulinemia in thoroughbreds, standardbreds, and quarter horses: Affected foals do not produce IgG or IgM because they lack B-lymphocytes, but they do have T-lymphocytes. Presuckle serum lacks IgM, and maternal IgG and IgM obtained from colostrum disappear over time to yield the agammaglobulinemia.
   c. Selective IgM deficiency: Affected foals (Arabian and quarter horses) have a marked decrease in serum [IgM] but do produce other immunoglobulins. B-lymphocyte concentrations are not decreased.
   d. Selective IgG deficiency: Affected foals have a marked decrease in serum [IgG] but do produce other immunoglobulins.
   e. Combined variable deficiency: An affected adult horse had very low serum [IgG], [IgM], [IgA], and [IgG(T)].[94] Blood, marrow, and spleen lacked B-lymphocytes, but lymph nodes contained occasional B-lymphocytes.
   f. *Fell pony syndrome* appears to be genetic disorder in which there is defective production of B-lymphocytes that causes a hypogammaglobulinemia because of decreased [IgG] and [IgM]. If IgG is detected in serum, it is maternal IgG. The disorder, which affects foals of the Fell pony breed, was first recognized in Europe and has been found in the United States.[95]
2. Cattle[92]
   a. Severe combined immunodeficiency in an Angus calf: IgM and IgA were not detected in the serum of the affected 6-wk-old calf; a very low [IgG] was considered to be of maternal origin. The calf lacked lymphocytes in its thymus, lymph nodes were not detected, and its spleen was small.
   b. Selective IgG$_2$ deficiency: About 1–2 % of red Danish cattle lack detectable IgG$_2$, but they do have other immunoglobulins. An IgG$_2$ deficiency has also been reported in a Holstein heifer.[96]
   c. Transient hypogammaglobulinemia: A Simmental heifer was reported to have a delayed production of immunoglobulins.
3. Dogs[92,93]
   a. Severe combined immunodeficiency in Jack Russell terriers (autosomal recessive): Affected dogs lack B- and T-lymphocytes and thus cannot produce immunoglobulins. They have lymphopenia and generalized lymphoid hypoplasia.
   b. Severe combined immunodeficiency in basset hounds and Cardigan Welsh corgis (X linked): Affected dogs lack IgG and IgA in serum but the [IgM] is WRI. The dogs have a marked reduction in CD8 lymphocytes and are lymphopenic. The defective mutations are different in the two breeds.
   c. Selective IgM deficiency in Doberman pinschers: Affected dogs had increased serum [IgA], decreased [IgG], and very low [IgM].
   d. Selective IgA deficiency in German shepherds: Affected dogs have decreased serum [IgA], but [IgG] and [IgM] were WRI.

       e. Selective IgA deficiency in shar-peis: Affected dogs have decreased serum [IgA].

       f. Selective IgA deficiency in beagles: Affected dogs had decreased serum [IgA], but [IgG] and [IgM] were each WRI.

       g. Selective IgG and IgA deficiency in Weimaraners: Affected pups have decreased serum [IgG] and [IgA] associated with chronic infections.[97]

  B. Analytical concepts

    1. Documenting a marked decrease in an immunoglobulin concentration requires species-specific assays that have an appropriate analytical range; that is, the capability of accurately measuring concentrations below reference intervals. Typically, these assays are radial immunodiffusion assays, but other immunologic assays can be used. Because immunoglobulins in healthy animals represent about a third of the total [globulin], a complete absence of immunoglobulins might create a hypoglobulinemia. However, there are many other more common reasons for hypoglobulinemia (see Hypoglobulinemia above).

    2. Because most of the γ-globulin fraction of SPE is composed of IgG, an IgG deficiency can be suspected when there is hypogammaglobulinemia. However, the suspicion should be confirmed with a species-specific quantitative assay for IgG or IgG subclasses. Because IgA and IgM represent only a small amount of the β- or γ-globulins in health, a deficiency in those immunoglobulins cannot be detected by routine SPE.

III.   Immunoglobulin excess

  A. Most hyperglobulinemias are caused by a chronic infection or dehydration, but a few are due to excessive production of an immunoglobulin by neoplastic B-lymphocytes. If not caused by dehydration (hemoconcentration), SPE determination of which immunoglobulin or immunoglobulins are contributing to the hyperglobulinemia will provide diagnostic evidence for either a chronic inflammatory state or B-lymphocyte neoplasia. In such cases, it typically is more important to characterize the type of immunoglobulin present than to measure immunoglobulin concentrations.

  B. An earlier section (Hyperproteinemia, sect. III.B) of this chapter described diagnostic methods that can be used to attempt to differentiate an inflammatory oligoclonal gammopathy from a B-lymphocyte neoplastic gammopathy. Most of those diagnostic assays target the heavy chain of the immunoglobulin class or subclass and do not prove clonality. Documenting that a gammopathy is caused by only one IgG subclass, or IgM, or IgA would be better evidence of a monoclonal state because it would be unlikely that the concentration of only one would be increased in an inflammatory state. Establishing that a neoplastic clone is producing a single antigen-specific immunoglobulin is nearly impossible.

  C. Most monoclonal gammopathies are diagnosed by association; that is, finding a probable monoclonal gammopathy by SPE and concurrent lymphoid neoplasia (e.g., lymphoma, lymphoid leukemia, plasmacytoma, or myeloma). Most polyclonal gammopathies are diagnosed by finding a probable polyclonal gammopathy by SPE and a concurrent chronic inflammatory state, typically caused by a chronic infection. These conclusions become more difficult and uncertain when these typical associations are not found; for example, possible monoclonal gammopathy in an animal with a chronic infection. Then, more definitive characterization of the immunoglobulins may establish the pathogenesis for the gammopathy.

COLLOIDAL OSMOTIC PRESSURE (COP) (ONCOTIC PRESSURE)

I.   Physiologic processes and concepts
  A. COP is also called oncotic pressure; the prefix *onco-* comes from the Greek for "bulk" or "swelling," which, in this context, refers to spaces containing colloidal particles that swell with fluid. A more common context refers to neoplasms; that is, oncology.
  B. Hydraulic pressure gradients and COP gradients force the movement of protein-poor fluids out of and into capillaries as described in Starling's law (Fig. 7.3 and Eq. 7.2). In health, these gradients are important for the maintenance of blood volume. In edematous, transudative, and exudative disorders, alterations in the gradients cause plasma H_2O to move into interstitial spaces (see Chapter 19).

Pressure gradient $= \Delta$ hydraulic pressure $- \Delta$ oncotic pressure   (7.2.)
$$= (P_{cap} - P_{if}) - (\pi_{cap} - \pi_{if})$$

  C. COP is caused by concentrations of colloidal solutes or particles. *Colloidal particles* in blood are macromolecules that are too small to settle out due to gravity but too large to permeate intact vascular membranes. They are generally 1 nm to 1 μm in diameter, with $M_r > 30,000$, though colloidal properties are affected by factors other than size (e.g., surface area). In normoproteinemic plasma, albumin contributes about 75–80 % of total COP.
    1. COP develops whenever two fluids with different concentrations of colloid particles are separated by a semipermeable membrane.
    2. Of a total capillary COP of 25 mmHg in human plasma, about 17 mmHg is directly related to plasma proteins and about 8 mmHg is due to the Gibbs-Donnan equilibrium.[98]
      a. The major concepts of the Gibbs-Donnan equilibrium are illustrated in Fig. 7.4. The proteins "trapped" in the intravascular space have a negative charge. For electroneutrality, there must be more diffusible cations (e.g., Na^+) in the plasma to balance the negative charges of the proteins. In the Gibbs-Donnan equilibrium, the product of the major diffusible cation charge concentration and major diffusible anion charge concentration of the plasma equals the product of the major diffusible cation charge concentration and major diffusible anion charge concentration of the interstitial fluid (Eq. 7.3 and Fig. 7.4).

$[Na^+]_{plasma} \times [Cl^-]_{plasma} = [Na^+]_{interstitial\ fluid} \times [Cl^-]_{interstitial\ fluid}$ (7.3.)

$[major\ cations^+]_{plasma} \times [major\ anions^-]_{plasma} = [major\ cations^+]_{interstitial\ fluid} \times$
  $[major\ anions^-]_{interstitial\ fluid}$

      b. This protein-induced imbalance of ions causes a greater osmolality in blood and augments the direct colloidal osmotic pressure. In health, plasma proteins contribute about 0.9 mmol/kg, and the Gibbs-Donnan effect contributes about 0.4 mmol/kg.[98]
  D. [Total protein] and [albumin] may suggest altered COP, but COP is influenced by pH and the spectrum of protein types present, so [total protein] may be misleading.

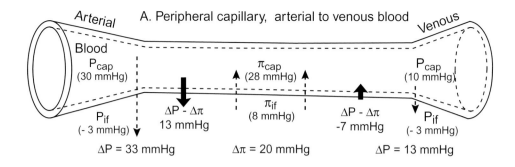

A. Peripheral capillary, arterial to venous blood

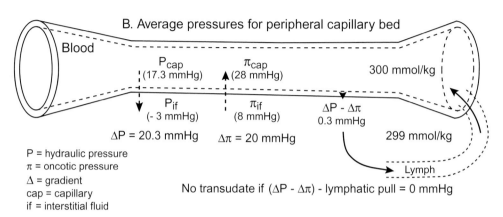

B. Average pressures for peripheral capillary bed

P = hydraulic pressure
π = oncotic pressure
Δ = gradient
cap = capillary
if = interstitial fluid

No transudate if (ΔP - Δπ) - lymphatic pull = 0 mmHg

Fig. 7.3. Illustration of fluid movements because of Starling's law in a typical capillary bed.
A. Peripheral capillary, arterial to venous blood.
- Hydraulic pressures in health
  - The plasma hydraulic pressure in the arterial side of the capillary bed is much higher than the hydraulic pressure in the interstitial fluid. The difference in the hydraulic pressure is called the hydraulic pressure gradient (Eq. 7.2). A typical hydraulic pressure gradient (ΔP) on the arterial side of the capillary is about 33 mmHg.
  - The plasma hydraulic pressure in the venous side of the capillary bed is higher than the hydraulic pressure in the interstitial fluid. A typical ΔP on the venous side of the capillary is about 13 mmHg.
  - The hydraulic pressure in the interstitial fluid is about −3 mmHg. The negative pressure is created by the actions of valves in the lymphatic vessels and pressure changes in vena cava vessels.
- Oncotic (colloidal osmotic) pressures in health.
  - The plasma oncotic pressure is greater than the interstitial oncotic pressure because the plasma [total protein] is greater than the interstitial fluid [total protein]. The [total protein] essentially does not change in the capillary beds, and thus the oncotic pressure gradient (Δπ) remains the same from the arterial side to the venous side of the capillary bed. For most capillaries, the Δπ is near 20 mmHg.
  - Most of the oncotic pressure (both in plasma and in interstitial fluid) is due to albumin, but globulins do contribute. See the text for more information about plasma oncotic pressure (colloidal osmotic pressure).
- The difference between the ΔP and Δπ (i.e., ΔP − Δπ) is a major factor that determines the rate of flow of fluid out of and into capillaries. On the arterial side, the difference is about 13 mmHg, and thus fluid leaves the capillary and enters the interstitial space. On the venous side, the difference is about −7 mmHg, and thus fluid leaves the interstitial space and enters the capillary.
B. Average pressures for peripheral capillary bed.
- Even though the ΔP on the arterial side is much greater than the ΔP on the venous side, the net difference in tissues is only about 0.3 mmHg. Most fluid returns to the capillaries because of two factors: (1) there are more venous capillaries (entering venules) than arterial capillaries (leaving arterioles), and (2) the venous capillaries are more permeable than arterial capillaries.[105]

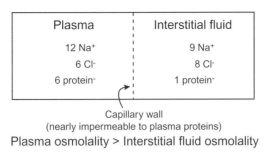

Fig. 7.4. Conceptual representation of the Gibbs-Donnan equilibrium.

The protein concentration in plasma is greater than in interstitial fluid, and most plasma proteins have a negative charge (at pH 7.4). The typical capillary wall is nearly impermeable to the proteins but is permeable to Na^+ and Cl^-. Movement of cations and anions is controlled by concentration and charge gradients. At equilibrium, electroneutrality occurs on each side of the capillary wall; for example, 12 cation charges and 12 anion charges in the plasma, and 9 cation charges and 9 anion charges in interstitial fluid. Because of the negatively charged protein molecules, there are more cations and fewer diffusible anions in plasma (12 and 6, respectively) than in interstitial fluid (9 and 8, respectively). Osmolality (determined by the number of solute molecules or ions) is greater in the plasma (24 particles) than in interstitial fluid (18 particles). The COP is generated by the presence of nondiffusible proteins, which causes a greater osmolality in plasma than interstitial fluid (Gibbs-Donnan effect). The Gibbs-Donnan effect increases with the square of the protein charge. Since the average protein molecule has > 1 negative charge, the Gibbs-Donnan effect is proportionately greater at greater protein concentrations.

II. Analytical Concepts
  A. The osmotic effect of proteins is used to measure COP with a colloid osmometer as illustrated in Fig. 7.5.
  B. The COP of blood, plasma, and serum will essentially be the same. Blood cells are not colloidal particles and thus do not contribute to COP. In theory, blood and plasma COP values will be slightly greater than serum COP values because serum lacks fibrinogen. Serum or plasma is typically the preferred sample because free Hgb can be more easily detected; also, whole blood may contain unseen small clots that can plug tubing.
  C. Units: 1 mmHg = 1 torr; 1 mmHg × 133.322 = 1 pascal
  D. Interferences
    1. Hgb in the sample increases the COP because Hgb is a colloidal particle. In a small study, Hgb increased the COP at a rate of nearly 4 mmHg per every 1 g/dL of Hgb.[99] This will falsely increase the COP if the Hgb is from in vitro hemolysis. Hemoglobinemia from in vivo hemolysis would also increase the COP.

Fig. 7.3. *continued*
  • As long as the lymphatic system removes the interstitial fluid, a transudate does not accumulate.
  • Even though the oncotic (colloidal osmotic) pressure is greater in plasma than in interstitial fluid, there is very little difference in the osmolalities of the fluids because proteins contribute very little to total osmolality, and the concentrations of major solutes (i.e., electrolytes, glucose, and urea) are nearly the same in the two fluids (see Chapter 9). The Gibbs-Donnan effect (see Fig. 7.4) creates differences in the osmolality.

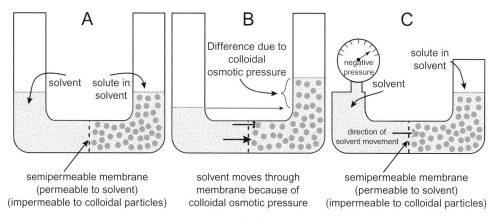

Fig. 7.5. Schematic representation of the principles of colloid osmometry.
A. Two fluids are present in an open-tube system: a solvent (such as isotonic saline) and a similar fluid that also contains large solute colloidal particles (e.g., proteins). The fluids are initially separated by a semipermeable membrane—a membrane that is permeable to the solvent and its small solute particles but not permeable to the large colloidal particles. The presence of large colloidal particles on one side results in a higher osmolality (see the Gibbs-Donnan effect in Fig. 7.4) and thus an osmotic gradient. This gradient creates osmotic pressure; thus the term *colloidal osmotic pressure*. The colloidal osmotic pressure initiates the movement of solvent towards the colloidal particles (movement from **A** to **B**).
B. When the system's pressures equilibrate, solvent has moved to the fluid that contained the colloidal particles. The difference in the fluid levels is primarily due to the colloidal osmotic pressure that was created by the colloidal particles. Other factors (such as bulging of the membrane in this open system and gravity) also affect the difference.
C. In the closed system of a colloid osmometer, the effects of membrane bulging and gravity are reduced. However, the same general principles apply and the colloidal particles attract the fluid. The colloidal osmotic pressure is measured by a pressure transducer.

      2. Plasma expanders (e.g., hetastarch and dextran) increase COP. In samples containing plasma expanders, the COP does not represent the concentration of colloidal proteins.
   E. Comments: Because the COP of plasma is typically due to plasma proteins, various formulas have been proposed for estimating or calculating COP by using measured concentrations of plasma proteins. Because of the differences in concentrations of each plasma protein among individuals of a species and among different species, these formulas may not provide a reliable estimate of plasma COP.[100–102] Also, the formulas will not be useful after treatment with synthetic colloids.

III. Increased COP
   A. By itself, an increased COP is not a common diagnostic problem for two reasons: (1) it typically will be due to hyperproteinemia, and this condition is more easily detected by other means; and (2) COP is rarely measured in samples that might have an increased COP.
   B. Increased COP can occur with increases in plasma colloidal particles.
      1. Increased plasma or serum Hgb concentration
         a. In plasma, free Hgb from in vivo or in vitro hemolysis can increase plasma COP.

b. Infusion of Hgb-based oxygen carriers (e.g., Oxyglobin and Biopure) quickly increases plasma COP. In one study, the Hgb-based oxygen carrier had a COP about twice that of canine plasma (43 mmHg vs 20 mmHg). Infusion increased the plasma COP quickly to about 36 mmHg, but the COP returned to baseline values after 3 h.[103]

2. Infusion of plasma expanders such as hetastarch can increase COP.[104] However, plasma expanders are typically administered to animals that have a decreased COP because of marked hypoproteinemia, and it is unlikely that enough hetastarch would be given to increase the plasma COP value to the reference interval. When given to dogs at a rate of 20 mL/kg body weight over 4 h, the plasma COP values typically increased 2–4 mmHg but returned to baseline values by 12 h.[99]

IV. Decreased COP
   A. Decreased COP values result from hypoproteinemia.
   B. The primary value of measuring COP is for the clinical management of severely hypoproteinemic animals. Because marked hypoproteinemia (especially if an acute onset) can result in the movement of water from blood to cause hypovolemia and edematous states, plasma or plasma expanders (such as hetastarch) may be administered to increase blood COP and thus reduce the pathologic consequences of hypoproteinemia.
      1. Hetastarch administration increases COP, but the duration of its effects depends on two major factors:
         a. The rate at which the hetastarch is degraded by the animal.
         b. The permeability of capillaries to hetastarch. During inflammatory states, increased vascular permeability will enable both plasma proteins and hetastarch to move from plasma to interstitial fluid.
      2. The degree that hetastarch increases the COP is somewhat less than one might expect. When hetastarch is first given, it quickly increases the plasma COP and thus alters the COP gradient in capillary beds. As a result, more water is pulled back into the plasma to expand blood volume, but this concurrently reduces [total protein]. Thus, the protein contribution to the measured COP is reduced.
      3. When there is a marked decrease in COP, administration of plasma has two major advantages over administration of hetastarch: (1) the circulating half-life of most plasma proteins (especially albumin) is much greater than that of hetastarch; and (2) the increase in COP is due to plasma proteins, and thus effects can be monitored by either COP or plasma protein concentrations.
   C. When an animal's blood has a decreased COP, the animal will be prone to develop edema or a transudate. However, other factors also influence the extravasation of fluid.
      1. Extravasation of a small amount of fluid to the interstitial space increases the hydraulic pressure in the interstitial space, thus limiting additional extravasation.
      2. Extravasation of protein to the interstitial space is less than the extravasation of H_2O (unless permeability is altered by inflammation), so the protein concentration in the interstitial fluid decreases and there is an increased colloidal osmotic gradient that limits additional extravasation.
      3. The lymphatic systemic can greatly increase its drainage of interstitial fluid in some tissues. Thus, even though fluid may be leaving the plasma faster, it may not accumulate in the interstitial space.

4. Retention of Na^+ and H_2O is largely responsible for most transudative states (e.g., cirrhosis, PLN, and heart failure) (see Chapter 19).

References

1. Dixon FJ, Maurer PH. 1953. Half-lives of homologous serum albumins in several species. Proc Soc Exp Biol Med 83:287–288.
2. Cornelius CE, Baker NF, Kaneko JJ, Douglas JR. 1962. Distribution and turnover of iodine-131–tagged bovine albumin in normal and parasitized cattle. Am J Vet Res 23:837–842.
3. Mattheeuws DR, Kaneko JJ, Loy RG, Cornelius CE, Wheat JD. 1966. Compartmentalization and turnover of 131-I–labeled albumin and gamma globulin in horses. Am J Vet Res 27:699–705.
4. Lavoie J-P, Spensley MS, Smith BP, Mihalyi J. 1989. Absorption of bovine colostral immunoglobulins G and M in newborn foals. Am J Vet Res 50:1598–1603.
5. Pollock PJ, Prendergast M, Schumacher J, Bellenger CR. 2005. Effects of surgery on the acute phase response in clinically normal and diseased horses. Vet Rec 156:538–542.
6. Ceron JJ, Eckersall PD, Martynez-Subiela S. 2005. Acute phase proteins in dogs and cats: Current knowledge and future perspectives. Vet Clin Pathol 34:85–99.
7. Petersen HH, Nielsen JP, Heegaard PM. 2004. Application of acute phase protein measurements in veterinary clinical chemistry. Vet Res 35:163–187.
8. Andrews GA, Smith JE. 2000. Iron metabolism. In: Feldman BF, Zinkl JG, Jain NC, eds. *Schalm's Veterinary Hematology*, 5th edition, 129–134. Philadelphia: Lippincott Williams & Wilkins.
9. Thomas JS. 2000. Overview of plasma proteins. In: Feldman BF, Zinkl JG, Jain NC, eds. *Schalm's Veterinary Hematology*, 5th edition, 891–898. Philadelphia: Lippincott Williams & Wilkins.
10. Silverman LM, Christenson RH. 1994. Amino acids and proteins. In: Burtis CA, Ashwood ER, eds. *Tietz Textbook of Clinical Chemistry*, 2nd edition, 625–734. Philadelphia: WB Saunders.
11. Sutton RH. 1976. The refractometric determination of the total protein concentration in some animal plasmas. NZ Vet J 24:141–148.
12. Lundberg GD, Iverson C, Radulescu G. 1986. Now read this: The SI units are here. J Am Med Assoc 255:2329–2339.
13. Cannon DC, Olitzky I, Inkpen JA. 1974. Proteins. In: Henry RJ, Cannon DC, Winkelman JW, eds. *Clinical Chemistry Principles and Technics*, 2nd edition, 405–502. Hagerstown, MD: Harper & Row.
14. Johnson AM, Rohlfs EM, Silverman LM. 1999. Proteins. In: Burtis CA, Ashwood ER, eds. *Tietz Textbook of Clinical Chemistry*, 3rd edition, 477–540. Philadelphia: WB Saunders.
15. Trivedi VD, Saxena I, Siddiqui MU, Qasim MA. 1997. Interaction of bromocresol green with different serum albumins studied by fluorescence quenching. Biochem Mol Biol Int 43:1–8.
16. Stokol T, Tarrant JM, Scarlett JM. 2001. Overestimation of canine albumin concentration with the bromcresol green method in heparinized plasma samples. Vet Clin Pathol 30:170–176.
17. Sinton E, Taylor T. 1972. The use of 2-(4′-hydroxyazobenzene)-benzoic acid (HABA) in determining canine albumin. J Am Anim Hosp Assoc 8:130–132.
18. Abate O, Zanatta R, Malisano T, Dotta U. 2000. Canine serum protein patterns using high-resolution electrophoresis (HRE). Vet J 159:154–160.
19. Ritzmann SE, Wolf RE, Lawrence MC, Hart JS, Levin WC. 1969. The Sia euglobulin test: A re-evaluation. J Lab Clin Med 73:698–705.
20. Gabay C, Kushner I. 1999. Acute-phase proteins and other systemic responses to inflammation. N Engl J Med 340:448–453.
21. MacEwen EG, Hurvitz AI. 1977. Diagnosis and management of monoclonal gammopathies. Vet Clin North Am 7:119–132.
22. Font A, Closa JM, Mascort J. 1994. Monoclonal gammopathy in a dog with visceral leishmaniasis. J Vet Intern Med 8:233–235.
23. Burkhard MJ, Meyer DJ, Rosychuk RA, O'Neil SP, Schultheiss PC. 1995. Monoclonal gammopathy in a dog with chronic pyoderma. J Vet Intern Med 9:357–360.
24. Diehl KJ, Lappin MR, Jones RL, Cayatte S. 1992. Monoclonal gammopathy in a dog with plasmacytic gastroenterocolitis. J Am Vet Med Assoc 201:1233–1236.
25. Giraudel JM, Pages JP, Guelfi JF. 2002. Monoclonal gammopathies in the dog: A retrospective study of 18 cases (1986–1999) and literature review. J Am Anim Hosp Assoc 38:135–147.

26. Kent JE, Roberts CA. 1990. Serum protein changes in four horses with monoclonal gammopathy. Equine Vet J 22:373–376.

27. Kyle RA, Greipp PR. 1978. The laboratory investigation of monoclonal gammopathies. Mayo Clin Proc 53:719–739.

28. Attaelmannan M, Levinson SS. 2000. Understanding and identifying monoclonal gammopathies. Clin Chem 46:1230–1238.

29. Stone MJ. 1982. Monoclonal gammopathies: Clinical aspects. In: Ritzmann SE, ed. *Protein Abnormalities*, volume 2: *Pathology of Immunoglobulins: Diagnostic and Clinical Aspects*, 161–236. New York: Alan R Liss.

30. Edwards DF, Parker JW, Wilkinson JE, Helman RG. 1993. Plasma cell myeloma in the horse: A case report and literature review. J Vet Intern Med 7:169–176.

31. Kato H, Momoi Y, Omori K, Youn HY, Yamada T, Goto N, Ono K, Watari T, Tsujimoto H, Hasegawa A. 1995. Gammopathy with two M-components in a dog with IgA-type multiple myeloma. Vet Immunol Immunopathol 49:161–168.

32. Bienzle D, Silverstein DC, Chaffin K. 2000. Multiple myeloma in cats: Variable presentation with different immunoglobulin isotypes in two cats. Vet Pathol 37:364–369.

33. Ramaiah SK, Seguin MA, Carwile HF, Raskin RE. 2002. Biclonal gammopathy associated with immunoglobulin A in a dog with multiple myeloma. Vet Clin Pathol 31:83–89.

34. Rothschild MA, Oratz M, Schreiber SS. 1988. Serum albumin. Hepatology 8:385–401.

35. Rogers KS, Forrester SD. 2000. Monoclonal gammopathy. In: Feldman BF, Zinkl JG, Jain NC, eds. *Schalm's Veterinary Hematology*, 5th edition, 932–936. Philadelphia: Lippincott Williams & Wilkins.

36. Werner LL, Turnwald GH, Willard MD. 2004. Immunologic and plasma protein disorders. In: Willard MD, Tvedten HW, eds. *Small Animal Clinical Diagnosis by Laboratory Methods*, 4th edition, 290–305. St Louis: WB Saunders.

37. Evans EW, Duncan JR. 2003. Proteins, lipids, and carbohydrates. In: Latimer KS, Mahaffey EA, Prasse KW, eds. *Duncan & Prasse's Veterinary Laboratory Medicine: Clinical Pathology*, 4th edition, 162–192. Ames: Iowa State Press.

38. Ritzmann SE. 1982. Immunoglobulin abnormalities. In: Ritzmann SE, Daniels JC, eds. *Serum Protein Abnormalities: Diagnostic and Clinical Aspects*, 351–486. New York: Alan R Liss.

39. Michels GM, Boon GD, Jones BD, Puget B. 1995. Hypergammaglobulinemia in a dog. J Am Vet Med Assoc 207:567–570.

40. Varela F, Font X, Valladares JE, Alberola J. 1997. Thrombocytopathia and light-chain proteinuria in a dog naturally infected with *Ehrlichia canis*. J Vet Intern Med 11:309–311.

41. Platz SJ, Breuer W, Pfleghaar S, Minkus G, Hermanns W. 1999. Prognostic value of histopathological grading in canine extramedullary plasmacytomas. Vet Pathol 36:23–27.

42. Majzoub M, Breuer W, Platz SJ, Linke RP, Linke W, Hermanns W. 2003. Histopathologic and immunophenotypic characterization of extramedullary plasmacytomas in nine cats. Vet Pathol 40:249–253.

43. Arun SS, Breuer W, Hermanns W. 1996. Immunohistochemical examination of light-chain expression (lambda/kappa ratio) in canine, feline, equine, bovine and porcine plasma cells. Zentralbl Veterinarmed [A] 43:573–576.

44. Kim DY, Taylor HW, Eades SC, Cho DY. 2005. Systemic AL amyloidosis associated with multiple myeloma in a horse. Vet Pathol 42:81–84.

45. Carothers MA, Johnson GC, DiBartola SP, Liepnicks J, Benson MD. 1989. Extramedullary plasmacytoma and immunoglobulin-associated amyloidosis in a cat. J Am Vet Med Assoc 195:1593–1597.

46. Werner JA, Woo JC, Vernau W, Graham PS, Grahn RA, Lyons LA, Moore PF. 2005. Characterization of feline immunoglobulin heavy chain variable region genes for the molecular diagnosis of B-cell neoplasia. Vet Pathol 42:596–607.

47. Iijima T, Inadome Y, Noguchi M. 2000. Clonal proliferation of B lymphocytes in the germinal centers of human reactive lymph nodes: Possibility of overdiagnosis of B cell clonal proliferation. Diagn Mol Pathol 9:132–136.

48. Zhou XG, Sandvej K, Gregersen N, Hamilton-Dutoit SJ. 1999. Detection of clonal B cells in microdissected reactive lymphoproliferations: Possible diagnostic pitfalls in PCR analysis of immunoglobulin heavy chain gene rearrangement. Mol Pathol 52:104–110.

49. Littman MP, Dambach DM, Vaden SL, Giger U. 2000. Familial protein-losing enteropathy and protein-losing nephropathy in soft coated Wheaten terriers: 222 cases (1983–1997). J Vet Intern Med 14:68–80.

50. Kern MR, Stockham SL, Coates JR. 1992. Analysis of serum protein concentrations after severe thermal injury in a dog. Vet Clin Pathol 21:19–22.

51. Hoover EA, Mullins JI, Quackenbush SL, Gasper PW. 1987. Experimental transmission and pathogenesis of immunodeficiency syndrome in cats. Blood 70:1880–1892.

52. Tyler JW, Hancock DD, Parish SM, Rea DE, Besser TE, Sanders SG, Wilson LK. 1996. Evaluation of 3 assays for failure of passive transfer in calves. J Vet Intern Med 10:304–307.

53. Harvey JW, West CL. 1987. Prednisone-induced increases in serum alpha-2-globulin and haptoglobin concentrations in dogs. Vet Pathol 24:90–92.

54. Moore GE, Mahaffey EA, Hoenig M. 1992. Hematologic and serum biochemical effects of long-term administration of anti-inflammatory doses of prednisone in dogs. Am J Vet Res 53:1033–1037.

55. Rothschild MA, Oratz M, Schreiber SS. 1980. Albumin synthesis. Int Rev Physiol 21:249–274.

56. Campbell J, Rastogi KS. 1968. Elevation in serum insulin, albumin, and FFA, with gains in liver lipid and protein, induced by glucocorticoid treatment in dogs. Can J Physiol Pharmacol 46:421–429.

57. Keay G, Doxey DL. 1984. A study of the interaction between bromocresol green dye and bovine, ovine and equine serum globulins. Vet Res Commun 8:25–32.

58. Gustafsson JE. 1976. Improved specificity of serum albumin determination and estimation of "acute phase reactants" by use of the bromcresol green reaction. Clin Chem 22:616–622.

59. Schalm OW, Smith R, Kaneko JJ. 1970. Plasma protein:fibrinogen ratios in dogs, cattle and horses. Part I. Influence of age on normal values and explanation of use in disease. Calif Vet 24:9–11.

60. Duncan JR, Prasse KW. 1977. *Veterinary Laboratory Medicine*, 1st edition. Ames: Iowa State University Press.

61. Schalm OW. 1970. Plasma protein:fibrinogen ratios in routine clinical material from cats, dogs, horses, and cattle. Part III. Calif Vet 24:6–10.

62. Schalm OW, Jain NC, Carroll EJ. 1975. *Veterinary Hematology*, 3rd edition. Philadelphia: Lea & Febiger.

63. Wilkerson MJ, Johnson GS, Stockham S, Riley L. 2005. Afibrinogenemia and a circulating antibody against fibrinogen in a bichon frise dog. Vet Clin Pathol 34:148–155.

64. Kammermann B, Gmür J, Stünzi H. 1971. Afibrinogenemia in dogs. Zentralbl Veterinarmed [A] 18:192–205.

65. Andrews GA, Smith JE, Gray M, Chavey PS, Weeks BR. 1992. An improved ferritin assay for canine sera. Vet Clin Pathol 21:57–60.

66. Andrews GA, Chavey PS, Smith JE. 1994. Enzyme-linked immunosorbent assay to measure serum ferritin and the relationship between serum ferritin and nonheme iron stores in cats. Vet Pathol 31:674–678.

67. Smith JE, Moore K, Cipriano JE, Morris PG. 1984. Serum ferritin as a measure of stored iron in horses. J Nutr 114:677–681.

68. Kuribayashi T, Shimada T, Matsumoto M, Kawato K, Honjyo T, Fukuyama M, Yamamoto Y, Yamamoto S. 2003. Determination of serum C-reactive protein (CRP) in healthy beagle dogs of various ages and pregnant beagle dogs. Exp Anim 52:387–390.

69. Martinez-Subiela S, Ginel PJ, Ceron JJ. 2004. Effects of different glucocorticoid treatments on serum acute phase proteins in dogs. Vet Rec 154:814–817.

70. Tosa N, Morimatsu M, Nakagawa M, Miyoshi F, Uchida E, Niiyama M, Syuto B, Saito M. 1993. Purification and identification of a serum protein increased by anthelmintic drugs for *Dirofilaria immitis* in dogs. J Vet Med Sci 55:27–31.

71. Hojo T, Ohno R, Shimoda M, Kokue E. 2002. Enzyme and plasma protein induction by multiple oral administrations of phenobarbital at a therapeutic dosage regimen in dogs. J Vet Pharmacol Ther 25:121–127.

72. Lee WC, Hsiao HC, Wu YL, Lin JH, Lee YP, Fung HP, Chen HH, Chen YH, Chu RM. 2003. Serum C-reactive protein in dairy herds. Can J Vet Res 67:102–107.

73. Hyyppa S, Hoyhtya M, Nevalainen M, Poso AR. 2002. Effect of exercise on plasma ferritin concentrations: Implications for the measurement of iron status. Equine Vet J Suppl 34:186–190.

74. Sellon DC. 2000. Secondary immunodeficiency of horses. Vet Clin North Am Equine Pract 16:117–130.

75. Porter P. 1972. Immunoglobulins in bovine mammary secretions: Quantitative changes in early lactation and absorption by the neonatal calf. Immunology 23:225–238.

76. Husband AJ, Brandon MR, Lascelles AK. 1972. Absorption and endogenous production of immunoglobulins in calves. Aust J Exp Biol Med Sci 50:491–498.

77. Larson MA, Weber A, Weber AT, McDonald TL. 2005. Differential expression and secretion of bovine serum amyloid A3 (SAA3) by mammary epithelial cells stimulated with prolactin or lipopolysaccharide. Vet Immunol Immunopathol 107:255–264.

78. Clawson ML, Heaton MP, Chitko-McKown CG, Fox JM, Smith TP, Snelling WM, Keele JW, Laegreid WW. 2004. Beta-2-microglobulin haplotypes in U.S. beef cattle and association with failure of passive transfer in newborn calves. Mamm Genome 15:227–236.

79. Bertone JJ, Jones RL, Curtis CR. 1988. Evaluation of a test kit for determination of serum immunoglobulin G concentration in foals. J Vet Intern Med 2:181–183.

80. Parish SM, Tyler JW, Besser TE, Gay CC, Krytenberg D. 1997. Prediction of serum IgG1 concentration in Holstein calves using serum gamma glutamyltransferase activity. J Vet Intern Med 11:344–347.

81. McGuire TC, Adams DS. 1982. Failure of colostral immunoglobulin transfer to calves: Prevalence and diagnosis. Compend Contin Educ Pract Vet 4:S35–S40.

82. Hopkins FM, Dean DF, Greene W. 1984. Failure of passive transfer in calves: Comparison of field diagnostic methods. Mod Vet Pract 65:625–628.

83. Di Terlizzi R, Stockham SL, Kempegowda R, Wilkerson MJ. 2005. Comparison of protein concentrations in precolostral and postcolostral bovine sera using spectrophotometric, refractometric, electrophoretic, and radial immunodiffusion methods. Vet Clin Pathol 34:283 (abstract).

84. Pfeiffer NE, McGuire TC, Bendel RB, Weikel JM. 1977. Quantitation of bovine immunoglobulins: Comparison of single radial immunodiffusion, zinc sulfate turbidity, serum electrophoresis, and refractometer methods. Am J Vet Res 38:693–698.

85. Clabough DL, Conboy HS, Roberts MC. 1989. Comparison of four screening techniques for the diagnosis of equine neonatal hypogammaglobulinemia. J Am Vet Med Assoc 194:1717–1720.

86. Beetson SA, Hilbert BJ, Mills JN. 1985. The use of the glutaraldehyde coagulation test for detection of hypogammaglobulinaemia in neonatal foals. Aust Vet J 62:279–281.

87. Tyler JW, Besser TE, Wilson L, Hancock DD, Sanders S, Rea DE. 1996. Evaluation of a whole blood glutaraldehyde coagulation test for the detection of failure of passive transfer in calves. J Vet Intern Med 10:82–84.

88. Rumbaugh GE, Ardans AA, Ginno D, Trommershausen-Smith A. 1979. Identification and treatment of colostrum-deficient foals. J Am Vet Med Assoc 174:273–276.

89. Hudgens KAR, Tyler JW, Besser TE, Krytenberg DS. 1996. Optimizing performance of a qualitative zinc sulfate turbidity test for passive transfer of immunoglobulin G in calves. Am J Vet Res 57:1711–1713.

90. Morris DD, Meirs DA, Merryman GS. 1985. Passive transfer failure in horses: Incidence and causative factors on a breeding farm. Am J Vet Res 46:2294–2299.

91. Davis R, Giguere S. 2005. Evaluation of five commercially available assays and measurement of serum total protein concentration via refractometry for the diagnosis of failure of passive transfer of immunity in foals. J Am Vet Med Assoc 227:1640–1645.

92. Tizard IR. 2000. Primary immunodeficiencies. *Veterinary Immunology: An Introduction*, 7th edition, 413–427. Philadelphia: WB Saunders.

93. Zoran D. 2000. Immunodeficiency disorders. In: Feldman BF, Zinkl JG, Jain NC, eds. *Schalm's Veterinary Hematology*, 5th edition, 941–946. Philadelphia: Lippincott Williams & Wilkins.

94. Flaminio MJ, LaCombe V, Kohn CW, Antczak DF. 2002. Common variable immunodeficiency in a horse. J Am Vet Med Assoc 221:1296–1302, 1267.

95. Gardner RB, Hart KA, Stokol T, Divers TJ, Flaminio MJ. 2006. Fell Pony syndrome in a pony in North America. J Vet Intern Med 20:198–203.

96. Francoz D, Lapointe JM, Wellemans V, Desrochers A, Caswell JL, Stott JL, Dubreuil P. 2004. Immunoglobulin G2 deficiency with transient hypogammaglobulinemia and chronic respiratory disease in a 6-month-old Holstein heifer. J Vet Diagn Invest 16:432–435.

97. Day MJ, Power C, Oleshko J, Rose M. 1997. Low serum immunoglobulin concentrations in related Weimaraner dogs. J Small Anim Pract 38:311–315.

98. Rose BD, Post TW. 2001. *Clinical Physiology of Acid-Base and Electrolyte Disorders*, 5th edition. New York: McGraw-Hill.

99. Szladovits B, Stockham SL, Moore LE. 2004. The effect of multiple doses of hetastarch and in vitro hemolysis on serum colloid osmotic pressure in hypoalbuminemic dogs. Vet Pathol 41:547 (abstract).

100. Brown SA, Dusza K, Boehmer J. 1994. Comparison of measured and calculated values for colloid osmotic pressure in hospitalized animals. Am J Vet Res 55:910–915.

101. Thomas LA, Brown SA. 1992. Relationship between colloid osmotic pressure and plasma protein concentration in cattle, horses, dogs, and cats. Am J Vet Res 53:2241–2244.

102. Runk DT, Madigan JE, Rahal CJ, Allison DN, Fredrickson K. 2000. Measurement of plasma colloid osmotic pressure in normal thoroughbred neonatal foals. J Vet Intern Med 14:475–478.

103. Driessen B, Jahr JS, Lurie F, Golkaryeh MS, Gunther RA. 2003. Arterial oxygenation and oxygen delivery after hemoglobin-based oxygen carrier infusion in canine hypovolemic shock: A dose-response study. Crit Care Med 31:1771–1779.

104. Moore LE, Garvey MS. 1996. The effect of hetastarch on serum colloid oncotic pressure in hypoalbuminemic dogs. J Vet Intern Med 10:300–303.

105. Guyton AC, Hall JE. 2000. *Textbook of Medical Physiology*, 10th edition. Philadelphia: WB Saunders.

106. Ritzmann SE, Daniels JC, eds. 1982. *Serum Protein Abnormalities: Diagnostic and Clinical Aspects*. New York: Alan R Liss.

Chapter 8

URINARY SYSTEM

Physiologic Processes 416
Chronic Renal Insufficiency or Failure 425
Acute Renal Failure 427
Azotemia and Uremia 429
Urea Nitrogen (UN) Concentration in Serum or Plasma 433
Creatinine (Crt) Concentration in Serum or Plasma 436
Urea Nitrogen (UN) Concentration versus Creatinine (Crt) Concentration in
    Serum or Plasma 437
Creatinine (Crt) Clearance Rate 438
Abnormal Routine Serum Chemistry Results in Azotemic Animals 439
Major Urinalysis (UA) Concepts 440
Physical Examination of Urine 441
Chemical Examination of Urine (Qualitative or Semiquantitative) 452
Urine Sediment Examination 469
Quantitative Urinalysis 475
    I.   Basic Concepts 475
    II.   24 h Excretion Studies 476
    III.   Analyte Urine to Plasma Ratios 476
    IV.   Quantitative Urine Total Protein Assays 477
    V.   Urinary Protein to Creatinine (Prot:Crt)$_u$ Ratio 478
    VI.   Microalbuminuria 480
    VII.   Fractional Excretion (FE) Ratios or Percentages 483
    VIII.   Urine Bile Acid to Creatinine Ratio 485
H$_2$O Deprivation and Antidiuretic Hormone (ADH) Response Tests in Animals
    with Polyuria and Polydipsia (PU/PD) 485
Urolith Analysis 487

Table 8.1. Abbreviations and symbols in this chapter

$(Prot:Crt)_u$	Urinary protein to creatinine
[x]	x concentration (x = analyte)
1,25-DHCC	1,25-Dihydroxycholecalciferol
ADH	Antidiuretic hormone (arginine vasopressin)
AMP	Adenosine monophosphate
AMS	Amylase
ATPase	Adenosine triphosphatase
Bc	Conjugated bilirubin
Bu	Unconjugated bilirubin
Ca^{2+}	Calcium
Crt	Creatinine
ELISA	Enzyme-linked immunosorbent assay
FE	Fractional excretion
fCa^{2+}	Free ionized calcium (not bound or complexed)
fMg^{2+}	Free ionized magnesium (not bound or complexed)
GFR	Glomerular filtration rate
GGT	γ-Glutamyltransferase
HCO_3^-	Bicarbonate
hpf	High-power field (400× magnification)
lpf	Low-power field (100× magnification)
LPS	Lipase
M_r	Relative molecular mass
NH_3	Ammonia
NH_4^+	Ammonium
PD	Polydipsia
PO_4	Phosphate including PO_4^{3-}, HPO_4^{2-}, or $H_2PO_4^-$
PTH	Parathyroid hormone
PU	Polyuria
RPF	Renal plasma flow
sd	Standard deviation
SDS-PAGE	Sodium dodecyl sulfate–polyacrylamide gel electrophoresis
SI	Système International d'Unités
SSA	Sulfosalicylic acid
tCa^{2+}	Total calcium
UA	Urinalysis (urine analysis)
UN	Urea nitrogen
UN:Crt	Urea nitrogen to creatinine
USG	Urine specific gravity
USG_{ref}	Refractometric urine specific gravity

PHYSIOLOGIC PROCESSES

I. Three major processes control renal excretion of H_2O and solutes: glomerular filtration (passive), tubular resorption (active or passive), and tubular secretion (active or passive). The net results of the renal functions on plasma in healthy animals are summarized in Table 8.2.

Table 8.2. Net result of normal renal function on plasma analytes

Conserved	Excreted
H_2O	Urea
Glucose	Creatinine
Amino acids	PO_4
Proteins	K^+
Na^+	$H^{+ \ a}$
Cl^-	NH_4^+
HCO_3^-	Lactate
$Ca^{2+ \ b}$	Acetoacetate
Mg^{2+}	β-Hydroxybutyrate
	Bilirubin
	Hemoglobin dimers
	Myoglobin

[a] Renal excretion of H^+ may result in either acidic or alkaline urine, depending on the amount of H^+ in urine. Most H^+ excreted by kidneys is bound to PO_4 ($HPO_4^{2-} + H^+ \rightarrow H_2PO_4^-$) or in NH_4^+ ($NH_3 + H^+ \rightarrow NH_4^+$).

[b] Except in horses in which kidneys excrete Ca^{2+} if consuming a Ca^{2+}-rich diet

II. Glomerular filtration
   A. A major route for solute and H_2O excretion from an animal is through renal glomeruli. The glomerular filtration barrier is composed of capillary endothelium, basement membrane, and glomerular epithelial cells (podocytes) with foot processes (Fig. 8.1). The filtering function of glomeruli is typically assessed by evaluating the renal excretion of substances that pass freely through the glomerular filtration barrier.
      1. The potential for a substance to pass through the healthy glomerular filtration barrier (from plasma to filtrate) depends on two major factors:
         a. Molecular size: Nearly 100 % of molecules with radius < 2.5 nm pass through. Almost no molecules with radius > 3.4 nm pass through.
         b. Electrical charge: Positively charged and electrically neutral substances pass through better than negatively charged substances because the glomerular basement membrane contains negatively charged molecules.
      2. In many species, albumin ($M_r \approx 69,000$; 3.5 nm radius) is near the threshold size of the filtration barrier; its negative charge also impedes transit. Albumin is not expected in the urine of cats, horses, or cattle. A small amount may be found in the urine of apparently healthy dogs. This albuminuria may represent a subclinical disease or a species variation.
   B. GFR
      1. *GFR* is the rate fluid moves from plasma to glomerular filtrate and is measured by determining the rate a substance is cleared from plasma.
      2. GFR depends primarily on the rate of RPF and varies proportionately with RPF. RPF depends on blood volume, cardiac output, number of functional glomeruli, and constriction or dilation of afferent and efferent glomerular arterioles. Other factors that affect GFR include intracapsular hydrostatic pressure in Bowman's space (if pressure is increased, GFR is decreased) and plasma colloidal osmotic (oncotic) pressure (if pressure is decreased, GFR is increased).

Glomerulus   Glomerular Filtration Barrier

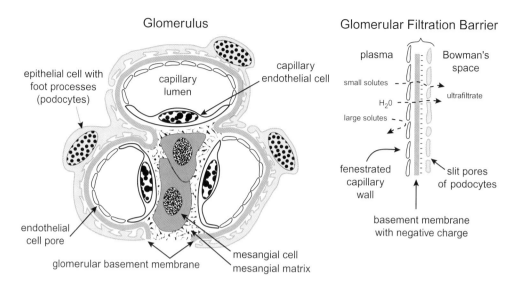

Fig. 8.1. Glomerular filtration barrier. The glomerular filtration barrier consists of the capillary endothelial cell, the glomerular basement membrane, and the epithelial cells (podocytes). H_2O and most solutes pass through fenestrations in the endothelial cells, through a semipermeable basement membrane, through the slit pores between the foot processes of the podocytes, into Bowman's space, and then into the proximal renal tubule.

3. The ideal solute for measuring GFR would not be protein bound, would pass freely through the filtration barrier, and would be neither secreted nor resorbed by renal tubules. Inulin, iohexol, and mannitol nearly meet these criteria. Crt is often used because very little is secreted by renal tubules in most animals, and it meets the other criteria. GFR can also be assessed by imaging methods: excretion of radioactive compounds (renal scintigraphy) or contrast media (contrast nephrography).

III. Functions of renal tubules are reflected by the rate of urinary excretion of a plasma substance compared to the rate of inulin excretion.
   A. If excretion of a solute is greater than excretion of inulin, there is a net solute secretion by tubules. Renal tubular secretion involves processes by which solutes from plasma, interstitial fluid, or tubular cells are transferred to tubular fluid.
   B. If excretion of a solute is less than excretion of inulin, there is a net solute resorption by tubules or the substance does not freely pass through the filtration barrier.

IV. Functions of tubules pertaining to major solutes[1] (Fig. 8.2)
   A. Na^+
      1. About 75 % of filtrate Na^+ is resorbed in the proximal tubules down a concentration gradient established by the Na^+-K^+-ATPase pump (basolateral membrane) and a Na^+-H^+ antiporter. Na^+ resorption is enhanced by an electrical gradient established by conservation of HCO_3^-; Na^+ is cotransported with glucose, amino acids, and phosphates. Angiotensin II stimulates the proximal tubular resorption of Na^+, Cl^-, and H_2O.
      2. Na^+ is passively resorbed into the descending limb of the loop of Henle to maintain Na^+ in the countercurrent system.

   3. Na^+ accompanies K^+ and Cl^- that are resorbed in the thick ascending limb of the loop of Henle via a Na^+-K^+-$2Cl^-$ cotransporter in the luminal membrane. The rate-limiting factor is Cl^- delivery to the loop. Furosemide diuretics block this process.
   4. ADH stimulates Na^+ and Cl^- resorption in the medullary thick limb of the loop of Henle through the Na^+-K^+-$2Cl^-$ cotransporter (a minor role for ADH).
   5. Aldosterone stimulates the active resorption of Na^+ in collecting tubules by opening Na^+ channels, enhancing Na^+-K^+-ATPase activity in the basolateral membrane, and opening luminal K^+ channels. Its actions are probably mediated through aldosterone-induced proteins (Na^+-K^+-ATPase may be one of the proteins) (see Fig. 9.3).
   6. Na^+ and Cl^- resorption in the distal nephron (distal tubule and collecting duct) also involves an aldosterone-independent Na^+-Cl^- cotransporter. This process varies directly with Na^+ delivery to the distal nephron. Thiazide diuretics block this cotransporter.
   7. Na^+ resorption in the distal nephron is reduced during volume expansion through the action of atrial natriuretic peptide, which reduces the number of open Na^+ channels by a guanylate cyclase pathway.
B. Cl^-
   1. About 75 % of filtered Cl^- is resorbed in the proximal tubules down a concentration gradient created by Na^+ and H_2O resorption and through a formate-Cl^- exchanger.
   2. Cl^- is resorbed via a Na^+-K^+-$2Cl^-$ cotransporter in the thick ascending limb of the loop of Henle.
   3. Cl^- is passively resorbed in the distal nephron by an electrochemical gradient established by Na^+ movement (through aldosterone and aldosterone-independent processes) (see Fig. 9.3).
   4. Cl^- is also secreted by the type A intercalated cells when they are stimulated to secrete H^+. Concurrent with the secretion of Cl^-, HCO_3^- is produced by the cells and enters the plasma (see Fig. 9.4).
C. HCO_3^-
   1. About 90 % of filtered HCO_3^- is conserved indirectly in the proximal tubules during H^+ secretion. H^+ secretion is mediated by the Na^+-H^+ antiporter and depends on Na^+ resorption. As Na^+ is resorbed, the secreted H^+ combines with HCO_3^- in the filtrate to form H_2CO_3, which then forms CO_2 and H_2O. The CO_2 and H_2O enter the proximal tubular cells in which they are converted to H^+ (which is again available for secretion) and HCO_3^-. The HCO_3^- is transported to the peritubular fluid via a Na^+-$3HCO_3^-$ cotransporter (see Fig. 9.7).
   2. In the collecting ducts, HCO_3^- produced by the type A intercalated cells enters the peritubular fluid through a Cl^--HCO_3^- exchanger (see Fig. 9.4). A reverse process in type B intercalated cells leads to HCO_3^- secretion when there is excess HCO_3^- (see Fig. 9.8).
D. K^+
   1. In health, most of the K^+ that enters the proximal tubule through the glomerular filtration barrier is resorbed prior to the distal tubule. K^+ is secreted primarily by the principal cells of the collecting tubules, and secretion is promoted by aldosterone (see Fig. 9.3). K^+ movement from cell to tubular lumen occurs through K^+ channels opened by aldosterone. The movement is enhanced when the urinary flow rate through the tubule is high. With high flow rates, the K^+ is washed away quickly, and

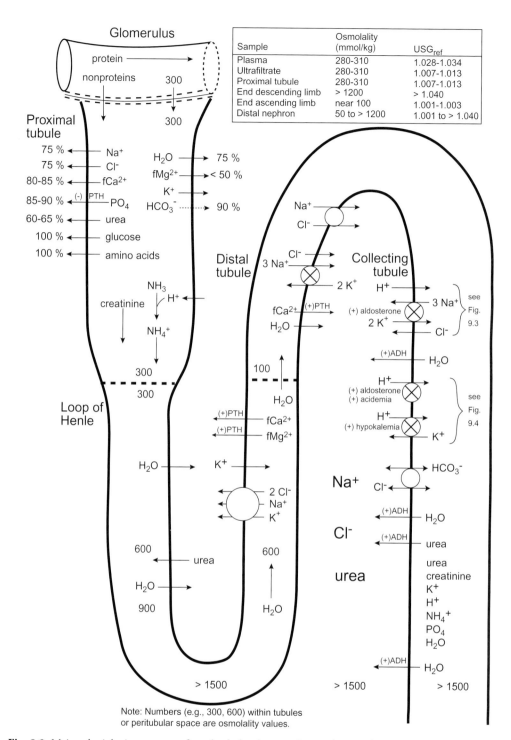

Fig. 8.2. Major physiologic processes of renal tubules that pertain to solutes and H_2O. The solute concentrations are provided to illustrate changes that occur as the fluid moves through the nephron (see Fig. 8.3). Actual solute concentrations would vary, depending on many physiologic and pathologic factors.

thus a concentration gradient is maintained. The movement is reduced when the urinary flow rate through the tubule is low because K^+ stays longer in the tubular fluid, and thus the concentration gradient is diminished.

2. ADH promotes K^+ secretion in the cortical collecting tubule, perhaps by opening K^+ channels in the luminal membrane. This process compensates for the reduced K^+ secretion that occurs with decreased urinary flow.

3. Type A intercalated cells conserve K^+ when hypokalemia is present (see Fig. 9.4).

E. H^+

1. H^+ is secreted from type A intercalated cells of the distal nephron through a H^+-ATPase pump that can work against a large concentration gradient (see Fig. 9.4). Aldosterone and acidemia promote this process. H^+ is also secreted, and K^+ is resorbed through H^+-K^+-ATPase pumps that appear to be most active when hypokalemia is present.

2. A limited amount of H^+ is secreted by the proximal tubular cells (see Fig. 9.7), after which it may be buffered by HCO_3^-, NH_3, or PO_4. Most of the renal excretion of H^+ is within NH_4^+ (see Fig. 9.6) and either HPO_4^{2-} or $H_2PO_4^-$. Very little is present as free H^+ ($\approx 10^{-8}$–10^{-6} mol/L).

Fig. 8.2. *continued*
- The osmolality of the plasma and the ultrafiltrate are equal (near 300 mmol/kg) as H_2O and nonprotein solutes pass through the glomerular filtration barrier.
- In the proximal tubules, a majority of the H_2O and solutes that enter the tubules are resorbed through active, facilitated, and passive processes. The osmolality of the tubular fluid leaving the proximal tubule is still near 300 mmol/kg, but the fluid volume is greatly diminished.
- In the descending limb of the loop of Henle, tubular fluid is concentrated and volume reduced by the passive movement of H_2O. Urea may diffuse from the interstitial fluid to the tubular fluid. At the bottom of the loop of Henle, the concentration of the tubular fluid will vary among species. The 1500 mmol/kg value is probably appropriate for horses and cattle, whereas the solute concentration in cats may be > 2400 mmol/kg.
- In the ascending limb of the loop of Henle, solutes (mostly Na^+, Cl^-, and K^+) passively leave the tubular fluid via a Na^+-K^+-2Cl^- carrier (energy provided the by Na^+-K^+-ATPase pump in the basolateral membrane), but H_2O remains. Thus, the tubular fluid becomes dilute, and the fluid leaving the diluting segment has an osmolality near 100 mmol/kg. Passive fCa^{2+} and fMg^{2+} resorption depends on an electrical gradient promoted by the Na^+-K^+-2Cl^- cotransporter and the recycling of K^+, whereas active fCa^{2+} and fMg^{2+} resorption is promoted by PTH.
- In the distal and collecting tubules, there are multiple processes involved in electrolyte balance, acid-base balance, and conservation of H_2O (see the text for specifics). The major actions of ADH are to promote resorption of H_2O and urea. The major actions of aldosterone are the resorption of Na^+ and Cl^- and the secretion of K^+ and H^+. The osmolality of the urine typically is > 600 mmol/kg and may be > 2000 mmol/kg.
- In most healthy domestic mammals, the net function of a nephron is to excrete urea, Crt, K^+, H^+, NH_4^+, and PO_4 and to conserve Na^+, Cl^-, HCO_3^-, fCa^{2+}, fMg^{2+}, glucose, amino acids, and H_2O. The equine nephron excretes fCa^{2+} instead of conserving it.

The table in the top of the figure shows a comparison of the approximate solute concentrations (in terms of osmolality and USG_{ref}) in different segments of a functional nephron. Note that the USG_{ref} for plasma (1.028–1.034) were determined by using a refractometer's urine specific gravity scale. The true specific gravity of the plasma would be nearer 1.018–1.022,[113] and such a range has little to no clinical relevance. $\otimes$, ATPase pump; and $\bigcirc$, transporter or shuttle.

F. Ca^{2+}

    1. About 80–85 % of filtrate Ca^{2+} is resorbed in the proximal tubules and loops of Henle through a passive process that depends on Na^+ and H_2O resorption. Ca^{2+} is passively resorbed in the ascending limb of the loop of Henle down an electrochemical gradient established by a Na^+-K^+-$2Cl^-$ cotransporter and a recycling of K^+.

    2. PTH promotes Ca^{2+} resorption by activating an adenylate cyclase pathway in the cortical thick ascending limb of the loop of Henle, the distal tubule, and the connecting segment between the distal tubule and the collecting ducts.

    3. Vitamin D promotes Ca^{2+} resorption in the distal nephron by inducing production of a calcium-binding protein. Calcitriol (1,25-DHCC) formation in the proximal renal tubules is stimulated by increased PTH activity and hypophosphatemia.

    4. Thiazide diuretics increase the resorption of Ca^{2+} in the distal nephron.

G. PO_4

    1. About 85–90 % of filtrate PO_4 is resorbed in the proximal tubule via the actions of a Na^+-PO_4 cotransporter.

    2. The cotransporter's activity is enhanced by hypophosphatemia and insulin, whereas it is diminished by hyperphosphatemia and increased PTH activity.

H. Mg^{2+}

    1. At physiologic concentrations, nearly all filtrate Mg^{2+} is resorbed (most in the cortical thick ascending limbs of loops of Henle, but also in the proximal tubules). Passive Mg^{2+} resorption is mostly down an electrochemical gradient established by the Na^+-K^+-$2Cl^-$ cotransporter and a recycling of K^+. There also may be specific transporters or channels whose activities depend on blood $[Mg^{2+}]$.

    2. ADH, PTH, glucagon, calcitonin, and β-adrenergic agonists stimulate Mg^{2+} resorption in the cortical thick ascending limb.

I. Glucose

    1. Typically, glucose passes freely through the glomerular filtration barrier, and all filtrate glucose is resorbed in the proximal tubules as Na^+ is resorbed by a Na^+-glucose cotransport system involving glucose transporter proteins. The glucose resorption process is called *secondary active transport* because it occurs *secondary* to Na^+ resorption and it is *active* because it is moving up a concentration gradient (with a higher concentration in cells than in tubular fluid in the healthy state).

    2. The transport process involves carrier proteins that can be saturated by excessive glucose from plasma, thus producing hyperglycemic glucosuria.

J. Proteins and amino acids

    1. Nearly all filtrate proteins and amino acids are resorbed in the proximal tubules.

    2. Amino acids are resorbed through carriers specific for seven amino acid groups. Small peptides are hydrolyzed at the brush border, and the amino acids are resorbed.

    3. Larger proteins (including albumin) enter the tubular cells through endocytosis and then are degraded to amino acids. In some apparently healthy dogs, some of the albumin is not resorbed and thus is present in urine in low concentrations. The urinary albumin may represent subclinical disease or a species variation.

    4. Megalin, aminionless, and cubilin, receptor proteins expressed in the apical part of proximal tubular epithelial cells, are important in mediating endocytosis of a wide variety of proteins. These include vitamin D–binding protein, which is required for renal formation of 1,25-DHCC. These proteins also mediate intrinsic factor–cobalamin uptake in the small intestine.

K. Urea
  1. About 60–65 % of filtrate urea is resorbed in the proximal tubules down a concentration gradient created by the movement of H_2O into the cells (which initially lowers cellular [urea] and raises tubular [urea]). This process is enhanced in hypovolemic states when there is greater proximal tubular resorption of Na^+ and H_2O, decreased urine flow rate, and thus more time for passive urea absorption.
  2. Urea is recycled in the remaining nephron by moving from interstitial fluid to fluid in the loop of Henle and then from medullary collecting duct fluid to medullary interstitial fluid.
  3. Urea resorption in the distal nephron is enhanced (nearly four times the baseline) by ADH activity and a concentration gradient established by H_2O resorption secondary to Na^+ and Cl^- resorption. ADH increases tubular permeability to urea.
  4. Urea contributes nearly 50 % of interstitial solute for the establishment of a hypertonic medulla that is necessary for renal concentrating ability.
L. Crt
  1. In some dogs, small amounts of Crt are secreted by the proximal tubules.[2,3] Crt secretion does not appear to occur in horses or cats.[4,5]
  2. In people, Crt secretion may occur through a pathway shared with organic cations. Serum [Crt] increases when other organic cations (such as cimetidine, trimethoprim, and quinidine) interfere with Crt secretion.
M. Resorption of H_2O by tubules
  1. About 30 % of RPF becomes ultrafiltrate. About 75 % of the ultrafiltrate H_2O is passively resorbed in the proximal tubules.
  2. H_2O is passively resorbed in the descending limb of the loop of Henle as the loop enters the hypertonic medulla.
  3. The ascending limb of the loop of Henle and connecting segments are impermeable to H_2O.
  4. The collecting tubules are permeable to H_2O in the presence of ADH. ADH binds to receptors on the basolateral membranes of principal epithelial cells of the collecting tubules, resulting in activation of a protein kinase that phosphorylates aquaporin 2 and enables it to be transported from vesicles to the apical membrane. Lack of ADH triggers endocytosis of aquaporin and its return to cytoplasmic vesicles. Water moves into cells through the pore at the center of the proteins. Water escapes to the interstitium through pores formed by aquaporin 3 in the basolateral membranes of the principal cells.

V. Renal concentrating ability and renal diluting ability
  A. Definitions
    1. *Concentrating ability*: the ability of kidneys to resorb filtrate H_2O in excess of filtrate solutes; ability to concentrate solutes
    2. *Diluting ability*: the ability of kidneys to resorb filtrate solute in excess of filtrate H_2O; ability to dilute solutes
  B. Terms used to describe the concentration of urine
    1. Many authors describe the solute concentration of urine with the terms hyposthenuria, isosthenuria, and hypersthenuria (*-sthen-* means "strength"). However, there is little agreement on the definitions for these terms. Isosthenuria should mean same (*iso-*) strength (*-sthen-*) urine (*-uria*).

2. Our definitions (see Fig. 8.8 for relationship of USG$_{ref}$ and urine osmolality)

   a. *Isosthenuria* (working definition) is the state in which urine osmolality is the same as plasma osmolality, whether plasma osmolality is low, normal, or high. We define "the same" as being within 100 mmol/kg of plasma osmolality; that is, osmolality$_u$ = osmolality$_p$ ± 100 mmol/kg. In most domestic mammals, such urine typically will have a USG$_{ref}$ from 1.007–1.013, inclusively (unpublished authors' data).

   b. *Hyposthenuria* is the state in which excreted urine has an osmolality that is less than the isosthenuric values; that is, osmolality$_u$ < (osmolality$_p$ − 100 mmol/kg). In most hyposthenuric animals, the USG$_{ref}$ will be less than 1.007. Such urine is dilute (the filtrate has been diluted by renal processes).

   c. To be consistent with terms, *eusthenuria* is the excretion of urine with the osmolality expected for an animal that has adequate renal function and normal hydration status, and *hypersthenuria* is the excretion of highly concentrated urine. However, the terms eusthenuria and hypersthenuria are rarely used.

C. Physiologic processes for concentrating or diluting glomerular filtrate

1. Functions of renal interstitium

   a. Provides a bridge between tubules and blood vessels to facilitate the movement of H$_2$O and solutes

   b. Helps maintain medullary hypertonicity to enable the concentration of tubular fluid

2. Functions of tubules

   a. Proximal tubule (proximal convoluted tubule)

      (1) Approximately 30 % of the plasma that enters glomeruli becomes glomerular filtrate (USG$_{ref}$ ≈ 1.010; osmolality ≈ 300 mmol/kg).

      (2) About 75 % of the H$_2$O in the ultrafiltrate is passively resorbed by the proximal tubules (independent of body needs). The remainder passes into the loop of Henle. The solute concentration does not change much in the proximal tubule, but fluid volume decreases markedly.

   b. Descending limb of the loop of Henle

      (1) The osmolality of tubular fluid increases because of the passive resorption of H$_2$O and the secretion of Na$^+$, Cl$^-$, and urea into the filtrate.

      (2) Fluid entering the loop of Henle has a USG$_{ref}$ ≈ 1.010 and an osmolality ≈ 300 mmol/kg. Tubular fluid at the distal end of the descending limb has a high concentration (USG$_{ref}$ > 1.050; osmolality > 1500 mmol/kg).

   c. Ascending limb of the loop of Henle (the diluting segment of the nephron)

      (1) The ascending limb is relatively impermeable to H$_2$O but actively pumps Cl$^-$ and Na$^+$ (also K$^+$, fCa^{2+}, and fMg^{2+}) from the tubular fluid to the interstitial fluid. Thus, tubular fluid loses solute and the interstitial fluid becomes more hypertonic. Fluid leaving the ascending limb for the distal tubule is dilute (USG$_{ref}$ < 1.007; osmolality < 200 mmol/kg).

      (2) A functional ascending limb is necessary to maintain a hypertonic interstitial fluid in the medullary region so that H$_2$O may be passively resorbed in the descending limb of the loop of Henle and in collecting tubules.

      (3) The ascending limb and the closely associated vasa recta are the major structures of the countercurrent system that maintain a hyperosmolar medullary interstitial fluid.

    d. Distal tubule (distal convoluted tubule)
      (1) The distal tubule has minimal H_2O permeability, and thus very little H_2O is resorbed in this segment.
      (2) The resorption of Na^+ and Cl^- in this segment lowers the tubular fluid osmolality.
    e. Collecting tubules
      (1) The collecting tubules of the distal nephron contain the concentrating processes of the nephron.
      (2) ADH controls permeability of the epithelium to H_2O. H_2O is resorbed in the presence of ADH if there is an osmolar gradient between the tubular fluid and medullary interstitial fluid. An osmolar gradient is created by high concentrations of urea, Na^+, and Cl^- in the interstitial fluid that are produced and maintained by segmental functions of the nephron.
      (3) The H_2O channels through the epithelial cells are created by membrane-associated proteins called *aquaporins*. When ADH binds to the renal epithelial cell basolateral membranes, it activates a cyclic adenosine monophosphate (cAMP)-dependent secondary messenger system by which aquaporins are transported to the apical membranes, and thus membranes become permeable to H_2O. ADH also appears to increase production of aquaporins.[6]
  3. For kidneys to concentrate the ultrafiltrate, the following are necessary:
    a. ADH must be present. Stimuli for ADH secretion include hyperosmolality, decreased cardiovascular pressures as seen with hypovolemia, and, to a lesser degree, increased [angiotensin].
    b. Epithelial cells of the distal nephron must be responsive to ADH.
    c. There must be a concentration gradient; that is, the osmolality of the interstitial fluid of the renal medulla must be greater than the osmolality of the fluid in the tubules.
  4. For kidneys to dilute the ultrafiltrate, the following are necessary:
    a. Na^+ and Cl^- must be actively transported from the tubular fluid to the interstitial fluid by epithelial cells of the ascending limb of the loop of Henle. This process requires delivery of Na^+ and Cl^- to the loop of Henle.
    b. Very little to no H_2O is removed from the tubular fluid by the distal nephron.
  D. The osmolality changes that occur in a nephron during the formation of urine are illustrated in Fig. 8.3.

CHRONIC RENAL INSUFFICIENCY OR FAILURE

I.   What is chronic renal insufficiency or failure?
  A. Many chronic diseases may damage kidneys sufficiently so that functional renal tissue is inadequate to maintain health. Then, the animal enters the pathophysiologic state of chronic renal insufficiency or failure.
  B. There are no universally accepted definitions or criteria for staging impaired renal function. One system seems to correlate with clinical findings seen in many domestic mammals.[7,8]
    1. Diminished renal reserve: The GFR is about 50 % of normal, and the animal is clinically healthy. Azotemia is not present, but the kidneys are less able to tolerate additional insult (e.g., disease, dehydration, or poor perfusion).

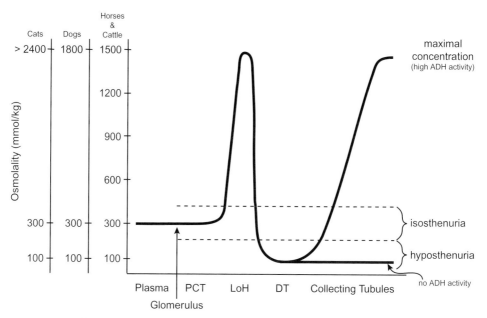

Fig. 8.3. Osmolality changes in a healthy mammal's nephron. (Details of the movement of solute and H_2O in nephrons are described in Fig. 8.2.)

The ultrafiltrate formed by glomerular filtration of plasma has an osmolality near 300 mmol/kg. As fluid moves through the proximal convoluted tubule (PCT), most of the H_2O and solutes are resorbed. Because resorption is isoosmotic, the tubular fluid's osmolality does not change. However, there are marked changes in osmolality during fluid transit through the loop of Henle (LoH). When fluid leaves the LoH, the tubular fluid's osmolality is near 100 mmol/kg. Minimal change in osmolality occurs in the distal tubule (DT) as electrolytes are resorbed. In the absence of ADH activity, H_2O remains in the collecting tubules, and thus the nephron produces hyposthenuric urine (typically $USG_{ref} < 1.007$). With minimal ADH activity in healthy mammals, the nephron produces isosthenuric urine (typically USG_{ref} of 1.007–1.013). With marked ADH activity in the collecting tubules, a large portion of the H_2O is resorbed to form maximal concentration. The maximal concentrating ability varies among domestic mammals. The right y-axis is probably appropriate for horses and cattle (i.e., maximum $USG_{ref} \approx 1.050$), whereas other y-axes are needed for dogs (≈ 1800 mmol/kg or $USG_{ref} \approx 1.060$) and cats (> 2400 mmol/kg or $USG_{ref} > 1.080$).

2. Chronic renal insufficiency: The GFR is approximately 20–50 % of normal. Azotemia and anemia appear. Polyuria occurs because of decreased concentrating ability.

3. Chronic renal failure: The GFR is < 20–25 % of normal. Azotemia and impaired concentrating ability (thus polyuria) are present. The kidneys cannot regulate extracellular fluid volume or electrolyte balance, and thus edema, hypocalcemia (generally not in horses), and metabolic acidosis will develop. Overt uremia with its neurologic, gastrointestinal and cardiovascular complications may develop.

4. End-stage renal disease: The GFR is < 5 % of normal. The terminal stages of uremia are present with either oliguria or anuria.

C. As a general concept, many authors write that more than two-thirds of functional renal mass must be lost before kidneys lose the ability to concentrate urine, and more than three-fourths must be lost before an animal becomes azotemic. Such fractions help develop major concepts but do not represent firmly established facts for all species. In one study in which renal function was reduced by nephrectomy and selective arterial ligation, cats became azotemic with only a 50 % reduction in functional mass, and most maintained renal concentrating ability (USG_{ref} > 1.040) with an estimated 83 % loss in renal function.[9]

II. Why do animals lose renal concentrating ability in chronic renal failure?
   A. More solute than usual is presented to the remaining functional nephrons, and the high solute content within the tubules contributes to solute diuresis.
   B. Medullary hypertonicity is not maintained because of three factors:
      1. Medullary tissue is damaged or medullary blood flow is abnormal.
      2. Na^+ and Cl^- transport is decreased from the ascending limb of the loop of Henle to the interstitial fluid.
      3. Damaged cells in the distal nephron are less responsive to ADH.

III. Polyuria in mammals with chronic renal insufficiency or failure
   A. The degree of polyuria in renal failure will not be as severe as with other diuretic states, such as diabetes insipidus, because the diminished GFR results in a decreased volume of filtered plasma H_2O. The urine volume produced in healthy people is about 1–2 L/d, about 3–4 L/d with polyuric renal failure, and about 6–8 L/d with other polyuric states (e.g., central and renal diabetes insipidus).
   B. Mammals with chronic renal disease typically lose concentrating ability (and thus have polyuria) before azotemia develops. Cats can concentrate glomerular filtrate to a greater degree than other domestic species and may, when azotemic, retain more concentrating ability than other species.
   C. Progression of renal disease and loss of additional nephrons will eventually cause either oliguric or anuric renal failure.

IV. Figure 8.4 illustrates the development of azotemia and abnormal urine volume caused by a progressive loss of nephrons.

V. Evidence of chronic renal insufficiency or failure
   A. Evidence of insufficiency or failure
      1. There is azotemia (increased [UN] and/or [Crt] in serum or plasma) because of inadequate renal ability to remove metabolic wastes from plasma.
      2. There is an inappropriately low USG_{ref} (often 1.007–1.013) because of a marked reduction in renal concentrating ability.
   B. Evidence of chronicity
      1. Clinical findings, including duration of signs
      2. Laboratory findings, including anemia and hypocalcemia (although hypocalcemia may also occur in acute renal failure and chronic renal failure may be associated with hypercalcemia, especially in horses)

ACUTE RENAL FAILURE

I. *Acute renal failure* is reversible or irreversible renal dysfunction resulting abruptly (within hours to days) from a renal disease or insult that markedly decreases GFR and leads to azotemia. Usual causes are toxicants, renal ischemia, or infections.

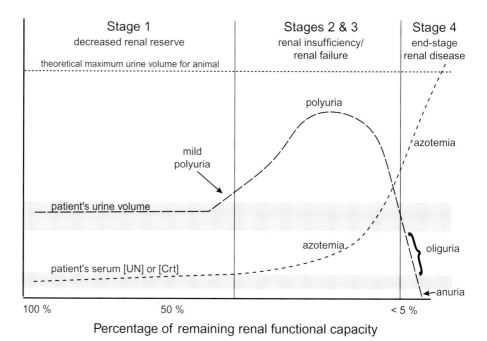

Fig. 8.4. Graphical representation of the effects of chronic renal disease and progressive dysfunction on an animal's urine volume and serum concentrations of UN or Crt. *Shaded grey areas* represent the reference intervals for urine volume (*top bar*) and for the [UN] or the [Crt] (*bottom bar*). The patient's urine volume and [UN] or [Crt] are represented by *labeled dashed lines*. A theoretical *maximal urine volume line* is shown to illustrate that animals with polyuric renal failure do not produce maximal urine volume.

- In *stage 1* (diminished renal reserve), progressive renal disease is destroying nephrons and thus GFR decreases. However, there is still sufficient function to clear urea and Crt adequately, and thus the animal is not azotemic. Also, there is sufficient ability to concentrate urine, and thus polyuria is absent or not detected. As the renal dysfunction approaches stage 2, a mild polyuria may develop because of impaired concentrating ability.
- In *stage 2* (renal insufficiency), there is sufficient loss of nephrons so that the renal concentrating ability is decreased (isosthenuria and polyuria develop) and the excretion of urea and Crt by the kidneys is insufficient (azotemia is present).
- In *stage 3* (renal failure), there is continued isosthenuria, polyuria, and azotemia but also inadequate control of H_2O balance or electrolyte concentrations. The animal has clinical signs of uremia and abnormal serum concentrations of Na^+, K^+, Cl^-, Ca^{2+}, PO_4, H^+, or HCO_3^-.
- In *stage 4* (end-stage renal disease, oliguric or anuric renal failure), only a few nephrons are filtering plasma, and thus a marked azotemia develops. The animal also becomes oliguric or anuric because very little plasma H_2O enters the kidney. The remaining tubules cannot concentrate or dilute the filtrate, and thus USG_{ref} will reflect isosthenuria.

II.   Azotemia
   A. The magnitude of the azotemia does not differentiate acute from chronic renal failure. Both can have mild to severe azotemias.
   B. The rates of increase of the [urea] and [Crt] are greater in acute renal failure than chronic renal failure; that is, a moderate to marked azotemia may develop within days in acute failure but take weeks to months with chronic failure.

III. Urine volume and USG_{ref}
   A. Because of the abrupt and severe decrease in GFR, with no time for compensatory hypertrophy of healthy nephrons, the kidneys may filter little blood and produce little or no urine (oliguria or anuria).
   B. The USG_{ref} can vary considerably.
      1. The urine may be unexpectedly concentrated if it was formed prior to the severe insult.
      2. The urine may be isosthenuric because of the same mechanisms that impair concentrating ability in chronic renal disease.
      3. The urine is not expected to be hyposthenuric because such a state would indicate loss of concentrating ability but retained diluting ability.

IV. Acid-base status and electrolyte concentrations can become acutely abnormal (e.g., hyperkalemia or acidemia).

AZOTEMIA AND UREMIA

I. Definitions
   A. *Azotemia* is increased nonprotein nitrogenous compounds in the blood that are routinely detected as increased serum [UN] and/or serum [Crt]
   B. *Uremia* is classically considered to mean "urinary constituents in blood" but now typically refers to the clinical signs reflecting renal failure (e.g., vomiting, diarrhea, coma, convulsions, and an ammoniacal odor of breath)

II. Azotemia classifications and disorders
   A. Decreased urinary excretion of urea or Crt
      1. *Prerenal azotemia*: The initiating cause of abnormal urea or Crt excretion involves reduced renal blood flow.
         a. Disorders (Table 8.3)
         b. Pathogeneses
            (1) Any process that diminishes RPF will directly decrease GFR and thus decrease clearance of urea and Crt. The volume (stretch) receptors in the juxtaglomerular apparatus of the afferent arteriole "sense" reduced blood flow and trigger the angiotensin-renin system. Angiotensin II constricts the afferent and efferent glomerular arterioles, which further reduces glomerular perfusion and thus GFR.
            (2) Hypovolemia enhances resorption of Na^+ and H_2O in proximal tubules, which in turn promotes passive proximal tubular resorption of urea (but not Crt) because the lower flow rate provides more time for resorption.
            (3) Hypovolemia also triggers release of ADH, which enhances resorption of urea (but not Crt) by medullary collecting tubules. (Aquaporin 2 transports urea, as well as H_2O.)
            (4) Azotemia occurring with a protein-losing nephropathy and marked hypoalbuminemia may be prerenal and related to decreased GFR caused by hypovolemia secondary to decreased colloidal osmotic pressure.
            (5) Azotemia is common in clinical hypoadrenocorticism. Aldosterone deficiency impairs renal excretion of K^+; the resulting hyperkalemia can cause bradycardia and thus decreased cardiac output. Concurrently, increased renal

Table 8.3. Diseases and conditions that cause azotemia[a]

Decreased urinary excretion of urea or Crt[b]
  Prerenal diseases or condition
    *Hypovolemia: dehydration (including hypoadrenocorticism), shock, blood loss
    Decreased cardiac output: cardiac insufficiency, shock, hypoadrenocorticism
    *Shock (hypovolemic, cardiogenic, anaphylactic, septic, neurogenic)
  Renal diseases or conditions
    *Inflammatory: glomerulonephritis, pyelonephritis, tubular-interstitial nephritis
    *Amyloidosis
    *Toxic nephroses: hypercalcemia, ethylene glycol, myoglobin, gentamicin,
       phenylbutazone
    *Renal ischemia or hypoxia: poor renal perfusion, infarction
    Congenital hypoplasia or aplasia
    Hydronephrosis
    Neoplasia (renal or metastatic)
  Postrenal diseases or conditions
    *Urinary tract obstruction: urolithiasis, urethral plugs in cats, neoplasia, prostatic disease
    *Leakage of urine from urinary tract: trauma, neoplasia
Increased urea or Crt production: intestinal hemorrhage, increased dietary urea or Crt,
       increased protein catabolism

* A relatively common disease or condition
[a] Greyhounds may have mildly increased Crt concentrations apparently related to high muscle mass.
[b] Decreased urinary excretion involves a decreased glomerular filtration of urea or Crt except when there is leakage of urine from urinary tract into the body.

loss of Na^+ reduces renal conservation of H_2O and sometimes results in hypovolemia. In some animals, there may be increased intestinal loss of H_2O (i.e., diarrhea) along with decreased H_2O intake to accentuate hypovolemia. Thus, a combination of factors can decrease renal blood flow and produce prerenal azotemia.

(6)   The prerenal azotemia developing in association with severe intestinal hemorrhage is partially due to hypovolemia, which leads to decreased renal excretion of Crt and urea (see Azotemia and Uremia sect. II.B4).

c. Decreased RPF that is severe and persistent may lead to renal hypoxia, acute renal damage, and thus acute renal failure. In such animals, the azotemia may be renal and prerenal.

2. *Renal azotemia*: The initiating cause is any renal disease that causes a major decrease in GFR. Any of the following may contribute: loss of nephrons, decreased vascular patency within the kidney, decreased glomerular permeability, increased renal interstitial pressure, or increased intratubular pressure.

a. Diseases or disorders (Table 8.3)

b. Pathogeneses

(1)   Renal disease (acute or chronic) causing the loss of at least 65–75 % of nephron functional capacity reduces the GFR sufficiently to produce azotemia. Reduced GFR causes inadequate renal excretion of urea and Crt

from plasma (without sufficient compensation by intestinal processes), and thus serum [UN] and [Crt] increase.

(2) Processes that contribute to a prerenal azotemia may also be present.

3. *Postrenal azotemia*: The initiating cause of defective urea or Crt excretion is distal to the nephron.

a. Diseases or disorders (Table 8.3)

b. Pathogenesis of obstructive azotemia

(1) Urinary tract obstruction causes the release of vasoactive substances (prostaglandins and angiotensin) that constrict the glomerular arterioles, thus reducing RPF and diminishing the GFR; reduced GFR impairs clearance of urea and Crt[10]

(2) Impaired outflow causes a transient increase in intracapsular hydrostatic pressure that decreases the GFR. The pressure diminishes with time as tubular fluid diffuses into tubular cells and less ultrafiltrate is formed.

c. Pathogenesis of azotemia caused by leakage of urine within the body

(1) If there is leakage into the peritoneal cavity, urea and Crt enter the plasma after passive absorption through the peritoneal epithelium. The peritoneal [UN] equilibrates faster with the plasma [UN] than the peritoneal [Crt] does with the plasma [Crt] (see Chapter 19).

(2) If there is leakage into tissue surrounding the urinary tract, urea and Crt diffuse from the extravascular to intravascular fluid and cause azotemia.

(3) In either case, if intestinal excretion of urea and Crt does not compensate for the diminished urinary excretion, then azotemia will occur. Glomerular filtration is not reduced initially, but a calculated GFR will be reduced if not all the urine produced during the test period is collected.

d. Processes that contribute to prerenal or renal azotemia may also be present.

B. Azotemia due to increased urea production, a form of prerenal azotemia

1. Disorders or conditions (Table 8.3)

2. Pathogenesis

a. Increased proteolysis generates more NH_4^+, which in turn increases the synthesis of urea by hepatocytes.

b. If the rate of urea synthesis exceeds the rate of urea excretion, then the serum [UN] will increase.

3. There is usually an adequate functional renal reserve, so increased urea production usually causes either mild or no azotemia in these disorders or conditions.

4. Experimental evidence indicates that intestinal hemorrhage will cause azotemia when there is a large amount of hemorrhage; concurrent hypovolemia also contributes to the azotemia (see Azotemia and Uremia, sect. II.A.1). The azotemia due to intestinal hemorrhage results from two processes: (1) increased urea production because the marked hemoglobin degradation increases NH_4^+ delivery to hepatocytes, and (2) decreased GFR associated with the hypovolemia.

a. Feeding whole blood at a rate nearly equal to 10 % of a dog's blood volume increased the [UN] by about 10 mg/dL, whereas feeding whole blood at a rate nearly equal to 25 % of a dog's blood volume increased the [UN] by about 20–30 mg/dL. The peak azotemia occurred by 12 h, and nearly all UN concentrations returned to baseline values by 24 h.[11]

b. Withholding H_2O for 24 h and feeding whole blood to six dogs at a rate near one-third of a dog's blood volume increased UN concentrations from

7–37 mg/dL in individual dogs. Peak concentrations occurred 4–7 h after feeding and returned to baseline values by 24–36 h. Removing from 52 % to 76 % of the blood volumes of seven dogs while restricting access to H_2O decreased blood pressures and caused concurrent azotemias. Concentrations of UN were increased 2–25 mg/dL in individual dogs from 12–24 h after bleeding. The combination of bleeding (near 50 % blood volume) during several hours and feeding blood (near 30 % blood volume) caused greater increases in [UN] (20–67 mg/dL increases in ten dogs). The authors concluded that hemorrhage causing decreased blood pressure, feeding a large amount of blood, or a combination of these processes can create azotemia.[12]

    c. In a retrospective study in which 52 dogs with upper gastrointestinal hemorrhage were compared to 52 dogs without upper gastrointestinal hemorrhage, the median [UN] was 14 mg/dL greater in the hemorrhage group. Also, the serum UN:Crt ratio was greater in the hemorrhage group. As the authors reported, however, they did not determine whether the hydration status of the hemorrhage group was similar to that of the control group. Thus, this study did not establish whether the azotemias associated with gastrointestinal hemorrhage were caused by increased urea production, decreased urea excretion, or both. In the data provided, some dogs with hemorrhage were not azotemic.[13]

III.   Guidelines for azotemia differentiation (Table 8.4)
    A. The cause of azotemia may be multifactorial. Both prerenal disorders (e.g., hypovolemia) and postrenal disorders (e.g., obstruction) can cause acute renal disease and thus

Table 8.4. Major criteria used to differentiate the three types of azotemia caused by decreased GFR

Type of azotemia	Expected USG_{ref}	Urine volume	Historical, physical exam, or other information
Prerenal	> 1.030[a]	↓[a]	Decreased GFR due to dehydration, acute hemorrhage, shock, or decreased cardiac output
Renal	1.007–1.013[b]	↑ Usually May be ↓	Other UA findings, electrolyte changes, or anemia that are suggestive of renal disease (acute or chronic)
Postrenal	?[c]	↓[c]	Dysuria, enlarged or ruptured urinary bladder, urine in abdomen

[a] This criterion is for dogs and is assuming there are not extrarenal disorders that are affecting the renal concentrating ability and urine volume. USG_{ref} guidelines for cats that have concentrating ability are > 1.040 instead of > 1.030; for horses and cattle > 1.025.

[b] Assuming there are not substances (such as protein and glucose) that interfere with USG_{ref} assessment of the urine solute concentration

[c] USG_{ref} depends on the animal's hydration status and presence or absence of concurrent renal disease. During postobstructive diuresis, the USG_{ref} will be low and urine volume will be increased.

Note: Prerenal, renal, and postrenal disorders may occur independently or may occur in combinations.

acute renal failure. Animals with renal failure may also be hypovolemic. Accordingly, at the time of presentation, an animal's azotemia may be the product of both renal and extrarenal factors.

B. The major laboratory criterion for differentiating azotemias involves the USG_{ref}. However, the diagnostician must consider the renal and extrarenal factors that may influence an animal's ability to concentrate and dilute urine.

   1. If azotemia is exclusively prerenal and related to decreased GFR, the USG_{ref} is expected to be > 1.030 (in dogs), > 1.040 (in cats), or > 1.025 (in cattle and horses) because the kidneys are being stimulated to conserve H_2O.

   2. If the USG_{ref} is below these values in azotemic animals and there is no evidence of increased urea production (e.g., gastrointestinal hemorrhage), there is impaired renal concentrating ability, but it may be due either to primary renal disease (renal azotemia) or to extrarenal disease (prerenal azotemia with impaired concentrating ability unrelated to primary renal disease, sometimes called *secondary renal disease*).

     a. Renal disease

       (1) The USG_{ref} is often 1.007–1.013 because of impaired tubulointerstitial function associated with nephron damage.

       (2) The USG_{ref} may be > 1.013 but still inappropriately low if:

         (a) The renal disease impairs glomerular function more than tubulointerstitial function (especially in cats or in any animal with acute renal failure).

         (b) High urine concentrations of protein or glucose affect the USG_{ref} such that the USG_{ref} overestimates urine osmolality (see Physical Examination of Urine, sect. IIIB.4.d.).

         (c) Plasma osmolality is increased, so urine osmolality is greater than expected despite failure to dilute or concentrate the filtrate.

     b. Extrarenal causes

       (1) Azotemia develops from hypovolemia.

       (2) Inappropriate renal concentrating ability is caused by one or more of the following:

         (a) Epithelial cells of the distal nephron are not responsive to ADH (nephrogenic diabetes insipidus). This may occur, for example, because of hypercalcemia.

         (b) Solute overload (too much solute entering the loop of Henle as occurs with osmotic diuresis) causes a high flow rate and decreases resorption of tubular fluid.

         (c) Decreased medullary hypertonicity because of the following:

           (i)   Prolonged hyponatremia or hypochloremia.

           (ii) Blocked Na^+ and Cl^- transport (e.g., loop diuretics).

           (iii) Decreased urea production because of liver disease.

           (iv) Solute overload or prolonged diuresis.

UREA NITROGEN (UN) CONCENTRATION IN SERUM OR PLASMA

I.   Physiologic processes or concepts regarding urea (Fig. 8.5)

II.   Analytical concepts

     A. Terms and units

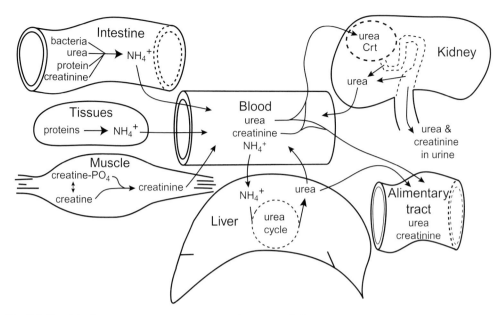

Fig. 8.5. Physiologic processes or concepts concerning urea and Crt.

Urea synthesis occurs in hepatocytes via the urea cycle, which is one method of incorporating NH_4^+ into molecules for excretion of excess NH_4^+ that is formed in tissues or intestine. After urea passively enters plasma from hepatocytes, it has two possible fates.

- Urea passes freely across the glomerular filtration barrier and is excreted in urine or resorbed by renal tubules: 50–65 % of urea present in glomerular filtrate is resorbed in proximal and collecting tubules. Urea resorption in proximal tubules is enhanced by H_2O resorption in proximal tubules and by increased ADH activity in the medullary collecting ducts.
- Urea enters the intestinal tract of monogastric mammals (via the blood or the biliary system), where it is degraded by enteric bacteria (with urease), passively absorbed into portal blood, or excreted in feces. In cattle, urea enters the rumen (via saliva and blood), where it is degraded to NH_4^+.[30]
- Crt is the product of creatine (not Crt) degradation. Creatine phosphate serves as a high-energy molecule for muscle contractions (creatine + ATP ↔ creatine PO_4 + ADP). Crt enters the plasma after the degradation of creatine or creatine PO_4 in muscle fibers (the animal's muscle or dietary meat). Crt is excreted from the body via the kidneys and intestine.
- Crt passes freely across the glomerular filtration barrier; it is not resorbed by tubules. Small quantities may be secreted by proximal tubules when there is increased plasma [Crt].
- Crt is also excreted or degraded in feces of people[114,115] and in saliva of cattle.[30] Alimentary tract excretion is suspected to occur in dogs, cats, and horses, as Crt is diffusible across most cell membranes.

1. Current clinical assays measure [urea] in serum, plasma, or whole blood, and some laboratories report [urea] directly. In many, though, the clinical custom is to express [urea] in terms of nitrogen content in the urea (i.e., urea nitrogen).

   a. Urea has a M_r of 60, so it weighs 60 g/mol. It is composed of one carbon, one oxygen, two nitrogen, and four hydrogen atoms. Therefore, 1 mol of urea contains 28 g of nitrogen. Accordingly, a [urea] of 1 mmol/dL = a [urea] of 60 mg/dL = a [UN] of 28 mg/dL.

   b. The [urea], reported as the concentration of UN, is commonly referred to as the *BUN* (blood urea nitrogen) concentration, although usually serum, not whole blood, is assayed. Because urea is a freely diffusible molecule for most cell membranes, the extracellular [UN] and intracellular [UN] in blood will usually be the same. Therefore, the [UN] in serum = [UN] in blood = [UN] in plasma (SUN = BUN = PUN).

   2. Unit conversion

      a. mg/dL of UN $\times$ 0.3570 = mmol/L of urea (SI unit, nearest 0.5 mmol/L)[14]

      b. mg/dL of urea $\times$ 0.1665 = mmol/L urea

B. Sample

   1. Serum or plasma may be used in most spectrophotometric assays.

   2. Urea is stable for 1 d at room temperature, several days at 4–6 °C, and at least 2–3 mo when frozen.[15]

C. Principles of urea assays

   1. Vitros dry reagent slide on the Vitros instrument

      a. In a reaction catalyzed by urease, urea is hydrolyzed to form NH_3 and CO_2. The NH_3 reacts with an indicator to generate a colored dye, which is detected by reflectance spectrophotometry.

      b. Positive interference

         (1) NH_4^+: Free NH_4^+ in the sample will react with the dye. Because the $[NH_4^+]$ in most plasma and serum samples is < 1 % of the [urea], the degree of interference should be clinically insignificant as long as the sample is not contaminated with NH_4^+ (e.g., with quaternary ammonium compounds).

         (2) Hemolysis: Hemoglobin at 50 mg/dL will increase the [UN] by about 1 mg/dL.

      c. Negative interference: Fluoride inhibits urease activity, so NaF tubes should not be used to collect blood samples for a urease assay.

   2. Roche Diagnostics wet reagents on the Hitachi instrument: In a reaction catalyzed by urease, urea is hydrolyzed to form NH_4^+ and CO_2. The NH_4^+ reacts in a coupled reaction that consumes reduced nicotinamide adenine dinucleotide (NADH) and thus decreases absorbance that is measured by kinetic spectrophotometry.

D. Increased [UN] in serum or plasma (azotemia) (Table 8.3)

E. Decreased [UN] in serum or plasma (Table 8.5)

   1. Disorders that decrease urea synthesis

      a. Hepatic insufficiency (see Chapter 13)

         (1) Extensive hepatocellular disease that markedly reduces functional hepatic mass (> 80 % loss) and thus sufficiently decreases urea synthesis to decrease [UN] and correspondingly increase $[NH_4^+]$

Table 8.5. Diseases and conditions that cause decreased serum or plasma [UN]

Disorders that cause decreased urea synthesis
  *Hepatic insufficiency: hepatocellular disease, portosystemic shunts
   Urea cycle enzyme deficiencies
Disorders that cause increased renal excretion of urea
  *Disorders that cause impaired proximal tubular resorption of urea: glucosuria
   Central or nephrogenic diabetes insipidus

  * A relatively common disease or condition

(2) Portosystemic shunt (congenital or acquired)
    (a) Less NH_4^+ is delivered to the hepatocytes from the intestines.
    (b) There is less uptake of NH_4^+ by hepatocytes because of decreased functional hepatic mass due to atrophy, necrosis, or fibrosis.
    b. Urea cycle enzyme deficiencies (congenital, extremely rare)
2. Disorders that increase renal excretion of urea
    a. When less H_2O is resorbed in the proximal tubules (e.g., because of glucosuria or expanded extracellular volume), less of the filtered urea is resorbed in the proximal tubules because the resorption of H_2O creates the concentration gradient for urea resorption.
    b. In central and nephrogenic diabetes insipidus, reduced ADH activity or response in the medullary collecting tubules decreases resorption of both urea and H_2O.
3. Consequence: The amount of urea in the renal interstitial fluid may diminish. Because about 50 % of the medullary hypertonicity is normally due to urea, the urea deficit may contribute to a reduced concentration gradient, impaired renal concentrating ability, and thus polyuria.

CREATININE (Crt) CONCENTRATION IN SERUM OR PLASMA

I.   Physiologic processes or concepts regarding Crt (Fig. 8.5)

II. Analytical concepts
    A. Terms and units
        1. Crt has a M_r of 113, about twice that of urea.
        2. Unit conversion: mg/dL × 88.4 = μmol/L (SI unit, nearest 10 μmol/L)[14]
    B. Sample
        1. Serum or plasma may be used in most spectrophotometric assays.
        2. Crt in serum is stable for up to 4 d at room temperature and longer (for 1–3 mo) when stored at −20 °C.[16]
    C. Principles of Crt assays
        1. Dry reagent slide on the Vitros instrument: Crt is enzymatically hydrolyzed to creatine, which then enters a series of reactions that result in H_2O_2 reacting with an indicator to generate a colored dye that is detected by reflectance spectrophotometry. Enzymatic methods may yield lower values than methods using Jaffe's reaction.[16]
        2. Roche Diagnostics wet reagents on the Hitachi instrument: Crt reacts with picric acid to form a colored complex (Jaffe's reaction). The rate of formation of the colored complex is measured by a spectrophotometer.
        3. In some assays using Jaffe's reaction, non-Crt chromogens interfere with the assay. However, modern modifications have reduced the interference, and interfering substances have less effect in kinetic than in end-point Crt assays. The non-Crt chromogens include proteins, glucose, acetoacetate, β-hydroxybutyrate, ascorbic acid, pyruvate, and cephalosporins.[17]
        4. In a study using domestic animal sera in a kinetic Jaffe assay, acetone, cephalosporins, and glucose caused a positive bias, whereas acetoacetic acid, bilirubin, and lipid produced a negative bias.[18] A [bilirubin] of 10 mg/dL reduces the [Crt] about 1 mg/dL.[19] Deproteinization of sera prior to the Jaffe reaction reduces the interference.
        5. In some assays (e.g., Roche Diagnostics reagents for the Hitachi 911), 0.3 mg/dL is subtracted from the assay result to remove the positive interference of serum

proteins. However, this correction factor is based on an assumption of a normoproteinemia. If there is a hyperproteinemia, the correction factor would be inadequate; if there is a hypoproteinemia, the correction factor would be excessive.

III. Increased [Crt] in serum or plasma (azotemia) (Table 8.3)
   A. [Crt] is typically increased by pathologic processes that cause decreased GFR; the initiating process may be prerenal, renal, or postrenal.
   B. Increased Crt production and release from damaged myocytes could contribute to increased serum [Crt] when renal function is impaired (e.g., myoglobinuric nephrosis secondary to rhabdomyolysis in horses), but Crt is quickly cleared from plasma if renal function is adequate. Baseline serum [Crt] may vary among individuals because of variations in total body muscle mass or meat intake, but these factors are not expected to cause more than a mild azotemia. Greyhounds have a greater mean serum [Crt] than the mean value for dogs in the general population, and some greyhounds have values mildly above the Crt upper reference limit.[20]
   C. Neonatal foals can have an increased serum [Crt] if born to dams with dysfunctional placentas that prevented normal clearance of fetal Crt by placental blood. In contrast to congenital renal failure, this azotemia should diminish quickly after birth and resolve over several days because Crt will be excreted via the urine.[21]

IV. Decreased [Crt] in serum or plasma
   A. A decreased [Crt] in serum or plasma is not clinically recognized or clinically significant. Animals with a decreased muscle mass would tend to have a lower [Crt], and the presence of a hypoproteinemia could yield a slightly lower [Crt] (see Creatinine Concentration in Serum or Plasma, sect. II.C.5).
   B. In most species, the lower reference limit for serum [Crt] is near the detection limit of Crt assays, so documenting a true decrease would be difficult.

UREA NITROGEN (UN) CONCENTRATION VERSUS CREATININE (Crt) CONCENTRATION IN SERUM OR PLASMA

I. Concepts
   A. In most mammals, increases in [Crt] and [UN] generally parallel each other, and thus the same information can usually be gained from either value alone. In horses, [Crt] tends to be more sensitive than [UN] to decreases in GFR, probably because of urea excretion into the alimentary tract. Similarly, in ruminants with renal failure, urea excretion into the alimentary tract may cause disproportionate increases in [Crt].
   B. In theory, [Crt] is a better indicator than [UN] of decreased GFR because the quantity of Crt presented to the kidneys is more constant and is not resorbed by the tubules, whereas urea is resorbed. Other factors that may affect [Crt] and [UN] include the following:
      1. Hypovolemia increases urea resorption in the tubules because of decreased flow rate in the tubules, which allows more time for urea diffusion, and ADH promotes urea resorption in the distal nephron.
      2. Increased protein in intestinal contents (high protein diet or massive intestinal hemorrhage) leads to increased generation of NH_4^+ and subsequently increased urea synthesis if digestive and absorptive processes are functioning.
      3. Intestinal excretion of urea and Crt may influence serum [UN] and [Crt].

Table 8.6. UN:Crt ratios in azotemic dogs and cats

Number of cases	Prerenal 6		Renal 78		Postrenal 17	
	Average	Range	Average	Range	Average	Range
[UN] (mg/dL)	89	21–183	140	38–470	194	85–340
[Crt] (mg/dL)	2.4	0.4–6.4	4.9	1.2–11.1	9.1	1.3–20
UN:Crt ratio	55.3	10–260	29.8	7–102	30.5	12–128

Source (adapted from): Finco and Duncan[22]

II. Serum UN:Crt ratio
   A. Clinical observations have suggested that a serum UN:Crt ratio can help differentiate prerenal and renal azotemias, and the following statements have been made:
      1. An increased serum [UN] and concurrent normal serum [Crt] is most likely a prerenal azotemia.
      2. If serum [Crt] is increased proportionately more than serum [UN], then the azotemia is probably renal or postrenal.
   B. Published serum UN:Crt ratios for azotemic dogs[22] are listed in Table 8.6. The authors' concluded the following:
      1. The most severe azotemias occur with renal or postrenal azotemias, whereas the greatest serum UN:Crt ratios are found in prerenal azotemias. However, renal azotemia cannot be consistently differentiated from extrarenal azotemias by means of the serum UN:Crt ratio because of the overlapping ranges.
      2. Concentrations of UN and Crt in serum should be regarded as crude indices of renal function because both lack diagnostic sensitivity and specificity for renal dysfunction caused by renal disease.

CREATININE (Crt) CLEARANCE RATE

I. *Crt clearance rate*, which is the rate Crt is cleared from plasma by the kidneys, is a good estimate of GFR in domestic animals but is not equivalent to GFR. A decreased Crt clearance rate (if a valid result) indicates the animal has a decreased GFR. However, the cause of the decreased GFR can be prerenal, renal, or postrenal.

II. Crt clearance rate formula (Eq. 8.1)

$$\text{Creatinine clearance rate} = \frac{[Crt]_u}{[Crt]_s} \times \text{volume}_u \div \text{time} \div \text{bw} \qquad (8.1.)$$

   $[Crt]_u$ = Crt concentration in collected urine during a timed collection period
   $[Crt]_s$ = Crt concentration in serum from a blood sample collected during the timed urine collection period
   volume_u = urine volume (in mL) collected during a timed collection period
   time = length of time (in min) during the urine collection period
   bw = body weight (in kg) of animal
   units = mL/min/kg = mL of plasma that were cleared of creatinine/min/kg

III. Endogenous Crt clearance rate
   A. Indications
      1. To assess GFR in nonazotemic, non-dehydrated animals that are suspected of having renal disease, usually because they are polyuric
      2. To obtain a more objective assessment of the degree of impaired GFR in azotemic animals, which may be helpful in predicting prognosis or monitoring response to therapy
   B. Basics of the procedure:[23] Adequate hydration must be established or confirmed. The urinary bladder must be emptied completely. All urine produced during a specified period (20 min to 24 h) is collected via a metabolism cage or catheterization, and the volume is recorded. A blood sample for serum [Crt] is collected during the urine collection period. The urine is mixed well, and the urine [Crt] is measured. It is critical that all urine produced is collected (with no spillage and minimal evaporation), especially when shorter collection periods are used.
   C. Potential technical problems include failure to empty the bladder completely before the procedure, failure to collect all the urine formed during the collection period, decreased GFR due to undetected patient dehydration, and assay interferents (effects of non-Crt chromogens).
   D. Reference intervals: Dogs: 3.7 ± 0.77 mL/min/kg (mean ± sd),[24] 3.64 ± 0.10 mL/min/kg (mean ± standard error of the mean).[23] Cats: 2.94 ± 0.32 mL/min/kg (mean ± sd),[9] 2.56 ± 0.61 mL/min/kg (mean ± sd).[25] Horses: 1.48 ± 0.043 mL/min/kg (mean ± standard error of the mean),[26] 1.92 ± 0.51 mL/min/kg (mean ± sd).[27]
   E. Endogenous Crt clearance rate is generally more sensitive than serum [Crt] for detecting decreased GFR because it is a direct assessment of renal excretion of Crt. Serum [Crt] depends on Crt production, renal excretion of Crt, and intestinal Crt excretion.

IV. Exogenous Crt clearance rate[28]
   A. Basics of the procedure: It is the same as the endogenous procedure except that Crt is injected into the patient and the urine collection period is routinely short.
   B. Advantages: There is increased plasma [Crt] and therefore increased challenge to the kidneys, so it is a better assessment of GFR. The procedure minimizes effects of assay interferents.
   C. Disadvantages: It may increase the percentage of excreted Crt from tubular secretion. There is a lack of standardization of methods.

ABNORMAL ROUTINE SERUM CHEMISTRY RESULTS IN AZOTEMIC ANIMALS

I. Serum [inorganic phosphorus]
   A. In dogs, cats, and horses, hyperphosphatemia occurs when renal clearance of plasma PO_4 is substantially reduced due to decreased GFR caused by renal disease (acute or chronic) or other pathologic states (e.g., prerenal or postrenal azotemic states).
   B. Some azotemic horses have a low-normal [inorganic phosphorus] or hypophosphatemia due to decreased renal conservation of PO_4 or to extrarenal excretion of PO_4.
   C. Cattle may or may not have hyperphosphatemia. Renal excretion of PO_4 is minor compared to excretion via saliva and the rumen.[29,30]

II. Serum [tCa^{2+}]
   A. The [tCa^{2+}] may be below, above, or within reference intervals in all species.

    B. Dogs, cats, and cattle usually have a low-normal [tCa^{2+}] or mild hypocalcemia in chronic renal failure because of decreased renal functional mass and therefore decreased renal formation of 1,25-DHCC. Hypercalcemia occurs in a minority of cases. In cattle, PO$_4$ excreted in saliva may bind with Ca^{2+} in the alimentary tract and make it less available for absorption.[30]

    C. In dogs with chronic renal failure, the [tCa^{2+}] may not reflect the regulation of the [fCa^{2+}] because the amount of Ca^{2+} bound to nonprotein anions is increased (see Chapter 11).[31]

    D. If their diet is relatively Ca^{2+} rich, horses are often hypercalcemic in acute or chronic renal disease because of decreased renal clearance of plasma Ca^{2+}; a major renal function of horses is to excrete excess dietary Ca^{2+}. Depending on the cause of the renal disease and the dietary intake of Ca^{2+}, horses can also be hypocalcemic during renal failure.

III.   Serum [K$^+$] and blood pH (or [H$^+$])
    A. Dogs, cats, and horses
       1. Acute decreases in renal function may cause hyperkalemia and acidemia because of impaired renal excretion of both cations. Also, inorganic acidemia accentuates hyperkalemia through the redistribution of ions between intracellular and extracellular compartments.
       2. Hyperkalemia and acidemia are seen primarily with oliguric or anuric renal failure and can be seen with either acute or terminal chronic renal failure.
       3. Many other factors influence serum [K$^+$] and blood pH, so expected changes may not occur.
    B. Cattle[32,33]
       1. Cattle tend to have hypokalemia due to alkalosis, decreased dietary potassium intake, or increased potassium excretion via saliva.[30]
       2. The animal's metabolic alkalosis and concurrent hypochloremia are often considered the result of H$^+$ and Cl$^-$ sequestration in the abomasum due to abomasal atony.
       3. Cattle tend to have concurrent hyponatremia, suggesting loss of Na$^+$ and Cl$^-$.

IV.   Serum AMS and LPS activities
    A. Dogs: Canine kidneys provide a major route of AMS and LPS excretion or inactivation. If renal perfusion or functional renal mass is decreased, there is less renal inactivation of AMS and LPS, and thus their long half-lives are increased. With time, mildly to moderately increased serum AMS and LPS activities may develop (see Chapter 12).
    B. Cats: The involvement of feline kidneys in the clearance or inactivation of AMS and LPS is not well documented. Of 32 cases of feline renal failure, hyperamylasemia (slight to threefold increase) was present in 10.[34]

MAJOR URINALYSIS (UA) CONCEPTS

I.   Components of a routine UA may vary from one laboratory to another; however, all procedures should be done on fresh urine (< 1 h old). Besides the potential for deterioration of cells and casts, delay of 6–24 h in completing the urinalysis may allow in vitro crystal formation, especially if the sample is stored at 4 °C.[35]

II.   Procedures for a routine urinalysis have been described.[36–39]

III. Common components of most routine urinalyses
   A. Physical examination: color, clarity, and USG_{ref}
   B. Chemical examination by reagent strip methods
      1. Common assays: pH, protein, glucose, ketone, heme (occult blood), bilirubin, and urobilinogen
      2. Other assays: nitrite, USG, and leukocyte esterase
   C. Sediment examination: microscopic examination to identify erythrocytes, leukocytes, bacteria, casts, crystals, epithelial cells, and other nondissolved material (may be done with nonstained or with stained urine sediment preparations)

IV. Urine composition is determined by three major factors. Because of these factors, the urine composition is affected by the entire urinary system and by other body systems.
   A. Quantity and composition of the plasma presented to kidneys
   B. Renal functions, including filtration, tubular secretion, and absorption
   C. Material (chemicals and cells) added to the glomerular filtrate as it flows through kidneys, ureters, urinary bladder, urethra, and prepuce or vagina/vulva

V. It is important to know the method of urine collection (i.e., voided, cystocentesis, catheterization, or "off-surface") when the UA results are being interpreted. Voided samples may have more bacteria, epithelial cells, and leukocytes from the distal urethra and genital tract. Cystocentesis samples may be affected by iatrogenic hemorrhage, but they localize abnormalities from the kidneys to the proximal urethra. Catheterized samples may have more epithelial cells, blood from iatrogenic hemorrhage, lubricant, and bacteria. And "off-surface" samples may be contaminated with a variety of microscopic particulates. Results expected in healthy dogs, cats, horses, and cattle are listed in Table 8.7.

PHYSICAL EXAMINATION OF URINE

I. Urine color (pigments)
   A. Physiologic processes
      1. The normal yellow to amber is due to *urochromes*, a group of poorly defined urine pigments of which one is riboflavin.
      2. Pale yellow urine is usually less concentrated than dark yellow urine, but not always (Plate 11A [for all plates, see the color section of this book]).
   B. Analytical concepts: Gross assessment of urine color is typically done on fresh, well-mixed urine.
   C. Abnormal urine color (*pigmenturia*)
      1. An abnormal color indicates the presence of abnormal pigments in the urine. Other parts of the urinalysis or other assays are needed to determine which pigment or pigments are present.
      2. Although concurrent pigmenturias may alter expected colors, the following are common abnormal colors and the substances that create them:
         a. Red: erythrocytes, hemoglobin, and myoglobin
         b. Red-brown: erythrocytes, hemoglobin, myoglobin, or methemoglobin
         c. Brown to black: methemoglobin from hemoglobin or myoglobin
         d. Yellow-orange: bilirubin
         e. Yellow-green or yellow-brown: bilirubin and biliverdin

Table 8.7. Expected UA results in healthy dogs, cats, horses, and cattle

	Dog	Cat	Horse	Cattle
Physical				
Color	Yellow[a]	Yellow[a]	Yellow[a]	Yellow[a]
Clarity	Clear	Clear	Hazy-turbid	Clear
USG$_{ref}$	1.015–1.045[b]	1.035–1.060[b]	1.020–1.050[b]	1.025–1.045[b]
Chemical				
pH	5.5–7.5	5.5–7.5	7.5–8.5	7.5–8.5
Protein	Neg–1+[c]	Neg	Neg	Neg
Glucose	Neg	Neg	Neg	Neg
Ketone	Neg	Neg	Neg	Neg
Heme	Neg	Neg	Neg	Neg
Bilirubin	Neg–1+[c]	Neg	Neg	Neg
Urobilinogen (EU)	0.2–1.0	0.2–1.0	0.2–1.0	0.2–1.0
Sediment (from centrifugation of 5 mL of fresh urine)				
Leukocytes/hpf	< 5[d]	< 5[d]	< 5[d]	< 5[d]
Erythrocytes/hpf	< 5	< 5	< 5	< 5
Bacteria/hpf	None	None	None	None
Casts/lpf	None[e]	None[e]	None[e]	None[e]
Epithelial cells/lpf	None to few[f]	None to few[f]	None to few[f]	None to few[f]
Crystals/lpf	None[g]	None[g]	None[g]	None[g]
Other	—	—	Mucus	—

[a] The intensity of yellow will typically vary proportionately with the USG$_{ref}$.

[b] Assuming normal hydration status and no treatments that alter water resorption by the kidneys

[c] Trace and 1+ reactions should be found in the more concentrated samples.

[d] The number of cells seen per microscopic field will differ when the diameter of the viewed field differs because of differences between microscope ocular lenses.

[e] A few hyaline casts usually are not associated with a pathologic state. Occasional granular casts can be found in healthy animals.

[f] This varies with the method of collection. Large round epithelial cells and squamous cells are expected in voided and some catheterized samples.

[g] Phosphate crystals in dogs and cats and carbonate crystals in horses and cattle are common, and their presence may not indicate a pathologic state (see Table 8.12).

      3. Horse urine may turn red or brown during storage or when exposed to snow. The pigmenturia is reported to be caused by pyrocatechin (pyrocatechol),[40] which is the aromatic portion of catecholamines. A pathologic state is not associated with this pigmenturia.

II. Urine clarity
    A. Physiologic processes
      1. Clear urine is expected, but it may have mild turbidity due to suspended particles (e.g., epithelial cells and crystals)
      2. Equine urine is frequently turbid or cloudy because of the presence of mucoprotein (produced by kidneys) or calcium carbonate crystals.
    B. Analytical concepts: Gross assessment of urine clarity is typically done on fresh, well-mixed urine.

C. Cloudiness or turbidity indicates the presence of formed elements, such as cells, crystals, bacteria, casts, and lipid droplets in the urine.

III. Solute concentration
   A. Physiologic processes
      1. The solutes in urine are the dissolved ions and molecules. Most of them, including electrolytes (Na^+, K^+, Cl^-, Ca^{2+}, PO_4, and NH_4^+) and metabolic products (urea and Crt), are being excreted by the kidneys.
      2. The concentrations of filtrate solutes are modified by the tubular resorption or secretion of solutes and by the resorption of filtrate H_2O.
      3. Urine solute concentrations are expected to increase when the kidneys are conserving H_2O and decrease when the kidneys are not conserving H_2O.
   B. Analytical concepts
      1. *Specific gravity* (also called *relative density*), a physical property of a solution, is the ratio of a solution's weight to the weight of an equal volume of H_2O (i.e., the ratio of their densities). Measurement of the true urine SG is an obsolete procedure. Specific gravity is a unitless ratio.
      2. Refractive index as an estimate of USG (USG_{ref})
         a. The refractive index of urine is measured with a refractometer and used as a routine clinical estimation of USG (USG_{ref}). The refractive index of a solution is the ratio of the speed of light in a vacuum to the speed of light in the solution. When light waves enter a solution, they slow down and bend (refract). As solute is added to H_2O, the degree to which the light slows and is refracted increases proportionately to the increase in solute concentration (i.e., the refractive index increases). Specific gravity also increases proportionately to the solute concentration, so specific gravity correlates with refractive index if the types and proportions of the solutes remain similar. If urine has relatively normal solute composition, USG_{ref} from a good-quality refractometer correlates very well with osmolality.
         b. The refractive index is highly dependent on three factors: solute concentration, chemical composition of the solute, and temperature. Refractometers measure the refractive index of the soluble solids in the fluid (i.e., solutes in the solvent); suspended particles (e.g., cells, casts, and most crystals) do not refract light and thus do not alter the refractive index of urine.[41] Because the suspended particles interfere with light transmission (thereby causing cloudiness or turbidity), they may make the demarcation line in the refractometer more difficult to read. The following are USG_{ref} values for ten cloudy urine samples (direct reading/supernatant reading): 1.043/1.043, 1.054/1.054, 1.028/1.028, 1.016/1.016, 1.083/1.083, 1.021/1.022, 1.051/1.052, 1.048/1.048, 1.061/1.062, and 1.051/1.052 (authors' unpublished data).
         c. Most temperature-compensated refractometers have USG_{ref} scales that are calibrated for the normal composition of human urine (Fig. 8.6).
         d. However, there are refractometers that are calibrated for constituents of canine, feline, and large animal urine (Fig. 8.7).
            (1) The calibration scale for dogs and large animals is slightly different from the calibration scale for people.
            (2) The calibration scale for cats is moderately different; for example, a 1.010 on the canine scale is about a 1.008 on the feline scale, a 1.025 on the

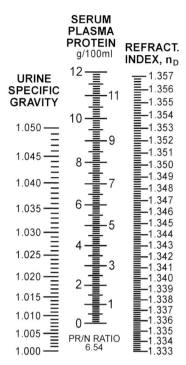

Fig. 8.6. Illustration of scales in a Leica TS400 hand-held refractometer. The refractometer measures the fluid's refractive index, and the *urine specific gravity* and *serum plasma protein* scales are used to estimate USG_{ref} or total protein concentrations, respectively. The refractometer scales were calibrated for human samples. Image used with permission from Leica Microsystems, Buffalo, NY. PR/N ratio 6.54, conversion factor—6.54 g of protein contains 1 g of nitrogen.

canine scale is about a 1.022 on the feline scale, and a 1.040 on the canine scale is about a 1.036 on the feline scale.

e. The amount of error in the feline USG_{ref} is mild when a refractometer calibrated for human urine is used. If refractive indices of human and feline urine were 1.3365, the USG_{ref} would be 1.010 and 1.008, respectively. If the refractive indices were 1.3420, the USG_{ref} would be 1.025 and 1.021, respectively.[42] Thus, if a refractometer calibrated for human urine is used for cat urine, the urine appears slightly more concentrated than it really is.

f. Non-temperature-compensated refractometers underestimate the USG value when ambient temperature increases above 68 °F (20 °C). The amount of error increases as the temperature increases.

g. When the USG_{ref} is greater than the upper end of the USG scale of the refractometer, a direct reading cannot be obtained. If a reading can be made on the refractive index scale, some labs convert the refractive index value to a USG based on tables generated experimentally. If the reading is also greater than the refractive index scale, the sample may be diluted 1:2 with distilled water, reevaluated, and reported after correcting for the dilution (a 1.026 result with the diluted sample would be reported as 1.052). However, diagnostically, it is usually

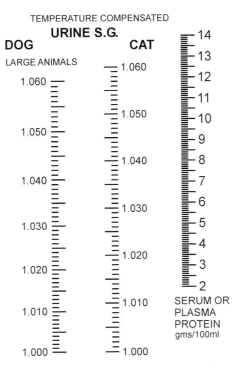

Fig. 8.7. Illustration of scales in a Leica VET 360 hand-held veterinary refractometer. The refractometer has a specific gravity scale for dog and large animal urine and a separate scale for cat urine. Note that, for a given refractive index, the specific gravity for cat urine is greater than the specific gravity for dog or large animal urine. Image used with permission from Leica Microsystems, Buffalo, NY.

    not necessary to know how concentrated the urine is when it is too concentrated to be read directly from the refractometer.

3. Osmolality (see Chapter 9 for interpretation of serum osmolality values)

    a. Principle (*freezing-point osmometry* method): The freezing point of a solution is inversely related to the solute concentration in the solution. As the solute concentration increases, the freezing point decreases. A freezing-point osmometer detects the freezing point of a solution and converts the value to osmolality.

    b. *Osmolality*, which is the solute concentration of a solution, can be expressed in osmoles of solute particles per kilogram of solvent (osmol/kg) or in moles of solute per kilogram of solvent (mol/kg): 1 osmol is 1 mol of osmotically active particles. For a substance that does not dissociate in solution, 1 mol equals 1 osmol. For a substance that completely dissociates into two ions per mole, each 1 mol of the substance generates 2 osmol of particles.

    c. Urine osmolality measurements are usually limited to specific cases where accurate assessment of renal concentrating or diluting abilities is critical. The gold standard for assessing urine solute concentration is freezing-point osmometry.

4. USG_{ref} as an estimate of osmolality

    a. Figure 8.8 illustrates the relationship between USG_{ref} and urine osmolality measurements.

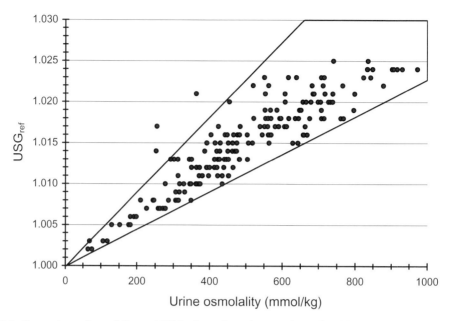

Fig. 8.8. Comparison of osmolality and USG_{ref} in canine urine samples with $USG_{ref} \leq 1.025$ (n = 185). There is a high correlation (r = 0.91) between the two methods of assessing urine solute concentration: freezing-point osmometry and refractive index. For these samples, the mean $Osm_u:USG_{ref}$ was 33 with a sd of 5; the mean ± 2 sd (or 95 % interval) is represented by the area between the *two diagonal lines*. The three values that fell above the 95 % interval had high protein concentrations (estimated concentration ≥ 500 mg/dL).

b. Conclusions from the comparison
   (1) In most urine samples, there is a good linear relationship between USG_{ref} and osmolality. Thus, the USG_{ref} is typically an accurate reflection of the urine solute concentration.
   (2) Because of this good correlation, the $Osm_u:USG_{ref}$ ratio is relatively constant (Eq. 8.2). In 185 canine urine samples with $USG_{ref} \leq 1.025$, the $Osm_u:USG_{ref}$ ratio was 33 ± 5 (mean ± sd). In 37 feline urine samples with $USG_{ref} \leq 1.025$ (using non-feline scale), the $Osm_u:USG_{ref}$ ratio was 35 ± 5 (mean ± sd).[43]

$$Osm_u:USG_{ref} = \frac{\text{Urine osmolality}}{1000\,(USG_{ref} - 1.000)} \qquad (8.2.)$$

Example: If urine osmolality = 600 mosm/kg and $USG_{ref} = 1.020$, then:

$$Osm_u:USG_{ref} = \frac{600}{1000\,(1.020 - 1.000)} = \frac{600}{1000\,(0.020)} = \frac{600}{20} = 30$$

OR

$$Osm_u:USG_{ref} = \frac{\text{Urine osmolality}}{\text{Last 2 digits of USG}}; Osm_u:USG_{ref} = \frac{600}{20} = 30$$

    c. When interpreting either the USG_{ref} value or urine osmolality, it may be impor-
tant to recognize the following relationships:

      (1) If urine 1 has an osmolality of 300 mmol/kg and urine 2 has an osmolality
of 600 mmol/kg, the solute concentration in urine 2 is twice the solute
concentration in urine 1.

      (2) If the USG_{ref} of urine 3 is 1.010 and the USG_{ref} of urine 4 is 1.020, the
solute concentration in urine 4 is approximately twice the solute concentration in urine 3.

    d. When there is either a marked proteinuria or marked glucosuria, the USG_{ref}
overestimates the concentration of urine solutes and thus renal concentrating
ability (Fig. 8.8). The Osm_u:USG_{ref} ratio will be decreased (in dogs, below 20).

      (1) A [protein] of 1 g/dL adds about 0.003–0.005 to USG_{ref} but has almost no
effect on osmolality.

      (2) A [glucose] of 1 g/dL adds about 0.004–0.005 to USG_{ref} and only slightly
increases urine osmolality (about 5 mmol/kg).

5. Reagent strip for estimating USG (Bayer Diagnostics)

    a. The reagent strip method is not recommended for estimation of urine solute
concentration or USG of domestic mammals.

    b. Principle: The ionic strength of urine is related to total solute concentration. The
reagent system has indicators that produce different colors when dipped in urine
samples of different ionic strengths.

    c. The semiquantitative scale is 1.000–1.030 at 0.005 intervals, with best accuracy
when the urine pH is < 6.5. Add 0.005 to the reading for a pH > 6.5.

    d. Falsely low results occur in alkaline urine; for example, most urines with a
pH $\geqslant$ 7.0 and a USG_{ref} of 1.025–1.035 had a dipstick USG of 1.015.[44]
Moderate quantities of protein can cause falsely high values, and glucosuria
can cause falsely low values.[45]

C. Expected USG_{ref}

1. One must have knowledge of an animal's H_2O balance and medications to properly
assess an animal's ability to concentrate or dilute urine.

    a. An animal that is dehydrated or has restricted access to H_2O should excrete a
relatively small volume of concentrated urine; that is, with a relatively high
USG_{ref}.

    b. After diuretic or fluid therapy, an animal should excrete a relatively high volume of
less concentrated, isosthenuric, or dilute urine; that is, urine with a lower USG_{ref}.

2. Healthy animals with normal or adequate renal function can excrete urine with a
broad USG_{ref} range, depending on what the kidneys are being challenged to do.

    a. Maximal urine dilution in domestic mammals as assessed by USG_{ref}: near 1.001

    b. Maximal urine concentration as assessed by USG_{ref}: cats > 1.080, dogs near
1.060, and horses and cattle near 1.050

    c. Usual USG_{ref} values when H_2O intake is adequate and hydration status is
normal: dogs (1.015–1.045), cats (1.035–1.065), horses (1.020–1.050), and
cattle (1.025–1.045). However, the USG_{ref} may be lower or higher in animals
with normal renal function.

D. Interpretation of USG_{ref} values

1. A USG_{ref} is usually needed for the assessment of renal concentrating ability when
animals are azotemic, polyuric, oliguric, or anuric. Because of the many variables
that change urine solute concentrations, it is difficult to formulate firm guidelines
for the interpretation of USG_{ref} in all cases.

Table 8.8. Major pathogenic mechanisms of polyuria

	Solute diuresis	↓ Tubular response to ADH	↓ Medullary tonicity	↓ ADH
Chronic renal failure	+[a]	+	+	−[b]
Acute renal failure	−	+[c]	−	−
Postobstructive diuresis[d]	+	+[c]	−	−
Diabetes mellitus	+	−	−[e]	−
Hypercalcemia	−	+	−[e]	−
Canine pyometra	−	+	−[e]	−
Hypokalemia	−	+	−[e]	−
Hypoadrenocorticism	−	−	+[f]	±[g]
Liver failure	−	−[h]	+	−
Central diabetes insipidus	−	−	−[e]	+
Hyperadrenocorticism	−	−	−[e]	+
Psychogenic polydipsia	−	−	−[e]	+[i]

[a] A *plus sign* indicates that mechanism can contribute to the polyuria.

[b] A *minus sign* indicates that mechanism does not contribute to the polyuria.

[c] Initially, there may be oliguria. If the animal survives the acute illness, the surviving but damaged tubules may not be able to respond to ADH adequately.

[d] Altered Na^+-regulatory hormone responses and other defective tubular functions may contribute.

[e] Persistent diuresis may decrease medullary tonicity because of decreased tubular resorption of solutes.

[f] Persistent hyponatremia and hypochloremia may result in loop of Henle failure.

[g] Hypoosmolality would decrease the stimulus for ADH release, but concurrent hypovolemia would stimulate ADH release.

[h] An increased NH_4^+ concentration may interfere with tubular response to ADH.

[i] An increased GFR may also contribute.

   2. Animals with impaired renal concentrating ability will have one or more of the following defects (mechanisms for the resulting polyuric states are listed in Table 8.8):
      a. ADH deficiency is present (central diabetes insipidus).
      b. Epithelial cells of distal nephrons are not responsive to ADH (nephrogenic diabetes insipidus).
      c. Solute overload was present (too much solute entering the loop as occurs with osmotic diuresis, renal failure, or increased GFR), causing a high flow rate and decreased resorption of tubular H_2O.
      d. Decreased medullary hypertonicity
         (1) Prolonged hyponatremia or hypochloremia
         (2) Defective Na^+ and Cl^- transport in the loop of Henle (e.g., loop diuretics)
         (3) Decreased urea production because of liver disease
         (4) Solute overload or prolonged diuresis
   3. General guidelines for USG_{ref} interpretation are in Table 8.9.
   4. USG_{ref} in various disorders or conditions
      a. USG_{ref} > 1.030 in an oliguric dog, > 1.040 in an oliguric cat, and > 1.025 in oliguric horses or cows

Table 8.9. Guidelines for interpretation of USG$_{ref}$ values in a dog

Case information	USG$_{ref}$[a]	Interpretation
Nothing known	1.001–1.060	Could be found in a clinically healthy or sick dog
Dehydrated	> 1.030	Reflects renal attempts to conserve H_2O appropriately
	1.014–1.030	Suggests impaired renal concentrating ability and possibly renal failure; could be seen with glucosuria, hyponatremia/hypochloremia, partial renal diabetes insipidus disorders, hypoadrenocorticism
	1.007–1.013	Strongly indicates defective renal concentrating ability; if azotemic, then renal insufficiency or failure until proven otherwise
	< 1.007	Strongly indicates defective renal concentrating ability but not due to renal failure, as kidneys have ability to dilute ultrafiltrate; consider central or renal diabetes insipidus disorders
Polyuria	> 1.020	Reflects renal attempts to conserve H_2O and thus not in renal insufficiency/failure; could be seen with glucosuria, hyponatremia/hypochloremia, partial central or renal diabetes insipidus disorders
	1.007–1.013	Strongly indicates defective renal concentrating ability; if azotemic, then renal insufficiency or failure until proven otherwise
	< 1.007	Strongly indicates defective renal concentrating ability but not due to renal failure, as kidneys have ability to dilute ultrafiltrate; consider central or renal diabetes insipidus disorders
Oliguria	> 1.030	Reflects renal attempts to conserve H_2O appropriately
	1.014–1.030	Uncommon; suspect acute renal failure
	1.007–1.013	Typical for oliguric renal failure; acute or chronic
Glucosuria	> 1.020	Reflects renal concentrating ability but may be partially impaired by solute diuresis or decreased medullary hypertonicity (medullary washout); USG$_{ref}$ may be falsely increased 0.004–0.005 for every 1 g/dL of glucose in urine)
	1.007–1.020	May reflect impaired concentrating ability caused by solute diuresis or medullary washout but could have concurrent renal insufficiency/failure
Hyponatremia and hypochloremia	> 1.020	Reflects renal concentrating ability but may be impaired by loop of Henle failure as may occur with hypoadrenocorticism
	1.007–1.013	May reflect greater impairment of concentrating ability because of the loop of Henle failure but also must consider renal insufficiency/failure
	< 1.007	Reflect renal diluting ability and thus not renal insufficiency/failure; defective ADH secretion probably present

[a] Assuming that the USG$_{ref}$ values are not falsely elevated by either protein or glucose

Note: Guidelines for cats would reflect the greater concentrating ability of the feline kidneys; guidelines for horses and cattle would reflect lesser concentrating ability when challenged or in health.

(1) Nonrenal processes (e.g., hypovolemia and decreased cardiac output) have led to decreased renal perfusion. Hypovolemia or plasma hyperosmolality stimulated the release of ADH.

(2) ADH promoted the resorption of H_2O in the collecting tubules, thus concentrating the tubular fluid and thus urine.

b. $USG_{ref} < 1.030$ in an obviously dehydrated dog, < 1.040 in a dehydrated cat, and < 1.025 in a dehydrated cow or horse

  (1) Such findings indicate a renal concentrating defect that could be caused by renal or extrarenal disease.

  (2) Pathogeneses of the specific causes vary with the pathologic states (see polyuric disorders in the next section).

c. $USG_{ref} = 1.020$–1.035 in a polyuric animal

  (1) Diabetes mellitus: Glucosuria causes an osmotic diuresis by inhibiting the passive resorption of H_2O in the proximal tubules. If it persists, the high flow rate may impair resorption of Na^+, Cl^-, and urea, and thus medullary tonicity decreases.

  (2) Potentially seen with renal glucosuria

  (3) Partial diabetes insipidus and hypoadrenocorticism: An animal may have polyuria and a corresponding low USG_{ref} on some days, but values in the 1.020–1.035 interval on other days.

  (4) Renal failure: Concentrating ability may be incompletely impaired when kidneys are failing, but a lower USG_{ref} is more typical of polyuric renal failure.

d. $USG_{ref} = 1.007$–1.013 in oliguric animal

  (1) This typically indicates renal failure or end-stage renal disease if the animal is azotemic, but it could represent acute renal disease or urinary tract obstruction.

  (2) Concentrating and diluting defects could be caused by solute diuresis, decreased tubular response to ADH, or impaired ability to maintain medullary solute gradient.

e. $USG_{ref} = 1.007$–1.013 in polyuric animal

  (1) If there is concurrent azotemia, such findings are essentially diagnostic of renal failure.

  (2) Concentrating and diluting defects are caused by solute diuresis, decreased tubular response to ADH, or impaired ability to maintain medullary solute gradient.

  (3) If there is not azotemia, the finding could represent earlier stages of renal insufficiency or extrarenal disorders that impair renal concentrating ability.

f. $USG_{ref} = 1.001$–1.015 in a polyuric animal that is not azotemic

  (1) Central diabetes insipidus: Hypothalamic or pituitary disease decreases the production of ADH, and thus collecting tubules cannot resorb H_2O and thus solutes are not concentrated in the distal nephron.

  (2) Hyperadrenocorticism: The pathogenesis of impaired concentrating ability is not firmly established.

    (a) Glucocorticoid hormones inhibited ADH secretion in some studies.[46,47] With lower ADH activity, there is less stimulation of collecting tubules to resorb H_2O.

(b) Cortisol may inhibit the responsiveness of renal tubules to ADH, and thus less H_2O is resorbed. However, some studies indicate that cortisol does not interfere with renal activity of ADH.[46,48]

(3) Hyperaldosteronism: The pathogenesis of a dog's polyuric state was not firmly established, but the evidence supported an impaired response to ADH and delayed ADH release after hypertonic stimulation.[49] Plasma cortisol concentrations were within reference intervals in the basal state and during a low-dose dexamethasone suppression test. Measurement of other adrenal steroid concentrations was not mentioned.

(4) *Nephrogenic diabetes insipidus* is a group of renal and extrarenal diseases in which ADH is present but renal tubules are not responsive to it. The group includes hypercalcemia, canine pyometra, liver failure, and hypokalemia.

(5) Hypercalcemia

(a) Increased $[fCa^{2+}]$ inhibits ADH activity via dysregulation of aquaporins. Aquaporin 2 translocation to apical membranes appears to be decreased. In addition, cellular aquaporin 2 appears to be decreased because of degradation by a calcium-sensitive protease.[50–52]

(b) There is also evidence that Ca^{2+} reduces resorption of Na^+ and Cl^- in the ascending limb of the loop of Henle, which reduces the osmotic gradient needed for H_2O resorption in the distal nephron.[51]

(c) A persistently increased $[fCa^{2+}]$ may cause mineralization of tubular basement membranes, which results in a calcium nephropathy and thus renal insufficiency or failure.

(6) Hypoadrenocorticism (Addison's disease)

(a) The USG_{ref} will be this low in only a small minority of hypoadrenocorticism patients.

(b) The pathogenesis is not well documented, but there may be failure of Na^+ and Cl^- delivery to the loop of Henle and thus failure to maintain medullary hypertonicity.

(c) Decreased effective plasma osmolality (because of hyponatremia and hypochloremia) will reduce the osmotic stimulus for ADH synthesis and release. Thus, ADH activity might be reduced (conversely, hypovolemia is probably stimulating ADH release).

(7) Canine pyometra: The specific pathogenesis is not clear, but the kidneys are refractory or poorly responsive to ADH. One potential mechanism is that bacterial endotoxins initiate the refractory state.

(8) Liver failure

(a) Decreased urea synthesis may lead to a decreased medullary [urea] and thus a decreased medullary concentration gradient (medullary washout).

(b) Other possibilities have been suggested: psychogenic polydipsia, defects in portal vein osmoreceptors, and impairment of renal concentrating mechanisms because of increased NH_4^+ excretion.

(9) Hypokalemia

(a) Hypokalemia makes collecting tubules less responsive to ADH, perhaps because of reduced generation of cyclic adenosine monophosphate (cAMP)[53] and down-regulated expression of aquaporin channels.[6,51]

        (b) K^+ is needed for Na^+ and Cl^- resorption in the ascending limb of the loop of Henle, and thus hypokalemia may impair countercurrent function.[51,54]

    (10) Hypoparathyroidism: The pathogenesis is not well understood.

    (11) Feline hyperthyroidism: The pathogenesis is not well understood.

    (12) Psychogenic polydipsia: Excessive H_2O consumption leads to expanded extracellular fluid volume and hypoosmolality. Polyuria results from increased GFR and decreased ADH secretion.

    (13) Others: diuretic therapy, alcohol administration, intravenous fluid administration, or dextrose or mannitol fluid therapy

    (14) Thyroiditis: Occasional dogs with thyroiditis (but not hypothyroidism) have polyuria and polydipsia. The pathogenesis is not known, but it may not be directly related to thyroiditis.[55]

  g. Variable USG_{ref} values (< 1.007 to > 1.020) with hyponatremia and hypochloremia

    (1) Because Na^+ and Cl^- are major contributors to the hypertonic interstitial fluid in renal medullae, any disorder that diminishes medullary resorption of Na^+ and Cl^- may diminish renal concentrating ability. The impairment of concentrating ability will vary with the degree of reduced medullary hypertonicity. Na^+ and Cl^- resorption in the ascending limb of the loop of Henle may be diminished through two major processes:

      (a) A defective transport system (e.g., inhibition of the Na^+-K^+-$2Cl^-$ cotransporter or Na^+-K^+-ATPase)

      (b) Decreased delivery of Na^+ or Cl^- to the loop of Henle (e.g., persistent hyponatremia or hypochloremia)

    (2) Hyponatremia and hypochloremia will also reduce plasma osmolality and thus reduce the stimulus for ADH secretion. Reduced ADH activity in the collecting tubules results in formation of more dilute urine.

CHEMICAL EXAMINATION OF URINE (QUALITATIVE OR SEMIQUANTITATIVE)

I.   Major concepts

  A. Semiquantitative results of urinalysis procedures (chemical and microscopic) are used to detect or characterize pathologic renal and extrarenal states or to monitor response to therapy. The concentration of a solute in urine will depend on two major factors: (1) the amount of solute excreted in the urine over time, and (2) the amount of H_2O excreted by the urinary system during the same time interval. Solutes from the reproductive tract may alter urine solute concentrations, particularly in voided samples.

    1. The semiquantitative results of the reagent pad systems are graded on scales provided by the manufacturers of the reagent strips (Table 8.10).

      a. A 1+ result indicates enough solute was present to give a 1+ reaction but not enough to give a 2+ reaction.

      b. When reactions are read by visual examination, distinguishing between a 1+ reaction and a 2+ reaction, or between 2+ and 3+ (etc.), may be difficult. Thus, the true concentration of a solute may be considerably different from the reported value.

      c. It is important to store reagent pad sticks per manufacturer's recommendations because atmospheric moisture, light, and temperature affect the stability of the

Table 8.10. Semiquantitative values or terms of solute concentrations estimated by urinalysis reagent strip reactions

	Glucose (mg/dL)	Bilirubin (mg/dL)	Ketone (mg/dL)	Heme[a] (mg/dL)	Protein (mg/dL)	Urobilinogen (mg/dL)
Multistix by Bayer						
Negative[b]	<75 to 125	<0.4 to 0.8	<5 to 10	<0.015 to 0.062	15–30	—
Trace	100	—	5	—	10	0.2–1.0
1+	250	Small	15	Small	30	2
2+	500	Moderate	40	Moderate	100	4
3+	1000	Large	80	Large	300	8
4+	2000	—	160	—	1000	—
Chemstrip by Roche						
Negative[c]	<40	<0.5	<9	<10	<6	—
Trace	50	—	—	—	6	—
1+	100	0.5	Small	10	30	1
2+	250–500	1.0	Moderate	50	100	4
3+	1000	2.0	Large	250	500	8
4+	—	—	—	—	—	12

[a] The heme test is commonly referred to as either the "blood" or "occult blood" test (see the text for explanation).

[b] Ranges are the reported analytical detection limits of the reactions in contrived urine. Reactions may vary in the actual samples. Bilirubin units are mg/dL. The ketone detection limit was measured with acetic acid. The heme detection limit was measured with hemoglobin (mg/dL). The protein detection limit was measured with albumin.

[c] These values were listed as the detection limits in the package insert.

Note: See the text for pH values.

reagents in the pads. Routine use of commercial urine control solutions is recommended to ascertain that the reactions are valid.

2. Automated reflectance photometers are available for photometric assessment of color changes (e.g., the Clinitek 100 Urine Chemistry Analyzer). A major advantage of the instruments is that they remove the person-to-person variation in the color changes on the pad.

   a. In a study involving canine urine samples, the authors reported good agreement between visual estimation and automatic measurements for most analytes. The USG reagent pad values were unreliable.[56]

   b. In another comparison of 40 canine urine samples, there was very good to excellent agreement for glucose and heme. Instrument readings for protein tended to be slightly lower, and ketone and bilirubin detection was slightly higher (i.e., some instrument reactions were positive when visual readings were negative).[57]

3. Relationship of urine solute concentration, urine volume, and daily urinary excretion of solutes (Eq. 8.3)

$$\text{Daily urinary solute excretion} = [\text{solute}]_u \times \text{urine volume/day} \qquad (8.3.)$$

For example for protein excretion:

$$\text{Daily urinary protein excretion} = 70 \text{ mg/dL} \times 1000 \text{ mL/d}$$
$$= 700 \text{ mg/d}$$

   a. If the urine solute concentration remained constant (e.g., 150 mg/dL) from one day to the next, but the urine volume doubled (e.g., from 100 mL/d to 200 mL/d), then the urinary excretion of the solute doubled from one day to the next (from 150 mg/d to 300 mg/d).

   b. If the urine solute concentration doubled (from 150 mg/dL to 300 mg/dL) from one day to the next, but the urine volume remained constant (100 mL/d), then the urinary excretion of the solute doubled from one day to the next (from 150 mg/d to 300 mg/d).

   c. If the urine solute concentration doubled (from 150 mg/dL to 300 mg/dL) from one day to the next, but the urine volume halved (from 100 mL/d to 50 mL/d), then the urinary excretion of the solute remained constant from one day to the next (150 mg/d).

4. Relationship of urine volume and USG_{ref} values

   a. If the animal is not in renal insufficiency or failure, urine volume is inversely proportional to USG_{ref}.

   b. If the urinary excretion of solutes remains constant (e.g., 1 g/d), but the urine volume doubles from one day to the next, the USG_{ref} is expected to "halve" from one day to the next (e.g., from 1.040 to 1.020).

   c. If the urinary excretion of solutes remains constant (e.g., 1 g/d), but the urine volume halves from one day to the next, the USG_{ref} is expected to "double" from one day to the next (e.g., from 1.020 to 1.040).

5. Use of concepts to interpret urinalysis results

   a. Dog 1 with a urine [glucose] of 500 mg/dL and a USG_{ref} of 1.015 is typically excreting just as much glucose per day as dog 2 that has a urine [glucose] of 1.0 g/dL and a USG_{ref} of 1.030.

   b. Dog 3 with a urine [protein] of 50 mg/dL and a USG_{ref} of 1.040 is probably not proteinuric. Healthy dogs may have urine protein concentrations of

4–65 mg/dL;[58] USG_{ref} is typically 1.020–1.045. However, dog 4 with a urine [protein] of 50 mg/dL and a USG_{ref} of 1.010 is proteinuric.

    c. Cat 1 with a urine [protein] of 50 mg/dL and a USG_{ref} of 1.010 is typically excreting just as much protein per day as cat 2 that has a urine [protein] of 200 mg/dL and a USG_{ref} of 1.040. Both cats are proteinuric.

6. Conclusions

    a. In results from routine urinalyses, the USG_{ref} helps determine the significance of estimated solute concentrations.

    b. A positive chemical reaction should first be considered a qualitative result (substance present), and then the significance of the positive reaction can be weighted according to the strength of the reaction and the USG_{ref}.

B. The physical and chemical properties of urine may be different after centrifugation if enough particles were suspended in the urine prior to centrifugation.

1. These following values may be the same prior to and after centrifugation (unless the heme pigment in erythrocytes interferes with the reading of color changes):

    a. Color (if due to pigmented solute and not pigmented cells or suspended particles)

    b. USG_{ref} (but the line may be more difficult to read if the urine is cloudy)

    c. pH

    d. Protein (unless hemoglobin is present in erythrocytes)

    e. Glucose

    f. Ketone

    g. Heme (if the positive reaction is due to free hemoglobin, free methemoglobin, or myoglobin rather than erythrocytes)

    h. Bilirubin

2. The following values may be different prior to and after centrifugation:

    a. Color (if due to pigmented cells or other suspended particles)

    b. Protein (if hemoglobin in the erythrocytes is reacting with the pad)

    c. Heme (if intact erythrocytes are present)

II.   pH (negative logarithm of free $[H^+]$) of urine

A. Physiologic processes

1. The pH of urine is affected by many renal and extrarenal factors. Carnivores usually have acidic urine, whereas herbivores usually have alkaline urine unless they are on milk diets.

2. Typical urine pH in healthy mammals vary among species: dogs and cats (6.0–7.5), and horses and cows (7.5–8.5).

3. Much of the H^+ that is excreted by kidneys is incorporated into other molecules (e.g., NH_4^+, $H_2PO_4^-$, and H_2O)

B. Analytical concepts

1. Principle: based on the double indicator system that is sensitive to change in $[H^+]$. The indicator does not detect H^+ being excreted in NH_4^+ or $H_2PO_4^-$

2. The reagent strip has a pH indicator pad with a range of 5.0–8.5. Results are reported to the nearest 0.5 units (except 5.5 reaction with some strips). The system is designed to provide an estimate of urine pH and does not replace the more precise pH meter when quantitative analysis is needed.[59]

3. Abnormal urine color (pigmenturia) may interfere with visual interpretation of the color change in the reagent pad.

Table 8.11. Major disorders or conditions which cause abnormal chemistry results in a routine UA

Aciduria
   *Expected in healthy carnivores, omnivores, and herbivores on a milk diet
   *Acidoses, some metabolic and potentially with respiratory
   *Associated with hypochloremic metabolic alkalosis (paradoxical aciduria)
   Hypokalemia
   H^+ production by bacteria
   Proximal tubular acidosis (if HCO_3^- is depleted)
Alkalinuria
   *Expected in healthy herbivores and after meals in monogastric mammals (alkaline tide)
   *Urea degradation: spontaneous in older samples, initiated by urease-containing bacteria
   Alkaloses, some metabolic and potentially with respiratory
   Proximal tubular acidosis (early)
Proteinuria
   Prerenal (overflow): hemoglobinuria, myoglobinuria, paraproteinuria
   *Glomerular: glomerulonephritis or amyloidosis
   Tubular: congenital or acquired proximal tubular diseases
   *Hemorrhagic or inflammatory proteinuria
   False-positive reaction (see the text)
Glucosuria (glycosuria)
   *Hyperglycemia
   Renal: congenital or acquired proximal tubular diseases
   False-positive reaction (see the text)
Ketonuria
   *Ketosis
   False-positive reaction (see the text)
Heme positive[a]
   *Hematuria (pathologic, iatrogenic, estral)
   *Hemoglobinuria
   Myoglobinuria
   Methemoglobinuria
   False-positive reaction (see the text)
Bilirubinuria
   *Expected in substantially concentrated urine of healthy dogs
   *Hemolytic diseases
   *Hepatobiliary diseases
   False-positive reaction (see the text)

   * A relatively common disease or condition
   [a] In most reagent systems, the heme test is called either the "blood" test or the "occult blood" test, although the assay is designed to detect heme.

    4. Contamination with buffer from an adjacent protein reagent pad may falsely decrease the urine pH result.
  C. Aciduria suggests an increased secretion of H^+ (Table 8.11)
    1. It is expected in carnivores, some omnivores, and herbivores on milk. H^+ is produced from protein diets.

2. Acidoses, respiratory and some metabolic: There is a net increase in H^+ secretion (H^+ and NH_4^+) by proximal and distal tubular cells; the secretion is enhanced by decreased extracellular pH.

3. Hypochloremic metabolic alkalosis (see pathogenesis in Chapter 9: Bicarbonate Concentration and Total Carbon Dioxide Concentration, sect. III).

4. Hypokalemia: H^+ is secreted, and type A intercalated cells resorb K^+ through H^+-K^+-ATPase pumps that appear to be most active when there is a state of K^+ depletion.

5. Furosemide therapy: The H^+ secretion may be increased because of hypokalemia or increased by other factors (secondary hyperaldosteronism or enhanced renal excretion of Na^+ and H^+ because the Na^+-K^+-$2Cl^-$ cotransporter in the loop of Henle is blocked by furosemide).[1]

6. Proximal renal tubular acidosis (if HCO_3^- depleted): A decreased conservation of HCO_3^- by proximal tubules provides more HCO_3^- to buffer more H^+ in tubular fluid, and thus the urine pH is greater than expected in an acidotic animal (which may be alkalinuric). However, when plasma $[HCO_3^-]$ decreases, the remaining tubular function may be enough to conserve the filtered HCO_3^-. Then, there will not be sufficient HCO_3^- in the tubular fluid to buffer the H^+, and aciduria may be present.

D. Alkalinuria suggests a decreased excretion of H^+ (Table 8.11)

1. Urea splitting or hydrolysis: Breakdown of urea releases two $-NH_2$ groups that each quickly accepts H^+ ion to form NH_4^+. Removal of free H^+ from urine makes the urine more alkaline.

   a. It may occur with the spontaneous degradation of urea that occurs with delayed completion of urinalyses.

   b. It may be caused by urease-containing bacteria (e.g., *Staphylococcus* and *Proteus*), either in vivo or in vitro.

2. Respiratory alkalosis: Probably less H^+ is secreted by the distal nephron because of less stimulation of the H^+-ATPase pump.

3. Distal renal tubular acidosis: Decreased H^+ secretion by the distal nephron can lead to an inappropriately high urine pH (> 6.0) in the face of acidosis. The pH may not be alkaline.

4. Proximal renal tubular acidosis (see the explanation in the preceding sect. C.6).

III. Protein in urine

A. Physiologic processes

1. Many small proteins (usually Mr < 68,000) can pass through the glomerular filtration barrier. In most healthy animals, the proteins are resorbed in the proximal tubules, and thus very little to no protein is detected in urine samples.

2. Urine of healthy dogs may contain a measurable [protein] without clear evidence of urinary tract disease.

   a. Most of the protein is albumin.

   b. Dogs (n = 145) with concentrated urine (1.020–1.045) and without evidence of urinary tract disease had negative, trace, or 1 + reactions with a dipstick reagent pad: 4–65 mg/dL with a Coomassie brilliant blue method and 4–95 mg/dL with a trichloroacetic acid method.[58]

3. *Tamm-Horsfall protein* is a mucoprotein that apparently is secreted by the thick ascending limb of the loop of Henle and part of the distal tubule and collecting ducts. It is soluble above pH 7 but insoluble below pH 7. It is a major component of hyaline casts and thought to be part of the matrix of granular casts.

B. Analytical concepts
   1. Reagent strip method
      a. Principle: The reagent pad contains a colorimetric pH indicator (tetrabromphenol blue) at acidic pH. Amino groups of negatively charged proteins bind the dye and change the pad's color.
      b. Changes in the color of the pad correspond to estimated [protein] (Table 8.10).
      c. Abnormal urine color (pigmenturia) may interfere with reagent pad color and therefore with estimation of [protein].
      d. Readings may be falsely increased in highly buffered alkaline urine (i.e., > 8.0), in moderately alkaline urine if highly concentrated,[60] or in urine that contains quaternary ammonium salts or chlorhexidine.
      e. Analytical sensitivity and specificity
         (1) The method detects albumin better than globulins, which are less negatively charged. Protein in cells (e.g., epithelial cells and leukocytes) reacts very poorly with reagents.
         (2) Protein concentrations needed to give a trace to 1 + reaction: albumin (14–21 mg/dL), α-globulin (20–30 mg/dL), β-globulin (40–50 mg/dL), γ-globulin (> 1,000 mg/dL), light-chain proteins (26–52 mg/dL), and hemoglobin (5–50 mg/dL)[61,62]
   2. SSA turbidity
      a. Principle: Proteins are denatured by acids and form a precipitate that is seen as increased solution turbidity. Urine that is hazy to cloudy should be centrifuged prior to SSA turbidity testing.
      b. Results may be expressed on a visual turbidity scale (1 + to 4 +) or visually compared against standard solutions to interpolate concentrations. There are also spectrophotometric SSA methods that provide more quantitative results. There is a lack of interlaboratory standardization for reporting SSA test results.
      c. SSA reacts with albumin better than globulins (reportedly 2–4 times as well) and will detect Bence Jones proteins if concentrations are sufficient.
      d. Falsely increased readings can be caused by X-ray contrast media, tolbutamide, penicillin (massive dose), sulfisoxazole, tolmetin sodium, and turbidity caused by coprecipitation of crystals because of the low pH of SSA.
      e. Falsely decreased readings can be caused by highly buffered alkaline urine.[37,63]
C. Proteinuria (Table 8.11 and Fig. 8.9)
   1. Prerenal (overflow, overload, and preglomerular) proteinuria
      a. A pathologic state increases the plasma concentration of a small protein that passes through the glomerular filtration barrier. If the amount of filtered protein exceeds the ability of proximal tubules to resorb it, the protein is excreted in the urine. Examples: paraproteinuria (light-chain proteins including monomers with $M_r \approx 23,000$ and dimers with $M_r \approx 46,000$), hemoglobinuria (dimer $M_r \approx 34,000$), myoglobinuria ($M_r \approx 17,000$), and postcolostral proteinuria (includes β-lactoglobulinuria) in food animals.
      b. Light-chain proteins, hemoglobin, and myoglobin molecules are detected by routine urine protein assays.
      c. Overflow proteinurias do not produce hypoproteinemia.
   2. Glomerular proteinuria
      a. Glomerular disease damages the filtration barrier and decreases selective permeability. The glomerulus becomes increasingly permeable to larger proteins or to

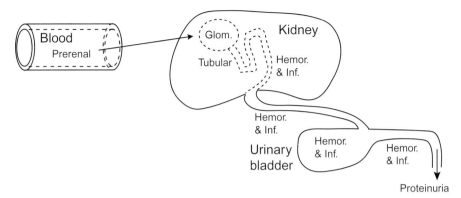

Fig. 8.9. Four major types of proteinuria.

- In prerenal proteinurias (*Prerenal*), small proteins (e.g., hemoglobin dimers, light chains, and myoglobin) present in the plasma at increased concentrations are excreted in the urine because they pass through the glomerular filtration barrier and are incompletely resorbed in tubules.
- In glomerular proteinurias (*Glom.*), glomerular disease damages the filtration barrier and decreases selective permeability. Glomeruli become increasingly permeable to larger or negatively charged plasma proteins. These proteins pass through the defective filtration barrier and are incompletely resorbed by tubules, so they are excreted in urine.
- In tubular proteinurias (*Tubular*), proximal renal tubules are defective, so proteins that normally are resorbed from ultrafiltrate (e.g., some albumin and smaller globulins) are not, and thus they are excreted in the urine.
- In hemorrhagic and inflammatory proteinurias (*Hemor. & Inf.*), plasma proteins or hemoglobin enter the urine because of hemorrhage or inflammation involving the renal tubules, renal pelvis, ureters, urinary bladder, urethra, or genital tract tissues.

---

negatively charged proteins. Prolonged mild or rapid severe glomerular proteinuria will cause a selective hypoproteinemia (loss of plasma proteins except for the largest forms) (see Chapter 7). Increased amounts of albumin and larger proteins are expected on SDS-PAGE of urine from dogs with glomerular proteinuria.[64,65]

  b. In people, a transient proteinuria that occurs after exercise is considered a form of glomerular proteinuria.

3. Tubular proteinuria

  a. Proximal renal tubules are defective, so proteins that normally are resorbed from ultrafiltrate (e.g., some albumin and smaller globulins) are not and thus are excreted in the urine. Increased numbers of protein bands representing proteins with a molecular mass less than that of albumin are expected with SDS-PAGE of urine from dogs with tubular proteinuria.[64,65]

  b. Tubular proteinurias are usually associated with acute renal diseases (toxicoses and hypoxia) but can be congenital. They do not produce hypoalbuminemia.

4. Hemorrhagic or inflammatory proteinuria (also called secretory or postrenal proteinuria, but hemorrhage and exudation may occur in kidneys and are not secretory processes)

  a. Hemorrhagic: hemorrhage into the genitourinary tract due to impaired hemostasis, including blood vessel damage by inflammation, trauma, neoplasia, or other necrosis

     b. Inflammatory: exudation of plasma proteins through vessel walls into the genitourinary tract due to inflammation

     c. The postrenal proteinurias are the most common proteinurias. The quantity of protein lost is usually not sufficient to cause hypoalbuminemia, but there may be mild hypoalbuminemia caused by inflammation or hemorrhage. Most proteins detected in the urine entered filtrate from the plasma. Proteins from leukocytes and epithelial cells are poorly detected by urine protein assays.

     d. Evidence to support this type of proteinuria is usually found in other urinalysis results: inflammation (pyuria) and hemorrhage (hematuria).

     e. One must consider reproductive tract sources (e.g., prostatitis and estral bleeding), especially in voided urine samples.

D. Other proteinuria classifications: The aforementioned classification system is not the only system. Some divide proteinurias into three types (prerenal, renal, and postrenal) in which the renal type includes both glomerular and tubular proteinurias. Another classification scheme based on prerenal, renal, and postrenal divisions includes functional and pathologic subdivisions of the renal proteinuria category, with glomerular, tubular, and interstitial subgroups of the pathological renal category.[66] In this scheme, functional proteinurias are considered to be mild and transient proteinurias caused by physiologically altered renal handling of normal plasma proteins in the absence of renal lesions (e.g., seen with exercise or fever).

E. Protein-losing nephropathy and renal failure concepts (Fig. 8.10)

    1. Urea and Crt are small molecules that pass freely through the glomerular filtration barrier (sieves). Some filtrate urea is resorbed by tubules. The remaining urea and Crt are excreted in urine and thus do not accumulate in blood. It has been presumed that albumin does not pass through the glomerular filtration barrier in health and thus remains in the blood (dogs may be an exception).

    2. With a protein-losing nephropathy, the glomerular "sieves" become more porous, and larger proteins or charged proteins that usually are repelled enter the renal filtrate via glomeruli. If the ability to resorb proteins is exceeded, then a proteinuria will be present. The continual loss of protein will lead to hypoalbuminemia. As long as the number of functional glomeruli is adequate, urea and Crt will be adequately removed from blood and azotemia will not develop.

    3. If the glomerular disease destroys more nephrons, then renal failure occurs. The few remaining functional glomeruli cannot remove urea and Crt fast enough from the blood, so azotemia develops. Proteinuria continues because the remaining functional glomeruli are permeable to proteins. The severity of hypoalbuminemia increases because of continued albumin loss, but defective excretion of H_2O (associated with Na^+ and H_2O retention) may contribute to hypoalbuminemia.

F. Bence Jones proteinuria (immunoglobulin light-chain proteinuria)

    1. Analysis of urine for Bence Jones proteins is not part of a routine urinalysis. It may be indicated to clarify the type of proteinuria or to investigate a possible lymphoproliferative disease.

    2. *Bence Jones proteins* are light chains (either κ or λ) of immunoglobulins that have unique thermal properties: they precipitate between 40 °C and 60 °C, return to a soluble state at 100 °C, and then precipitate again when cooled. The thermal properties of Bence Jones proteins are due to the variable portions of the light-chain proteins.[67] As described by Ritzman and Daniels,[68] these proteins were first recognized by William MacIntyre in 1845. Dr. MacIntyre sent the urine sample to Dr.

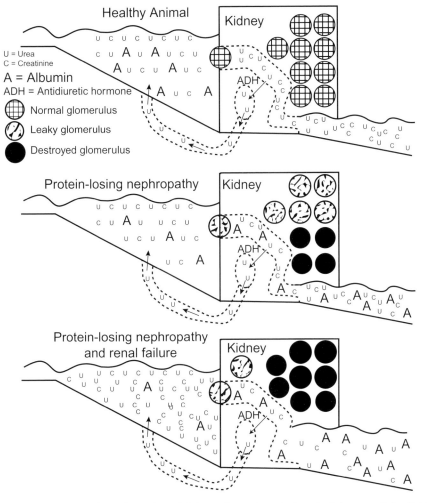

Fig. 8.10. Protein-losing nephropathy and renal failure. Illustrations depict a body's extracellular fluid as a lake, kidneys as a dam, and the urine as the river below the dam. Urea and Crt molecules are small fish in the lake, and albumin molecules are big fish. The nephron consists of the sieve or filter at the lake outlet and the tubes that run through the dam. Some H_2O and urea are reclaimed to maintain extracellular fluid H_2O and urea content. Only one of ten nephrons is shown as a filter with a connected tubular system.

- In healthy animals, urea and Crt pass freely through ten functional filters, into the dam's tubes, and into the river. Some urea (and H_2O) is reclaimed from the dam's tubes in a process enhanced by ADH. Albumin is too big to pass through the filters, so it stays in the lake.
- In the protein-losing nephropathy illustration, 40 % of the filters (and nephrons) have been destroyed. The remaining 60 % are damaged, more porous, and allow albumin to enter the dam and river. The loss of albumin from the lake causes hypoalbuminemia and proteinuria. The remaining filters are sufficient to keep urea and Crt removed from the lake, and thus azotemia does not develop.
- In protein-losing nephropathy and renal failure, 80 % of the filters (and nephrons) have been destroyed. The remaining 20 % are damaged, more porous, and allow albumin to enter the dam and river. The loss of albumin from the lake causes hypoalbuminemia and proteinuria. The remaining filters are insufficient to keep urea and Crt removed from the lake, and thus azotemia develops. Also, the remaining nephrons cannot adequately conserve H_2O, and thus polyuria develops.

Henry Bence Jones, who confirmed the findings. These proteins are known as "Bence Jones proteins" and not "MacIntyre proteins," perhaps because Bence Jones published the case data first (1847) and MacIntyre's publication was in 1850.

3. The unique thermal properties of light-chain proteins are used as the basis of the Bence Jones test.

   a. Basics of the positive heat test:[39] (1) Urine is acidified to a pH near 4.9. (2) Acidified urine is heated to 56 °C for 15 min and observed for flocculence or precipitates. (3) If flocculence or precipitates are present (the test is negative if they are absent), the urine sample is placed in a boiling water bath for 3 min and examined for a decreased amount of precipitate. A decrease in flocculence suggests Bence Jones proteinuria. (4) Filter the hot urine through a funnel with filter paper into a tube containing a thermometer. If Bence Jones proteins are present, they should precipitate at about 60 °C and redissolve at about 40 °C. Variations in the heat test acidifying solutions, filtrations, and time intervals have been described.

   b. The concentration of Bence Jones proteins needs to be > 145 mg/dL to get a positive result, and regulation of the pH is very important.[67]

   c. Other proteins may precipitate during heating (e.g., fibrinogen precipitates at 56–58 °C), which makes interpretation difficult without the filtering and assessment of precipitation during cooling.

4. Other methods of detecting light-chain proteinuria

   a. The Bence Jones proteins react better in the SSA protein method than they do in the protein reagent pad method of routine urinalysis procedures.[67] The reagent pad test may fail to detect light-chain proteinuria if the proteinuria is minimal.

   b. If urine proteins are concentrated prior to electrophoresis, normal light-chain proteins can be found in the β_2-globulin fraction (Plate 12J.2).

   c. Immunoelectrophoresis for κ- or λ-light-chain proteins is the preferred method of documenting light-chain proteinuria, but species-specific antisera are not readily available for individual species. Results from immunohistochemical studies suggest that antibodies against human light-chain proteins cross-react with light-chain proteins of domestic mammals (see Chapter 7).

5. Bence Jones proteinuria may occur because the formation of κ- or λ-light-chain proteins by lymphocytes or plasma cells is increased.

   a. Typically, their presence is associated with B-lymphocyte or plasma cell neoplasia. One study reported that about 30 % of the dogs with myeloma had a Bence Jones proteinuria, though the authors did not state how the presence of the Bence Jones proteins was detected or confirmed.[69]

   b. Bence Jones proteinuria can also be caused by B-lymphocyte hyperplasia. By means of SDS-PAGE and immunofixation methods, light-chain proteinurias were found in dogs with leishmaniasis, ehrlichiosis, and babesiosis.[70]

6. Light-chain proteins ($M_r \approx 23,000$ monomer or 46,000 dimer) pass through the glomerular filtration barrier, and small quantities are resorbed by the proximal tubules. If renal resorptive capacity is exceeded or if renal disease develops, light-chain proteins are excreted in the urine.

IV. Glucose in urine

   A. Physiologic processes

      1. Glucose is a relatively small molecule ($M_r = 180$) that passes freely through the glomerular filtration barrier and enters the ultrafiltrate.

2. Glucose is resorbed in the proximal tubules via a Na^+-glucose cotransport system that depends on a favorable gradient established by active Na^+ transport from tubular cells to the peritubular fluid. The gradient promotes Na^+ resorption from the tubular fluid, and glucose is resorbed secondarily (indirect active transport or secondary active transport).

3. The renal tubular transport maximum for glucose varies among domestic mammals. The approximate transport maximums are 180–220 mg/dL in dogs,[71] about 290 mg/dL in cats,[71] about 150 mg/dL in horses[72] and calves,[73] and probably lower in mature cattle.

B. Analytical concepts
   1. Reagent strip method
      a. Principle: Conversion of glucose to gluconic acid is catalyzed by glucose oxidase with liberation of H_2O_2, which reacts with an indicator to give a color change in the reagent pad. The degree of color change is proportional to the [glucose] (Table 8.10). Indicators vary with different products.
      b. Falsely increased reactions may be caused by H_2O_2 and sodium hypochlorite. Such contamination may occur when samples are obtained from an examination table or cage floor.
      c. Falsely decreased reactions may be caused by ascorbic acid, ketones, and very concentrated urine samples. Cold urine, especially when reaction times are very brief (e.g., 10 s), and marked bilirubinuria may also inhibit reactions.
   2. Copper-reduction method (Clinitest)
      a. Principle: Cu^{2+} reacts with a reducing substance (e.g., glucose, fructose, lactose, galactose, maltose, or pentose) to produce cuprous (Cu^+) oxide and cuprous hydroxide and thus a color change.
      b. Semiquantitative results for the standard method are negative, ≈ 250, ≈ 500, ≈ 750, ≈ 1000, or ≈ 2000 mg/dL. The method is probably more accurate than the reagent strip method but requires a greater concentration for detection; that is, the detection limit is higher.
      c. The method may be used to confirm questionable positive reagent strip results such as when urine color interferes with interpretation of the reagent pad color.
      d. False-positive reactions may be caused by cephalosporins, formaldehyde, and ascorbic acid (if concentrations are high enough). Reactions with sugars other than glucose might be considered false-positive reactions.

C. Glucosuria (glycosuria) disorders (Table 8.11)
   1. Hyperglycemic glucosuria
      a. Transient or persistent hyperglycemia results in more glucose in the ultrafiltrate than can be resorbed by proximal tubules.
      b. Hyperglycemia is typically concurrent with the glucosuria, but a transient hyperglycemia and delay in bladder emptying may mask concurrence.
   2. Renal glucosuria (normoglycemic glucosuria)
      a. Transient or persistent glucosuria results from defective resorption of glucose caused by damaged or abnormal proximal tubules.
      b. Tubular abnormalities can be acquired or congenital
         (1) Acquired: proximal renal tubular toxicosis or ischemia (sometimes referred to as *acquired Fanconi syndrome*)
         (2) Congenital: Fanconi syndrome and pure primary renal glucosuria (basenji, Norwegian elkhound, and Shetland sheepdog)[74]

3. Glucose in tubular fluid will cause osmotic diuresis (H_2O is "held" by the glucose in the tubular fluid, especially in the proximal tubules) and thus cause decreased renal concentrating ability and increased urine volume (polyuria).

V. Ketones in urine
   A. Physiologic processes
      1. Acetoacetate, β-hydroxybutyrate, and acetone are ketone bodies, but only acetoacetate and acetone have the chemical structure of ketones. Acetoacetic acid and β-hydroxybutyric acid are ketoacids that are produced by hepatocytes but dissociate at physiologic pH to their anionic form and H^+.
      2. Ketone bodies are not expected in the urine of healthy mammals that have an adequate intake of nutrients.
      3. Ketone bodies may enter the urine by both glomerular filtration of plasma and by tubular secretion. The tubular secretion process probably shares a transport process with other organic anions. After entering the tubular fluid, acetoacetate and β-hydroxybutyrate are nonresorbable.[1]
   B. Analytical concepts
      1. Reagent strip method (Bayer Diagnostics)
         a. Principle: Acetoacetate (mostly) and acetone (about 10 % as reactive as acetoacetate) form colored complexes with nitroprusside. The amount of color change reflects the amount of ketones present (Table 8.10). The reagent system does not react with β-hydroxybutyrate, the ketone body that does not have a ketone chemical structure.
         b. False-positive reactions may be caused by highly pigmented urine, levodopa metabolites, and some compounds that have sulfhydryl groups (e.g., captopril and cystine).[75] Trace reactions may occur in urine with high USG and low pH.
         c. In theory, β-hydroxybutyrate can be converted with H_2O_2 to acetoacetate so that nitroprusside methods can be used to detect β-hydroxybutyrate. However, urine concentrations of β-hydroxybutyrate must be > 200 mmol/L (using 3 % H_2O_2) or > 50 mmol/L (using 30 % H_2O_2) to produce more than a trace reaction. At such concentrations, the [acetoacetate] would probably be great enough to be detected routinely.[76]
      2. Acetest tablet method (Bayer Diagnostics)
         a. Principle: It is the same as with the reagent strip method. Color change is easier to detect, so it has a lower detection limit than some reagent pads (about 5 mg/dL in urine) and thus may be used to confirm trace or questionable reactions on reagent pads.
         b. The method may be used as a qualitative assay for blood, plasma, urine, and milk.
   C. Ketonuria (Table 8.11)
      1. *Ketonuria* occurs when the mobilization of lipids is increased because of a shift in energy production from carbohydrates to lipids (e.g., in diabetes mellitus, starvation, and hypoglycemic disorders). Excessive β-oxidation of fatty acids in hepatocytes generates more acetyl-coenzyme A than can be used for gluconeogenesis and triglyceride synthesis. Excess acetyl-coenzyme A stimulates hepatic ketogenesis and thus increased formation of ketoacids, leading to increased ketone bodies in blood *(ketonemia)*. Ketone bodies are easily cleared from blood and are excreted in urine.

2. Decreased insulin activity and increased glucagon activity promote ketogenesis. Such changes may result from either physiologic or pathologic processes.

D. The pathologic state caused by excess ketogenesis is called *ketosis* or, if laboratory data indicate a concurrent acidosis, *ketoacidosis*. In ketosis, primarily β-hydroxybutyrate (which is not detected by the assay) is excreted in urine, but acetoacetate and acetone (detected by the assay) are also excreted.

E. Renal excretion of acetoacetate and β-hydroxybutyrate (both of which are anions) obligates excretion of cations (e.g., Na^+ or K^+) by the kidneys. Prolonged ketonuria may cause Na^+ or K^+ depletion that contributes to hyponatremia and hypokalemia.

VI. Heme in urine (test frequently labeled *blood* or *occult blood*)
   A. Physiologic concepts: Heme-containing compounds are not expected to be present at detectable amounts in the urine of healthy mammals.
   B. Analytical concepts
      1. Reagent strip method
         a. Principle: In some systems, the peroxidase activity of heme catalyzes the oxidation of *o*-toluidine to a blue compound. In other systems, the peroxidase activity of heme catalyzes the oxidation of a chromogen (e.g., tetramethylbenzadine) to a colored compound.
         b. Heme may be from hemoglobin, methemoglobin, or myoglobin. If intact erythrocytes are present, the cells are lysed in the reagent pad to produce either speckled or solid color changes in the pad. Results may be described in semi-quantitative terms or as an estimated [hemoglobin] (Table 8.10).
         c. Falsely increased reactions may occur with oxidizing compounds such as hypochlorite (bleach) and microbial or leukocyte peroxidase.
         d. Falsely decreased reactions may occur with a high USG or with urine that contains captopril, ascorbic acid, or formaldehyde. Erythrocytes may not be detected if they are not suspended in the test sample.
      2. Hematest tablet method
         a. Principle: It is the same as with the reagent pad, with modifications.
         b. The method may be used as a confirmatory test and also to test for fecal occult blood.
      3. Unfortunately, there is not a widely available laboratory assay for differentiating myoglobin from hemoglobin in domestic mammals. Differentiation is usually accomplished by clinical deductive reasoning (see Table 3.12).
         a. A simple precipitant test using ammonium sulfate is considered unreliable. In theory, hemoglobin, but not myoglobin, precipitates in 80 % ammonium sulfate solution, whereas myoglobin precipitates in a 100 % ammonium sulfate solution. However, denatured myoglobin will precipitate in the 80 % soultion and thus be incorrectly classified as hemoglobin.[77] Also, a similar erroneous classification will occur if the urine pH is not adjusted to 7.0–7.5.[78]
         b. Immunologic methods require species-specific antibodies. Electrophoretic and spectrophotometric procedures may be employed.
      4. The heme assay is more sensitive than the protein assay. Therefore, when small amounts of blood are in the urine, there may be marked heme positivity without the hemoglobin causing a positive protein reaction.
   C. Heme-positive reaction in urine (Tables 8.11 and 3.12)
      1. Hematuria

a. Erythrocytes enter the urine via hemorrhage into the urogenital tract. Hemorrhage may be caused by a pathologic process (trauma, inflammation, neoplasia, coagulation defect, etc.) or the urine collection process (e.g., cystocentesis, catheterization, or bladder palpation pressure).

b. An [erythrocyte] near 5–20/μL is needed to produce a positive heme reaction.[63] Erythrocytes should be microscopically identified in the urine sediment to confirm hematuria. Erythrocytes tend to lyse if urine is very alkaline or unconcentrated (e.g., $USG_{ref} < 1.015$), so they may not be seen on examination of the sediment.

2. Hemoglobinuria

a. During clinical intravascular hemolysis, plasma hemoglobin dimers ($M_r \approx$ 32,000) may form from hemoglobin ($M_r \approx$ 64,000), pass through the glomerular filtration barriers, and enter the ultrafiltrate when haptoglobin is saturated (see Chapter 3). If not completely resorbed by the renal tubules, the hemoglobin dimers are excreted in the urine.

b. Intravascular hemolysis of sufficient severity to cause hemoglobinemia and hemoglobinuria can be caused by a variety of disorders that cause anemia (see Table 3.10). Hemoglobinuria may also be created by lysis of erythrocytes after they enter urine. In such cases, hemoglobinemia should not be present (unless erythrocytes were lysed during blood collection or handling).

3. Myoglobinuria

a. Myocyte necrosis or damage can release myoglobin ($M_r \approx$ 17,000) from the myocyte into the interstitial fluid, lymph, and finally blood, from which the small protein easily passes into the glomerular filtrate. If not completely resorbed by the renal tubules, myoglobin is excreted in the urine.

b. Myoglobin is rapidly cleared from plasma, and thus pink plasma is not expected. Myoglobinuria is associated with acute myopathies caused by trauma, excessive exertion, or exertional or paralytic rhabdomyolysis of horses (azoturia).

4. Methemoglobinuria

a. Methemoglobinuria may contribute to a positive urine heme reaction in the following situations (concurrent hemoglobinuria is expected):

   (1) When hemoglobin (or hemoglobin dimer) molecules are in the urine, some of the ferrous heme will undergo spontaneous oxidation to ferric heme (forming methemoglobin).

   (2) When there is an intravascular hemolytic anemia caused by an overwhelming exposure to oxidants, some of the lysed erythrocytes will release methemoglobin to plasma. Then, methemoglobin dimers can enter the glomerular filtrate.

b. Both metheme and heme have peroxidase activity, so either molecule will give a positive heme (occult blood) reaction.[79]

VII. Bilirubin in urine

A. Physiologic processes

1. Bilirubin is not expected in the urine of domestic mammals other than the dog.

2. Bu forms from the degradation of heme, primarily from hemoglobin degradation in macrophages. After conjugation in hepatocytes, Bc is excreted via the biliary system.

If regurgitated to the plasma, Bc passes freely through the glomerular filtration barrier and is excreted in urine (see Fig. 3.3 or 13.1).

3. Renal tubular cells in at least some species (e.g., dogs) can convert heme (from resorbed hemoglobin of hemoglobinuria) to Bu and then Bc, which can be excreted in the urine.

4. Usually, Bu is thought not to be in urine because it is bound to plasma albumin, which is not filtered by most glomeruli. However, because apparently healthy dogs may have mild albuminuria and glomerular diseases can cause proteinuria, Bu bound to albumin may be present in urine. Also, Bc may hydrolyze to Bu in urine.

B. Analytical concepts

1. Reagent strip method

a. Principle: Bilirubin becomes coupled with a diazonium salt in a strongly acid medium, and the coupling produces color changes that reflect the amount of bilirubin present (Table 8.10). Biliverdin (an intermediate breakdown product between heme and bilirubin) is not detected.

b. Falsely increased reactions may be caused by *indican* (a product of tryptophan degradation by intestinal bacteria) and metabolites of etodolac (a nonsteroidal anti-inflammatory drug).

c. Falsely decreased reactions may be caused by ascorbic acid if the animal is being given ascorbic acid.[39]

2. Ictotest method: Although based on the same analytical principle, it has a lower detection limit (about 0.1 that of reagent strips) and may be used to confirm trace reactions on reagent sticks. Reagent pad results should be reported when the Ictotest confirms positivity.

3. Bilirubin molecules are degraded to biliverdin by exposure to ultraviolet light. Biliverdin is not detected by the bilirubin reaction. Before analysis, urine should not be directly exposed to ultraviolet light for more than 30 min.

C. Bilirubinuria (Table 8.11)

1. Excessive bilirubin formation (in hemolytic states) or impaired hepatobiliary excretion of Bc increases plasma [Bc]. Bc passes easily through the glomerular filtration barrier and is excreted by the kidneys.

2. In dogs, a positive bilirubin reaction must be interpreted based on knowledge of the USG_{ref}. Concentrated urine (1.025–1.040) of healthy dogs frequently produces a small bilirubin reaction. Moderate reactions occasionally occur with more concentrated urine (> 1.040).

3. Because of the low renal threshold for bilirubin in most animals, especially dogs, bilirubinuria may be detected before hyperbilirubinemia or icterus is detected in hemolytic and hepatobiliary disorders. Hyperbilirubinemia without bilirubinuria suggests a false-negative urine bilirubin reaction or the degradation of urine bilirubin before sample analysis.

VIII. Urobilinogen in urine

A. Physiologic processes

1. *Urobilinogen*, a colorless compound formed from the degradation of bilirubin in the intestine, is passively absorbed by intestinal mucosa.

2. Urobilinogen that is not removed from portal blood by hepatocytes enters the systemic blood, from which it is excreted in the urine.

B. Analytical concepts for the reagent strip method
   1. Principle: Urobilinogen reacts with *p*-dimethylaminobenzaldehyde to form a red pigment via a modified Ehrlich's aldehyde reaction. The degree of color change reflects the [urobilinogen] (Table 8.10).
   2. Units: Ehrlich units (EU) or mg/dL; 1 EU = 1 mg/dL
   3. The assay cannot be used to detect decreased urobilinogen concentrations because the lowest reading is 0.2 mg/dL (Multistix) or 1.0 mg/dL (Chemstrip), the concentration expected in urine of healthy animals. There is not a negative reaction pad on the reagent strip, so this method cannot be used to detect decreased urobilinogen concentrations in urine.
   4. Falsely increased results may be caused by aminosalicylic acid, sulfonamides, and aminobenzoic acid.
   5. Falsely decreased reactions may be caused by formalin. In addition, urobilinogen degrades easily when urine is exposed to ultraviolet light.
C. Increased urobilinogenuria
   1. Hemolytic diseases will cause the increased formation, biliary excretion, and degradation of bilirubin. Thus, increased urobilinogen formation and excretion are expected. However, increased urobilinogenuria is not consistently found.
   2. Mammals with hepatic or biliary diseases may occasionally have increased urinary excretion of urobilinogen, perhaps from the degradation of bilirubin in the urinary system.
   3. Most veterinarians do not find the assessment of urine [urobilinogen] to be diagnostically fruitful.

IX. Nitrite in the urine
   A. Physiologic processes: Certain Gram-negative bacteria can reduce nitrate to nitrite.
   B. Analytical concepts for the reagent strip method
      1. Principle: Nitrite reacts with *p*-arsanilic acid to form a diazonium compound that couples with N-1-naphthyl ethylenediamine to form a pink product.
      2. Falsely increased reactions may result from analysis of stale urine containing contaminant bacteria.
      3. Falsely decreased reactions may occur if there is insufficient time (< 4 h) for bacterial reduction of nitrates. Ascorbic acid (especially when USG is high) may produce falsely decreased reactions in dog and cat urine.[37]
   C. Nitrite-positive reaction
      1. Suggestive of a Gram-negative bacterial infection in the urinary tract
      2. Detection of nitrites in urine is a screening procedure for Gram-negative bacterial urinary infections. Significant bacteriuria may be present but undetected with the nitrite assay.
   D. Most veterinarians do not find the urine nitrite test to be diagnostically valuable because it does not detect significant bacteriuria consistently.

X. Leukocyte esterase in the urine
   A. Physiologic processes: Leukocytes in the urine release an esterase.
   B. Analytical concept: The assay is considered to be inadequate for the chemical detection of pyuria in dogs because of false-negative results,[80] and false-positive reactions are a problem in cats.[39]

URINE SEDIMENT EXAMINATION

I. General concepts
    A. Consistently using the same urine volume for sediment preparation will enable a more critical assessment of the semiquantitative results. The quantity of urine used may vary between laboratories but is usually 5–10 mL. About twice the amount of sediment would be expected from 10 mL than from 5 mL. Expected findings in this chapter are based on the sedimentation of 5 mL of urine.
    B. The contents of urine are not stable, so urine should be analyzed within a few hours (ideally within 1 h) of collection. During sample storage, cells and casts deteriorate, crystals may dissolve or form, and bacteria may die or proliferate.
    C. The method of urine collection should be considered when urinalysis and especially urine sediment results are interpreted. A voided sample may contain cells and bacteria from the genital tract. A catheterized sample may contain more epithelial cells or erythrocytes because of urethral trauma. A cystocentesis sample may contain blood because the needle damaged blood vessels.
    D. Samples should be well mixed before the aliquots are removed for centrifugation in standardized conical based tubes at about $450 \times g$ for 5 min. The supernatant is poured off or removed by pipette to leave a residual urine volume in which the sedimented material should be thoroughly resuspended before a standardized drop is placed on a slide with a pipette and overlaid with a glass coverslip. The sediment should be analyzed after a few minutes (to let cells settle and lipid float) by using 10× and 40× or 45× objectives with the microscope condenser lowered to increase refraction. Systems designed for more standardized evaluation of urine sediment are commercially available (e.g., the Petstix 8).
    E. Most sediment findings are quantified by the number of structures seen per microscopic field (i.e., per lpf or hpf). The width of the viewed field can vary because of differences in the microscope objective and ocular lens. For example, the viewed area of a 25 mm ocular is about 50 % larger than the viewed area of a 20 mm ocular. Thus, in the same sediment, 15 leukocytes/hpf would be seen with a 25 mm ocular, and 10 leukocytes/hpf would be seen with a 20 mm ocular.
    F. Sediment stains may be used but could affect concentrations via dilution and may introduce organisms or particulate debris. Evaluation of stained and unstained preparations may be helpful.

II. Leukocytes in urine sediment (Plate 11B, D, and E)
    A. Physiologic processes: A few leukocytes (fewer than about 5/hpf) may be found in the urine of healthy mammals.
    B. Analytical concepts
        1. Leukocytes in urine sediment are enumerated as the range or mean of leukocytes seen in most 400× fields (hpf)
        2. Leukocytes are not routinely differentiated when found in urine. On stained slides prepared from fresh urine, most of the leukocytes will be neutrophils and macrophages, though eosinophils may occasionally be prominent. Small epithelial cells may look similar to leukocytes.
        3. Leukocytes deteriorate in urine within a few hours; thus, numbers diminish with time.
    C. Pyuria: increased [leukocyte] (number/hpf) in urine sediment (Table 8.12)

Table 8.12. Major disorders or conditions that cause abnormal findings in urine sediment examinations

Pyuria (Plate 11B)
  *Urinary tract inflammation, infectious and noninfectious
  Genital tract inflammation
Hematuria (Plate 11C)
  *Urinary tract hemorrhage: pathologic (damaged vessels or coagulation defect), iatrogenic
  Genital tract hemorrhage: pathologic, estrus
Bacteriuria (Plate 11D and E)
  *Infection in urinary or genital tract
  *In vitro growth or contamination
Cylindruria (Plate 11F–H)
  Can be found in low numbers in healthy animals
  Associated with glomerular proteinuria (especially hyaline casts)
  *Active renal tubular cell degeneration inflammation, or hemorrhage: nephroses, nephritis
Epithelial cells in sediment (Plate 11I and J)
  *Can be found in low numbers in healthy animals
  *Inflammation/hyperplasia in genitourinary tract
  Neoplasia in genitourinary tract
Crystalluria (urine pH in which crystals tend to occur)
  Ammonium (bi)urate (pH usually ≤ 7) (Plate 11K): seen in healthy mammals; common in Dalmatian dogs and English bulldogs; suggest liver dysfunction and portosystemic shunts in dogs and cats
  *Bilirubin (pH < 7) (Plate 11L): seen with bilirubinuria
  *Calcium carbonate (pH ≥ 7) (Plate 13A): healthy herbivores; not seen in dogs and cats
  Calcium oxalate dihydrate (pH usually ≤ 7) (Plate 13B): seen in healthy mammals, suggest possible hypercalciuria or hyperoxaluria (including ethylene glycol toxicosis or ingestion of oxalate-rich plants such as *Halogeton* and *Amaranthus* in ruminants)
  Calcium oxalate monohydrate (pH usually ≤ 7) (Plate 13C): suggest possible hypercalciuria or hyperoxaluria, especially ethylene glycol toxicosis
  Calcium phosphate (pH usually ≥ 7): seen in healthy dogs, dogs with calcium phosphate uroliths, or dogs with persistent alkalinuria
  Cholesterol (pH ≤ 7) (Plate 13D): uncommon; seen in healthy dogs; suggest hypercholesterolemia and proteinuria as seen with protein-losing nephropathy
  Cystine (pH usually ≤ 7): rare; seen with cystinuria and suggest liver disease
  Drug crystals (sulfa, ampicillin, contrast media, primidone) (Plate 13F): reflect presence of compound in urine
  Hippuric acid (pH usually ≤ 7): very rare, are confused with calcium oxalate monohydrate crystals
  Leucine (pH < 7): rare; suggest liver disease
  *Magnesium ammonium phosphate (struvite) (pH usually ≥ 7) (Plate 13E): common in dogs and cats with alkalinuria, may be associated with urease-producing bacteria
  Tyrosine (pH < 7): rare; suggest liver disease
  Urate, sodium (pH ≤ 7) or ammonium (pH variable): seen in healthy mammals; common in Dalmatians and English bulldogs; suggest liver dysfunction and portosystemic shunts in dogs and cats
  Uric acid (pH < 7) (Plate 13G): same significance as urates
  Xanthine (pH ≤ 7): rare; may reflect treatment with allopurinol or metabolic defect
Other organisms
  Fungi, yeast (*Candida* sp., *Blastomyces* sp., *Cryptococcus* sp.) and hyphal forms (Plate 13H and I)
  Nematode ova (*Dioctophyma renale, Capillaria plica*) (Plate 13J)
  Microfilaria (with hematuria)

* A relatively common disease or condition

1. Urinary tract inflammation
   a. Inflammation of mucosal or submucosal tissues or renal parenchyma may cause leukocytes (mostly neutrophils and monocytes) to migrate from blood to urine. Inflammation can be caused by infections (by bacteria, fungi, or parasites) or noninfectious processes (neoplasia, urolithiasis, or necrosis).
   b. The method of sample collection (voided, cystocentesis, or catheterization) may help determine the site of the inflammatory process; that is, leukocytes might be from anywhere in the genitourinary tract in a voided specimen, but their presence in a cystocentesis sample indicates the source is somewhere from the kidneys to, and including, the proximal urethra. Other clinical information may also help determine the site of the inflammation; for example, pollakiuria and stranguria would suggest lower urinary tract involvement, whereas fever, neutrophilia, or azotemia would suggest nephritis. Leukocyte casts indicate inflammation associated with renal tubules.
2. Genital tract inflammation
   a. Leukocytes may enter urine from the male or female genital tract before (e.g., prostate) or during (e.g., a preputial or vaginal source) micturition. The chance of contamination during micturition is reduced if the sample is collected midway through micturition.
   b. The inflammatory process may or may not be of clinical significance (e.g., mild posthitis).

III.   Erythrocytes in urine sediment (Plate 11C)
   A. Physiologic processes: A few erythrocytes (fewer than about 5/hpf) may be found in the urine of healthy mammals.
   B. Analytical concepts
      1. Erythrocytes in urine sediment are enumerated as the range or mean of erythrocytes seen in most 400× fields (hpf).
      2. Erythrocytes may crenate in urine and can be confused with leukocytes in nonstained sediment. They may swell in hypotonic urine.
      3. Erythrocytes may lyse in urine either before or after urine is collected and appear as ghost cells. Lysis tends to occur in unconcentrated or mildly concentrated urine ($USG_{ref} < 1.015$) or very alkaline urine, especially if analysis is delayed.
      4. If erythrocytes are seen in the urine sediment, the heme reaction should be positive.
   C. Hematuria: increased [erythrocyte] (number/hpf) in urine sediment (Table 8.12)
      1. Pathologic hemorrhage
         a. Vascular damage caused by trauma, inflammation, renal infarcts, or other processes; common in animals with urinary tract infections
         b. Thrombocytopenia, thrombocytopathia, or von Willebrand disease and the resultant poor repair of small vessels
         c. Coagulopathies (acquired or congenital)
         d. Abnormal erythrocyte shapes have been reported in human patients with glomerular hemorrhage, but differentiation of glomerular and nonglomerular hemorrhage by urine erythrocyte appearance has not been reported in veterinary species.
      2. Iatrogenic hemorrhage
         a. Blood vessels may be damaged during bladder palpation, cystocentesis, or catheterization.

         b. Animals with hemostasis defects or urinary mucosal disease may be more prone to iatrogenic hemorrhage.

      3. Genital tract hemorrhage (associated with estrus) in voided samples

IV.   Bacteria in urine sediment (Plate 11D and E)

     A. Physiologic processes: Urine formed by the kidneys should be sterile. Low numbers of bacteria may access the urine via the distal urinary tract or genital tissues.

     B. Analytical concepts

      1. Bacteria in urine sediment are enumerated as a relative density of bacteria seen in most 400× fields (hpf).

      2. Bacteria (especially cocci) may be difficult or impossible to differentiate from small particulate debris by routine sediment examination. Rods and chains of cocci are more easily identified with certainty than are single cocci.

      3. If bacteria are of clinical significance, pyuria is expected but not always found.

      4. Bacteria may multiply in urine after it is collected.

      5. There is no standard method of reporting the concentration of bacteria in urine sediment. Bacterial numbers may be graded (from few to many) or bacteria may simply be reported as present or absent. Routine centrifugation of urine does not concentrate bacteria appreciably in the sediment because they do not "spin down."[81] This is in contrast to other suspended particulates such as cells.

      6. The use of stained air-dried urine preparations for microscopic examination has been suggested as a better way to detect bacteriuria than the use of routine wet-mount preparations.[82]

     C. Bacteriuria (Table 8.12)

      1. Determining the clinical significance of bacteriuria involves consideration of the presence or absence of pyuria, the source of the sample, the concentration of bacteria, and other evidence of a urinary tract infection.

      2. The absence of detectable bacteria in urine sediment does not exclude the possibility of an infection. One should use quantitative urine culture methods whenever a urinary tract infection is suspected. As many as 10,000 rods/mL or 100,000 cocci/mL may be required for detection by routine urinalysis, but as few as 1000 bacteria/mL may be significant in a cystocentesis sample. The decision threshold (based on quantitative culture) between significant bacteriuria and contamination depends on the species of animal and the urine collection method used.[83]

V.   Casts in urine sediment (Plate 11F–H)

     A. Physiologic processes

      1. Casts are cylindrical concretions with round, square, irregular, or tapered ends and of varying widths that mirror the tubular segments in which they formed. They are formed in renal tubular lumens from proteins, intact cells, or cellular debris. Most are thought to have a matrix composed of Tamm-Horsfall mucoproteins secreted by epithelial cells of the loops of Henle, distal tubules, and collecting ducts.

      2. A few casts may form during the normal sloughing of tubular epithelial cells that occurs daily. Casts seen in healthy mammals typically are hyaline casts or fine granular casts. Typically, only a few hyaline or granular casts are found (< 2/lpf), but a shower of casts may occur after physical activity.

B. Analytical concepts
1. Casts in urine sediment are enumerated as the range or mean of casts seen in most 100× fields (lpf).
2. Casts are classified by their appearance, which reflects their content: fine and coarse granular (cell debris and plasma protein), epithelial cell (tubular epithelial cells), erythrocyte, leukocyte, fatty (lipid droplets or lipid accumulation within deteriorated cells), waxy (perhaps deterioration of granular cast), or mixed (combinations of the previously mentioned types).
3. Casts deteriorate in urine (especially alkaline urine) and thus are best detected in fresh urine samples.
4. Casts may be pigmented by bilirubin, hemoglobin, or myoglobin.

C. Cylindruria (casts in urine) (Table 8.12)
1. Casts may form in renal tubules but may not be flushed into urine, or they may be discharged intermittently in showers. Therefore, the absence of cylindruria does not exclude the possibility of active renal tubular disease.
2. Hyaline casts may be found in healthy animals and occur more commonly in animals with glomerular proteinurias.
3. Epithelial or fatty casts typically reflect active tubular degeneration or necrosis. They may be evidence of toxic nephrosis (e.g., gentamicin induced, or hemoglobinuric and myoglobinuric nephropathies) or renal ischemia.
4. Granular casts may similarly form from cellular degeneration and reflect tubular degeneration, necrosis, or inflammation. They may also form from the precipitation of plasma proteins. They can be found in the urine of healthy mammals, possibly related to normal cell turnover or to entrapped proteins.
5. Leukocyte casts reflect inflammation involving renal tubules (e.g., in tubular nephrosis and pyelonephritis).
6. Erythrocyte casts reflect glomerular or tubular hemorrhage.
7. Waxy casts are uncommon and seen primarily with chronic renal disease.
8. Hemoglobin and myoglobin casts are red- to brown-pigmented, granular casts and may be seen with hemoglobinuria or myoglobinuria.

D. Pathogenesis (prevailing theory)
1. Hyaline casts form from the conglutination of the Tamm-Horsfall mucoprotein that is secreted by tubular cells of the loop of Henle, distal tubules, and collecting ducts. The reason for the conglutination is not understood.
2. Granular, lipid, and cellular casts form when cellular debris or cells are trapped in the Tamm-Horsfall mucoprotein. Granular casts may also be formed by the incorporation of plasma proteins into the Tamm-Horsfall mucoprotein matrix. Waxy casts are formed by the deterioration and solidification of granular casts.

VI. Epithelial cells in urine sediment (Plate 11I and J)
A. Physiologic processes
1. Epithelial cells are constantly sloughing from the urinary tract mucosa and are replaced by new cells. Thus, epithelial cells are expected in the urine of healthy animals.
2. Types of epithelial cells vary within the urinary tract. Renal tubular epithelial cells are cuboidal in situ but may be round in suspension, transitional epithelial cells lining the mucosa from the renal pelvis through most of the urethra appear round, and squamous epithelial cells lining the distal urethra appear round or polygonal.

B. Analytical concepts
1. Epithelial cells in urine sediment are enumerated as the range or mean of epithelial cells seen in most $100 \times$ fields (lpf).
2. Some laboratory reports separate epithelial cell populations by origin, but differentiation is problematic:
   a. Superficial squamous epithelial cells are difficult or impossible to differentiate from the occasional transitional epithelial cells that have angular borders.
   b. Round transitional epithelial cells are difficult or impossible to differentiate from the round cells that occur in the intermediate layers of squamous epithelium.
   c. In nonstained sediment, individual renal tubular epithelial cells are difficult or impossible to differentiate from macrophages or small transitional epithelial cells, and clumps of renal tubular epithelium may look similar to transitional epithelium.
3. All cells deteriorate in urine and thus are best examined in fresh urine.
C. Clinical significance of epithelial cells in urine
1. Epithelial cells may be found in the urine of healthy animals, especially in catheterized samples.
2. More transitional epithelial cells may slough from inflamed or hyperplastic mucosa.
3. Neoplastic epithelial cells may be detected in urine sediment. Differentiation of malignant from nonmalignant cells is best accomplished by microscopic examination of stained, air-dried preparations of cells collected by traumatic catheterization or needle biopsy, but preparations of centrifuged, fresh, newly formed urine may also be useful. However, differentiation may be impossible. Dysplastic and proplastic (reactive) cells are common in urine from animals with cystitis and reactive hyperplasia.

VII. Crystals (Plates 11K and L and 13A–G)
A. Physiologic concepts
1. Crystals represent the precipitation of salts (cation + anion).
2. Some salts tend to form at an alkaline pH but dissolve at an acidic pH, whereas others tend to form at an acidic pH but dissolve at an alkaline pH. A salt that is soluble at a certain pH may form crystals if the concentration of the ions is high enough (saturation point) and the materials are present to begin crystal formation (nucleation).
B. Analytical concepts
1. Crystals are enumerated as the number of crystals seen in most $100 \times$ fields (lpf)
2. Enhanced crystal formation may occur in stored urine because of evaporation or because of changes in temperature (especially refrigeration) or pH.[35] Conversely, in other stored samples, some crystals may dissolve.
3. Crystals are routinely identified by their microscopic appearance. Chemical and crystallographic techniques can be used for further characterization (see the Urolith Analysis section).
C. Crystalluria (Table 8.12)
1. The degree of crystalluria depends on the pH, concentration of ions, and temperature of the urine.
2. Most urine crystals can be found in healthy animals. However, increased numbers in the urine sediment may suggest the presence of certain pathologic states that are causing changes in either urine pH or ion concentration.

   3. Presence or absence of crystalluria is not a reliable indicator for the presence or
      absence of urolithiasis (see the Urolith Analysis section), but crystalluria is a risk
      factor for urolithiasis.

VIII. Organisms other than bacteria (Plate 13H–J)
   A. Yeast structures (e.g., *Candida*, *Blastomyces*), hyphal structures (e.g., *Aspergillus* and
      various contaminants), algae (*Prototheca*), and parasitic structures (e.g., *Dioctophyma*,
      Capillaria, and *Stephanurus* ova; and *Dirofilaria* microfilaria) can be found in urine
      (Table 8.12). Identification of fungal structures may require culturing methods.
   B. Parasitic structures may be present because of sample contamination with fecal material.
      Ova of *Capillaria* species may be confused with ova of *Trichuris* species.

IX. Other sediment findings that are of little or no diagnostic significance
   A. Lipid droplets (Plate 13K)
      1. Probably from renal tubular epithelium
      2. Most common in cats, which normally store triglycerides in renal tubular cells
      3. May represent contaminating lubricants used during sample collection
   B. Mucus strands represent urogenital secretions and are abundant in urine of horses
   C. Spermatozoa (Plate 13L)
      1. Spermatozoa are an expected finding in urine from intact male animals, especially in
         voided samples.
      2. Occasionally, spermatozoa are found in urine of female animals after breeding.

QUANTITATIVE URINALYSIS

I. Basic concepts
   A. Quantitative urinalysis includes procedures in which chemical or physical properties
      of urine are measured with quantitative assays. In routine urinalyses, the assays are
      qualitative or semiquantitative. Typically, the purpose of a quantitative UA is to
      quantify the amount of a substance that is excreted by kidneys in a defined time period
      (e.g., 1 d).
   B. Analyte concentrations can be difficult to interpret because concentrations will depend
      on two major variables: the amount of analyte excreted per day and the amount of
      H_2O excreted per day. The relationship of these variables is expressed in Eq. 8.3. Please
      note that an animal would excrete the same amount of analyte per day if there were a
      doubling of the analyte concentration but a halving of the urine volume. An analyte's
      urine concentration can be assessed by considering the USG_{ref} because changes in
      USG_{ref} typically are inversely related to changes in urine volume (except in renal
      failure). More precise assessments usually are accomplished by either timed urine
      collections or by calculating clearance ratios.
   C. Examples of analytes whose renal excretion is assessed via quantitative assays.
      1. Electrolytes: Na^+, K^+, Cl^-, Ca^{2+}, and PO_4
      2. Protein: usually total protein; also albumin and occasionally other individual
         proteins
      3. All solutes combined: total solute excretion via urinary system assessed by osmolality
   D. Assay methods used to quantify the analyte concentration in serum may or may
      not accurately measure an analyte concentration in urine. Assay modifications or
      considerations include the following:

1. To measure urine [Crt], the urine sample needs to be diluted to get the [Crt] into the assay's analytical range. This process can cause inaccuracies.[84] Non-Crt chromogens may give positive interference with some Crt assays. Kinetic Crt assays are designed to minimize the interference of non-Crt chromogens.
2. To measure urine [tCa^{2+}], the urine sample must be acidified before analysis so that Ca^{2+} is in a soluble form and thus able to react with reagents.
3. To measure [K^+] in equine, bovine, and feline urine, a flame photometer should be used. The urine of those species contains a substance that inhibits the reaction of K^+ with ion-selective electrodes.[85]

E. These other factors may need to be considered when interpreting quantitative urinalysis results:
1. Are there appropriate reference intervals for your patient? For some analytes, body weight, diet, age-related factors, or treatments can alter urinary excretion of substances.
2. Is an analyte's urinary excretion decreased because the kidneys are trying to conserve the analyte or because less analyte is being presented to the kidneys?

II. 24 h Excretion studies
A. This is the most definitive method of determining urinary excretion of an analyte but is not frequently used in veterinary medicine because of several factors. First, it requires complete and timed urine collection that is difficult in most domestic mammals. Second, reference intervals are not always available for each species, for different assay methods, and for different diets.
B. Procedure: Begin the urine collection period by completely emptying the urinary bladder and discarding the urine. Collect all urine that is produced in 24 h. End the collection period by emptying the bladder. Measure the total volume of urine collected in 24 h. Measure the analyte's concentration in the collected urine. Finally, calculate the quantity of substance excreted (e.g., Eq. 8.4a). Because of the marked variation in the sizes of domestic mammals, results are usually expressed per kilogram of body weight (Eq. 8.4b).

Amount of analyte excreted in 24 h = analyte concentration × 24 h-urine volume   **(8.4a.)**
Example: analyte concentration = 50 mg/dL; 24 h-urine volume = 300 mL
Amount of analytes excreted in 24 h = 50 mg/dL × 300 mL = 150 mg

Amount of analyte excreted in 24 h per kg body weight =
   analyte concentration ÷ kg × 24 h-urine volume ÷ body wgt   **(8.4b.)**
Example: analyte concentration = 50 mg/dL; 24 h-urine volume = 300 mL; body wgt = 5 kg
Amount of analytes excreted in 24 h per kg body weight =
   50 mg/dL × 300 mL ÷ 5 kg = 30 mg/kg

C. Because a 24 h excretion study is difficult, more convenient methods to assess urinary excretion are usually used. These include urine to plasma ratios or analyte to Crt ratios. Although more convenient, they may be less accurate.

III. Analyte urine to plasma ratios
A. Theory
1. The rate of urinary excretion or clearance of a substance can be calculated by using an excretion rate formula (Eq. 8.5a).

$$\text{Analyte excretion rate} = \frac{[\text{Analyte}]_u}{[\text{Analyte}]_p} \times \text{volume}_u \div \text{time} \div \text{bw} \qquad \textbf{(8.5a.)}$$

$$\text{Analyte excretion rate} \propto \frac{[\text{Analyte}]_u}{[\text{Analyte}]_p} \qquad \textbf{(8.5b.)}$$

2. If urine volume, time, and body weight are considered constants for a given animal, then the urine to plasma ratio is proportional to the rate of urinary excretion of a substance (Eq. 8.5b). Those factors are not constants, but the ratio does tend to reflect the urinary excretion of a substance (analyte) or solutes.

B. Analyte urine to plasma ratios for differentiation of prerenal azotemia and renal azotemia

1. The urine osmolality to plasma osmolality ratio reflects the kidneys' ability to conserve H_2O.

   a. A high ratio reflects an ability to concentrate solutes. An animal with prerenal azotemia caused by dehydration should have a high ratio.

   b. A ratio near 1.0 indicates isosthenuria and thus failure to concentrate or dilute the ultrafiltrate solutes. In an animal with renal azotemia, the ratio should be near 1.0.

   c. A ratio much below 1.0 is not expected in most azotemic animals because the ratio would indicate renal diluting ability is present. Azotemic animals usually either form hypersthenuric urine (a high ratio in prerenal azotemia) or cannot concentrate or dilute their urine (a ratio near 1.0 in renal azotemia).

2. The urine UN to plasma UN and urine Crt to plasma Crt ratios assess the renal ability to excrete nitrogenous wastes.

   a. Higher ratios reflect the kidneys' ability to excrete nitrogenous waste via urine and thus are evidence of adequate renal function.

   b. Lower ratios reflect decreased renal excretion of urea or Crt (i.e., a decreased GFR) and would support the conclusion of renal azotemia, but they also may occur with prerenal and postrenal azotemias.

3. Published ratios for horses illustrate the application of the ratios (also called *urinary indices*) (Table 8.13). The ratios would vary between species, but the general concepts apply across species.

IV. Quantitative urine total protein assays: These are typically not part of a routine urinalysis but are used to determine a more accurate urine [protein] for protein to Crt ratios, for urine electrophoresis calculations, or for 24 h excretion studies.

A. Trichloroacetic acid method

1. Principle: Proteins are denatured by acids and form a precipitate that is seen as increased solution turbidity.

2. The trichloroacetic acid method is less affected by the albumin to globulin ratio in the sample than is the SSA method. The trichloroacetic acid method is temperature sensitive and needs to be completed at 20–25 °C.[86]

B. Coomassie brilliant blue assay

1. Principle: The amount of dye binding to amine groups of amino acids is proportional to the quantity of protein present.

Table 8.13. Urinary indices for differentiation of prerenal and renal azotemia in horses

	Healthy horses	Prerenal azotemia	Renal azotemia
Number of horses	6	6	10
Osmolality$_u$ (mmol/kg)	727–1456	458–961	226–495
Osm$_u$:Osm$_p$[a] ratio	2.5–5.2	1.7–3.4	0.8–1.7
[UN]$_u$:[UN]$_p$[b] ratio	34–100	15–44	2–14
[Crt]$_u$:[Crt]$_p$[c] ratio	2–344	51–242	3–37
FE of Na$^+$	0.0–0.70	0.0–0.5	0.8–10.1

Source: (adapted from): Grossman et al.[116]

[a] Urine osmolality to plasma osmolality

[b] Urine concentration of UN to plasma concentration of UN

[c] Urine concentration of Crt to plasma concentration of Crt

    2. This assay is minimally affected by albumin to globulin ratios in the urine and will detect Bence Jones proteins.

  C. Benzethonium chloride assay

    1. Principle: Benzethonium chloride reacts with proteins to produce a turbidity that is proportional to the amount of protein present.

    2. This quantitative turbidimetric assay is reported to react similarly with albumin and γ-globulins. Hemoglobin will react with the reagent.

  D. Quantitative urine albumin assays: Species-specific immunologic assays are used to measure low concentrations of albumin in urine (see Quantitative Urinalysis, sect. VI).

V.   Urinary protein to creatinine (Prot:Crt)$_u$ ratio

  A. Theory

    1. Increased protein loss via the urinary system is best determined by a 24 h protein excretion study; that is, determining the milligrams of protein lost per day per kilogram of body weight. However, such a study requires a timed and complete urine collection.

    2. Crt clearance via the urinary system is considered to be relatively constant in health. In addition, if urinary Crt clearance is decreased, then the rate of glomerular protein loss should be decreased because Crt passes more easily through the glomerular filtration barrier than do protein molecules. However, if more protein enters the urine through damaged glomeruli or through other processes, then the rate of protein excretion compared to Crt excretion will be increased.

    3. Considering the aforementioned concepts, comparing the rate of urinary protein loss to the Crt excretion should reflect true changes in protein loss via the urinary system. This concept can be seen in the comparison of urinary excretion formulas and the derivation of the (Prot:Crt)$_u$ ratio (Eq. 8.6).

$$\frac{\text{Protein excretion rate}}{\text{Creatinine excretion rate}} = \frac{\dfrac{[\text{Prot}]_u}{[\text{Prot}]_s} \times \text{volume}_u \div \text{time} \div \text{bw}}{\dfrac{[\text{Crt}]_u}{[\text{Crt}]_s} \times \text{volume}_u \div \text{time} \div \text{bw}} \qquad (8.6.)$$

For a randomly collected urine sample, some factors in the numerator and denominator formulas are either the same or remain relatively constant.
- The urine volume, the time over which the urine formed, and the body weight values are the same in both formulas.
- The serum [Prot] and [Crt] probably remained constant during the time the collected urine was formed.

Therefore, the relative rate of protein excretion compared to creatinine excretion can be estimated as follows.

$$\frac{\text{Protein excretion rate}}{\text{Creatinine excretion rate}} = \frac{\dfrac{[\text{Prot}]_u}{\text{constant}}}{\dfrac{[\text{Crt}]_u}{\text{constant}}} \quad or \quad \frac{\text{Protein excretion rate}}{\text{Creatinine excretion rate}} \propto \frac{[\text{Prot}]_u}{[\text{Crt}]_u} = (\text{Prot:Crt})_u \text{ ratio}$$

B. Analytical concepts
   1. Unless there is severe proteinuria, urine protein concentrations are below the analytical range of serum protein assays. Thus, different assays (collectively called *microprotein assays*) are needed to measure [protein] in most urine samples. Besides having an appropriate analytical range, a good microprotein assay will be minimally affected by types of proteins in the urine; that is, it should detect nearly all proteins equally.
   2. Most analytical methods designed for measuring serum [Crt] can be used for measuring urine [Crt]. However, for most urine samples, the urine must be diluted to produce a [Crt] that is within the analytical range of the assay, and varying the dilution ratio can cause inaccuracies.[84] Some benchtop analyzers have been shown to undermeasure urine [Crt] (especially at high concentrations) and thus produce higher (Prot:Crt)$_u$ ratios.[84]
C. Published data
   1. When dogs with potential nonrenal proteinuria were excluded, there was good correlation between the (Prot:Crt)$_u$ ratio and the quantity of urinary protein excreted per day (either mg/d or mg/kg/d).[87-89] Results of three studies are compared in Table 8.14. Note that the highest ratios for healthy dogs in the three studies were 0.54, 0.17, and 0.38 with two different protein assays, and the 0.54 and 0.38 values were from the same type of assay. Although differences in reference sample groups may have contributed to differences in the ratios, method differences also likely affected the results. Most recommended guidelines do not acknowledge the need for specific decision thresholds for different protein and Crt methods.
   2. Interpretation guidelines for the (Prot:Crt)$_u$ ratio based on these studies
      a. Healthy dogs: (Prot:Crt)$_u$ ratio < 0.5
      b. Borderline values: (Prot:Crt)$_u$ ratio = 0.5–1.0
      c. Dogs with glomerular proteinuria: (Prot:Crt)$_u$ ratio > 1.0 (Note: Other forms of proteinuria could give similar results but were excluded from the studies that were cited.)
   3. (Prot:Crt)$_u$ ratios were not influenced by collection period (day or night) or gender of animal.[90]
D. Diagnostic significance of increased (Prot:Crt)$_u$ ratio

Table 8.14. (Prot:Crt)$_u$ ratios and 24 h urinary protein excretion studies in dogs

	Group	White et al.[a,b 87]	Grauer et al.[b,c 112]	Center et al.[a,b 89]
(Prot:Crt)$_u$ ratio	Healthy	0.08–0.54 (8)[d]	0.02–0.17 (16)	0.01–0.38 (19)
	Proteinuric[e]	1.09–8.63 (10)	0.48–15.1 (14)	0.47–46.65 (38)
24 h Urinary protein	Healthy	1.9–11.7 (8)	0.6–5.1 (16)	0.2–7.7 (19)
excretion (mg/kg)	Proteinuric	32.2–271.1 (10)	12.2–287.5 (14)	7.5–533.7 (38)[f]

[a] Protein method: trichloroacetic acid protein method

[b] Crt method: alkaline picric acid

[c] Protein method: Coomassie brilliant blue

[d] The number in parenthesis is the number of dogs in a study group.

[e] Dogs with or suspected of having either prerenal or postrenal proteinuria were excluded from the studies.

[f] The dog with a protein loss of 7.5 mg/kg was included in the proteinuric group because it had glomerulonephritis and its (Prot:Crt)$_u$ ratio was increased (0.47).

1. The (Prot:Crt)$_u$ ratio should be increased in any animal with proteinuria, including prerenal (overflow), glomerular, tubular, and inflammatory/hemorrhagic proteinurias. Other clinical information is used to differentiate the proteinurias (see Chemical Examination of Urine, sect. III.C).

2. Glomerular proteinurias tend to be more severe and cause hypoalbuminemia or hypoproteinemia. However, earlier stages of glomerular damage may cause only mild proteinuria. In the absence of hyperproteinemia and increased cell concentrations in the urine, large increases in the (Prot:Crt)$_u$ ratio (e.g., > 5.0) suggest glomerular proteinuria. The ratios in cases of renal amyloidosis typically are higher than the ratios in cases of glomerulonephritis, but the observed values overlap considerably.[91]

3. Estimated (Prot:Crt)$_u$ ratio

    a. A semiquantitative method of estimating a (Prot:Crt)$_u$ ratio is available (Petstix 8 reagent strips).

    b. Until critical studies are available that assess the predictive values of the system with veterinary samples, the method probably should be considered to be another subjective assessment of urinary protein excretion and similar to interpreting the relationship between urine [protein] and USG$_{ref}$.

E. Comparison of urine [protein] to urine [Crt] reduces the variability caused by the amount of H_2O excreted by kidneys. If all else is equal, renal conservation of H_2O will cause a proportional increase in urine [protein] and urine [Crt]. Similar information could be obtained for less expense by dividing the urine [protein] by a factor derived from the USG$_{ref}$ (such as the last two digits or USG$_{ref}$ − 1). Diluting urine samples to a consistent USG$_{ref}$ of 1.010 prior to analysis, as is done with immunologic microalbuminuria assays (see the next section), standardizes the solute concentration so that protein concentrations can be compared without using calculations to correct for differences in urine concentration.

VI. Microalbuminuria

    A. General concepts

        1. In the classic view of renal functions, mammalian glomeruli are not permeable to albumin because it has a strong negative charge and the albumin molecular diameter

(36 Å) is close to the diameter of a glomerular pore (42 Å).[51] However, the glomerular filtration barrier does allow slightly smaller proteins to pass into the ultrafiltrate, from which they are resorbed by the proximal tubules. If there is minor damage to the barrier (a reduced negative charge or damaged podocytes), then albumin enters the tubular fluid. Incomplete resorption of the albumin causes albuminuria. With increasing damage, larger proteins (various globulins) also pass into the tubular fluid.

2. In random urine samples from healthy people, renal excretion of albumin results in a urine [albumin] < 3 mg/dL or < 20 mg excreted per day.[92] In this context, microalbuminuria is defined as a urinary albumin loss greater than those values but less than 20 mg/dL.[93] Using regular urinalysis reagent strips, such albumin concentrations might create trace protein reactions.

3. For many years, the protein reaction of a typical urinalysis was expected to be negative in the urine of healthy cats, horses, and cattle. However, a trace or 1 + reaction in concentrated canine urine was accepted as a species variation and not evidence of a pathologic state.[58] Moreover, bands corresponding to albumin are often present in electrophoresis gels of urine from clinically normal dogs.[64,94,95] However more recently, some have considered that the mild proteinurias in clinical healthy dogs represent evidence of subclinical glomerular disease.[96] Consequently, assays have been developed to measure low urine albumin concentrations; that is, to detect microalbuminuria.

4. The current working definition of *microalbuminuria* in dogs and cats is urine albumin concentrations from 1 mg/dL to 30 mg/dL in urine adjusted to a USG_{ref} of 1.010.[96,97] Concentrations > 30 mg/dL are referred to as *albuminuria* or *overt albuminuria*. It is important to remember that a urine [albumin] of 30 mg/dL in urine with a USG_{ref} of 1.010 would have an [albumin] of 60 mg/dL if the USG_{ref} was 1.020, or 120 mg/dL if the USG_{ref} was 1.040.

5. Some authors state that 30 mg/dL is the decision threshold for microalbuminuria because common urinalysis methods do not detect protein concentrations < 30 mg/dL. However, the Chemstrip package insert states that, in 90 % of urines tested, protein concentrations ≥ 6 mg/dL produced a color change. For the Multistix system, a trace reaction corresponds with an estimated [protein] of 10 mg/dL. When turbidity standard solutions are used with the SSA test, increased turbidity can be detected when [protein] is 5 mg/dL.

B. Analytical concepts

1. Quantitative immunologic assay

a. The immunologic microalbumin assays are species specific because of the species differences in albumin molecules. Enzyme-linked immunosorbent assays (ELISAs) and nephelometric assays have been developed for canine and feline urine.[93]

b. The standard solutions for the assays are canine or feline albumin. For one ELISA, standard solutions were diluted to create an analytical range of 1.9–30 ng/mL (0.19–3.00 μg/dL).[93] Urine samples were diluted (up to 1 : 3200) to obtain urine albumin concentrations within the analytical range of the assay, but such marked dilutions can be a source of analytical error.[98]

2. Semiquantitative immunologic assays

a. Commercial assays are marketed as ImmunoDip Canine and ImmunoDip Feline; both are called E.R.D.-HealthScreen Urine Tests (E.R.D. is an abbreviation for early renal disease). These assays are similar to an assay developed for human urine (Immunodip, Diagnostic Chemicals).

  b. After the urine solute concentration has been adjusted to a specific gravity near 1.010, the device is dipped into the urine, and then the reaction is graded visually. A negative reaction is expected if the [albumin] is < 1 mg/dL. Higher concentrations are graded from low positive to very high positive based on color changes in the device.

3. Albumin to creatinine ratio

  a. Bayer Diagnostics markets a reagent pad method of estimating an albumin to Crt ratio (Clinitek Microalbumin). The albumin reaction is a dye-binding method with color changes representing 0, 1, 3, 8, 15, and 50 mg/dL. The Crt reaction is a peroxidase-like assay with color changes corresponding to 30, 100, 200, and 300 mg/dL. When the color changes are read by reflectance photometry in a Bayer instrument (Clinitek), an estimated albumin to Crt ratio is calculated. The reported units of the ratios vary: 300 mg/g = 300 µg/mg = 0.3 mg/mg (or just 0.3).

  b. The albumin assay is not specific for albumin. Many other proteins will react with the dye including light chains, immunoglobulins, β_2-microglobulin, Tamm-Horsfall protein, hemoglobin, and myoglobin.[92] However, other than hemoglobin and myoglobin, most of these proteins are not expected to be in urine at sufficient concentrations to produce a false-positive albumin reaction.

  c. In one comparison using canine urine samples, the authors concluded that the available dipstick method (Clinitek Microalbumin) was not reliable for detection of microalbuminuria. The results of a dipstick method were compared to the results of a canine albumin-capture ELISA; albumin concentrations were normalized to a specific gravity of 1.010.[93] The Bayer albumin to Crt ratio method correctly classified 48 % of the microalbuminuric samples (i.e., those with albumin concentrations of 1–30 mg/dL). Some samples were hematuric (erythrocytes > 5/hpf, > 1+ heme reaction), and hemoglobin can bind to the reagent dye.[92] Thus, some discrepancies may have been due to proteins other than albumin binding to the reagent in the dipstick.

4. Comparison to other urine protein assays

  a. [Protein] estimated by routine protein assays of urinalyses (i.e., the reagent pad method and SSA turbidity) represents the sum of albumin and globulin concentrations. Both methods detect albumin better than most globulins, but globulins do contribute to the reactions. The detection limits of these assays vary (Table 8.10).

  b. The SSA assay is also called the *bumintest* because it detects albumin better than globulins. When a sample's result is compared to standard solutions, turbidity can be detected at an [albumin] of 5 mg/dL. If a very mild proteinuria is caused by glomerular disease, albumin will be the dominant protein in the urine.

  c. The results of these routine protein assays are typically not normalized to a specific gravity of 1.010. However, their results should be interpreted with knowledge of the sample's USG_{ref} so that an estimated adjustment can be made. In a concentrated urine sample in which microalbuminuria is detected after normalization to 1.010, it would not be unusual for common protein dipstick

reactions to produce a trace or 1 + reaction or for the SSA assay to have 1+
turbidity.

C. Canine microalbuminuria

1. There have been several published abstracts pertaining to the use of the ImmunoDip
   Canine test, but very few peer review publications. Because the abstracts did not
   contain complete information about materials and methods, it is difficult to
   critically review the available data.[99–101]

2. It is important to remember that microalbuminuria is not unique to glomerular
   disease. Microalbuminuria may be caused by any of the diseases and conditions that
   cause proteinuria (prerenal, glomerular, tubular, or hemorrhagic/inflammatory).
   Thus, the presence of microalbuminuria should be interpreted in the context of
   other clinical information. Clinical information (history, physical examination
   findings, urinalysis, and other routine laboratory results) typically enables one to
   recognize prerenal and hemorrhagic/inflammatory proteinurias. It is more difficult to
   differentiate glomerular from tubular proteinurias.[66]

3. The effects of urinary tract inflammation or hemorrhage on the urine [albumin]
   were explored by using a capture ELISA for canine [albumin] that the authors
   acknowledged was not fully validated.[97] The measured albumin concentrations were
   < 1 mg/dL in about two-thirds of the samples that had pyuria and in about half of
   the samples that had hematuria and pyuria.

4. In contrast to findings in people, exercise did not increase the urinary excretion of
   albumin in 26 dogs.[102]

VII. Fractional excretion (FE) ratios or percentages

A. Theory

1. In a random urine sample, the FE of substance X will reflect the relative rate of
   urinary excretion of substance X compared to Crt. If substance X passes freely
   through the glomerular filtration barrier and is neither secreted nor resorbed (like
   Crt), the FE would be 1.0. If some of substance X were resorbed after freely
   entering the filtrate, the FE would be < 1.0. Therefore, for solutes that freely pass
   the glomerular filtration barrier (e.g., electrolytes), FE is the fraction of the solute
   entering the filtrate or tubular fluid that is ultimately excreted. Substance X can be
   an electrolyte, an enzyme, or another solute. For the derivation of the FE formula
   (Eq. 8.7), substance X is Na^+.

$$\frac{\text{Urinary } Na^+ \text{ excretion rate}}{\text{Urinary creatinine excretion rate}} = \frac{\dfrac{\left[Na^+\right]_u}{\left[Na^+\right]_s} \times \text{volume}_u \div \text{time} \div \text{bw}}{\dfrac{\left[Crt\right]_u}{\left[Crt\right]_s} \times \text{volume}_u \div \text{time} \div \text{bw}} \qquad (8.7.)$$

For a randomly collected urine sample:

• Urine volume, time the over which urine formed, and the body weight values are
  the same in both formulas and thus cancel out.
• Serum [Na^+] and [Crt] will probably be nearly the same but can vary.
• Urine [Na^+] and [Crt] are expected to vary because of multiple factors.

Considering these factors, the relative rates of Na^+ and Crt urinary excretion can be
expressed as follows:

$$\frac{\text{Urinary Na}^+ \text{ excretion}}{\text{Urinary creatinine excretion}} = \frac{\dfrac{[Na^+]_u}{[Na^+]_s}}{\dfrac{[Crt]_u}{[Crt]_s}} = \frac{[Na^+]_u}{[Na^+]_s} \times \frac{[Crt]_s}{[Crt]_u}$$

$$\text{Therefore, fractional excretion of Na}^+ \left(\text{F.E. of Na}^+\right) = \frac{[Na^+]_u}{[Na^+]_s} \times \frac{[Crt]_s}{[Crt]_u}$$

$$\text{Or expressed as a percentage, percent excretion of Na}^+ = \frac{[Na^+]_u}{[Na^+]_s} \times \frac{[Crt]_s}{[Crt]_u} \times 100$$

      2. A major advantage of the FE study over a 24 h excretion study is that the assessment can be done on a random single urine sample. However, the urine and serum (or plasma) samples for the assessment should be collected near the same time. A FE value typically will be a better assessment of renal functions than a simple ratio of urine analyte concentration to plasma analyte concentration because FE considers variations in renal excretions caused by altered GFR.

B. Interpretive concepts

      1. A FE ratio provides the relative rate of excretion of an analyte compared to Crt. For a FE ratio to reflect the 24 h urinary excretion of an analyte accurately, Crt excretion needs to be within the reference interval and relatively constant.

      2. An increased FE ratio may reflect increased urinary excretion of an analyte.

         a. Plasma analyte concentrations are increased (resulting in increased filtered load), and the kidneys are attempting to excrete the excess. This may occur with increased dietary intake of the analyte.

         b. Increased tubular secretion of the analyte

         c. Decreased tubular resorption of the analyte

      3. Decreased FE ratio of an analyte may result from the opposite processes.

         a. Plasma analyte concentrations are decreased (resulting in decreased filtered load), and the kidneys are attempting to conserve the analyte. This may occur with decreased dietary intake of the analyte.

         b. Decreased tubular secretion of the analyte

         c. Increased tubular resorption of the analyte

      4. An increased FE ratio may also occur with decreased Crt excretion.

         a. An increased FE of K^+ would occur if the renal excretion of K^+ is maintained through secretion of K^+ but Crt excretion is decreased because of decreased GFR.

         b. FE of PO_4 may be increased because of decreased GFR (thus less filtration of Crt and PO_4) and decreased tubular resorption of filtered PO_4 because of increased PTH activity.

C. The assays used to measure analyte concentrations in serum or plasma may not provide accurate results for urine samples.

      1. Urine can contain an inhibitor that interferes with the ion-selective electrode assay for $[K^+]$.[85]

      2. Urine may need to be acidified to promote dissociation of ion complexes; for example, Ca^{2+} dissociation from PO_4 or other anions.

      3. Some assay systems require the protein matrix of serum or plasma, and the nearly protein-free fluid (urine) may not be acceptable.

    D. Clinical uses of fractional excretion studies
1. FE of Na^+
    a. In a hyponatremic animal, an increased FE of Na^+ indicates that renal excretion of Na^+ is contributing to the hyponatremia. Such a process may reflect decreased aldosterone activity, increased atrial natriuretic peptide, or renal tubular disease.
    b. In a hyponatremic animal, a decreased FE of Na^+ indicates that extrarenal factors are causing the hyponatremia and that the kidneys are attempting to conserve Na^+ through the actions of aldosterone, angiotensin II, or ADH.
    c. FE of Na^+ increases in renal failure and decreases with prerenal azotemia, whereas GFR is decreased in both conditions.
2. FE of PO_4
    a. In a hypocalcemic animal, an increased FE of PO_4 suggests increased PTH activity as may occur with nutritional or renal secondary hyperparathyroidism.
    b. In a hypocalcemic animal, a decreased FE of PO_4 suggests that decreased PTH activity may be contributing to the hypocalcemic state.
    c. In a patient with hypercalcemia caused by primary hyperparathyroidism, the FE of PO_4 is increased.
3. FE of GGT
    a. GGT is part of renal tubular cell membranes, so more GGT is excreted in urine when there is renal tubular cell damage. GGT activity in a random urine sample may or may not be increased with renal tubular disease. GGT activity should reflect the [GGT] in the urine, which is determined by relative amounts of GGT and H_2O in the urine. Thus, dilute urine would be expected to have lower GGT activity than does concentrated urine.
    b. An increased FE of GGT indicates active renal tubular damage or necrosis. It does not determine whether there is or is not renal insufficiency or failure, and it does not reflect GFR.[103]

    E. FE studies are not commonly used in veterinary medicine because information obtained may not be required for diagnosis and case management. Also, appropriate reference intervals are difficult to obtain for each species, especially when one considers that separate reference intervals may be needed for different assay systems and different diets.

VIII. Urine bile acid to creatinine ratio

Determining the urinary excretion of bile acids relative to Crt excretion is used as a method to detect abnormal bile acid metabolism by the liver. Details of this diagnostic method are presented in Chapter 13.

H_2O DEPRIVATION AND ANTIDIURETIC HORMONE (ADH) RESPONSE TESTS IN ANIMALS WITH POLYURIA AND POLYDIPSIA (PU/PD)

I. Renal concentrating ability is assessed in a routine urinalysis by determining the USG_{ref}. Typically, the USG_{ref} along with other case information (historical and physical findings and other laboratory data) enables veterinarians to identify the probable causes of a PU/PD disorder (see Tables 8.8 and 8.9). When a more critical assessment of renal concentrating ability is needed, and especially if central diabetes insipidus is suspected, either H_2O

deprivation or ADH response tests may be considered. Because interpretation guidelines may differ when specific aspects of the challenges vary, the following provides the major concepts (reference articles or texts should be consulted for specific interpretation guidelines):

II.   Abrupt H_2O deprivation test[23]
   A. General concepts
      1. The basic purpose is to assess the ability of the kidneys to concentrate the ultrafiltrate by inducing an abrupt stimulus (hypovolemia or hyperosmolality) for renal H_2O retention. The test may be used to evaluate undiagnosed PU/PD patients that consistently have urine with $USG_{ref} < 1.020$.
      2. The test is contraindicated in azotemic animals (or those known to have decreased GFR) or in dehydrated patients (already challenged to concentrate). The procedure can be dangerous in severe PU states, because the animal can quickly become severely hypovolemic.
   B. Basics of the procedure
      1. Baseline information is collected and may include body weight, USG_{ref}, urine and serum osmolality, and serum $[Na^+]$.
      2. Access to H_2O is abruptly removed, the animal is monitored, and the findings are compared with baseline information until they indicate one of the following:
         a. The animal has become dangerously dehydrated.
         b. The kidneys can concentrate urine.
         c. The animal was adequately challenged, and its kidneys did not adequately concentrate urine.
   C. Basic interpretations
      1. If the animal demonstrates ability to concentrate urine (the USG_{ref} or urine osmolality criteria are exceeded), the PU/PD state is a primary PD disorder.
      2. If the animal does not demonstrate ability to concentrate urine, several possibilities exist.
         a. The procedure had to be halted before renal concentrating mechanisms produced concentrated urine.
         b. Secondary medullary hypotonicity (medullary washout) may be present because of persistent polyuria from a variety of disorders.
         c. A disorder that causes nephrogenic diabetes insipidus is present.
         d. Central diabetes insipidus is present.

III. Gradual H_2O deprivation test[23]
   A. The purpose, indications, and contraindications are the same as for the abrupt H_2O deprivation test. The gradual H_2O deprivation test is indicated if medullary washout from prolonged PU is expected or if there is failure to concentrate urine after abrupt H_2O deprivation. The gradual decrease in H_2O intake will enable the kidneys to reestablish a medullary concentration gradient. It tends to be a less dangerous procedure in severely PU animals, but animals still must be monitored thoroughly for development of dehydration.
   B. The major difference between the gradual and the abrupt procedures is that H_2O intake and urine output are measured and recorded over 2 or more days. Then, H_2O availability is decreased by 10 % each day. Like the abrupt test, the animal must be monitored for evidence of dangerous dehydration and ability to concentrate urine.

    C. Advantages of the gradual H_2O deprivation are that it tends to be less dangerous and allows time for reestablishment of medullary hypertonicity. The major disadvantage is the time requirement; it may take over a week to complete the test.

IV. ADH (vasopressin) response test[23]
    A. The basic purposes are to assess the ability of the kidneys to respond to exogenous ADH and to confirm a complete or partial absence of ADH (diabetes insipidus) in a PU/PD patient. It may be more justified when H_2O deprivation does not lead to concentrated urine.
    B. Basics of the procedure
       1. H_2O access is ad libitum during the study.
       2. After administration of aqueous vasopressin or deamino-D-arginine vasopressin (DDAVP), renal concentrating ability is assessed by measuring the USG_{ref} or urine osmolality.
    C. Expected findings
       1. Central diabetes insipidus: The kidneys did not concentrate urine during H_2O deprivation but did when stimulated by exogenous ADH.
       2. Nephrogenic diabetes insipidus: The kidneys did not concentrate urine during H_2O deprivation or after stimulation by exogenous ADH. The same results may occur with "medullary washout" caused by any primary PU or PD disorder.

V. Modified H_2O deprivation test[104]
    A. Combination of H_2O deprivation test and ADH response test
    B. Procedure
       1. Abruptly deprive the animal of H_2O and then measure urine osmolality hourly until the increase in urine osmolality between consecutive hourly samples is < 5 %.
       2. ADH administered and urine collected 1 h after injection
    C. Expected results
       1. Healthy dogs: urine osmolality after H_2O deprivation > 1000 mmol/kg, and a 0 % increase in urine osmolality after ADH administration
       2. Partial central diabetes insipidus and partial renal diabetes insipidus cases (including dogs with hyperadrenocorticism): urine osmolality after H_2O deprivation < 600 mmol/kg, and a 20–50 % increase in urine osmolality after ADH administration
       3. Central diabetes insipidus cases: urine osmolality after H_2O deprivation < 300 mmol/kg, and a > 100 % increase in urine osmolality after ADH administration
       4. Primary polydipsia cases: The response should be similar to that of healthy dogs if the kidneys have medullary hypertonicity, but there may be a poor response if "medullary washout" is present.

UROLITH ANALYSIS

I. A *urolith* (or *urinary calculus*) is a solid concretion (stone) that forms within the urinary tract and typically is found in a renal pelvis, urinary bladder, urethra, or voided urine. Learning the composition of a urolith provides evidence for the pathogenesis of its formation and aids in developing therapeutic plans to remove or to reduce chances for recurrence. Uroliths are found most commonly in dogs and are relatively uncommon in cats,

Table 8.15. Inorganic composition of uroliths[a]

Group	Chemical name	Formula	Mineralogic name
Carbonate	Calcium carbonate	$CaCO_3$	Calcite, aragonite, vaterite
Cystine	Cystine	$S\ CH_2\ CH(NH_2)COOH$	Cystine
Oxalates	Calcium oxalate monohydrate	$CaC_2O_4 \cdot H_2O$	Whewellite
	Calcium oxalate dihydrate	$CaC_2O_4 \cdot 2H_2O$	Weddellite
Phosphates	Basic calcium phosphate	$Ca_5(PO_4)_3(OH)$	Apatite
	Hydroxyapatite	$Ca_{10}(PO_4)_6(OH)_2$	Hydroxyapatite
	Carbonate-apatite	$Ca_{10}(PO_4, CO_3OH)_6(OH)_2$	Carbonate-apatite
	Calcium hydrogen phosphate dihydrate	$CaHPO_4 \cdot 2H_2O$	Brushite
	Tricalcium phosphate	$Ca_3(PO_4)_2$	Whitlockite
	Octacalcium phosphate	$CaH(PO_4)_3 \cdot 2 \cdot 5H_2O$	—
	Magnesium ammonium phosphate hexahydrate	$MgNH_4PO_4 \cdot 6H_2O$	Struvite
	Magnesium hydrogen phosphate trihydrate	$MgHPO_4 \cdot 3H_2O$	Newberyite
Silica	Silicone dioxide	SiO_2	Silica
Uric acids	Anhydrous uric acid	$C_5H_4N_4O_3$	—
	Uric acid dihydrate	$C_5H_4N_4O_3 \cdot 2H_2O$	—
Urates	Ammonium acid urate[b]	$C_5H_3N_4O_3NH_4$	—
	Sodium acid urate monohydrate	$C_5H_3N_4O_3Na \cdot H_2O$	—

[a] A urolith is classified as to a specific type if at least 70 % of its composition is composed of that mineral. If it does not meet that criterion, it is referred to as a mixed urolith.

[b] Also known as ammonium hydrogen urate or ammonium biurate

horses, and cattle. Most urinary tract obstructions in cats are not caused by uroliths but by plugs consisting of phosphate crystals and mucoid material. Uroliths are not large urine crystals but consist of aggregated crystals and an organic matrix. Crystals form with a unique three-dimensional structure. The chemical compositions of uroliths are listed in Table 8.15.

II. Two issues of the *Veterinary Clinics of North America* contain valuable information regarding the detection, analysis, treatment, and management of canine uroliths.[105,106] Updated information can be found in medicine textbooks for individual species.

III. Analytical concepts
   A. For many years, uroliths were analyzed chemically with a series of qualitative chemical reactions to detect the presence of certain cations and anions. These chemical methods are nearly obsolete because (1) they did not agree well with results of quantitative crystallographic methods, (2) they did not provide a relative amount of each constituent, (3) significant amounts of some ions were missed, (4) they lacked methods for detecting silica and cystine, (5) false-positive results occurred for some compounds, and (6) mixed uroliths could not be classified.[107]

B. The chemical methods have been replaced by physical analytical methods. These analyses are offered by a few specialized laboratories (e.g., the Minnesota Urolith Center, the Urolithiasis Laboratory at Baylor College of Medicine, the Urinary Stone Analysis Laboratory at the University of California–Davis, and the Canadian Veterinary Urolith Centre at the University of Guelph).[108–110]

1. Optical crystallography: Ground urolith material is examined with a polarizing microscope after the material is placed in a series of oils with different refractive indices. Each crystal is identified when its refractive index is matched with one of the oils (i.e., it disappears). Different layers of the urolith are analyzed to determine the composition of each layer.

2. X-ray diffraction: Ground urolith material is bombarded with X-rays. As the X-rays hit a crystal, they are diffracted (scattered) in a unique way for each crystal. The diffractions are recorded to determine the chemical composition of the urolith.

3. Other less common methods: electron microprobe, scanning electron microscopy, and infrared spectroscopy

IV. Pathogenesis of urolith formation: Urolith formation is a complex process that involves many factors that promote and others that inhibit formation. The major steps of urolith formation are as follows:[111]

A. The cations and anions of the urolith are present at supersaturated concentrations in urine.

B. The cations and anions combine into a unique crystalline structure. Factors such as pH, temperature, and flow rate influence crystallization. This process occurs more easily when it occurs on the surface of debris, casts, or other urine particles, a process called *heterogeneous nucleation*. These crystals may be seen in urine sediment and usually do not grow fast enough to become lodged in the urinary tract; instead, they are flushed out via the urine.

C. The crystals can combine into aggregates relatively quickly. If the small aggregates are not passed, then they provide a surface for additional crystallization and aggregation.

D. The formation of crystals and aggregates is naturally inhibited by a variety of substances. For example, citrate binds Ca^{2+} and thus limits its availability for crystal formation. Tamm-Horsfall protein is produced by the renal tubular cells and is a natural inhibitor of aggregation.

E. During the formation of many uroliths, variable amounts of matrix are incorporated into the urolith. In people, the matrix is composed mostly of hexosamine, which might be a product of Tamm-Horsfall (uromucoid) degeneration.

V. Predisposing or contributing factors for urolith formation: Factors that contribute to crystalluria typically also contribute to urolith formation. In addition, increased amounts of the noncrystalline matrix and lower amounts of inhibitors will promote aggregation.

A. Struvite uroliths are associated with urinary tract infections, especially by urease-producing bacteria, which degrade urea and increase the urine's alkalinity.

B. Calcium phosphate uroliths are associated with urinary tract infections (see struvite) and hypercalciuria caused by hypercalcemia.

C. Calcium oxalate uroliths occur with increased urinary excretion of Ca^{2+} associated with hypercalcemia, increased intake of Ca^{2+} or vitamin D. They also occur with increased urinary excretion of oxalate because of ingestion of material with high oxalate content (chocolate, nuts, spinach, sweet potatoes, wheat germ, and oxalate-containing plants such as halogeton).

D. Urate uroliths are found primarily in Dalmatians and English bulldogs because of their excretion of urate via kidneys, but they are also found in dogs with portosystemic shunts or hepatic insufficiency.

E. Cystine uroliths are found in dogs that have defective metabolic pathways that lead to cystinuria, including English bulldogs, Newfoundlands, dachshunds, mastiffs, bullmastiffs, Australian cattle dogs, and Scottish deerhounds.

F. Xanthine uroliths are found in dogs treated with xanthine oxidase to control urate urolithiasis and in dogs with xanthinuria (cavalier King Charles spaniels and dachshunds).

G. Silica urolith formation in dogs has been associated with ingestion of diets containing corn gluten feed or soybean hulls. Silica uroliths may form in cattle grazing silica-rich soils.

References

1. Rose BD. 1994. *Clinical Physiology of Acid-Base and Electrolyte Disorders*, 4th edition. New York: McGraw-Hill.
2. O'Connell JMB, Romeo JA, Mudge GH. 1962. Renal tubular secretion of creatinine in the dog. Am J Physiol 203:985–990.
3. Robinson T, Harbison M, Bovee KC. 1974. Influence of reduced renal mass on tubular secretion of creatinine in the dog. Am J Vet Res 35:487–491.
4. Finco DR, Groves C. 1985. Mechanism of renal excretion of creatinine by the pony. Am J Vet Res 46:1625–1628.
5. Finco DR, Barsanti JA. 1982. Mechanism of urinary excretion of creatinine by the cat. Am J Vet Res 43:2207–2209.
6. Frøkiaer J, Marples D, Knepper MA, Nielsen S. 1998. Pathophysiology of aquaporin-2 in water balance disorders. Am J Med Sci 316:291–299.
7. Cotran RS, Kumar V, Collins T. 1999. *Robbins Pathologic Basis of Disease*, 6th edition. Philadelphia: WB Saunders.
8. Foreman JW, Tsuru N, Chan JCM. 1990. Pathophysiology and management of chronic renal failure. In: Chan JCM, Gill JR Jr, eds. *Kidney Electrolyte Disorders*, 457–489. New York: Churchill Livingston.
9. Ross LA, Finco DR. 1981. Relationship of selected clinical renal function tests to glomerular filtration rate and renal blood flow in cats. Am J Vet Res 42:1704–1710.
10. Sheehan SJ, Moran KT, Dowsett DJ, Fitzpatrick JM. 1994. Renal haemodynamics and prostaglandin synthesis in partial unilateral ureteric obstruction. Urol Res 22:279–285.
11. Yuile CL, Hawkins WB. 1941. Azotemia due to ingestion of blood proteins. Am J Med Sci 201:162–167.
12. Gregory R, Ewing PL, Levine H. 1945. Azotemia associated with gastrointestinal hemorrhage. Arch Intern Med 75:381–394.
13. Prause LC, Grauer GF. 1998. Association of gastrointestinal hemorrhage with increased blood urea nitrogen and BUN/creatinine ratio in dogs: A literature review and retrospective study. Vet Clin Pathol 27:107–111.
14. Lundberg GD, Iverson C, Radulescu G. 1986. Now read this: The SI units are here. J Am Med Assoc 255:2329–2339.
15. Tietz NW. 1995. *Clinical Guide to Laboratory Tests*, 3rd edition. Philadelphia: WB Saunders.
16. Braun JP, Lefebvre HP, Watson AD. 2003. Creatinine in the dog: A review. Vet Clin Pathol 32:162–179.
17. Newman DJ, Price CP. 1999. Renal function and nitrogen metabolites. In: Burtis CA, Ashwood ER, eds. *Tietz Textbook of Clinical Chemistry*, 3rd edition, 1204–1270. Philadelphia: WB Saunders.
18. Jacobs RM, Lumsden JH, Taylor JA, Grift E. 1991. Effects of interferents on the kinetic Jaffæ reaction and an enzymatic colorimetric test for serum creatinine concentration determination in cats, cows, dogs, and horses. Can J Vet Res 55:150–154.
19. Lolekha PH, Jaruthunyaluck S, Srisawasdi P. 2001. Deproteinization of serum: Another best approach to eliminate all forms of bilirubin interference on serum creatinine by the kinetic Jaffe reaction. J Clin Lab Anal 15:116–121.
20. Feeman WE III, Couto CG, Gray TL. 2003. Serum creatinine concentrations in retired racing Greyhounds. Vet Clin Pathol 32:40–42.
21. Brewer BD. 1990. The urogenital system. Section 2: Renal diseases. In: Koterba AM, Drummond WH, Kosch PC, eds. *Equine Clinical Neonatology*, 446–458. Philadelphia: Lea & Febiger.

22. Finco DR, Duncan JR. 1976. Evaluation of blood urea nitrogen and serum creatinine concentrations as indicators of renal dysfunction: A study of 111 cases and a review of related literature. J Am Vet Med Assoc 168:593–601.

23. Finco DR. 1995. Evaluation of renal functions. In: Osborne CA, Finco DR, eds. *Canine and Feline Nephrology and Urology*, 1st edition, 216–229. Baltimore: Williams & Wilkins.

24. Bovæ KC, Joyce T. 1979. Clinical evaluation of glomerular function: 24-hour creatinine clearance in dogs. J Am Vet Med Assoc 174:488–491.

25. Rogers KS, Komkov A, Brown SA, Lees GE, Hightower D, Russo EA. 1991. Comparison of four methods of estimating glomerular filtration rate in cats. Am J Vet Res 52:961–964.

26. Gronwall R. 1985. Effect of diuresis on urinary excretion and creatinine clearance in the horse. Am J Vet Res 46:1616–1618.

27. Kohn CW, Strasser SL. 1986. 24-Hour renal clearance and excretion of endogenous substances in the mare. Am J Vet Res 47:1332–1337.

28. Finco DR, Coulter DB, Barsanti JA. 1982. Procedure for a simple method of measuring glomerular filtration rate in the dog. J Am Anim Hosp Assoc 18:804–806.

29. Watts C, Campbell JR. 1970. Biochemical changes following bilateral nephrectomy in the bovine. Res Vet Sci 11:508–514.

30. Watts C, Campbell JR. 1971. Further studies on the effect of total nephrectomy in the bovine. Res Vet Sci 12:234–245.

31. Schenck PA, Chew DJ. 2003. Determination of calcium fractionation in dogs with chronic renal failure. Am J Vet Res 64:1181–1184.

32. Brobst DF, Parish SM, Torbeck RL, Frost OL, Bracken FK. 1978. Azotemia in cattle. J Am Vet Med Assoc 173:481–486.

33. Divers TJ, Crowell WA, Duncan JR, Whitlock RH. 1982. Acute renal disorders in cattle: A retrospective study of 22 cases. J Am Vet Med Assoc 181:694–699.

34. Lulich JP, Osborne CA, O'Brien TD, Polzin DJ. 1992. Feline renal failure: Questions, answers, questions. Compend Contin Educ Small Anim Pract 14:127–153.

35. Albasan H, Lulich JP, Osborne CA, Lekcharoensuk C, Ulrich LK, Carpenter KA. 2003. Effects of storage time and temperature on pH, specific gravity, and crystal formation in urine samples from dogs and cats. J Am Vet Med Assoc 222:176–179.

36. Graff L. 1983. *A Handbook of Routine Urinalysis*. Philadelphia: JB Lippincott.

37. Macdougall DF, Curd GJ. 2000. Urine collection and complete analysis. In: Bainbridge J, Elliott J, eds. *BSAVA Manual of Canine and Feline Nephrology and Urology*, 1st edition, 86–106. Ames: Iowa State University Press.

38. McBride LJ. 1998. *Textbook of Urinalysis and Body Fluids*. Philadelphia: Lippincott-Raven.

39. Osborne CA, Stevens JB. 1999. *Urinalysis: A Clinical Guide to Compassionate Patient Care*. Shawnee Mission, KS: Bayer.

40. Coffman JR. 1981. *Equine Clinical Chemistry and Pathophysiology*. Bonner Springs, KS: Veterinary Medicine.

41. Goldberg HE. 1997. *Principles of Refractometry*. Buffalo, NY: Leica.

42. Wolf AV. 1966. *Aqueous Solutions and Body Fluids: Their Concentrative Properties and Conversion Tables*, New York: Hoeber.

43. Stockham SL, Scott MA. 2000. Unpublished data.

44. McCrossin T, Roy LP. 1985. Comparison of hydrometry, refractometry, osmometry, and Ames N-Multistix SG in estimation of urinary concentration. Aust Paediatr J 21:185–188.

45. Chu SY, Sparks D. 1984. Assessment of a solid-phase reagent for urinary specific gravity determination. Clin Biochem 17:34–36.

46. Raff H. 1987. Glucocorticoid inhibition of neurohypophysial vasopressin secretion. Am J Physiol 252:R635–R644.

47. Dingman JF, DesPointes RH. 1960. Adrenal steroid inhibition of vasopressin release from the neurohypophysis of normal subjects and patients with Addison's disease. J Clin Invest 39:1851–1863.

48. Lindeman RD, Van Buren HC, Raisz LG. 1961. Effect of steroids on water diuresis and vasopressin sensitivity. J Clin Invest 40:152–158.

49. Rijnberk A, Kooistra HS, van Vonderen IK, Mol JA, Voorhout G, van Sluijs FJ, Ijzer J, van den Ingh TS, Boer P, Boer WH. 2001. Aldosteronoma in a dog with polyuria as the leading symptom. Domest Anim Endocrinol 20:227–240.

50. Earm JH, Christensen BM, Frøkiær J, Marples D, Han JS, Knepper MA, Nielsen S. 1998. Decreased aquaporin-2 expression and apical plasma membrane delivery in kidney collecting ducts of polyuric hypercalcemic rats. J Am Soc Nephrol 9:2181–2193.

51. Rose BD, Post TW. 2001. *Clinical Physiology of Acid-Base and Electrolyte Disorders*, 5th edition. New York: McGraw-Hill.

52. Puliyanda DP, Ward DT, Baum MA, Hammond TG, Harris HW Jr. 2003. Calpain-mediated AQP2 proteolysis in inner medullary collecting duct. Biochem Biophys Res Commun 303:52–58.

53. Raymond KH, Lifschitz MD, McKinney TD. 1987. Prostaglandins and the urinary concentrating defect in potassium-depleted rabbits. Am J Physiol 253:F1113–F1119.

54. Luke RG, Wright FS, Fowler N, Kashgarian M, Giebisch GH. 1978. Effects of potassium depletion on renal tubular chloride transport in the rat. Kidney Int 14:414–427.

55. Belshaw BE. 1983. Thyroid diseases. In: Ettinger SJ, ed. *Textbook of Veterinary Internal Medicine: Diseases of the Dog and Cat*, 2nd edition, 1592–1614. Philadelphia: WB Saunders.

56. Paquignon A, Tran G, Provost JP. 1993. Evaluation of the Clinitek 200 urinary test-strip reader in the analysis of dog and rat urines in pre-clinical toxicology studies. Lab Anim 27:240–246.

57. Wilkerson MJ, Stockham SL. 2002. Assessing agreement of results of urine reagent strip assays: Visual assessment versus Clinitek 100 Urine Chemistry Analyzer. In: Teaching Clinical Pathology, Annual Meeting of the American Society for Veterinary Clinical Pathology, New Orleans.

58. Barsanti JA, Finco DR. 1979. Protein concentration in urine of normal dogs. Am J Vet Res 40:1583–1588.

59. Heuter KJ, Buffington CAT, Chew DJ. 1998. Agreement between two methods for measuring urine pH in cats and dogs. J Am Vet Med Assoc 213:996–998.

60. Moore FM, Brum SL, Brown L. 1991. Urine protein determination in dogs and cats: Comparison of dipstick and sulfasalicylic acid procedures. Vet Clin Pathol 20:95–97.

61. Hinberg IH, Katz L, Waddell L. 1978. Sensitivity of in vitro diagnostic dipstick tests to urinary protein. Clin Biochem 11:62–64.

62. Jansen BS, Lumsden JH. 1985. Sensitivity of routine tests for urine protein to hemoglobin. Can Vet J 26:221–223.

63. Schumann GB, Schweitzer SC. 1996. Examination of urine. In: Kaplan LA, Pesce AJ, Kazmierczak SC, eds. *Clinical Chemistry: Theory, Analysis, and Correlation*, 3rd edition, 1114–1139. St Louis: CV Mosby.

64. Schultze AE, Jensen RK. 1989. Sodium dodecyl sulfate polyacrylamide gel electrophoresis of canine urinary proteins for the analysis and differentiation of tubular and glomerular diseases. Vet Clin Pathol 18:93–97.

65. Zini E, Bonfanti U, Zatelli A. 2004. Diagnostic relevance of qualitative proteinuria evaluated by use of sodium dodecyl sulfate–agarose gel electrophoresis and comparison with renal histologic findings in dogs. Am J Vet Res 65:964–971.

66. Lees GE, Brown SA, Elliott J, Grauer GF, Vaden SL. 2005. Assessment and management of proteinuria in dogs and cats: 2004 ACVIM Forum Consensus Statement (small animal). J Vet Intern Med 19:377–385.

67. Stone MJ. 1982. Monoclonal gammopathies: Clinical aspects. In: Ritzmann SE, ed. *Protein Abnormalities*, volume 2: *Pathology of Immunoglobulins: Diagnostic and Clinical Aspects*, 161–236. New York: Alan R Liss.

68. Ritzmann SE, Daniels JC. 1982. *Serum Protein Abnormalities: Diagnostic and Clinical Aspects*. New York: Alan R Liss.

69. MacEwen EG, Hurvitz AI. 1977. Diagnosis and management of monoclonal gammopathies. Vet Clin North Am 7:119–132.

70. Bonfanti U, Zini E, Minetti E, Zatelli A. 2004. Free light-chain proteinuria and normal renal histopathology and function in 11 dogs exposed to *Leishmania infantum*, *Ehrlichia canis*, and *Babesia canis*. J Vet Intern Med 18:618–624.

71. Feldman EC, Nelson RW. 1996. Diabetes mellitus. In: *Canine and Feline Endocrinology and Reproduction*, 2nd edition, 339–391. Philadelphia: WB Saunders.

72. Link RP. 1940. Glucose tolerance in horses. J Am Vet Med Assoc 97:261–262.

73. Hostettler-Allen RL, Tappy L, Blum JW. 1994. Insulin resistance, hyperglycemia, and glucosuria in intensively milk-fed calves. J Anim Sci 72:160–173.

74. Bovæe KC, Joyce T, Blazer-Yost B, Goldschmidt MS, Segal S. 1979. Characterization of renal defects in dogs with a syndrome similar to the Fanconi syndrome in man. J Am Vet Med Assoc 174:1094–1104.

75. Bayer. 2005. Package insert for Bayer reagent strips. Elkhart, IN.

76. Oster JR, Rietberg B, Taylor AL, Perez GO, Chandra R, Gardner LB. 1984. Can beta-hydroxybutyrate be detected at the bedside by in vitro oxidation with hydrogen peroxide. Diabetes Care 7:80–82.

77. Adams EC. 1971. Differentiaton of myoglobin and hemoglobin in biological fluids. Ann Clin Lab Sci 1:208–221.

78. Chu SY, Curtis C, Turkington VE. 1978. Influence of pH on the simple solubility test for myoglobinuria. Clin Biochem 11:230–231.

79. Waugh WH. 2003. Simplified method to assay total plasma peroxidase activity and ferriheme products in sickle cell anemia, with initial results in assessing clinical severity in a trial with citrulline therapy. J Pediatr Hematol Oncol 25:831–834.

80. Vail DM, Allen TA, Weiser G. 1986. Applicability of leukocyte esterase test strip in detection of canine pyuria. J Am Vet Med Assoc 189:1451–1453.

81. Osborne CA, Stevens JB, Lulich JP, Ulrich LK, Bird KA, Koehler LA, Swanson LL. 1995. A clinician's analysis of urinalysis. In: Osborne CA, Finco DR, eds. *Canine and Feline Nephrology and Urology*, 136–205. Baltimore: Williams & Wilkins.

82. Swenson CL, Boisvert AM, Kruger JM, Gibbons-Burgener SN. 2004. Evaluation of modified Wright-staining of urine sediment as a method for accurate detection of bacteriuria in dogs. J Am Vet Med Assoc 224:1282–1289.

83. Osborne CA, Lees GE. 1995. Bacterial infections of the canine and feline urinary tract. In: Osborne CA, Finco DR, eds. *Canine and Feline Nephrology and Urology*, 759–797. Baltimore: Williams & Wilkins.

84. Trumel C, Diquelou A, Lefebvre H, Braun JP. 2004. Inaccuracy of routine creatinine measurement in canine urine. Vet Clin Pathol 33:128–132.

85. Brooks CL, Garry F, Swartout MS. 1988. Effect of an interfering substance on determination of potassium by ion-specific potentiometry in animal urine. Am J Vet Res 49:710–714.

86. Schriever H, Gambino SR. 1965. Protein turbidity produced by trichloracetic acid and sulfosalicylic acid at varying temperatures and varying ratios of albumin and globulin. Am J Clin Pathol 44:667–672.

87. White JV, Olivier NB, Reimann K, Johnson C. 1984. Use of protein-to-creatinine ratio in a single urine specimen for quantitative estimation of canine proteinuria. J Am Vet Med Assoc 185:882–885.

88. Dilena BA, Penberthy LA, Fraser CG. 1983. Six methods for determining urinary protein compared. Clin Chem 29:553–557.

89. Center SA, Wilkinson E, Smith CA, Erb H, Lewis RM. 1985. 24-Hour urine protein/creatinine ratio in dogs with protein-losing nephropathies. J Am Vet Med Assoc 187:820–824.

90. McCaw DL, Knapp DW, Hewett JE. 1985. Effect of collection time and exercise restriction on the prediction of urine protein excretion, using urine protein/creatinine ratio in dogs. Am J Vet Res 46:1665–1669.

91. Cook AK, Cowgill LD. 1996. Clinical and pathological features of protein-losing glomerular disease in the dog: A review of 137 cases (1985–1992). J Am Anim Hosp Assoc 32:313–322.

92. Pugia MJ, Lott JA, Clark LW, Parker DR, Wallace JF, Willis TW. 1997. Comparison of urine dipsticks with quantitative methods for microalbuminuria. Eur J Clin Chem Clin Biochem 35:693–700.

93. Pressler BM, Vaden SL, Jensen WA, Simpson D. 2002. Detection of canine microalbuminuria using semiquantitative test strips designed for use with human urine. Vet Clin Pathol 31:56–60.

94. Zaragoza C, Barrera R, Centeno F, Tapia JA, Duran E, Gonzalez M, Mane MC. 2003. SDS-PAGE and Western blot of urinary proteins in dogs with leishmaniasis. Vet Res 34:137–151.

95. Zaragoza C, Barrera R, Centeno F, Tapia JA, Mane MC. 2004. Canine pyometra: A study of the urinary proteins by SDS-PAGE and Western blot. Theriogenology 61:1259–1272.

96. Grauer GF. 2005. Early detection of renal damage and disease in dogs and cats. Vet Clin North Am Small Anim Pract 35:581–596.

97. Vaden SL, Pressler BM, Lappin MR, Jensen WA. 2004. Effects of urinary tract inflammation and sample blood contamination on urine albumin and total protein concentrations in canine urine samples. Vet Clin Pathol 33:14–19.

98. Gaines Das RE. 1980. Dilution as a source of error: Implications for preparation and calibration of laboratory standards and for quality control of radioimmunoassays. Clin Chem 26:1726–1729.

99. Whittemore JC, Jensen WA, Prause L, Radecki S, Gill V, Lappin MR. 2003. Comparison of microalbuminuria, urine protein dipstick, and urine protein creatinine ratio results in clinically ill dogs. J Vet Intern Med 17:437 (abstract).

100. Grauer GF, Oberhauser EB, Basaraba RJ, Lappin MR, Simpson DF, Jensen WA. 2002. Development of microalbuminuria in dogs with heartworm disease. J Vet Intern Med 16:352 (abstract).

101. Lees GE, Jensen WA, Simpson DF, Kashtan CE. 2002. Persistent albuminuria precedes onset of overt proteinuria in male dogs with X-linked hereditary nephropathy. J Vet Intern Med 16:353 (abstract).

102. Gary AT, Cohn LA, Kerl ME, Jensen WA. 2004. The effects of exercise on urinary albumin excretion in dogs. J Vet Intern Med 18:52–55.

103. Gossett KA, Turnwald GH, Kearney MT, Greco DS, Cleghorn B. 1987. Evaluation of γ-glutamyl transpeptidase-to-creatinine ratio from spot samples of urine supernatant, as an indicator of urinary enzyme excretion in dogs. Am J Vet Res 48:455–457.

104. Mulnix JA, Rijnberk A, Hendriks HJ. 1976. Evaluation of a modified water-deprivation test for diagnosis of polyuric disorders in dogs. J Am Vet Med Assoc 169:1327–1330.

105. Osborne CA. 1986. Canine urolithiasis I. Vet Clin North Am Small Anim Pract 16:1–207.

106. Osborne CA. 1986. Canine urolithiasis II. Vet Clin North Am Small Anim Pract 16:209–415.

107. Bovee KC, McGuire T. 1984. Qualitative and quantitative analysis of uroliths in dogs: Definitive determination of chemical type. J Am Vet Med Assoc 185:983–987.

108. Ling GV, Thurmond MC, Choi YK, Franti CE, Ruby AL, Johnson DL. 2003. Changes in proportion of canine urinary calculi composed of calcium oxalate or struvite in specimens analyzed from 1981 through 2001. J Vet Intern Med 17:817–823.

109. Houston DM, Moore AE, Favrin MG, Hoff B. 2004. Canine urolithiasis: A look at over 16,000 urolith submissions to the Canadian Veterinary Urolith Centre from February 1998 to April 2003. Can Vet J 45:225–230.

110. Kyles AE, Hardie EM, Wooden BG, Adin CA, Stone EA, Gregory CR, Mathews KG, Cowgill LD, Vaden S, Nyland TG, Ling GV. 2005. Clinical, clinicopathologic, radiographic, and ultrasonographic abnormalities in cats with ureteral calculi: 163 cases (1984–2002). J Am Vet Med Assoc 226:932–936.

111. Menon M, Resnick MI. 2005. Urinary lithiasis: Etiology, diagnosis, and medical management. In: Walsh PC, Retik AB, Vaughan ED Jr, Wein AJ, eds. *Campbell's Urology*, 8th edition, 3229–3305. Philadelphia: WB Saunders.

112. Grauer GF, Thomas CB, Eicker SW. 1985. Estimation of quantitative proteinuria in the dog, using the urine protein-to-creatinine ratio from a random, voided sample. Am J Vet Res 46:2116–2119

113. American Optical. 1976. *Instructions for use and care of the AO TS meter (a Goldberg refractometer)*. Buffalo, NY: American Optical, Scientific Instrument Division.

114. Wrong O. 1978. Nitrogen metabolism in the gut. Am J Clin Nutr 31:1587–1593.

115. Jones JD, Burnett PC. 1974. Creatinine metabolism in humans with decreased renal function: Creatinine deficit. Clin Chem 20:1204–1212.

116. Grossman BS, Brobst DF, Kramer JW, Bayly WM, Reed SM. 1982. Urinary indices for differentiation of prerenal azotemia and renal azotemia in horses. J Am Vet Med Assoc 180:284–288.

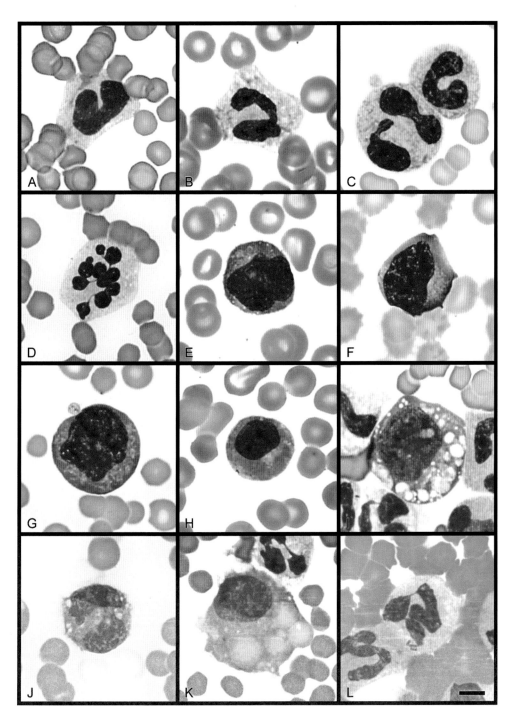

Plate 1. Photomicrographs of leukocyte abnormalities (all blood films stained with Wright stain) (5 μm bar in *L* applies to each frame).

    A. Toxic band neutrophil with foamy cytoplasm that contains Döhle bodies, horse. **B.** Toxic neutrophil, dog. **C.** Toxic giant neutrophil with double nucleus and toxic band neutrophil, cat. **D.** Hypersegmented neutrophil, horse. **E.** Reactive lymphocyte, dog. **F.** Reactive lymphocyte, dog. **G.** Reactive lymphocyte, horse. **H.** Reactive plasmacytoid lymphocyte, cat. **I.** Activated monocyte or macrophage, cat. **J.** Sideroleukocyte, dog. **K.** Erythrophage, foal with neonatal isoerythrolysis. **L.** Neutrophil containing bacterial bacilli, cat.

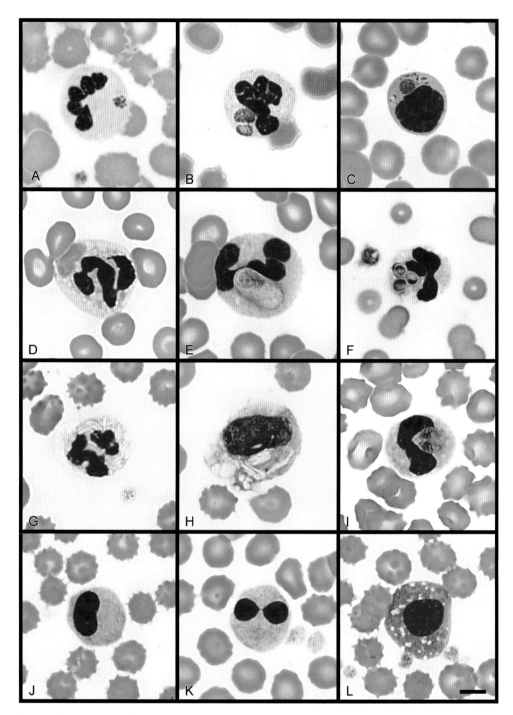

Plate 2. Photomicrographs of leukocyte abnormalities (all Wright-stained blood films unless otherwise stated) (5 μm bar in *L* applies to each frame).

A. Morula of *Ehrlichia ewingii* in a neutrophil, dog. **B.** Morulae of *Anaplasma phagocytophilum* in a neutrophil, horse (from ASVCP slide contributed by J.W. Harvey, 1983). **C.** Morula of *Ehrlichia canis* in a granular lymphocyte, Panótico Rápido dip stain, Brazilian dog, (blood film courtesy of Camilo Bulla, Michigan State University). **D.** Distemper inclusions in a neutrophil, dog (from ASVCP slide contributed by J.C. Tobey, 1993). **E.** Gametocyte of *Hepatozoon americanum* in a monocyte, dog (from ASVCP slide contributed by C.J. LeBlanc et al., 2002). **F.** Yeast stages of *Histoplasma capsulatum* in a neutrophil, cat. **G.** Negative-staining *Mycobacterium* sp. in a neutrophil, dog (from ASVCP slide contributed by H.W. Tvedten, 1988). **H.** Negative-staining *Mycobacterium* sp. in a monocyte, dog (from same slide as *G*). **I.** Tachyzoites of *Toxoplasma gondii* in a neutrophil, dog. **J.** Pelger-Huët neutrophil, dog. **K.** Spectacle form of Pelger-Huët neutrophil, dog. **L.** Pelger-Huët eosinophil, dog.

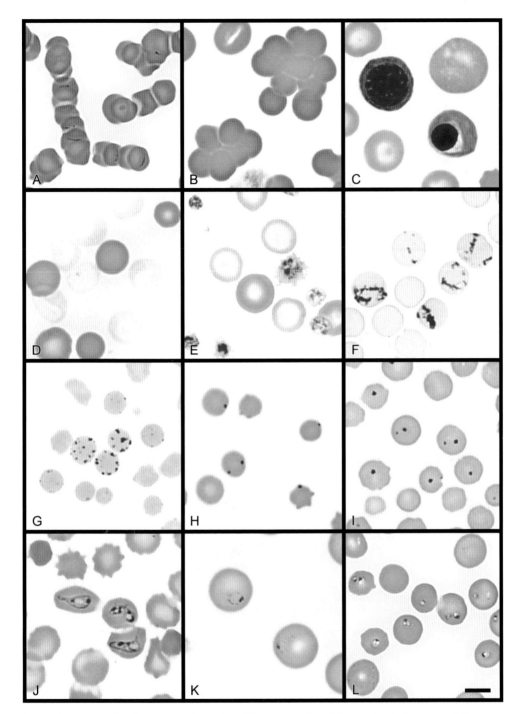

Plate 3. Photomicrographs of erythrocyte abnormalities (all Wright-stained blood films unless otherwise stated) (5 μm bar in *L* applies to each frame).

A. Rouleaux, horse. **B.** Agglutination, dog. **C.** Rubricytosis (metarubricyte and rubricyte) and polychromatophilic erythrocyte, dog. **D.** Ghost erythrocytes, dog. **E.** Hypochromic eryth-rocytes of Fe deficiency, dog. **F.** Aggregate reticulocytes, new methylene blue vital stain, dog. **G.** Reticulocytes (coarse and fine punctate), new methylene blue vital stain, cat. **H.** *Anaplasma marginale*, cow. **I.** *Anaplasma centrale*, cow. **J.** *Babesia canis*, dog. **K.** *Babesia gibsoni*, dog (from ASVCP slide contributed by A.R. Irizarry-Rovira et al., 1999). **L.** *Cytauxzoon felis*, cat.

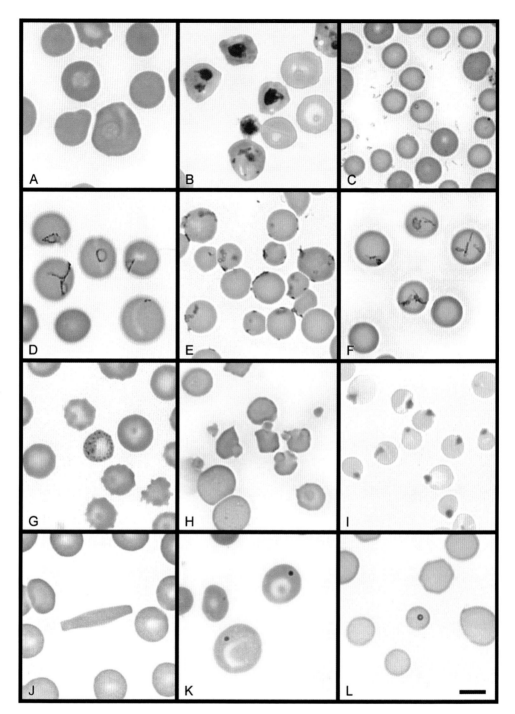

Plate 4. Photomicrographs of erythrocyte abnormalities (all Wright-stained blood films unless otherwise stated) (5 μm bar in *L* applies to each frame).

A. Distemper inclusions, dog (from ASVCP slide contributed by D.C. Bernreuter, 1981). **B.** Distemper inclusions, Diff-Quik stain, dog (from ASVCP slide contributed by J.R. Duncan, 1981). **C.** *Mycoplasma wenyonii*, most detached from erythro-cytes, cow (from ASVCP slide contributed by E.G. Welles et al., 1993). **D.** *Mycoplasma haemocanis*, dog. **E.** *Mycoplasma haemofelis*, cat. **F.** *Theileria buffeli*, cow. **G.** Basophilic stippling of plumbism, dog. **H.** Heinz bodies, cat. **I.** Heinz bodies, new methylene blue vital stain, cat. **J.** Hemoglobin crystal, dog. **K.** Howell-Jolly bodies, dog. **L.** Howell-Jolly body, ring variant, horse.

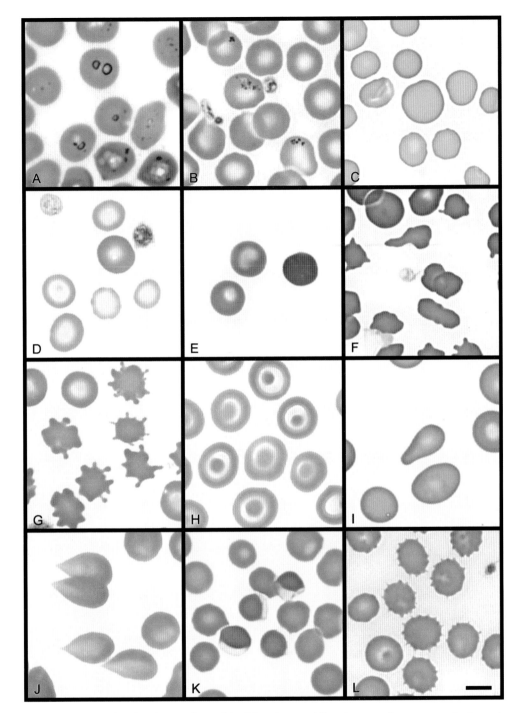

Plate 5. Photomicrographs of erythrocyte abnormalities (all Wright-stained blood films unless otherwise stated) (5 μm bar in *L* applies to each frame).

A. Refractile artifact, Diff-Quik stain with water in fixative, dog. **B.** Siderocytes with siderotic granules, dog. **C.** Macrocyte and resulting anisocytosis, horse. **D.** Leptocytic, hypochromic microcytes of Fe deficiency, dog. **E.** Normochromic and poly- chromatophilic microcytes of a portosystemic shunt, dog. **F.** Poikilocytes including an elongated form (*lower center*) and a cell with a broad appendage (*upper center*), cat. **G.** Acanthocytes, splenic hemangiosarcoma, dog. **H.** Codocytes, dog. **I.** Dacryo- cyte, dog. **J.** Artifactual dacryocytes, dog. **K.** Eccentrocytes, horse. **L.** Echinocytes, dog.

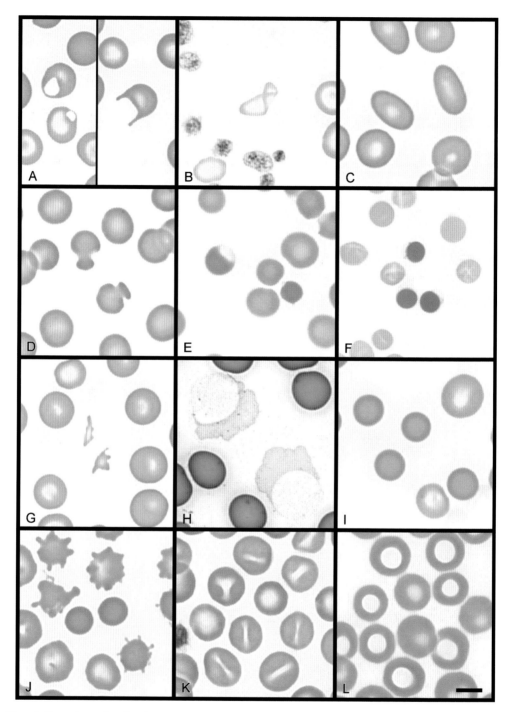

Plate 6. Photomicrographs of erythrocyte abnormalities (all Wright-stained blood films unless otherwise stated) (5 μm bar in *L* applies to each frame).

A. Prekeratocytes (*left*) and keratocyte (*right*), dog. **B.** Folded, hypochromic, microcytic leptocyte of Fe deficiency, dog. **C.** Ovalocytes, dog. **D.** Pincered cells, dog. **E.** Pyknocyte (4 o'clock), horse. **F.** Pyknocytes, new methylene blue vital stain, horse. **G.** Schizocytes, dog. **H.** Selenocytes (artifacts), Diff-Quik stain, dog. **I.** Spherocytes, immune-mediated hemolytic anemia, dog. **J.** Acanthocytes and fragmentation-derived spherocytes, dog. **K.** Stomatocytes, dog (from ASVCP slide contributed by D.E. Brown et al., 1992). **L.** Torocytes (artifact), dog.

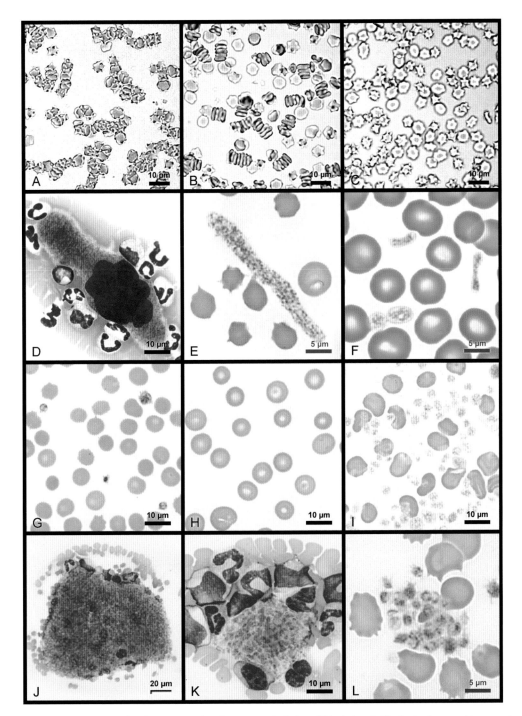

Plate 7. Photomicrographs of erythrocytes in a saline dispersion test, and platelet abnormalities in Wright-stained blood films (scale bar in each frame).

A. Marked rouleaux, 1 part blood to 1 part saline, nonstained wet preparation, dog. **B.** Rouleaux, 1 part blood in *A* to 3 parts saline, nonstained wet preparation. **C.** Absence of rouleaux, 1 part blood in *A* to 9 parts saline, nonstained wet preparation. **D.** Megakaryocyte in feathered edge of blood film, dog. **E.** Elongated platelet (proplatelet), cow. **F.** Oval and elongated platelets,

fresh citrated blood, dog. **G.** Platelet density seen with a normal platelet concentration, dog. **H.** Platelet density seen with thrombocytopenia, dog. **I.** Platelet density seen with marked thrombocytosis due to essential thrombocythemia, dog (from ASVCP slide contributed by C.P. Mandell et al., 1987). **J.** Large platelet clump in feathered edge of blood film, cow. **K.** Smaller platelet clump surrounded by leukocytes and erythrocytes in feathered edge of blood film, cow. **L.** Small platelet clump in body of blood film, dog.

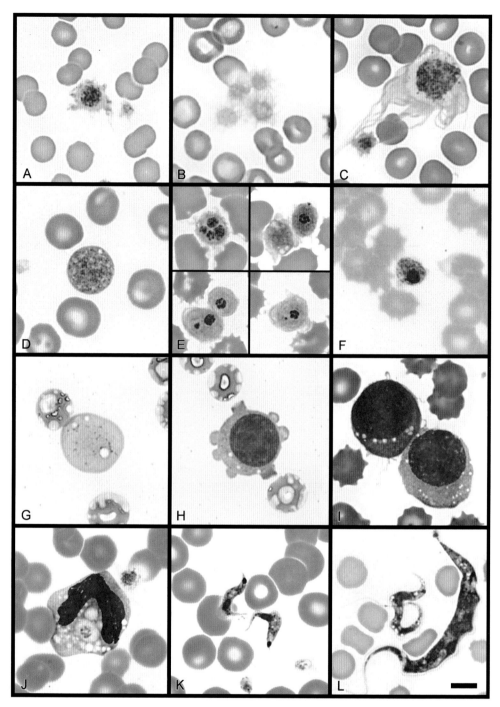

Plate 8. Photomicrographs of platelet abnormalities in Wright-stained blood films (5 μm bar in *L* applies to each frame).
  A. Activated giant platelet with pseudopods and centralized granules, cat. **B.** Cluster of four activated, degranulated platelets, cat. **C.** Giant activated platelet with pseudopods and centralized granules, Cavalier King Charles spaniel. **D.** Giant platelet, unactivated, dog. **E.** *Anaplasma platys* morulae in platelets, Panótico Rápido dip stain (*all four quarters*), dog (slide courtesy of C. Lucidi, Universidade Estadual Paulista, Botucatu, Brazil). **F.** Platelet containing a probable fragment of nuclear material that can be mistaken for an organism, dog. **G.** Abnormal giant and hypogranular platelet associated with megakaryocytic leukemia (M7), dog (from ASVCP slide contributed by J. Messick et al., 1989). **H.** Megakaryoblast with cytoplasmic blebs, megakaryocytic leukemia (M7), dog (from same slide as *G*). **I.** Megakaryoblasts, megakaryocytic leukemia M7), dog (from ASVCP slide contributed by M. Ameri et al., 2006). **J.** Monocyte containing phagocytized platelet (rare finding), immune-mediated thrombocytopenia, dog. **K.** *Trypanosoma cruzi*, dog (from slide contributed by P.K. Penny et al., 2006). **L.** *Trypanosoma theileri*, cow (from ASVCP slide contributed by H. Bender et al., 1989).

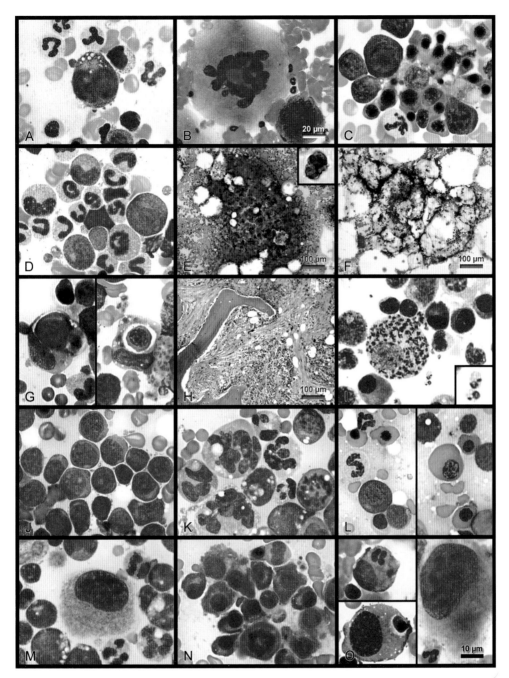

Plate 9. Photomicrographs of cells and other microscopic findings in marrow samples; major reason for image is provided (all Wright-stained films of marrow aspirates unless otherwise stated) (scale bar in *O* applies to all frames except inserts and frames with separate scale bars).

A. Promegakaryocyte, dog. **B.** Mature megakaryocyte and smaller immature megakaryocyte, dog. **C.** Erythroid 'island' of nucleated erythroid series, dog. **D.** Granulocytic series from late myeloblasts to segmented neutrophil, dog. **E.** Hypercellular marrow fragment with darkly stained hemosiderin, high magnification insert with nonstained golden hemosiderin, dog. **F.** Marrow fragment with decreased hematopoietic cellularity, dog. **G.** Macrophages with engulfed rubriblast and degraded cell (*left*) and polychromatophilic rubricyte (*right*) associated with immune-mediated nonregenerative anemias, dogs. **H.** Myelofibrosis with bundles of fibrocytes and collagen, marrow core, hematoxylin and eosin stain, dog. **I.** Macrophage laden with amastigotes of *Leishmania* sp., insert with high magnification of amastigotes and their rod-shaped kinetoplasts, dog. **J.** Undifferentiated blast cells of acute leukemia, dog. **K.** Dysplastic myelomonocytic cells, cat. **L.** Dysplastic erythroid cells (*left* and *right*), cat. **M.** Dysplastic megakaryocyte with hyposegmented nucleus and mature cytoplasm (micromegakaryocyte), cat. **N.** Pleomorphic neoplastic plasma cells, multiple myeloma, dog. **O.** Neoplastic histiocytic cells with phagocytized neutrophil (*top left*), phagocytized rubricyte (*bottom left*), and large cell with atypical nucleoli (*right*), histiocytic sarcoma, dog.

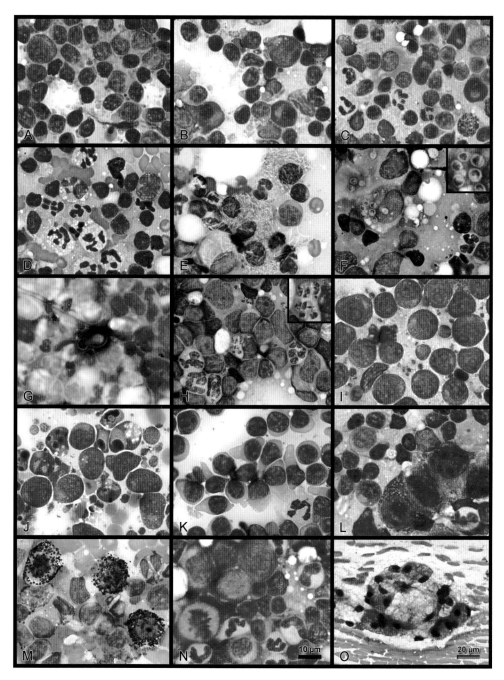

Plate 10. Photomicrographs of cells and other microscopic findings in lymph node aspirates or imprints (except *O*); major reason for image is provided (all Wright-stained films of aspirates or imprints unless otherwise stated) (scale bar in *N* applies to all frames except *O*).

A. Predominantly small and intermediate lymphocytes, expected findings in health, dog. **B.** Plasma cells, large lymphocyte, and small lymphocytes, reactive lymph node, dog. **C.** Plasma cells, neutrophils, eosinophil, and small lymphocytes, reactive lymphadenitis, dog. **D.** Neutrophils, reactive intermediate lymphocyte, small lymphocytes, neutrophilic lymphadenitis, dog. **E.** Macrophages and neutrophils laden with nonstaining *Mycobacterium* sp., mycobacterial lymphadenitis, cat. **F.** *Histoplasma capsulatum* in a macrophage and extracellularly, high magnification insert of *Histoplasma* yeasts, fungal lymphadenitis.

G. Budding yeast of *Blastomyces dermatitidis* and many neutrophils in different focal plane, fungal lymphadenitis, dog. **H.** *Leishmania* sp. amastigotes in neutrophils and macrophages, high magnification insert shows intracellular amastigotes with rod-shaped kinetoplasts, protozoal lymphadenitis, dog. **I.** Intermediate and large neoplastic lymphocytes, lymphoma, dog. **J.** Cell death of neoplastic lymphocytes 1 d after glucocorticoid therapy, lymphoma, dog. **K.** Small to intermediate neoplastic lymphocytes, lymphoma, dog. **L.** Small raft of pleomorphic epithelial cells, metastatic carcinoma, dog. **M.** Metastatic mast cells, eosinophils, and lymphocytes, dog. **N.** Neoplastic myeloid cells, metastatic myeloid leukemia (granulocytic sarcoma), dog. **O.** Secretory epithelial cells of mandibular salivary gland and windrowing of erythrocytes in the mucoid salivary fluid, salivary gland aspirate (attempted lymph node aspirate), dog.

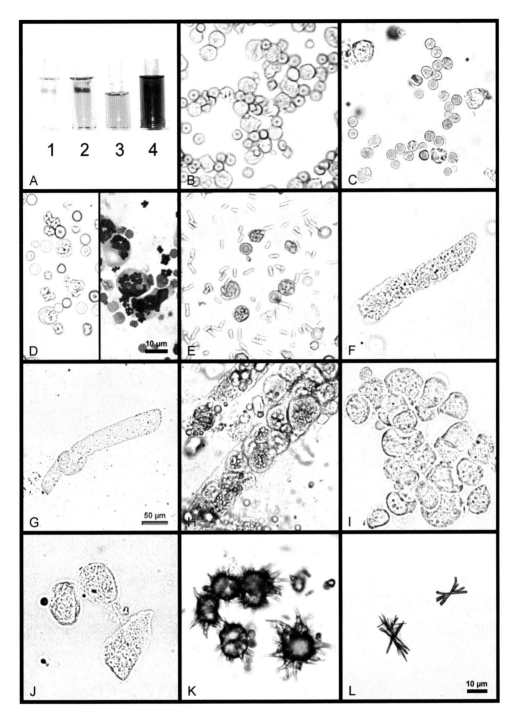

Plate 11. Photograph of urine (*A*) and photomicrographs of urine sediment findings (*B–L*). Sediment was unstained except when air-dried (*D*). All wet sediment photomicrographs were taken using a high-dry objective (use scale bar in frame *L*) except for *G*, which was taken using a 10× objective (grey scale bar).

A. USG_ref and osmolality of urine samples with different gross appearances and colors demonstrating that appearance does not necessarily predict USG_ref or solute concentration: (*1*) colorless, USG_ref = 1.014, osmolality = 410 mmol/kg; (*2*) light yellow, USG_ref = 1.014, osmolality = 531 mmol/kg; (*3*) yellow, USG_ref = 1.013, osmolality = 292 mmol/kg; and (*4*) dark yellow, USG_ref = 1.023, osmolality = 551 mmol/kg. **B.** Leukocytes and erythrocytes. **C.** Erythrocytes. **D.** Erythrocytes, three leukocytes, and clusters of bacterial cocci, no stain (*left*); erythrocytes and neutrophils with intracellular and extracellular clusters of bacterial cocci, air-dried cytocentrifuge preparation of sediment, Wright-stain (*right*), dog. **E.** Large bacterial rods and several leukocytes (courtesy of Don Schmidt, University of Missouri). **F.** Granular cast. **G.** Hyaline cast. **H.** Epithelial cell cast. **I.** Epithelial cell cluster (probably transitional epithelial cells). **J.** Squamous epithelial cells. **K.** Ammonium biurate crystals. **L.** Bilirubin crystals.

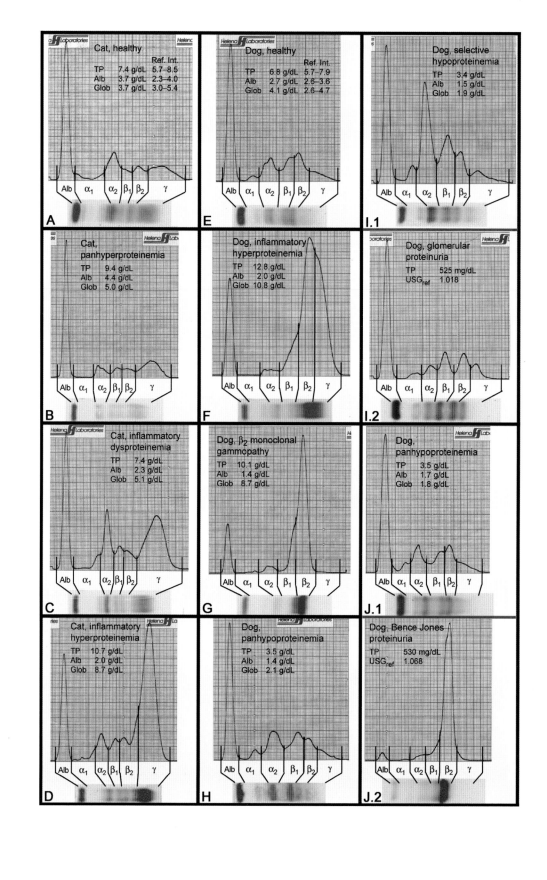

Plate 12. Serum protein electrophoresis densitometer tracings, cellulose acetate strips, and serum protein concentrations from dogs and cats. Reference intervals for total protein, albumin, and globulin concentrations for cats and dogs are in sections A and E, respectively.

A. Cat, healthy: The densitometer tracing is within expected results for healthy cats and is provided as a reference pattern; minor variations in the distribution of protein fractions would be found in other healthy cats.

B. Cat, panhyperproteinemia: The densitometer tracing is within expected results for a healthy cat but is found in a hyperproteinemic sample. Thus, protein concentrations are increased proportionately (panhyperproteinemia) and are consistent with hemoconcentration due to dehydration.

C. Cat, inflammatory dysproteinemia: The densitometer tracing shows a selective pattern—relatively less albumin compared to the globulin regions. Even though total globulin concentration is WRI, there are relatively more of α_2-globulin and γ-globulin fractions compared to the other globulin fractions. The increased α_2-globulin region is probably due to increased concentrations of haptoglobin or α_2-macroglobulin (positive acute-phase proteins). The increased γ-globulin region is broad-based and is thus due to a polyclonal gammopathy (probably mostly IgG). Overall, the dysproteinemia is a delayed-response pattern caused by an inflammatory process of more than 7 d duration.

D. Cat, inflammatory hyperproteinemia: The densitometer tracing shows a selective pattern—relatively less albumin compared to the globulin regions. The hyperglobulinemia is due to increased γ-globulin concentration. The increased γ-globulin region is narrow and thus could be a monoclonal gammopathy or a polyclonal gammopathy with restricted migration. In this case, a post mortem diagnosis of feline infectious peritonitis and the absence of B-lymphocyte neoplasia indicated that the hyperproteinemia, hypoalbuminemia, and hyperglobulinemia were due to chronic inflammation.

E. Dog, healthy: The densitometer tracing is within expected results for healthy dogs and is provided as a reference pattern; minor variations in the distribution of protein fractions would be found in other healthy dogs.

F. Dog, inflammatory hyperproteinemia: The densitometer tracing shows a selective pattern—relatively less albumin compared to the globulin regions. The hyperglobulinemia is due to increased β_2- and γ-globulin concentrations. This broad-based region represents a pronounced polyclonal gammopathy. In this case, clinical signs and an extremely high titer to *Ehrlichia canis* indicated that the hyperproteinemia was due to a chronic rickettsial (bacterial) infection.

G. Dog, β_2-monoclonal gammopathy: The densitometer tracing shows a selective pattern—relatively less albumin compared to the globulin regions. The hyperglobulinemia is due to increased β_2-globulin concentration. The β_2-globulin region is contains a narrow peak and an anodal shoulder. The combination of narrow β_2-globulin region and an apparent decrease in the γ-globulin concentration is indicative of a monoclonal gammopathy of a non-IgG immunoglobulin. This dog's hyperproteinemia was due to a myeloma and the serum IgA concentration was markedly increased.

H. Dog, panhypoproteinemia: The densitometer tracing is within expected results for a healthy dog but is found in a hypoproteinemic sample. Thus, protein concentrations are decreased proportionately (panhypoproteinemia). Causes of panhypoproteinemia include acute blood loss, maldigestive and malabsorptive disorders, starvation, cachexia, and occasionally hepatic failure. This dog had intestinal lymphoma.

I. Dog, selective hypoproteinemia and glomerular proteinuria
1. Serum: The densitometer tracing shows a selective pattern—relatively less albumin compared to the globulin regions. In a hypoproteinemic sample, this selective pattern indicates that albumin concentration is decreased more than some globulin concentrations. Even though the total globulins concentration is decreased, the relative excess of α_2-globulin region indicates that concentrations of other globulin fractions decreased more than the α_2-globulin concentration. This pattern is indicative of protein-losing nephropathy in which the glomerular filtration barrier has become more permeable to plasma proteins because of glomerulonephritis or glomerular amyloidosis. In such cases, there is a relative excess of the α_2-globulin region because α_2-macroglobulin is too large to pass through the filtration barrier but smaller proteins can. Note that even though there is hypoproteinemia, hypoalbuminemia, and hypoglobulinemia, there was not truly a panhypoproteinemia because the concentration of α_2-globulins was not decreased.
2. Urine: The densitometer tracing shows that most urine proteins are in the albumin region, consistent with a protein-losing nephropathy with a glomerular proteinuria. Note that the proteinuria is a selective proteinuria as the urine protein pattern is not the same as the dog's serum protein pattern.

J. Dog, non-selective hypoproteinemia and Bence Jones proteinuria
1. Serum: The densitometer tracing is within expected results for a healthy dog but is found in a hypoproteinemic sample. Thus, protein concentrations are decreased proportionately (panhypoproteinemia). Causes of panhypoproteinemia include acute blood loss, maldigestive and malabsorptive disorders, starvation, cachexia, and occasionally hepatic failure. This dog had multicentric lymphoma with Mott cells and its hypoproteinemia was probably due to multiple processes.
2. Urine: Most urine proteins are in the β_2-globulin region, consistent with migration of immunoglobulin light chains. The Bence Jones urine test was positive; that is, urine supernatant was initially clear, formed precipitate at 40–60 °C, cleared at 100 °C, and then appearances reversed as the sample returned to room temperature. Note that the proteinuria is a selective proteinuria as the urine protein pattern is not the same as the dog's serum protein pattern and represents one type of a prerenal proteinuria (see Chapter 8).

Note: The serum total protein and albumin concentrations were measured by biuret and BCG methods, respectively. The serum globulin concentrations were calculated by subtraction from the measured values. When the electrophoresis strips were scanned, the densitometer was set so that the darkest protein band in the sample caused the maximum deflection of the tracing pen. Hyperproteinemic samples were diluted (either 1 part serum to 1 part saline or 3 parts saline) prior to electrophoresis so that there was a more linear relationship between quantity of protein in the darkest band and the amount of light that passes through the strip. The urine total protein concentrations were measured by the Coomassie brilliant blue assay. The urine samples were concentrated 10-fold prior to electrophoresis.

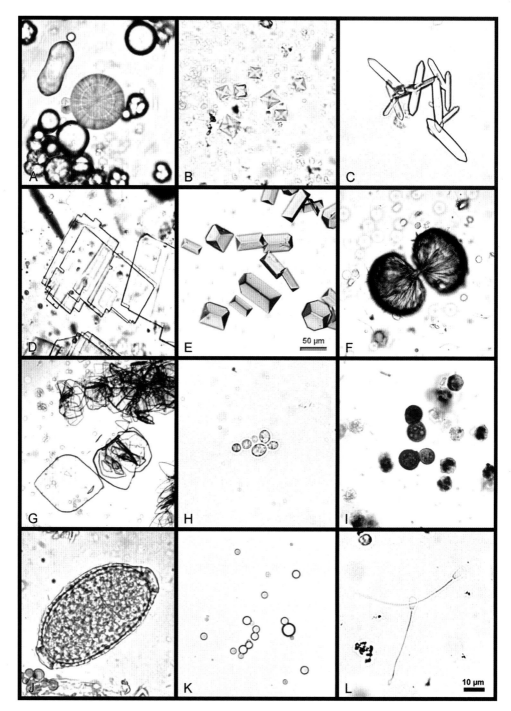

Plate 13. Photomicrographs of direct urine sediment findings. Sediment was unstained except where noted (*I*). All photomicrographs were taken using a high-dry objective (use scale bar in frame *L*) except for *E*, which was taken using a 10× objective (grey scale bar).

A. Calcium carbonate crystals. **B.** Calcium oxalate dihydrate crystals and bacteria. **C.** Calcium oxalate monohydrate crystals.

D. Cholesterol crystals (courtesy of Don Schmidt). **E.** Struvite crystals. **F.** Sulfa crystals and erythrocytes (courtesy of Don Schmidt). **G.** Uric acid crystals. **H.** Yeast. **I.** *Blastomyces* sp. and several neutrophils, new methylene blue stain. **J.** *Capillaria* sp. ovum (courtesy of Don Schmidt). **K.** Lipid droplets. **L.** Sperm.

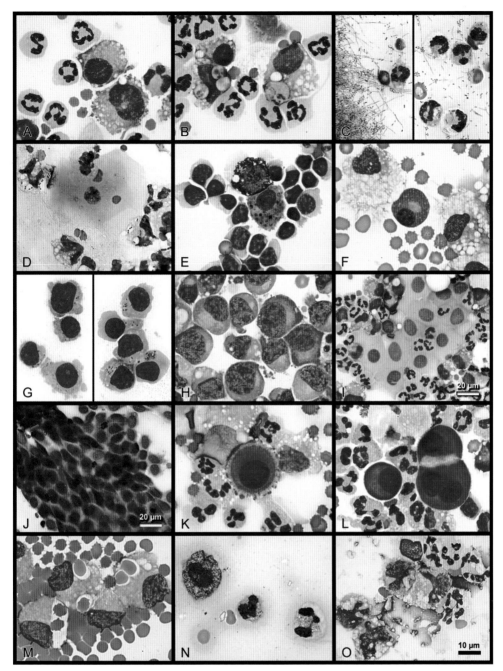

Plate 14. Photomicrographs of cells and other microscopic findings in direct smears (*C, G, J,* and *N*) or cytocentrifuge preparations of cavitary effusions; erythrocytes are not described unless of major significance (all Wright-stained unless otherwise stated) (scale bar in *O* applies to all frames unless a frame has a separate scale bar).

A. Nondegenerate neutrophils and macrophages, peritoneal fluid, horse. **B.** Nondegenerate neutrophils and macrophages including two leukophages, peritoneal fluid, horse. **C.** Filamentous, beaded, branching (*upper area*) bacilli and small bacilli, consistent with *Actinomyces* sp. or *Nocardia* sp. (*left*), mildly degenerate neutrophils with phagocytized bacteria (*right*), pleural bacterial exudate, dog. **D.** Degenerate neutrophils (some containing short chains of cocci) and mature squamous cell, peritoneal bacterial exudate, ruptured stomach, foal. **E.** Small lymphocytes, mast cell, and macrophage containing hemosiderin (siderophage), lymphoid pleural effusion, dog. **F.** Plasma cell and vacuolated macrophages, pleural effusion, dog. **G.** Neoplastic granular lymphocytes (*left* and *right*), neoplastic lymphoid peritoneal effusion, cat. **H.** Intermediate and large neoplastic lymphocytes, neoplastic lymphoid pleural effusion, dog. **I.** Small sheet of non-reactive mesothelial cells, neutrophils, and macrophages, peritoneal fluid, horse. **J.** Sheet of mesothelial cells, ox. **K.** Reactive mesothelial cell, nondegenerate neutrophils, and macrophage, pleural fluid, dog. **L.** Reactive mesothelial cells and nondegenerate neutrophils, pleural fluid, dog. **M.** Erythrophages and many erythrocytes, hemorrhagic peritoneal effusion, dog. **N.** Neutrophils and macrophage containing barium, foreign body peritoneal exudate, cat (slide courtesy of Jenny Thomas, Michigan State University). **O.** Nondegenerate neutrophils and macrophages with intracellular and extracellular particulate clot activator from collecting fluid into an activator-containing clot tube (in vitro phagocytosis), peritoneal fluid, cat.

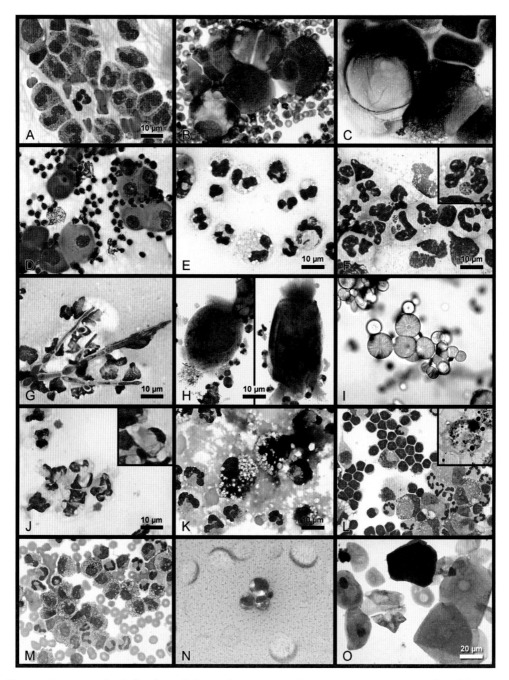

Plate 15. Photomicrographs of cells and other findings in direct or cytocentrifuge (*A, H, K–M* and *O*) preparations of cavitary effusions; erythrocytes are not described (Wright-stained unless otherwise stated) (scale bar in *O* applies to all frames unless a frame has a separate scale bar).

A. Mostly eosinophils and blue fibrinous material consistent with clotting, eosinophilic exudate, cat. **B.** Pleomorphic large cells, neoplastic effusion, metastatic mammary carcinoma, dog. **C.** Pleomorphic large mesothelial cells, neoplastic effusion, mesothelioma, horse. **D.** Squamous epithelial cells and neutrophils, neoplastic effusion with exudation, gastric squamous cell carcinoma, horse (ASVCP slide contributed by M.J. Burkhard et al., 1995). **E.** Mostly degenerate neutrophils (one containing bacilli), bacterial exudate, dog. **F.** Mostly neutrophils (one containing morulae—another morula magnified in inserted image), exudate with *Anaplasma phagocytophilum*, horse (ASVCP slide contributed by

D. Wood et al., 2001). **G.** Pseudohyphae of *Candida* sp. and damaged adherent cells, pericardial mycotic exudate, dog. **H.** Intestinal protozoa (*left* and *right*), bacterial peritoneal exudate due to intestinal rupture, horse. **I.** Calcium carbonate crystals and nucleated cells (out of focus), equine uroperitonium (ASVCP slide contributed by L. Vap et al., 1994). **J.** Sperm heads in neutrophils, exudate of seminoperitoneum, mare (ASVCP slide contributed by P. McWilliams, 1992). **K.** Bile pigment, neutrophils, and macrophages, bile peritonitis, dog. **L.** Small lymphocytes, nondegenerate neutrophils, and macrophages, insert with Sudanophilic lipid in and adjacent to macrophage, chylous effusion, cat. **M.** Vacuolated macrophages and nondegenerate neutrophils, exudate, pancreatitis, dog. **N.** Macrophages, granular protein and protein crescents, proteinaceous exudate, feline infectious peritonitis, cat. **O.** Nucleated and anucleated squamous epithelial cells, amnionic fluid collected during attempted abdominocentesis, alpaca.

Chapter 9

MONOVALENT ELECTROLYTES AND OSMOLALITY

Basic Concepts for the Interpretation of Electrolyte Concentrations 497
Sodium (Na$^+$) Concentration 498
    I.   Physiologic Processes 498
    II. Analytical Concepts 500
    III. Hypernatremia. 501
    IV. Normonatremia in Dehydrated or Edematous Animals. 503
    V. Hyponatremia 505
Potassium (K$^+$) Concentration 509
    I.   Physiologic Processes 509
    II. Analytical Concepts 510
    III. Hyperkalemia. 511
    IV. Normokalemia in Acidotic or Alkalotic Animals 516
    V. Hypokalemia 516
Sodium to Potassium (Na$^+$:K$^+$) Ratio 519
Chloride (Cl$^-$) Concentration 520
    I.   Physiologic Processes 520
    II. Analytical Concepts 521
    III. Hyperchloremia. 522
    IV. Normochloremia. 523
    V. Hypochloremia 523
Bicarbonate (HCO$_3^-$) Concentration and Total Carbon Dioxide (tCO$_2$)
  Concentration 525
    I.   Physiologic Processes 525
    II. Analytical Concepts 527
    III. Increased Bicarbonate (HCO$_3^-$) Concentration or Total Carbon
        Dioxide (tCO$_2$) Concentration. 529
    IV. Decreased Bicarbonate (HCO$_3^-$) Concentration or Total Carbon
        Dioxide (tCO$_2$) Concentration. 531
Anion Gap. 534
Lactate Concentration (L-lactate and D-lactate) 538
β-Hydroxybutyrate (BHB) and Acetoacetate (AcAc) Concentrations. 543
Osmolality and Osmo. Gap. 545

Table 9.1. Abbreviations and symbols in this chapter

$Na^+:K^+$	Sodium to potassium
[x]	x concentration (x = analyte)
AcAc	Acetoacetate
AcCoA	Acetyl-coenzyme A
ADH	Antidiuretic hormone
ANP	Atrial natriuretic peptide
ATP	Adenosine triphosphate
ATPase	Adenosine triphosphatase
BHB	β-Hydroxybutyrate
ECF	Extracellular fluid
EDTA	Ethylenediaminetetraacetic acid
fCa^{2+}	Free ionized calcium
fMg^{2+}	Free ionized magnesium
HCl	Hydrochloric acid
HCO_3^-	Bicarbonate
ICF	Intracellular fluid
IV	Intravenous
LD	L-lactate dehydrogenase
mA^-	Measured anion charge
mC^+	Measured cation charge
M_r	Relative molecular mass
NAD^+	Nicotinamide adenine dinucleotide
NADH	Reduced nicotinamide adenine dinucleotide
NH_4^+	Ammonium
Osm_c	Calculated osmolality
Osm_m	Measured osmolality
Osmo. Gap	Difference between measured osmolality and calculated osmolarity
Pco_2	Partial pressure of carbon dioxide
pH	$-\log [H^+]$
pK_a	$-\log (K_a)$ where K_a is the ionization constant for a partially ionized acid
PO_4	Phosphate, all forms
RAS	Renin-angiotensin system
SI	Système International d'Unités
SID	Strong ion difference
SO_4	Sulfate, all forms
tA^-	Total anionic charge
tbH_2O	Total body water content
tbK^+	Total body potassium content
$tbNa^+$	Total body sodium content
tC^+	Total cationic charge
tCO_2	Total carbon dioxide content
uA^-	Unmeasured anion charge
uC^+	Unmeasured cation charge
WRI	Within the reference interval

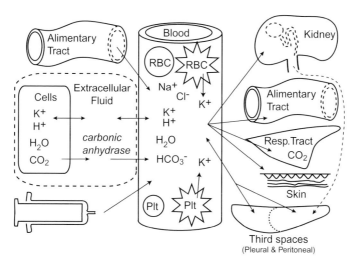

Fig. 9.1. Basic concepts for electrolyte and H_2O movements into and out of plasma. Electrolytes and H_2O enter plasma from the alimentary tract, from cells, and by injections or infusions. In vitro lysis of blood cells and platelet activation may add K^+ to the plasma or serum. Electrolytes and H_2O may leave the plasma and the body via kidneys, alimentary tract, respiratory tract, or skin, and they may enter extravascular sites within the body in the form of third-space loss (e.g., to pleural and peritoneal cavities). In some pathologic states involving muscle, H_2O or electrolytes shift between the ICF and ECF spaces (see the text for details). Fluids (e.g., plasma or urine) can enter pleural or peritoneal cavities and, if not removed via centesis, electrolytes and H_2O will be absorbed (see the text for details). Plt, platelet; and RBC, erythrocyte.

BASIC CONCEPTS FOR THE INTERPRETATION OF ELECTROLYTE CONCENTRATIONS

I.   Electrolyte concentrations in serum or plasma are the net result of intake, excretion, and shifts between ICF and ECF. Shifts may occur in vivo or in vitro. The basic concepts for electrolyte and H_2O movements in and out of plasma are shown in Fig. 9.1. Electrolyte concentrations in serum or plasma essentially represent the electrolyte concentrations in all ECF.

  A. Na^+, K^+, and Cl^- typically enter the body via oral intake of food or fluids. HCO_3^- typically is generated by carbonic anhydrase reactions in lungs, gastric mucosa, kidneys, and erythrocytes.

  B. Outside the vascular system, metabolic processes govern the movement of electrolytes into and out of cells.

   1. In health, ECF is relatively rich in Na^+ and Cl^- but poor in K^+, whereas ICF is relatively rich in K^+ but poor in Na^+ and Cl^- (except in erythrocytes of some species and breeds).

   2. Electrolyte shifts from or to the ECF will alter plasma or serum concentrations of those electrolytes.

  C. Cells within blood may alter plasma or serum electrolyte concentrations if they release electrolytes.

   1. In vitro lysis of K^+-rich erythrocytes will result in falsely elevated plasma $[K^+]$. However, erythrocytes are K^+-rich in only some species and breeds (see Potassium Concentration, sect. III.B.1.h).

      2. The $[K^+]$ is slightly greater in serum than in plasma because platelets release K^+ during clotting. The magnitude of the increase can be clinically significant when there is a thrombocytosis.

  D. Electrolytes and H_2O are excreted or lost from the ECF via kidneys, alimentary tract, skin, and airways. ECF tends to become hypotonic with loss of hypertonic fluids or hypertonic with loss of hypotonic fluids. Drinking H_2O after the loss of ECF will dilute the remaining ECF.

  E. HCO_3^- concentrations are altered by changes in the concentrations of other electrolytes and by changes in acid-base balance.

II.   Abnormal electrolyte concentrations in plasma or serum result from one or more of these basic processes involving electrolytes or H_2O:
  A. Decreased or increased intake
  B. Shifts to and from ICF
  C. Increased renal retention
  D. Increased loss via the kidneys, alimentary tract, skin, or airways (HCO_3^- indirectly)

III.   Electrolyte concentrations and acid-base abnormalities
  A. The regulation of acid-base status in an animal involves physiologic processes that may alter plasma (serum) concentrations of Na^+, Cl^-, K^+, and HCO_3^-, the major topics of this chapter.
  B. Pathologic states that first alter electrolyte concentrations can create acid-base abnormalities, the major topics of Chapter 10. Thus, it is difficult to completely separate electrolyte concepts from acid-base concepts. The early sections of Chapter 10 contain the major definitions and classifications of acid-base abnormalities. The end of Chapter 10 contains a section on SID. The SID approach uses electrolyte concentrations to define metabolic acid-base disorders.

SODIUM (Na^+) CONCENTRATION

I.   Physiologic processes
  A. Plasma $[Na^+]$ is nearly equivalent to ECF $[Na^+]$, which is dependent on the ratio of $tbNa^+$ to tbH_2O (Eq. 9.1a–c). Therefore, plasma or serum $[Na^+]$ must be interpreted with knowledge of the patient's tbH_2O (i.e., state of hydration) and consideration of the patient's ECF volume (i.e., normovolemic, hypovolemic, or hypervolemic). Although not completely accurate, this basic conceptual relationship assists in the understanding of most disorders that affect plasma or serum $[Na^+]$.

$$\text{Normonatremia} \Rightarrow \text{normal} \frac{tbNa^+}{tbH_2O} \Rightarrow \frac{\text{normal}}{\text{normal}} \; or \; \frac{\uparrow}{\uparrow} \; or \; \frac{\downarrow}{\downarrow} \tag{9.1a.}$$

$$\text{Hypernatremia} \Rightarrow \uparrow \frac{tbNa^+}{tbH_2O} \Rightarrow \frac{\uparrow}{\text{normal}} \; or \; \frac{\text{normal}}{\downarrow} \; or \; \frac{\downarrow}{\downarrow\downarrow} \tag{9.1b.}$$

$$\text{Hyponatremia} \Rightarrow \downarrow \frac{tbNa^+}{tbH_2O} \Rightarrow \frac{\downarrow}{\text{normal}} \; or \; \frac{\text{normal}}{\uparrow} \; or \; \frac{\downarrow\downarrow}{\downarrow} \tag{9.1c.}$$

$$\text{Plasma}\,[Na^+] \cong \frac{[Na_e^+] + [K_e^+]}{tbH_2O} \tag{9.1d.}$$

B. A more accurate relationship is shown in Eq. 9.1d, in which Na^+_e and K^+_e represent the exchangeable Na^+ and K^+ in the body (ions bound in molecules are not exchangeable).[1] From this equation, it can be seen that the total body exchangeable K^+ content influences plasma $[Na^+]$. Thus, when hypokalemia is present because of K^+ depletion, plasma $[Na^+]$ decreases. The change occurs as K^+ leaves cells and Na^+ enters to maintain electrical neutrality (see Sodium Concentration, Sect. V.B.6). Hyperkalemia tends not to cause a significant hypernatremia for two reasons: (1) a marked hyperkalemia would be necessary to create changes in $[Na^+]$, but marked hyperkalemia is life-threatening; and (2) increasing $[Na^+]$ stimulates thirst centers so that intake of H_2O reduces that magnitude of change.

C. Movement of Na^+ frequently is associated with movement of H_2O in response to Na^+-induced changes in osmotic pressure. Na^+ retention tends to cause H_2O retention (edema or ascites), and Na^+ wasting tends to cause loss of H_2O (hypovolemia or dehydration). However, H_2O does not follow Na^+ across tubular cell membranes of the distal nephron in the absence of ADH or across membranes of the ascending limb of the loop of Henle.

D. Serum $[Na^+]$ is controlled through two major mechanisms: regulation of blood volume and regulation of plasma osmolality.
   1. Regulation of blood volume
      a. When hypovolemia or, more specifically, decreased effective blood volume is sensed by juxtaglomerular cells in kidneys, the RAS is activated, which promotes formation of angiotensin II in the lungs and aldosterone in the adrenal cortices. Angiotensin II stimulates the proximal tubular resorption of Na^+, Cl^-, and H_2O. Aldosterone stimulates the active resorption of Na^+ in collecting tubules by opening Na^+ channels, enhancing Na^+-K^+-ATPase activity, and opening luminal K^+ channels. Its actions are probably mediated through aldosterone-induced proteins. Na^+-K^+-ATPase may be one of the proteins.
      b. If hypovolemia is detected by carotid sinus baroreceptors, ADH is secreted.
      c. If hypervolemia is sensed by atrial baroreceptors, Na^+ resorption in the distal nephron is reduced through the action of ANP, which reduces the number of open Na^+ channels via the guanylate cyclase pathway.
   2. Regulation of plasma osmolality
      a. If hyperosmolality is sensed by hypothalamic osmoreceptors, thirst centers are stimulated to promote drinking of H_2O and ADH is released to promote H_2O resorption by the kidney. In a relatively minor role, ADH stimulates Na^+ and Cl^- resorption in the medullary thick limb through the Na^+-K^+-$2Cl^-$ carrier.
      b. Conversely, hypoosmolality leads to decreased H_2O intake and increased urinary H_2O excretion.
   3. Plasma $[Na^+]$ is also somewhat self-regulated in that hyponatremia promotes aldosterone secretion and thus Na^+ retention, whereas hypernatremia inhibits aldosterone secretion and thus reduces Na^+ retention. However, plasma $[K^+]$ and alterations in effective blood volume are the major factors that control aldosterone secretion.[1]

E. Na^+ and Cl^- resorption in the distal nephron also involves an aldosterone-independent Na^+-Cl^- cotransporter; the resorption via this cotransporter increases with increased Na^+ delivery to the distal nephron. Thiazide diuretics block this cotransporter by binding to the Cl^- receptor.

F. The pathologic state of dehydration is equivalent to decreased tbH_2O.
1. Dehydrated animals have either a H_2O deficit or a H_2O and Na^+ deficit.
   a. Causes of a H_2O deficit (without Na^+ deficit) include decreased H_2O intake and loss of free H_2O (central diabetes insipidus, nephrogenic diabetes insipidus, or insensible respiratory losses).
   b. Causes of H_2O and Na^+ deficits include alimentary losses (vomiting, diarrhea, sequestration, or excessive salivation), renal losses (most polyuric states), and cutaneous losses (sweating).
2. Types of dehydration
   a. Hypernatremic, hyperosmolar, or hypertonic dehydration is caused by net hypoosmolar or hypotonic fluid loss; that is, H_2O loss > Na^+ loss.
   b. Normonatremic, isoosmolar, or isotonic dehydration is caused by net isoosmolar or isotonic fluid loss; that is, H_2O loss $\approx$ Na^+ loss.
   c. Hyponatremic, hypoosmolar, or hypotonic dehydration is caused by net hyperosmolar or hypertonic fluid loss; that is, H_2O loss < Na^+ loss.

II. Analytical concepts
A. Terms and units
   1. Assays measure the electrical potential of Na^+ by direct or indirect potentiometry, and then the electrical potential is converted to concentration units.[2] Na^+ is mostly a free ion in the plasma or serum H_2O.
      a. In direct potentiometry, Na^+ ion activity (electrical potential) is measured in a *nondiluted* sample by the interaction of Na^+ with the surface of an ion-selective electrode. The resultant $[Na^+]$ represents the $[Na^+]$ in the sample's H_2O. If the sample contained less H_2O than normal because of increased protein or lipid, the result would be the same because only the activity in the H_2O phase is measured.
      b. In indirect potentiometry, the sample is *diluted* (sometimes greatly) before Na^+ ion activity is measured by the interaction of Na^+ with the surface of an ion-selective electrode. The Na^+ ion activity measured depends on the $[Na^+]$ in the H_2O portion of the diluted sample. The sample $[Na^+]$ is determined by multiplying the measured $[Na^+]$ by the dilution factor. If the sample contains increased lipids or proteins and therefore a lower percentage of H_2O, the H_2O portion will be diluted more than usual by the diluent added. The measured Na^+ activity will therefore be falsely decreased. When the measured value is multiplied by the sample dilution factor (rather than the H_2O-phase dilution factor), the result will also be a falsely decreased value for $[Na^+]$. Results reflect mmol/L *of sample* rather than mmol/L *of H_2O*, as for direct potentiometry values.
      c. Flame photometric methods have the same problem as the indirect potentiometric methods in that high concentrations of solids in the sample that displace H_2O (e.g., lipidemia or hyperproteinemia) cause falsely decreased $[Na^+]$.
   2. Unit conversion: mEq/L $\times$ 1 = mmol/L, and mg/dL $\div$ 2.3 = mmol/L (SI unit, nearest 1 mmol/L)[3]
B. Sample for $[Na^+]$ quantitation
   1. Serum is preferred. $[Na^+]$ is stable for months if the sample does not dehydrate.
   2. Na_2EDTA plasma should not be used because the anticoagulant's Na^+ will be in the plasma. The amount of Na^+ in Na-heparin is too small to cause clinically relevant changes in heparinized plasma $[Na^+]$.

Table 9.2. Diseases and conditions that cause hypernatremia

H_2O-deficit group (decreased total body H_2O, hypertonic dehydration)

    Inadequate H_2O intake

        *H_2O deprivation

        Defective thirst response (hypothalamic defect)

    Pure H_2O loss (without adequate H_2O replacement)

        *Insensible loss: panting, hyperventilation, or fever

        Diabetes insipidus (central or nephrogenic)

    H_2O loss > Na^+ loss

        Renal: osmotic diuresis

        Alimentary: osmotic diarrhea, osmotic sequestration, phosphate enemas, or paintball toxicosis

Na^+-excess group (increased total body Na^+)

    Excess Na^+ with concurrent restricted H_2O intake

        Salt poisoning

        Administration of hypertonic saline or sodium bicarbonate

    Decreased renal excretion of sodium

        Hyperaldosteronism

Other or unknown mechanism

    Severe exercise in greyhounds

* A relatively common disease or condition

Note: Sample evaporation or sublimation will cause spurious hypernatremia.

  C. Assays

    1. Ion-selective electrode assays are the most common.

    2. Flame photometers for measuring $[Na^+]$ used to be the gold standard, but the instruments are no longer used for routine patient screening.

III. Hypernatremia

  A. This occurs when the ratio of $tbNa^+$ to tbH_2O is increased (Eq. 9.1b) or with the shifting of H_2O from ECF to ICF.

  B. Disorders and pathogeneses (Table 9.2)

    1. H_2O-deficit group (decreased tbH_2O, hypertonic dehydration): Dehydration may cause hypernatremia directly via hemoconcentration (pure H_2O loss) and indirectly by activating the RAS, which stimulates renal Na^+ retention via actions of aldosterone and angiotensin II. In most nephron segments, Na^+ resorption promotes H_2O resorption. But since the distal nephron is permeable to H_2O only in the presence of ADH, Na^+ retention without sufficient ADH activity results in hypernatremia.

      a. Inadequate H_2O intake

        (1) H_2O deprivation: Access to H_2O may be restricted because of accidents (water bowl turned over on a hot day), weather (frozen water tank), or other situations. Without H_2O intake, physiologic H_2O losses via kidneys, lungs, skin, or intestine may produce dehydration.

        (2) Defective thirst response: Hypothalamic disease may damage the osmoreceptor that triggers a thirst response, or the thirst center itself may be damaged. Hypodipsic hypernatremia in miniature schnauzers may be caused by lobar holoprosencephaly.[4]

    b. Pure H_2O loss without H_2O replacement

        (1) Insensible loss of H_2O by panting, hyperventilation, or fever: The animal becomes H_2O depleted by losing H_2O via the respiratory system or skin.

        (2) Diabetes insipidus (central or nephrogenic)

            (a) In the diabetes insipidus disorders, diminished ADH activity or response in the collecting ducts may result in pure H_2O loss (i.e., urine with very low concentrations of Na^+ and other solutes; urine specific gravity approaches 1.000).

            (b) Animals with diabetes insipidus that have unrestricted access to H_2O may drink sufficiently to prevent the hypernatremia.

        (3) Adrenocortical neoplasm secreting corticosterone and aldosterone in a dog[5]

            (a) This disorder is uncommon, and the laboratory features of the case were hypernatremia, hyperchloremia, hypokalemia, hyposthenuria, and abnormal results of adrenocorticotropic hormone stimulation tests (inadequate increase in serum [cortisol], exaggerated increase in [corticosterone], and exaggerated increase in [aldosterone]).

            (b) This hypernatremia probably is related to the renal loss of free H_2O because of the inhibition of ADH release by corticosterone.

    c. H_2O loss > Na^+ loss

        (1) Osmotic diuretic agents (e.g., glucose and mannitol) in renal tubular fluid inhibit passive H_2O resorption.

        (2) In the alimentary system:

            (a) Accumulation of osmotic agents (as occurs in some diarrheas) will inhibit H_2O absorption.

            (b) A phosphate enema will pull H_2O from ECF spaces to the colon. Concurrent colonic absorption of Na^+ may augment the hypernatremia.[6]

            (c) In ruminal acidosis (grain overload), accumulation of solutes (including lactic acid) in the rumen causes the osmotic movement of H_2O into the rumen to produce hypernatremia.[7]

            (d) Dogs with paintball toxicosis (after ingestion of paintballs) may develop hypernatremia because the paintballs contain osmotic molecules (e.g., glycerol and sorbitol) that pull H_2O from plasma to intestines.[8]

        (3) The H_2O that moves during osmosis contains a small amount of Na^+ because of solute drag, but the net result is greater loss of H_2O than Na^+, and thus hypernatremia occurs.

        (4) Unrestricted access to H_2O may prevent this hypernatremia. Also, other processes in such cases (e.g., ketosis) may increase renal Na^+ loss and counteract hypernatremic tendencies.

2. Na^+-excess group (increased $tbNa^+$)

    a. Excess Na^+ with concurrent restricted H_2O intake (rare)

        (1) Salt poisoning: Cattle with excessive Na^+ (and Cl^- intake) and with concurrent restricted access to H_2O may develop an increased $tbNa^+$ (and total body Cl^- content) and thus hypernatremia (and hyperchloremia).[9] Extreme hypernatremia and hyperchloremia occurred in a dog that ingested a salt-flour mixture that was used as modeling clay.[10]

        (2) Administration of hypertonic saline or sodium bicarbonate can lead to increased $tbNa^+$ and thus hypernatremia (and hyperchloremia or increased HCO_3^-).

      b. Decreased renal excretion of Na^+ (hyperaldosteronism) (rare)
        (1) Excessive aldosterone promotes excessive renal Na^+ (and Cl^-) retention. Hypernatremia (and hyperchloremia) may occur if there is H_2O restriction or defective ADH activity.
        (2) The Na^+-retaining activity of aldosterone may play a role, but, because of a mechanism referred to as aldosterone escape, hyperaldosteronism does not typically cause hypernatremia. Once Na^+ retention begins, and there is corresponding H_2O retention, natriuresis prevents the development of hypernatremia. The natriuresis may be promoted by ANP.[1]

   3. Other or unknown mechanisms
      a. Severe exercise (racing greyhounds):[11-13] During and immediately after a race, the $[Na^+]$ in plasma may be 10–20 mmol/L above prerace concentrations. There is a concurrent hypovolemia and lactic acidosis; thus, the hypernatremia may be caused by the shifting of H_2O from ECF to ICF. The accumulation of L-lactate in muscle fibers may create the osmotic gradient.[1]
      b. Sample dehydration: Exposure of serum or plasma to air may allow evaporation that causes hypernatremia. This is especially true of air-conditioning systems that blow cool, dry air over the sample processing or analysis areas. Sublimation of H_2O from frozen samples may cause hypernatremia if the storage container is not adequately sealed or if it is too large for the sample size.

IV. Normonatremia in dehydrated or edematous animals
  A. Normonatremia does not necessarily indicate that the Na^+ balance is normal (Eq. 9.1a). Recognizing the possibility of altered Na^+ regulation in normonatremic animals is important in the management and treatment of these cases. (That is, do you need to administer Na^+ or restrict Na^+ intake?)
  B. Disorders and pathogeneses (Table 9.3)
    1. Net loss of isotonic fluids that causes dehydration
      a. Alimentary loss of isotonic fluid may occur with vomiting, diarrhea, or sequestration.
      b. Renal loss of Na^+ and H_2O may occur in several situations.
        (1) Many polyuric renal diseases cause Na^+ and H_2O loss because of defective tubular functions.
        (2) Osmotic diuresis impairs resorption of H_2O in tubules. A high tubular flow rate also contributes to Na^+ loss.

Table 9.3. Diseases and conditions that cause normonatremia in dehydrated or edematous animals

Net loss of isotonic fluids causing dehydration
*Alimentary losses: vomiting, diarrhea, sequestration
*Renal losses: renal disease, osmotic diuresis, diuretics
Skin loss: sweating in horses
Net retention of isotonic fluids causing edema or transudate
*Congestive heart failure
*Hepatic cirrhosis
*Nephrotic syndrome

  * A relatively common disease or condition

(3) Most diuretic agents (e.g., furosemide or thiazides) cause Na^+ and H_2O loss through interference with Cl^- resorption.

c. Cutaneous loss in horses: The $[Na^+]$ in sweat is about the same as the $[Na^+]$ in serum or plasma. Thus, profuse sweating without increased H_2O intake could cause normonatremic dehydration.

2. Net retention of isotonic fluids that causes edema or transudation (Note: Edematous disorders may create either normonatremia or hyponatremia, depending on the relative retention of Na^+ and H_2O.)

a. Congestive heart failure (caused by valvular disease or cardiomyopathies)

(1) "Forward" hypothesis: Cardiac disease decreases cardiac output, which is sensed by baroreceptors as decreased effective blood volume, and thus the sympathetic nervous system and the RAS are stimulated. If these responses do not reestablish the effective blood volume, continued activation of the RAS promotes renal resorption of Na^+ and Cl^-, which increases plasma osmolality. Hyperosmolality stimulates release of ADH and the thirst center, which may cause retention of H_2O and increased blood volume. If the hypervolemia increases venous hydraulic pressure sufficiently, it promotes movement of isotonic fluid to extravascular spaces and thus formation of edema (pulmonary or dependent) or accumulation of H_2O in the pleural or peritoneal cavities (transudation).

(2) Retention of Na^+ and H_2O is a compensatory process that helps maintain an effective blood volume. If effective blood volume is not achieved, the hypovolemic stimulus may promote thirst and thus increase H_2O intake. Mammals with a cardiac disease that decreases cardiac output will have increased $tbNa^+$ and tbH_2O even without clinical edema.

b. Hepatic cirrhosis with abdominal transudation

(1) Three theories (underfilling, overflow, and peripheral arterial vasodilation) attempt to explain the peritoneal transudation that occurs with hepatic cirrhosis.[14,15]

(a) In the *underfilling theory*, the initiating event is the loss of plasma H_2O caused by increased hydraulic pressure in hepatic sinusoids (caused by fibrosis or venous congestion) and loss of protein-rich plasma into the space of Disse (sinusoids are highly permeable to albumin). This causes splanchnic pooling of blood and loss of H_2O across the hepatic capsule to the peritoneal cavity and thus underfilling of vascular spaces. Movement of fluid from vessels decreases the effective blood volume, which activates the RAS, stimulates the release of aldosterone, promotes the retention of Na^+ and, subsequently, H_2O. The expanded blood volume accentuates vascular hydraulic pressures and thus promotes more loss of plasma H_2O and more attempts to compensate. At the time of clinical transudation, the animal will have increased $tbNa^+$ and tbH_2O; increased concentrations of renin, norepinephrine, and ADH; and reduced renal excretion of Na^+.

(b) In the *overflow theory*, the initiating event is renal retention of Na^+ and H_2O, but the factors involved are poorly understood.

(c) In the *peripheral arterial vasodilation theory*, peripheral vasodilation decreases the effective blood volume, which activates the RAS. This increases hydraulic pressure in hepatic sinusoids, which leads to transudation.

(2) Hypoalbuminemia and hypoproteinemia play secondary roles in ascites formation.

(a) In health, plasma proteins create colloidal osmotic (oncotic) pressure (about 80 % from albumin and 20 % from globulins) that helps retain H_2O in vessels that are impermeable to proteins. When hypoprotein-emia is present with hepatic cirrhosis, the increases in vascular hydraulic pressure have more effect in promoting movement of H_2O from some vessels (hepatic or pulmonary) to extravascular spaces.

(b) Hypoalbuminemia alone will not cause the transudation. People with analbuminemia may have mild dependent edema but do not have generalized transudation, because of compensatory processes (increased globulins, altered capillary hydraulic pressure, or altered renal blood flow).[16,17] Also, hepatic sinusoids are freely permeable to albumin and H_2O, so plasma H_2O moves out of the sinusoids in either the presence or the absence of hypoalbuminemia.

c. Nephrotic syndrome (protein-losing nephropathy that leads to abdominal transudation)[1,18]

(1) The pathogenesis of Na^+ and H_2O retention is not established but involves several processes: increased activity of the RAS, decreased renal responsive-ness to ANP, decreased plasma protein concentration, inappropriate neural reflexes involving the kidneys, and glomerular disease.

(2) If the renal disease also causes loss of tubular functions, the kidneys have less ability to retain Na^+ and H_2O, and thus the edematous state may not develop in some cases of protein-losing nephropathy.

V. Hyponatremia

A. This typically occurs when the ratio of $tbNa^+$ to tbH_2O is decreased (Eq. 9.1c) or with the shifting of H_2O from ICF to ECF.

B. Disorders and pathogeneses (Table 9.4)

1. Na^+-deficit group: net Na^+ loss > H_2O loss (hypotonic dehydration). In the follow-ing disorders, the $[Na^+]$ in lost fluid is usually not greater than the plasma $[Na^+]$, but loss of Na^+-containing fluid followed by drinking of H_2O may cause hyponatremia.

a. Alimentary loss of Na^+-containing H_2O may occur with vomiting, diarrhea, sequestration, excess salivation, canine whipworm infections, and bovine hemor-rhagic bowel syndrome.[19] For these conditions to cause hyponatremia, there probably is a loss of isotonic ECF followed by drinking H_2O and renal H_2O retention (ADH response) that dilute the remaining plasma Na^+.

b. Renal loss

(1) Hypoadrenocorticism:[1] Adrenal insufficiency decreases the [aldosterone], which causes less resorption of Na^+ and subsequently Cl^- by the renal principal cells. Decreased Na^+ and Cl^- resorption leads to decreased plasma osmolality and decreased renal medullary hypertonicity. The latter leads to a decreased ability to resorb H_2O, so hypovolemia ensues. Hypovolemia stimulates ADH release and thirst centers. Increased ADH activity and increased H_2O intake dilute ECF Na^+ and thus cause hyponatremia (and hypochloremia). Hypocortisolemia promotes the hypothalamic release of

Table 9.4. Diseases and conditions that cause hyponatremia

Na^+-deficit group: net Na^+ loss > H_2O loss (loss of Na^+-containing fluid followed by increased H_2O intake, hypotonic dehydration)

  *Alimentary loss: vomiting, diarrhea, sequestration, canine whipworm infection, excess salivation, bovine hemorrhagic bowel syndrome

  *Renal loss: hypoadrenocorticism, prolonged diuresis, ketonuria, Na^+-wasting nephropathies, hypoaldosteronism

  Cutaneous loss: sweating in horses

  Third-space loss: repeated drainage of chylous effusion, acute hemorrhage or exudation

H_2O-excess groups (with or without edema)

  Edematous disorders

    *Congestive heart failure

    Hepatic cirrhosis

    Nephrotic syndrome

  Expanded ECF volume (but without edema)

    Syndrome of inappropriate ADH secretion

    Excess administration of Na^+-poor fluids

Shifting of H_2O from ICF to ECF

  *Hyperglycemia

  Mannitol infusion (IV)

Shifting of Na^+ from ECF to ICF

  Acute muscle damage

Shifting of Na^+ from intravascular to extravascular fluid

  Uroperitoneum

K^+ depletion causing shifts in Na^+ and H_2O

* A relatively common disease or condition

Note: Pseudo-hyponatremia may be caused by displacement of serum or plasma H_2O (see the text).

ADH (multiple theories), which causes defective excretion of H_2O (retention of free H_2O in the presence of hypoosmolality) and a dilutional hyponatremia.[1,20] In people with hypoaldosteronism and lack of hypocortisolemia, normonatremia is maintained by enhanced tubular resorption of Na^+ caused by increased angiotensin II, decreased ANP, and enhanced passive resorption.[1]

(2) Prolonged diuresis

  (a) Prolonged osmotic diuresis with Na^+-poor fluid[21] or other forms of diuresis (e.g., caused by furosemide administration)[22] tend to deplete Na^+ and H_2O, cause hypovolemia, and stimulate ADH release and thirst centers. H_2O drinking tends to dilute the Na^+ in the ECF and thus cause hyponatremia.

  (b) Thiazide diuretics cause Na^+, Cl^-, and K^+ loss in excess of H_2O loss, and thus hyponatremia, hypochloremia, and hypokalemia may develop. Urinary Na^+ and Cl^- loss is increased because thiazides inhibit a Na^+-Cl^- cotransporter in distal nephrons. Urinary K^+ loss is increased because of an increased flow rate in distal nephrons and hypovolemia-induced release of aldosterone, which opens K^+ channels. The hypovolemia also stimulates ADH release, which promotes resorption of free H_2O and thus dilution of the remaining Na^+, Cl^-, and K^+.

- (3) Ketonuria
    - (a) During ketonuria, the excretion of ketone bodies (AcAc and BHB) is increased. The presence of these nonabsorbable anions in the tubular lumen obligates the excretion of cations and thus increased renal excretion of Na^+.
    - (b) Concurrent osmotic diuresis (from glucosuria) may compound the Na^+ loss associated with ketonuria in patients with diabetes mellitus.
- (4) Na^+-wasting nephropathies: Some renal diseases (especially tubular diseases or pyelonephritis) cause an excess excretion of Na^+ because of decreased Na^+ resorption. This is seen more in horses than other domestic mammals.
- (5) Hyperreninemic hypoaldosteronism (see hyperkalemia)

- c. Cutaneous loss by sweating
    - (1) Among the domestic mammals, only horses sweat sufficiently to cause electrolyte and H_2O imbalances.
    - (2) Equine sweat is a Na^+-, K^+-, Cl^--rich fluid (concentrations are greater than plasma concentrations but evaporation may contribute to the increases).[23,24] Drinking of H_2O or the ADH-stimulated retention of H_2O after sweating may lead to dilutional hyponatremia.

- d. Third-space loss (typically loss to pleural cavity or peritoneal cavity)
    - (1) Repeated drainage of chylous thoracic effusions
        - (a) Repeated removal of isotonic fluid from the thoracic cavity probably results in a Na^+- and H_2O-depleted state that is followed by intake of H_2O and an ADH response to cause dilutional hyponatremia.[25,26]
        - (b) This type of hyponatremia would probably also result from repeated removal of other cavitary effusions, but such removal is not as common as it is for chylous effusions.
    - (2) Acute internal hemorrhage or acute exudation
        - (a) Acute loss of ECF from the vascular space to other extracellular sites in the body (third-space loss) causes an isotonic hypovolemia. If followed by increased intake of H_2O and an ADH response, dilutional hyponatremia may develop.
        - (b) This type of hyponatremia is rare, since hypovolemia would also stimulate renal Na^+ retention.

2. H_2O-excess group (H_2O retention > Na^+ retention) with or without edema
    - a. Edematous disorders
        - (1) Congestive heart failure, hepatic cirrhosis, and nephrotic syndrome
        - (2) Although these conditions are often associated with normonatremia (see the preceding sect. IV.B.2), hyponatremia (typically mild) may also occur if the ratio of tbNa^+ to tbH_2O is decreased.
    - b. Expanded ECF volume (but without edema)
        - (1) Syndrome of inappropriate ADH secretion (SIADH)
            - (a) This is characterized by nonphysiologic release of ADH in the presence of hypoosmolality and hypervolemia. Excess ADH with unrestricted H_2O intake leads to free-H_2O resorption and dilutional hyponatremia. Renal Na^+ excretion (perhaps due to ANP) is increased because of activation of volume receptors.[1]

       (b) Neurologic, pulmonary, and thyroid disorders are associated with the syndrome of inappropriate ADH secretion, as are many drugs. A few cases have been reported in domestic mammals.[27]

    (2) Excessive administration of Na^+-poor fluids: Administration of 5 % dextrose or 0.45 % saline could lead to a dilutional hyponatremia.

    (3) Primary polydipsia may cause hyponatremia but typically is a minor abnormality because functional kidneys can excrete the consumed H_2O.[28]

3. Shifting of H_2O from ICF to ECF

   a. A marked or persistent increase in effective plasma osmolality (e.g., because of hyperglycemia or mannitol infusion) creates an osmolar gradient between ECF and ICF. This draws H_2O into the blood by osmosis, thus diluting the plasma $[Na^+]$. In people, if glucose concentrations increase by 100 mg/dL, the serum $[Na^+]$ is reported to decrease 1.6 mmol/L for glucose concentrations < 400 mg/dL and 4 mmol/L for glucose concentrations > 400 mg/dL.[29]

   b. Concurrent processes (osmotic diuresis and ketonuria) also contribute to the Na^+ loss and thus hyponatremia.

4. Shifting of Na^+ from ECF to ICF

   a. Acute damage to the cell membrane of muscle fibers allows Na^+ to move from a high concentration in ECF to a lower concentration in ICF.[30]

   b. In this condition, there is a concurrent influx of H_2O and fCa^{2+} and efflux of K^+ and PO_4 to cause hypovolemia, hypocalcemia, hyperkalemia, and hyperphosphatemia.

5. Shift of Na^+ from intravascular to extravascular space

   a. When urine, typically a Na^+ and Cl^- poor fluid, is in the abdominal cavity (*uroperitoneum*), diffusion of Na^+ and Cl^- from the plasma to the peritoneal fluid may cause hyponatremia and hypochloremia.[31]

   b. Experimentally in dogs, hyponatremia and hypochloremia were detected within 1–2 d of the onset of uroperitoneum and were marked after 4 d.[32]

6. K^+ depletion causing shifts in Na^+ and H_2O[1] (see Eq. 9.1d)

   a. As described later in this chapter (see Potassium Concentration, sect. V.B.2), K^+ can be lost from the body during a variety of gastrointestinal and renal disorders. If these losses are not replaced by intake, the body will become K^+ depleted.

   b. These K^+ losses decrease the extracellular $[K^+]$, which creates a gradient for K^+ movement from cells to the ECF. Because proteins and other large anions cannot leave the cells, the electrical neutrality is maintained by one or more of the following—each contributes to the development of hyponatremia:

    (1) Na^+ ions shift from the ECF to the intracellular fluid.

    (2) Cl^- leaves the cell with K^+ and thus lowers the intracellular osmolality. The resulting osmotic gradient causes H_2O to move from cells to the ECF, thus diluting the ECF $[Na^+]$.

    (3) H^+ ions enter the cell as K^+ leaves, but the H^+ ions bind with intracellular buffers and thus do not add to the intracellular osmolality. However, the K^+ loss from the cells lowers the intracellular osmolality, and thus H_2O moves from cells to the ECF, thus diluting the ECF $[Na^+]$.

7. Pseudo-hyponatremia

   a. This may occur when the serum $[Na^+]$ is determined by flame photometry or indirect potentiometry (see Sodium Concentration, sect. II.A.1). The same principles apply to the $[Cl^-]$ and the resultant pseudo-hypochloremia.

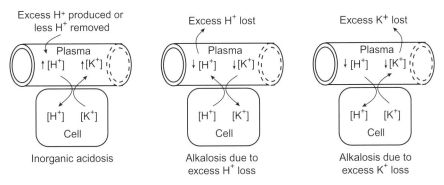

Fig. 9.2. H^+ and K^+ shift in acid-base disorders.

- In an inorganic acidosis, there is an accumulation of H^+ in ECF. As H^+ shifts into cells to equilibrate concentrations, K^+ shifts out of cells to maintain electrical neutrality and enters plasma (hyperkalemia occurs).[33] In an organic acidosis, hyperkalemia is not expected because additional factors influence plasma $[K^+]$(see the text).
- In an alkalosis, $[H^+]$ in ECF is reduced. As H^+ shifts out of cells to equilibrate concentrations, K^+ enters cells (leaves the plasma; hypokalemia occurs). The illustration shows the alkalotic state beginning with H^+ loss; the H^+ depletion may be due to other processes.
- Conversely, if K^+ depletion causes hypokalemia, K^+ shifts out of the cells and H^+ enters and thus lowers blood $[H^+]$ (alkalemia). The illustration shows the alkalotic state beginning with K^+ loss; the K^+ depletion may be due to other processes.

    b. Laboratories may measure serum or plasma $[Na^+]$ by direct potentiometry by using ion-selective electrodes. Such assays do not require sample dilution, so excess solids in the plasma do not affect them. The electrodes detect the Na^+ activity in the aqueous phase only.

POTASSIUM (K^+) CONCENTRATION

I.   Physiologic processes
   A. Serum $[K^+]$ is nearly equivalent to ECF $[K^+]$, which is mostly dependent on tbK^+ and movement of K^+ into and out of K^+-rich cells in response to changes in acid-base status. Therefore, serum $[K^+]$ should be interpreted with consideration of acid-base status and potential variations in tbK^+ status.
   B. Most cells are rich in K^+ because of a Na^+-K^+-ATPase pump that constantly pumps K^+ into cells against a concentration gradient.
   C. Acidoses and alkaloses alter the serum $[K^+]$ (Fig. 9.2).
       1. An inorganic or mineral acidosis (caused by renal failure, some diarrheas, or administration of NH_4Cl) may cause hyperkalemia because of the shifting of K^+ out of cells.
       2. An organic acidosis (e.g., lactic acidosis and ketoacidosis) typically does not cause hyperkalemia, but the reasons may vary.[33]
           a. If an anion (such as L-lactate or ketone body) enters a cell when H^+ does, electroneutrality is maintained and thus K^+ does not need to leave the cell.

      b. Acidemia may promote the loss of K^+ from cells, but the K^+ is excreted in urine with the organic anions (e.g., L-lactate or AcAc) that are also excreted during lactic acidosis and ketoacidosis, respectively.

  3. Treatment of a normokalemic acidotic state may cause hypokalemia that reflects tbK^+ depletion in an animal.

  4. Metabolic alkalosis may cause mild hypokalemia.

  5. Respiratory acidoses and alkaloses are not associated with altered serum $[K^+]$,[1] maybe because other regulatory systems are still functional.

D. If the acid-base status is normal, then serum or plasma $[K^+]$ tends to reflect tbK^+; that is, hyperkalemia tends to occur with increased tbK^+, whereas hypokalemia tends to occur with decreased tbK^+. However, a K^+-depleted state may occur before hypokalemia develops.[34]

E. Plasma $[K^+]$ is regulated through two major processes: (1) distribution between ECF and ICF, and (2) renal excretion.

  1. K^+ distribution between ECF and ICF

      a. Epinephrine and insulin promote the uptake of K^+ into cells through the action of a Na^+-K^+-ATPase pump. This effect of insulin is independent of its actions on glucose uptake.

      b. Hyperkalemia promotes the cellular uptake of K^+, whereas hypokalemia promotes the loss of K^+ from cells.

  2. Renal excretion of K^+

      a. Typically, K^+ is resorbed before the renal tubular fluid reaches the distal nephron. Therefore, the $[K^+]$ in tubular fluid entering the distal nephron is near zero.

      b. K^+ is secreted primarily by the principal cells of the collecting tubules (Fig. 9.3). Aldosterone promotes this process by stimulating Na^+-K^+-ATPase in the basolateral membrane and opening luminal K^+ channels. Hyperkalemia and angiotensin II are the major stimulants of aldosterone secretion. Adrenocorticotropic hormone (ACTH) and hyponatremia also stimulate aldosterone release, but the effect of hyponatremia is diminished if the effective blood volume is adequate.[1]

      c. A high flow rate of tubular fluid also promotes K^+ secretion because secreted K^+ is quickly washed away and thus does not inhibit the passive movement of K^+ from cells to tubular fluid. Conversely, a low flow rate inhibits K^+ secretion.

      d. Resorption of Na^+ without Cl^- (e.g., hypochloremic states) establishes an electrochemical gradient (tubular fluid more negative than cell) that promotes the secretion of K^+.

  3. K^+ is conserved by type A intercalated cells of the distal nephron through H^+-K^+-ATPase pump activity when hypokalemia is caused by decreased total body K^+ (Fig. 9.4).

  4. ADH promotes K^+ secretion that counterbalances the reduced K^+ secretion that occurs with decreased urinary flow. The enhanced secretion prevents the hyperkalemia that might be caused by dehydration-induced oliguria.

  5. Plasma $[K^+]$ is also influenced by intestinal and cutaneous processes: absorption of dietary K^+ by the intestine, loss of K^+ via feces, and loss of K^+ via sweat.

II. Analytical concepts

A. Terms and units

  1. Assays measure the electrical potential of K^+ (potentiometry) and convert it to concentrations, or they measure $[K^+]$ (flame photometry) in plasma, serum, or whole blood. The K^+ is mostly a free ion in the plasma or serum H_2O.

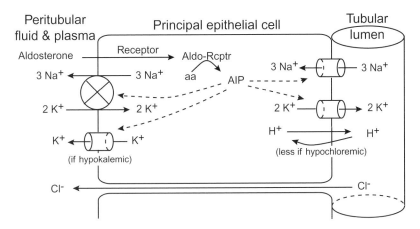

Fig. 9.3. Actions of aldosterone on principal epithelial cells in cortical collecting tubules. Aldosterone enters the principal cells and binds to receptor proteins. The aldosterone-receptor complex (Aldo-Rcptr) stimulates the synthesis of aldosterone-induced proteins (AIP), which may include components of the Na^+-K^+-ATPase pump and membrane channels for Na^+ and K^+. Through the actions on the pump or channels, aldosterone promotes the following:

1. Na^+ is pumped from the cell to the peritubular fluid, and the resulting luminal cell gradient promotes the resorption of Na^+ through an opened Na^+ channel.
2. K^+ is pumped into the cell from the peritubular fluid and typically exits to the tubular fluid through an opened K^+ channel. When hypokalemia is present, K^+ may return to the peritubular fluid via an opened basolateral membrane channel (K^+ is recycled).
3. Typically, the Na^+-K^+-ATPase pump results in a net negative charge in the tubular fluid (3 Na^+ resorbed and two K^+ secreted). The negative charge promotes the resorption of Cl^- through a paracellular route. When there is less Cl^- available (as occurs with hypochloremia), the negative charge promotes the retention of H^+ in the tubular fluid (the H^+ that passively leaves and reenters the principal cells) and thus increases renal secretion of H^+.

The net result of aldosterone actions in health is the resorption of Na^+ and Cl^- and secretion of K^+. In the presence of hypochloremia, there is increased secretion of H^+, which can promote aciduria or a metabolic alkalosis. ⊗, ATPase pump; and aa, amino acids.

---

      2. Unit conversion: mEq/L × 1 = mmol/L, and mg/dL ÷ 3.9 = mmol/L (SI unit, nearest 0.1 mmol/L)[3]

  B. Sample for [K^+] quantitation
      1. Serum is preferred. The [K^+] is stable for months if the sample does not dehydrate.
      2. K_3EDTA should not be used as an anticoagulant for testing plasma [K^+] because the anticoagulant's K^+ will be added to the plasma and be measured.

  C. Assays
      1. Ion-selective electrode assays are the most common.
      2. Flame photometers for measuring [K^+] were the gold standard but are no longer used for routine patient screening.

III.   Hyperkalemia
  A. This typically occurs when the renal excretion of K^+ decreases or K^+ shifts from ICF to ECF. Hyperkalemia may also occur with increased intake of K^+ or treatment with K^+, especially if there is renal compromise. If the acid-base status is normal, then serum [K^+] tends to reflect tbK$^+$.

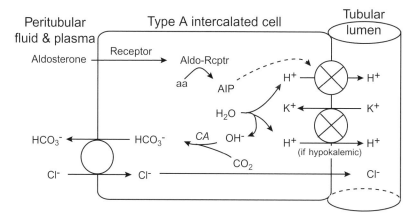

Fig. 9.4. Secretion of H^+ by type A intercalated cells of the distal nephron. Aldosterone enters the type A intercalated cells and binds to receptor proteins. The aldosterone-receptor complex (Aldo-Rcptr) stimulates the synthesis of aldosterone-induced proteins (AIP) that may include components of H^+-ATPase pump. Through the actions of the pump, which is more active during systemic acidemia, aldosterone causes the secretion of H^+ and formation of HCO_3^- through the following processes:

1. H^+ released from the dissociation of H_2O is pumped into the tubular lumen.
2. OH^- released from the dissociation of H_2O combines with CO_2 in the presence of carbonic anhydrase (*CA*) to form HCO_3^-, which is exchanged for Cl^- in the peritubular fluid.
3. Cl^- that enters the cell in the Cl^--HCO_3^- exchanger is secreted into the tubular lumen to maintain electrical neutrality (balance the H^+ secretion).

The net result if stimulated by acidemia or aldosterone is increased H^+ and Cl^- secretion and increased HCO_3^- in plasma. In an independent process but in the same cells, a H^+-K^+-ATPase promotes the resorption of K^+ and secretion of H^+; this pump is more active when hypokalemia is present. Thus, hypokalemia promotes increased H^+ secretion, HCO_3^- production, and thus alkalosis.

$\otimes$, ATPase pump; $\bigcirc$, cotransporter or counter transporter (antiporter); and aa, amino acids.

B. Disorders and pathogeneses (Table 9.5)
  1. Shifting of K^+ from ICF to ECF
     a. Metabolic inorganic acidoses causing acidemia: shifting of K^+ out of cells when H^+ moves in (see Fig. 9.2)
     b. Rhabdomyolysis or other muscle damage (release of K^+ from muscle fibers)
        (1) Acquired disorders: selenium deficiency,[30] malignant hyperthermia,[35] and seizures
        (2) Congenital disorders: They can be induced by stress or anesthetic in dystrophin-deficient cats[36] and include hyperkalemic periodic paralysis in quarter horses[37] and possibly hyperkalemic periodic paralysis in a dog (the dog's serum $[K^+]$ was never documented at > 5 mmol/L but did increase from 3.9 mmol/L to 4.9 mmol/L after exercise).[38]
     c. Strenuous exercise may cause hyperkalemia. Hyperkalemia is caused by K^+ release from active myocytes. The K^+ release might be related to ion shifts caused by a decrease in nondiffusible intracellular anions that occur as phosphocreatine, a highly dissociated acid, hydrolyzes to neutral creatine.[39] Also, myocytes may be damaged.

Table 9.5. Diseases and conditions that cause hyperkalemia

Shifting of K^+ from ICF to ECF (no change in total body K^+)
  *Metabolic acidoses caused by accumulation of inorganic acids
  Rhabdomyolysis or other muscle damage
    Acquired: strenuous exercise, seizures, selenium deficiency
    Congenital: hyperkalemic periodic paralysis in quarter horses and perhaps dogs
  Massive intravascular hemolysis in animals with K^+ rich erythrocytes
  Other massive tissue necrosis
  After exercise in hypothyroid dogs
Increased total body K^+
  Decreased renal excretion of K^+
    *Renal insufficiency or failure (primarily oliguric or anuric)
    *Urinary tract obstruction or leakage into body
    Hypoaldosteronism
      *Hypoadrenocorticism (Addison's)
      Angiotensin-converting enzyme inhibitors
      Hyperreninemic hypoaldosteronism
    Trimethoprim-induced K^+ retention
  Increased intake
    Administration of K^+-rich fluid
Other or unknown mechanism
  Repeated drainage of chylous thoracic effusions
  Peritoneal effusions in cats

  * A relatively common disease or condition
  Note: Also consider pseudo-hyperkalemia (see the text)

   d. Massive intravascular hemolysis in animals with K^+-rich erythrocytes: English
      springer spaniels with phosphofructokinase deficiency have hyperkalemia
      concurrent with their hemolytic episodes which might involve K^+-rich young
      erythrocytes.[40]
   e. Massive tissue necrosis (in tissues other than muscle or blood), which is caused
      by the release of K^+-rich ICF from dead cells, is seen with tumor necrosis, arterial
      thrombosis with tissue ischemia, and sometimes just prior to death.
   f. Hypertonicity (e.g., caused by hyperglycemia in diabetes mellitus) leads to an
      osmotic shift of H_2O from cells to ECF, thereby increasing the intracellular $[K^+]$
      (but not total K^+ content). K^+ then shifts down a concentration gradient into
      ECF. Although the K^+ shift decreases the intracellular $[K^+]$, the net effect on
      the plasma $[K^+]$ depends on many other factors (e.g., renal loss of K^+ due to
      ketonuria and osmotic diuresis in diabetes mellitus), and thus hyperkalemia may
      not be present.
   g. Plasma $[K^+]$ increased, but only slightly exceeded the upper reference limit, when
      dogs with experimentally induced hypothyroidism were exercised (running for
      5 min); the increase did not occur in euthyroid dogs. The hyperkalemia may
      have been caused by an ICF to ECF shift of K^+ related to reduced Na^+-K^+-
      ATPase activity in skeletal muscle.[41] Hyperkalemia is not expected in
      nonexercised hypothyroid dogs.

   h. Pseudo-hyperkalemia
       (1) In vitro hemolysis or leakage of K^+ because of delayed removal of serum or
            plasma from erythrocytes
            (a) If the $[K^+]$ in erythrocytes is greater than the $[K^+]$ in plasma, then the
                 loss of K^+ from erythrocytes may cause pseudo-hyperkalemia. The ratio
                 of erythrocyte $[K^+]$ to plasma $[K^+]$ varies among species and among
                 breeds of dogs.
            (b) This form of pseudo-hyperkalemia may occur in horses,[42] some dogs
                 (i.e., Japanese Akitas[43], Japanese Shibas, and rarely others), and cattle.
                 Serum or plasma may not appear hemolyzed despite substantial K^+
                 leakage from erythrocytes.
            (c) Hemolysis is not expected to cause hyperkalemia in cats or other breeds
                 of dogs.
       (2) Thrombocytosis[44]
            (a) K^+ is released from platelets in the clotted blood sample. The released
                 K^+ is part of the $[K^+]$ used to establish serum reference intervals.
                 Without a thrombocytosis, serum $[K^+]$ is about 0.3–0.5 mmol/L greater
                 than plasma $[K^+]$ in samples collected from the same blood draw.[45]
            (b) When thrombocytosis is marked (> 1,000,000/μL), more K^+ is added to
                 the serum during clotting than normally occurs and thus the measured
                 serum $[K^+]$ may be increased.
       (3) Leakage of K^+ from leukemic cells[46]
2. Increased total body K^+
    a. Decreased renal excretion of K^+
        (1) Renal insufficiency or failure (primarily oliguric or anuric; acute renal
             disease or the terminal stages of chronic renal disease)
             (a) In oliguric or anuric phases of acute or chronic renal failure, K^+
                  excretion is diminished because of decreased flow of tubular fluid to the
                  distal nephron. When the rate of tubular fluid flow is low in the
                  collecting tubules, secreted K^+ accumulates in the tubular fluid and thus
                  the K^+ concentration gradient is diminished. Because the movement of
                  K^+ from cells is a passive process, K^+ secretion from the distal tubular
                  cells is diminished. When renal K^+ secretion is impaired, dietary K^+ or
                  K^+ released from cells accumulates in plasma.
             (b) A reduction in renal blood flow will reduce the amount of K^+ presented
                  to the kidney for excretion and thus contribute to the hyperkalemia.
             (c) The metabolic acidosis of renal failure may contribute to the hyperkale-
                  mia (a shifting of K^+ from cells to plasma). In chronic polyuric renal
                  failure, the number of functional nephrons decreases, but the K^+
                  excretion per functioning nephron increases. Therefore, hyperkalemia is
                  not expected in polyuric chronic renal failure.
        (2) Urinary tract obstruction or leakage
             (a) With urinary tract leakage (ruptured bladder or leakage from ureter or
                  urethra), K^+ enters the ECF and thus is not removed from the body.
                  With time, hyperkalemia may develop. In experimentally produced
                  uroperitoneum, some dogs developed hyperkalemia within 2 d, and all
                  dogs were hyperkalemic after 4 d.[32] Hyperkalemia is not always seen in
                  spontaneous canine and feline cases of uroperitoneum, probably because

of the variable durations and variable amounts of urine in the peritoneal cavities.

    (b) Urinary tract obstruction may cause a similar hyperkalemia because of the defective excretion of K^+ and the development of an acidosis.

  (3) Hypoaldosteronism

    (a) Hypoadrenocorticism (Addison's disease)

      (i) Bilateral adrenocortical hypoplasia decreases the production of aldosterone and cortisol.

      (ii) Hypoaldosteronemia decreases the activity of Na^+-K^+-ATPase pumps in the basolateral membranes of the principal cells of collecting tubules. This leads to decreased resorption of Na^+ and therefore decreased movement of K^+ into the tubular epithelial cells for passive secretion to the tubular lumen. This process is further inhibited because the number of luminal K^+ channels decreases with decreased aldosterone.

    (b) Inhibitors of angiotensin-converting enzyme might cause hyperkalemia because of the development of hypoaldosteronism. However, if renal function is adequate, K^+ is secreted through aldosterone-independent processes, and thus only mild hyperkalemia occurs.[1]

    (c) In primary hypoaldosteronism of people, hyperkalemia is present, but normonatremia is maintained by the actions of increased angiotensin II and decreased ANP.[1]

    (d) Hyperreninemic hypoaldosteronism was diagnosed in a 9-yr-old dog that had marked hyperkalemia, mild hyponatremia, mild hypochloremia, normocortisolemia, hypoaldosteronemia, and increased plasma renin activity.[47] The defect that led to the hypoaldosteronemia was not determined.

  (4) Trimethoprim-induced K^+ retention[48]

    (a) Trimethoprim (especially when protonated in acidic urine) blocks the luminal Na^+ channels of the collecting ducts and thus acts like a K^+-sparing diuretic.[49,50] With reduced Na^+ resorption, the electrical gradient that promotes K^+ secretion is reduced.

    (b) Effects of trimethoprim would be enhanced if the flow rate in the tubules were decreased, because K^+ secretion depends on a K^+ gradient maintained by high urine flow rates that carry secreted K^+ away, thus increasing the intracellular to lumen K^+ gradient.

  b. Increased intake of K^+: administration of K^+-rich fluid,[51] especially if there is renal compromise

3. Repeated drainage of chylous thoracic effusions:[25,26] Pathogenesis of hyperkalemia is not established but may be related to concurrent hyponatremia. In the presence of hyponatremia and hypovolemia, much of the filtrate Na^+ is resorbed in the proximal tubules and ascending loop of Henle. If Na^+ is not delivered to the distal nephron, less Na^+ is resorbed distally and thus less K^+ secretion occurs.

4. Peritoneal effusions: Four cats with peritoneal effusions had hyperkalemias and either mild or marked hyponatremias.[52] The effusions were caused by abdominal carcinomatosis (one cat) and feline infectious peritonitis (two and possibly three cats; firm diagnosis not made in the last cat). The hyperkalemia may be caused by impaired renal secretion of K^+ because of decreased distal tubular flow rate and

concurrent hyponatremia. The hyponatremia was considered a dilutional one that resulted from H_2O retention caused by stimulation of ADH release and thirst centers by a decreased effective blood volume.

IV. Normokalemia in acidotic or alkalotic animals
   A. Normokalemia in an acidotic animal
      1. Because inorganic acidemia is expected to increase serum $[K^+]$, normokalemia in the presence of inorganic acidemia suggests an animal has a decreased tbK^+. Therapeutic correction of the inorganic acidemia may lower the serum $[K^+]$ into the hypokalemic range. Disorders that may produce this pathophysiologic state include renal failure and some cases of diarrhea.
      2. As mentioned earlier (see Potassium Concentration, sect. I.C), animals with an organic metabolic acidosis may not be hyperkalemic. This is because either the K^+ shift into cells is accompanied by an organic anion shift, or renal excretion of K^+ is increased to maintain electroneutrality as organic anions are excreted.
   B. Normokalemia in an alkalotic animal
      1. Because alkalemia is expected to decrease serum $[K^+]$, normokalemia in the presence of alkalemia suggests an animal has an increased tbK^+. Therapeutic correction of the alkalemia may raise the serum $[K^+]$ into the hyperkalemic range.
      2. This combination of findings is not expected because disorders that cause metabolic alkalosis typically do not concurrently increase tbK^+.

V. Hypokalemia
   A. This typically occurs when there is a shift of K^+ from ECF to ICF, a decreased dietary intake of K^+, or an increased K^+ loss via kidneys, alimentary tract, or skin. If the acid-base status is normal, then the serum $[K^+]$ tends to reflect tbK^+.
   B. Disorders and pathogeneses (Table 9.6)
      1. Shifting of K^+ from ECF to ICF
         a. Metabolic alkalosis causing alkalemia: A general concept for the hypokalemia of alkalosis is that K^+ shifts into cells when H^+ moves out (see Potassium Concentration, sect. I.C). However, this process may play a minor role. Most metabolic alkaloses have three other reasons for hypokalemia: (1) concurrent hypovolemia activates the renin-angiotensin-aldosterone system and thus increases the renal secretion of K^+, (2) bicarbonaturia obligates the renal excretion of cations including K^+, and (3) dietary intake of K^+ decreases because of anorexia or vomiting.
         b. Increased insulin activity: Insulin promotes the cellular uptake of K^+, probably through the activation of a Na^+-K^+-ATPase. Administration of exogenous insulin or a sudden release of endogenous insulin after IV glucose administration may cause hypokalemia. A ketotic diabetic animal would more likely develop hypokalemia because it might have decreased tbK^+ (see Potassium Concentration, sect. V.B.2).
         c. Experimental endotoxemia causes a hypokalemia.[53,54] The hypokalemia may develop because endotoxin stimulates the Na^+-K^+-ATPase of skeletal muscle, which causes K^+ to shift from the ECF to muscle fibers.[53] The endotoxin-induced release of insulin may also contribute to the K^+ shift.
      2. Decreased total body K^+
         a. Decreased K^+ intake
            (1) Because most diets are K^+ rich, anorexia or prolonged food restriction can contribute to decreased tbK^+.

Table 9.6. Diseases and conditions that cause hypokalemia

Shifting of K^+ from ECF to ICF (no change in total body K^+)
   Metabolic alkalosis with alkalemia
   Increased insulin activity (rapid increase)
   Endotoxemia
Decreased total body K^+
   *Decreased K^+ intake: anorexia or other reasons for not eating
   Increased excretion of K^+
      Increased renal loss
         *Increased fluid flow in distal nephron: osmotic, Na^+-losing nephropathies,
            therapeutic diuresis (including loop and thiazide diuretics)
         *Increased renal excretion of anions (ketonuria, lactaturia, bicarbonaturia)
         *Vomiting or sequestration of H^+ and Cl^- causing hypochloremic metabolic
            alkalosis
          Hyperaldosteronism, primary
       *Increased alimentary loss: vomiting, diarrhea, sequestration, excess salivation
       Increased cutaneous loss: sweating in horses
Other or unknown mechanisms
   *Hypokalemic renal failure in cats
   Hypokalemic myopathy of Burmese kittens

* A relatively common disease or condition

   (2) The severity of hypokalemia will be enhanced if other processes are leading
       to K^+ loss or shifting to ICF.
   b. Increased excretion of K^+
      (1) Increased renal loss
         (a) Increased tubular flow
             (i) Increased flow of fluid through the collecting tubules allows for
                 increased secretion of K^+ from the tubular cells. Rapid flushing of
                 K^+ maintains a low tubular $[K^+]$, which allows the passive move-
                 ment of K^+ out of the cells.
             (ii) Polyuric states that promote hypokalemia include glucosuria,
                  Na^+-losing nephropathies (pyelonephritis, tubular interstitial
                  nephritis, and possibly hypercalcemic nephropathy), and diuretic
                  use (loop diuretics and thiazide).
         (b) Increased renal excretion of anions
             (i) Ketonuria: AcAc and BHB (ketone bodies) are anions that are not
                 resorbed in the tubules. Their negative charges add to the electro-
                 chemical gradient that promotes K^+ excretion, especially when there
                 is concurrent stimulation of Na^+ resorption. Animals with ketoaci-
                 dotic diabetes mellitus tend to be hypokalemic; however, the net K^+
                 balance is the result of multiple concurrent processes.
             (ii) Lactaturia: Lactate is a poorly resorbed by renal tubules. Thus,
                  increased renal excretion of L-lactate (in lactic acidosis) obligates
                  the loss of cations such as Na^+ and K^+.

        (iii) Bicarbonaturia: When plasma [HCO_3^-] exceeds the renal capacity to conserve HCO_3^- (renal threshold) or if there is a tubular acidosis, the HCO_3^- that remains in the tubular fluid obligates the renal excretion of cations such as Na^+ and K^+.

    (c) Vomiting or sequestration of H^+ and Cl^- that causes hypochloremic metabolic alkalosis (e.g., displaced abomasum, bovine hemorrhagic bowel syndrome, or other disorders causing upper gastrointestinal obstruction)

        (i) During the development of this metabolic alkalosis, plasma [HCO_3^-] may increase sufficiently that the tubular maximum for HCO_3^- is exceeded and thus HCO_3^- is presented to the distal nephron. Because HCO_3^- is not resorbed in the distal nephron, its presence adds to the electrochemical gradient that promotes tubular K^+ secretion.

        (ii) Renal secretion of K^+ (and concurrently H^+) is promoted through the actions of aldosterone if an animal is hypovolemic.

        (iii) Some K^+ in gastric secretions may be lost via vomiting.

    (d) Hyperaldosteronism, primary[55]

        (i) Dogs with hyperaldosteronism caused by adrenal neoplasms may have hypokalemia.[5,56] A similar pathologic state has been reported in cats.[57–60]

        (ii) Cats also have been reported to have a primary hyperaldosteronism that is associated with adrenal hyperplasia and not neoplasia.[61] These cats had a high-normal to increased [aldosterone] concurrent with hypokalemia and an increased aldosterone to plasma renin activity ratio. The cats were considered to have *primary* hyperaldosteronism because hyperkalemia and hyperreninemia were not present. However, hyperplasia may have been secondary to incomplete suppression of renin secretion because of renal disease. Some of the cats did develop renal failure.

        (iii) The increased aldosterone concentrations would promote renal K^+ secretion by stimulating Na^+-K^+-ATPase and opening K^+ channels in the collecting tubules (Fig. 9.3).

(2) Increased alimentary loss of K^+ via vomiting, diarrhea, sequestration, or excess salivation

    (a) Vomiting may cause loss of K^+-rich fluid and reduced intestinal absorption of K^+ and thus lead to hypokalemia. Also, enhanced renal excretion of K^+ (due to response to increased aldosterone activity and decreased availability of Cl^-) may add to a decreased tbK^+.

    (b) With diarrheas, loss of electrolytes and H_2O may be massive. H_2O intake may contribute a dilutional component to the hypokalemia. In addition, lack of absorption of dietary K^+ may augment the severity of the tbK^+ depletion and thus hypokalemia.

    (c) K^+-rich fluid may be sequestered in the intestines of animals with ileus, especially in horses.

    (d) Because saliva is a K^+-rich fluid, loss of large volumes of saliva (because of choking, a lacerated salivary gland, dysphagia, or ptyalism) in horses and cattle can produce hypokalemia.[62] Initially, the concurrent loss of HCO_3^- may produce a mild acidosis. If the animals also become hyponatremic, hypochloremic, and hypovolemic, then renal compensations (conservation of Na^+ and HCO_3^-, and excretion of K^+ and H^+) may lead to a hypokalemic metabolic alkalosis.

   (3) Increased cutaneous loss: sweating in horses

      (a) Equine sweat is relatively K^+ rich as compared to plasma. Thus, profuse sweating can lead to K^+ loss, tbK^+ depletion, and hypokalemia.[23,24]

      (b) If the horse is drinking, H_2O intake would promote dilution of the remaining K^+.

  c. Other or unknown mechanisms

    (1) Hypokalemic renal failure in cats

      (a) Cats with progressive renal disease that cause chronic renal failure are prone to tbK^+ depletion (*kaliopenia*) and thus develop hypokalemia.

      (b) The exact pathogenesis of the hypokalemia of chronic renal failure is unknown and may be due to multiple factors: increased renal K^+ excretion, increased colonic K^+ excretion, and decreased dietary K^+ intake. Because cats retain renal concentrating ability much longer in renal disease than other domestic mammals, possibly their distal tubules remain responsive to aldosterone during hypovolemia and thus retain Na^+ and secrete K^+. In experimental conditions, a NaCl-restricted diet did result in hypokalemia and inappropriate kaliuresis when the glomerular filtration rate was reduced.[63]

    (2) Hypokalemic myopathy in Burmese kittens[64–66]

      (a) The Burmese kittens had hypokalemia, muscle weakness, and high serum creatine kinase activities. The myopathy was precipitated by stress or exercise.

      (b) The pathogenesis of the hypokalemia is not established but may be due to a sudden shift of K^+ from the ECF to ICF.

SODIUM TO POTASSIUM (Na^+:K^+) RATIO

I.   Because several physiologic processes involve both Na^+ and K^+, it's not surprising that [Na^+] and [K^+] may change concurrently in the same animal. Calculating a Na^+:K^+ ratio may enhance detection of electrolyte disorders.

  A. The Na^+:K^+ ratio is obtained by dividing a measured serum or plasma [Na^+] by a measured serum or plasma [K^+] (both expressions in mmol/L or mEq/L).

  B. A low Na^+:K^+ ratio is common and expected in hypoadrenocorticism. It has been written that a Na^+:K^+ ratio < 27 (or 25 or 22) is diagnostic of hypoadrenocorticism in dogs. The lowest ratios will be found when hyponatremia and hyperkalemia are concurrent, but a low ratio is not unique to hypoadrenocorticism.

II.   Causes of a decreased Na^+:K^+ ratio:[67,68] A decreased Na^+:K^+ ratio is not required to detect the following disorders but suggests possible abnormalities in Na^+ or K^+ concentrations:

  A. Hypoadrenocorticism (Addison's disease)

    1. Hyponatremia is caused by increased renal excretion of Na^+ (due to decreased aldosterone) and retention of H_2O (due to increased ADH secondary to hypocortisolemia).

    2. Hyperkalemia is caused by decreased renal secretion of K^+ (due to decreased aldosterone).

B. Diarrhea (dogs, cats, and horses)
   1. Hyponatremia is caused by increased intestinal loss of Na^+, perhaps accompanied by increased H_2O intake. Horses with severe diarrhea are more prone to low Na^+:K^+ ratios than are dogs and cats.
   2. Hyperkalemia may occur because of acidemia associated with HCO_3^- loss.
   3. When seen with a whipworm (*Trichuris vulpus*) infection, the disorder has been called pseudo–Addison's disease. Neither adrenocortical hypoplasia nor hypoaldosteronism are present, and responsive hyperaldosteronism is expected.
C. Renal failure (dogs and cats)
   1. Hyponatremia is caused by decreased ability of tubules to resorb Na^+.
   2. Hyperkalemia is caused by decreased ability to secrete K^+ (primarily in oliguric states).
D. Urinary tract obstruction (dogs and cats) or uroperitoneum
   1. Mild hyponatremia might be found during obstruction. If uroperitoneum is present, Na^+ may diffuse into peritoneal fluid to create hyponatremia.
   2. Hyperkalemia caused by obstruction occurs primarily because of acute oliguria or anuria leading to decreased tubular secretion of K^+. Uroperitoneum may cause hyperkalemia via K^+ diffusion from the peritoneal cavity to blood. Acidosis may contribute in both types of cases.
E. Diabetes mellitus with ketonuria (dogs and cats)
   1. Hyponatremia is caused by increased renal Na^+ excretion (due to osmotic diuresis and obligated cation excretion) and plasma dilution (a shift of H_2O from ICF to ECF because of marked hyperglycemia).
   2. Hyperkalemia is not expected with ketoacidosis. It is more common for $[K^+]$ to be WRI or decreased.
F. Third-space loss (pleural or peritoneal effusions) (dogs and cats)[26,52]
   1. Hyponatremia may result from the dilution of ECF $[Na^+]$ by the H_2O that is retained through hypovolemic ADH and thirst responses. Drainage of effusions—for example, repeated drainage of chylous effusions—would remove ECF Na^+ and thus enhance the severity of the hyponatremia.
   2. Hyperkalemia may result from one or more processes, including decreased renal excretion of K^+ (caused by decreased distal tubular flow rate or hyponatremia) or a shift from ICF to ECF because of an associated acidosis.
G. Others
   1. Any disorder that causes hyponatremia without a corresponding decrease in serum $[K^+]$ will lower the Na^+:K^+ ratio.
   2. Any disorder that causes hyperkalemia without a corresponding increase in serum $[Na^+]$ will lower the Na^+:K^+ ratio.

CHLORIDE (Cl^-) CONCENTRATION

I. Physiologic processes
   A. Serum $[Cl^-]$ is nearly equivalent to ECF $[Cl^-]$, which is influenced by ECF concentrations of Na^+ and HCO_3^-. Therefore, complete interpretation of serum $[Cl^-]$ requires knowledge of serum $[Na^+]$ and at least a consideration of an animal's acid-base status.
   B. Control of serum $[Cl^-]$
      1. Renal resorption and secretion of Cl^{-1}
         a. About 75 % of filtered Cl^- is resorbed in the proximal tubules down a concentration gradient created by Na^+ and H_2O resorption and through a formate-Cl^-

exchanger. Angiotensin II stimulates the proximal tubular resorption of Na^+, Cl^-, and H_2O.

    b. Cl^- is actively resorbed in the thick ascending limb of the loop of Henle via a Na^+-K^+-$2Cl^-$ transporter in the luminal membrane. The rate-limiting factor is Cl^- delivery to the loop. This process is blocked by loop diuretics (e.g., furosemide) and is stimulated by ADH.

    c. Cl^- is passively resorbed in the distal nephron by an electrochemical gradient established by Na^+ movement through Na^+ channels. Aldosterone promotes Na^+ resorption in the distal nephron.

    d. Na^+ and Cl^- resorption in the distal nephron also involves an aldosterone-independent Na^+-Cl^- cotransporter. This process varies directly with Na^+ delivery to the distal nephron. Thiazide diuretics block this cotransporter.

    e. Type A intercalated cells of the distal nephron secrete Cl^- when H^+ is secreted. The process is stimulated by acidemia (Fig. 9.4). Conversely, when there is an alkalemia or HCO_3^- excess, Cl^- is conserved and HCO_3^- is secreted by type B intercalated cells (see Fig. 9.8).

  2. Alimentary tract functions pertaining to Cl^-

    a. Gastric (or abomasal) mucosa secretes HCl as part of the digestive process. In healthy animals, the secreted Cl^- is resorbed after it passes into the intestinal tract.

    b. Secretion of Cl^- requires the generation of HCO_3^- (see Fig. 9.5).

II.   Analytical concepts

  A. Terms and units

    1. Assays measure the electrical potential of Cl^- (potentiometry) or $[Cl^-]$ (spectrophotometry or coulometric/amperometric titration) in plasma, serum, or whole blood. The Cl^- is mostly a free ion in the plasma or serum H_2O.

    2. Unit conversion: $mEq/L \times 1 = mmol/L$, and $mg/dL \div 3.55 = mmol/L$ (SI unit, nearest 1 mmol/L)[3]

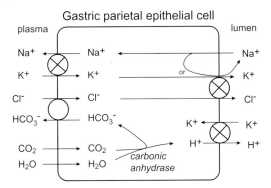

Fig. 9.5. Gastric or abomasal secretion of H^+ and Cl^-. H^+ and HCO_3^- are formed from the combination of OH^- (from H_2O) and CO_2 in a reaction catalyzed by carbonic anhydrase. H^+ (from H_2O) is secreted into the lumen via a H^+—K^+-ATPase pump. The generated HCO_3^- is transported to the ECF via a Cl^--HCO_3^- exchanger. Cl^- is actively pumped into the lumen with Na^+ and K^+, but most Na^+ and K^+ ions are resorbed, thus leaving H^+ and Cl^- in the lumen. The major results of the process are gastric secretion of H^+ and Cl^-, a lesser plasma $[Cl^-]$, and greater plasma $[HCO_3^-]$.

   $\otimes$, ATPase pump; and $\bigcirc$, cotransporter or counter transporter (antiporter).

B. Sample for [Cl⁻] quantitation
1. Serum is preferred. [Cl⁻] is stable for months if the sample does not dehydrate.
2. Plasma may be used.
C. Principles of assays
1. Ion-selective electrode assays are the most common. Other halides (e.g., bromide and iodide) will react with the electrode to give a falsely increased [Cl⁻], sometimes markedly so. Bromide may be present when potassium bromide is used as an anticonvulsant. Other anions (e.g., lactate and BHB) may react to give mildly increased values; that is, the Cl⁻ value is increased about 3 mmol/L by lactate at 10 mmol/L and BHB at 16 mmol/L (i-STAT literature).
2. Coulometric/amperometric titration assays were common but have mostly been replaced by ion-selective electrode assays.

III. Hyperchloremia
A. This typically occurs when there is hypernatremia but occasionally is found concurrently with a decreased [HCO₃⁻] (i.e., hyperchloremic metabolic acidoses). Conceptually, changes in [Cl⁻] are related to attempts to maintain electrical neutrality. As [Na⁺] increases, so does [Cl⁻]. As [HCO₃⁻] decreases, [Cl⁻] increases.
B. Disorders and pathogeneses (Table 9.7)

Table 9.7. Diseases and conditions that cause hyperchloremia

H₂O-deficit group (with hyperchloremia and hypernatremia)
  Inadequate H₂O intake
    *H₂O deprivation
    Defective thirst response (hypothalamic defect)
  Pure H₂O loss (without adequate H₂O replacement)
    *Insensible loss: panting, hyperventilation, or fever
    Diabetes insipidus (central or nephrogenic)
  H₂O loss > Na⁺ and Cl⁻ loss
    Renal: osmotic diuresis
    Alimentary: osmotic diarrhea, osmotic sequestration, or phosphate enemas
Cl⁻-excess group (increased total body Cl⁻)
  Excess Cl⁻ with concurrent restricted H₂O intake
    Salt poisoning
    Administration of hypertonic saline, KCl, or NH₄Cl
  Decreased renal excretion of Na⁺ and Cl⁻
    Hyperaldosteronism
Hyperchloremic metabolic acidosis
  *Alimentary loss of HCO₃⁻
  Renal loss of HCO₃⁻
    Proximal renal tubular acidosis
    Distal renal tubular acidosis
Respiratory alkalosis (chronic)

* A relatively common disease or condition

1. H_2O-deficit group (hyperchloremic and hypernatremic disorders): Because Cl^- is the major anion that helps maintain electrical neutrality in the ECF, disorders that cause hypernatremic dehydration also tend to create hyperchloremia (see Sodium Concentration, sect. III.B.1).
2. Cl^--excess group (and usually concurrent Na^+ excess)
   a. Increased intake of Cl^- via oral or IV administration of solutions containing Cl^- may also lead to hyperchloremia.
   b. Decreased renal excretion of Na^+ (hyperaldosteronism) (rare)
      (1) Excessive aldosterone promotes excessive renal Cl^- (and Na^+) retention.
      (2) Hyperchloremia (and hypernatremia) may occur if H_2O is restricted or ADH activity is reduced. Aldosterone escape may prevent hyperchloremia (see Sodium Concentration, sect. III.B.2b).
3. Hyperchloremic metabolic acidosis
   a. Alimentary loss of HCO_3^-
      (1) Vomiting or diarrhea that causes a loss of HCO_3^--rich intestinal secretions may lead to HCO_3^- depletion and metabolic acidosis. Cattle that do not ingest saliva (because of an esophageal obstruction) become HCO_3^- depleted because their saliva is rich in HCO_3^-.
      (2) The HCO_3^- secretions are also Na^+ rich but Cl^- poor. Therefore, the ECF left behind becomes Cl^- rich, and thus hyperchloremia develops.
   b. Renal loss of HCO_3^-
      (1) In proximal renal tubular acidosis, the reduced reclamation of HCO_3^- may allow more Cl^- to be resorbed with Na^+, and thus hyperchloremic metabolic acidosis develops.
      (2) In distal renal tubular acidosis, the impaired ability to secrete H^+ might be linked to the failure of a Cl^--HCO_3^- shuttle, thus impairing secretion of Cl^- and reclamation of HCO_3^-.
4. Respiratory alkalosis (chronic)
   a. As a compensatory change to prolonged hypocapnia and alkalemia, the renal retention of H^+ is increased and thus the renal conservation of HCO_3^- is reduced.
   b. The fall in HCO_3^- is balanced by an increase in Cl^- and other anions that are not identified.[69]
5. Dehydration of the sample (evaporation or sublimation): Exposure of serum or plasma to air may allow evaporation that causes hyperchloremia. This is especially true of air-conditioning systems that blow cool dry air over the sample processing or analysis areas. Sublimation of H_2O from frozen samples may cause hyperchloremia.

IV. Normochloremia: Recognizing the presence of normochloremia may be important when either hypernatremia or decreased serum $[HCO_3^-]$ is present, because it suggests the presence of an increased anion gap (see the Anion Gap section).

V. Hypochloremia
   A. This typically occurs when there is hyponatremia (and pseudo-hypochloremia when there is pseudo-hyponatremia) or an increased serum $[HCO_3^-]$ (as occurs with metabolic alkaloses). It may also occur in a metabolic acidosis because Cl^- excretion accompanies the enhanced renal excretion of H^+ either via NH_4^+ excretion (Fig. 9.6) or via type A intercalated cells (Fig. 9.4).

Table 9.8. Diseases and conditions that cause hypochloremia

Cl⁻-deficit group: net Cl⁻ loss > H₂O loss (loss of Cl⁻-containing fluid followed by increased
    H₂O intake)
  Concurrent loss of Na⁺ (see the Na⁺-deficit group in Table 9.4)
  Metabolic alkaloses
    *Loss or sequestration of HCl: vomiting, displaced abomasum, pyloric obstruction,
      bovine hemorrhagic bowel syndrome
    *Bovine renal failure
    Furosemide toxicosis
    Thiazide diuretics
  Metabolic acidoses with an increased anion gap
    *Ketoacidosis
    *Lactic acidosis
    Ingestion of foreign substance (e.g., ethylene glycol) that generates anions
H₂O-excess groups (with or without edema) (see the same group in Table 9.4)
Shifting of H₂O from ICF to ECF (see the same group in Table 9.4)
Shifting of Cl⁻ from intravascular to extravascular fluid (see the same group in Table 9.4)

  * A relatively common disease or condition
  Note: Pseudo-hypochloremia may be caused by displacement of serum or plasma H₂O (see the text).

B. Disorders and pathogeneses (Table 9.8)
  1. Cl⁻-deficit group (Cl⁻ loss > H₂O loss)
    a. Because Cl⁻ is the major anion that helps maintain electrical neutrality in the
       ECF, disorders that cause hyponatremic dehydration (via gastrointestinal, urinary,
       or cutaneous loss) tend to also create hypochloremia (see Sodium Concentration,
       sect. V.B.1).
    b. Hypochloremia in the absence of hyponatremia suggests the presence of meta-
       bolic alkalosis (with an increased [HCO₃⁻]) or an increased anion gap (with an
       increased concentration of an anion other than Cl⁻ or HCO₃⁻) because electrical
       neutrality must be maintained. Interpretation of HCO₃⁻ (or tCO₂) and anion
       gap values should be sufficient to identify these conditions, but calculations for
       corrected [Cl⁻] and SID may be used (see the section on Strong Ion Difference
       and Stewart's Method of Acid-Base Analysis in Chapter 10).
      (1) Metabolic alkaloses
        (a) Loss or sequestration of HCl (e.g., vomiting, displaced abomasum,
            other upper gastrointestinal tract obstruction, gastric reflux in horses, or
            bovine hemorrhagic bowel syndrome): Loss of Cl⁻-rich secretions leads
            to depletion of Cl⁻ in the ECF and thus hypochloremia.
        (b) Bovine renal failure: Cattle with renal insufficiency tend to become
            alkalotic. The acid-base changes may result from abomasal atony, which
            creates a functional obstruction and thus sequestration of Cl⁻ (see
            Bicarbonate Concentration, sect. III.B.1). Also, cattle excrete more K⁺
            via saliva during renal failure. When swallowed, the K⁺ may limit the
            absorption of Cl⁻.[70]
        (c) Furosemide: This competes for the Cl⁻-binding site in the Na⁺-K⁺-2Cl⁻
            transporter of the luminal membrane of the thick ascending limb of the
            loop of Henle and thus inhibits Cl⁻ resorption. Excess excretion of Cl⁻

(relative to H_2O) causes hypochloremia. Concurrent hypokalemic metabolic alkalosis may occur (see Bicarbonate Concentration, sect. III.B.1.b).

(d) Thiazide diuretics act in the distal tubule by interfering with Cl^- resorption in a Na^+-K^+ cotransporter. Because this process occurs in the cortical nephron, it does not diminish medullary hypertonicity and thus the kidneys maintain concentrating ability. Thus, when stimulated by ADH, H_2O resorption will cause hyponatremia and hypochloremia by dilution.

(2) Metabolic acidoses with increased anion gaps

(a) In ketoacidosis and lactic acidosis, there is an increased filtration of unresorbable anions (ketone bodies and L-lactate, respectively) from plasma. These anions obligate the renal excretion of Na^+ to maintain electrical neutrality. Thus, less Na^+ is resorbed in the proximal and collecting tubules. Because Cl^- resorption in those tubules depends on the electrochemical gradient established by Na^+ resorption, the diminished Na^+ resorption diminishes the Cl^- resorption.[1]

(b) Ingestion of a foreign substance that generates anions (e.g., ethylene glycol): Pathogenesis of the hypochloremia parallels that found with ketoacidosis and lactic acidosis, because the filtration of unresorbable anions obligates Na^+ loss. As Cl^- resorption depends frequently on Na^+ resorption, Na^+ loss leads to Cl^- loss. Other examples of exogenous anionic substances are listed in the Anion Gap section.

(c) If there is adequate renal function, the renal response to an acidemia is to increase the excretion of H^+ by the following processes that increase the excretion of H^+ and Cl^- and the production of HCO_3^-. The net effect is to reduce the severity of the acidemia (excretion of H^+ and generation of HCO_3^- for buffering) and reduce plasma $[Cl^-]$.

(i) Acidemia stimulates the type A intercalated cells (Fig. 9.4).

(ii) Acidemia stimulates the increased renal excretion of NH_4^+ in both the proximal and collecting tubular epithelial cells (Fig. 9.6). This mechanism of acid excretion in the distal nephron may be impaired with anorexia, possibly to help maintain muscle mass.[71]

2. H_2O-excess group (see Sodium Concentration, sect. V.B.2)
3. Shifting of H_2O from ICF to ECF (see Sodium Concentration, sect. V.B.3)
4. Shifting of Cl^- from intravascular to extravascular space (see Sodium Concentration, sect. V.B.5)
5. Pseudo-hypochloremia: The same factors (e.g., lipemia and hyperproteinemia) that cause pseudo-hyponatremia will also cause a pseudo-hypochloremia if the $[Cl^-]$ is measured by indirect potentiometry or coulometric/amperometric titration assays (see Sodium Concentration, sect. V.B.7).

BICARBONATE (HCO_3^-) CONCENTRATION AND TOTAL CARBON DIOXIDE (tCO_2) CONCENTRATION

I. Physiologic processes

A. HCO_3^- in the body is a major buffer that helps maintain blood pH at physiologic concentrations. HCO_3^- is produced from H_2O and CO_2 in cells that have carbonic

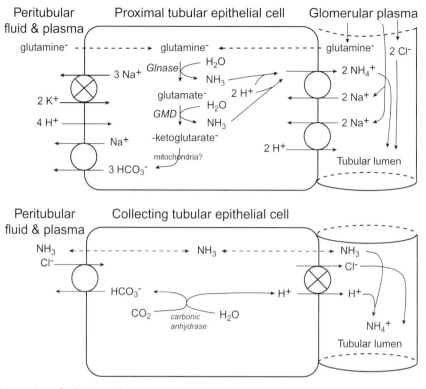

Fig. 9.6. Excretion of H^+ via NH_4^+.

- Proximal renal tubular epithelial cells: Acidemia results in the increased uptake and degradation of glutamine. Energy for electrolyte transport is provided by the $3Na^+$-$2K^+$-ATPase and involves the increased activity of glutaminase (*Glnase*) and glutamate dehydrogenase (*GMD*). These processes reduce the severity of acidemia by (1) H^+ combining with NH_3 to form NH_4^+ and (2) the generation of HCO_3^-, which can buffer ECF H^+. The increased renal excretion of NH_4^+ obligates the excretion of anions (primarily Cl^-) to maintain electrical neutrality.
- Collecting tubular epithelial cells: In the collecting tubules, NH_3 diffuses into the tubular fluid and combines with H^+ that is secreted with Cl^-. This renal compensation for an acidemia increases the renal excretion of H^+ (in NH_4^+), increases the renal excretion of Cl^-, generates HCO_3^-, and thus produces a compensatory hypochloremic metabolic alkalosis.

$\otimes$, ATPase pump; and $\bigcirc$, cotransporter or counter transporter (antiporter).

anhydrase: erythrocytes, proximal renal tubular cells (luminal and intracellular), parietal cells of the gastric and abomasal epithelium, intercalated cells (type A and B) of the collecting tubules, and exocrine pancreatic epithelial cells.

B. In gastric or abomasal mucosal cells, HCl secretion is accomplished by the utilization of Cl^- from the ECF and by the generation of HCO_3^- (Fig. 9.5).

C. In the proximal nephron, 90 % of filtered HCO_3^- is conserved (not directly resorbed) (Fig. 9.7). This occurs during the H^+ secretion that is mediated through the Na^+-H^+ antiporter and is dependent on Na^+ resorption.

D. Distal nephron
1. HCO_3^- produced by the type A intercalated cells of the collecting tubules enters the peritubular fluid through a Cl^--HCO_3^- exchanger. This process is linked to H^+ secretion by H^+-ATPase and is promoted by aldosterone (Fig. 9.4).

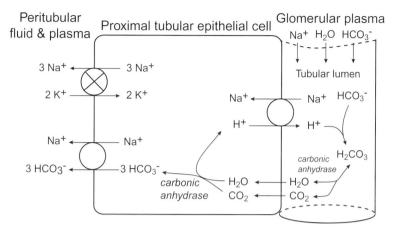

Fig. 9.7. Proximal tubular conservation of HCO_3^-. H^+ secreted by a luminal border Na^+-H^+ exchanger combines with filtrate HCO_3^- to form H_2CO_3. Dissociation of H_2CO_3 into CO_2 and H_2O is facilitated by luminal carbonic anhydrase. After passive absorption, cellular carbonic anhydrase helps CO_2 and OH^- (from H_2O) combine to form HCO_3^-, which is transported to the peritubular fluid via a Na^+-$3HCO_3^-$ cotransporter. The H^+ released from the H_2O is available for secretion in the next cycle. The energy for the HCO_3^- conservation is provided by a Na^+-K^+-ATPase pump in the basolateral membrane. The electrolyte movement in the figure is not balanced; movement of other electrolytes (K^+, Cl^-, and NH_4^+) are involved to maintain electrical neutrality. The net result of the process is HCO_3^- conservation and Na^+ resorption, but the HCO_3^- that enters the peritubular fluid is not the same HCO_3^- molecule that entered the ultrafiltrate. Thus HCO_3^- is not directly resorbed (HCO_3^- is a not a resorbable anion). $\otimes$, ATPase pump; and $\bigcirc$, cotransporter or counter transporter (antiporter).

       2. HCO_3^- can be secreted (when there is a metabolic alkalosis) through a Cl^--HCO_3^- exchanger in type B intercalated cells of the distal nephron (Fig. 9.8).

II.   Analytical concepts
    A. Terms and units
       1. The $[HCO_3^-]$ is calculated during blood gas analysis of heparinized blood (see Eq. 10.1a), but estimates may be obtained from serum samples.
       2. The $[HCO_3^-]$ in serum can be estimated indirectly by measuring the $[tCO_2]$. tCO_2 reflects the total amount of CO_2 gas that can be liberated from serum. At a physiologic pH of 7.4, about 95 % of the potential CO_2 gas is in the form of HCO_3^-, about 5 % is in dissolved CO_2, and < 1 % is in carbamino compounds. Therefore, the $[tCO_2]$ is nearly equal to the $[HCO_3^-]$. tCO_2 is also called *total carbon dioxide content* ($tcCO_2$).
       3. Unit conversion: mEq/L × 1 = mmol/L (SI unit, nearest 1 mmol/L)[3]
    B. Sample for $[HCO_3^-]$ quantitation
       1. Serum is preferred, but plasma may be used.
       2. Samples should have minimal exposure to air before and after serum is harvested (a few minutes is acceptable). Because the Pco_2 of air is near 0 mmHg, $CO_{2(g)}$ will diffuse from the sample to air. The lowering of the Pco_2 in the sample "pulls HCO_3^- out of solution" (shifts the equilibrium toward CO_2 and away from HCO_3^-, thus lowering the $[HCO_3^-]$ and $[H^+]$ of the sample) (Eq. 9.2). The same reaction occurs in vivo during expiration (as shown in Fig. 10.1) to remove H^+ from blood, but the

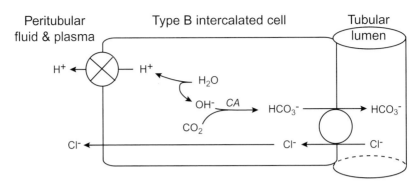

Fig. 9.8. Secretion of HCO_3^- by type B intercalated cells of the distal nephron. When there is metabolic alkalosis (increased plasma $[HCO_3^-]$ and alkalemia), type B intercalated cells can secrete HCO_3^- into the tubular lumen and concurrently generate H^+. In respect to HCO_3^- and H^+, type B intercalated cells essentially have the opposite function of type A intercalated cells. The net result is increased renal excretion of HCO_3^- and increased H^+ and Cl^- in plasma. $\otimes$, ATPase pump; and $\bigcirc$, cotransporter or counter transporter (antiporter).

$[HCO_3^-]$ decrease is not detected in physiologic states because there is relatively much more HCO_3^- than H^+ (mmol/L vs nmol/L, respectively) and the HCO_3^- that is used is replaced.

$$H^+ + HCO_3^- \rightarrow H_2CO_3 \rightarrow H_2O + CO_2 \rightarrow CO_2 \text{ lost to air} \tag{9.2.}$$

   3. The $[tCO_2]$ in underfilled blood collection tubes (e.g., 3 mL of blood into a 10 mL tube) is less than in filled tubes after contact with erythrocytes for about 20 min.[72] Erythrocytes may contribute to loss of CO_2 into underfilled tubes' dead spaces (which initially would be devoid of CO_2), because carbonic anhydrase in erythrocytes accelerates the conversion of HCO_3^- to CO_2. Even greater loss of CO_2 occurs with exposure to air before or after centrifugation.
C. Principles of assays (three variations provided)
   1. Vitros enzymatic tCO_2
      a. In a very alkaline environment, nearly all CO_2 is in the form of HCO_3^-. HCO_3^- reacts with phosphoenolpyruvate to form oxaloacetate, which is coupled to a reaction that consumes NADH. The disappearance of NADH is measured by reflectance spectrophotometry.
      b. Positive interference: L-lactate dehydrogenase (LD) activity of 4500 U/L will increase the $[tCO_2]$ by 3 mmol/L because it promotes consumption of NADH as it catalyzes the conversion of serum L-lactate to pyruvate (Vitros method package insert). Oxamate is incorporated into some assays to inhibit LD and reduce the interference.
   2. Beckman analyzer: In an acid environment, nearly all forms of CO_2 are converted to gaseous CO_2. The liberated CO_2 diffuses into a HCO_3^- solution with a pH electrode. Changes in pH relate to the amount of liberated CO_2.
   3. Hitachi and Olympus analyzers
      a. HCO_3^- reacts with phosphoenolpyruvate in the presence of NADH to produce oxaloacetate, PO_4, and NAD^+ in the presence of catalytic enzymes. The

Table 9.9. Diseases and conditions that cause increased serum [HCO$_3^-$] or [tCO$_2$] (metabolic alkalosis)

Loss of H$^+$ from body
   *Gastric loss: vomiting, pyloric obstruction (functional or mechanical)
   Renal loss
     Loop or thiazide diuretics
     Secondary to respiratory acidosis
     *Hypokalemia
   Secondary to endurance races or intestinal disorders in horses
Shift of H$^+$ from ECF to ICF due to hypokalemia
Administration of sodium bicarbonate, lactate, citrate, or magnesium hydroxide
*Contraction alkalosis: vomiting

  * A relatively common disease or condition
  Note: Spurious increase may be caused by increased serum lactate dehydrogenase activity (see the text).

         consumption of NADH is proportional to [HCO$_3^-$] and is measured via spectrophotometry.
    b. LD activity also converts NADH to NAD$^+$. Extreme increases in serum LD activity caused by rhabdomyolysis can result in falsely increased [HCO$_3^-$].[73]

III. Increased bicarbonate (HCO$_3^-$) concentration or total carbon dioxide (tCO$_2$) concentration
    A. Increased [HCO$_3^-$] is usually associated with a metabolic alkalosis, either primary or as compensation for a respiratory acidosis. Metabolic alkaloses are typically produced by the loss of H$^+$ from the ECF (which causes alkalemia) (see Fig. 10.1). For each H$^+$ that is lost, there is an equimolar generation of HCO$_3^-$.
    B. Disorders and pathogeneses (Table 9.9)
      1. Loss of H$^+$ from the body
        a. Gastric loss (vomiting, or physical or functional pyloric obstruction)
          (1) Secretion of H$^+$ by gastric mucosa generates HCO$_3^-$ (Fig. 9.5). If the H$^+$ is lost by vomiting, drainage of stomach contents (horses), or sequestration proximal to the intestine, it is not resorbed in the intestine. Therefore, the generated HCO$_3^-$ is not used to buffer the H$^+$ (that would otherwise have been resorbed), and thus it accumulates in plasma.
          (2) Concurrent hypovolemia and hypochloremia lead to increased renal conservation of HCO$_3^-$. Hypovolemia stimulates the RAS to cause the tubular resorption of Na$^+$ and Cl$^-$. If the animal is Cl$^-$ depleted, resorption of Na$^+$ without Cl$^-$ in the distal nephron increases the electrochemical gradient, which promotes H$^+$ secretion and thus the generation of HCO$_3^-$ (Fig. 9.3).
          (3) Cattle in renal failure may develop a metabolic alkalosis. The prevailing theory is that the cattle develop abomasal atony that leads to HCl sequestration, which generates the alkalosis.
        b. Renal loss of H$^+$
          (1) Loop of Henle diuretics: Furosemide and other loop diuretics (bumetanide and ethacrynic acid) block the action of a Na$^+$-K$^+$-2Cl$^-$ transporter; thus, the

resorption of Na^+, K^+, and Cl^- by the ascending limb of the loop of Henle is decreased. The resulting impaired H_2O resorption and increased fluid flow in the distal nephron promote H^+ secretion by maintaining a favorable H^+ gradient. Also, hypovolemia and hypochloremia lead to increased secretion of H^+ and thus increased HCO_3^- generation. In addition, increased renal excretion of K^+ may lead to hypokalemia that also promotes alkalosis (Figs. 9.2 and 9.4).

(2) Thiazide diuretics inhibit a Na^+-Cl^- cotransporter in the distal nephron by competing for the Cl^--binding site. As noted in the preceding paragraph, hypovolemia and hypochloremia promote the formation of metabolic alkalosis.

(3) Secondary to respiratory acidosis: Chronic respiratory acidosis allows time (3–5 d) for renal compensation consisting of increased H^+ secretion by tubular cells (proximal primarily) and thus increased HCO_3^- generation (Fig. 9.7). The increased H^+ secretion is probably stimulated by the acidemia.

(4) Hypokalemia stimulates H^+-K^+-ATPase in the distal nephron, thereby promoting K^+ retention, H^+ secretion, and HCO_3^- generation (Fig. 9.4). Hypokalemia may also promote alkalosis by shifting of H^+ into cells in exchange for K^+ (Fig. 9.2).

(5) After endurance races or during intestinal disorders (e.g., colitis), horses can develop metabolic alkalosis. Sometimes these alkaloses are explained as being caused by contraction alkalosis (see Bicarbonate Concentration and Total Carbon Dioxide Concentration, sect. III.B.4) or gastric sequestration of HCl; such mechanisms may be present, but such statements are typically not referenced. Because both conditions produce electrolyte changes that could cause the renal secretion of H^+ and the corresponding generation of HCO_3^-, other mechanisms may be involved.

   (a) Extensive sweating may occur during endurance races. Equine sweat is K^+ rich and Cl^- rich compared to plasma, so sweating results in hypertonic loss of these electrolytes in addition to the loss of body H_2O that may not be replaced by drinking.

   (b) Watery diarrhea depletes Cl^- and H_2O. If the horse is not eating, lack of feed intake would reduce tbK^+.

   (c) As explained in the foregoing section B.1.a and in Fig. 9.4, the concurrent states of hypovolemia, hypochloremia, and hypokalemia increase renal secretion of H^+ and thus increase production of HCO_3^-. These processes create a metabolic alkalosis.

2. Shift of H^+ from ECF to ICF due to hypokalemia
   a. Alkalosis can lead to hypokalemia, but hypokalemia can also contribute to an alkalosis.
   b. If there is tbK^+ depletion, a fall in $[K^+]$ in the ECF promotes the movement of K^+ out of the cell and the movement of H^+ into cells. The higher intracellular $[H^+]$ also promotes H^+ secretion by renal tubular cells and increased generation of HCO_3^-, thus promoting alkalemia.

3. Administration of sodium bicarbonate, organic anions that generate HCO_3^-, or magnesium hydroxide in ruminants or horses
   a. Excess administration of sodium bicarbonate (while treating acidemia) may increase serum $[HCO_3^-]$.

       b. Metabolism of some organic anions (e.g., L-lactate and citrate) by hepatocytes leads to the production of HCO_3^-. Alkalosis is not expected unless large quantities of organic anions are given.

       c. Magnesium hydroxide administered orally in ruminants causes a metabolic alkalosis, probably because of the alkalinizing effects in the rumen.[74] In monogastric animals, there is less of an alkalinizing effect, because of gastric secretion of H^+.

       d. Administration of bicarbonate solutions ("milkshakes") to horses prior to races will increase serum $[HCO_3^-]$.[75]

  4. Contraction alkalosis

       a. When Cl^--rich but HCO_3^--poor ECF is lost (as may occur with vomiting, HCl sequestration, and loop diuretics), there is ECF volume contraction without a corresponding drop in HCO_3^- content. Therefore, the $[HCO_3^-]$ in the remaining ECF increases. The magnitude of increase is minimal because H^+ is released from other buffers in the body (e.g., PO_4, bone, and Hgb) and combines with the HCO_3^-.

       b. Volume contraction also helps maintain the alkalosis by decreasing renal HCO_3^- excretion. In response to hypovolemia, aldosterone promotes the renal secretion of H^+ and Cl^- by the intercalated cells and concurrent production of HCO_3^- (Fig. 9.4).

       c. The primary processes that result in the loss of Cl^- (vomiting, sequestration, diuretics, and sweating) may also cause the loss of H^+ and produce HCO_3^- and thus contribute to metabolic alkalosis. When there is a loss of Cl^- and accumulation of HCO_3^-, then the Cl^--HCO_3^- exchanger in the gastric parietal epithelial cells (Fig 9.5) or the Type A intercalated cells (Fig. 9.4) are probably involved in the pathogenesis of the hypochloremic metabolic alkalosis.

IV. Decreased bicarbonate (HCO_3^-) concentration or total carbon dioxide (tCO_2) concentration

  A. Decreased $[HCO_3^-]$ is usually associated with metabolic acidosis, either primary or as compensation for respiratory alkalosis. The generation of excess H^+ or a loss of HCO_3^- typically produces metabolic acidosis (see Fig. 10.1). The loss of HCO_3^- (or other body buffers) reduces the buffering capacity of the body and thus allows H^+ to accumulate.

  B. Disorders and pathogeneses (Table 9.10)

    1. Generation of excess H^+: If metabolic pathways generate sufficient acid to exceed the buffering capacity of blood, then H^+ accumulates to create acidemia. HCO_3^- is depleted when it is used to buffer the generated H^+; therefore, these conditions may be referred to as *titration acidoses*.

       a. Lactic acidosis occurs when cellular metabolism switches to anaerobic glycolysis. The resultant increased degradation of ATP causes excessive release of H^+ (see Lactate Concentration, sect. III.A.1b). In neonatal calf diarrhea, ruminal and enteric fermentation of lactose may be the source of D-lactate and H^+.[76]

       b. Ketoacidosis occurs when there is excessive β-oxidation of triglycerides in hepatocytes.

       c. Ingestion of certain compounds (e.g., ethylene glycol) creates an acidemia because the catabolism of the compound generates acid (see Table 9.12).

    2. Decreased renal excretion of H^+: As with excess generation of acid, $[HCO_3^-]$ decreases as HCO_3^- (and other buffers) is used to buffer H^+ that accumulates in plasma.

Table 9.10. Diseases and conditions that cause decreased serum [HCO$_3$$^-$] or [tCO$_2$] (metabolic acidosis)

Generation of excess H$^+$
  *Lactic acidosis
  *Ketoacidosis
  Ingestion of certain compounds (see Table 9.12)
Decreased renal excretion of H$^+$
  *Renal failure
  *Uroperitoneum or urinary tract obstruction
  Distal renal tubular acidosis (type 1)
  Hypoaldosteronism
Increased HCO$_3$$^-$ loss
  *Alimentary losses: diarrhea, sequestration, or vomiting of pancreatic secretions
  Renal losses: proximal renal tubular acidosis (type 2)
Dilutional acidosis (rapid infusion of saline)

* A relatively common disease or condition
Note: Spurious decrease may occur due to aerobic sample handling.

a. Renal failure creates an acidemia because of the kidneys' inability to excrete the daily acid load produced by metabolic pathways. With progressive renal disease, less NH$_4$$^+$ is excreted because there are fewer functional nephrons to form NH$_4$$^+$. Abnormalities in HCO$_3$$^-$ and PO$_4$ excretion may also play a role in the development of acidemia.
b. Urinary tract obstruction also produces an acidemia because of impaired urinary excretion of H$^+$.
c. With uroperitoneum, H$^+$ is excreted by the kidneys but not from the body. Also, urine is typically a HCO$_3$$^-$-poor fluid, so when the H$_2$O in urine is resorbed by lymphatic vessels, it dilutes the plasma [HCO$_3$$^-$].
d. Distal renal tubular acidosis (type 1) occurs when the H$^+$ secretion by the distal tubules is decreased because of tubular disease. It may also occur with urinary tract obstruction and hyperkalemia.
e. Hypoaldosteronism (as seen with hypoadrenocorticism) may promote acidemia through multiple mechanisms. Hypoaldosteronism is also called *type 4 renal tubular acidosis.*
  (1) Reduced H$^+$ (and K$^+$) secretion by principal epithelial cells (see Fig. 9.3).
  (2) Reduced H$^+$ secretion by type A intercalated cells (see Fig. 9.4).
  (3) The resulting hyperkalemia inhibits NH$_4$$^+$ excretion (Fig. 9.6). Also, hyperkalemia may cause shifts of H$^+$ from ICF to ECF (related to concepts in Fig. 9.2).
3. Increased HCO$_3$$^-$ loss
  a. Alimentary losses
    (1) Intestinal and pancreatic secretions are relatively HCO$_3$$^-$-rich fluids. Thus, diarrhea, vomiting (if pancreatic secretions are included), and intestinal sequestration can cause HCO$_3$$^-$ depletion and thus a loss of buffering capacity.
    (2) With time, H$^+$ produced by metabolic pathways accumulates and promotes acidemia.

b. Renal losses
   (1) In proximal renal tubular acidosis (type 2), there is a defect in HCO_3^- conservation in the proximal tubules. The defect may be due to abnormal Na^+ resorption or to the presence of a carbonic anhydrase inhibitor. The defect may be part of either an inherited or acquired Fanconi's syndrome. Besides proximal renal tubular acidosis, other findings in Fanconi's syndrome include renal glucosuria, aminoaciduria, hypokalemia, and hypophosphatemia.
   (2) Acquired proximal renal tubular acidosis has been seen with multiple myeloma, hypocalcemia, and a variety of drugs in people. In dogs, the disorder has been seen with hypocalcemia (due to hypoparathyroidism and hypovitaminosis D), streptozotocin and maleic acid treatments, and an overdose of amoxicillin.[77-80] Acquired proximal renal tubular acidosis was reported in a mare, but the cause was not determined.[81]
4. Dilutional acidosis may occur with rapid saline infusion, which may decrease $[HCO_3^-]$ by diluting ECF HCO_3^-. However, absolute change caused by dilution is expected to be minor and thus cause a minor change in blood pH.
5. In vitro loss of HCO_3^- from the sample (see Bicarbonate Concentration Sect. II.B.2)
C. Decreased $[HCO_3^-]$ or $[tCO_2]$ with hyperchloremia: Hyperchloremic metabolic acidosis strongly suggests the presence of renal tubular acidosis, either the proximal or distal form.
   1. For proximal renal tubular acidosis, proximal tubular disease reduces tubular secretion of H^+ and decreases conservation of HCO_3^-. As shown in Fig. 9.7, proximal tubular HCO_3^- conservation normally leads to the movement of HCO_3^- and Na^+ ions from the cells into the interstitial fluid and blood. If HCO_3^- ions are not being formed in the proximal tubular cells because of inhibition of carbonic anhydrase, the Na^+-K^+-ATPase pump creates an electrical gradient that enhances Cl^- resorption. The net result is decreased $[HCO_3^-]$, increased $[Cl^-]$, and therefore hyperchloremic metabolic acidosis.
   2. For distal renal tubular acidosis, distal tubular disease impairs the secretion of H^+ and thus decreases the generation of HCO_3^- by the carbonic anhydrase reaction. As shown in Fig. 9.4, decreased generation of HCO_3^- by the type A intercalated epithelial cells decreases the renal secretion of Cl^-. The net result is decreased plasma $[HCO_3^-]$, increased plasma $[Cl^-]$, and therefore hyperchloremic metabolic acidosis.
   3. There is confusion in the literature regarding when it is appropriate to characterize an acidosis as a renal tubular acidosis.
      a. One view is that the classification of renal tubular acidosis should be limited to those disorders in which a renal tubular disorder produces a hyperchloremic metabolic acidosis without an increased anion gap and there is no evidence of decreased glomerular filtration rate (i.e., the animal is not azotemic). Others do not restrict this classification to nonazotemic animals and thus include renal failure patients that might have an increased anion gap.[82,83]
      b. These differences may be considered relatively unimportant, but the lack of consistency results in confusion and perhaps incorrect case management.
         (1) By the more restrictive definition, the acidosis is created by a tubular dysfunction. That is, either the proximal or distal tubules are not adequately secreting H^+ and conserving or producing HCO_3^-. In these animals, plenty of functional glomeruli are providing filtrate to the tubules.

(2) In renal failure, the defective renal excretion of H^+ is because of too few functional nephrons. Those nephrons that are still functional may still be able to secrete H^+. Because the excretion of PO_4 and other anions is also impaired, these animals may have an increased anion gap.

(3) Unfortunately, some animals may shift from the restrictive group to the nonrestrictive group; that is, acute proximal tubular disease (e.g., toxicosis) may create proximal renal tubular acidosis, but if the damage is severe enough, the disease may also damage enough nephrons that an animal enters acute renal failure.

ANION GAP

I. Definitions
   A. *Cation*: an atom or molecule with a positive charge. Monovalent cations have one positive charge, divalent cations have two.
   B. *Measured cation charge* (mC^+): the charge concentration of the major monovalent cations (Na^+ and K^+) whose serum activities or concentrations are directly measured. Because these ions are monovalent and measured as free ions, their ion concentrations are equivalent to their charge concentrations.
   C. *Unmeasured cation charge* (uC^+): the charge concentration of all other cations in blood, including fCa^{2+}, fMg^{2+}, and cationic globulins, for which concentrations are not measured for the anion gap calculation. Charge concentrations for cations that are not monovalent are greater than their ion concentrations.
   D. *Total cation charge* (tC^+): total charge concentration of all cations in the blood ($tC^+ = mC^+ + uC^+$)
   E. *Anion*: an atom or molecule with a negative charge. Monovalent anions have one negative charge, divalent anions have two, and trivalent anions (e.g., PO_4^{3-}) have three.
   F. *Measured anion charge* (mA^-): the charge concentration of the major monovalent anions (Cl^- and HCO_3^-) whose serum activities or concentrations are measured. Because these ions are monovalent and measured as free ions, their ion concentrations are equivalent to their charge concentrations. $[HCO_3^-]$ may be estimated from $[tCO_2]$.
   G. *Unmeasured anion charge* (uA^-): the charge concentration of all other anions in serum, including PO_4, albumin, anions of organic acids, and SO_4, for which concentrations are not measured for the anion gap calculation. Charge concentrations for anions that are not monovalent are greater than their ion concentrations.
   H. *Total anion charge* (tA^-): total charge concentration of all anions in the blood ($tA^- = mA^- + uA^-$)
   I. *Anion gap*: the difference (gap) in the charge concentrations (not ion concentrations) between uA^- and uC^+ (anion gap = $uA^- - uC^+$). The anion gap can be calculated because this is also equal to the difference between mC^+ and mA^- concentrations (Eq. 9.3).

$$\text{Anion gap} = mC^+ - mA^- = ([Na^+] + [K^+]) - ([Cl^-] + [HCO_3^-]) \tag{9.3.}$$

II. Physiologic processes
   A. Serum is always electrically neutral; that is, total positive charges equal total negative charges. The major contributors to the electrical neutrality and their relative contributions are listed in Table 9.11. In the example, 150 of the 157 mmol/L of cation charge

Table 9.11. Cations and anions of serum in health (approximate concentrations provided to simplify concept)

Cations	mmol/L ion charge	Anions	mmol/L ion charge
Na^+	146	Cl^-	110
K^+	4.0	HCO_3^-	24
fCa^{2+}	5.0	Proteins	16[a]
fMg^{2+}	2.0	Organic anions	3.5[b]
H^+	10^{-7}	PO_4	2.5
		SO_4	1.0
Total	157	Total	157

[a] Molar concentrations of proteins are not measured because of variations in molecular weights of proteins. (Note: Using the common anion gap formulas, proteins are the major component of the anion gap in healthy animals.)

[b] In health, organic anions (e.g., lactate, AcAc, BHB, and citrate) contribute very little to total anionic charge. However, they are frequently the reason for an increased anion gap when they accumulate in plasma.

is from Na^+ and K^+ (the mC^+), and 134 of the 157 mmol/L of anion charge is from Cl^- and HCO_3^- (mA^-).

B. Anion gap formula derivation (Eq. 9.4)

As serum is electrically neutral, $tC^+ = tA^-$.   (9.4.)

As $tC^+ = mC^+ + uC^+$ and $tA^- = mA^- + uA^-$,

  then $mC^+ + uC^+ = mA^- + uA^-$.

As $mC^+ = ([Na^+] + [K^+])$ and $mA^- = [Cl^-] + [HCO_3^-]$,

  then $([Na^+] + [K^+]) + uC^+ = ([Cl^-] + [HCO_3^-]) + uA^-$.

Rearranging the equation, $uA^- - uC^+ = ([Na^+] + [K^+]) - ([Cl^-] + [HCO_3^-])$.

As anion gap $= uA^- - uC^+$,

  then anion gap $= ([Na^+] + [K^+]) - ([Cl^-] + [HCO_3^-])$.

C. The major purpose of calculating anion gaps is to identify increased $[uA^-]$ and therefore an increase in circulating anionic molecules (e.g., L-lactate and ketone bodies) in states of metabolic acidosis (Fig. 9.9).

1. As shown in Table 9.11, $uA^- > uC^+$ in health; that is, the sum of charges due to proteins, organic ions, PO_4, and SO_4 is greater than the sum of charges due to fCa^{2+}, fMg^{2+}, and H^+. Also, the "unmeasured" anion concentrations can change more markedly than can the "unmeasured" cation concentrations.

2. Clinically significant changes in the anion gap are usually the result of changes in uA^-. Major changes in $[fCa^{2+}]$ and $[fMg^{2+}]$ are life-threatening. Only minor changes in $[fCa^{2+}]$ and $[fMg^{2+}]$ are seen clinically, and these cause only minor changes in anion gap.

3. Most changes in anion gap are due to increased concentrations of the anions of organic acids. These organic acids may be endogenous substances (e.g., L-lactate and ketone bodies), or they may be generated from exogenous substances (e.g., ethylene glycol).

4. Increases and decreases in protein concentrations, especially albumin, cause mild increases and decreases, respectively, in the anion gap. Most plasma proteins are in the uA^- group.

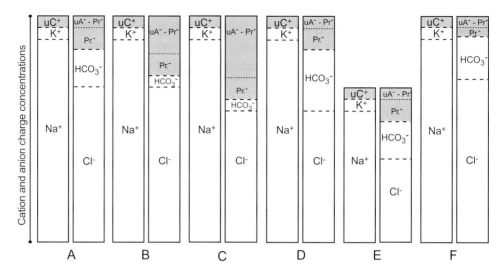

Fig. 9.9. Bar diagrams of anion gap concepts. In all cases, total cation charge concentration equals total anion charge concentration. The uC^+ is due mostly to charges from fCa^{2+}, fMg^{2+}, and some globulins, whereas the uA^- is due mostly to charges from PO_4, SO_4, and anions of organic acids and proteins (Pr^-). Proteins are separated in the diagrams to illustrate their relative contributions to total anionic charge. Cations and anions that contribute to the anion gap are within the *grey-shaded areas*. In these examples, the uC^+ concentrations remain constant but may not be in pathologic states.

A. In healthy animals, the anion gap is almost equivalent to the combined physiologic concentrations of anions of organic acids and proteins, PO_4, and SO_4.

B. In a normochloremic metabolic acidosis (therefore low $[HCO_3^-]$), the increased anion gap represents increased concentrations of uA^- (organic acid anions, PO_4, SO_4, or other anions of the acids). These acidoses may be organic (e.g., lactic acidosis) or inorganic (e.g., renal failure).

C. In a hypochloremic metabolic acidosis (therefore low $[HCO_3^-]$ and low $[Cl^-]$), the increased anion gap represents increased concentrations of uA^- (organic acid anions, PO_4, SO_4, or anions other than Cl^- or HCO_3^-). These acidoses may be organic (e.g., lactic acidosis) or inorganic (e.g., renal failure).

D. In a hypochloremic metabolic alkalosis (therefore high $[HCO_3^-]$), the anion gap is not increased because the sum of $[Cl^-]$ and $[HCO_3^-]$ and the sum of $[Na^+]$ and $[K^+]$ have not changed. These alkaloses may occur with vomiting or gastrointestinal sequestration of H^+ and Cl^-.

E. With concurrent hyponatremia and hypochloremia, the anion gap has not changed because the $[Na^+]$ and $[Cl^-]$ decreased proportionally and other concentrations did not change. These findings are more common when there is concurrent loss of Na^+ and Cl^-; for example, intestinal loss via diarrhea or renal loss in hypoadrenocorticism.

F. With hypoproteinemia, the anion gap is decreased because there is a lower concentration of proteins, an increased sum of $[Cl^-] + [HCO_3^-]$, and no change in the sum of $[Na^+] + [K^+]$. These findings occur in hypoproteinemic disorders when there are not concurrent acid-base disorders (e.g., hepatic failure).

     5. With hyperphosphatemia, each 1 mg/dL increase in $[PO_4]$ is associated with about a 0.6 mmol ion charge/L increase in uA^- and therefore in anion gap (1 mg/dL PO_4 = 0.323 mmol/L PO_4, at an average negative valence of about 1.8).

III.   Analytical concepts
     A. Units: mmol ion charge/L (same as mmol/L of ion or mEq/L of ion for monovalent ions, but not equivalent to ion concentration for multivalent ions like PO_4, fCa^{2+}, and albumin)

   B. As with any calculated value, the anion gap will be only as accurate as the measured values. If needed, refer to prior sections on the individual electrolytes.

   C. The $[HCO_3^-]$ used in the formula may be either $[tCO_2]$ or a calculated $[HCO_3^-]$. Even with marked elevations in P_{CO_2} values, the tCO_2 and HCO_3^- values do not differ by more than 2 mmol/L (2 mEq/L) if both values are accurate. Laboratory reference intervals should be based on the measured values used in the calculation.

   D. The anion gap is sometimes calculated without inclusion of $[K^+]$ because $[K^+]$ contributes relatively little to the mC^+ and is maintained within relatively narrow bounds. Reference values used to interpret these values should also be based on calculations that do not include $[K^+]$.

IV. Increased anion gap

   A. This typically is seen with certain metabolic acidoses (especially normochloremic and hypochloremic), but an increased anion gap is not specific for a particular cause. Hyperchloremic metabolic acidoses will typically not have an increased anion gap. Minor increases in the anion gap can be seen in nonacidotic disorders that cause hyperalbuminemia or reduce the concentration of fCa^{2+} and fMg^{2+}.

   B. Because the anion gap is a calculated value, the value may be erroneous if the values used to calculate it are erroneous.

      1. Pseudo-hyponatremia and pseudo-hypochloremia would lead to unreliable anion gap values. Depending on the cause of the H_2O displacement, $[K^+]$ and $[HCO_3^-]$ may also be erroneous.

      2. The anion gap will be falsely decreased if the $[Cl^-]$ is falsely increased because of the presence of bromide in the sample.

      3. The anion gap will be falsely increased when $[HCO_3^-]$ is falsely decreased because of escape of CO_2 from serum samples excessively exposed to air.

   C. Disorders: Diseases and conditions that increase the anion gap are listed in Table 9.12.

Table 9.12. Diseases and conditions that cause an increased anion gap

Metabolic acidoses
   *Lactic acidosis: increased lactate (either L-lactate or D-lactate)
   *Ketoacidosis: increased ketone bodies (BHB or AcAc)
   *Renal failure: increased PO_4, sulfate, or citrate
   Massive rhabdomyolysis: probably increased lactate and PO_4
   Ingestion of certain compounds
      *Ethylene glycol (antifreeze): increased glycolate or oxalate
      Methanol poisoning (antifreeze): formate
      Paraldehyde (sedative or anesthetic): increased acetate and chloroacetate
      Metaldehyde poisoning (snail bait)
      Penicillin (very high doses)
Hyperalbuminemia (minor changes)

   * A relatively common disease or condition

   Note: A spurious increase in anion gap may occur when decreased $[HCO_3^-]$ is caused by aerobic sample handling.

Table 9.13. Diseases and conditions that cause a decreased anion gap

Decreases in uA⁻
  *Hypoalbuminemia
Increases in uC⁺
  Hypercalcemia (minor changes)
  Hypermagnesemia (minor changes)
  Multiple myeloma that is producing cationic proteins

* A relatively common disease or condition

Note: A spurious decrease in anion gap may occur when there is a pseudo-hyperchloremia caused by bromide. Pseudo-hyponatremia will cause unreliable anion gap values that may be decreased (see the text).

V.   Decreased anion gap
     A. A decreased anion gap has minimal clinical significance, since it does not relate to specific pathologic states. Decreased anion gaps often accompany hypoalbuminemia (decreased uA⁻). They may also accompany increased uC⁺, but such changes are mild.
     B. Recognizing that hypoalbuminemia lowers the anion gap aids in the interpretation of anion gap values that are WRI or increased; that is, the anion gap value would have been greater if the animal had not had hypoalbuminemia.
     C. Disorders: Diseases and conditions that decrease the anion gap are presented in Table 9.13.

VI. Strong ion difference (SID)
     A. Evaluation of SID assesses acid-base abnormalities in the context of abnormal concentrations of ions (strong cations and strong anions). SID concepts are similar to anion gap concepts but also consider other factors.
     B. Complete explanation of SID is beyond the scope of this book, but major aspects are presented in Chapter 10.

LACTATE CONCENTRATION (L-LACTATE AND D-LACTATE)

I.   Physiologic processes
     A. The glycolytic pathway anaerobically converts glucose into energy (ATP) and generates pyruvate, which may be converted into L-lactate (Fig. 9.10).
     B. The major tissue source of L-lactate is skeletal muscle. L-lactate diffuses from the muscle fibers to plasma and is taken up by hepatocytes as part of the Cori cycle: glucose to L-lactate via anaerobic glycolysis in peripheral tissues, and L-lactate to glucose via gluconeogenesis in hepatocytes. Hepatocytes can also use L-lactate for ATP production via the Krebs cycle.
     C. Because mammalian erythrocytes lack mitochondria, glycolysis in erythrocytes produces L-lactate. Also, L-lactate from muscle enters erythrocytes via three methods: (1) diffusion across cell membranes, (2) transportation via a monocarboxylate transporter, and (3) transportation via the inorganic anion-exchange transporter (band-3 protein).[84] Erythrocytes may serve as a transporter of L-lactate and also a "lactate sink" that enhances L-lactate diffusion from muscle to plasma (i.e., muscle to plasma to erythrocytes).

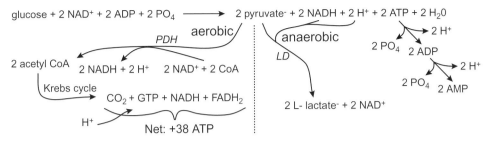

Fig. 9.10. Products of aerobic and anaerobic glycolysis. Catabolism of each glucose molecule results in two pyruvate molecules, two H^+ ions, and a net production of two ATP molecules. When there is adequate oxygenation of cells and after pyruvate enters mitochondria, pyruvate enters the Krebs citric acid cycle (tricarboxylic acid cycle) with pyruvate dehydrogenase (PDH) promoting the breakdown of pyruvate to form CO_2, GTP, NADH, and $FADH_2$. GTP, NADH, and $FADH_2$ are used to generate 36 molecules of ATP in other reactions (therefore a net 38 molecules of ATP). However, if tissue hypoxia is present, pyruvate is instead converted to L-lactate in a reaction promoted by LD. This reaction uses H^+ and thus increases the pH in the cells (or uses the H^+ produced by catabolism of glucose). The pK_a of lactic acid is 3.1, so nearly all of the lactate produced remains in the anionic form; very little buffers H^+ to form lactic acid at physiologic pH values. As explained in the text, the acidemia in lactic acidosis caused by anaerobic conditions comes from the use of ATP (which produces H^+) for energy because ATP production (which consumes H^+; reactions not shown) is not efficient in anaerobic conditions. ADP, adenosine diphosphate; AMP, adenosine monophosphate; CoA, coenzyme A; $FADH_2$, reduced flavin adenine dinucleotide; GTP, guanosine triphosphate; NAD^+, nicotinamide adenine dinucleotide; and NADH, reduced nicotinamide adenine dinucleotide.

Fig. 9.11. Chemical structure of pyruvate, lactate, and ketone body molecules. Knowing the chemical composition of molecules can facilitate an understanding of the relationships of those molecules in pathologic states. The reduction of pyruvate by LD increases the formation of L-lactate in lactic acidosis. L-lactate and D-lactate are optical isomers (mirror images). L-lactate is the major form produced by mammalian cells, and D-lactate is produced by bacteria. Of the three ketone bodies, only AcAc and acetone are truly ketones. AcAc can be converted to either acetone or BHB. (Note: *Solid wedges* extend forward, and *dashed wedges* extend backward.)

D. Bacteria produce D-lactate, and some produce L-lactate. The stereoisomer of L-lactate (Fig. 9.11), D-lactate can also be produced in mammalian cells via the *glyoxalase pathway*, which metabolizes methylglyoxal produced during glycolysis or via conversion from acetone.[85] In health, plasma concentrations of D-lactate are very small compared to those of L-lactate.

II. Analytical concepts
   A. L-lactate
      1. Common clinical assays for lactate measure the L-lactate produced by animal cells. L-lactate assays use either LD (spectrophotometric methods) or L-lactate oxidase (e.g., i-STAT and NOVA).
      2. L-lactate concentrations are measured by many blood gas analyzers, but, depending on the analytical method, either whole blood or plasma is the preferred sample. In the NOVA instruments, a plasma [L-lactate] is measured in a whole blood sample by allowing only plasma to enter the reaction chamber.
   B. D-lactate concentrations can be measured by high-performance liquid chromatography or by D-lactate dehydrogenase enzymatic methods. These assays are not commonly available in clinical laboratories.
   C. Unit: mg/dL × 0.112 = mmol/L (SI unit) (Note: This is a conversion for the analyte lactate. The conversion factor for lactic acid is 0.111.)
   D. Sample for [L-lactate]
      1. Blood samples should be processed or analyzed quickly so that L-lactate produced by erythrocytes does not increase the plasma [L-lactate]. If the sample cannot be processed immediately, L-lactate production can be reduced by collecting blood into a tube containing sodium fluoride and chilling the blood until the plasma is separated from the erythrocytes; fluoride inhibits phosphopyruvate hydratase (synonym: enolase) of the glycolytic pathway.
      2. Ideally, blood should be collected from free-flowing blood (without a tourniquet) so that blood stagnation does not result in increased L-lactate production.
      3. L-lactate concentrations are also measured in bovine milk, as in indicator of ruminal acidosis, and in body cavity effusions as evidence of bacterial infection (see Chapter 19).
      4. Special collection methods for D-lactate samples were not found.
   E. Substances that interfere with the measurement of [L-lactate] will vary with the method used.
      1. Bromide falsely decreases the [L-lactate] determined by the i-STAT L-lactate oxidase method, but similar interference is not described for the NOVA L-lactate oxidase method.
      2. The presence of free hemoglobin and hemoglobin-based oxygen carriers in the sample will result in falsely low L-lactate concentrations if measured by the L-lactate oxidase assay, probably because the peroxidase activity of heme removes the H_2O_2 produced by the L-lactate oxidase reaction.[86,87]

III. Increased plasma L-lactate concentrations (*hyperlactatemia*)
   A. L-lactate accumulates in plasma when its formation exceeds the removal by tissues (primarily by hepatocytic uptake and glomerular filtration).
      1. The primary reason for increased L-lactate production is hypoxia.
         a. During anaerobic (hypoxic) conditions, catabolism of pyruvate switches from entry into the Krebs cycle to L-lactate production (Fig. 9.10). It should be noted that this process generates L-lactate and not lactic acid and that the conversion of pyruvate to L-lactate results in the use of H^+ (thus increased pH).
         b. Concurrently, changes in other metabolic pathways result in the accumulation of H^+ in the blood (acidemia).[88] In aerobic conditions and via the Krebs cycle, cells consume H^+ while producing large amounts of ATP. However, in anaerobic conditions, the negative energy status causes a net degradation of ATP and thus

Table 9.14. Diseases and conditions that cause hyperlactatemia (L-lactate)

Inadequate delivery of O_2 to tissues
    *Stagnant hypoxia: shock, blood vessel occlusion
    *Demand hypoxia: strenuous exercise, struggling during restraint
    Hypoxemia: respiratory disorders
    Hemoglobic hypoxia: anemia, methemoglobinemia
Increase production by metabolic pathways
    Grain overload
    Defective metabolic pathways for aerobic glycolysis
        Hyperammonemia: urea toxicosis, ammoniated forage toxicosis
        Pyruvate dehydrogenase deficiency
Other or unknown mechanisms
    Sepsis
    Canine babesiosis
    Liver disease
    Transfusion of stored blood or packed erythrocytes

  * A relatively common disease or condition

        production of H^+ (Fig. 9.10). Other metabolic changes also add to the accumulation of H^+ (e.g., altered lipid metabolism).

  2. Increased L-lactate production may also be due to defective metabolic pathways (see the following sect. B.2.b).

  3. Potentially, decreased removal of L-lactate from plasma can contribute to hyperlactatemia, but it is uncommon for this process to occur alone.

  B. Disorders and pathogeneses (Table 9.14)

    1. Inadequate delivery of O_2 to tissues: Such disorders vary from recent muscular exercise to those causing hypoxemia, hemoglobic hypoxia, or stagnation hypoxia (see Chapter 10).

      a. Stagnant hypoxia

        (1) Shock: The redistribution of blood results in poor perfusion of peripheral tissues, which causes stagnation hypoxia and increased generation of L-lactate.

        (2) Equine colic caused by gastrointestinal disorders (e.g., torsion, strangulation, and infarction): The excessive L-lactate production may be due to poor perfusion of tissues, but absorbed endotoxins may also stimulate L-lactate production, and intestinal bacteria may contribute D-lactate and L-lactate. In one study involving 14 horses with increased anion gaps, L-lactate concentrations were increased much more than D-lactate concentrations.[89] Generally, the severity of the hyperlactatemia is inversely proportional to the prognosis in colicky horses.[90]

      b. Demand hypoxia

        (1) Strenuous exercise: Excessive muscular activity increases anaerobic glycolysis and thus increases L-lactate production and release from muscle.[91]

        (2) Struggling cats: In experimental studies of stress-induced hyperglycemia, struggling associated with harness restraint for blood collection increased plasma L-lactate concentrations. The hyperlactatemia was considered to be caused by increased muscular activity.[92] Similar changes in other animals would be expected with similar conditions.

    c. Hypoxemia: Poor oxygenation of blood could produce sufficient hypoxia to cause a hyperlactatemia, but this situation is not commonly recognized.

    d. Hemoglobic hypoxia: Defective transport of O_2 to tissues could produce hyperlactatemia, but this situation is not commonly recognized.

2. Increased production by metabolic pathways

    a. Grain overload (in ruminants, horses, and ponies): Excess intake of starch (grain or other sources) increases the formation of L-lactate and D-lactate by rumen (ruminants) or hindgut (equids) bacteria. Increased lumen acidity alters the microbial environment, which intensifies lactate production and diminishes lactate use by flora. The lactate is absorbed by the mucosa, thus increasing plasma lactate concentrations.

    b. Defective glycolytic pathways

       (1) Hyperammonemia

          (a) This may occur from excessive production of ammonium (e.g., urea toxicosis or ammoniated forage toxicosis), from various causes of hepatic insufficiency, and from urea cycle defect.

          (b) High $[NH_4^+]$ may interfere with the Krebs cycle such that the aerobic production of ATP is defective. Generation of ATP switches to anaerobic glycolysis, which produces L-lactate.[93,94]

       (2) Pyruvate dehydrogenase deficiency in Sussex spaniels and Clumber spaniels results in excess formation of L-lactate.[95,96] Pyruvate dehydrogenase catalyzes the conversion of pyruvate to AcCoA, which then enters the Krebs cycle. With pyruvate dehydrogenase deficiency, the conversion of pyruvate to L-lactate by LD is increased.

3. Other or unknown mechanism

    a. Sepsis: The mechanism of hyperlactatemia (L-lactate) is frequently considered to be caused by poor tissue perfusion,[97] but endotoxemia by itself has been reported to cause hyperlactatemia in people.[53] Also, experiments in dogs indicate that the use of L-lactate by liver and other tissues during sepsis is decreased.[98]

    b. Canine babesiosis: Hyperlactatemia (L-lactate) occurs in some dogs with acute babesiosis, but the pathogenesis of the hyperlactatemia is not established.[99] It does not appear to be related to the degree of anemia and thus is not caused by hemoglobic hypoxia. Because of the concurrent hypoglycemia, the hyperlactatemia is likely caused by accelerated anaerobic glycolysis that consumes glucose and produces L-lactate. This consumption of glucose is a feature of sepsis-induced hypoglycemia (see Glucose Concentration, sect. I.V.C.1.f, in Chapter 14).

    c. Liver disease: Severe liver disease may cause hyperlactatemia (L-lactate), but the pathogenesis is not established. The hyperlactatemia might be due to excessive lactate production (hepatic hypoxia or decreased mitochondrial function) and not due to defective utilization.

    d. Transfusion of stored blood or packed erythrocytes: During storage, erythrocytes continue glycolysis to produce L-lactate, and thus L-lactate–rich blood is administered IV.

IV. Increased plasma D-lactate concentrations

   A. [D-lactate] may be increased in animals with diabetes mellitus.[85]

    1. D-lactate concentrations were greater in cats with ketotic diabetes mellitus (mean ≈ 340 μmol/L) than in cats with nonketotic diabetes mellitus (mean ≈ 140 μmol/L)

or in healthy cats (mean ≈ 25 µmol/L). D-lactate may have been formed through a pathway involving acetone or methylglyoxal.

2. Even though there was a significant difference in D-lactate concentrations among the groups, the increase was < 1 mmol/L and thus would not contribute clinically to increased anion gap values. Also, the D-lactate concentrations are much less than found in mammals with L-lactate acidosis (e.g., 10–20 mmol/L).

B. Absorption of D-lactate (produced by enteric bacteria) can increase [D-lactate] (not measured by routine lactate assays but may be contributory to increased anion gaps).

   1. D-lactate is a major contributor to total [lactate] in neonatal calves with diarrhea.[76,100,101]

   2. A cat with exocrine pancreatic insufficiency had metabolic acidosis and a concurrent increase in plasma [D-lactate]. The authors concluded that the uncommon maldigestive disorder caused enteric production of D-lactate by bacteria.[102]

   3. In milk-fed calves, failure of esophageal groove reflex allows milk to enter the reticuloruminal cavity (called *ruminal* drinking) in which bacterial fermentation of lactose results in the formation of D-lactic and L-lactic acids. After the ions are absorbed (probably in intestine), a metabolic acidosis with increased plasma concentrations of D-lactate may develop. The rapid metabolism of L-lactate prevents it from accumulating in the plasma.[103]

   4. In a group of 50 colicky horses with mild lactic acidosis, none had increased D-lactate concentrations.[104]

C. Ingestion of propylene glycol may result in increased [D-lactate].[105]

   1. Cats that ingested diets of 12 % and 41 % propylene glycol on a dry weight basis had an increased [D-lactate]. The lower percentage, which is near that found in some commercial cat food, produced nearly a 2 mmol/L increase in [D-lactate], whereas the higher dose produced nearly a 7 mmol/L increase by 20 d. Corresponding with the increased [D-lactate], the anion gap values increased. [L-lactate] decreased slightly from the preexisting small concentrations during the study.

   2. Propylene glycol is converted to D-lactate. This probably occurs via the actions of alcohol dehydrogenase and through methylglyoxal.

V.   Relationship to the anion gap

A. Both L-lactate and D-lactate will contribute to an anion gap (see the Anion Gap section). Each mmol/L increase in the [lactate] can account for each mmol/L increase in the anion gap.

B. If there is an increased anion gap in serum or plasma and the [L-lactate] is not increased sufficiently to account for the anion gap's magnitude, the increased anion gap could be due to D-lactate or other unmeasured anions (Table 9.12).

β-HYDROXYBUTYRATE (BHB) AND ACETOACETATE (AcAc) CONCENTRATIONS

I.   Physiologic processes

A. Ketogenesis occurs in hepatocytes through a series of reactions that convert AcCoA into BHB, AcAc, and acetone; the two anions (BHB and AcAc) and acetone are collectively called *ketone bodies*, but BHB does not have the chemical structure of a ketone (Fig. 9.11). The amounts of AcAc and BHB in hepatocytes are in equilibrium. The equilibrium shifts toward BHB when NADH is abundant in hepatocytes (e.g., in diabetes mellitus), whereas the equilibrium shifts toward AcAc when NAD^+ is abundant. The pK_a of acetoacetic acid is 3.6, and the pK_a of β-hydroxybutyric acid is 4.7. Therefore, at physiologic pH values, nearly all of these molecules are in their anionic forms.

B. Ketogenesis is promoted by glucagon and inhibited by insulin.

C. Renal excretion of BHB helps with the excretion of H^+ because the pK_a of BHB is near that of acidic urine, and thus it binds more H^+ at a urine pH of 5 than at a plasma pH of 7.4. Similarly, AcAc aids in the excretion of H^+.

II. Analytical concepts

    A. Units (Note: Conversion factors are for anions and not the corresponding acids.)

        1. AcAc: mg/dL × 99 = μmol/L or mg/dL × 0.099 = mmol/L (SI unit)

        2. BHB: mg/dL × 97 = μmol/L or mg/dL × 0.097 = mmol/L (SI unit)

    B. Assays: There are three types of assays for ketone bodies.

        1. Spectrophotometric quantitative assays use BHB dehydrogenase to measure serum [BHB] by catalyzing the conversion of BHB to AcAc. In some assays, a high [AcAc] may interfere with the reaction to produce a falsely low [BHB].[106] Hemolysis can decrease the measured values.

        2. The common nitroprusside methods (Ketostix strip, Acetest tablet, and Ketocheck powder) are used for blood, serum, milk, and urine for the detection of AcAc and acetone. BHB does not react.[107]

        3. Relatively uncommon qualitative or semiquantitative methods are designed to detect BHB. The KetoTest strip is used for urine or milk. The Ketolac BHB strip is used to detect BHB in milk.[107,108]

    C. BHB stability: BHB is reported to be stable in serum for 1 wk at 4 °C and longer if kept at −20 °C.[109]

    D. When ketone bodies are detected in blood or serum, they should also be in urine. However, when comparing results, the type of assay and its analytic properties should be considered. For example, the BHB might be increased in serum and urine, but the urine test for ketones (AcAc) may not be positive. However, typically the urinary excretion of both BHB and AcAc is sufficient so that the nitroprusside method will provide a positive ketone reaction.

    E. In theory, BHB can be converted with H_2O_2 to AcAc so that nitroprusside methods can be used to detect BHB. However, BHB concentrations must be > 50 mmol/L in urine or > 100 mmol/L in serum (using 30 % H_2O_2) to produce more than a trace reaction. Such concentrations are not clinically relevant for serum samples, and if urine BHB concentrations were this great, AcAc concentrations would probably be great enough to be detected routinely (see Chemical Examination of Urine, sect. V, in Chapter 8).[110]

III. Increased ketone body concentration

    A. An increased concentration of ketone bodies in blood is *ketonemia*. The clinical disorder is called *ketosis*. Ketosis occurs primarily for two reasons:

        1. Excessive β-oxidation of fatty acids results in the production of more AcCoA than can be used by the Krebs cycle. The excess AcCoA, especially with glucagon excess or insulin deficiency, enters the ketogenic pathway to form AcAc, which can be converted to either acetone or BHB. This occurs during diabetes mellitus and starvation.

        2. The AcCoA produced from oxidation of lipids typically combines with oxaloacetate as it enters the Krebs cycle, which eventually results in ATP production. When an

animal is in a negative energy status, oxaloacetate is used for gluconeogenesis, so there may be an inadequate amount of oxaloacetate to react with AcCoA. The accumulation of AcCoA promotes ketogenesis.

B. Conditions and disorders with ketonemia
  1. All mammals: starvation, prolonged anorexia, and diabetes mellitus
  2. Cattle: bovine ketosis associated with freshening and the high-energy demands of lactation, diabetes mellitus, displaced abomasum, and hepatic lipidosis
  3. Dogs: diabetes mellitus, starvation, lactation, and endurance racing
  4. Horses: diabetes mellitus and endurance racing

C. Three cowside tests have been evaluated for detecting bovine ketosis: Ketocheck for AcAc in milk, Ketostix for AcAc in urine, and KetoTest for BHB in milk.[107]
  1. The gold standard in the study was serum [BHB]: Ketosis was considered to be present if the serum [BHB] was > 1.4 mmol/L.
  2. The diagnostic properties varied with the decision thresholds, but generally the diagnostic sensitivity and diagnostic specificity of the Ketostix and KetoTest methods were good. The diagnostic sensitivity of the Ketocheck was considered inadequate for use a screening test for subclinical ketosis.

OSMOLALITY AND OSMO. GAP

I. Definitions
  A. *Osmolality*: the concentration of a solute expressed in moles of solute per *kilogram* of solvent (mol/kg). In the clinical assessment of body fluids, osmolality is expressed as mmol/kg or mOsm/kg (the authors prefer the simpler SI unit of mmol/kg).
  B. *Osmolarity*: the concentration of a solute expressed in moles of solute per *liter* of solution (mol/L). In clinical assessments, it is also expressed as mOsm/L. Serum osmolality does not equal serum osmolarity, because 1 L of normal serum will contain about 930 mL of H_2O (0.93 kg of H_2O). In the absence of postprandial lipemia, the remaining volume ($\approx$ 70 mL) is occupied mostly by proteins.
  C. *Osmole*: 1 mole of osmotically active particles. For a substance that does not dissociate in solution, 1 mole equals 1 osmole. For a substance that completely dissociates into two ions per mole, there are 2 osmoles of dissociated solute particles per 1 mole of undissociated substance. Most dissociable solutes do not dissociate completely.
  D. *Mole*: the SI unit for the amount of substance present when there are 6.023×10^{23} (Avogadro's number) identical particles of it (based on the number of particles in 0.012 kg of carbon 12). One mole of a substance weighs its gram molecular weight (e.g., 1 mole of glucose weighs 180 g and 1 mole of Na^+ weighs 23 g).
  E. *Osmotic pressure*: the force required to counterbalance the force of osmotic solvent flow through a semipermeable membrane, such as cell membranes. It is also referred to as *total osmotic pressure* to differentiate it from colloidal osmotic pressure (Fig. 9.12).
  F. *Osmosis*: the passage of solvent (e.g., H_2O) from a solution of lesser solute concentration (greater [H_2O]) through a semipermeable membrane (one that does not permit passage of some solute particles) to a solution of greater solute concentration (lesser [H_2O])
  G. *Osmometry*: any technique for measuring the osmolality or osmotic pressure of a solution
  H. *Osmometer*: a device or instrument that measures the osmolality (osmotic concentration) or osmotic pressure of a solution. A freezing-point osmometer measures osmolality, and a membrane osmometer measures colloidal osmotic pressure.

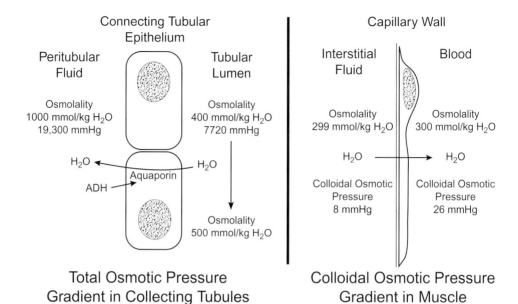

Connecting Tubular Epithelium

Peritubular Fluid

Tubular Lumen

Osmolality 1000 mmol/kg H_2O 19,300 mmHg

Osmolality 400 mmol/kg H_2O 7720 mmHg

H_2O ← Aquaporin ← H_2O

ADH →

Osmolality 500 mmol/kg H_2O

Capillary Wall

Interstitial Fluid

Blood

Osmolality 299 mmol/kg H_2O

Osmolality 300 mmol/kg H_2O

H_2O → H_2O

Colloidal Osmotic Pressure 8 mmHg

Colloidal Osmotic Pressure 26 mmHg

Total Osmotic Pressure Gradient in Collecting Tubules

Colloidal Osmotic Pressure Gradient in Muscle

Fig. 9.12. Schematic comparison of osmotic pressure and colloidal osmotic pressure.

- In the **left** drawing of the renal collecting tubule, under phyisiologic conditions, the peritubular fluid has a much greater osmolality than the tubular fluid. Osmotic pressure can be calculated from osmolality (each 1 mmol/kg of osmolality is equivalent to 19.3 mmHg of osmotic pressure). Therefore, an osmolality of 1000 mmol/kg equates to an osmotic pressure of 19,300 mmHg, and an osmolality of 400 mmol/kg creates 7720 mmHg of osmotic pressure. The large difference in osmolality creates a large osmotic pressure gradient (almost 12,000 mmHg in this example). The peritubular fluid's hypertonicity is mostly due to high concentrations of Na^+, Cl^-, and urea. When ADH is present, it increases the permeability of the tubular epithelium (via aquaporin) to H_2O so that H_2O is resorbed and thus increases the solute concentration in the tubular fluid).

- In the **right** drawing of a capillary wall in skeletal muscle, the colloidal osmotic pressure (synonym: oncotic pressure) is greater in the blood than in the interstitial fluid because the protein concentration is greater in plasma than in interstitial fluid and because of the related Gibbs-Donnan equilibrium. The colloidal osmotic pressure gradient (18 mmHg in this example) tends to cause the movement of H_2O (and small solutes) from interstitial fluid to plasma. The movement of H_2O out of or into the plasma is determined by the hydraulic pressure gradient across the semipermeable membrane (see the Colloidal Osmotic Pressure section in Chapter 7, and General Concepts and Definitions, sect. V, in Chapter 19).

Note: The osmotic pressure gradient in the distal nephron is more than 600 times the colloidal osmotic pressure in the capillary bed. The pressure values are provided to illustrate the magnitude of the differences between the forces of osmotic pressure gradients and colloidal osmotic pressure gradients.

I. *Tonicity*: the *effective* osmolality of a solution; that is, that solute concentration that can contribute to movement of H_2O across a semipermeable membrane

J. *Solute*: a substance dissolved in a solvent

K. *Colloidal osmotic pressure* (oncotic pressure): the osmotic pressure exerted by colloidal particles suspended in a solvent at a capillary membrane. Colloidal particles are macromolecules that are too small (1 nm to 1 μm) to be settled out by gravity. Most oncotic pressure of plasma is caused by plasma proteins (about 80 % albumin and 20 % globulins). Part of the colloidal osmotic pressure is attributed to cations (e.g., Na^+) that are attracted to the negatively charged proteins (*Donnan equilibrium effect*).

Table 9.15. Solutes that contribute to serum osmolarity (approximate concentrations provided to simplify concept)

Solute	Measured concentration	Factor to convert to mmol/L	Contribution to osmolarity	Contribution to total osmolality in serum of healthy animal
Na^+	146 mmol/L	× 1	146 mmol/L ⎫	
K^+	4 mmol/L	× 1	4 mmol/L ⎪	281 mmol/L
Cl^-	107 mmol/L	× 1	107 mmol/L ⎬	94 % of total solute
HCO_3^-	24 mmol/L	× 1	24 mmol/L ⎭	
UN	20 mg/dL	÷ 2.8	7 mmol/L ⎫	12 mmol/L
Glucose	100 mg/dL	÷ 18	5.5 mmol/L ⎬	4 % of total solute
PO_4	4 mg/dL	× 0.32	1.3 mmol/L ⎫	5 mmol/L
tCa^{2+}	10 mg/dL	× 0.25	2.5 mmol/L ⎬	2 % of total solute
Mg^{2+}	1 mmol/L	× 1	1.0 mmol/L ⎭	
Protein	7 g/dL	Varies with protein	< 1.0 mmol/L	No significant contribution
Total			299.3 mmol/L	

Most nonprotein solutes do not contribute to osmotic pressure in capillaries, because the capillaries are permeable to H_2O and the small solutes. Chapter 7 contains information regarding the measurement and interpretation of colloidal osmotic pressures.

II. Physiologic processes
    A. As stated in the foregoing definitions, osmolality is the concentration of solutes per kilogram of solvent and depends on the number of molecules or ions in the solution. The major contributors to serum osmolality and their relative contributions are listed in Table 9.15.
    B. Major concepts of relative contributions of solutes to serum osmolality
        1. Na^+ is the major solute in serum. About half of the solute (moles, not mass) in serum is actually Na^+ ions.
        2. Cl^- runs a close second. Because Cl^- frequently follows Na^+, changes in $[Na^+]$ are frequently accompanied by changes in $[Cl^-]$, which approximately doubles the changes in osmolality.
        3. At physiologic concentrations, urea and glucose are small contributors to total osmolality. However, marked azotemia or hyperglycemia will cause hyperosmolality.
        4. Protein contributes very little (< 1 mmol/kg) to osmolality. Protein molecules are relatively very large but extremely rare (compared to electrolytes, urea, and glucose).
        5. Hypothalamic osmoreceptors are sensitive to increases and decreases in effective plasma osmolality (tonicity).
           a. If effective osmolality is increased, ADH is released to stimulate the renal collecting tubules to resorb H_2O. In addition, the thirst center is stimulated to increase the intake of H_2O. Both processes cause a dilutional correction of the plasma solute concentration.

  b. If the effective osmolality is decreased, ADH secretion is diminished, and thus there is less H_2O resorption by the collecting tubules, increased H_2O loss, and thus a correctional increase in concentration of plasma solutes.

6. Effective osmolality (tonicity)
  a. When different concentrations of solute are on two sides of a membrane that is H_2O permeable, the solutes establish an osmolar gradient that promotes osmosis (movement of H_2O to diminish the gradient). If the membrane is impermeable to a solute, then that solute contributes to the effective osmolality.
  b. Urea is a small molecule that is freely diffusible across most cell membranes (the major exception is the epithelial cell of collecting tubules). Wherever urea ($M_r = 60$) is freely diffusible, it does not contribute to an osmolar gradient and thus does not contribute to the effective osmolality.
  c. Methanol ($M_r = 32$), ethanol ($M_r = 46$), and ethylene glycol ($M_r = 62$) are ineffective osmoles for the same reason, and thus they increase osmolality without changing H_2O distribution or [Na^+]. Mannitol ($M_r = 182$), glycerol ($M_r = 92$), sorbitol ($M_r = 182$), and glucose ($M_r = 180$) do contribute to effective osmolality because they are not freely diffusible across most cell membranes.
  d. If urea is contributing to an increased serum osmolality and other data do not suggest the presence of other ineffective solutes (e.g., ethylene glycol), effective osmolality of serum (or plasma) may be estimated (Eq. 9.5).

$$\text{effective osmolality} = \text{measured osmolality} - \frac{[UN]}{2.8}\,(\text{if UN in mg/dL}) \qquad \textbf{(9.5.)}$$
$$= \text{measured osmolality} - [urea]\,(\text{if urea in mmol/L})$$

  e. Knowledge of effective osmolality is useful in two clinical situations:
    (1) Determining the presence of hyperosmolar syndrome
      (a) When the effective plasma osmolality rapidly rises (> 350 mmol/kg or [Na^+] > 170 mmol/L),[111] H_2O leaves cells, including neurons. Consequently, the animal can be depressed, stuporous, or even die from the hyperosmolar state.
      (b) However, if the hyperosmolar state develops slowly, then intracellular production of organic molecules such as taurine, glycine, glutamine, sorbitol and inositol (so-called idiogenic osmoles) diminishes the osmotic gradient, and thus less H_2O leaves the cell. If hypotonic fluids are then administered to reduce the plasma osmolality, there can be a rapid influx of H_2O into neurons and development of cerebral edema.
    (2) Determining physiologic responses that are expected in azotemic animals
      (a) If the hyperosmolality is caused by increased urea concentrations only (i.e., effective osmolality is not increased), there should not be a stimulus to drink H_2O or release ADH (unless hypovolemia is present).
      (b) If the hyperosmolality is due to effective solutes and not urea, the hyperosmolality is expected to stimulate thirst and ADH release.

III. Analytical concepts for osmolality (see Chapter 7 for colloidal osmotic pressure)
  A. Osm_m
    1. Osmometry is based on physiochemical properties (called *colligative properties*) that depend on the number of particles in a solution. Two colligative properties are used in clinical osmometry:

  a. Freezing-point depression: A 1 mol/kg solution of a solute in H_2O (1 molal) will have a freezing point 1.86 °C lower than that of pure H_2O.

  b. Vapor pressure (or dew point) depression: A 1 mol/kg solution of a solute in H_2O (1 molal) will have a vapor pressure 0.03 mmHg lower than that of pure H_2O.

2. Freezing-point osmometers are more common, more precise, and more accurate than vapor pressure osmometers. Vapor pressure osmometers do not measure the contribution of volatile solutes (e.g., alcohols) to total osmolality. (Note: Colloid osmometers measure colloidal osmotic pressure and not osmolality; see the Colloidal Osmotic Pressure section in Chapter 7.)

3. Osm_m indicates the total concentration of solutes in the serum but does not indicate which solutes are present.

4. Serum is the required sample for measuring osmolality; the addition of anticoagulants for plasma samples would be adding solute to the plasma. The stability of a serum osmolality will depend on the stability of the individual solutes in the sample (see sections for Na^+, K^+, Cl^-, HCO_3^-, glucose, urea, or other solutes that can be present).

B. Osm_c

1. Because there is a direct correlation between molality and osmolality and there is a relationship between molality and molarity, knowing the millimolar concentrations of solutes enables us to estimate the osmolality that is expected due to those solutes. However, this conversion is not exact because of three factors:

  a. Osmolality and osmolarity of plasma solutes are not equal because 1 L of plasma contains about 0.93 kg H_2O and about 0.07 kg solids. Most plasma solids are proteins.

  b. The concentrations of some plasma solutes are not measured, and thus their contributions to total osmolality are not included in calculations.

  c. Some plasma solutes are not completely dissociated (e.g., small amounts of Na^+ and Cl^- are present in plasma as NaCl).

2. At least 14 formulas have been used to calculate an estimate (Osm_c) of the true osmolality (Osm_m) of serum.[112] Each formula includes measured values for some of the major solutes contributing to osmolality, and constants or factors to estimate the effects of the other solutes. The formulas vary because of the following:

  a. Different investigators attempted to estimate true osmolality by using different solutes and conversion factors.

  b. Method variations for some of the analytes produce different results, which require different mathematical manipulations to best estimate true osmolality.

  c. The dissociation of ionic compounds may vary among species.

  d. The conversion of serum osmolarity to serum osmolality is imperfect.

3. Ideally, each laboratory would determine a best-fit equation to predict Osm_m for that laboratory's assays. However, most use one of four equations (Eq. 9.6a–d).

In all formulas, Na^+ and K^+ concentrations are in mmol/L or mEq/L.
If UN and glucose concentrations are in mg/dL, then

$$Osm_c = 1.86\,([Na^+]+[K^+]) + \frac{[UN]}{2.8} + \frac{[glucose]}{18} \tag{9.6a.}$$

$$Osm_c = 2\,[Na^+] + \frac{[UN]}{3} + \frac{[glucose]}{20} \tag{9.6b.}$$

If UN and glucose concentrations are in mmol/L, then

$$Osm_c = 1.86\ ([Na^+] + [K^+]) + [urea] + [glucose] \tag{9.6c.}$$

$$Osm_c = 2\ [Na^+] + [urea] + [glucose] \tag{9.6d.}$$

4. What are the components of the equations?
   a. $1.86 \times ([Na^+] + [K^+])$ or $2 \times [Na^+]$: an estimate of the osmolality due to the major four electrolytes; that is, the sum of Na^+, K^+, Cl^-, and HCO_3^- concentrations
      (1) Because serum must remain electrically neutral, increased concentrations of other anions will be associated with lower $[Cl^-]$ or $[HCO_3^-]$ if cation concentrations remain constant. Thus, the expression estimates the osmolality due to electrolytes even when there is an increased anion gap.
      (2) The inclusion of K^+ tends to yield a more accurate estimate of osmolality, especially if there is hyponatremia and hyperkalemia. However, because serum $[K^+]$ cannot change much (± 2 mmol/L) without serious medical consequences, major changes in serum $[K^+]$ cause only minor changes in total serum osmolality.
      (3) Others approach the conceptual contributions of the electrolytes with the concept that 1 mmol of NaCl contributes only about 1.75 mmol because NaCl, like other plasma salts, is not completely dissociated in plasma.[1] With the assumption that plasma is 93 % H_2O, the osmolality due to Na^+ salts is about $1.88 \times$ plasma $[Na^+]$; $1.88 = 1.75 \div 0.93$. The osmolality due to other salts (i.e., K^+, Ca^{2+}, and Mg^{2+} salts) is about $0.12 \times$ plasma $[Na^+]$. Thus, $2 \times$ plasma $[Na^+]$ estimates the osmolality due to the electrolytes if the ratios of Na^+ to other electrolytes are physiologic.
      (4) When considering the calculated osmolality, it is important to recognize that the first part of the formula (that which contains Na^+ or $Na^+ + K^+$) represents the contributions of all ions, not just Na^+ or just Na^+ and K^+.
   b. $[UN] \div 2.8$: conversion of $[UN]$ from mg/dL to mmol/L of urea (M_r of UN = 28, and there are 10 dL in 1 L)
   c. $[UN] \div 3$: approximate conversion of $[UN]$ from mg/dL to mmol/L of urea
   d. $[Glucose] \div 18$: conversion of $[glucose]$ from mg/dL to mmol/L (M_r of glucose = 180, and there are 10 dL in 1 L)
   e. $[Glucose] \div 20$: approximate conversion of $[glucose]$ from mg/dL to mmol/L
5. An Osm_c is of little value by itself; it is simply an estimate of the osmolality due to commonly measured solute concentrations. If a measured solute concentration (i.e., Na^+, urea, or glucose) is increased, then the Osm_c will be increased proportionately and it may or may not estimate the true serum osmolality.

C. Osmo. gap
   1. There is not a correct unit for the osmo. gap because the Osm_m is expressed as mmol/kg (molality) and the Osm_c is expressed as mmol/L (molarity). Since neither osmolar gap nor osmolal gap is a correct term, the term *osmo. gap* is used.
   2. Osmo. gap formula (Eq. 9.7)

$$Osmo.\ gap = Osm_m - Osm_c \tag{9.7.}$$

   a. *Osm_m* represents the total solute concentration in the sample. *Osm_c* estimates the solute concentration by use of some combination of Na^+, K^+, urea, and glucose concentrations.

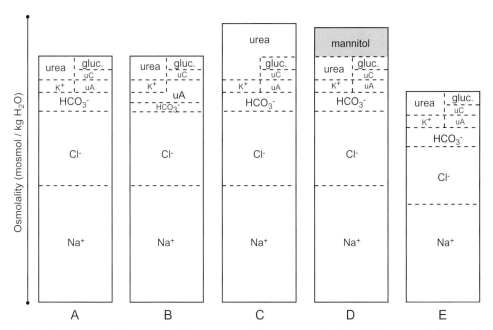

Fig. 9.13. Bar diagrams of serum osmolality concepts. The unmeasured cations (uC) are mostly fCa^{2+} and fMg^{2+}, whereas the unmeasured anions (uA) are mostly PO_4, SO_4, and anions of organic acids. Proteins are not included because they do not contribute significantly to osmolality. Solutes that contribute to the osmo. gap are within the *grey-shaded area*.

A. In healthy animals, nearly all nonprotein solutes are monovalent electrolytes except for urea and glucose (gluc.). The osmo. gap should be near 0 if an appropriate formula for Osm_c is used.

B. In a normochloremic metabolic acidosis (therefore low $[HCO_3^-]$), the osmo. gap is not increased, because the 1.86 ($Na^+ + K^+$) should account for the sum of all cations and anions. Because electrical neutrality must be maintained, increases in the concentration of unmeasured anions must be accompanied by either increases in cations, decreases in other anions, or both. In any case, the 1.86 ($Na^+ + K^+$) should account for the sum of all cations and anions.

C. When hyperosmolality is caused by azotemia, the osmo. gap is not increased, because both the Osm_m and the Osm_c are increased proportionately by the higher [urea]. The same concept applies for hyperosmolality caused by hyperglycemia or hypernatremia.

D. When hyperosmolality is caused by an abnormal nonionic solute (e.g., mannitol), the osmo. gap is increased, because the exogenous solute increases the Osm_m but is not included in the Osm_c formula.

E. When hypoosmolality is caused by hyponatremia and hypochloremia, the osmo. gap is not changed, because the Osm_m and the Osm_c are decreased by the same amount.

    b. If the formula used for Osm_c is optimized to match Osm_m values, the osmo. gap reference interval would be near zero.

    c. One cannot reliably interpret osmo. gap values if a laboratory has not determined the relationship between paired values for Osm_c and Osm_m for values determined by that laboratory, although marked increases may be readily apparent.

IV.   Evaluation of serum osmolality and osmo. gap. The major concepts are shown in Fig. 9.13.

Table 9.16. Disorders and conditions that cause abnormal serum osmolality or increased osmo. gaps

Osm_m	Osmo. gap	Abnormal [solute]	Disorders, conditions
*Increased	WRI	Increases in Na^+, urea, or glucose concentrations	See the Hypernatremia section See the Azotemia section in Chapter 8 See the Hyperglycemia section in Chapter 14
Increased	Increased	Increased concentration of a nonanionic compound other than urea or glucose	Mannitol infusion (IV) Radiographic contrast media (IV) Ethanol, methanol, ethylene glycol
*Decreased	WRI	Indicates a true hyponatremia	See Sodium Concentration, sect. V

* A relatively common disease or condition.

Note: A spurious increase in osmo. gap will occur if there is a pseudo-hyponatremia (see Sodium Concentration, sect. V.B.7).

V. Interpretation of osmolality data (Table 9.16)

A. Serum hyperosmolality and osmo. gap WRI: An increased Osm_m indicates the concentration of one or more solutes is increased. Since the osmo. gap is WRI, there is a proportionate increase in Osm_c and Osm_m. Because an increased Osm_c results from increased concentrations of Na^+, urea, or glucose, then the increased Osm_m is due to increased Na^+, urea, or glucose concentrations.

B. Serum hyperosmolality and increased osmo. gap: An increased Osm_m indicates the concentration of one or more solutes is increased. Because the osmo. gap is increased, the Osm_c is not increased or not increased as much as the increase in Osm_m. In this situation, substantial increases in the osmo. gap are associated with poisonings by nonelectrolytes (e.g., ethylene glycol, methanol, or paraldehyde) or IV administration of mannitol or radiographic contrast media. The increased osmo. gap is due to a nonionic solute other than urea or glucose for the following reasons:

1. Increases in $[Na^+]$, $[K^+]$, or anions (Cl^-, HCO_3^-, or others) would result in increased Osm_m and the same increase in the Osm_c. The Osm_m increases because there are more particles in solution. The Osm_c increases because the "1.86 $([Na^+] + [K^+])$" and "2 $[Na^+]$" expressions estimate the concentration of all ions, assuming that Eq. 9.6a and b provide reliable estimates of the serum osmolality. Because the expressions do not account for biologic variation in ion concentrations (within an animal, between animals, or between species), we must remember that the expressions provide only estimates.

2. With an increase in unmeasured anions and the requirement of electroneutrality, there will be either a concomitant increase in cations or a concomitant decrease in other anions.

   a. If cations (Na^+ and/or K^+) increase to the same degree that the unmeasured anions increase, the Osm_c will be increased along with Osm_m, so the osmo. gap will not be increased.

   b. If other anions (Cl^- and/or HCO_3^-) decrease to the same degree that the unmeasured anions increase, the Osm_m and Osm_c will remain unchanged.

   c. Either way, and because of electroneutrality, the osmo. gap should not increase with an increased concentration of anionic compounds in circulation.

3. The 1.86 ($[Na^+]$ + $[K^+]$) and 2 × $[Na^+]$ expressions would underestimate the total ion concentration if there were increases in cation concentrations other than $[Na^+]$ or $[K^+]$. However, increases in $[fCa^{2+}]$ or $[fMg^{2+}]$ of 2–3 mmol/L would create pathologic states but increase the serum osmolality by no more than 4–6 mmol/kg. (The increase in cation charge concentration could be matched by an increase in anion charge concentration, or by a reduction in $[Na^+]$ and/or $[K^+]$.) A change in osmo. gap of 4–6 units would typically be considered clinically insignificant because it could represent physiologic or analytical variation.

4. Even though the osmo. gap will increase because of an increased concentration of a nonionic solute, there can be a concurrent increase in anions to create an anion gap.[1] Methanol can contribute to an osmo. gap, and its metabolite (formate) can contribute to an anion gap. Ethylene glycol can contribute to an osmo. gap, and its metabolites (glycolate or oxalate) can contribute to an anion gap. In ketoacidosis, acetone might contribute to osmo. gap, but AcAc and BHB contribute to the anion gap.

C. Serum hypoosmolality and osmo. gap WRI: A decreased Osm_m indicates that the concentration of one or more solutes is decreased. Because the osmo. gap is WRI, there is a proportionate decrease in Osm_c and Osm_m, and thus there must be decreased concentrations of Na^+, UN, or glucose. As UN and glucose contribute about 7 and 5 mmol/kg, respectively, in health, and a marked decrease in either (e.g., from 7 to 3 or 5 to 2) causes only a minor decrease in total osmolality, any clinically significant hypoosmolality will be caused by hyponatremia.

D. If there is a pseudo-hyponatremia (and pseudo-hypochloremia), the Osm_m will be an accurate value because lipids or proteins do not affect the concentration of major osmoles in plasma H_2O. However, the Osm_c will be decreased because of the spuriously low $[Na^+]$. Therefore, the osmo. gap will be artifactually increased.

References

1. Rose BD, Post TW. 2001. *Clinical Physiology of Acid-Base and Electrolyte Disorders*, 5th edition. New York: McGraw-Hill.
2. Scott MG, Heusel JW, LeGrys VA. 1999. Electrolytes and blood gases. In: Burtis CA, Ashwood ER, eds. *Tietz Textbook of Clinical Chemistry*, 3rd edition, 1056–1092. Philadelphia: WB Saunders.
3. Lundberg GD, Iverson C, Radulescu G. 1986. Now read this: The SI units are here. J Am Med Assoc 255:2329–2339.
4. Sullivan SA, Harmon BG, Purinton PT, Greene CE, Glerum LE. 2003. Lobar holoprosencephaly in a Miniature Schnauzer with hypodipsic hypernatremia. J Am Vet Med Assoc 223:1783–1787.
5. Behrend EN, Weigand CM, Whitley EM, Refsal KR, Young DW, Kemppainen RJ. 2005. Corticosterone- and aldosterone-secreting adrenocortical tumor in a dog. J Am Vet Med Assoc 226:1662–1666.
6. Jorgensen LS, Center SA, Randolph JF, Brum D. 1985. Electrolyte abnormalities induced by hypertonic phosphate enemas in two cats. J Am Vet Med Assoc 187:1367–1368.
7. Patra RC, Lal SB, Swarup D. 1993. Physicochemical alterations in blood, cerebrospinal fluid and urine in experimental lactic acidosis in sheep. Res Vet Sci 54:217–220.
8. Donaldson CW. 2003. Paintball toxicosis in dogs. Vet Med 995–997.
9. Senturk S, Huseyin C. 2004. Salt poisoning in beef cattle. Vet Hum Toxicol 46:26–27.
10. Khanna C, Boermans HJ, Wilcock B. 1997. Fatal hypernatremia in a dog from salt ingestion. J Am Anim Hosp Assoc 33:113–117.
11. Toll PW, Gaehtgens P, Neuhaus D, Pieschl RL, Fedde MR. 1995. Fluid, electrolyte, and packed cell volume shifts in racing greyhounds. Am J Vet Res 56:227–232.
12. Pieschl RL, Toll PW, Leith DE, Peterson LJ, Fedde MR. 1992. Acid-base changes in the running greyhound: Contributing variables. J Appl Physiol 73:2297–2304.

13. Rose RJ, Bloomberg MS. 1989. Responses to sprint exercise in the greyhound: Effects on haematology, serum biochemistry and muscle metabolites. Res Vet Sci 47:212–218.

14. Gentilini P, Laffi G. 1992. Pathophysiology and treatment of ascites and the hepatorenal syndrome. Baillieres Clin Gastroenterol 6:581–607.

15. Arroyo V, Ginès P. 1993. Mechanism of sodium retention and ascites formation in cirrhosis. J Hepatol 17(Suppl 2): S24–S28.

16. Watkins S, Madison J, Galliano M, Minchiotti L, Putnam FW. 1994. Analbuminemia: Three cases resulting from different point mutations in the albumin gene. Proc Natl Acad Sci USA 91:9417–9421.

17. Cormode EJ, Lyster DM, Israels S. 1975. Analbuminemia in a neonate. J Pediatr 86:862–867.

18. Orth SR, Ritz E. 1998. The nephrotic syndrome. N Engl J Med 338:1202–1211.

19. Dennison AC, VanMetre DC, Callan RJ, Dinsmore P, Mason GL, Ellis RP. 2002. Hemorrhagic bowel syndrome in dairy cattle: 22 cases (1997–2000). J Am Vet Med Assoc 221:686–689.

20. Schmale H, Fehr S, Richter D. 1987. Vasopressin biosynthesis: From gene to peptide hormone. Kidney Int 32(Suppl 21):S8–S13.

21. Roussel AJ, Cohen ND, Ruoff WW, Brumbaugh GW, Schmitz DG, Kuesis BS. 1993. Urinary indices of horses after intravenous administration of crystalloid solutions. J Vet Intern Med 7:241–246.

22. Weiss DJ, Geor R, Smith CM II, McClay CB. 1992. Furosemide-induced electrolyte depletion associated with echinocytosis in horses. Am J Vet Res 53:1769–1772.

23. Rose RJ, Arnold KS, Church S, Paris R. 1980. Plasma and sweat electrolyte concentrations in the horse during long distance exercise. Equine Vet J 12:19–22.

24. Kerr MG, Snow DH. 1983. Composition of sweat of the horse during prolonged epinephrine (adrenaline) infusion, heat exposure, and exercise. Am J Vet Res 44:1571–1577.

25. Willard MD, Fossum TW, Torrance A, Lippert A. 1991. Hyponatremia and hyperkalemia associated with idiopathic or experimentally induced chylothorax in four dogs. J Am Vet Med Assoc 199:353–358.

26. Thompson MD, Carr AP. 2002. Hyponatremia and hyperkalemia associated with chylous pleural and peritoneal effusion in a cat. Can Vet J 43:610–613.

27. Breitschwerdt EB, Root CR. 1979. Inappropriate secretion of antidiuretic hormone in a dog. J Am Vet Med Assoc 175:181–186.

28. van Vonderen IK, Kooistra HS, Timmermans-Sprang EP, Meij BP, Rijnberk A. 2004. Vasopressin response to osmotic stimulation in 18 young dogs with polyuria and polydipsia. J Vet Intern Med 18:800–806.

29. Hillier TA, Abbott RD, Barrett EJ. 1999. Hyponatremia: Evaluating the correction factor for hyperglycemia. Am J Med 106:399–403.

30. Perkins G, Valberg SJ, Madigan JM, Carlson GP, Jones SL. 1998. Electrolyte disturbances in foals with severe rhabdomyolysis. J Vet Intern Med 12:173–177.

31. Richardson DW, Kohn CW. 1983. Uroperitoneum in the foal. J Am Vet Med Assoc 182:267–271.

32. Burrows CF, Bovee KC. 1974. Metabolic changes due to experimentally induced rupture of the canine urinary bladder. Am J Vet Res 35:1083–1088.

33. Perez GO, Oster JR, Vaamonde CA. 1981. Serum potassium concentration in acidemic states. Nephron 27:233–243.

34. Johnson PJ, Goetz TE, Foreman JH, Vogel RS, Hoffmann WE, Baker GJ. 1991. Effect of whole-body potassium depletion on plasma, erythrocyte, and middle gluteal muscle potassium concentration of healthy, adult horses. Am J Vet Res 52:1676–1683.

35. Waldron-Mease E, Klein LV, Rosenberg H, Leitch M. 1981. Malignant hyperthermia in a halothane-anesthetized horse. J Am Vet Med Assoc 179:896–898.

36. Gaschen F, Gaschen L, Seiler G, Welle M, Bornand Jaunin V, Gonin Jmaa D, Neiger-Aeschbacher G, Adæ-Damilano M. 1998. Lethal peracute rhabdomyolysis associated with stress and general anesthesia in three dystrophin-deficient cats. Vet Pathol 35:117–123.

37. Spier SJ, Carlson GP, Holliday TA, Cardinet GH III, Pickar JG. 1990. Hyperkalemic periodic paralysis in horses. J Am Vet Med Assoc 197:1009–1017.

38. Jezyk PF. 1982. Hyperkalemic periodic paralysis in a dog. J Am Anim Hosp Assoc 18:977–980.

39. Wasserman K, Stringer WW, Casaburi R, Zhang YY. 1997. Mechanism of the exercise hyperkalemia: An alternate hypothesis. J Appl Physiol 83:631–643.

40. Giger U, Harvey JW. 1987. Hemolysis caused by phosphofructokinase deficiency in English springer spaniels: Seven cases (1983–1986). J Am Vet Med Assoc 191:453–459.

41. Schaafsma IA, van Emst MG, Kooistra HS, Verkleij CB, Peeters ME, Boer P, Rijnberk A, Everts ME. 2002. Exercise-induced hyperkalemia in hypothyroid dogs. Domest Anim Endocrinol 22:113–125.

42. Muylle E, van den Hende C, Nuytten J, Deprez P, Vlaminck K, Oyaert W. 1984. Potassium concentration in equine red blood cells: Normal values and correlation with potassium levels in plasma. Equine Vet J 16:447–449.

43. Degen M. 1987. Pseudohyperkalemia in Akitas. J Am Vet Med Assoc 190:541–543.

44. Reimann KA, Knowlen GG, Tvedten HW. 1989. Factitious hyperkalemia in dogs with thrombocytosis: The effect of platelets on serum potassium concentration. J Vet Intern Med 3:47–52.

45. Gunn-Moore DA, Reed N, Simpson KE, Milne EM. 2006. Effect of sample type, and timing of assay, on feline blood potassium concentration. J Feline Med Surg 8:192–196.

46. Henry CJ, Lanevschi A, Marks SL, Beyer JC, Nitschelm SH, Barnes S. 1996. Acute lymphoblastic leukemia, hypercalcemia, and pseudohyperkalemia in a dog. J Am Vet Med Assoc 208:237–239.

47. Lobetti RG. 1998. Hyperreninaemic hypoaldosteronism in a dog. J S Afr Vet Assoc 69:33–35.

48. Rubin SI, Toolan L, Halperin ML. 1998. Trimethoprim-induced exacerbation of hyperkalemia in a dog with hypoadrenocorticism. J Vet Intern Med 12:186–188.

49. Choi MJ, Fernandez PC, Patnaik A, Coupaye-Gerard B, D'Andrea D, Szerlip H, Kleyman TR. 1993. Brief report: Trimethoprim-induced hyperkalemia in a patient with AIDS. N Engl J Med 328:703–706.

50. Muto S, Tsuruoka S, Miyata Y, Fujimura A, Kusano E. 2006. Effect of trimethoprim-sulfamethoxazole on Na^+ and K^+ transport properties in the rabbit cortical collecting duct perfused in vitro. Nephron Physiol 102:51–60.

51. Dhein CR, Wardrop KJ. 1995. Hyperkalemia associated with potassium chloride administration in a cat. J Am Vet Med Assoc 206:1565–1566.

52. Bissett SA, Lamb M, Ward CR. 2001. Hyponatremia and hyperkalemia associated with peritoneal effusion in four cats. J Am Vet Med Assoc 218:1590–1592.

53. Bundgaard H, Kjeldsen K, Suarez KK, van HG, Simonsen L, Qvist J, Hansen CM, Moller K, Fonsmark L, Lav MP, Klarlund PB. 2003. Endotoxemia stimulates skeletal muscle Na^+—K^+-ATPase and raises blood lactate under aerobic conditions in humans. Am J Physiol Heart Circ Physiol 284:H1028–H1034.

54. Toribio RE, Kohn CW, Hardy J, Rosol TJ. 2005. Alterations in serum parathyroid hormone and electrolyte concentrations and urinary excretion of electrolytes in horses with induced endotoxemia. J Vet Intern Med 19:223–231.

55. Ahn A. 1994. Hyperaldosteronism in cats. Semin Vet Med Surg (Small Anim) 9:153–157.

56. Feldman EC, Nelson RW. 1996. Hyperadrenocorticism (Cushing's syndrome). In: *Canine and Feline Endocrinology and Reproduction*, 2nd edition, 187–265. Philadelphia: WB Saunders.

57. Flood SM, Randolph JF, Gelzer ARM, Refsal K. 1999. Primary hyperaldosteronism in two cats. J Am Anim Hosp Assoc 35:411–416.

58. Eger CE, Robinson WF, Huxtable CRR. 1983. Primary aldosteronism (Conn's syndrome) in a cat: A case report and review of comparative aspects. J Small Anim Pract 24:293–307.

59. Ash RA, Harvey AM, Tasker S. 2005. Primary hyperaldosteronism in the cat: A series of 13 cases. J Feline Med Surg 7:173–182.

60. Rijnberk A, Voorhout G, Kooistra HS, van der Waarden RJ, van Sluijs FJ, IJzer J, Boer P, Boer WH. 2001. Hyperaldosteronism in a cat with metastasised adrenocortical tumour. Vet Q 23:38–43.

61. Javadi S, Djajadiningrat-Laanen SC, Kooistra HS, van Dongen AM, Voorhout G, van Sluijs FJ, van den Ingh TSGAM, Boer WH, Rijnberk A. 2005. Primary hyperaldosteronism, a mediator of progressive renal disease in cats. Domest Anim Endocrinol 28:85–104.

62. Stick JA, Robinson NE, Krehbiel JD. 1981. Acid-base and electrolyte alterations associated with salivary loss in the pony. Am J Vet Res 42:733–737.

63. Buranakarl C, Mathur S, Brown SA. 2004. Effects of dietary sodium chloride intake on renal function and blood pressure in cats with normal and reduced renal function. Am J Vet Res 65:620–627.

64. Jones BR, Gruffydd-Jones TJ. 1990. Hypokalemia in the cat. Cornell Vet 80:13–16.

65. Blaxter A, Lievesley P, Gruffydd-Jones T, Wotton P. 1986. Periodic muscle weakness in Burmese kittens. Vet Rec 118:619–620.

66. Jones BR, Swinney GW, Alley MR. 1988. Hypokalaemic myopathy in Burmese kittens. N Z Vet J 36:150–151.

67. Roth L, Tyler RD. 1999. Evaluation of low sodium:potassium ratios in dogs. J Vet Diagn Invest 11:60–64.

68. Bell R, Mellor DJ, Ramsey I, Knottenbelt C. 2005. Decreased sodium:potassium ratios in cats: 49 cases. Vet Clin Pathol 34:110–114.

69. Gennari FJ, Goldstein MB, Schwartz WB. 1972. The nature of the renal adaptation to chronic hypocapnia. J Clin Invest 51:1722–1730.

70. Watts C, Campbell JR. 1971. Further studies on the effect of total nephrectomy in the bovine. Res Vet Sci 12:234–245.

71. Halperin ML, Cheema-Dhadli S, Chen CB. 2002. Effect of fasting for two days on the excretion of ammonium in dogs with chronic metabolic acidosis. Nephron 91:695–700.

72. James KM, Polzin DJ, Osborne CA, Olson JK. 1997. Effects of sample handling on total carbon dioxide concentrations in canine and feline serum and blood. Am J Vet Res 58:343–347.

73. Collins ND, LeRoy BE, Vap L. 1998. Artifactually increased serum bicarbonate values in two horses and a calf with severe rhabdomyolysis. Vet Clin Pathol 27:85–90.

74. Kasari TR, Woodbury AH, Morcom-Karsari E. 1990. Adverse effect of orally administered magnesium hydroxide on serum magnesium concentration and systemic acid-base balance in adult cattle. J Am Vet Med Assoc 196:735–742.

75. Auer DE, Skelton KV, Tay S, Baldock FC. 1993. Detection of bicarbonate administration (milkshake) in standard-bred horses. Aust Vet J 70:336–340.

76. Ewaschuk JB, Naylor JM, Palmer R, Whiting SJ, Zello GA. 2004. D-lactate production and excretion in diarrheic calves. J Vet Intern Med 18:744–747.

77. Freeman LM, Breitschwerdt EB, Keene BW, Hansen B. 1994. Fanconi's syndrome in a dog with primary hypoparathyroidism. J Vet Intern Med 8:349–354.

78. Meyer DJ. 1977. Temporary remission of hypoglycemia in a dog with an insulinoma after treatment with streptozotocin. Am J Vet Res 38:1201–1204.

79. Al-Bander HA, Weiss RA, Humphreys MH, Morris RC Jr. 1982. Dysfunction of the proximal tubule underlies maleic acid–induced type II renal tubular acidosis. Am J Physiol 243:F604–F611.

80. Bark H, Perk R. 1995. Fanconi syndrome associated with amoxicillin therapy in the dog. Canine Pract 20:19–22.

81. van der Kolk JH, Kalsbeek HC. 1993. Renal tubular acidosis in a mare. Vet Rec 133:43–44.

82. Aleman MR, Kuesis B, Schott HC, Carlson GP. 2001. Renal tubular acidosis in horses (1980–1999). J Vet Intern Med 15:136–143.

83. Hostutler RA, DiBartola SP, Eaton KA. 2004. Transient proximal renal tubular acidosis and Fanconi syndrome in a dog. J Am Vet Med Assoc 224:1611–1614.

84. Vaihkonen LK, Heinonen OJ, Hyyppa S, Nieminen M, Poso AR. 2001. Lactate-transport activity in RBCs of trained and untrained individuals from four racing species. Am J Physiol Regul Integr Comp Physiol 281: R19–R24.

85. Christopher MM, Broussard JD, Fallin CW, Drost NJ, Peterson ME. 1995. Increased serum D-lactate associated with diabetic ketoacidosis. Metabolism 44:287–290.

86. Osgood SL, Jahr JS, Desai P, Tsukamoto J, Driessen B. 2005. Does methemoglobin from oxidized hemoglobin-based oxygen carrier (Hemoglobin Glutamer-200) interfere with lactate measurement (YSI 2700 SELECT Biochemistry Analyzer)? Anesth Analg 100:437–439.

87. Jahr JS, Osgood S, Rothenberg SJ, Li QL, Butch AW, Gunther R, Cheung A, Driessen B. 2005. Lactate measurement interference by hemoglobin-based oxygen carriers (Oxyglobin, Hemopure, and Hemolink). Anesth Analg 100:431–436.

88. Dennis SC, Gevers W, Opie LH. 1991. Protons in ischemia: Where do they come from; where do they go to? J Mol Cell Cardiol 23:1077–1086.

89. Gossett KA, Cleghorn B, Adams R, Church GE, McCoy DJ, Carakostas MC, Flory W. 1987. Contribution of whole blood L-lactate, pyruvate, D-lactate, acetoacetate, and 3-hydroxyutyrate concentrations to the plasma anion gap in horses with intestinal disorders. Am J Vet Res 48:72–75.

90. Orsini JA, Elser AH, Galligan DT, Donawick WJ, Kronfeld DS. 1988. Prognostic index for acute abdominal crisis (colic) in horses. Am J Vet Res 49:1969–1971.

91. Koho NM, Vaihkonen LK, Poso AR. 2002. Lactate transport in red blood cells by monocarboxylate transporters. Equine Vet J Suppl 555–559.

92. Rand JS, Kinnaird E, Baglioni A, Blackshaw J, Priest J. 2002. Acute stress hyperglycemia in cats is associated with struggling and increased concentrations of lactate and norepinephrine. J Vet Intern Med 16:123–132.

93. Visek WJ. 1979. Ammonia metabolism, urea cycle capacity and their biochemical assessment. Nutr Rev 37:273–282.

94. Kitamura SS, Antonelli AC, Maruta CA, Soares PC, Sucupira MC, Mori CS, Mirandola RM, Ortolani EL. 2003. A model for ammonia poisoning in cattle. Vet Hum Toxicol 45:274–277.

95. Abramson CJ, Platt SR, Shelton GD. 2004. Pyruvate dehydrogenase deficiency in a Sussex spaniel. J Small Anim Pract 45:162–165.

96. Shelton GD, Van Ham L, Bhatti S, Cook-Olson S, Johnson K, Barshop B, Toone J, Applegarth D. 2006. Pyruvate dehydrogenase deficiency in Clumber Sussex spaniels in the United States and Belgium. J Vet Intern Med 14:342 (abstract).

97. Corley KT, Donaldson LL, Furr MO. 2005. Arterial lactate concentration, hospital survival, sepsis and SIRS in critically ill neonatal foals. Equine Vet J 37:53–59.

98. Chrusch C, Bautista E, Jacobs HK, Light RB, Bose D, Duke K, Mink SN. 2002. Blood pH level modulates organ metabolism of lactate in septic shock in dogs. J Crit Care 17:188–202.

99. Jacobson LS, Lobetti RG. 2005. Glucose, lactate, and pyruvate concentrations in dogs with babesiosis. Am J Vet Res 66:244–250.

100. Omole OO, Nappert G, Naylor JM, Zello GA. 2001. Both L- and D-lactate contribute to metabolic acidosis in diarrheic calves. J Nutr 131:2128–2131.

101. Ewaschuk JB, Naylor JM, Zello GA. 2003. Anion gap correlates with serum D- and DL-lactate concentration in diarrheic neonatal calves. J Vet Intern Med 17:940–942.

102. Packer RA, Cohn LA, Wohlstadter DR, Shelton GD, Naylor JM, Zello GA, Ewaschuk JB, Williams DA, Ruaux CG, O'Brien DP. 2005. D-lactic acidosis secondary to exocrine pancreatic insufficiency in a cat. J Vet Intern Med 19:106–110.

103. Gentile A, Sconza S, Lorenz I, Otranto G, Rademacher G, Famigli-Bergamini P, Klee W. 2004. D-Lactic acidosis in calves as a consequence of experimentally induced ruminal acidosis. J Vet Med [A] 51:64–70.

104. Nappert G, Johnson PJ. 2001. Determination of the acid-base status in 50 horses admitted with colic between December 1998 and May 1999. Can Vet J 42:703–707.

105. Christopher MM, Eckfeldt JH, Eaton JW. 1990. Propylene glycol ingestion causes D-lactic acidosis. Lab Invest 62:114–118.

106. Sacks DB. 1999. Carbohydrates. In: Burtis CA, Ashwood ER, eds. *Tietz Textbook of Clinical Chemistry*, 3rd edition, 750–808. Philadelphia: WB Saunders.

107. Carrier J, Stewart S, Godden S, Fetrow J, Rapnicki P. 2004. Evaluation and use of three cowside tests for detection of subclinical ketosis in early postpartum cows. J Dairy Sci 87:3725–3735.

108. Geishauser T, Leslie K, Tenhag J, Bashiri A. 2000. Evaluation of eight cow-side ketone tests in milk for detection of subclinical ketosis in dairy cows. J Dairy Sci 83:296–299.

109. Hsu WS, Kao JT, Tsai KS. 1993. Fully automated assay of blood D-3-hydroxybutyrate for ketosis. J Formos Med Assoc 92:336–340.

110. Oster JR, Rietberg B, Taylor AL, Perez GO, Chandra R, Gardner LB. 1984. Can beta-hydroxybutyrate be detected at the bedside by in vitro oxidation with hydrogen peroxide. Diabetes Care 7:80–82.

111. Chrisman CL. 1982. Coma and altered states of consciousness. In: Chrisman CL, ed. *Problems in Small Animal Neurology*, 199–214. Philadelphia: Lea & Febiger.

112. Weisberg HF, for the American Association of Clinical Pathologists Commission on Continuing Education. 1971. Osmolality. Clinical Chemistry Check sample no. CC-71:1–49.

Chapter 10

BLOOD GASES, BLOOD pH, AND STRONG ION DIFFERENCE

Definitions 561
Physiologic Processes 561
Analytical Concepts 565
Acid-Base Abnormalities 574
    I.   Metabolic (Nonrespiratory) Acidosis 574
    II. Respiratory Acidosis. 575
    III. Metabolic (Nonrespiratory) Alkalosis 576
    IV. Respiratory Alkalosis 576
    V. Classification of Acid-Base Disorders. 578
Hypoxemia and Hypoxia 581
Strong Ion Difference (SID) and Stewart's Method of Acid-Base Analysis 584

Table 10.1. Abbreviations and symbols in this chapter

[x]	Concentration of x (x = analyte)
2,3-DPG	2,3-Diphosphoglycerate
$AaDO_2$	Arterial alveolar oxygen tension gradient
A_{TOT}	Sum or total of nonvolatile weak acids
BE_B	Base excess in blood
BE_{ECF}	Base excess in extracellular fluid
BE_P	Base excess in plasma
CO	Carbon monoxide
$CO_{2(g)}$	Gaseous carbon dioxide
CO_3^{2-}	Carbonate
COHgb	Carboxyhemoglobin
ECF	Extracellular fluid
fCa^{2+}	Free ionized calcium
FIo_2	Fractional concentration of oxygen in inspired gas
fMg^{2+}	Free ionized magnesium
FO_2Hgb	Fraction of oxyhemoglobin in total hemoglobin
H_2CO_3	Carbonic acid
H_2O	Water
$H_2PO_4^-$	Dihydrogen phosphate
HCO_3^-	Bicarbonate
Hct	Hematocrit
Hgb	Hemoglobin
HHgb	Deoxyhemoglobin (reduced hemoglobin)
HPO_4^{2-}	Hydrogen phosphate
O_2ct	Oxygen content
P_aCO_2	Partial pressure of carbon dioxide in arterial blood
P_ACO_2	Partial pressure of alveolar carbon dioxide
P_aO_2	Partial pressure of oxygen in arterial blood
P_AO_2	Partial pressure of alveolar oxygen
PCO_2	Partial pressure of carbon dioxide
pH	$-\log [H^+]$
PIo_2	Partial pressure of inspired oxygen
Po_2	Partial pressure of oxygen
PO_4	Phosphate including PO_4^{3-}, HPO_4^{2-}, or $H_2PO_4^-$
PO_4^{3-}	Phosphate
P_vCO_2	Partial pressure of carbon dioxide in venous blood
P_vO_2	Partial pressure of oxygen in venous blood
S_aO_2	Percent hemoglobin saturation with oxygen in arterial blood
SID	Strong ion difference
$SID_{Cl^-corrected}$	Strong ion difference using corrected chloride concentration
SID_{true}	True strong ion difference
SID_x	Strong ion difference calculated using x strong ions
So_2	Percent hemoglobin saturation with oxygen
Spo_2	Percent hemoglobin saturation with oxygen of arterial blood by pulse oximetry ("p" is for "pulse" oximetry)
tCO_2	Total carbon dioxide
uSA	Unidentified strong anion
WRI	Within reference interval

DEFINITIONS

Definitions of important terms in this chapter:

Acidemia is a decreased blood pH (increased [H$^+$]).
Alkalemia is an increased blood pH (decreased [H$^+$]).
Acidosis is a condition in which acidemia tends to occur. An animal may not be acidemic because of compensating mechanisms or because of the width of the reference interval.
Alkalosis is a condition in which alkalemia tends to occur. An animal may not be alkalemic because of compensating mechanisms or because of the width of the reference interval.
Hypercapnia is excess CO_2 in blood (increased P_{CO_2}). It is also called *hypercarbia*.
Hypocapnia is a deficiency of CO_2 in blood (decreased P_{CO_2}). It is also called *hypocarbia*.
Hypoxemia is a deficiency of dissolved O_2 in blood (decreased P_{O_2}).
Hypoxia is a deficiency of O_2 reaching the tissues, cells, or organelles of the body.
Hyperventilation is an excessive rate and/or depth of respiration leading to abnormal loss of CO_2 from the blood because of increased movement of new air to (and from) the gas-exchange regions of the lung. Because hypocapnia can be the consequence of hyperventilation, sometimes hypocapnia and hyperventilation are considered synonyms.
Hypoventilation is deficient ventilation of the lungs that causes reduction in the O_2 content of the blood, increase in the CO_2 content of the blood, or both, because of decreased movement of new air to (and from) the gas-exchange regions of the lung. Because hypercapnia can be the consequence of hypoventilation, sometimes hypercapnia and hypoventilation are considered synonyms.
Tachypnea is an increased rate of respiration. The increased rate may or may not cause hyperventilation.
Bradypnea is a decreased rate of respiration. The decreased rate may or may not cause hypoventilation.

PHYSIOLOGIC PROCESSES

I.   Several respiratory and nonrespiratory processes help maintain [H$^+$] at a minute, but stable, concentration (about 40 nmol/L). Metabolic processes continually produce H$^+$, and it is either excreted (via kidneys) or bound to buffers (HCO_3^-, PO_4, ammonia, sulfates, Hgb, and other proteins, such as albumin). Of the total buffering capacity in health, HCO_3^- contributes over 20 mmol/L, whereas the nonbicarbonate buffers contribute less than 10 mmol/L.[1]

II.   As the buffers work together, changes in one buffering system reflect changes in the others. In clinical medicine, the bicarbonate buffering system is used to monitor control of [H$^+$] and therefore acid-base status.

    A. The relationship of [H$^+$], [HCO_3^-], and P_{CO_2} in normal blood at 37 °C can be expressed with the Henderson-Hasselbalch equation or a nonlogarithmic version (Eq. 10.1a). The [H_2CO_3] is calculated from a measured P_{CO_2} value and the solubility coefficient of CO_2 in an aqueous solution (Eq. 10.1b).

$$pH = 6.1 + \log\frac{[HCO_3^-]}{[H_2CO_3]} \quad or \quad [H^+] = 24 \times \frac{P_{CO_2}}{[HCO_3^-]} \qquad \textbf{(10.1a.)}$$

$$P_{CO_2} \times 0.0307 = [H_2CO_3] \qquad \textbf{(10.1b.)}$$

[H$^+$] in nmol/L; [HCO_3^-] & [HCO_3] in mmol/L; P_{CO_2} in mmHg

B. As seen in the nonlogarithmic equation, $[H^+]$ is clearly related to the ratio of P_{CO_2} to $[HCO_3^-]$. When the ratio increases in an animal, the animal becomes acidemic. When the ratio decreases in an animal, the animal becomes alkalemic.

III. Pulmonary functions related to blood gases and acid-base status
    A. Expiration of CO_2 leads to the elimination of free H^+ (Fig. 10.1A).

A. Healthy animal

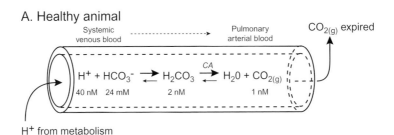

B. Metabolic acidosis

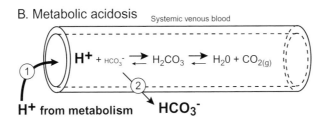

C. Respiratory acidosis

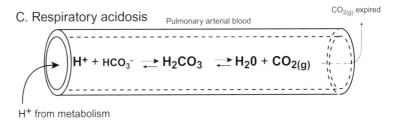

D. Metabolic alkalosis

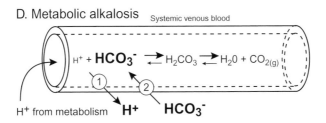

E. Respiratory alkalosis

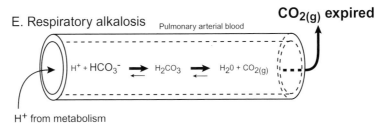

1. Because blood $[H^+]$ is very low compared to $[HCO_3^-]$ (ratio $\approx 1:600,000$), this process does not lower $[HCO_3^-]$ unless there is excessive generation of H^+.
2. It may be helpful to consider the bicarbonate system going through H_2CO_3 (Eq. 10.2a), but the actual reaction catalyzed by carbonic anhydrase involves the dissociation of H_2O, release of H^+, and reaction of hydroxide ion (OH^-) with CO_2 to form HCO_3^- without a H_2CO_3 intermediate (Eq. 10.2b). The reaction is reversible.

$$H^+ + HCO_3^- \leftrightarrow H_2CO_3 \leftrightarrow H_2O + CO_{2(g)} \qquad \textbf{(10.2a.)}$$

$$H^+ + HCO_3^- \xleftrightarrow{\textit{carbonic anhydrase}} H_2O + CO_{2(g)} \qquad \textbf{(10.2b.)}$$

B. Hyperventilation increases expiration of CO_2 and tends to cause alkalemia. Hypoventilation decreases expiration of CO_2 and tends to cause acidemia. Two types of chemoreceptors control respiration:
   1. Central chemoreceptors (in the brain stem) are stimulated by increased $[H^+]$ in surrounding fluid.
   2. Peripheral chemoreceptors (carotid and aortic bodies) are stimulated primarily by hypoxemia but also by acidemia (increased $[H^+]$).
C. Oxygenation of blood and pulmonary ventilation
   1. The basic physiologic aspects of the interchange of O_2 and CO_2 are described in Fig. 10.2.

Fig. 10.1. Schematic representation of the basic concepts of the bicarbonate buffering system in health and in acid-base disorders. Respiratory disorders involve removal of CO_2 from pulmonary arterial (capillary) blood. Metabolic disorders cause abnormal concentrations of H^+ and HCO_3^- in systemic venous blood.
A. In health, H^+ from metabolism is buffered by HCO_3^- to form H_2CO_3, which dissociates to H_2O and $CO_{2(g)}$. The $CO_{2(g)}$ is expired via the respiratory system. In the presence of carbonic anhydrase (*CA*), the reactions are reversible but the net flow is to the right (toward $CO_{2(g)}$ expiration). The approximate molar concentrations of H^+, HCO_3^-, H_2CO_3, and dissolved $CO_{2(g)}$ in plasma show that a large excess of HCO_3^- is available to buffer H^+.
B. In a metabolic acidosis, acidosis occurs because of one of two basic processes. Without compensation, P_{CO_2} remains WRI. However, $\uparrow [H^+]$ will stimulate respiration and result in increased removal of CO_2 from pulmonary blood and thus a $\downarrow P_{CO_2}$.
   1. Excess H^+ accumulates because of increased production of organic acids, increased H^+ release from ATP usage, or decreased renal excretion of H^+. The excess H^+ drives the equation to the right and thus leads to consumption of HCO_3^-.
   2. Excess loss of HCO_3^- via the alimentary or urinary system reduces the buffering capacity and allows H^+ to accumulate.
C. In a respiratory acidosis, hypoventilation causes reduced expiration of $CO_{2(g)}$, which leads to an $\uparrow P_aCO_2$ and an $\uparrow [H^+]$ ($\downarrow$ pH). Without compensation, $[HCO_3^-]$ is insignificantly increased and remains WRI. Given time, the kidneys will compensate for acidemia and conserve HCO_3^-.
D. In a metabolic alkalosis, alkalosis occurs because of one of two basic processes. Without compensation, P_{CO_2} remains WRI.
   1. Excess H^+ is lost via gastric or renal secretion. The secretion of H^+ results in a generation of HCO_3^- that accumulates in plasma.
   2. Excess HCO_3^- is formed, conserved, or administered and results in more removal of H^+ from blood and thus an alkalemia.
E. In a respiratory alkalosis, hyperventilation causes excessive expiration of $CO_{2(g)}$, which leads to a $\downarrow P_aCO_2$ and a $\downarrow [H^+]$ ($\uparrow$ pH). Without compensation, $[HCO_3^-]$ remains WRI.

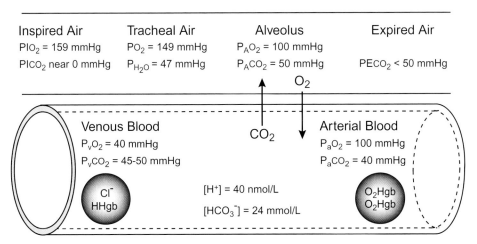

Fig. 10.2. Schematic drawing of the exchange of O_2 and CO_2 at the alveolus-capillary junction. Pressure values are included in the figure to illustrate the magnitude of changes that occur. Actual pressures will vary because of several factors (e.g., total atmospheric pressure is 760 mmHg at sea level but near 735 mmHg at 1000 ft elevation).

- Atmosphere to alveolus: Inspired air has a P_{O_2} (PI_{O_2}) of 159 mmHg. With the contribution of P_{H_2O} (47 mmHg) in the warm trachea, the P_{O_2} drops to 149 mmHg [0.209(760 − 47)]. In the alveolus, the P_{AO_2} is lower, near 100 mmHg, because of the interchange of O_2 with the blood and because of the increased P_ACO_2 (50 mmHg) from the blood.
- Alveolus to blood: In health, O_2 quickly diffuses from the alveolus to the capillary blood (P_{O_2} near 40 mmHg) to give a P_{O_2} of 100 mmHg, which represents the pressure exerted by the dissolved O_2 in plasma. The O_2 also diffuses into erythrocytes and binds to Hgb (O_2Hgb) to saturate the oxygen-binding sites of ferrous heme (S_{O_2} = 100 %). With a normal [Hgb], 1 L of blood contains about 200 mL O_2 bound to Hgb (i.e., 1.31 mL O_2/g Hgb) and 3 mL of dissolved O_2.
- Blood to alveolus: Reversal of the carbonic anhydrase reaction produces CO_2 (not shown) which quickly diffuses from blood to alveolus and thus lowers the P_vCO_2 to P_aCO_2 near 40 mmHg. The [H^+] decreases slightly because it combines with HCO_3^- to form CO_2 and H_2O. In the healthy lung, CO_2 diffuses from blood to alveoli at 20 times the rate that O_2 diffuses from alveoli to blood.
- Alveolus to atmosphere: When breathing air, the PE_{CO_2} will be less than the P_ACO_2 because the PE_{CO_2} represents a mixture of alveolar gases and the gases in the airways. During anesthesia, measuring the expired P_{CO_2} (capnography) provides information to assess CO_2 production, pulmonary gas exchange, and elimination of CO_2 by the anesthetic equipment.

PE_{CO_2}, partial pressure of expired carbon dioxide; P_{H_2O}, partial pressure of water vapor.

2. For there to be adequate oxygenation of blood, several processes must be functional.
   a. The inspired air must have adequate O_2.
   b. The inspired air must be delivered to alveoli.
   c. The inspired O_2 must diffuse from alveoli to the capillary blood quickly.
   d. The alveoli must be perfused with blood.
3. For there to be adequate gas exchange, alveoli must be perfused with blood, CO_2 must diffuse from blood to alveoli quickly, and CO_2 must be expired. Because the solubility of CO_2 in H_2O is greater than that of O_2, the diffusion coefficient of CO_2 is greater, and it can diffuse from blood to alveoli much faster than O_2 can diffuse

from alveoli to blood; the diffusion coefficient for CO_2 is 20 times the diffusion coefficient for O_2.
D. Transport of O_2 to tissues
   1. Once O_2 has diffused into pulmonary blood, most of it enters erythrocytes and binds to Hgb. The processes involved in the oxygenation and deoxygenation of Hgb are illustrated in Fig. 10.3.
   2. For there to be adequate oxygenation of tissues, several processes must be functional.
      a. The lungs must oxygenate the blood.
      b. The blood must have sufficient amounts of functional Hgb.
      c. The blood must perfuse the tissues.

IV. Renal functions related to acid-base balance
   A. The kidneys have key roles in maintaining acid-base status (see Chapters 8 and 9).
   B. Their major functions that pertain to acid-base status in health are to excrete H^+, either directly or by incorporation into ammonium (NH_4^+), dihydrogen phosphate ($H_2PO_4^-$), or bisulfate (HSO_4^-), and to conserve HCO_3^-.
   C. Hormonal and other factors that alter Na^+, Cl^-, and K^+ excretion will typically influence renal excretion of H^+ and HCO_3^-.

ANALYTICAL CONCEPTS

I. Blood gas instruments
   A. Blood gas instruments measure the $[H^+]$, Po_2, and Pco_2 in blood.
      1. Descriptions of measured analytes
         a. *$[H^+]$* is the free H^+ concentration in blood. It reflects the net effect of bodily processes on blood $[H^+]$ and is reported as pH, the unitless negative log of $[H^+]$.
         b. *Po_2* (mmHg) is the partial pressure of O_2 in the blood. It reflects the amount of dissolved O_2 but does not measure O_2 associated with Hgb. It is useful in assessing pulmonary gas exchange.
         c. *Pco_2* (mmHg) is the partial pressure of CO_2 in blood. It reflects the amount of dissolved CO_2 in blood and is useful to assess alveolar ventilation.
      2. Blood gas analyzers used in veterinary patients were designed to be used for human samples. Therefore, measurements are made at 37 °C rather than at the temperatures of typical veterinary patients, and values are not accurate reflections of the in vivo values (see the following sect. C, Temperature Correction Factors).
      3. Selective membranes allow only H^+, O_2, or CO_2 to pass from the blood to cause reactions with specific electrodes. In the Pco_2 system, the CO_2 reacts in a bicarbonate buffer to change the pH; the change in pH is detected by a pH (H^+-selective) electrode.
      4. The membranes also protect the electrodes from proteins and other substances in the blood. Maintenance of blood gas instruments involves maintenance (cleaning and replacement) of the membranes.
      5. Some blood gas instruments can measure So_2 by reflectance photometry based on the differences in the absorption of different wavelengths of light by oxyhemoglobin and deoxyhemoglobin.
      6. Point-of-care testing: Small hand-held or portable chemical analyzers that use a disposable cartridge containing ion-selective electrodes can do the following: (1) measure blood gas values (pH, Pco_2, and Po_2), (2) measure common blood analyte

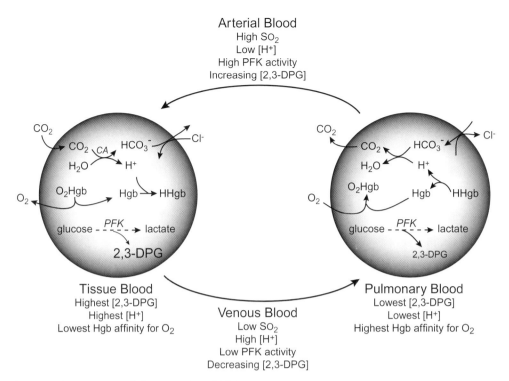

Fig. 10.3. Oxygenation and deoxygenation of Hgb.

Erythrocytes in peripheral tissue blood

- Because erythrocytes have their greatest [2,3-DPG] and greatest [H$^+$] while moving through peripheral capillaries, their Hgb molecules have the lowest affinity for O$_2$ and thus release O$_2$ to plasma. The O$_2$ is then able to diffuse into tissue and participate in metabolic pathways.
- CO$_2$ (from metabolic pathways) diffuses into plasma and then into erythrocytes. Via the carbonic anhydrase (*CA*) reaction, CO$_2$ and H$_2$O are converted to HCO$_3$$^-$ and H$^+$. The HCO$_3$$^-$ moves to plasma in exchange for Cl$^-$. Most of the H$^+$ is buffered by the deoxygenated Hgb. The CO$_2$ produced in tissues is carried in blood in two forms: (1) as dissolved CO$_2$ with a P$_v$co$_2$ near 45–50 mmHg, and (2) as HCO$_3$$^-$ in erythrocytes after reacting with H$_2$O in the presence of carbonic anhydrase.
- Erythrocytes enter in peripheral tissues with high [2,3-DPG], but the more acidic environment (increased [H$^+$]) inhibits phosphofructokinase (*PFK*) in the glycolytic pathway, and thus the rate of 2,3-DPG formation decreases.

Erythrocytes in pulmonary blood

- O$_2$ diffuses from alveoli to pulmonary plasma and into erythrocytes. Because erythrocytes have their least [2,3-DPG] and least [H$^+$] in the pulmonary vessels, their Hgb molecules have the greatest affinity for O$_2$ and thus become saturated with O$_2$ (So$_2$ = 100 %) to form O$_2$Hgb. With a normal [Hgb], 1 L of blood contains about 200 mL O$_2$ bound to Hgb (i.e., 1.31 mL O$_2$/g Hgb) and 3 mL of dissolved O$_2$.
- HCO$_3$$^-$ moves into erythrocytes (in exchange for Cl$^-$) and combines with H$^+$ to form CO$_2$ and H$_2$O. The CO$_2$ diffuses into plasma and then to alveoli from which it is exhaled.
- Most of the H$^+$ is buffered by the HCO$_3$$^-$.
- Erythrocytes enter pulmonary blood with low [2,3-DPG], but the more alkaline environment (lowest [H$^+$]) stimulates PFK in the glycolytic pathway, and thus the rate of 2,3-DPG formation increases.

concentrations (Na^+, K^+, Cl^-, urea, glucose, fCa^{2+}, and Hgb), and (3) calculate several concentrations or values (HCO_3^-, tCO_2, anion gap, So_2, BE_{ecf}, BE_B, and hematocrit).

B. Calculated acid-base and blood gas values: The following values can be calculated from the measured pH, Pco_2, and Po_2 by using other known factors (e.g., body temperature or [Hgb]):

1. *[HCO$_3^-$]$_{actual}$* (in mmol/L) is calculated via the Henderson-Hasselbalch equation by using the measured pH and measured Pco_2 (Eq. 10.1a).

2. *[tCO$_2$]* (in mmol/L) is calculated from the calculated [HCO_3^-]$_{actual}$ and measured Pco_2 (Eq. 10.3). The Pco_2 is multiplied by 0.0307 (a solubility coefficient) to calculate the amount of dissolved CO_2 in the blood sample. The [tCO_2] generated by routine serum chemistry analysis is based on different methods.

$$[tCO_2] = [HCO_3^-] + [H_2CO_3] = [HCO_3^-] + (Pco_2 \times 0.0307) \qquad \textbf{(10.3.)}$$

3. *[HCO$_3^-$]$_{standard}$* (in mmol/L) is also called standard bicarbonate concentration (SBC).

   a. *[HCO$_3^-$]$_{standard}$* is the [HCO_3^-] in plasma when fully oxygenated blood from a "normal" animal is equilibrated at 37 °C to a P_aco_2 of 40 mmHg. The calculated [HCO_3^-]$_{standard}$ is an estimate of the [HCO_3^-] in the sample if the Pco_2 were 40 mmHg.

   b. The [HCO_3^-]$_{standard}$ is theoretically a better estimate of buffer base in a blood sample because it is independent of changes in Pco_2, whereas a [HCO_3^-]$_{actual}$ depends on Pco_2 values (e.g., when Pco_2 increases, [HCO_3^-] increases in plasma).[2]

   c. The calculation for [HCO_3^-]$_{standard}$ requires the use of several assumed values that may not be accurate for particular species or individuals.

4. BE_{ecf} or BE_P (in mmol/L)[1]

   a. *BE$_{ecf}$* or *BE$_P$* is the amount of strong acid (mmol/L) that is needed to titrate extracellular fluid or plasma to a pH of 7.4 if the Pco_2 is 40 mmHg at 37 °C.

   b. The calculation uses the measured pH, calculated [HCO_3^-], an assumed normal [HCO_3^-] (e.g., 24–25 mmol/L), and an assumed normal plasma protein concentration.

   c. Changes in BE_{ecf}

      (1) A positive BE_{ecf} indicates an excess of plasma buffer (e.g., HCO_3^-, proteins) and thus a metabolic alkalosis.

      (2) A negative BE_{ecf} indicates a deficit of plasma buffer (e.g., HCO_3^-, proteins) and thus a metabolic acidosis.

      (3) If blood pH changes because of a change in Pco_2 but the [HCO_3^-] is WRI, then the BE_{ecf} will remain WRI.

5. BE_B (in mmol/L)

   a. The *BE$_B$* value is the amount of strong acid (mmol/L) that is needed to titrate blood to a pH of 7.4 if the Pco_2 is 40 mmHg at 37 °C.

   b. The calculation involves the same values as BE_{ecf} plus the contribution of Hgb to the buffer base. Erythrocyte 2,3-DPG contributes to the buffer base but is not specifically included in the calculation. The Hgb value may be inaccurate because of the mean cell hemoglobin concentration (MCHC) assumptions when calculated from measured hematocrit values or because of inaccuracies of the blood gas analyzer's hematocrit measurement (see Chapter 3).

c. Positive and negative BE_B values provide essentially the same information about the patient as does the BE_{ecf}. The BE_B values should approach the BE_{ecf} as an animal becomes more anemic.

6. Buffer base (or total buffer base) (in mmol/L)

a. *Buffer base* is the sum of "buffer ions" of blood, including HCO_3^-, Hgb, and plasma proteins.

b. Buffer base is related to base excess as follows: buffer base$_{actual}$ = buffer base$_{normal}$ + base excess. Buffer base$_{actual}$ is the calculated sum of the "buffer ions" in a patient's sample. Buffer base$_{normal}$ is the expected sum of the "buffer ions" in a healthy human. Base excess (if positive) is the amount of excess "buffer ions" compared to normal.

7. So_2 (in %)

a. *So_2* is the amount of oxyhemoglobin in blood expressed as a percentage of the total amount of hemoglobin able to bind O_2. (See sects. II [Pulse oximetry] and III [CO-oximeter] for methods of measuring the percentage.)

b. The So_2 depends primarily on the Po_2 as described by the sigmoid O_2-Hgb dissociation curve (Fig. 10.4). At a Po_2 of 100 mmHg, the So_2 is expected to be about 97 %. Acidemia, increased erythrocyte [2,3-DPG], hyperthermia, and hypercarbia shift the dissociation curve to the right (So_2 decreases for a given Po_2).

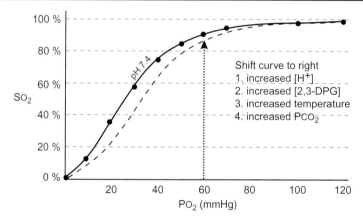

Fig. 10.4. Oxygen-hemoglobin dissociation curve. With a typical P_aO_2 of 95 mmHg and at a pH of 7.4, the So_2 is near 96 %. Because of the high affinity of Hgb for O_2, So_2 values remain at > 90 % as long as the Po_2 remains at > 60 mmHg (dashed arrow). When Po_2 values are > 100 mmHg, the So_2 will be near 100 %. Increased [H+], increased erythrocyte [2,3-DPG], hyperthermia, and hypercarbia will shift the curve to the right. If Po_2 stays constant, shifting the curve to the right will result in a lower So_2. The displayed dissociation curve was constructed from human data. Dissociation curves for other species are slightly different because of differences in Hgb molecules, [2,3-DPG] differences, and other factors. Accordingly, the average P_{50} values (P_aO_2 when hemoglobin is 50 % saturated with oxygen at pH 7.4, 37 °C, and 40 mmHg P_aCO_2) differ: horses ≈ 25 mmHg, cattle ≈ 26 mmHg, people ≈ 27 mmHg, dogs ≈ 30 mmHg, and cats ≈ 34 mmHg.[43,44]

    c. Some blood gas instruments calculate the So_2 from measured pH, P_aco_2, and P_ao_2 values by using formulas that attempt to correct for temperature variations and a complex formula that attempts to describe the O_2 dissociation curve.[3] The calculated So_2 may be erroneous because of assumed normal O_2 affinity for Hgb and assumed normal [2,3-DPG].[4]

      (1) If the pH is constant, but the Po_2 decreases, then So_2 decreases.

      (2) If the Po_2 is constant, but the pH decreases (acidemia), then So_2 decreases. If Po_2 is constant, but pH increases (alkalemia), then So_2 increases.

8. P_ao_2 (in mmHg): alveolar O_2 pressure (sometimes abbreviated as A)

    a. $P_{A}o_2$ is the partial pressure of O_2 in the alveolar air (gas). Two formulas incorporating FIo_2 and P_aco_2 can be used to calculate the value (Eq. 10.4a).[3] FIo_2 is the fractional percentage of inspired O_2 in a gas. The FIo_2 of air is 0.2093 (or about 21 %), and the PIo_2 of air is about 159 mmHg (21 % of 760 mmHg). During gas anesthesia, the FIo_2 could be 1.0 (100 % O_2).

Simplified: $P_A O_2 = PIo_2 - \dfrac{P_a CO_2}{R}$ **(10.4a.)**

Complete: $P_A O_2 = PIo_2 - \dfrac{P_a CO_2}{R}(1 - FIo_2(1 - R))$

where P_Ao_2 is partial pressure of alveolar oxygen, PIo_2 is the partial pressure of inspired oxygen, P_aco_2 is the partial pressure of CO_2 in arterial blood, R is the average metabolic respiratory quotient, and FIo_2 is the fractional concentration of oxygen in inspired air (gas).

Arterial alveolar oxygen tension gradient: $AaDo_2 = P_Ao_2 - P_ao_2$ **(10.4b.)**

Arterial alveolar oxygen tension ratio: $a/A = \dfrac{P_a O_2}{P_A O_2}$ **(10.4c.)**

Inspired oxygen fraction ratio: $P_a o_2/FI = \dfrac{P_a O_2}{FIo_2}$ **(10.4d.)**

    b. The respiratory quotient (R) is the ratio of the volume of CO_2 produced to the volume of O_2 consumed by a body. In other words, R is the ratio of the amount of CO_2 diffusing from blood into alveoli to the amount of O_2 diffusing in the opposite direction. The respiratory quotient varies with the type of fuels the body is using (e.g., fats versus carbohydrates). Generally, the average ratio is 0.8; that is, 0.8 L of CO_2 is formed when 1 L of O_2 is consumed by metabolic pathways. However, the value for R can vary considerably.

    c. The concentration of alveolar O_2 for a given concentration of O_2 in inspired air is determined by a balance between alveolar ventilation and amount of O_2 diffusing into capillary blood.

    d. The P_Ao_2 calculation assumes that $P_aco_2 = P_Aco_2$, an assumption that may not be true if there is a mismatch in ventilation-perfusion.

9. *AaDO_2* (in mmHg) is the arterial alveolar O_2 tension gradient (Eq. 10.4b). The value is used as an index of the exchange of O_2 in lungs.

10. *a/A* (unitless) is the arterial alveolar O_2 tension ratio (Eq. 10.4c). The value is used as an index of the exchange of O_2 in lungs and remains relatively stable with changes in FIo_2.

11. *P_aO_2/FI* (unitless) is the inspired O_2 fraction ratio (Eq. 10.4d). The value is used as an index of the delivery of O_2 to alveoli and exchange of O_2 in lungs.

12. *O_2ct* (mL/dL) is the O_2 content. The O_2ct represents the total amount (volume) of O_2 in a given blood volume (100 mL), including that dissolved in plasma and that bound to hemoglobin.

13. P_{50} or Po_2 (0.5) (in mmHg): The P_{50} is defined as the P_aO_2 of a sample when hemoglobin is 50 % saturated with O_2 at pH 7.4, 37 °C, and 40 mmHg P_aco_2.

C. Temperature correction factors for blood pH and gas values with variations in body temperature

1. Partial pressures of dissolved gases vary with the temperature of the solvent. For example, if O_2 and CO_2 content remain constant in a sample but temperature increases, the Po_2 and Pco_2 values increase (hot gas expands and thus exerts more pressure).

2. Blood gas instruments measure pH, Po_2, and Pco_2 in a 37 °C chamber. If the patient's temperature is 40 °C, then the in vivo values will be different from those determined by the instrument. Correction factors for increasing temperatures are in Table 10.2. For example, if the Pco_2 were 40 mmHg at 37 °C, then the Pco_2 would be 44 mmHg (40 + 10 % of 40 mmHg) at 39 °C and 48 mmHg (40 + 20 % of 40 mmHg) at 41 °C.

3. There are differences of opinion and unanswered questions regarding the need for temperature correction of blood gas.

   a. For example, lowering blood's temperature (as in hypothermia) will lower the Po_2, but the O_2 content of blood will not change. In the hypothermic state, is the lower P_aO_2 value desired for the lower metabolic rate or should the P_aO_2 be increased by increasing the FIo_2?

   b. If temperature-corrected values are used to monitor a patient, and if the patient's body temperature changes, will changes in pH, Po_2, or Pco_2 be caused by changes in body temperature or other factors?

4. If a laboratory reports temperature-corrected values, it should also report the values measured at 37 °C. If all in vitro values are reported at 37 °C regardless of the body temperature, then changes in Po_2 and Pco_2 values will reflect changes in O_2 and CO_2 content of blood.

Table 10.2. Correction of blood gas and pH values for variations in body temperature

°C	°F	pH	Pco_2	Po_2
41	105.8	− 0.06	+ 20 %	+ 33 %
40	104.0	− 0.04	+ 15 %	+ 24 %
39	102.2	− 0.03	+ 10 %	+ 15 %
38	100.4	− 0.01	+ 5 %	+ 7 %
37	98.6	None	None	None

Note: Correction factors calculated from established formulas[42]

II. Pulse oximetry
   A. An *oximeter* is a device that measures arterial So_2, denoted here as Spo_2. During the 1980s, the pulse oximeter became an accepted instrument in human medicine for monitoring Hgb oxygenation during anesthesia and is common in the monitoring of critical care patients.
   B. The pulse oximeter determines the Spo_2 by a spectrophotometric method.[5]
      1. Light at two wavelengths (e.g., 660 and 940 nm) is passed through tissue that contains arterial blood (e.g., the ear lobe or finger in people; the tongue, lip, ear, toe, or tail in dogs; and the tongue in horses).[6,7] In dogs, the best agreement of Spo_2 with S_aO_2 occurred with the lip and tongue placements.[8]
      2. At the higher wavelength (e.g., 940 nm), oxyhemoglobin absorbs more light than does deoxyhemoglobin (reduced Hgb). At the lower wavelength (e.g., 660 nm), oxyhemoglobin absorbs less light than does deoxyhemoglobin. From the measured absorbance values, a ratio can be calculated that reflects the S_aO_2 (Eq. 10.5a).

$$S_aO_2 = \frac{[O_2Hgb]}{[O_2Hgb]+[HHgb]} \times 100 \qquad \textbf{(10.5a.)}$$

$$O_2Hgb\% = \frac{[O_2Hgb]}{[O_2Hgb]+[HHgb]+[COHgb]+[MetHgb]} \times 100 \qquad \textbf{(10.5b.)}$$

   O_2Hgb (oxyhemoglobin), HHgb (reduced hemoglobin), COHgb (carboxyhemoglobin), MetHgb (methemoglobin)

      3. The interference caused by other light-absorbing substances in the tissues is removed by measuring the light while arterial blood pulses through the tissue. In pulse oximetry, it is assumed that the changes in absorbance values occur when O_2-rich blood pulsates through the tissue. The pulse quality can be evaluated graphically.
      4. COHgb and methemoglobin also absorb light at the measurement wavelengths and thus interfere with measurements of $[O_2Hgb]$ if they are present (see Hypoxemia and Hypoxia, sect. II.D) and give falsely increased S_aO_2 and $O_2Hgb\%$ values (Eq. 10.5b)

III. CO-oximeter values
   A. A CO-oximeter determines the different types of Hgb by measuring the absorbance of several wavelengths of light. Each type of Hgb has a unique absorbance spectrum, and the concentration of each type is determined. The CO-oximeter can be used to identify methemoglobinemia or CO poisoning.
   B. Calculated values (Eq. 10.6)

$$[tHgb] = [O_2Hgb] + [HHgb] + [COHgb] + [MetHgb] \qquad \textbf{(10.6.)}$$

$$O_2Hgb\% = \frac{[O_2Hgb]}{[tHgb]} \times 100$$

$$HHgb\% = \frac{[HHgb]}{[tHgb]} \times 100$$

$$COHgb\% = \frac{[COHgb]}{[tHgb]} \times 100$$

$$MetHgb\% = \frac{[MetHgb]}{[tHgb]} \times 100$$

$$SO_2 = \frac{[O_2Hgb]}{[O_2Hgb] + [HHgb]} \times 100$$

$$FO_2Hgb = \frac{[O_2Hgb]}{[tHgb]}$$

$$O_2ct = \frac{1.31\,mL\,O_2}{g\,Hgb} \times [tHgb]\left(\frac{SO_2}{100}\right)$$

O_2Hgb (oxyhemoglobin), HHgb (reduced hemoglobin), COHgb (carboxyhemoglobin), MetHgb (methemoglobin), FO_2Hgb (fraction of oxyhemoglobin in total hemoglobin), O_2ct (oxygen content)

1. Total Hgb (tHgb) concentration represents the sum of the hemoglobin types as determined by absorbance photometry.
2. The percentages of each type of Hgb are calculated from the concentrations determined by absorbance photometry.
3. O_2ct is also calculated from the oximeter's measured values.

C. Blood substitutes may interfere with CO-oximetry values.
1. The NOVA CO-Oximeter provided accurate values for O_2 saturation with various concentrations of hemoglobin-based O_2 carriers, but the i-STAT provided accurate values with only low concentrations of the carriers.[9]
2. Compared to results obtained from an O_2-selective electrode assay, the O_2 content measured by an Instrumentation Laboratories CO-oximeter differed more than 20 % 1 h after infusion with a hemoglobin-based O_2 carrier. The differences were greater with the larger dosage of the blood substitute.[10]

IV. Sample for blood gas and pH analysis
A. Heparinized whole blood: 0.05–0.1 mL of heparin (1,000 units/mL) per mL of blood, or 50–100 units/mL of blood
1. Arterial blood is the preferred sample for all blood gas and pH analyses and is required for the assessment of oxygenation of blood or pulmonary function.
2. Venous blood may give adequate results for assessment of metabolic disorders but will have lower pH, higher P_{CO_2}, and lower P_{O_2} values. The P_{O_2} of venous blood is not an accurate reflection of pulmonary function. The source of the venous blood may affect the P_{CO_2} value. Venous blood from a hypoxic leg will have a different P_{CO_2} value than venous blood from a well-perfused head.
3. Mixed venous blood contains blood from all venous sources and is collected from either the right ventricle or pulmonary artery. The P_{O_2} in the mixed venous sample reflects the O_2 remaining in blood after the blood returns from all tissues and before it is oxygenated in the pulmonary capillaries.

4. Blood may be collected in either glass or quality plastic syringes, though Po_2 may decrease more quickly in glass syringes. To prevent exposure to air, the needle must be sealed with cork or rubber immediately after collection. Air should not be in the syringe during or after the collection of a sample.

5. Optimally, a heparinized blood sample should be tested (point-of-care testing) or transported to the laboratory immediately after collection. If not possible, acceptable blood gas and pH results can be obtained if the heparinized blood is immersed in an ice bath and analyzed within 1 h. Placement of the sample in a refrigerator will not cool the sample as quickly; do not place a sample in a freezer, because erythrocytes will lyse.

6. Excessive heparin in the collecting syringe can result in erroneous values; there should only be enough heparin to coat the needle and a 3 mL syringe. This can be accomplished by drawing 0.5 mL heparin into a 3 mL syringe to the 3 mL mark and then forcefully expelling it by using 3 mL air in the syringe. Leaving heparin in the hub of the syringe creates minimal alterations in blood gas values but may cause significantly decreased $[fCa^{2+}]$ and significantly increased $[Cl^-]$. Larger amounts also cause lower Pco_2, $[HCO_3^-]$, $[K^+]$, and lactate concentrations and higher Po_2 (if breathing air) and $[Na^+]$.[11]

B. Erroneous blood gas and pH values because of poor sample collection or handling

1. Exposure to air (including air bubbles) or excess heparin in the sample[12]

a. The Po_2 and Pco_2 values for arterial blood and room air are different (Table 10.3). The Po_2 and Pco_2 of heparin will be the same as room air if heparin is exposed to air.

b. The Po_2 and Pco_2 of blood and air quickly equilibrate; the blood Po_2 increases (unless the patient is on O_2 therapy) and blood Pco_2 decreases. The loss of CO_2 from blood causes decreases in the $[HCO_3^-]$ and $[H^+]$ of the sample.

c. Net result: ↑ pH, ↑ Po_2, ↓ Pco_2, and ↓ $[HCO_3^-]$

2. Delay in sample analysis or failure to chill the sample adequately (but no air exposure)

a. Aerobic metabolism of leukocytes and platelets causes decreased Po_2. Based on stability studies for equine blood P_aO_2, arterial blood should be analyzed within 10 min (if kept at room temperature) or within 2 h (if stored in ice bath). The P_aCO_2 and pH were stable for up to 1 h at room temperature.[13]

b. Glycolysis in leukocytes, erythrocytes, and platelets causes increased H^+ production and thus decreased pH.

c. Net result: ↓ pH and ↓ Po_2

Table 10.3. Differences in Po_2 and Pco_2 values (mmHg) between air and blood (samples from healthy animal inspiring room air)

	Room air	Arterial blood	Venous blood
Po_2	≈ 150	≈ 90	≈ 40
Pco_2	< 1	≈ 40	≈ 46

Source: Muir and Hubbell.[20]

ACID-BASE ABNORMALITIES

I. Metabolic (nonrespiratory) acidosis

    A. *Metabolic acidosis* is a pathophysiologic state in which a nonrespiratory process causes the accumulation of H^+ in blood and a decrease in plasma or serum $[HCO_3^-]$.

    B. Metabolic acidoses are typically produced by the excess generation of H^+ or a loss of HCO_3^-. The loss of HCO_3^- (or other body buffers) reduces the buffering capacity of the body and thus allows H^+ to accumulate (Fig. 10.1B).

    C. Disorders and pathogeneses (see Table 9.10 and the associated text)

        1. Excess generation of H^+: lactic acidosis (including rumen overload), ketoacidosis, and ingestion and metabolism of certain compounds (e.g., ethylene glycol)

        2. Decreased renal excretion of H^+: renal failure, uroperitoneum, distal renal tubular acidosis (type 1), and hypoaldosteronism

        3. Increased HCO_3^- loss: gastrointestinal losses (diarrhea or saliva loss in ruminants), renal losses (proximal renal tubular acidosis, type 2)

    D. The metabolic acidoses are sometimes classified into one of five groups:

        1. *Titrational acidosis*: $[HCO_3^-]$ decreases because it is being used to buffer H^+ that is either being produced excessively (e.g., lactic acidosis) or not being adequately excreted by kidneys (e.g., renal failure). *Titrational* is somewhat of a misnomer because *titrating* is the chemistry laboratory process of adding a reagent to produce a given effect (e.g., adding acid to determine the concentration of a base). The decreased $[HCO_3^-]$ is caused by buffering, not by titrating. HCO_3^- is one of several buffers in blood and is used to assess alterations in the concentrations of buffers.

        2. *Secretory acidosis*: $[HCO_3^-]$ decreases because it is being lost from the body (e.g., excess salivary loss or proximal tubular acidosis) or not being produced (distal tubular acidosis). The hallmark of these acidoses is the concurrent hyperchloremia. *Secretory* is an appropriate adjective when HCO_3^- is being secreted (e.g., in saliva). However, in the context of the tubular acidoses, *secretory* is not an appropriate adjective because the decreased $[HCO_3^-]$ is not caused by the secretion of HCO_3^- into the tubular fluid.

        3. *Organic acidosis*: The decrease in $[HCO_3^-]$ is linked to the accumulation of an organic anion (e.g., lactate, acetoacetate, β-hydroxybutyrate, or citrate). The organic anion may represent the increased production of an organic acid (e.g., acetoacetic acid) by metabolic pathways, but sometimes the organic anion and the H^+ are being produced by different pathways (see the L-lactate section in Chapter 9).

        4. *Inorganic acidosis*: The decrease in $[HCO_3^-]$ is linked to the accumulation of an inorganic anion (e.g., PO_4 or sulfate). The metabolic acidosis of renal failure is sometimes called an inorganic acidosis (due to ↑ $[PO_4]$), but there also may be increased concentrations of organic anions (e.g., citrate).

        5. *Dilutional acidosis*: In the SID approach to acid-base disorders (see the Strong Ion Difference section), a *dilutional acidosis* occurs when an excess of free H_2O in plasma dilutes the electrolytes proportionately (e.g., decreases both $[Na^+]$ and $[Cl^-]$ by 20 %). However, a 20 % decrease in $[Na^+]$ (e.g., from 150 mmol/L to 120 mmol/L) results in a greater absolute decrease than the 20 % decrease in $[Cl^-]$ (e.g., from 110 mmol/L to 88 mmol/L), and thus the SID decreases. In the traditional approach to acid-base disorders, the excess of free H_2O also dilutes the $[HCO_3^-]$ and thus causes a metabolic acidosis (e.g., from 24.0 mmol/L to 19.2 mmol/L).

Some people also consider the hyperchloremic acidosis that is caused by the rapid infusion of saline ([Na^+] + [Cl^-] = 154 mmol/L, but [HCO_3^-] = 0 mmol/L) to be a dilutional acidosis. Saline is not free H_2O but does contain a higher percentage of H_2O (100 %) per unit volume than does plasma (about 93 %).

   E. Physiologic compensation for metabolic acidosis

     1. Acidemia stimulates the central respiratory chemoreceptors to cause hyperventilation. Hyperventilation increases the excretion of CO_2 (thus reducing the blood P_{CO_2}) and thus reduces the [H^+] (compensatory respiratory alkalosis).

     2. In nonrenal disorders, the kidneys increase the secretion of H^+ (see Figs. 9.3, 9.4, and 9.6).

II. Respiratory acidosis

   A. *Respiratory acidosis* is a pathophysiologic state in which a respiratory disorder causes the accumulation of H^+ in blood and an increase in blood P_{CO_2} values (hypercapnia).

   B. Respiratory acidoses occur because of alveolar hypoventilation and thus an impaired excretion of CO_2. Metabolism continues to generate H^+, but the animal cannot remove it adequately via the bicarbonate buffering system (Fig. 10.1C).

   C. Hypoxemia will accompany (and typically precede) hypercapnia if patients are breathing room air.

   D. Disorders or conditions (Table 10.4)

   E. Physiologic compensation for respiratory acidosis

     1. In response to acidemia, kidneys will increase the secretion of H^+ and, in doing so, increase the plasma [HCO_3^-] (compensatory metabolic alkalosis).

     2. The renal response takes about 2–5 d to raise the blood pH during chronic hypercapnia.[14,15]

Table 10.4. Diseases and conditions that cause respiratory acidosis (hypoventilation)[a]

Inhibition or dysfunction of medullary respiratory center
   *Drugs: anesthetics, sedatives, and narcotics
   Brain stem disease (trauma, infection, neoplasia, etc.)
   Alkalemia due to a metabolic alkalosis
Inhibition or dysfunction of respiratory muscles (diaphragm, chest wall): tick paralysis, tetanus, botulism, myasthenia gravis, hypokalemia, and succinylcholine
Upper airway dysfunction: foreign body, vomitus, and mechanical hypoventilation
Impaired gas exchange at pulmonary capillaries
   *Pulmonary disease: infection, allergy, edema, fibrosis, neoplasia, and hyaline membrane disease in neonates
   *Restrictive disease: pneumothorax, pleural effusions, and diaphragmatic hernia
   Vascular disorders: right-to-left shunts (e.g., patent ductus arteriosus)

---

  * A relatively common disease or condition

  [a] Disorders that cause respiratory acidosis (↑ P_aCO_2) because of reduced gas exchange in the lungs will likely also result in ↓ P_aO_2, but the decrease may not be sufficient for the disorder to be classified as a hypoxemic disorder (Table 10.9).

  Note: During their first few days of life, neonatal foals and calves may have greater P_{CO_2} values than adult animals.[23,24]

III. Metabolic (nonrespiratory) alkalosis
   A. *Metabolic alkalosis* is a pathophysiologic state in which a nonrespiratory process causes the depletion of H^+ from blood and an increase in serum and plasma $[HCO_3^-]$.
   B. Metabolic alkaloses are typically produced by loss of H^+ (renal secretion or gastric/abomasal secretion) and the resultant generation of HCO_3^- (Fig. 10.1D). The loss of H^+ and the concurrent production of HCO_3^- are illustrated in Fig. 9.4 (type A intercalated renal tubular cells) and Fig. 9.5 (gastric parietal epithelial cell). Note that the H^+ secreted by the gastric mucosa is produced in the epithelial cell; it is not lost from plasma.
   C. Disorders and pathogeneses (see Table 9.9 and the associated text)
     1. Loss of H^+ from body
       a. Gastric loss: vomiting or pyloric obstruction (functional or mechanical)
       b. Renal loss
         (1) Loop or thiazide diuretics
         (2) Secondary to respiratory acidosis
         (3) Hypokalemia
     2. Shift of H^+ from ECF to intracellular fluid because of hypokalemia
     3. Administration of sodium bicarbonate or organic anions that generate HCO_3^-
     4. Contraction alkalosis: loss of HCO_3^--poor fluid, which causes hypovolemia and increased plasma $[HCO_3^-]$ (see Chapter 9)
   D. Physiologic response
     1. In nonrenal disorders associated with metabolic alkalosis, the kidneys are expected to decrease the secretion of H^+ (exception: see "paradoxical" aciduria [discussed in the following sect. 3]) and conserve less HCO_3^-.
       a. With increased plasma $[HCO_3^-]$, the amount of HCO_3^- that enters the filtrate may exceed the capacity of the proximal tubules to conserve it.
       b. Excess HCO_3^- will be secreted by intercalated cells (type B) of the distal nephron.
     2. Alkalemia inhibits the central respiratory chemoreceptors and thus causes hypoventilation. Hypoventilation decreases the excretion of CO_2 (thus elevating the blood Pco_2) and increases the $[H^+]$ (compensatory respiratory acidosis).
     3. *"Paradoxical" aciduria*
       a. It is called *paradoxical* because the aciduria is concurrent with an alkalosis.
       b. When an animal has concurrent alkalosis, hypochloremia, and hypovolemia, the kidneys may produce acidic urine (see Figs. 9.3 and 9.4).
         (1) Hypovolemia stimulates the resorption of Na^+ and Cl^- in the tubules through the actions of aldosterone and angiotensin II.
         (2) Na^+ resorption is not always accompanied by Cl^- (because of Cl^- depletion), and thus an electrochemical gradient is established that promotes the secretion of H^+ (thus aciduria) and K^+ (thus contributing to a concurrent hypokalemia).
         (3) The secretion of H^+ by tubules also increases the generation of HCO_3^-, which adds to the severity of the metabolic alkalosis.
       c. It is seen most frequently in cattle but also may be seen in other mammals.

IV. Respiratory alkalosis
   A. *Respiratory alkalosis* is a pathophysiologic state in which a respiratory disorder causes depletion of H^+ in blood and a decrease in blood Pco_2 values (hypocapnia).

Table 10.5. Diseases and conditions that cause respiratory alkalosis (hyperventilation)

Hypoxemia (stimulation of peripheral chemoreceptors) (see Table 10.9)

Pulmonary disease (stimulation of nociceptive receptors)

Stimulation of respiratory center

    *Metabolic acidosis

    Septicemia (Gram negative)

    Heat stroke or fever

    Drugs: salicylates and aminophylline

    Central neurologic disease: trauma, neoplasia, inflammation, cerebrovascular accident,
      and hepatic encephalopathy

Mechanical hyperventilation

Pain or anxiety

* A relatively common disease or condition

Note: When determined by the i-STAT, the P_{CO_2} can be falsely decreased by the presence of thiopental in the blood sample.

Source: de Morais and DiBartola.[15]

B. Respiratory alkaloses occur because of alveolar hyperventilation; respirations remove CO_2 and thus H^+ at a rate faster than H^+ is being made (Fig. 10.1E).
C. Disorders or conditions (Table 10.5)
   1. Hypoxemia disorders: Peripheral chemoreceptors (carotid and aortic bodies) stimulated by hypoxemia initiate hyperventilation that causes the increased loss of CO_2 and thus loss of H^+. (See Table 10.9 for diseases and conditions that cause hypoxemia.) Pulmonary disease may result in poor oxygenation of blood (hypoxemia), which stimulates hyperventilation. Because CO_2 diffuses more easily than O_2, hyperventilation may cause excess loss of CO_2 and thus a respiratory alkalosis. If there is acute hypoxemia, loss of CO_2 may be somewhat self-limiting because the resultant alkalemia inhibits respiration. However, with chronic hypoxemia and respiratory alkalosis, the resulting compensatory metabolic acidosis reduces the degree of alkalemia, and thus hypoxemia continues to stimulate hyperventilation.[16]
   2. Stimulation of the respiratory center: Acidemia and other factors, including central nervous system disease, may stimulate the central respiratory center to cause hyperventilation and thus a loss of H^+.
   3. Mechanical ventilation: Animals assisted by mechanical ventilators may develop alkalemia if there is excessive loss of CO_2.
   4. Interferent: When determined by the i-STAT, the P_{CO_2} can be falsely decreased by the presence of thiopental in the blood sample.[17]
D. Physiologic compensation
   1. In response to alkalemia, healthy kidneys decrease the secretion of H^+ and, in doing so, reduce the conservation of HCO_3^- (compensatory metabolic acidosis). Also, metabolic alkalosis stimulates type B intercalated cells to secrete HCO_3^- (see Fig. 9.8).[16]
   2. The renal response takes about 2–5 d to raise the $[H^+]$.

Table 10.6. Blood gas data in simple acid-base disorders

Disorder	pH	P_aCO_2	$[HCO_3^-]$
Respiratory acidosis	↓	↑	WRI
Respiratory acidosis with compensatory metabolic alkalosis	↓–WRI	↑	↑
Metabolic acidosis	↓	WRI	↓
Metabolic acidosis with compensatory respiratory alkalosis	↓–WRI	↓	↓
Respiratory alkalosis	↑	↓	WRI
Respiratory alkalosis with compensatory metabolic acidosis	↑–WRI	↓	↓
Metabolic alkalosis	↑	WRI	↑
Metabolic alkalosis with compensatory respiratory acidosis	↑–WRI	↑	↑

V. Classification of acid-base disorders
   A. The major patterns for the simple acid-base disorders are listed in Table 10.6.
      1. Simple acid-base disorders are those in which the pathophysiologic state is limited to a primary disturbance (e.g., lactic acidosis) and the expected compensatory process (e.g., hyperventilation). Figure 10.5 includes an algorithm for the classification of simple acid-base disorders.
      2. When two or more simple acid-base disorders are present (e.g., vomiting causing a metabolic alkalosis, and renal failure causing a metabolic acidosis), there is a *mixed acid-base disorder*. Physical examination and laboratory findings may contain clues that an animal has a mixed acid-base disorder. Such clues include the following: (1) an unexpected blood pH (WRI or opposite change) for a given clinical state, (2) P_aCO_2 and $[HCO_3^-]$ changes are in opposite directions (e.g., ↓ $[HCO_3^-]$, and ↑ P_aCO_2 would indicate both metabolic and respiratory acidoses), and (3) lack of any expected compensation (see the next section). Additional information on mixed acid-base disorders is available.[18]
   B. Expected compensatory changes in acid-base disorders
      1. Compensation for respiratory acidosis or alkalosis: If there is not renal disease, the kidneys are expected to alter their excretions of H^+ and HCO_3^- (also other electrolytes) to compensate for the acidemia or alkalemia.
      2. Compensation for metabolic acidosis or alkalosis: If there is not renal disease and the acid-base disturbance is not of renal origin, then the kidneys are expected to alter their excretions of H^+ and HCO_3^- accordingly to compensate for the acidemia or alkalemia. The respiratory system is also expected to alter its excretion of CO_2 to compensate appropriately for acidemias or alkalemias.
      3. When there is either respiratory or metabolic compensation, there is never complete compensation. Blood pH may return to the reference interval, but it will never return to the normal pH for that animal as long as the disorder causing the acid-base balance remains.
      4. How much can these systems compensate if given time to do so? One aspect of the interpretation of blood gas data is attempting to determine whether the animal's

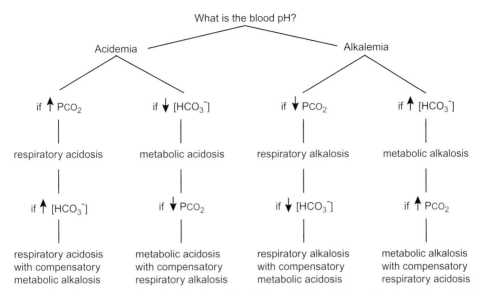

Fig. 10.5. Algorithmic approach to classification of simple (not mixed) acid-base disorders. Refer to Tables 10.7 and 10.8 for expected compensatory responses.

respiratory or metabolic systems have compensated appropriately. If the data indicate that an animal has not achieved expected compensation, they may indicate the following:

a. The animal has not had time to compensate. This is especially true of renal compensation for acute respiratory disorders.

b. The animal has more than one disorder that is altering the acid-base status, and this disorder is preventing an expected compensation.

5. To attempt to determine expected compensations in dogs, experimental acid-base disorders were created and changes were monitored. The findings from several experiments were summarized in a review article;[19] data were extracted from that article for Table 10.7. The proposed purpose of the correction factors is to determine whether the changes in $[HCO_3^-]$ or P_aCO_2 represent a physiologic compensation to a single acid-base disorder or whether other factors are affecting the $[HCO_3^-]$ or P_aCO_2.

6. A formula for calculating an expected P_aCO_2 is provided in Eq. 10.7. The expected P_aCO_2 value is frequently calculated using average values for healthy dogs; that is, average P_aCO_2, average $[HCO_3^-]$, and an average compensation factor. Because of the biologic differences in dogs and the analytical differences in blood gas methods, those average values may or may not be appropriate for a given patient. Some people recommend that the expected P_aCO_2 value be considered a rough estimate ± 3 mmHg. However, Table 10.8 provides examples showing that a greater amount of variation in the expected P_aCO_2 values is obtained if one considers the interindividual variation in $[HCO_3^-]$ and P_aCO_2 values.

Table 10.7. Expected compensations for acid-base disorders in dogs

Disorder	Expected [HCO$_3^-$] change (mmol/L)[a,b]	Expected P$_a$co$_2$ change (mmHg)[a,c]
For each mmHg ↑ in P$_a$co$_2$ in:		
Acute respiratory acidosis (< 24 h)	↑ 0.15 (0.04–0.20)	—
Chronic respiratory acidosis (> 3–5 d)	↑ 0.35 (0.29–0.43)	—
For each mmHg ↓ in P$_a$co$_2$ in:		
Acute respiratory alkalosis	↓ 0.25 (0.14–0.36)	—
Chronic respiratory alkalosis	↓ 0.55 (0.43–0.76)	—
For each mmol/L ↓ in [HCO$_3^-$] in:		
Metabolic acidosis	—	↓ 0.7 (0.5–1.1)
For each mmol/L ↑ in [HCO$_3^-$] in:		
Metabolic alkalosis	—	↑ 0.7 (0.5–1.3)

[a] Expected compensations were reported in a review article.[19] The first number is the recommended guideline value. The numbers in parentheses represent the interval of values reported in various experimental conditions that produced the acid-base disorders.

[b] The HCO$_3^-$ methods (either measured or calculated from blood gas data) are not precise enough to justify reporting [HCO$_3^-$] to the nearest hundredth but may be precise enough to justify reporting concentrations to the nearest tenth. Therefore, instead of expected changes of ↑ 0.15 (0.04–0.20), consideration of significant figures should result in an expected change of ↑ 0.2 (0.0–0.2).

[c] The P$_a$co$_2$ methods are not precise enough to justify reporting them to the nearest tenth but may be precise enough to justify reporting concentrations to the whole number. Therefore, instead of expected changes of ↓ 0.7 (0.5–1.1), consideration of significant figures should result in an expected change of ↓ 1 (0–1).

$$\begin{pmatrix} \text{Expected} \\ \text{P}_a\text{CO}_2 \end{pmatrix} = \begin{pmatrix} \text{P}_a\text{CO}_2 \\ \text{in healthy dog} \end{pmatrix} + \begin{pmatrix} \text{HCO}_3^- \\ \text{in patient} - \frac{\text{HCO}_3^-}{\text{in healthy dog}} \end{pmatrix} \times \begin{pmatrix} \text{compensation} \\ \text{factor} \end{pmatrix} \qquad \textbf{(10.7.)}$$

Example:
Patient results: pH = 7.146; P$_a$co$_2$ = 36 mmHg; [HCO$_3^-$] = 12 mmol/L
Average values for healthy dog (Table 10.8): P$_a$co$_2$ = 40 mmHg; [HCO$_3^-$] = 21 mmol/L

$$\begin{pmatrix} \text{Expected} \\ \text{P}_a\text{CO}_2 \end{pmatrix} = (40 \text{ mmHg}) + (12 \text{ mmol/L} - 21 \text{ mmol/L}) \times \left(\frac{0.7 \text{ mmHg}}{\text{mmol/L}} \right)$$
$$= 34 \text{ mmHg}$$

7. The calculation of expected compensatory changes in blood gas data should be considered an estimate. If the goal of the interpretation of the data is to determine whether the animal has more than one disorder affecting the acid-base status, sometimes there are other ways of arriving at the conclusion.
   a. If a dog has ketoacidotic diabetes mellitus and is vomiting, the dog very likely has both a metabolic acidosis (caused by ketosis) and a metabolic alkalosis (due to vomiting).
   b. If a dog has a pulmonary disorder that is causing a respiratory acidosis and also has evidence of renal failure, the dog very likely has both a respiratory acidosis and a metabolic acidosis.

Table 10.8 Examples of expected compensation calculation for metabolic acidosis in dogs; expected P_aCO_2 calculated using Eq. 10.7

Blood gas data for a dog:
pH = 7.146 (7.310–7.420) P_aCO_2 = 36 mmHg (35–45) $[HCO_3^-]$ = 12 mmol/L (17–24)

Example	$[HCO_3^-]$ in patient (mmol/L)	$[HCO_3^-]$ in health (mmol/L)	Compensation factor mmHg/ (mmol/L)	P_aCO_2 in health (mmHg)	Expected P_aCO_2 (mmHg)	Difference between measured and expected P_aCO_2 (mmHg)
A	12	21	0.7	40	34	2
B	12	21	1.1	40	30	6
C	12	24	1.1	35	22	14

Example A: Expected P_aCO_2 was calculated using average P_aCO_2, average $[HCO_3^-]$, and average compensation factor for healthy dogs (see Table 10.7). The difference between measured and expected P_aCO_2 values is 2 mmHg and thus within the ± 3 guideline. Therefore, the measured P_aCO_2 of 36 mmHg represents an expected respiratory compensation (i.e., compensatory respiratory alkalosis) for the metabolic acidosis.

Example B: Expected P_aCO_2 was calculated using average P_aCO_2, average $[HCO_3^-]$, and higher compensation factor (1.1) for healthy dogs (see Table 10.7). The difference between measured and expected P_aCO_2 values is 6 mmHg and thus greater than the ± 3 guideline. This value suggests that there has not been an appropriate respiratory compensation for the metabolic acidosis, and thus there may be a concurrent respiratory acidosis. However, the 6 mmHg was calculated using values found in experimental healthy dogs, and thus the compensation might be appropriate.

Example C: Expected P_aCO_2 was calculated using the lower reference limit P_aCO_2 (i.e., 35 mmHg), the upper reference limit $[HCO_3^-]$ (i.e., 24 mmol/L), and the higher compensation factor (1.1) for healthy dogs (see Table 10.7). The difference between measured and expected P_aCO_2 values is 14 mmHg and thus much greater than the ± 3 guideline. This value suggests that there has not been an appropriate respiratory compensation for the metabolic acidosis, and thus there may be a concurrent respiratory acidosis. However, the 14 mmHg was calculated using values found in experimental healthy dogs, and thus the compensation might be appropriate.

8. The estimated compensatory factors in this section are for dogs and were determined during experimental conditions. Experiments for cats, horses, and cattle would probably yield different compensatory factors. Results in spontaneous diseases with multisystem involvement would probably also be different.

HYPOXEMIA AND HYPOXIA

I.   Expected P_{O_2}
    A. Arterial blood is the only acceptable sample for the assessment of oxygenation of blood by the respiratory system. The expected P_aO_2 varies with the FIo_2, the O_2 content of the inhaled gas (FIo_2 in decimal fraction, P_aO_2 in mmHg): (0.2, 95–100), (0.3, 150), (0.4, 200), (0.5, 250), (0.8, 400), and (1.0, 500).[20]
    B. For room air, the FIo_2 is near 0.2, and thus a P_aO_2 of 90–100 mmHg is expected. Some authors consider a P_aO_2 of < 80 mmHg to be hypoxemia,[20] although one could also consider hypoxemia to be present whenever P_aO_2 falls below a valid lower reference limit. Hypoxemic stimulus of chemoreceptors is reported to occur when P_aO_2 is < 70 mmHg[21] or < 60 mmHg.[22]

Table 10.9. Diseases and conditions that cause hypoxemia[a]

Decreased inhaled O_2 content: high altitude or closed ventilation area
Inhibition or dysfunction of the medullary respiratory center (see Table 10.4)
Inhibition or dysfunction of the respiratory muscles (see Table 10.4)
Upper airway dysfunction: foreign body, vomitus, or mechanical hypoventilation
*Impaired gas exchange at pulmonary capillaries (see Table 10.4)

* A relatively common disease or condition
[a] Disorders that cause respiratory acidosis ($\uparrow P_aco_2$) because of reduced gas exchange in the lungs (Table 10.4) will likely also result in $\downarrow P_ao_2$, but the decrease may not be sufficient to be classified a hypoxemia.

Notes: Compared to adult horses, neonatal foals have lower P_ao_2, higher P_aco_2, higher $[HCO_3^-]$, and slightly lower pH values because of underdeveloped lungs. Similar patterns occur in calves and possibly other species.

   C. With the increased use of point-of-care instruments that have O_2 electrodes, more P_vo_2 values are being measured. In free-flowing venous blood in an animal with a P_ao_2 near 95 mmHg, the P_vo_2 will be near 40 mmHg. If the sample is collected from an occluded vein, the P_vo_2 will be lower. If collected from capillary blood, the Po_2 should be between the P_ao_2 and P_vo_2 values.

   D. Blood gas data in neonates are different from those of adult animals.[23,24]

     1. Compared to the adult horse, a foal at birth has lower P_ao_2 (< 40 mmHg) and higher P_aco_2 values (> 50 mmHg) during its first few hours. The P_ao_2 increases quickly to near adult values by 1 d of age, and the P_aco_2 slowly changes to adult values by 4–7 d of age.

     2. Similar patterns are seen in neonatal calves. The P_ao_2 approaches adult values by 1 d of age, and the P_aco_2 approaches adult values by 2 d of age.

     3. Plasma $[HCO_3^-]$ values are also greater initially, corresponding to the greater P_aco_2 pressures.

II. *Hypoxemia* (decreased dissolved O_2 in blood; decreased P_ao_2) may cause *hypoxia* (decreased O_2 delivery or utilization of O_2 by tissues), but there are other disorders in which there is hypoxia but not hypoxemia. The different types of hypoxia can be divided into seven groups.[25] Hypoxemic and hypoxic disorders or conditions and the expected laboratory data for hypoxia disorders are listed in Tables 10.9 and 10.10.

   A. *Atmospheric hypoxia*: inhalation of atmosphere that has decreased O_2 content (e.g., high altitude, anesthetic problem, or in an airtight box)

     1. The inhalation of atmosphere that has decreased O_2 content causes a decreased P_Ao_2, and thus less O_2 diffuses to blood ($\downarrow P_ao_2$) and less O_2 binds to Hgb ($\downarrow So_2$). The combination of $\downarrow P_ao_2$ and $\downarrow So_2$ results in a decreased amount of O_2 in the blood ($\downarrow O_2ct$).

     2. If the hypoxemia stimulates the peripheral chemoreceptors (carotid or aortic bodies), increased respirations result in hyperventilation and thus $\downarrow P_aco_2$ (respiratory alkalosis) if the CO_2 is actually exhaled (see tidal hypoxia in the next section).

   B. *Tidal hypoxia*: decreased O_2 uptake because of impaired respiratory exchange (e.g., respiratory obstruction, or hypoventilation caused by anesthetic agents)

     1. The impaired delivery of air to the alveoli has the same effect on the oxygenation of blood as conditions that cause atmospheric hypoxia; that is, $\downarrow P_ao_2$, $\downarrow So_2$, and $\downarrow O_2ct$.

Table 10.10. Blood gas results expected for each general type of hypoxia

Hypoxia	Atmospheric	Tidal	Alveolar	Hemoglobic	Stagnant	Histotoxic	Demand
P_aO_2	↓	↓	↓	WRI	WRI	WRI	WRI
So_2	↓	↓	↓	?[a]	WRI	WRI	WRI
Spo_2	↓	↓	↓	WRI	WRI	WRI	WRI
P_{50}	WRI	WRI	WRI	WRI	WRI	WRI	WRI
O_2ct	↓	↓	↓	↓	WRI	WRI	WRI
$P_{A}O_2$	↓	↓	↓	WRI	WRI	WRI	WRI
a/A	WRI	WRI	↓	WRI	WRI	WRI	WRI
$AaDO_2$	WRI	WRI	↑	WRI	WRI	WRI	WRI
P_aO_2/FI	WRI	WRI	↓	WRI	WRI	WRI	WRI
P_aCO_2	↓[b]	↑[c]	↑[c]	WRI	WRI	WRI	WRI
pH	WRI–↑[b]	WRI–↓[c]	WRI–↓[c]	WRI	WRI	WRI	WRI

[a] If the hemoglobic hypoxia is caused by anemia, the So_2 will be WRI. If the hemoglobic hypoxia is caused by methemoglobinemia or carboxyhemoglobinemia, the So_2 will be decreased.

[b] If the hypoxemia results in the stimulation of respiration, hyperventilation would result in decreased P_aCO_2 and a respiratory alkalosis.

[c] If there is inadequate ventilation, there would be an increased P_aCO_2 and a respiratory acidosis.

    2. The impaired respiratory exchange causes impaired excretion of CO_2. Thus, there may be ↑ P_aCO_2 and a respiratory acidosis.

C. *Alveolar hypoxia*: decreased O_2 uptake because of decreased alveolar function (e.g., pneumonia, emphysema, pleural effusion, intrapulmonary exudates, right-to-left shunts, ventilation-perfusion mismatch, pulmonary edema, or pulmonary fibrosis)

    1. The impaired diffusion of O_2 has the same effect on the oxygenation of blood as do conditions that cause atmospheric hypoxia; that is, ↓ P_aO_2, ↓ So_2, and ↓ O_2ct. However, the arterial alveolar O_2 tension gradient ($AaDO_2$) and arterial alveolar O_2 tension ratio (a/A) identify the defective diffusion of O_2 from the alveolus to blood.

    2. The impaired respiratory exchange results in impaired excretion of CO_2. Thus, there may be ↑ P_aCO_2 and a respiratory acidosis.

    3. A right-to-left shunt results in ↓ P_aO_2 because venous blood with a P_vO_2 of 45–50 mmHg is mixed with arterial blood with a P_aO_2 of 95–100 mmHg (if breathing air).

    4. A ventilation-perfusion mismatch occurs when blood is perfusing nonfunctional alveoli; that is, blood is available for gas exchange, but the gas exchange does not occur. Thus, blood from those vessels is not oxygenated (remains as "venous" blood) and then mixes with oxygenated arterial blood from other pulmonary tissue.

D. *Hemoglobic hypoxia*: decreased O_2 bound to Hgb (e.g., methemoglobinemia or CO poisoning) or decreased Hgb (e.g., anemia)

    1. For these disorders, there is not a defect in the delivery of O_2 to the blood; thus, the P_aO_2 will not be decreased. Po_2 is a measure of the tension created by dissolved O_2 in the plasma and is not dependent on blood [Hgb].

    2. If an animal is anemic, the O_2ct will be decreased because most of the O_2 in blood is bound to Hgb. If there is not a concurrent defective Hgb, the So_2 will not be decreased. If an anemic animal's blood contains metHgb or COHgb, the So_2 will also be decreased.

3. With methemoglobinemia, both ferrous (Fe^{2+}) and ferric (Fe^{3+}) heme molecules are present. In this state, the ferric heme cannot bind O_2, and the ferrous heme has greater affinity for O_2. Both processes result in hypoxia.[26]

4. CO has a much greater affinity for Hgb than does O_2, and thus even small amounts of CO interfere with delivery of O_2 to tissues.

E. *Stagnant hypoxia* is decreased delivery of O_2 to tissue because of poor blood circulation (e.g., shock, blood vessel occlusion, or hyperviscosity syndrome). Blood gas data will not detect an abnormality.

F. *Histotoxic hypoxia* is defective O_2 use by tissues because of interference with metabolic pathways (e.g., some drugs or alcohol). Blood gas data will not detect an abnormality.

G. *Demand hypoxia* is increased O_2 demand by hyperfunctioning cells (e.g., hyperthyroidism, pyrexia). Blood gas data will not detect an abnormality.

III. SpO_2

A. A decreasing SpO_2 typically indicates the development of hypoxemia but only when the P_aO_2 is < 90 mmHg. With greater FIO_2 such as occurs during anesthesia, greater P_aO_2 values are expected. Because of the shape of the oxyhemoglobin dissociation curve (Fig. 10.4), falling S_aO_2 values may not be detected until the P_aO_2 is < 60 mmHg, which might be considerably less than expected for high FIO_2 values.

B. Erroneous values:[5] With increasing concentrations of COHgb (as in CO poisoning), the SpO_2 remained at > 90 % even when O_2Hgb percentage decreased to 30 %, because the oximeter does not differentiate COHgb from O_2Hgb. Similar but less severe, false positive interference was seen with increasing concentrations of methemoglobin. As shown in Eq. 10.5b, the O_2Hgb percentage will decrease with increased concentrations of COHgb or methemoglobin.

C. In horses, the SpO_2 underestimated the S_aO_2 by an average of 4.4 % when S_aO_2 was ≥ 90 % and overestimated the S_aO_2 by an average of 4.1 % when S_aO_2 was ≤ 90 %.[27] The errors might be due to different properties of equine blood compared to human blood.

D. In dogs with S_aO_2 of ≥ 70 %, the average difference between SpO_2 and S_aO_2 was about 3–4 % (e.g., SpO_2 of 87 % and S_aO_2 of 90 %), depending on application site (tongue or tail) and type of probe (ear or finger). The reason for the difference is not known.[6] As with the equine data, pulse oximetry underestimated the S_aO_2 when it was high and overestimated the S_aO_2 when it was low.

STRONG ION DIFFERENCE (SID) AND STEWART'S METHOD OF ACID-BASE ANALYSIS

I. Evaluation of electrolyte relationships led to an alternate method of assessing metabolic (nonrespiratory) acid-base disturbances (Stewart's quantitative analysis of acid-base chemistry) and the calculation of SID. A complete description of Stewart's method and SID concepts is beyond the scope of this book, but major aspects and a comparison with more traditional assessment of acid-base disorders is presented. For a complete analysis of Stewart's method and SID, additional references should be studied.[28–33]

In Stewart's method:

A. Electrolyte disturbances are approached in the context of physiochemistry with consideration of equilibrium equations, conservation of mass, and balance of charge.

    B. Nontraditional definitions of acids and bases are used.

    C. All electrolytes in biologic fluids are considered to be involved in acid-base balance, and maintenance of electrical neutrality is expected (Eq. 10.8a).

$$[Na^+] + [K^+] + [fCa^{2+}] + [fMg^{2+}] + [H^+] + [NH_4^+] = \qquad \text{(10.8a.)}$$
$$[OH^-] + [Cl^-] + [HCO_3^-] + [CO_3^{2-}] + [Alb^{x-}] + [PO_4^{y-}] + [uSA]$$

        where x and y represent the variable charges on albumin and phosphates, respectively, and uSA includes SO_4^{2-}, lactate, acetoacetate, β-hydroxybutyrate, other acidic anions of metabolism, and exogenous anions.

$$([Na^+] + [K^+] + [fCa^{2+}] + [fMg^{2+}]) - ([Cl^-] + [uSA]) = \qquad \text{(10.8b.)}$$
$$([OH^-] + [HCO_3^-] + [CO_3^{2-}] + [Alb^{x-}] + [PO_4^{y-}]) - ([H^+] + [NH_4^+])$$

        strong cations − strong anions = weak anions − weak cations
        If SID_{true} = strong cations − strong anions
        Then SID_{true} = weak anions − weak cations

$$SID_{true} = ([OH^-] + [HCO_3^-] + [CO_3^{2-}] + [Alb^{x-}] + [PO_4^{y-}]) - ([H^+] + [NH_4^+]) \qquad \text{(10.8c.)}$$

    D. Analytes involved in acid-base balance are considered to be either independent or dependent variables.

        1. The independent variables are those analytes that are regulated or changed independently of others: Pco_2, SID, and A_{TOT} (see the definitions in the next section).

        2. The dependent variables are those analytes that change if and only if one of the independent variables changes. The dependent variables include H^+, OH^-, HCO_3^-, and tCO_2.

    E. Changes in $[H^+]$ are predicted from changes in concentrations of strong ions. The actual blood $[H^+]$ (i.e., pH) is not measured.

    F. Albumin is included as a contributor to acid-base balance, whereas it is not a formalized part of the classic traditional approach. However, albumin concentrations do affect anion gaps and are considered in base excess calculations.

    G. Hgb is not included as a contributor to acid-base balance, whereas it is a part of the calculated BE_B value that is common in blood gas data.

II.   Differences in definitions between the two systems can lead to confusion.[2]

    A. Definitions in the traditional assessment of acid-base disorders by using pH, Pco_2, and HCO_3^-

        1. An *acid* is a substance that can give off a H^+ (a proton) at a given pH (e.g., hydrochloric acid is capable of giving off H^+).

        2. A *base* is a substance that can bind a H^+ (e.g., HCO_3^- is capable of binding H^+).

        3. An *acidosis* is a condition in which acidemia (lower pH and higher $[H^+]$) tends to occur.

        4. An *alkalosis* is a condition in which alkalemia (higher pH and lower $[H^+]$) tends to occur.

    B. Definitions in the Stewart's method

        1. *Strong cations* or *strong anions* are those ions that are completely dissociated in physiologic fluids. (Note that the definition does not consider the ions that are complexed with protein or nonprotein ions; for example, most serum calcium ions

are complexed with anions and are not free or completely dissociated ions. Also, Na^+ and Cl^- behave as though they are only 75 % dissociated in plasma.)[16]

   a. Strong cations (Na^+, K^+, fCa^{2+}, and fMg^{2+}): Strong cations (e.g., Na^+) are considered bases because when added to ECF, and if there is not a balancing shift of a strong ion (e.g., removal of K^+ or addition of Cl^-), H^+ shifts out of the ECF to make it more alkaline.

   b. Strong anions (Cl^-, sulfate, lactate, acetoacetate, β-hydroxybutyrate, and other acidic products of metabolism): Strong anions (e.g., Cl^-) are considered acids because when added to ECF, and if there is not a balancing shift of a strong ion (e.g., addition of Na^+ or removal of lactate), H^+ shifts into the ECF to make it more acidic.

2. An *acidosis* is a condition in which there is an excess of strong anions ("acids") or a deficit of strong cations ("bases"). In the SID approach, an acidosis is present if SID is decreased.

3. An *alkalosis* is a condition in which there is an excess of strong cations ("bases") or a deficit of strong anions ("acids"). In the SID approach, an alkalosis is present if SID is increased.

4. *Weak electrolytes* are those electrolytes that are in equilibria in physiologic fluids.
   a. Weak cations: NH_4^+, H^+, and some γ-globulins
   b. Weak anions: HCO_3^-, CO_3^{2-}, PO_4^{3-}, HPO_4^{2-}, $H_2PO_4^-$, and proteins (mostly albumin)

5. A_{TOT} is the sum of the nonvolatile weak acids ($HA + A^-$). In plasma, these occur as various anionic forms of PO_4 and proteins (albumin and globulins).

6. SID_{true} is the difference between the sum of strong ion concentrations; that is, the difference between the sum of strong cation concentrations and the sum of strong anion concentrations. By rearranging Eq. 10.8a, it is shown that SID_{true} (i.e., strong cations minus strong anions) also equals the difference between the sum of weak anion concentrations and the sum of weak cation concentrations (Eq. 10.8b). This is an important concept for interpreting calculated SID values. Thus, SID_{true} could be calculated if the analyte concentrations in Eq. 10.8c could be measured.

C. Using the same concepts as Stewart,[28] Singer and Hastings[34] defined buffer base, which is identical to Stewart's SID.[2]

III. SID equations: Several SID equations have been proposed. Other than the SID_{true}, these SID equations yield values that are estimates based on assumptions. If the assumptions are not correct, the estimates will not be correct. The naming of the equations in this edition differs from the previous edition and is patterned after some of the recent SID publications.

A. SID_{true} (Eq. 10.9a):[29] This equation is consistent with the SID definition but is not useful because concentrations of many analytes in the formula are not measured in clinical laboratories.

$$SID_{true} = \text{(sum of strong cations)} - \text{(sum of strong anions)} \quad \text{(10.9a.)}$$
$$= ([Na^+] + [K^+] + [fCa^{2+}] + [[fMg^{2+}]) - ([Cl^-] + [uSA])$$

uSA includes SO_4^{3-}, lactate, acetoacetate, β-hydroxybutyrate, other acidic anions of metabolism, and exogenous anions.

$$SID_3 = ([Na^+] + [K^+]) - [Cl^-] \tag{10.9b.}$$

$$SID_4 = ([Na^+] + [K^+]) - ([Cl^-] + [L\text{-lactate}^-]) \tag{10.9c.}$$

$$SID_5 = ([Na^+] + [K^+] + [fCa^{2+}]) - ([Cl^-] + [L\text{-lactate}^-]) \tag{10.9d.}$$

$$SID_6 = ([Na^+] + [K^+] + [fCa^{2+}] + [fMg^{2+}]) - ([Cl^-] + [L\text{-lactate}^-]) \tag{10.9e.}$$

$$SID_{Cl^-corrected} = [Na^+]_{mean\ normal} - [Cl^-]_{corrected} \tag{10.9f.}$$

$$\text{where}\ [Cl^-]_{corrected} = [Cl^-]_{patient} \times \frac{[Na^+]_{mean\ normal}}{[Na^+]_{patient}}$$

and the "mean normal" concentrations of Na^+ and Cl^- are for the appropriate reference intervals for the patient's values.

B. *SID₃* (Eq. 10.9b):[33] This equation estimates the SID by using three strong ion concentrations that are routinely measured in serum or plasma; this is probably one of the more common clinical SID formulas. Note that it does not include the concentrations of fCa^{2+}, fMg^{2+}, or uSA; thus, changes in those analyte concentrations would cause the estimate of SID to be inaccurate.

C. *SID₄* (Eq. 10.9c):[33,35] This equation estimates the SID by using four strong ion concentrations (the three for SID₃ plus L-lactate). Note that it does not include the concentrations of fCa^{2+}, fMg^{2+}, or uSA other than L-lactate (such as D-lactate); thus, changes in those analyte concentrations would cause the estimate of SID to be inaccurate.

D. *SID₅* (Eq. 10.9d):[35] This equation estimates the SID by using five strong ions (the four for SID₄ plus fCa^{2+}). Note that it does not include the concentrations of fMg^{2+} or uSA other than L-lactate (such as D-lactate); thus, changes in those analyte concentrations would cause the estimate of SID to be inaccurate.

E. *SID₆* (Eq. 10.9e):[35] This equation estimates the SID by using six strong ion concentrations (those used for SID₅ plus fMg^{2+}). Note that it does not include the concentrations of uSA other than L-lactate (such as D-lactate); thus, changes in those analyte concentrations would cause the estimate of SID to be inaccurate.

F. *SID₍Cl⁻corrected₎* (Eq. 10.9f)[32]

1. The basis of the $[Cl^-]_{corrected}$ is that changes in $[Na^+]$ are expected to be matched by proportional changes in $[Cl^-]$ if there is either hemoconcentration or hemodilution; for example, a 10 % increase in $[Na^+]$ should be accompanied by a 10 % increase in $[Cl^-]$. However, the absolute change in $[Na^+]$ would be greater than the absolute change in $[Cl^-]$; for example, 150–165 versus 110–121. By calculating a $[Cl^-]_{corrected}$ based on relative changes in $[Na^+]$, one assumes that any additional change in $SID_{Cl^-corrected}$ is due to changes in other anions (i.e., HCO_3^-, albumin, PO_4, or "other strong anions").

2. The equation is based on assumptions and estimations and thus is prone to be inaccurate. A major assumption is that all animals start with a mean $[Na^+]$ of a "normal" animal. Based on actual distribution of $[Na^+]$ in healthy animals, the assumption is rarely true. There is also an assumption that a "mean normal" concentration for one laboratory will apply to other laboratories. Again, this assumption is typically not true. If the formula is used, then a "mean normal"

concentration appropriate for the laboratory method (the same as used for patient's [Na$^+$]) should be used.

G. Other SID formulas have been proposed that include some but not all of the strong ions.[29,36] Also, there are not standardized names for SID formulas, and thus SID information should be interpreted carefully. For example, some formulas contain [fCa^{2+}], [fMg^{2+}], or [L-lactate], but not [acetoacetate] or [β-hydroxybutyrate]. Reference intervals for estimated SID values and possible causes for abnormal estimated SID values vary depending on the analytes that are or are not used in the formulas and the methods used to measure analyte concentrations.

IV. Comparison of SID formulas
   A. The relationship between SID$_{true}$ and SID$_3$ is shown in Eq. 10.10. SID$_3$ is a good approximation of SID$_{true}$ if concentrations of fCa^{2+}, fMg^{2+}, and uSA are small. However, when there is a high [uSA] such as occurs in lactic acidosis or ketoacidosis, the SID$_3$ value will be greater than the SID$_{true}$; that is, the SID$_3$ overestimates the SID$_{true}$.

Given Eq. 10.9a and 10.9b,   **(10.10.)**

$$SID_{true} = SID_3 + ([fCa^{2+}] + [fMg^{2+}]) - [uSA]$$

$$\text{or } SID_3 = SID_{true} - [fCa^{2+}] - [fMg^{2+}] + [uSA]$$

   B. The relationship between SID$_{true}$ and the other formulas used to estimate SID (Eq. 10.9b–e) varies with the analytes that are or are not included in the formulas. It is more difficult to compare SID$_{Cl^-corrected}$ with the other SID formulas. However, the SID$_{Cl^-corrected}$ would also overestimate the SID$_{true}$ if there were an increased [uSA].
   C. The changes in SID values that are caused by changes in weak ion concentrations can be seen by examining Eq. 10.11a–f (Eq. 10.11a is the same as Eq. 10.8c). As shown in Eq. 10.11e, changes in SID$_3$ occur when the sum of [HCO$_3^-$], [Alb^{x-}], [PO$_4^{y-}$], and [uSA] changes.
      1. If [Alb^{x-}], [PO$_4^{y-}$], and [uSA] stay constant, changes in SID$_3$ reflect changes in [HCO$_3^-$]; that is, ↑ SID$_3$ reflects ↑ [HCO$_3^-$] and thus a metabolic alkalosis, or ↓ SID$_3$ reflects ↓ [HCO$_3^-$] and thus a metabolic acidosis. However, the relationship between SID$_3$ and [HCO$_3^-$] is less predictable, or is not present, when there are changes in [Alb^{x-}], [PO$_4^{y-}$], and [uSA].
      2. Equation 10.11c also shows that SID$_{true}$ depends on two major factors: [HCO$_3^-$] and [A$_{TOT}$]. Thus, if PO$_4$ and protein concentrations do not change, changes in [HCO$_3^-$] change the SID$_{true}$. This is where the traditional approach and SID approach to acid-base balances have commonality.
         a. Metabolic alkalosis = ↑ [HCO$_3^-$] = ↑ SID$_{true}$
         b. Metabolic acidosis = ↓ [HCO$_3^-$] = ↓ SID$_{true}$
      3. Another way to examine Eq. 10.11a and b is in terms of the buffering capacity of plasma. The electrolytes in those equations that can buffer H$^+$ are HCO$_3^-$, PO$_4^{y-}$, and Alb^{x-}. Thus, in terms of the weak electrolytes, an increase in SID$_{true}$ indicates an increase in the plasma buffer concentration (i.e., traditional metabolic alkalosis). Conversely, a decrease in SID$_{true}$ indicates a decrease in the plasma buffer concentration (i.e., traditional metabolic acidosis).

Given Eq. 10.8b. and 10.9a.,   (**10.11a.**)
$$SID_{true} = ([OH^-] + [HCO_3^-] + [CO_3^{2-}] + [Alb^{x-}] + [PO_4^{y-}]) - ([H^+] + [NH_4^+])$$

Because typical plasma concentrations of OH^-, CO_3^{2-}, H^+, and NH_4^+ are relatively small,
$$SID_{true} \approx [HCO_3^-] + [Alb^{x-}] + [PO_4^{y-}]$$ (**10.11b.**)

Given $[Alb^{x-}] + [PO_4^{y-}] \approx [A_{TOT}]$,   (**10.11c.**)
$$SID_{true} \approx [HCO_3^-] + [A_{TOT}]$$

Given Eq. 10.10 and that typical plasma $[fCa^{2+}]$ and $[fMg^{2+}]$ are relatively small,
$$SID_{true} \approx SID_3 - [uSA]$$ (**10.11d.**)

Given Eq. 10.11c and 10.11d,   (**10.11e.**)
$$SID_3 - [uSA] \approx [HCO_3^-] + [A_{TOT}]$$
$$\text{or } SID_3 \approx [HCO_3^-] + [A_{TOT}] + [uSA]$$

Considering Eq. 10.9b, Eq. 10.11e, and that   (**10.11f.**)
anion gap = $([Na^+] + [K^+]) - ([Cl^-] + [HCO_3^-])$,
anion gap = $SID_3 - [HCO_3^-] \approx [A_{TOT}] + [uSA]$

D. For those who are accustomed to interpretation of anion gaps (see Chapter 9), Eq. 10.11f shows the relationship between anion gap and SID_3. As described in Chapter 9, the anion gap is mostly due to the ionic charge of proteins if there are not increased concentrations of organic anions.

E. The anion gap calculation can also be used to calculate a SID value (Eq. 10.12c). Because an increased anion gap typically indicates an increased concentration of anions other than HCO_3^- or Cl^-, the increase in anion gap can be used to estimate the [uSA]. This formula would provide a more accurate estimate of SID than does the SID_3 formula when there is a metabolic acidosis. However, the need to calculate a SID is minimal if a decreased $[HCO_3^-]$ has already been recognized.

Given that SID_{true} = (sum of strong cations) − (sum of strong anions)   (**10.12a.**)
$SID_{true} = ([Na^+] + [K^+] + [fCa^{2+}] + [fMg^{2+}]) - ([Cl^-] + [uSA])$
where uSA includes SO_4^{3-}, lactate, acetoacetate, β-hydroxybutyrate, other acidic anions of metabolism, and exogenous anions.

And that an increased anion gap (AG) $\approx$ [uSA]   (**10.12b.**)

Then $SID_{AG} = ([Na^+] + [K^+]) - ([Cl^-] + (AG_{patient} - AG_{normal}))$ (**10.12c.**)

V. Interpretation of abnormal SID_3 values
   A. According to Stewart's method and definitions, changes in SID_{true} create either an alkalosis or an acidosis. Based on the definitions and the calculation of SID_3, the major types of acid-base disorders are listed in Table 10.11. Note that the expected changes in the dependent variables (i.e., $[HCO_3^-]$ and pH) are those expected in the traditional approach to acid-base disorders; ↑ $[HCO_3^-]$ in metabolic alkaloses, and ↓ $[HCO_3^-]$ in metabolic acidoses.

Table 10.11. Classification of acid-base disorders from P_aCO_2, $A_{TOT,}$ and SID

Change in independent variable		Change in measured analyte	Classification	Expected dependent variable change	
				[HCO_3^-]	pH
P_aCO_2	↓	↓ P_aCO_2	Respiratory alkalosis	WRI	↑
	↑	↑ P_aCO_2	Respiratory acidosis	WRI	↓
A_{TOT}	↑	↑ Albumin[a]	Hyperalbuminemic acidosis	↓	↓
	↑	↑ PO_4	Hyperphosphatemic acidosis	↓	↓
	↓	↓ Albumin[b]	Hypoalbuminemic alkalosis	↑	↑
SID_t/SID_3[c]	↑/↑	↑ Na^+	Hypernatremic or contraction alkalosis[d]	↑	↑
	↑/↑	↓ Cl^-	Hypochloremic alkalosis	↑	↑
	↓/↓	↓ Na^+	Hyponatremic or dilutional acidosis[e]	↓	↓
	↓/↓	↑ Cl^-	Hyperchloremic acidosis	↓	↓
	↓/WRI	None[f]	Metabolic acidosis and ↑ [uSA][g]	↓	↓
	↓/↑	Variable[h]	Metabolic acidosis and ↑ [uSA][i]	↓	↓

[a] If hyperproteinemia, then hyperproteinemic acidosis

[b] If hypoproteinemia, then hypoproteinemic alkalosis

[c] $SID_t = SID_{true}$

[d] With loss of free water, [Na^+] and [Cl^-] increase proportionately, but [Na^+] increases more than [Cl^-] on an absolute basis. Therefore, SID increases (but mildly).

[e] Opposite explanation of hypernatremic alkalosis

[f] Concentrations of Na^+, K^+, and Cl^- are all WRI.

[g] Because the SID_3 is WRI, the acidosis would be recognized if it is known that either a ↓ [HCO_3^-] or an ↑ anion gap (which indicates ↑ [uSA]) is present.

[h] Could be found in hyponatremia, normonatremic, or hypernatremic animals. The SID_3 is increased because the difference between [$Na^+ + K^+$] and [Cl^-] is increased.

[i] The acidosis would be recognized if it is known that either a ↓ [HCO_3^-] or an ↑ anion gap (which indicates ↑ [uSA]) is present.

    B. Based on the definitions, changes in concentrations of two ions may cause a mixed acid-base disorder; for example, loss of plasma H_2O could result in concurrent hypernatremic alkalosis and hyperalbuminemic acidosis. The concurrent alkalosis and acidosis in the Stewart method raises the question of whether there is noSIDosis.☺

VI. As recommended by some authors, SID values should be interpreted with routine blood gas values (pH, Pco_2, and [HCO_3^-]) to determine whether the animal has an acid-base problem and whether the problem is respiratory or nonrespiratory (metabolic).[31,32] If the problem is a nonrespiratory acid-base disturbance, then the contributions of nonbicarbonate electrolytes can be explored with Stewart's method.

VII. Prior to the proposed use of the strong ion theory, an understanding of an animal's acid-base and electrolyte disorder was obtained through the interpretation of pH, Pco_2, [HCO_3^-], BE_B, [Na^+], [K^+], [Cl^-], anion gap, and albumin concentration (see the preceding

Acid-Base Abnormalities section and Chapter 9). Evaluation of such information has provided and will continue to provide an understanding of an animal's pathologic state.

VIII. Those who study SID theory and its application state that the SID approach requires species-specific values for A_{TOT}; that is, the sum of the concentrations of nonvolatile buffers, serum or plasma proteins, and PO_4.[35] As stated earlier (in the preceding sect. II.B.5) and in Eq. 10.11c, plasma A_{TOT} consists primarily of the various anionic forms of PO_4 and proteins (albumin and globulins).

A. There have been attempts to calculate plasma A_{TOT} values for healthy cattle,[37,38] dogs,[39] cats,[40] and birds.[41] The calculated values (mean ± sd) were obtained by using results from only 10 dogs, 10 cats, 12 pigeons, and 9 calves (or pooled bovine and ovine plasma). For most of the data, the variations in the calculated plasma A_{TOT} values represent the expected variations in plasma protein and PO_4 concentrations in such samples from healthy animals.

B. Using those calculated mean plasma A_{TOT} values and measured $[HCO_3^-]$, an SID value can be calculated (Eq. 10.11c). However because there are biologic variations in the serum concentrations of PO_4 and proteins, a mean A_{TOT} value may not be appropriate for all healthy animals and will definitely not be appropriate for animals that have abnormal protein and PO_4 concentrations. Also because of the lack of agreement in many clinical assays, plasma A_{TOT} values calculated for one set of assays may not be appropriate for another set of assays.

References

1. Heusel JW, Scott MG. 1999. Physiology and disorders of water, electrolytes, and acid-base metabolism. In: Burtis CA, Ashwood ER, eds. *Tietz Textbook of Clinical Chemistry*, 3rd edition, 1095–1120. Philadelphia: WB Saunders.
2. Siggaard-Andersen O, Fogh-Andersen N. 1995. Base excess or buffer base (strong ion difference) as measure of a non-respiratory acid-base disturbance. Acta Anaesthesiol Scand 39(Suppl 107):123–128.
3. Jones NL. 1987. *Blood Gases and Acid-Base Physiology*. New York: Thieme Medical.
4. Salyer JW, Chatburn RL, Dolcini DM. 1989. Measured vs calculated oxygen saturation in a population of pediatric intensive care patients. Respir Care 34:342–348.
5. Barker SJ, Tremper KK. 1993. Pulse oximetry. In: Ehrenwerth J, Eisenkraft JB, eds. *Anesthesia Equipment: Principles and Applications*, 249–263. St Louis: CV Mosby.
6. Jacobson JD, Miller MW, Matthews NS, Hartsfield SM, Knauer KW. 1992. Evaluation of accuracy of pulse oximetry in dogs. Am J Vet Res 53:537–540.
7. Whitehair KJ, Watney GCG, Leith DE, DeBowes RM. 1990. Pulse oximetry in horses. Vet Surg 19:243–248.
8. Huss BT, Anderson MA, Branson KR, Wagner-Mann CC, Mann FA. 1995. Evaluation of pulse oximeter probes and probe placement in healthy dogs. J Am Anim Hosp Assoc 31:9–14.
9. Jahr JS, Lurie F, Driessen B, Tang Z, Louie RF, Kullar R, Kost G. 2000. Validation of oxygen saturation measurements in a canine model of hemoglobin based oxygen carrier (HBOC) infusion. Clin Lab Sci 13:173–179.
10. Lurie F, Driessen B, Jahr JS, Reynoso R, Gunther RA. 2003. Validity of arterial and mixed venous oxygen saturation measurements in a canine hemorrhage model after resuscitation with varying concentrations of hemoglobin-based oxygen carrier. Anesth Analg 96:46–50.
11. Hopper K, Rezende ML, Haskins SC. 2005. Assessment of the effect of dilution of blood samples with sodium heparin on blood gas, electrolyte, and lactate measurements in dogs. Am J Vet Res 66:656–660.
12. Scott MG, Heusel JW, LeGrys VA. 1999. Electrolytes and blood gases. In: Burtis CA, Ashwood ER, eds. *Tietz Textbook of Clinical Chemistry*, 3rd edition, 1056–1092. Philadelphia: WB Saunders.
13. Deane JC, Dagleish MP, Benamou AE, Wolf BT, Marlin D. 2004. Effects of syringe material and temperature and duration of storage on the stability of equine arterial blood gas variables. Vet Anaesth Analg 31:250–257.
14. DiBartola SP, de Morais HSA. 1992. Respiratory acid-base disorders. In: DiBartola SP, ed. *Fluid Therapy in Small Animal Practice*, 1st edition, 258–275. Philadelphia: WB Saunders.
15. de Morais HA, DiBartola SP. 2000. Respiratory acid-base disorders. In: DiBartola SP, ed. *Fluid Therapy in Small Animal Practice*, 2nd edition, 241–250. Philadelphia: WB Saunders.

16. Rose BD, Post TW. 2001. *Clinical Physiology of Acid-Base and Electrolyte Disorders*, 5th edition. New York: McGraw-Hill.

17. i-STAT Corporation. 2000. Decreased PCO_2 results associated with thiopental sodium. East Windsor, NJ: i-STAT.

18. de Morais HS. 2000. Mixed acid-base disorders. In: DiBartola SP, ed. *Fluid Therapy in Small Animal Practice*, 2nd edition, 251–261. Philadelphia: WB Saunders.

19. de Morais HSA, DiBartola SP. 1991. Ventilatory and metabolic compensation in dogs with various diseases and signs of disease. J Vet Emerg Crit Care 1:39–49.

20. Muir WW III, Hubbell JAE. 1989. Acid-base balance and blood gases. In: *Handbook of Veterinary Anesthesia*, 191–201. St Louis: CV Mosby.

21. Lumb WV, Johns EW. 1984. *Veterinary Anesthesia*, 2nd edition. Philadelphia: Lea & Febiger.

22. Nunn JF. 1987. *Applied Respiratory Physiology*, 3rd edition. Boston: Butterworth.

23. Vaala WE, House JK. 2002. Manifestations of disease in the neonate. In: Smith BP, ed. *Large Animal Internal Medicine*, 3rd edition, 319–381. St Louis: CV Mosby.

24. Stewart JH, Rose RJ, Barko AM. 1984. Respiratory studies in foals from birth to seven days old. Equine Vet J 16:323–328.

25. Saklad M. 1953. Classification of hypoxia. In: Saklad M, ed. *Inhalation Therapy and Resuscitation*, 29–34. Springfield, IL: Charles C Thomas.

26. Ranney HM, Sharma V. 2001. Structure and function of hemoglobin. In: Beutler E, Lichtman MA, Coller BS, Kipps TJ, Seligsohn U, eds. *Williams Hematology*, 6th edition, 345–353. New York: McGraw-Hill.

27. Gootjes P, Moens Y, Lagerweij E. 1994. Pulse oximetry in horses: A study with the aid of an *in vitro* blood circuit. In: Proceedings of the Fifth International Congress of Veterinary Anesthesia, American College of Veterinary Anesthesiologists, Guelph, Canada, 135.

28. Stewart PA. 1983. Modern quantitative acid-base chemistry. Can J Physiol Pharmacol 61:1444–1461.

29. Fencl V, Leith DE. 1993. Stewart's quantitative acid-base chemistry: Applications in biology and medicine. Respir Physiol 91:1–16.

30. Eicker SW. 1990. An introduction to strong ion difference. Vet Clin North Am Food Anim Pract 6:45–49.

31. de Morais HSA. 1992. A nontraditional approach to acid-base disorders. In: DiBartola SP, ed. *Fluid Therapy in Small Animal Practice*, 1st edition, 297–316. Philadelphia: WB Saunders.

32. Russell KE, Hansen BD, Stevens JB. 1996. Strong ion difference approach to acid-base imbalances with clinical applications to dogs and cats. Vet Clin North Am Small Anim Pract 26:1185–1201.

33. Constable PD. 1999. Clinical assessment of acid-base status: Strong ion difference theory. Vet Clin North Am Food Anim Pract 15:447–471.

34. Singer RB, Hastings AB. 1948. An improved clinical method for the estimation of disturbances of the acid-base balance of human blood. Medicine (Baltimore) 27:223–242.

35. McCullough SM, Constable PD. 2003. Calculation of the total plasma concentration of nonvolatile weak acids and the effective dissociation constant of nonvolatile buffers in plasma for use in the strong ion approach to acid-base balance in cats. Am J Vet Res 64:1047–1051.

36. Constable PD. 1997. A simplified strong ion model for acid-base equilibria: Application to horse plasma. J Appl Physiol 83:297–311.

37. Constable PD, Stämpfli HR, Navetat H, Berchtold J, Schelcher F. 2005. Use of a quantitative strong ion approach to determine the mechanism for acid-base abnormalities in sick calves with or without diarrhea. J Vet Intern Med 19:581–589.

38. Constable PD. 2002. Calculation of variables describing plasma nonvolatile weak acids for use in the strong ion approach to acid-base balance in cattle. Am J Vet Res 63:482–490.

39. Constable PD, Stämpfli HR. 2005. Experimental determination of net protein charge and A(tot) and K(a) of nonvolatile buffers in canine plasma. J Vet Intern Med 19:507–514.

40. McCullough SM, Constable PD. 2003. Calculation of the total plasma concentration of nonvolatile weak acids and the effective dissociation constant of nonvolatile buffers in plasma for use in the strong ion approach to acid-base balance in cats. Am J Vet Res 64:1047–1051.

41. Stämpfli H, Taylor M, McNicoll C, Gancz AY, Constable PD. 2006. Experimental determination of net protein charge, [A]tot, and Ka of nonvolatile buffers in bird plasma. J Appl Physiol 100:1831–1836.

42. Ashwood ER, Kost G, Kenny M. 1983. Temperature correction of blood-gas and pH measurements. Clin Chem 29:1877–1885.

43. Cambier C, Wierinckx M, Clerbaux T, Detry B, Liardet MP, Marville V, Frans A, Gustin P. 2004. Haemoglobin oxygen affinity and regulating factors of the blood oxygen transport in canine and feline blood. Res Vet Sci 77:83–88.

44. Cambier C, Di PN, Clerbaux T, Amory H, Marville V, Detry B, Frans A, Gustin P. 2005. Blood-oxygen binding in healthy Standardbred horses. Vet J 169:251–256.

Chapter 11

CALCIUM, PHOSPHORUS, MAGNESIUM, AND THEIR REGULATORY HORMONES

Total Calcium (tCa^{2+}) Concentration 594
    I.   Physiologic Processes 594
    II. Analytical Concepts of $[tCa^{2+}]$ 596
    III. Hypercalcemia. 598
    IV. Hypocalcemia 602
Free Calcium (fCa^{2+}) Concentration 610
    I.   Physiologic Processes 610
    II. Analytical Concepts of $[fCa^{2+}]$ 610
    III. Abnormal Concentrations 613
    IV. Conceptual relationships of $[tCa^{2+}]$ and $[fCa^{2+}]$ 614
Inorganic Phosphorus (Pi) Concentration 615
    I.   Physiologic Processes 615
    II. Analytical Concepts of [Pi]. 617
    III. Hyperphosphatemia 618
    IV. Hypophosphatemia. 619
Total Magnesium (tMg^{2+}) Concentration 621
    I.   Physiologic Processes 621
    II. Analytical Concepts of $[tMg^{2+}]$. 622
    III. Hypermagnesemia 622
    IV. Hypomagnesemia. 623
Free Magnesium (fMg^{2+}) Concentration. 625
Immunoreactive Parathyroid Hormone (iPTH) Concentration. 626
Parathyroid Hormone–Related Protein (PTHrp) Concentration 628
Vitamin D Concentration 628
Calcitonin Concentration 630
Major Patterns for Calcium (Ca^{2+}) and Inorganic Phosphorus (Pi) Disorders 631

Table 11.1. Abbreviations and symbols in this chapter

[x]	x concentration (x = analyte)
1,25-DHCC	1,25-Dihydroxycholecalciferol (calcitriol)
24,25-DHCC	24,25-Dihydroxycholecalciferol
25-HCC	25-Hydroxycholecalciferol (calcidiol)
Ca^{2+}	Calcium
ECF	Extracellular fluid
EDTA	Ethylenediaminetetraacetic acid
fCa^{2+}	Free ionized calcium
fMg^{2+}	Free ionized magnesium
GFR	Glomerular filtration rate
GH	Growth hormone
HHM	Humoral hypercalcemia of malignancy
ICF	Intracellular fluid
iPTH	Immunoreactive parathyroid hormone
Mg^{2+}	Magnesium
Pi	Inorganic phosphorus
PO_4	Phosphate including PO_4^{3-}, HPO_4^{2-}, or $H_2PO_4^-$
PTH	Parathyroid hormone
PTHrp	Parathyroid hormone–related protein
RIA	Radioimmunoassay
SI	Système International d'Unités
tCa^{2+}	Total calcium
tMg^{2+}	Total magnesium
WRI	Within reference interval

TOTAL CALCIUM (tCa^{2+}) CONCENTRATION

I.   Physiologic processes

    A. Serum or plasma Ca^{2+} is distributed into three major fractions. *All Ca^{2+} in body fluids is ionized*, but some is free and some is bound to anionic molecules.

        1. General concepts

           a. fCa^{2+} (often referred to as *ionized calcium*): About 50 % of $[tCa^{2+}]$ is *fCa^{2+}*, which is present as free ions in plasma H_2O. The $[fCa^{2+}]$ is the portion of $[tCa^{2+}]$ that is hormonally regulated and contributes to pathologic states.

           b. Anion-bound Ca^{2+}

               (1) Bound to anionic proteins: About 40–45 % of tCa^{2+} is bound to negatively charged sites on proteins (80 % to albumin and 20 % to globulins).[1] Since binding is charge dependent, changes in blood pH slightly alter Ca^{2+} binding and thus slightly alter distribution of Ca^{2+} between bound and free fractions.

               (2) Bound to nonprotein anions: About 5–10 % of tCa^{2+} is bound to citrates, PO_4, lactate, and other small, diffusible anions.

        2. Using a filtration system to separate protein-bound Ca^{2+} from other Ca^{2+} fractions and measuring $[fCa^{2+}]$, the distribution of Ca^{2+} fractions in 13 dogs averaged 56 %

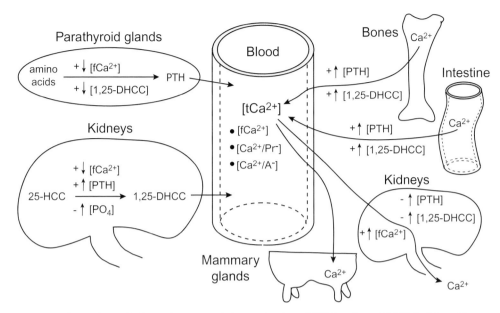

Fig. 11.1. Relationships of calcium kinetics and the production of PTH and 1,25-DHCC. (Note: Horse kidneys lack 1α-hydroxylase and thus do not form 1,25-DHCC.)

- PTH production in parathyroid glands is stimulated by ↓ [fCa²⁺] and ↓ [1,25-DHCC] and inhibited by ↑ [fCa²⁺] and ↑ [1,25-DHCC].
- Conversion of 25-HCC to 1,25-DHCC in kidneys is catalyzed by 1α-hydroxylase. The activity of 1α-hydroxylase is promoted by ↓ [fCa²⁺] and ↑ PTH and inhibited by ↑ [fCa²⁺] and ↑ [PO₄].
- Ca²⁺ mobilization from bone and Ca²⁺ absorption in intestine are promoted by ↑ [1,25-DHCC] and ↑ PTH. Less Ca²⁺ mobilization and absorption occur if there is ↓ [1,25-DHCC] or ↓ PTH.
- Urinary excretion of Ca²⁺ is enhanced by ↑ [fCa²⁺], and excretion is reduced by ↓ [fCa²⁺], ↑ PTH, and ↑ 1,25-DHCC. Increased excretion of anions may obligate Ca²⁺ excretion and thus decreases in [fCa²⁺].
- During lactation, a large amount of Ca²⁺ is excreted via milk.
- Ca²⁺ is present in plasma in three forms: fCa²⁺, Ca²⁺ bound to proteins, and Ca²⁺ bound to small anions such as citrate and PO₄.

+, positive effector or stimulates the process; −, negative effector or inhibits the process; Ca²⁺/Pr⁻, calcium bound to protein; and Ca²⁺/A⁻, calcium bound to nonprotein anions.

---

fCa²⁺, 34 % protein bound, and 10 % bound to other anions.[2] In a group of 20 horses, the [fCa²⁺] averaged 51 % of the [tCa²⁺].[3]

 B. Major factors that determine serum [tCa²⁺] (Fig. 11.1)

  1. Age: Young dogs (6–24 wk old) have serum [tCa²⁺] about 1–2 mg/dL greater than mature dogs.[4,5] Young foals (1–60 d) have serum [tCa²⁺] similar to adult values.[6] Kittens (4–6 wk to 20–24 wk) have serum [tCa²⁺] similar to adult values.[7] Age-related data were not found for calves.

  2. Because serum Ca²⁺ concentrations in common chemistry profiles represent the [tCa²⁺], a decrease in serum protein concentration (especially hypoalbuminemia) causes a decrease in the bound Ca²⁺ and thus may cause hypocalcemia.

  3. Absorption of Ca²⁺ in intestine (mostly in ileum, but from duodenum to colon)

   a. In dogs, cats, and cattle, intestinal Ca²⁺ absorption requires vitamin D to induce mucosal epithelial cell synthesis of Ca²⁺-binding proteins. PTH activity augments vitamin D actions to increase Ca^{2+} absorption, mostly by stimulating 1,25-DHCC production.

b. Based on renal failure studies in horses, Ca^{2+} absorption in the equine intestine depends less on vitamin D and more on the amount of dietary Ca^{2+}.[8] Equine kidneys lack 1α-hydroxylase (and thus do not convert 25-HCC to 1,25-DHCC) but can produce small quantities of 24,25-DHCC.[9]

4. Resorption from or deposition of Ca^{2+} in bone[10]

   a. PTH stimulates Ca^{2+} pumps in the osteocyte membrane system that promote Ca^{2+} movement from bone to bone fluid to ECF. Secondarily, PTH induces osteoblasts to change shape and enables osteoclasts to contact bone matrix, or to release substances that stimulate osteoclasts to degrade bone by enzymatic digestion and acidification.[11]

   b. Vitamin D enhances Ca^{2+} resorption from bone by promoting osteoclastic activity and by enhancing response to PTH.[12]

   c. Calcitonin blocks osteoclastic osteolysis through direct changes in osteoclasts and by reducing activation of osteoprogenitor cells. However, with continuous PTH stimulation, osteoclasts escape from the suppressive effects of calcitonin.

5. Resorption of fCa^{2+} from tubular fluid in kidney tubules[13]

   a. Ca^{2+} (free and bound to small anions) passes freely through the glomerular filtration barrier, but protein-bound Ca^{2+} should not pass through. About 66 % of filtered Ca^{2+} is resorbed passively in proximal tubules with a Na^+-Ca^{2+} cotransport system, 25 % in the ascending limb of the loop of Henle, and the remainder is resorbed in the distal tubules. PTH regulates the Ca^{2+} resorption in the ascending limb of the loop of Henle and in the distal tubule by activating a hormone-specific adenylate cyclase system. Vitamin D plays a relatively minor role by promoting Ca^{2+} resorption through the formation of calbindin, a Ca^{2+}-binding protein in the distal nephron.

   b. Angiotensin II stimulates the resorption of Na^+ in the proximal tubules via a Na^+-Ca^{2+} cotransport system. Ca^{2+} is concurrently resorbed.

C. Ca^{2+} and PO_4 interaction.

1. The $[fCa^{2+}]$ and $[PO_4]$ in plasma are great enough in healthy animals that $Ca_3(PO_4)_2$ complexes would form if inhibitors were not present.[14]

2. $Ca^{2+} \times PO_4$: When the product of the $[tCa^{2+}]$ and the [Pi] (both in mg/dL) exceeds 70, metastatic mineralization of tissues (kidneys and lungs) tends to occur. However, precipitation may not occur, because it may depend on other factors such as variations in inhibitors of precipitation and relative amounts of Ca^{2+} and PO_4.

II. Analytical concepts of $[tCa^{2+}]$

A. Sample

1. Serum is the preferred sample for $[tCa^{2+}]$. Heparinized plasma may be used in some assays.

2. Blood anticoagulants that bind Ca^{2+} (EDTA, citrate, and oxalate) should not be used in samples for Ca^{2+} assays.

3. In people, prolonged venous occlusion during blood collection may increase the $[tCa^{2+}]$ by 0.5–1.0 mg/dL.[1]

B. Common clinical assays are photometric assays that measure $[tCa^{2+}]$ (free + bound).

1. o-Cresolphthalein assay: o-Cresolphthalein reacts with Ca^{2+} to form a red complex.

2. Arsenazo III dye colorimetric assay: Bound Ca^{2+} is liberated from anions and then Ca^{2+} reacts with Arsenazo III dye to produce a colored complex. In some systems, aerobic sample handling may increase measured $[tCa^{2+}]$ by 0.4 mg/dL when the sample's pH increases because of the loss of CO_2 (see Chapter 10).

C. Unit conversion: mg/dL × 0.2495 = mmol/L, and mEq/L × 0.5 = mmol/L (SI unit, nearest 0.02 mmol/L)[15]

D. Because a large portion of tCa^{2+} is protein bound but the body regulates the $[fCa^{2+}]$, the $[tCa^{2+}]$ may be decreased because of hypoproteinemia or hypoalbuminemia when the animal does not have a defect in regulating the $[fCa^{2+}]$. To estimate the effect of lower protein and albumin concentrations, correction or adjusting formulas have been proposed.

1. Canine adjusted $[tCa^{2+}]$ considering albumin concentration (Eq. 11.1a)[4]

$$\text{Canine adjusted } [tCa^{2+}] = \text{measured } [tCa^{2+}] - \text{measured [albumin]} + 3.5 \ (\pm 1.3) \qquad \textbf{(11.1a.)}$$

Example: If $[tCa^{2+}]$ = 8.0 mg/dL & [albumin] = 1.0 g/dL;
Canine adjusted $[tCa^{2+}]$ = 8.0 − 1.0 + 3.5 (± 1.3) = 10.5 ± 1.3
   = 9.2 to 11.8 mg/dL
Interpretation: If the dog was not hypoalbuminemic, its serum $[tCa^{2+}]$ would be from 9.2 to 11.8 mg/dL in 95 % of canine samples.

$$\text{Canine adjusted } [tCa^{2+}] = \text{measured } [tCa^{2+}] - (0.4 \times \text{measured [TP]}) + 3.3 \ (\pm 1.6) \qquad \textbf{(11.1b.)}$$

Example: If $[tCa^{2+}]$ = 8.0 mg/dL & [TP] = 4.0 g/dL;
Canine adjusted $[tCa^{2+}]$ = 8.0 − (0.4 × 4.0) + 3.3 (± 1.6) = 9.7 ± 1.6
   = 8.1 to 11.3 mg/dL
Interpretation: If the dog was not hypoproteinemic, its serum $[tCa^{2+}]$ would be from 8.1 to 11.3 mg/dL in 95 % of canine samples.

a. Some authors do not include the "± 1.3," which is an estimate of the 95 % confidence interval of the published data.

b. The formula should be used cautiously for three reasons: (1) the adjusted $[tCa^{2+}]$ is at best an estimate; (2) the formula was generated using canine tCa^{2+} and albumin concentrations determined by one set of assays, and an identical formula would probably not be obtained if other assays were used; and (3) the formula does not consider the variations in Ca^{2+} binding to globulins. Ca^{2+} is bound to albumin and some globulins. The relative amount of Ca^{2+} bound to albumin and globulins varies with different albumin to globulin ratios; for example, samples with panhypoproteinemia versus those with hypoalbuminemia and hyperglobulinemia.

2. Canine adjusted $[tCa^{2+}]$ considering total protein concentration (Eq. 11.1b)

a. Some authors do not include the "± 1.6," which is an estimate of the 95 % confidence interval of the published data.

b. Even though the formula does include total protein concentration, it should be used cautiously for the aforementioned reasons.

3. Other investigators have found statistically significant correlations between [albumin] and $[tCa^{2+}]$ in dogs, cats, horses, and cattle, but the correlations were weak, especially in cattle.[16,17] Although the general principle that $[tCa^{2+}]$ varies with [albumin] is true, the weakness and variation in the relationship among

individuals suggest that rigid correction formulas may not be appropriate, especially in cattle.

4. In a retrospective analysis of 1633 canine samples, it was concluded that these adjusted [tCa^{2+}] equations do not reliably predict whether a dog has either an increased or decreased serum [fCa^{2+}].[18] This report did not indicate whether there was analytical agreement between the methods used for these samples and the methods used in the original 1982 study on which the equations were based.[4] Also, the basis for the reference intervals used to classify results as increased or decreased was not provided, and the magnitude of the discrepancies between measured and calculated values was not evaluated.

5. It is recommended that the potential effects of dysproteinemia be considered when interpreting [tCa^{2+}]. If the formulas for adjusting the measured concentrations in canine sera are used, the calculated values should be considered only rough approximations.

III. Hypercalcemia (Table 11.2)
A. Increased Ca^{2+} mobilization from bone or absorption in intestine
1. Increased PTH or PTHrp activity
a. Primary hyperparathyroidism[19-21]
(1) Parathyroid adenomas or carcinomas secrete PTH that stimulates Ca^{2+} resorption from bone and increases Ca^{2+} absorption in the intestine. Renal excretion of Ca^{2+} may be increased because hypercalcemia causes an increased filtered load (more filtered than can be resorbed even with increased PTH activity) but not enough to prevent hypercalcemia.
(2) Hypophosphatemia is expected because PTH is a potent phosphaturic agent. If GFR is decreased, there may be normophosphatemia or hyperphosphatemia because PTH cannot promote phosphaturia if PO$_4$ does not enter the tubular fluid.
(3) The [iPTH] is expected to be WRI to increased. Of 210 hypercalcemic dogs with primary hyperparathyroidism, 73 % had an [iPTH] WRI and 27 % had an increased [iPTH].[22] In the presence of hypercalcemia, an appropriate physiologic response would be a decreased [iPTH]. Thus, a [iPTH] that is WRI, particularly in the upper range of the reference interval concurrent with hypercalcemia, indicates an inappropriate release of PTH.
b. Humoral hypercalcemia of malignancy (HHM) (pseudo-hyperparathyroidism)
(1) In some paraendocrine neoplasms, a hypercalcemic agent is produced by cells that normally do not produce the agent. Nearly all neoplasms and especially carcinomas have the potential to be paraendocrine.
(2) Some paraendocrine neoplasms produce PTHrp. *PTHrp* is a polypeptide; its first 13 N-terminal amino acids are very similar to those of the N-terminal of PTH. It has bone osteoclastic and renal resorptive effects similar to PTH. Many normal cells produce PTHrp, but very little of the PTHrp produced by healthy cells enters blood.[10] PTHrp plays important roles in fetal development, but PTH governs systemic Ca^{2+} homeostasis after birth.
(3) Neoplasms known to produce PTHrp (Note: Only some neoplasms of each type are associated with hypercalcemia, and hypercalcemia without increased PTHrp does not exclude lymphoma or other neoplasms.)

Table 11.2. Diseases and conditions that cause hypercalcemia

Increased Ca^{2+} mobilization from bone or absorption in intestine
  Increased PTH or PTHrp activity
    Primary hyperparathyroidism (parathyroid neoplasia)
    *Humoral hypercalcemia of malignancy (HHM): lymphoma, several carcinomas
    Humoral hypercalcemia of benign disorders (canine schistosomiasis)
  Increased vitamin D activity (hypervitaminosis D)
    Exogenous vitamin D
      Rodenticides containing cholecalciferol
      Compounds containing tacalcitol or calcipotriol
      Plants containing ergocalciferol (vitamin D_2)
      Excess dietary supplementation
    Endogenous vitamin D
      Granulomatous inflammation: blastomycosis, histoplasmosis, cryptococcosis,
        pulmonary angiostrongylosis
      Neoplasm-associated hypervitaminosis D
  Neoplasia in bone: myeloma, lymphoma, metastatic neoplasm
Decreased urinary excretion of Ca^{2+}
  Renal failure
    *Horses (common in both acute and chronic)
    Dogs and cats (uncommon in acute and chronic)
  Hypoadrenocorticism in dogs and cats (other theories: increased Ca^{2+} bound to protein or
    citrate)
  Thiazide diuretics
Increased protein-bound Ca^{2+}: hyperglobulinemia in multiple myeloma
Other or unknown mechanisms
  Excess intravenous infusion of Ca^{2+}
  Hemoconcentration
  Hypothyroidism (juvenile onset)
  Retained fetus and endometritis in a dog
  Idiopathic hypercalcemia in cats

* A relatively common disease or condition
Note: The $[tCa^{2+}]$ in healthy young dogs (< 1 yr old, especially in large breeds) may be up to
2 mg/dL higher than the $[tCa^{2+}]$ reference intervals for mature dogs.

    (a) In dogs, these neoplasms include lymphoma (usually T cell),[23,24] apocrine gland carcinoma,[24] other carcinomas (pulmonary, nasal, mammary, squamous cell, thyroid, and thymic),[24] and malignant melanoma.[25] Lymphoma is the most common neoplasm associated with hypercalcemia in dogs, followed by apocrine gland carcinoma.
    (b) In cats, these neoplasms include pulmonary carcinoma, undifferentiated carcinoma, thyroid carcinoma, and lymphoma.[26]
    (c) In horses, myeloma has been reported to produce PTHrp.[27]
  (4) Documentation of PTHrp involvement was limited by availability of valid assays for many years. Other hypercalcemia-inducing neoplasms that have been reported without documented increases in [PTHrp] include the following:

(a) In dogs, these neoplasms include epidermoid carcinoma[28] and metastatic adenocarcinoma.[29]

(b) In cats, these neoplasms include feline myeloproliferative disease[30] and squamous cell carcinoma.[31]

(c) In horses, these neoplasms include gastric carcinoma,[32] lymphoma,[33–35] and adrenocortical carcinoma.[36]

(5) Other expected findings

(a) Hypophosphatemia may be present. Its presence depends on the phosphaturic action of the agent relative to GFR. Decreased GFR reduces the amount of PO_4 that enters the tubular fluid and thus reduces the amount of PO_4 that is influenced by PTH activity.

(b) Serum [iPTH] determined by an N-terminal assay is often WRI for reasons that are not understood. Increased $[fCa^{2+}]$ should decrease PTH production.[24] In people, intact PTH assays are used to detect suppressed PTH production associated with HHM.

(c) Serum [PTHrp] should be increased if PTHrp is the hypercalcemic agent.

c. Humoral hypercalcemia of benign disorders

(1) In people, increased PTHrp production by benign neoplasms has been recognized and has been called *humoral hypercalcemia of benignancy.*[37]

(2) Two dogs with schistosomiasis caused by *Heterobilharzia americana* had hypercalcemia, normophosphatemia, increased [PTHrp], and decreased [iPTH].[38] It was concluded that the increased [PTHrp] was caused by the associated granulomatous inflammation. Necropsy failed to detect evidence of neoplasia.

2. Increased vitamin D activity (hypervitaminosis D)

a. Excessive vitamin D activity causes hypercalcemia through multiple processes. Hyperphosphatemia may be a concurrent finding because vitamin D promotes intestinal absorption of PO_4.

(1) It stimulates formation of Ca^{2+}-binding proteins (*calbindins*)[39] in intestinal mucosa so that more dietary Ca^{2+} is absorbed.

(2) It enhances bone resorption by making osteolytic cells more responsive to PTH.

(3) It decreases renal excretion of Ca^{2+} (perhaps through increased calbindin synthesis).

b. Sources of exogenous vitamin D

(1) Ingestion of a rodenticide containing cholecalciferol (Quintox, Rampage, or Rat-Be-Gone), which is converted to 25-HCC.[40]

(2) Ingestion of tacalcitol or calcipotriol by dogs,[41–43] the latter (also known as calcipotriene) being present in a topical ointment (Dovonex) that is used for human psoriasis

(3) Ingestion of plants containing ergocalciferol (vitamin D_2)[44,45] including *Cestrum diurnum* (day-blooming jessamine) in Florida[46] or *Solanum* in Hawaii, Brazil, and Argentina[10]

(4) Excessive dietary intake of vitamin D,[45,47–49] including ingestion of misformulated commercial feeds

c. Sources of endogenous vitamin D

(1) Granulomatous inflammation

(a) Hypercalcemia is reported in cases of blastomycosis,[50] histoplasmosis,[51] cryptococcosis,[52] and pulmonary angiostrongylosis.[53]

      (b) The hypercalcemia is produced when stimulated histiocytes or macrophages produce vitamin D (1,25-DHCC).

    (2) Neoplasm-associated hypervitaminosis D: Inappropriately high vitamin D concentrations have been reported with canine apocrine gland adenocarcinoma and lymphoma.[24] The neoplastic cells may be producing vitamin D or stimulating vitamin D synthesis in other cells.

  3. Neoplasia (hemic or nonhemic) in bone

    a. Hypercalcemic agents other than PTH, PTHrp, or vitamin D have been associated with malignancies in bone. Some dogs with lymphoma and myeloma have localized bone resorption and corresponding hypercalcemia.[10] The hypercalcemic agents may be working locally or systemically and may include interleukin 1, interleukin 6, tumor growth factor, tumor necrosis factor, and prostaglandins.[10,24]

    b. The [Pi] may be within reference intervals or increased.

B. Decreased urinary excretion of Ca^{2+}

  1. Renal insufficiency or failure

    a. Horses with some acute or chronic renal diseases

      (1) In health, equine kidneys excrete excess dietary Ca^{2+}. Renal diseases that decrease GFR impair renal excretion of Ca^{2+} and thus cause or contribute to hypercalcemia.[54] Lowering dietary Ca^{2+} intake by switching from alfalfa hay to grass hay can reduce or eliminate the hypercalcemia, but the impaired GFR persists.[55] Alfalfa hay can contain 2–10 times the Ca^{2+} content of grass or mixed hay.[56]

      (2) Hypophosphatemia may be present.

      (3) Horses with hypercalcemic renal failure have a decreased [iPTH].[57]

    b. Dogs and cats with acute or chronic renal disease

      (1) Occasional dogs and cats with acute renal failure are hypercalcemic. Hypercalcemia may be due to an increased concentration of Ca^{2+} bound to citrate or PO_4. Raisin and grape toxicoses frequently result in hypercalcemic acute renal failure.[58]

      (2) Of dogs with chronic renal failure, 10–15 % are reported to be hypercalcemic, which appears to be primarily due to binding of Ca^{2+} to retained anions.[59] However, most dogs with chronic renal failure have a low-normal to mildly decreased $[tCa^{2+}]$. Binding of Ca^{2+} to retained anions may also yield normocalcemia ($[tCa^{2+}]$ WRI) that masks a decrease in $[fCa^{2+}]$.

  2. Hypoadrenocorticism (Addison's disease) in dogs and cats

    a. About 30 % of dogs with hypoadrenocorticism are hypercalcemic.[10,60] Hypercalcemia has also been described in cats with hypoadrenocorticism.[61,62] The reason for the hypercalcemia is not established but probably is at least partially caused by decreased renal excretion and might be caused by increased Ca^{2+} binding to protein or citrate.

    b. Renal Ca^{2+} excretion in adrenalectomized dogs is decreased by excessive tubular resorption of Ca^{2+}.[63] The reason for enhanced tubular resorption is not established but may involve angiotensin II or cortisol deficiency.

      (1) When dogs with hypoadrenocorticism become hypovolemic because of vomiting, diarrhea, or impaired renal concentrating ability, angiotensin II activity increases. Angiotensin II promotes Na^+ resorption in proximal renal tubules via a Na^+-Ca^{2+} cotransport system.[13] Thus, enhanced resorption of

Na^+ may also promote the proximal tubular resorption of Ca^{2+} and cause hypercalcemia. Concurrent hemoconcentration itself may slightly increase the serum $[tCa^{2+}]$.

   (2) Administration of glucocorticoids does increase renal excretion of Ca^{2+}. Thus, a deficiency in cortisol may allow more Ca^{2+} to be resorbed.

   3. Ruptured urinary bladder in foals: These foals may develop hypercalcemia (authors' unpublished data), but most do not. When present, the hypercalcemia is probably caused by the resorption of urinary Ca^{2+} from the peritoneal cavity.

   4. Thiazide diuretics: These act in the distal nephron to promote hypernatruria and, secondarily, volume depletion. Hypovolemia promotes enhanced proximal tubular resorption of Na^+ and, secondarily, proximal tubular resorption of Ca^{2+}.[13] Thiazides also promote the resorption of Ca^{2+} in the distal tubules.[13] This form of hypercalcemia is rarely reported in domestic animals but does occur in dogs.[64]

C. Increased protein-bound Ca^{2+}: In some cases of marked hyperproteinemia associated with multiple myeloma, there is an increase in negatively charged globulins that bind cations including Ca^{2+}. When fCa^{2+} associates with proteins, the $[fCa^{2+}]$ transiently decreases and there is compensatory release of PTH to increase $[fCa^{2+}]$. The net result is increased $[tCa^{2+}]$ and $[fCa^{2+}]$ WRI.

D. Other or unknown mechanisms
   1. Intravenous infusion of Ca^{2+}: This can be a mechanism if the rate of administration exceeds the rate of renal excretion.
   2. Hemoconcentration: If hypercalcemia occurs, expect it to be mild and associated with increased protein-bound or small anion-bound Ca^{2+}. It may also be related to angiotensin II–stimulated transport of Na^+ and Ca^{2+} in proximal tubules.
   3. Juvenile-onset hypothyroidism:[65] This may be caused by increased intestinal absorption and decreased renal excretion of Ca^{2+}.
   4. A retained fetus and endometritis in a dog[66]
   5. Idiopathic hypercalcemia: This was found in a group of cats that did not have recognized hypercalcemic disorders. Some of the cats had calcium oxalate urolithiasis.[67]

IV. Hypocalcemia (Table 11.3)
   A. Hypoalbuminemic hypocalcemia (hypoproteinemic hypocalcemia)[4]
      1. Hypocalcemia results from a decreased concentration of negatively charged proteins and therefore of protein-bound Ca^{2+}. The regulation of the $[fCa^{2+}]$ would be adequate in these animals unless there is a concurrent defect in the regulation of the $[fCa^{2+}]$.
      2. It has been called *pseudo-hypocalcemia* because the $[fCa^{2+}]$ does not decrease and clinical signs of hypocalcemia do not occur. However, the animal truly has hypocalcemia when the $[tCa^{2+}]$ is lower than the appropriate reference interval.
   B. Decreased PTH activity
      1. Primary hypoparathyroidism
         a. Parathyroid glands are damaged (by trauma, surgery, neoplasia, or inflammation) and do not respond to hypocalcemia or do not release adequate quantities of PTH to prevent hypocalcemia.
         b. Hypocalcemia is caused by decreased resorption of Ca^{2+} from bone and/or decreased Ca^{2+} absorption in the intestine. Renal excretion of Ca^{2+} should be increased initially because of decreased PTH-stimulated resorption, but it may decrease due to the low filtered Ca^{2+} load when hypocalcemia is present.

Table 11.3. Diseases and conditions that cause hypocalcemia

*Hypoalbuminemia (hypoproteinemia)
Decreased PTH activity
    Primary hypoparathyroidism (damaged parathyroid gland)
    Pseudo-hypoparathyroidism (decreased PTH receptor responsiveness)
    Hypomagnesemia (bovine grass tetany)
Inadequate Ca^{2+} mobilization from bone or absorption in intestine
    Hypovitaminosis D
      *Chronic renal disease or failure in dogs, cats, and cattle
      Protein-losing enteropathy in dogs
      Dietary vitamin D deficiency (rare)
    Vitamin D–receptor defect rickets (vitamin D–dependent rickets, type II)
    Exocrine pancreatic insufficiency (dogs)
  *Pregnancy, parturient, or lactational hypocalcemia (milk fever, puerperal tetany)
    Hypercalcitonism: thyroid C-cell neoplasia, iatrogenic (calcitonin therapy)
    Nutritional hypocalcemia (rare)
    Oxalate toxicity
Excess urinary excretion of Ca^{2+}
    Ethylene glycol toxicosis (dogs and cats)
    Intravenous HCO_3^- infusions
    Furosemide treatment
Ca^{2+} binding with diffusible anions
    Ca^{2+}-binding anticoagulants: EDTA, citrate, oxalate (in vivo or in vitro)
    Tetracycline administration
Ca^{2+} deposition during fracture healing
Other or unknown mechanisms
    *Acute pancreatitis in dogs and cats
    Urinary tract obstruction
    Acute renal failure
    Phosphate enemas
    Blister beetle poisoning (cantharidiasis) in horses
    Myopathies: transport tetany, exertional rhabdomyolysis, malignant hypothermia,
      endurance-type exercise
    Acute tumor lysis syndrome
    Rumen overload (acute carbohydrate ruminal engorgement)

* A relatively common disease or condition
Note: The [tCa^{2+}] may be falsely decreased if the sample contains EDTA (wrong tube or contamination of clot tube). A concurrent false hyperkalemia would be expected with the potassium salt of EDTA.

    c. The serum [iPTH] will be decreased or low-normal. In the presence of hypocalcemia and functional parathyroid glands, the [iPTH] should be increased as a physiologic response.

    d. Hyperphosphatemia is expected because of increased resorption of PO_4 by renal tubules (because of less PTH to promote phosphaturia), and thus renal excretion of PO_4 is decreased. However, renal excretion of PO_4 may increase later because hyperphosphatemia causes an increased filtered PO_4 load.

e. Hyperphosphatemia enhances hypocalcemia by inhibiting renal formation of 1,25-DHCC (except in horses).

2. Pseudo-hypoparathyroidism
   a. In this rare disorder, PTH receptors or post-PTH receptor pathways are unresponsive. Therefore, the [fCa^{2+}] decreases because of diminished PTH effects on intestine, bone, and kidneys.
   b. The [Pi] may be increased because of inadequate renal excretion of PO$_4$.
   c. The [iPTH] should be increased because of the hypocalcemia.

3. Hypomagnesemia
   a. Hypomagnesemia caused by Mg^{2+} depletion may produce a functional hypoparathyroid state and hypocalcemia. The dysfunction may be due to two processes:
      (1) Mg^{2+}-depleted cells may be resistant to PTH. PTH cellular responses are mediated by adenylate cyclase, which requires Mg^{2+}.
      (2) Parathyroid cells secrete less PTH either because of diminished cyclic adenosine monophosphate (cAMP) formation (impaired adenylate cyclase) or because of diminished competitive inhibition of Ca^{2+} binding to parathyroid cells. In the presence of hypomagnesemia, there may be more available binding sites for Ca^{2+} on the parathyroid cells and thus a lesser [fCa^{2+}] is able to inhibit PTH secretion.[68]
   b. These mechanisms may explain the hypocalcemia of bovine grass tetany. Also a dog with a protein-losing enteropathy had a marked hypomagnesemia, hypocalcemia, decreased [fCa^{2+}], and a [iPTH] WRI. The [iPTH] was considered to be inappropriate in the presence of a decreased [fCa^{2+}] and thus reflected a functional hypoparathyroid state.[69]

C. Inadequate Ca^{2+} mobilization from bone or absorption in intestine
   1. Hypovitaminosis D
      a. Chronic renal disease and failure in dogs, cats, and cattle.
         (1) Dogs, cats, and cattle with chronic renal disease may have a low-normal [tCa^{2+}] or mild hypocalcemia because of abnormal vitamin D metabolism. To compensate for hypocalcemia or low vitamin D concentration, dogs, cats, and cattle develop secondary hyperparathyroidism. Similar changes are not expected in horses because equine kidneys lack 1α-hydroxylase activity[9] and decreased GFR in horses tends to cause hypercalcemia, not hypocalcemia.
         (2) The pathogenesis of secondary renal hyperparathyroidism is illustrated in Fig. 11.2. Sequential steps of the progressive state are shown in Fig. 11.3.
         (3) Tissue mineralization occurring secondary to hyperphosphatemia may contribute to hypocalcemia in renal failure.
      b. Protein-losing enteropathy in dogs[70]
         (1) Dogs with lymphangiectasia and lymphocytic or plasmacytic enteritis had concurrent findings of hypocalcemia, decreased [fCa^{2+}], decreased [25-HCC], and decreased [1,25-DHCC].
         (2) The vitamin D deficiency may be due to decreased absorption of vitamin D because of extensive intestinal mucosal disease.
      c. Dietary vitamin D deficiency (experimental)[71,72]
   2. Vitamin D–receptor defect rickets (vitamin D–dependent rickets, type II)
      a. The clinical manifestations of vitamin D–receptor defect rickets are produced by defective target-organ receptors and response to vitamin D (1,25-DHCC). The

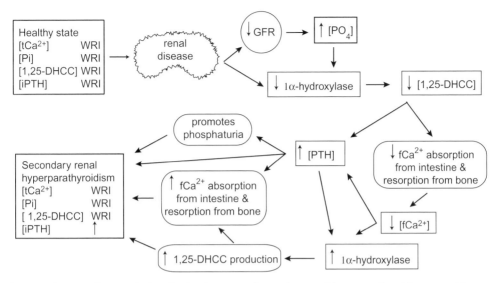

Fig. 11.2. Sequential events during the development of secondary renal hyperparathyroidism caused by chronic renal disease in dogs, cats, and cattle. Eventually, tCa²⁺, Pi, and 1,25-DHCC concentrations may be abnormal (see Fig. 11.3).

- Renal disease causes a loss of nephrons and a decrease in GFR, which causes less PO_4 to be filtered from plasma and a mild hyperphosphatemia develops.
- Damaged tubular epithelial cells may result in less endocytic resorption of 25-HCC and vitamin D–binding protein.
- Either because of the damaged tubular cells or inhibition of 1α-hydroxylase by increased $[PO_4]$, there is less conversion of 25-HCC to 1,25-DHCC, and thus less vitamin D is available for Ca^{2+} metabolism.
- Decreased [1,25-DHCC] leads to ↓ [fCa²⁺] and perhaps ↓ [tCa²⁺] because of ↓ intestinal Ca^{2+} absorption and ↓ Ca^{2+} resorption from bone.
- Decreased [1,25-DHCC] also reduces the 1,25-DHCC inhibition of PTH synthesis, and thus PTH synthesis increases.
- Decreased [fCa²⁺] causes ↑ PTH production, ↓ calcitonin release, and ↑1α-hydroxylase activity.
- Increased PTH promotes vitamin D–dependent Ca^{2+} absorption in intestine, stimulates Ca^{2+} and PO_4 resorption from bone, stimulates 1α-hydroxylase activity in kidneys, and inhibits renal PO_4 resorption (promotes phosphaturia).
- Actions of increased PTH due to parathyroid hyperplasia tend to correct the hypocalcemia, hyperphosphatemia, and decreased [1,25-DHCC]. At this point, secondary renal hyperparathyroidism is present.

defective intestinal absorption of Ca^{2+} and defective responses in bone and kidneys cause hypocalcemia, a compensatory increase in [1,25-DHCC], and secondary hyperparathyroidism (with increased [iPTH]).

    b. A young cat that had this disorder had hypocalcemia (3.9 mg/dL), increased [iPTH], and increased [1,25-DHCC].[73] It was presented because of vomiting, diarrhea, muscle tremors, and mydriasis.

  3. Exocrine pancreatic insufficiency (dogs)

    a. Idiopathic pancreatic acinar atrophy, chronic pancreatitis, pancreatic neoplasia, or pancreatic surgery may lead to exocrine pancreatic insufficiency and thus cause incomplete digestion of dietary lipids and other ingesta.

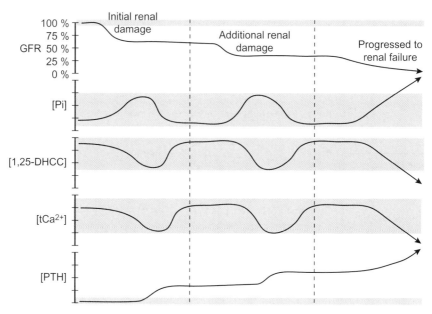

Fig. 11.3. Schematic pathogenesis of secondary renal hyperparathyroidism in dogs, cats, and cattle. *Shaded areas* represent reference intervals for GFR or each analyte concentration.

- Initial renal damage: The sequence of events described in Fig. 11.2 initially compensates for the decreased clearance of PO_4 and inadequate activation of vitamin D. A new homeostasis in Ca^{2+} and PO_4 balance is maintained by ↑ PTH secretion.
- Additional renal damage: As renal disease progresses and more nephrons are lost, pathophysiologic responses recur that stimulate more PTH synthesis in an attempt to maintain physiologic concentrations of fCa^{2+}, PO_4, and 1,25-DHCC.
- Progressed to renal failure: Eventually, renal disease reduces GFR sufficiently for serum [Pi] to remain increased, and insufficient 1,25-DHCC and PTH are made to maintain $[fCa^{2+}]$. The animal is presented with clinical signs of renal insufficiency or failure, azotemia, impaired ability to concentrate or dilute urine, mild hypocalcemia, and hyperphosphatemia. The $[tCa^{2+}]$ may not reflect the abnormal regulation of the $[fCa^{2+}]$ because of the Ca^{2+} that is bound to anions that are not excreted in renal failure.

      b. Dietary Ca^{2+} may be less available for intestinal absorption because of its binding to partially digested lipids. Also, maldigestion of lipids may reduce absorption of fat-soluble vitamins, including vitamin D.

      c. Dogs with exocrine pancreatic insufficiency frequently develop hypoalbuminemia that also would contribute to the hypocalcemia.

    4. Pregnancy, parturient, or lactational hypocalcemia

      a. Parturient hypocalcemia (milk fever) in cattle

        (1) Hypocalcemia results from excess Ca^{2+} loss (via milk or fetal bone development) relative to intestinal absorption and bone resorption. Because most paretic cattle have an increased [iPTH] and an increased [1,25-DHCC], the disorder involves an inadequate response of target cells (e.g., decreased receptors or defective biochemical pathways).[74,75] Dietary factors that promote metabolic alkalosis may decrease the target cell response to PTH.[76]

(2) A decreased $[fCa^{2+}]$ leads to clinical signs of hypocalcemia (hyperesthesia and tetany early, and paresis to flaccid paralysis later) because of defective neural transmissions and muscle contractions.

(3) Hypophosphatemia may occur because of lactation, poor bone resorption, and the phosphaturic action of PTH.

b. Puerperal tetany or eclampsia (bitches, mares, and ewes)[77]
   (1) It is associated with peak lactation and corresponding peak loss of Ca^{2+} in milk.
   (2) An animal may have concurrent hypomagnesemia and hypophosphatemia or hyperphosphatemia.

c. Preparturient hypocalcemia in queens[78]
   (1) Clinical signs (anorexia, depression, and lethargy) occurred 3–17 d prior to parturition.
   (2) Three queens had a decreased $[tCa^{2+}]$. The $[fCa^{2+}]$ was decreased in the one cat in which it was measured.

5. Hypercalcitonism
   a. This is usually caused by thyroid C-cell neoplasms (medullary thyroid carcinomas), which are relatively uncommon neoplasms reported most often in older bulls.[79] When associated with C-cell neoplasms, hypercalcitonism usually causes only mild hypocalcemia because of the following:
      (1) Neoplasms are seen in older animals, and their bones are relatively refractory to calcitonin (calcitonin does not inhibit PTH-stimulated osteoclastic activity).
      (2) Lowering of the $[fCa^{2+}]$ causes a compensatory increase in PTH production that attempts to maintain a physiologic $[fCa^{2+}]$.
   b. Marked hypocalcemia may occur if a C-cell neoplasm destroys parathyroid glands, which causes hypercalcitonism and concurrent primary hypoparathyroidism.
   c. Excess administration of salmon calcitonin (used to lower the $[tCa^{2+}]$ in hypervitaminosis D or HHM) may cause hypocalcemia.

6. Nutritional hypocalcemia (nutritional secondary hyperparathyroidism)
   a. Occurs with vitamin D–deficient diets and when diets are not balanced for Ca^{2+} and PO_4; that is, the dietary $Ca^{2+}:PO_4$ ratio is lower than the desired ratio for the species. The diet causes the hypocalcemia, which stimulates parathyroid gland hyperplasia. Imbalanced diets may include excessive PO_4 (carnivores' meat diet) and/or a relative or absolute deficiency of Ca^{2+}. The net effect is too much PO_4 in the body and too little Ca^{2+}.
   b. A decrease in the $[fCa^{2+}]$ stimulates parathyroid glands to cause secondary hyperparathyroidism. The increased PTH release tends to keep the $[fCa^{2+}]$ near normal at the expense of the Ca^{2+} content of bones, and thus osteomalacia may be present, especially in young animals (the bones of older animals are relatively refractory to PTH-stimulated osteoclastic activity).
   c. The degree of hypocalcemia depends on the severity of dietary imbalance and the availability of Ca^{2+} from bones (with Ca^{2+} being more available in young animals initially).
   d. Renal PO_4 excretion is increased because of the phosphaturic actions of PTH and, in some cases, the high dietary intake of PO_4. If the renal PO_4 excretion is measured, one should expect increased 24 h PO_4 clearance and increased fractional excretion of PO_4.

7. Oxalate toxicity[80]
   a. Horses that eat plants that have high oxalate content but low Ca^{2+} content absorb less dietary Ca^{2+}, and develop hypocalcemia. Such plants include fuffel, pangola, *Setaria*, kikuyu, rhubarb, halogeton, greasewood, and soursob (*Oxalis pes-caprae*).
   b. In ruminants, *Halogeton* and curly dock (*Rumex crispus*) may cause hypocalcemia.[81]
   c. Alfalfa has high oxalate content, but ingestion does not cause hypocalcemia because alfalfa also has high Ca^{2+} content.
D. Excess urinary excretion of Ca^{2+}
   1. Ethylene glycol toxicosis
      a. Products of ethylene glycol metabolism (including oxalates) bind Ca^{2+} in renal tubular fluid and thus cause hypercalciuria. Also, a high plasma oxalate concentration may cause intravascular formation of calcium oxalate crystals.[82]
      b. Acute nephrosis of the disorder may decrease tubular resorption of Ca^{2+}.[83,84]
   2. Metabolic alkalosis
      a. If an animal has a persistent metabolic alkalosis resulting in a plasma $[HCO_3^-]$ above the renal threshold for HCO_3^-, the resultant bicarbonaturia would obligate the renal loss of cations such as Ca^{2+}.
      b. Intravenous HCO_3^- infusions in cats[85]
         (1) Both the $[tCa^{2+}]$ and the $[fCa^{2+}]$ are reported to be decreased in some cats receiving intravenous HCO_3^-.
         (2) The pathogenesis of the hypocalcemia was not explained, but possible mechanisms include decreased Ca^{2+} resorption in proximal tubules because of Ca^{2+} complexing with excess HCO_3^-, alkalemia resulting in decreased $[fCa^{2+}]$, or increased renal Na^+ excretion causing concurrent hypercalciuria.
      c. Metabolic alkalosis contributes to the hypocalcemia of parturient hypocalcemia in cattle by reducing target cell response to PTH.[76]
   3. Furosemide treatment: Furosemide directly inhibits Na^+ and Cl^- resorption in the ascending limb of the loop of Henle and thus secondarily inhibits Ca^{2+} resorption in the ascending limb because the passive resorption of Ca^{2+} depends on gradients established by Na^+ resorption.[13,86] Thus, when furosemide is used to promote diuresis, hypocalcemia can develop. This calciuric effect of furosemide is used therapeutically to treat hypercalcemia. Thiazide diuretics should not be used in such cases because they actually promote Ca^{2+} resorption in the distal tubules.
E. Ca^{2+} binding with diffusible anions
   1. Ca^{2+} binds with EDTA, oxalate, or citrates given systemically or present in blood collection systems.
   2. Tetracycline is a Ca^{2+}-binding agent, and its rapid intravenous infusion may lower the $[fCa^{2+}]$, but the $[tCa^{2+}]$ remains WRI.[80]
F. Ca^{2+} deposition during fracture healing: Serum calcium concentrations decreased slightly (about 0.6 mg/dL) during the early stages of fracture healing in dogs.[87] The decrease may not be enough to cause hypocalcemia by itself, but the Ca^{2+} deposition during fracture healing could contribute to hypocalcemia.
G. Other or unknown mechanisms
   1. Acute pancreatitis (dogs and cats)
      a. Hypocalcemia may be present in acute edematous or hemorrhagic pancreatitis in dogs. Hypocalcemia is common in cats with acute pancreatitis, with a decreased

[fCa^{2+}] being more common than a decreased [tCa^{2+}]; a low [fCa^{2+}] was associated with a poorer prognosis.[88]

b. The pathogeneses of the hypocalcemia and decreased [fCa^{2+}] are not clearly identified and may involve multiple mechanisms.

    (1) Historically, the hypocalcemia was attributed to the binding of Ca^{2+} to fatty acids in the peritoneal cavity (forming Ca^{2+} soaps); fatty acids were liberated from necrotic peritoneal fat because of actions of pancreatic lipase. However, there is little evidence to support the soap theory, and there is evidence to refute it.[89]

    (2) Other theories with variable support include abnormal hormonal regulation of the [fCa^{2+}] (involving glucagon, calcitonin, or PTH), entry of Ca^{2+} into cells because of damaged membranes, binding of fCa^{2+} to plasma fatty acids, and extravasation of protein-bound Ca^{2+} because of increased vascular permeability.[89–91]

2. Urinary tract obstruction[92]

a. Mild to moderate hypocalcemia may be present; the [fCa^{2+}] is decreased more than the [tCa^{2+}].

b. The pathogenesis of this hypocalcemia is not clearly understood but may be related to increased [Pi] and the resultant binding of fCa^{2+}. Also, the renal tubular damage that occurred during obstruction may increase the renal excretion of Ca^{2+} after the obstruction has been cleared.

3. Acute renal failure

a. Hypocalcemia may occur in animals with acute renal failure, but the cause of the hypocalcemia may be either the renal failure or the concurrent pathologic states.[93]

b. If the acute renal failure is primarily due to ischemia, then perhaps a rapid-onset hyperphosphatemia leads to Ca^{2+} binding and hypocalcemia, or the acute nephrosis reduces the tubular resorption of Ca^{2+}.

c. Other concurrent pathologic states that may be contributing to the hypocalcemia include acute pancreatitis, ethylene glycol poisoning, and hypoalbuminemia.

4. Phosphate enemas

a. In reported feline cases, authors proposed that the hypocalcemia developed because of hyperphosphatemia.[94]

b. Hyperphosphatemia may produce hypocalcemia through three processes:

    (1) Acutely, the high PO$_4$ load drives the following equation to the right in plasma, thus lowering the [fCa^{2+}]: $Ca^{2+} + PO_4 \rightarrow Ca^{2+} - PO_4$ compounds. There also may be more Ca^{2+}-PO$_4$ complexes in tissues.[13]

    (2) Increased renal excretion of anionic PO$_4$ may obligate increased excretion of cations, including Ca^{2+}.

    (3) PO$_4$ inhibits the renal formation of 1,25-DHCC.[13] However, the 1,25-DHCC deficiency would develop slowly and thus not contribute to the acute-onset hypocalcemia of this disorder.

5. Gastrointestinal disorders in colicky horses

a. Colicky horses with a variety of gastrointestinal disorders frequently are hypocalcemic; the [fCa^{2+}] is decreased more frequently than the [tCa^{2+}].[95,96] A pathogenesis that is common to all disorders has not been established.

b. Horses with blister beetle poisoning (cantharidiasis) are typically hypocalcemic. Blister beetles produce cantharidin, a toxicant that interferes with mitochondrial respiration and protein phosphorylation. The pathogenesis of hypocalcemia is not understood, but loss of protein-bound Ca^{2+} into the intestinal tract may contribute.[97,98]

6. Myopathies
    a. Hypocalcemia may occur in a variety of equine myopathies (e.g., transport tetany, exertional rhabdomyolysis, endurance-type exercise, monensin toxicosis, postanesthetic myositis, exhausted horse syndrome, atypical myoglobinuria, malignant hyperthermia, and selenium myopathy).[80,99–102]
    b. The pathogenesis of the hypocalcemia may be multifactorial (e.g., decreased intake, increased renal loss, increased movement of Ca^{2+} into damaged cells, and profuse sweating).
    c. Sweating in horses can create an alkalemia (hypochloremic alkalosis) that may increase Ca^{2+} binding to albumin and thus lower the $[fCa^{2+}]$. Also, there may be direct loss of Ca^{2+} in sweat.[103]

7. Acute tumor lysis syndrome
    a. PO_4 released from lysed cells may bind Ca^{2+}, and the Ca^{2+}-PO_4 complexes deposit in tissues.
    b. PO_4 and lactate (produced by hypoxic neoplastic cells) may bind Ca^{2+} in renal tubular fluid and thus inhibit tubular resorption of Ca^{2+}.[104]

8. Rumen overload (acute carbohydrate ruminal engorgement)
    a. Ruminants that ingest large amounts of fermentable carbohydrate may develop acute lactic acidosis, hypovolemia, azotemia, hyperphosphatemia, and hypocalcemia.[105]
    b. The pathogenesis of the hypocalcemia is not established but may relate to increased renal excretion, because Ca^{2+} may be bound to PO_4 or lactate in the tubular fluid. It may also relate to deposition of Ca^{2+}-PO_4 complexes in tissues.

9. Hyperadrenocorticism in dogs.
    a. Hypocalcemia is present in a small percentage of dogs with hyperadrenocorticism.[106]
    b. Alterations in Ca^{2+} concentrations are probably related to increased glucocorticoid activity, but the exact mechanisms have not been established.

FREE CALCIUM (fCa^{2+}) CONCENTRATION

I. Physiologic processes (see Total Calcium Concentration, sect. I)

II. Analytical concepts of $[fCa^{2+}]$
    A. Terms
        1. In clinical jargon and in many veterinary publications, fCa^{2+} is often called *ionized calcium* and is abbreviated as iCa, iCa^{2+}, or just Ca^{2+}. However, all calcium in body fluids is present in an ionized state either as a free ion (i.e., fCa^{2+}) or as anion-bound ionized Ca^{2+}. Anions that bind Ca^{2+} include proteins, citrate, and PO_4.
        2. In this book, these abbreviations are used: calcium ion (Ca^{2+}), free calcium ion (fCa^{2+}), and total calcium ion (tCa^{2+}). Referring to the unbound Ca^{2+} as fCa^{2+} is also preferred by other clinical chemists[1] and is analogous to using tT_4 and fT_4 for total and free thyroxine, respectively.
    B. Sample
        1. Because of the potential changes in $[fCa^{2+}]$ caused by preanalytical variations, it is essential that patient samples and samples for determination of reference intervals be

collected and processed by using uniform and stringent criteria. Because changes in $[fCa^{2+}]$ may be related to dietary intake and postprandial alkalosis, samples should be collected from dogs after the dogs have been fasted overnight.[107] Similar changes would be expected in cats and horses.

2. Acceptable samples include serum, heparinized whole blood, and heparinized plasma. However, special conditions apply to all samples. For accurate results, blood samples should be collected and processed anaerobically to reduce changes in pH caused by loss of CO_2 to air. Serum and plasma should be harvested within 1 h of blood collection to reduce potential errors created by lactate and H^+ generation by blood cells. An excess amount of heparin should be avoided.

3. Sample storage
   a. $[fCa^{2+}]$ is more stable in serum than in plasma or whole blood.[108] However, silicone-separator tubes should not be used because the gel contains Ca^{2+}.[109]
   b. The $[fCa^{2+}]$ did not change significantly in equine sera or heparinized plasma that was stored anaerobically for 4 d at room temperature.[3] Serum and plasma $[fCa^{2+}]$ is reported to be stable in glass tubes for 1 wk at 4 °C and for 6 wk at −20 °C.[110]
   c. $[fCa^{2+}]$ in heparinized whole blood is reported to be stable for 9 h at 4 °C.

4. Samples should be processed anaerobically and quickly to avoid the effect of pH changes on $[fCa^{2+}]$: raising the pH decreases $[fCa^{2+}]$, whereas lowering the pH increases $[fCa^{2+}]$.[1] The $[fCa^{2+}]$ changes by about 5 % for each 0.1 change in pH. Exposing sera to air by simply inverting tubes containing sera and air lowered the $[fCa^{2+}]$ (average 0.1 mmol/L lower) and raised the pH values (average, 0.35 higher).[111]
   a. Albumin and other protein molecules have negatively charged surfaces that enable them to bind cations, including Ca^{2+} and H^+. Even though an albumin molecule has a surplus of binding sites, changes in plasma or serum pH alter the binding of Ca^{2+} to plasma or serum proteins. This relationship is illustrated in Fig. 11.4.
      (1) A higher pH increases the available negative-charge sites on albumin and other proteins because fewer H^+ ions are present to bind them. This leads to increased protein-bound Ca^{2+} and thus decreased $[fCa^{2+}]$. Aerobic sample handling leads to escape of CO_2 to air, an increase in pH, and thus a falsely low $[fCa^{2+}]$.
      (2) A lower pH induces the opposite changes and thus increases $[fCa^{2+}]$. Delayed sample analysis will allow blood cell metabolic pathways to produce H^+, causing a falsely increased $[fCa^{2+}]$.
   b. Some assays assume a blood pH of 7.4. Others normalize the fCa^{2+} to pH 7.4 if the pH is abnormal. If so, results should be reported as normalized or adjusted $[fCa^{2+}]$. If a patient is either acidemic or alkalemic, a normalized or adjusted $[fCa^{2+}]$ may be misleading because it does not represent the true $[fCa^{2+}]$ in the sample.

5. Anticoagulants for whole blood and plasma samples
   a. Heparin is the only acceptable anticoagulant for measuring $[fCa^{2+}]$ in blood or plasma samples, but heparin (a polyanion) does bind Ca^{2+}. To minimize preanalytical error, the use of special calcium-titrated heparin tubes is recommended. If the special tubes are unavailable, then the heparin concentration should not exceed 15 U/mL of blood.[110]

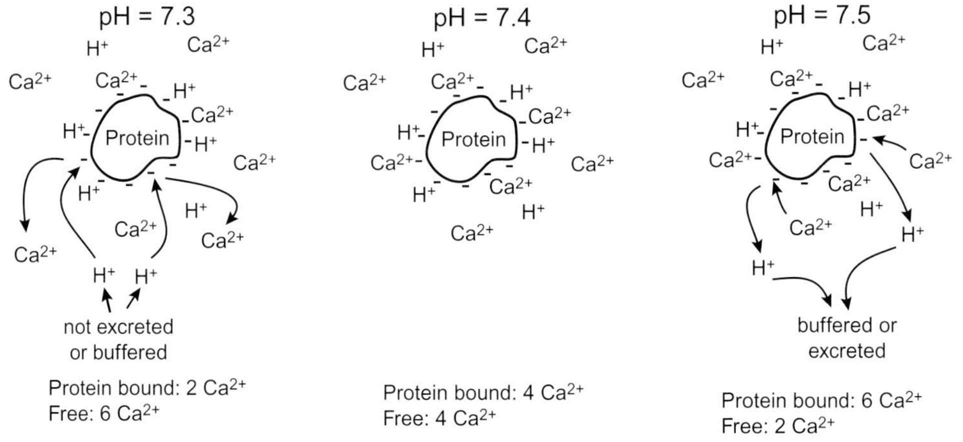

Fig. 11.4. Conceptual illustration of the effects of plasma or serum pH on the [fCa^{2+}]. The drawing illustrates the effect of the [H^+] in plasma on the binding of Ca^{2+} to negatively charged proteins. A similar effect occurs with Mg^{2+}.

- At a pH of 7.4, there are Ca^{2+} and H^+ ions bound to plasma or serum proteins and Ca^{2+} and H^+ ions that are free in the plasma or serum water. The free ions create the [fCa^{2+}] and pH of the fluid. In this illustration, there are four protein-bound and four free Ca^{2+} ions.
- If sample handling, respiratory disorders, or metabolic disorders cause an ↑ [H^+], then more H^+ and less Ca^{2+} bind to the proteins. The release of Ca^{2+} from the proteins increases the [fCa^{2+}]. In this illustration with a pH of 7.3, the sample contains six free Ca^{2+} ions.
- If either sample handling, respiratory disorders, or metabolic disorders cause a ↓ [H^+], then less H^+ and more Ca^{2+} bind to the proteins. The binding of Ca^{2+} to the proteins decreases the [fCa^{2+}]. In this illustration with a pH of 7.5, the sample contains two free Ca^{2+} ions.

(1) The [fCa^{2+}] may decrease from 5 % to 50 % by varying the amount of sodium heparinate (commonly called heparin) in the sample.[112] In an experiment, canine blood was collected into syringes (to the 1 mL mark) that contained varying amounts of heparin. The [fCa^{2+}] in samples collected after heparin was forcibly expelled three times was considered the most accurate value. The [fCa^{2+}] decreased by 0.2 mmol/L with about 0.1 mL of excess heparin (the amount in the syringe dead space and needle), decreased 0.5 mmol/L with about 0.2 mL of excess heparin (heparin in the dead space plus 0.1 mL in the syringe), and decreased 0.7 mmol/L with about 0.35 mL of excess heparin (heparin in the dead space plus 0.25 mL in the syringe).[113]

(2) The Ca^{2+} content in the calcium-titrated heparin approximates the expected midpoint concentration of fCa^{2+} in human plasma and should reduce the binding of patient fCa^{2+} to heparin. However, the measured [fCa^{2+}] represents Ca^{2+} from the calcium-titrated heparin and Ca^{2+} in the patient's plasma, and thus appropriate reference intervals must be available.

(3) The use of zinc heparinate was attempted as an anticoagulant, but the zinc interfered with the fCa^{2+} assay.[114]

b. Other anticoagulants that bind Ca^{2+} (EDTA, citrate, and oxalate) cannot be used in samples for fCa^{2+} or tCa^{2+} assays.

6. It is recommended that the $[fCa^{2+}]$ be reported with special information: type of sample, site of collection, measured $[fCa^{2+}]$, measured pH, and $[fCa^{2+}]$ converted to a sample pH of 7.4.[110]

C. Common clinical assays.

1. Special instruments measure $[fCa^{2+}]$ by using Ca^{2+}-selective electrodes via potentiometry. If the instrument also contains a pH electrode, it may measure pH and adjust the measured $[fCa^{2+}]$ to a calculated $[fCa^{2+}]$ that would be expected if the pH of the sample was 7.4.

2. Different sources of standard solutions may result in different measured $[fCa^{2+}]$.

D. Unit conversion: mg/dL × 0.2495 = mmol/L, and mEq/L × 0.5 = mmol/L (SI unit, nearest 0.01 mmol/L).[15]

III. Abnormal concentrations.

A. $[fCa^{2+}]$ is tightly controlled by hormones. Abnormalities in $[fCa^{2+}]$ indicate abnormal Ca^{2+} regulation and may cause clinical signs or pathologic events. Although $[tCa^{2+}]$ often parallels $[fCa^{2+}]$ and is a good screening test for disorders of Ca^{2+} homeostasis, $[tCa^{2+}]$ does not necessarily reflect the more relevant $[fCa^{2+}]$ as illustrated by the following conditions:

1. Hypocalcemia caused by hypoproteinemia or hypoalbuminemia: The $[tCa^{2+}]$ is decreased because of less protein-bound Ca^{2+}. The $[fCa^{2+}]$ may be WRI.

2. Hypercalcemia in renal failure or multiple myeloma: The $[tCa^{2+}]$ is increased because of more bound Ca^{2+} (Ca^{2+} bound to citrate, PO_4, or abnormal globulins). The $[fCa^{2+}]$ may be WRI.

3. In urinary tract obstruction in cats, decreases in $[fCa^{2+}]$ may be greater and more common than decreases in $[tCa^{2+}]$. Ca^{2+} may be bound to PO_4 or other anions not excreted by the urinary system.[92]

4. In a study involving 1633 samples from dogs with chronic renal failure or a variety of other disorders, the same percentage of samples had both increased $[tCa^{2+}]$ and $[fCa^{2+}]$ (19 %) and nearly the same percentages of decreased $[tCa^{2+}]$ and $[fCa^{2+}]$ (27 % and 31 %, respectively). However, when only the dogs with chronic renal failure (n = 490) were considered, a higher percentage of dogs had increased $[tCa^{2+}]$ (22 %) than increased $[fCa^{2+}]$ (9 %), and a lower percentage of dogs had decreased $[tCa^{2+}]$ (19 %) than decreased $[fCa^{2+}]$ (36 %).[18] The data from the renal failure group suggest that a higher percentage of $[tCa^{2+}]$ was the bound-Ca^{2+} fraction (probably not protein bound) and the $[tCa^{2+}]$ does not reflect changes in the $[fCa^{2+}]$ in canine chronic renal failure.

5. Hyperthyroid cats may have a decreased $[fCa^{2+}]$ but $[tCa^{2+}]$ WRI. The pathogenesis of the decreased $[fCa^{2+}]$ is not understood. The cats do have secondary hyperparathyroidism.[115]

6. Horses after a cross-country race had decreased $[fCa^{2+}]$ but $[tCa^{2+}]$ WRI.[116] In another study involving endurance rides (80 km), the average decrease in plasma $[fCa^{2+}]$ was near 0.8 mg/dL; concurrently, the concentrations of lactate, Pi, and albumin increased; data for $[tCa^{2+}]$ were not reported.[117] The lower $[fCa^{2+}]$ may have been due to several factors, including increased binding to albumin, increased binding to lactate, movement of Ca^{2+} from ECF to ICF, or loss of Ca^{2+} in sweat.

7. A massive transfusion of blood or plasma containing citrate as the anticoagulant can cause a decreased $[fCa^{2+}]$. In one study in which dogs were transfused with either a volume of blood product equal to their estimated blood volume over 24 h or a

volume > 50 % of their estimated blood volume in 3 h, the average decrease in [fCa^{2+}] was near 0.3 mmol/L (1.2 mg/dL).[118]

8. In hypocalcemic, 5- to 10-d-old calves that were acidotic because of diarrhea, the [fCa^{2+}] was not decreased as much as the [tCa^{2+}] prior to treatments. Both [tCa^{2+}] and [fCa^{2+}] decreased after fluid therapy that reduced the severity of acidosis.[119] The relationships between blood pH and [fCa^{2+}] should be considered when acidemic animals are administered NaHCO$_3$ intravenously, because such therapy can rapidly decrease the [fCa^{2+}].[119]

B. The acid-base status of an animal can affect the [fCa^{2+}] by three processes:
1. As explained in the analytical section (Free Calcium Concentration, sect. II) changing the blood pH affects the binding of Ca^{2+} to proteins and other anions. Acidemia increases the [fCa^{2+}] and alkalemia decreases the [fCa^{2+}].

2. When there is an organic acidosis (e.g., lactic acidosis or ketoacidosis), the organic ion (e.g., lactate or acetoacetate) in the plasma may bind Ca^{2+} to lower the [fCa^{2+}], whereas concurrent acidemia would raise the [fCa^{2+}]. Also, the presence of the organic anion in renal tubular fluid would decrease the tubular resorption of Ca^{2+}. With these multiple factors, the actual alteration in [fCa^{2+}] may depend on the severity and duration of the organic acidosis.

3. The blood pH also affects plasma concentrations of PTH independently of [fCa^{2+}]. The [iPTH] increased during experimentally induced metabolic and respiratory acidoses if [fCa^{2+}] was kept constant.[120] Conversely, the [iPTH] decreased during experimentally induced metabolic and respiratory alkaloses if [fCa^{2+}] was kept constant.[121] Thus, in clinical acid-base disorders, changes in [fCa^{2+}] could also be related to changes in PTH. The altered [iPTH] in acid-base disorders may reflect its roles in maintaining acid-base status. The PO$_4$ released from bone acts as a buffer in blood, and the PO$_4$ participates in the renal excretion of H$^+$. Also, persistently increased PTH activity reduces the renal excretion of HCO$_3$$^-$.[122]

IV. Conceptual relationships of [tCa^{2+}] and [fCa^{2+}].
A. Three major concepts must be remembered when interpreting Ca^{2+} concentrations:
1. The routine assays of a serum chemistry profile measure [tCa^{2+}], which includes three Ca^{2+} fractions: free, protein bound, and bound to anions other than proteins.

2. The body regulates the [fCa^{2+}] through the actions of several hormones.

3. Serum [fCa^{2+}] values may be inaccurate when blood is not handled anaerobically, when serum separation from blood clot is delayed, and when serum-separator tubes are used.

B. With these concepts in mind, Fig. 11.5 illustrates potential relationships of the three Ca^{2+} fractions. Major points that should be understood include the following:
1. An animal may have hypocalcemia because of hypoproteinemia or hypoalbuminemia, but the systems that regulate [fCa^{2+}] are not defective (Fig. 11.5B).

2. If serum protein concentrations are WRI, then hypocalcemia typically indicates that the [fCa^{2+}] is decreased (Fig. 11.5C).

3. Most hypercalcemic samples have an increased [fCa^{2+}] (Fig. 11.5D)

4. Normocalcemia in the presence of hypoproteinemia suggests an increased [fCa^{2+}] (Fig 11.5E).

5. The severity of decreased [fCa^{2+}] may not be evident from the [tCa^{2+}] if the concentrations of the bound-Ca^{2+} fractions are increased (Fig. 11.5F)

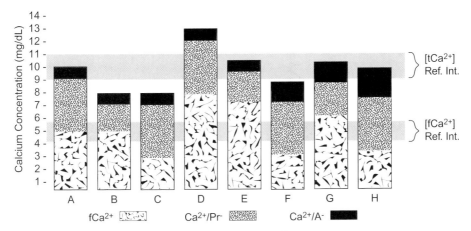

Fig. 11.5. Conceptual relationships of total, free, and bound Ca^{2+} fractions in serum or plasma.

A. Healthy animal: The $[tCa^{2+}]$ and $[fCa^{2+}]$ are within respective reference intervals.

B. Hypoproteinemia (hypoalbuminemia): The hypocalcemia is caused by a decreased concentration of protein-bound Ca^{2+}. The $[fCa^{2+}]$ (the regulated concentration) is within its reference interval.

C. Primary hypoparathyroidism, hypovitaminosis D: The hypocalcemia is primarily caused by a decreased $[fCa^{2+}]$ because of either inadequate PTH or vitamin D activity. In this schematic example, the bound Ca^{2+} concentration is unchanged.

D. Primary hyperparathyroidism, hypervitaminosis D, humoral hypercalcemia of malignancy, humoral hypercalcemia of benign disorders: The hypercalcemia is primarily caused by increased $[fCa^{2+}]$ because of increased activity of PTH, PTHrp, or vitamin D activity. In this schematic example, the bound-Ca^{2+} concentration is unchanged.

E. HHM and concurrent hypoproteinemia: The $[fCa^{2+}]$ is increased because of the increased PTHrp activity, but the protein-bound Ca^{2+} concentration is decreased because of concurrent hypoproteinemia. The net result is a $[tCa^{2+}]$ within its reference interval.

F. Chronic renal failure: The $[fCa^{2+}]$ is mildly decreased because of the inadequate formation of 1,25-DHCC. Concurrently, the concentration of Ca^{2+} bound to nonprotein anions (e.g., Ca^{2+} bound to citrate or PO_4) is increased. In this schematic example, the protein-bound Ca^{2+} concentration is unchanged and the net result is a mild hypocalcemia. The protein-bound Ca^{2+} concentration would be decreased with hypoalbuminemia caused by a protein-losing nephropathy.

G. Lactic acidosis: The acidemia promotes Ca^{2+} detaching from proteins (thus, a decreased protein-bound $[Ca^{2+}]$). Some of the released Ca^{2+} binds to lactate to increase the Ca^{2+} bound to nonprotein anions. In this schematic example, the $[tCa^{2+}]$ is within its reference interval.

H. Excess heparin in plasma: Collection of blood with an inappropriate amount of heparin (an anion) results in some of the fCa^{2+} binding to heparin and thus a decreased $[fCa^{2+}]$. The $[tCa^{2+}]$ does not change.

6. The $[fCa^{2+}]$ is affected by altered plasma pH and the presence of nonprotein anions in the plasma (Fig. 11.5G)

7. Excess heparin in a blood sample can cause a falsely decreased $[fCa^{2+}]$ (Fig. 11.5H).

INORGANIC PHOSPHORUS (Pi) CONCENTRATION

I. Physiologic processes

   A. Pi exists in different forms, depending on pH: $H_3PO_4 \leftrightarrow H^+ + H_2PO_4^- \leftrightarrow 2 H^+ + HPO_4^{2-} \leftrightarrow 3 H^+ + PO_4^{3-}$. At a pH of 7.4, predominant forms are $H_2PO_4^-$ and HPO_4^{2-}

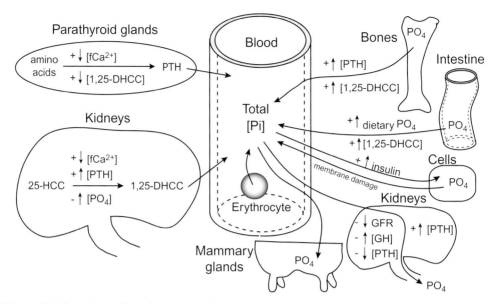

Fig. 11.6. Relationships of PO_4 kinetics and the production of PTH and 1,25-DHCC. (Note: Horse kidneys lack 1α-hydroxylase and thus do not form 1,25-DHCC.)

- PTH production in parathyroid glands is stimulated by ↓ $[fCa^{2+}]$ and ↓ [1,25-DHCC] and inhibited by ↑ $[fCa^{2+}]$ and ↑ [1,25-DHCC].
- Conversion of 25-HCC to 1,25-DHCC in kidneys is catalyzed by 1α-hydroxylase. The activity of 1α-hydroxylase is promoted by ↓ $[fCa^{2+}]$ and ↑ PTH and inhibited by ↑ $[fCa^{2+}]$ and ↑ $[PO_4]$.
- PO_4 mobilization from bone is promoted by ↑ [1,25-DHCC] and ↑ PTH. Less PO_4 mobilization occurs with ↓ [1,25-DHCC] and ↓ PTH.
- PO_4 absorption in intestine is promoted by ↑ [1,25-DHCC] and ↑ dietary PO_4. Less PO_4 absorption occurs with ↓ [1,25-DHCC] and ↓ dietary PO_4.
- Urinary excretion of PO_4 is enhanced by ↑ PTH, and excretion is reduced by ↓ GFR, ↓ PTH, and ↑ GH activity.
- Insulin promotes the uptake of PO_4 by cells. However, cell damage will allow PO_4 to escape from the cells and enter plasma.
- During lactation, a large amount of PO_4 is excreted via milk.
- PO_4 present in plasma is mostly in two forms (HPO_4^{2-} and $H_2PO_4^{-}$), but the measured phosphorus is reported in terms of inorganic phosphorus (Pi).
- In vitro hemolysis or delayed removal of serum or plasma allows PO_4 in erythrocytes to enter serum or plasma and thus cause an erroneous $[PO_4]$.

+, positive effector (stimulates the process); and −, negative effector (inhibits the process).

in a 1:4 ratio. Unless stated otherwise, all forms in this chapter are designated as PO_4. About 10 % of Pi is bound to cationic proteins, 35 % is bound to nonprotein cations, and 55 % is free.[1]

  B. Major factors that determine serum [Pi] (Fig. 11.6)

    1. Renal clearance of PO_4

      a. A major route of PO_4 excretion is via kidneys in most mammals, so disorders that cause decreased GFR tend to increase the serum [Pi].

      b. PTH is a potent phosphaturic agent. In the presence of PTH, less of filtered PO_4 is resorbed in the distal tubules. PTH acts through a cyclic adenosine monophosphate messenger system to inhibit the cotransport of Na^+ and PO_4.

  2. Absorption of PO_4 in intestines

      a. If animals are eating, then they will typically consume large quantities of PO_4 that are absorbed in intestines.

      b. Absorption is enhanced by 1,25-DHCC, either directly or through Ca^{2+} complexes.

  3. Resorption from bone: PTH stimulates osteocytes (rapid effect) and osteoclasts (delayed effect) to release PO_4 from bone. Because of the potent phosphaturic action of PTH, the release of PO_4 does not increase the [Pi] as long as renal function is adequate.

  4. Shifting of PO_4 between ICF and ECF compartments

      a. Intracellular biochemical processes that involve phosphorylation need PO_4 from ECF.

      b. Insulin promotes PO_4 entry into cells by enhancing the movement of glucose into cells. Once in cells, glucose is phosphorylated to enter glycolytic or glycogen synthesis pathways. The binding of free PO_4^{3-} to glucose or other organic molecules reduces the ICF concentration of free PO_4^{3-} and allows more PO_4 to enter cells from the ECF.

  5. Animal age

      a. GH is reported to be largely responsible for the increased [Pi] in young, growing animals. GH increases the renal tubular resorption of PO_4.[123]

      b. Serum [Pi] is typically greater in young, growing animals than in the adult animals used to establish most reference intervals.[5,7] In pups (< 12 wk), serum [Pi] reference intervals were about 5.7–10.8 mg/dL, whereas adult dog intervals were about 2.5–5.5 mg/dL. In kittens (4–6 wk to 20–24 wk), serum [Pi] reference intervals were about 5.0–10.0 mg/dL, whereas adult cat intervals were about 1.8–6.4 mg/dL. A corresponding age-related difference is that these young animals have greater serum alkaline phosphatase activity than mature animals (usually < 3 × the upper reference limit for adults).

      c. Metastatic mineralization of tissues tends to occur when the product of $[tCa^{2+}]$ and [Pi] (both in mg/dL) exceeds 70 in adult animals. The same does not seem to occur in young animals.

II.   Analytical concepts of [Pi]

  A. Sample.

    1. Serum is the preferred sample, but plasma may be used.

    2. In vitro hemolysis or delayed removal of serum from a blood clot may increase serum [Pi] because PO_4 is liberated into serum from erythrocytes (cytoplasmic PO_4 and membrane PO_4 released from phospholipids).

  B. Assays

    1. In most common assays, PO_4 reacts with ammonium molybdate to form a colored complex that is measured by photometry.

    2. In some systems, conjugated bilirubin may interfere with the assay to produce falsely decreased results (*pseudo-hypophosphatemia*),[124] whereas, in other assay systems, bilirubin has no effect or may produce falsely increased values.

    3. In spectrophotometric assays that use the strongly acidic ammonium molybdate reagent, the reagent can precipitate immunoglobulins to produce a turbidity that

results in a falsely increased [Pi] by 1–2 mmol/L (≈ 3–6 mg/dL).[125] This positive interference has been seen in samples with monoclonal gammopathies despite assay modifications such as the addition of detergent to prevent protein precipitation.

C. Methods of expressing concentrations

1. [Pi] is often referred to as the phosphorus concentration. More accurately, [Pi] is the serum PO_4 reported as phosphorus in mg/dL. It is not reported as a PO_4 concentration in mg/dL because the amount of each form of PO_4 changes with pH, and each form has a different relative molecular mass (M_r). This problem is overcome by reporting phosphate in SI units of mmol/L.

2. Relationship between [PO_4] and [Pi]

   a. 1 mmol of $H_2PO_4^-$ weighs 97 mg. In 1 mmol of $H_2PO_4^-$ there are 31 mg of P. Therefore, a solution of 97 mg/dL of $H_2PO_4^-$ contains 31 mg/dL of P.

   b. 1 mmol of HPO_4^{2-} weighs 96 mg. In 1 mmol of HPO_4^{2-} there are 31 mg of P. Therefore, a solution of 96 mg/dL of HPO_4^{2-} contains 31 mg/dL of P.

   c. Because of the equilibrium among the different PO_4 molecules at a pH of 7.4, 1 mmol of PO_4 averages about 96.2 mg/dL.

D. Unit conversion for [Pi]: mg/dL × 0.3229 = mmol/L (SI unit, nearest 0.05 mmol/L)[15]

III. Hyperphosphatemia (Table 11.4)

A. Decreased urinary PO_4 excretion.

   1. Disorders that decrease GFR (see prerenal, renal, and postrenal azotemias in Chapter 8): Hyperphosphatemia occurs because PO_4 is not filtered adequately from plasma.

Table 11.4. Diseases and conditions that cause hyperphosphatemia

Decreased urinary PO_4 excretion
  *Decreased GFR (see prerenal, renal, and postrenal azotemias in Chapter 8)
  Urinary bladder rupture or urine leakage into tissues
  Decreased [PTH] or activity (hypoparathyroidism)
  Acromegaly
Increased PO_4 absorption from intestine
  Phosphate enema or ingestion of phosphate urinary acidifier
  Increased vitamin D (see Table 11.2)
  Ischemic intestinal lesions (maybe also shift from ICF to ECF)
  Diet with a low Ca^{2+}:PO_4 ratio (rare)
Shift of PO_4 from ICF to ECF
  Myopathies: endurance rides in horses, exertional rhabdomyolysis, malignant hyperthermia
  Acute tumor lysis syndrome
Other or unknown mechanisms
  Hyperthyroidism in cats
  Lactic acidosis
  Hyperadrenocorticism in dogs

* A relatively common disease or condition

Note: The [Pi] in growing mammals may be up to 3 mg/dL higher than Pi reference intervals for adults of the species. In vitro hemolysis or delayed removal of serum or plasma from blood samples will allow PO_4 from erythrocytes to increase the [Pi] in the serum or plasma. Also, a falsely increased [Pi] can be found in samples with hyperbilirubinemia or monoclonal gammopathies.

The magnitude tends to parallel the severity of azotemia in dogs, cats, and cattle, but it may not in horses.

2. Urinary bladder rupture or leakage of urine into tissues: Hyperphosphatemia results from decreased urinary excretion of PO_4 from the body.
3. Decreased [iPTH] or activity (primary hypoparathyroidism or pseudo-hypoparathyroidism) (see Total Calcium Concentration, sect. IV.B).
4. Acromegaly: GH increases tubular PO_4 resorption.[123]

B. Increased PO_4 absorption from intestine
1. Phosphate enema[126,127] or ingestion of a phosphate urinary acidifier[128]
2. Increased vitamin D
   a. Hypervitaminosis D in ruminants: perhaps increased intestinal absorption of PO_4 or increased bone resorption
   b. Cholecalciferol intoxication in dogs (see Total Calcium Concentration, sect. III.A.2).
3. Intestinal lesions requiring intestinal resection: Devitalized intestinal mucosa allows PO_4 to enter plasma (and peritoneal fluid). Also, shifting of PO_4 from ICF to ECF may be involved.[129]
4. Diets with low Ca^{2+}:PO_4 ratio

C. Shift of PO_4 from ICF to ECF
1. Myopathies (endurance rides in horses, exertional rhabdomyolysis, and malignant hyperthermia): release of PO_4 from damaged muscle fibers[100–102,130]
2. Acute tumor lysis syndrome: release of PO_4 from necrotic neoplastic cells[104]

D. Other or unknown mechanisms
1. Hyperthyroidism in cats: Thyroxine may promote osteoclastic activity to cause release of Ca^{2+} and PO_4 from bone. Hyperthyroid cats may have hyperphosphatemia, a decreased [fCa^{2+}], and an increased [iPTH].[115] The reason for the decreased [fCa^{2+}] has not been established but has been considered the stimulus for the increased [iPTH].
2. Lactic acidosis:[131] This causes hyperphosphatemia more frequently than other metabolic acidoses, but the mechanisms have not been completely explained. The hyperphosphatemia might be linked to the acidemia mechanism; that is, anaerobic glycolysis causes a net degradation of adenosine triphosphate (ATP) and thus increases cellular production of H^+ and PO_4 (see Fig. 9.10).[132]
3. Hyperadrenocorticism in dogs: The serum [Pi] in 68 dogs with hyperadrenocorticism was significantly greater than in 20 hospitalized dogs without clinical signs of hyperadrenocorticism. The dogs with hyperadrenocorticism also had significantly greater plasma [iPTH], but no significant differences for [tCa^{2+}] or [fCa^{2+}] were found between the groups.[106]

E. Pseudo-hyperphosphatemia: As noted in the analytical section (Inorganic Phosphorus Concentration, sect. II) the presence of hyperbilirubinemia, a monoclonal gammopathy, or in vitro hemolysis can result in a falsely increased [Pi].

IV. Hypophosphatemia (Table 11.5)
A. Increased urinary PO_4 excretion
1. Prolonged diuresis: Less filtered PO_4 is resorbed.
2. Increased [iPTH] or [PTHrp] (Table 11.2).
3. Fanconi syndrome: Animals with *Fanconi syndrome* have a proximal tubular defect that decreases tubular resorption of glucose, amino acids, and PO_4. Some people

Table 11.5. Diseases and conditions that cause hypophosphatemia

Increased urinary PO_4 excretion
    Prolonged diuresis
    Increased PTH or PTHrp activity (see Table 11.2)
    Fanconi syndrome (dogs)
Decreased intestinal PO_4 absorption
    *Prolonged anorexia or PO_4-deficient diet
    PO_4-binding agents
    Hypovitaminosis D
    Intestinal malabsorption
Shift of PO_4 from ECF to ICF
    Hyperinsulinism (endogenous or exogenous)
    Glucose infusion
    Respiratory alkalosis
Defective mobilization of PO_4 from bone
    Postparturient paresis (milk fever) and eclampsia in bitches
Other or unknown mechanisms
    *Equine renal disease (failure)
    Halothane anesthesia in horses

* A relatively common disease or condition
Note: Conjugated bilirubin may interfere with some Pi assays to produce falsely increased or decreased results.

restrict the term *Fanconi syndrome* to inherited or congenital forms, whereas others include acquired disorders. The decreased resorption of PO_4 in dogs with Fanconi syndrome may cause hypophosphatemia and phosphaturia in some dogs[133,134] but not others.[135]

B. Decreased intestinal PO_4 absorption
  1. Prolonged anorexia or a PO_4-deficient diet: less dietary PO_4 available for absorption
  2. PO_4-binding agents: interference with PO_4 absorption
  3. Hypovitaminosis D: absence of a promoter of PO_4 absorption
  4. Intestinal malabsorption: decreased PO_4 absorption
C. Shift of PO_4 from ECF to ICF
  1. Hyperinsulinism (endogenous or exogenous)
    a. Insulin promotes entry of PO_4 into cells to phosphorylate the glucose that enters the cells.
    b. High insulin activity could result from insulin injections, an insulin-secreting neoplasm, or in response to glucose infusion.
  2. Glucose infusion (in horses) led to a hypophosphatemia.[136] The hypophosphatemia may be due to increased renal excretion of PO_4 secondary to solute diuresis and also due to insulin-induced movement of PO_4 from ECF to ICF secondary to glucose uptake.
  3. Respiratory alkalosis: Experimentally induced respiratory alkalosis caused hypophosphatemia and increased muscle glycolysis.[137] Phosphofructokinase is the rate-limiting enzyme in glycolysis, and alkalemia stimulates its activity. Thus, alkalemia promotes PO_4 movement into erythrocytes because of the increased phosphorylation during accelerated glycolysis.

    D. Defective mobilization of PO_4 from bone
        1. Postparturient paresis (milk fever): Cows cannot mobilize sufficient Ca^{2+} and PO_4 from bones to replace the Ca^{2+} and PO_4 that are lost in milk.
        2. Eclampsia in bitches: the same mechanism as milk fever
    E. Other or unknown mechanisms
        1. Equine renal disease (failure): Hypophosphatemia may be seen in equine renal disease that causes concurrent hypercalcemia.[138] However, it is not a consistent finding and the pathogenesis is not known.
        2. Halothane anesthesia in horses:[139] After prolonged halothane anesthesia (12 h), six horses had mild hyperphosphatemia for the first hour, but then hypophosphatemia developed and persisted for 3–4 d. The pathogenesis of the hypophosphatemia was not determined.
    F. Pseudo-hypophosphatemia: As noted in the analytical section (Inorganic Phosphorus Concentration, sect. II) the presence of conjugated hyperbilirubinemia can result in a falsely decreased [Pi].

TOTAL MAGNESIUM (tMg^{2+}) CONCENTRATION

I.   Physiologic processes
    A. Serum or plasma magnesium is distributed into three major fractions. *All Mg^{2+} in body fluids is ionized*, but some is free and some is bound to anionic molecules.
        1. *Free magnesium (fMg^{2+})*: About 55 % of tMg^{2+} is fMg^{2+} present as free ions in plasma H_2O. fMg^{2+} is the portion of tMg^{2+} that is hormonally regulated and contributes to pathologic states.
        2. Bound magnesium
           a. About 30 % of tMg^{2+} is bound to negatively charged sites on proteins (albumin and globulins).
           b. About 15 % of tMg^{2+} is bound to anions such as citrate and PO_4.
    B. Mg^{2+} is located in bones (about 60 %), in soft tissues (about 38 %), and in the extracellular fluid, including blood (1–2 %). Except in cattle, the $[tMg^{2+}]$ in erythrocytes is greater than in plasma (or serum).
    C. Major factors that determine the serum $[tMg^{2+}]$
        1. Hypoproteinemia decreases the amount of bound Mg^{2+} and thus may cause hypomagnesemia (decreased $[tMg^{2+}]$).
        2. Absorption of Mg^{2+} in the gastrointestinal tract[10]
           a. In ruminants, Mg^{2+} is absorbed by the rumen (and maybe intestine) in a process linked to Na^+-K^+-adenosine triphosphatase.
           b. In monogastric animals, Mg^{2+} absorption occurs in the distal small intestine and colon and is enhanced by vitamin D and inhibited by high dietary Ca^{2+} or PO_4.
        3. Excretion
           a. Mg^{2+} in feces may represent unabsorbed dietary Mg^{2+} but also loss of endogenous Mg^{2+}.
           b. Kidneys
             (1) Mg^{2+} not bound to proteins passes freely through the glomerular filtration barrier. Thus, a decreased GFR can reduce renal excretion of Mg^{2+} and cause hypermagnesemia.
             (2) If the amount of Mg^{2+} entering the proximal tubules exceeds the tubular resorptive capacity, excess Mg^{2+} is excreted. Osmotic diuresis and loop diuretics increase renal excretion of Mg^{2+}.

(3) If Mg^{2+} is present in bovine urine, then the cow is not expected to be hypomagnesemic because the presence of Mg^{2+} typically indicates that the transport maximum has been exceeded. Thus, finding Mg^{2+} in urine indicates that a cow does not have hypomagnesemic tetany (grass tetany) unless there is a defect in the resorption of Mg^{2+}.

  c. Mammary gland during lactation: The ratio of milk $[tMg^{2+}]$ to serum $[tMg^{2+}]$ is about 5.

 D. Hormonal regulation

  1. Antidiuretic hormone (arginine vasopressin), PTH, glucagon, calcitonin, and β-adrenergic agonists can stimulate Mg^{2+} absorption in the cortical thick ascending limb of the loop of Henle.[13]

  2. PTH can increase serum $[tMg^{2+}]$ by increasing intestinal Mg^{2+} absorption and increasing Mg^{2+} resorption in renal tubules and bone.[140]

  3. Administration of 1,25-DHCC reduces the plasma $[tMg^{2+}]$, perhaps secondarily to decreased PTH activity.[140]

  4. Thyroxine tends to decrease the plasma $[tMg^{2+}]$ by increasing Mg^{2+} excretion in urine and feces.[141]

  5. Aldosterone promotes increased fecal and urinary Mg^{2+} excretion. Experimentally, aldosterone infusions decreased ruminal Mg^{2+} absorption.[142] Decreased aldosterone activity increases the serum $[tMg^{2+}]$.

II. Analytical concepts of $[tMg^{2+}]$

 A. Sample.

  1. Serum is the preferred sample, but heparinized plasma may be used in some assays.

  2. Blood anticoagulants that bind Mg^{2+} (e.g., EDTA, citrate, and oxalate) should not be used in samples for $[tMg^{2+}]$ assays.

  3. Except in cattle, in vitro hemolysis or delayed removal of serum from a blood clot will increase serum $[tMg^{2+}]$ because Mg^{2+} is liberated into the serum from the erythrocytes. In cattle, plasma and erythrocyte concentrations of Mg^{2+} are similar.

  4. Postmortem aqueous humor and vitreous humor samples can be used to reflect the antemortem $[tMg^{2+}]$. The $[tMg^{2+}]$ was more stable in vitreous humor (up to 48 h) than in aqueous humor (up to 24 h).[143]

 B. Clinical assays

  1. Common assays are photometric and measure $[tMg^{2+}]$. In these assays, metallochromic indicators or dyes change colors when they selectively bind Mg^{2+}. Atomic absorption spectrometry is the reference method but is not used in most clinical laboratories.

  2. The $[fMg^{2+}]$ can be measured by ion-selective electrodes or it can be calculated from tMg^{2+} measurements before and after dialysis of serum to remove bound Mg^{2+}. However, there is currently very little clinical use of the results of $[fMg^{2+}]$ measurements.

 C. Unit conversion: $mg/dL \times 0.4114 = mmol/L$; and $mEq/L \times 0.500 = mmol/L$ (SI unit, nearest 0.02 mmol/L).[15]

III. Hypermagnesemia (Table 11.6)

 A. Decreased urinary excretion: renal failure and other causes of decreased GFR

 B. Shift of Mg^{2+} from ICF to ECF: Except in cattle, in vitro hemolysis, active in vivo hemolysis, or the delayed removal of serum from a blood clot will allow erythrocyte Mg^{2+} to be added to the serum concentration.

Table 11.6. Diseases or conditions that cause hypermagnesemia

Decreased urinary excretion
    *Renal failure and other causes of decreased GFR
Shift of fMg^{2+} from ICF to ECF
    Active in vivo hemolysis
Increased [PTH]
    Milk fever
Increased intestinal absorption of Mg^{2+} without increased PTH or PTHrp
    MgO, $Mg(OH)_2$, or similar antacids or cathartics (cattle)
    $MgSO_4$ (horses)
Other mechanisms
    Excess intravenous infusion of Mg^{2+}

    * A relatively common disease or condition
    Note: Pseudo-hypermagnesemia may occur from in vitro hemolysis or delayed removal of serum from blood clot (not in cattle).

C. Increased intestinal absorption of Mg^{2+} without increased PTH
    1. Excess oral administration of MgO (magnesium oxide) and $Mg(OH)_2$ (magnesium hydroxide) to cattle[144]
    2. Excess oral administration of $MgSO_4$ (magnesium sulfate) to horses[145]
D. Other or unknown mechanisms
    1. Milk fever: Increased PTH may induce increased renal resorption of Mg^{2+}, leading to hypermagnesemia.[146]
    2. A transient increase in $[tMg^{2+}]$ and $[fMg^{2+}]$ occurs in cattle postpartum. The increase may be related to increased PTH activity causing increased renal resorption of Mg^{2+} and increased Mg^{2+} mobilization from bone.[146]
    3. Excess intravenous infusion of Mg^{2+}
    4. In people, Addison's disease and hypothyroidism may cause hypermagnesemia. Similar findings have not been reported in domestic mammals.

IV. Hypomagnesemia (Table 11.7)
    A. Hypoproteinemia: decreased Mg^{2+} bound to proteins (decreased $[tMg^{2+}]$).
    B. Inadequate ruminal or intestinal absorption of Mg^{2+}
        1. Prolonged anorexia or poor feed intake (especially in lactating cattle): In one study that involved the death of 55 dairy cows, marked hypomagnesemia was present with clinical tetany (except in one cow).[147] For tetany to be associated with hypomagnesemia, concurrent hypocalcemia may be required.
        2. Calves on a whole milk diet can develop hypomagnesemia because the dietary Mg^{2+} requirement of growing calves is about 50 % greater than the amount of Mg^{2+} in milk.[10]
        3. Grass tetany in cattle[10,140]
            a. The hypomagnesemia is considered to result from decreased ruminal absorption of Mg^{2+}, but there are multiple theories for the absorption defect.
            b. A lush grass diet is high in PO_4 and K^+ content and low in Mg^{2+} and Na^+. In some studies, the combination of high K^+ and low Mg^{2+} was the key factor that led to hypomagnesemia. Other contributing factors in some cows include high nitrogen forage, increased dietary organic anions, and high aluminum forage.

Table 11.7. Diseases or conditions that cause hypomagnesemia

*Hypoproteinemia
Inadequate ruminal or intestinal absorption of Mg^{2+}
   *Prolonged anorexia or poor feed intake
   Calves on whole milk diet
   *Grass tetany in cattle
   Enteric diseases
Excess urinary excretion of Mg^{2+}
   *Osmotic diuresis
   *Ketonuria
Other or unknown mechanisms
   Blister beetle poisoning in horses
   Lactation tetany in Shetland mares

   * A relatively common disease or condition

     c. The roles of aldosterone in the process are not established, but aldosterone might be the link between K^+ and Mg^{2+}. Mg^{2+} absorption may be reduced by factors independent of aldosterone, such as the low $Na^+:K^+$ ratio of rumen contents.[142]
     d. Grass tetany is difficult to diagnose postmortem because of the lack of gross or microscopic lesions. Also, the postmortem plasma samples cannot be used for detecting hypomagnesemia because the release of Mg^{2+} from cells (other than erythrocytes) will falsely elevate the postmortem concentration. However, the $[tMg^{2+}]$ in aqueous and vitreous humor also decreases in animals with Mg^{2+} depletion, and the postmortem $[tMg^{2+}]$ in those fluids is more stable than in plasma.
       (1) If the aqueous or vitreous fluids are to be analyzed, they should be centrifuged soon after collection to remove contaminant cells and then stored at 4 °C. The viscosity of vitreous humor can interfere with accurate pipetting.
       (2) The $[tMg^{2+}]$ in vitreous humor was stable up to 48 h postmortem in bovine eyes, and, with one assay, a $[tMg^{2+}] < 0.55$ mmol/L (1.3 mg/dL) was associated with antemortem hypomagnesemic tetany. If a concurrent $[K^+]$ in the vitreous humor is > 10 mmol/L, then there has been too much postmortem change to consider the $[tMg^{2+}]$ a reliable indicator of antemortem concentrations.[143]
       (3) The $[tMg^{2+}]$ in aqueous humor was stable up to 24 h postmortem in bovine eyes, and, with one assay, a $[tMg^{2+}] < 0.25$ mmol/L (0.6 mg/dL) was associated with antemortem hypomagnesemic tetany.[143]
   4. Enteric diseases
     a. Dogs with enteric diseases may develop hypomagnesemia because of increased fecal loss or concurrent hypoproteinemia.[148,149]
     b. Horses with enterocolitis[150] and colicky horses[151] frequently have hypomagnesemia, which could be caused by decreased intake or increased intestinal loss.
  C. Excess urinary excretion of Mg^{2+}.[152]
   1. Osmotic diuresis: decreased tubular resorption due to solvent drag
   2. Ketonuria: decreased tubular resorption because of complexing with ketone bodies (β-hydroxybutyrate and acetoacetate).

D. Other or unknown mechanisms
1. Blister beetle poisoning in horses:[98,153] The pathogenesis has not been documented, but possibly a loss of protein-bound Mg^{2+} may contribute.
2. Lactation tetany in Shetland mares[77]
3. Endotoxemia in horses causes hypomagnesemia. The decrease is caused by the shifting of Mg^{2+} into cells and might be mediated by vasopressin or insulin.[154]

FREE MAGNESIUM (fMg^{2+}) CONCENTRATION

I. Physiologic processes (see Total Magnesium Concentration, sect. I)

II. Analytical concepts of [fMg^{2+}]
A. Terms: Most of the statements in the fCa^{2+} section also apply to terms used for Mg^{2+} concentrations. For consistency, these abbreviations are used: magnesium ion (Mg^{2+}), free magnesium ion (fMg^{2+}), and total magnesium ion (tMg^{2+}). In clinical jargon and in many veterinary publications, fMg^{2+} is often called *ionized magnesium* and is abbreviated as iMg, iMg^{2+}, or just Mg^{2+}, and thus there is a potential for miscommunication.
B. Sample: Most statements for [fCa^{2+}] also apply to [fMg^{2+}] because fCa^{2+} and fMg^{2+} are both divalent cations that bind to anions. Heparin is a polyanion and may complex fMg^{2+}, especially with excessive amounts of heparin. However, there are few published data about factors that alter [fMg^{2+}].
C. Clinical assays for [fMg^{2+}] are not common. Special instruments measure [fMg^{2+}] by using Mg^{2+}-selective electrodes via potentiometry. If the instrument also contains a pH electrode, it may measure pH and adjust the measured [fMg^{2+}] to a calculated [fMg^{2+}] that would be expected if the pH of the sample was 7.4.
D. Unit conversion: mg/dL × 0.4114 = mmol/L, and mEq/L × 0.5 = mmol/L (SI unit, nearest 0.01 mmol/L)[15]

III. Abnormal concentrations.
A. Disorders of tMg^{2+} homeostasis may be disorders of fMg^{2+} homeostasis or disorders affecting anions that bind fMg^{2+}. More studies are needed to establish the pathologic consequences of altered [fMg^{2+}].
B. A few published studies have explored the potential value of measuring [fMg^{2+}].[155,156] At this time, the many factors influencing [fMg^{2+}] limit the useful interpretation of altered concentrations.
1. In horses, both increased [fMg^{2+}] and decreased [fMg^{2+}] were common prior to and after colic surgery, but the reasons for the variations were not determined.[95] During experimental endotoxemia, both [tMg^{2+}] and [fMg^{2+}] were decreased. The changes occurred quickly and were thought to be due to movement of Mg^{2+} from plasma to cells.[154]
2. Serum [fMg^{2+}] remained unchanged when horses were fed a reduced-Mg^{2+} diet even though there was decreased renal Mg^{2+} excretion and decreased Mg^{2+} content in muscles.[157]
3. Both [tMg^{2+}] and [fMg^{2+}] in sera decreased in cats fed Mg^{2+}-deficient diets.[158]
4. In cats with nonketotic diabetes mellitus or ketotic diabetes mellitus, the [fMg^{2+}] was decreased more frequently than the [tMg^{2+}].[152] However, dogs with diabetic ketoacidosis tended to have a greater [fMg^{2+}] than did dogs with uncomplicated diabetes mellitus or healthy dogs; the reason for the greater [fMg^{2+}] was not

determined.[155] As a group, the [fMg^{2+}] in the dogs with uncomplicated diabetes mellitus was much more variable (some low and some high) than the [fMg^{2+}] in the healthy dogs.

IMMUNOREACTIVE PARATHYROID HORMONE (iPTH) CONCENTRATION

I.   Physiologic processes
    A.   *PTH* is a polypeptide hormone (84 amino acids) produced by parathyroid glands and inactivated or degraded by kidneys and liver. PTH is secreted by parathyroid glands in response to a decreased [fCa^{2+}] in blood, whereas vitamin D and an increased [fCa^{2+}] inhibit synthesis of PTH.
       1.   PTH secretion is primarily mediated by fCa^{2+} binding to the parathyroid gland chief cell calcium-sensing receptor (CaSR). This receptor is linked to a series of intracellular signaling pathways that inhibit PTH secretion.[159,160] Mutations in the CaSR gene can cause increased or decreased receptor activity and hypocalcemia or hypercalcemia, respectively.
       2.   Mg^{2+} may influence PTH responses by interfering with fCa^{2+} binding. Therefore, hypomagnesemia may inhibit PTH secretion at a lower [fCa^{2+}].[68]
       3.   The acid-base status of an animal also affects the secretion of PTH. Acidoses (metabolic and respiratory) stimulate PTH secretion, although, in metabolic acidosis, the increase in [fCa^{2+}] due to pH-induced shifts can be sufficient to inhibit increases in PTH. Alkaloses (metabolic and respiratory) inhibit PTH secretion.[120,121]
    B.   Primary target organs: bone, intestine, and kidney
       1.   PTH promotes increased Ca^{2+} absorption by intestine (in the presence of vitamin D) and increased resorption in renal tubules.
       2.   PTH promotes mobilization of Ca^{2+} and PO$_4$ from bone.
       3.   PTH promotes renal PO$_4$ excretion by inhibiting resorption of PO$_4$ by tubules (a potent phosphaturic action).
    C.   The net effect of PTH activity is to increase plasma [fCa^{2+}] by Ca^{2+} mobilization and decrease plasma [Pi] by promoting phosphaturia.

II.   Analytical concepts for iPTH assays
    A.   RIAs developed for human PTH have sufficient species cross-reactivity to be valid for domestic mammals.[23]
       1.   iPTH values generated by RIAs for intact PTH or N-terminal fragments correlate well with expected biologic PTH activity. Because some immunoassays may react with preproparathyroid hormone, proparathyroid hormone, intact PTH, or a PTH fragment, the analyte of these assays can collectively be called *immunoreactive PTH* (iPTH). Only if the assay was 100 % specific for intact PTH would [PTH] equal [iPTH].
       2.   iPTH assays tend to be limited to endocrinology and larger reference laboratories.
       3.   iPTH assays do not detect PTHrp.
    B.   A human immunoradiometric assay for active whole PTH has been validated for equine iPTH[161] and canine iPTH.[162]
    C.   Samples for [iPTH] should be collected from dogs after an overnight fast. Postprandial alkalosis and variations in the [fCa^{2+}] after meals can alter the [iPTH] in dogs.[107] Similar changes might occur in cats and horses.

    D. Because PTH is susceptible to proteolysis, the preferred sample for PTH is EDTA-plasma that contains a protease inhibitor (aprotinin). If the sample is not analyzed on the day of collection, some investigators write that plasma or serum without aprotinin is acceptable if the sample remains frozen during storage or transit.[108] In a stability study at 21 °C and 37 °C, the serum [iPTH] remained stable for 2 d with two protease inhibitors (Pefabloc SC and 4-[2-aminoethyl]-benzenesulfonyl fluoride), but the serum [iPTH] decreased with other protease inhibitors.[163] Equine [iPTH] in EDTA plasma was stable for up to 3 mo when stored at −20 °C.[164]

    E. The serum [tCa^{2+}] and ideally [fCa^{2+}] of the same sample should be known when interpreting the [iPTH]. For example, a high-normal or increased [iPTH] in the presence of hypercalcemia would represent a pathologic state, whereas, in the presence of hypocalcemia, it may represent a physiologic response.

III.   Increased serum or plasma [iPTH] (Table 11.8)

    A. Most disorders that cause increased serum or plasma [iPTH] are due to excessive production of PTH by neoplastic parathyroid cells or by hyperplastic parathyroid cells (secondary to decreased [fCa^{2+}]).

    B. However, many dogs with hypercalcemia due to primary hyperparathyroidism do not have an increased [iPTH]. Instead, the [iPTH] is WRI but inappropriately high in relation to an increased [fCa^{2+}], thus reflecting a defective negative feedback on PTH secretion

    C. In one study, many dogs with hyperadrenocorticism had unexplained increases in plasma [iPTH] and concurrent normocalcemia.[106]

IV.   Decreased serum or plasma [iPTH] (Table 11.9)

Table 11.8. Diseases or conditions that cause increased [iPTH]

Increased PTH production by neoplastic cells
   Neoplastic parathyroid gland (primary hyperparathyroidism)
   Multiple endocrine neoplasia (type 1 or 2A)
Increased PTH production by hyperplastic parathyroid glands (idiopathic or secondary hyperparathyroidism)
  *Chronic renal disease
   Diet with a low $Ca^{2+}:PO_4$ ratio
   Hypocalcemic disorders (with a decreased [fCa^{2+}]), other than hypoparathyroidism
   Pseudo-hypoparathyroidism (decreased PTH receptor responsiveness)
   Hyperadrenocorticism in dogs

  * A relatively common disease or condition

Table 11.9. Diseases or conditions that cause decreased [iPTH]

Decreased PTH production due to damaged or removed parathyroid glands (hypoparathyroidism)
Decreased PTH production due to inhibition
  Hypervitaminosis D
  Hypercalcemic disorders (with an increased [fCa^{2+}]) except primary hyperparathyroidism
  Hypomagnesemia due to Mg^{2+} depletion

PARATHYROID HORMONE–RELATED PROTEIN (PTHrp) CONCENTRATION

I.   Physiologic processes
     A. PTHrp promotes Ca^{2+} balance in the fetus and modulates cartilage and bone development. After birth, the control of Ca^{2+} balance switches from PTHrp to PTH.[23]
     B. PTHrp is produced by many cells in fetuses and adults, but plasma [PTHrp] is very low in healthy adults.

II. Analytical concepts
     A. Sample
         1. Because of rapid proteolysis of PTHrp, it has been recommended that blood be collected into EDTA tubes with an added protease inhibitor (aprotinin or leupeptin). Separated plasma is analyzed fresh or shipped frozen to reference laboratories.[165]
         2. Some laboratories, however, request serum samples be shipped on ice.
     B. Assays designed to measure human [PTHrp] (N terminal) are used for measuring canine [PTHrp]; however, the same assay is not valid for equine [PTHrp].[23] One human PTHrp assay also can be used for measuring feline [PTHrp].[26]

III. Increased [PTHrp] in serum
     A. Some neoplasms (especially lymphomas and carcinomas) can produce enough PTHrp to cause an increase in serum [PTHrp]; the increased PTHrp activity can result in a hypercalcemia. There also are rare reports of increased [PTHrp] in dogs with granulomatous diseases.
     B. More information about these hypercalcemic disorders is presented in the Total Calcium Concentration section of this chapter.

VITAMIN D CONCENTRATION

I.   Physiologic processes
     A. Formation of vitamin D
         1. Cholesterol is converted to 7-dehydrocholesterol, which is converted by ultraviolet light to cholecalciferol (vitamin D_3). Vitamin D_3 can also be of dietary origin. Vitamin D_2 (ergocalciferol) can be ingested in plants.
         2. 25-Hydroxylase in hepatocytes catalyzes the formation of 25-HCC from cholecalciferol. 25-HCC circulates bound to vitamin D–binding protein.
         3. Megalin, amnionless, and cubilin receptors on proximal renal tubular epithelial cells mediate endocytic uptake of 25-HCC and vitamin D–binding protein that pass through the glomerular filtration barrier. This receptor-mediated uptake prevents loss of 25-HCC in the urine and delivers it to renal tubular epithelial cells. Uptake of cobalamin/intrinsic factor complexes by the intestine is also mediated by cubilin, amnionless, and megalin.[166]
         4. 1α-Hydroxylase in renal tubular cells catalyzes the formation of 1,25-DHCC from 25-HCC in most mammals. Studies have shown that horses lack renal 1α-hydroxylase and have low concentrations of 25-HCC, 24,25-DHCC, and 1,25-DHCC in plasma.[9]
         5. 1,25-DHCC (also called calcitriol) has 25 times the biologic activity of 25-HCC, which has 3–5 times the activity of cholecalciferol.

      6. PTH activity and $[Ca^{2+}]$ affect the formation of 1,25-DHCC, but $[Ca^{2+}]$ appears to be the major factor controlling 1,25-DHCC concentrations. One study indicated that when there is increased PTH activity, low $[tCa^{2+}]$ leads to an increased 1,25-DHCC concentration, whereas high $[tCa^{2+}]$ leads to a decreased 1,25-DHCC concentration.[167] In that study, the $[tCa^{2+}]$ was measured, but the altered $[tCa^{2+}]$ probably reflected a change in the $[fCa^{2+}]$.

   B. Actions of vitamin D in dogs, cats, and cattle. (Roles of vitamin D in horses in regulation of $[fCa^{2+}]$ appear to be minor).[9]

      1. Vitamin D promotes intestinal uptake of Ca^{2+} by stimulating the formation of a Ca^{2+}-binding protein (calbindin) in the mucosal epithelial cells. It also stimulates absorption of PO_4.

      2. Vitamin D promotes Ca^{2+} and PO_4 liberation from bone by stimulating osteoclastic activity.

      3. Vitamin D promotes resorption of fCa^{2+} by proximal renal tubules by stimulating the formation of calbindin.

      4. Vitamin D inhibits PTH synthesis in parathyroid glands by inhibiting transcription of the PTH mRNA.

      5. Net effect of vitamin D: promotes hypercalcemia

II.   Analytical concepts

   A. Sample

      1. Serum is the common sample but plasma (with either heparin or EDTA) is acceptable. Concentrations of 1,25-DHCC and 25-HCC are stable for 3 d at 24 °C.[168] Samples should be frozen if analysis is delayed.

      2. Prior to most assays, the sample is deproteinized or extracted to free vitamin D metabolites from vitamin D–binding proteins (specific α-globulins and albumin). Nearly all vitamin D molecules are protein bound in serum.

   B. Assays

      1. The [1,25-DHCC] can be measured by a radioreceptor assay.[169] The assay uses a vitamin D receptor from calf thymus. The [1,25-DHCC] can be measured also by a RIA.[170,171]

      2. [25-HCC] can be measured by RIAs, though the antibody might cross-react with 1,25-DHCC.[1] It can also be measured by a protein-binding assay.[171]

III. Because of the limited availability of 1,25-DHCC assays, there are few reports of abnormal [1,25-DHCC] in domestic mammals. The following lists are based on reported or expected concentrations in various disorders.[1] Possible related defects in 1,25-DHCC pathways are within parentheses.

   A. Increased [1,25-DHCC] expected or reported

      1. Granulomatous disease: Macrophages may produce 1,25-DHCC.

      2. Primary hyperparathyroidism:[170] PTH promotes 1α-hydroxylase activity, which results in increased 1,25-DHCC production.

      3. Lymphoma and other HHM disorders:[24,170] Either PTHrp promotes 1α-hydroxylase activity or neoplastic cells produce 1,25-DHCC.

      4. Vitamin D intoxication:[49,172] increased intake.

      5. Vitamin D–receptor defect rickets: vitamin D–dependent rickets, type II[73]

      6. Bovine parturient paresis (milk fever):[74] Decreased $[fCa^{2+}]$ and increased PTH activity promote 1α-hydroxylase activity, which increases 1,25-DHCC production.

      7. Chronic renal failure in hypercalcemic dogs: This was reported in 2 of 10 hypercalcemic dogs diagnosed with chronic renal failure, whereas 4 of 10 had decreased [1,25-DHCC]. Reasons for the increased [1,25-DHCC] were not determined or proposed.[170]

   B. Decreased [1,25-DHCC] expected or reported.
      1. Renal failure, including protein-losing nephropathy: This may be caused by decreased functional renal tissue and therefore decreased production of 1,25-DHCC, or by a loss of the vitamin D–binding proteins.[170,171]
      2. Hyperphosphatemia not caused by increased vitamin D: Increased [PO_4] inhibits 1α-hydroxylase activity, which decreases 1,25-DHCC production.
      3. Hypomagnesemia: This may create a pseudo-hypoparathyroidism, which decreases 1,25-DHCC production, or hypomagnesemia may impair PTH secretion.
      4. Hypoparathyroidism: Less PTH activity causes less 1α-hydroxylase activity, which decreases 1,25-DHCC production.
      5. Pseudo-hypoparathyroidism: Less response to PTH causes less 1α-hydroxylase activity, which decreases 1,25-DHCC production.
      6. HHM[24,170] (This is perhaps caused by hypercalcemia, reduced [iPTH], hyperkalemic nephropathy, or the presence of an inhibitor of 1α-hydroxylase.)
      7. Protein-losing enteropathies in dogs[70] (probably decreased intestinal absorption).
      8. Vitamin D-deficient diet[71] (decreased intake)
      9. Dogs with cubilin, amnionless, or megalin dysfunction and diminished renal tubular resorption of 25-HCC and vitamin D–binding protein had decreased plasma concentrations of 25-HCC and 1,25-DHCC.[166]

CALCITONIN CONCENTRATION

I. Physiologic processes
   A. Calcitonin is a polypeptide hormone synthesized by thyroid C cells that are part of the APUD family of cells. (APUD is the acronym for endocrine cells that have a role in *a*mine *p*recursor *u*ptake, and *d*ecarboxylation.)
   B. The regulation of secretion is not thoroughly understood
      1. Calcitonin secretion is stimulated by increased concentrations of fCa^{2+} (major), fMg^{2+}, α- and β-adrenergic hormones, gastrin, and cholecystokinin.
      2. Calcitonin secretion is inhibited by decreased [fCa^{2+}] and increased somatostatin concentration.

II. Actions
   A. Calcitonin inhibits osteoclastic activity in bone.
   B. Calcitonin inhibits renal tubular resorption of Ca^{2+} and PO_4.
   C. The net effect of calcitonin activity is to decrease serum [tCa^{2+}], [fCa^{2+}], and [Pi]

III. Analytical concepts
   A. Marked differences in amino acid sequences between species may limit the cross-species immunoreactivity in RIAs.
   B. RIAs for canine calcitonin have been developed.[173,174]

IV. Increased immunoreactive calcitonin concentrations
   A. Medullary thyroid carcinoma[175]
   B. Nonthyroid cancer, especially from neural crest tissue

Table 11.10. Expected hormone and mineral patterns for major diseases or conditions (without complications)

	[tCa^{2+}]	[Pi]	[iPTH]	[PTHrp]	[vitamin D]
Primary hyperparathyroidism	↑[a]	↓[b]–WRI	WRI–↑[c]	WRI	WRI
Humoral hypercalcemia of malignancy[d]	↑	↓	↓–WRI	↑	WRI
Excess vitamin D	↑	WRI–↑	↓–WRI	WRI	↑
Canine hypoadrenocorticism	↑	WRI–↑	↓–WRI	WRI	WRI
Renal failure, hypercalcemic[e]	↑	WRI–↓	↓[f]	WRI	?[g]
Renal failure, chronic[h]	WRI–↓	↑	↑	WRI	↓–WRI
Hypoalbuminemia	↓	WRI	WRI	WRI	WRI
Primary hypoparathyroidism	↓	WRI–↑	↓–WRI	WRI	WRI
Vitamin D–receptor defect rickets	↓	↓	↑	WRI	↑
Milk fever	↓	↓	WRI–↑	WRI	WRI–↑
Prolonged anorexia	WRI	↓	WRI	WRI	WRI

[a] ↑, above the reference interval

[b] ↓, below the reference interval

[c] The value may not be increased but is inappropriately high for the hypercalcemic status.

[d] Due to increased PHTrp production by neoplastic cells (different patterns with other hypercalcemic agents)

[e] More common in horses than other species; can be either acute or chronic renal failure.

[f] [iPTH] is decreased in hypercalcemic renal failure in horses; similar data were not found for other animals.

[g] A question mark (?) indicates that the expected result is not known in most mammals. Healthy horses have very little vitamin D, and one would expect less in the presence of hypercalcemia.

[h] More common than hypercalcemic renal failure in most domestic species

[i] The expected result is not known in most mammals, but decreases are expected in the human condition.

Note: Secondary pathologic states may alter patterns. For example, prolonged or severe hypercalcemia may cause renal failure that might change the serum [Pi] from hypophosphatemia to hyperphosphatemia.

MAJOR PATTERNS FOR CALCIUM (Ca^{2+}) AND INORGANIC PHOSPHORUS (Pi) DISORDERS

Because of the physiologic relationships among Ca^{2+}, PO$_4$, PTH, PTHrp, and vitamin D, some diseases are expected to cause certain patterns of abnormal analyte concentrations suggestive of those diseases. Patterns for major diseases or conditions are listed in Table 11.10. Because of compensation, some analyte concentrations may remain WRI but be inappropriately located near either the upper or lower limits of the reference interval. Findings in clinical cases may represent a combination of factors; for example, an animal with primary hyperparathyroidism may have hypercalcemia because of excess PTH activity, and hyperphosphatemia because of hypercalcemic nephrosis that produced renal failure.

References

1. Endres DB, Rude RK. 1999. Mineral and bone metabolism. In: Burtis CA, Ashwood ER, eds. *Tietz Textbook of Clinical Chemistry*, 3rd edition, 1395–1457. Philadelphia: WB Saunders.

2. Schenck PA, Chew DJ, Brooks CL. 1996. Fractionation of canine serum calcium, using a micropartition system. Am J Vet Res 57:268–271.

3. van der Kolk JH, Nachreiner RF, Refsal KR, Brouillet D, Wensing T. 2002. Heparinised blood ionised calcium concentrations in horses with colic or diarrhoea compared to normal subjects. Equine Vet J 34:528–531.

4. Meuten DJ, Chew DJ, Capen CC, Kociba GJ. 1982. Relationship of serum total calcium to albumin and total protein in dogs. J Am Vet Med Assoc 180:63–67.

5. Harper EJ, Hackett RM, Wilkinson J, Heaton PR. 2003. Age-related variations in hematologic and plasma biochemical test results in beagles and Labrador retrievers. J Am Vet Med Assoc 223:1436–1442.

6. Fenger CK. 1998. Neonatal and perinatal diseases. In: Reed SM, Bayly WM, eds. *Equine Internal Medicine*, 938–970. Philadelphia: WB Saunders.

7. Meyer DJ, Coles EH, Rich LJ. 1992. *Veterinary Laboratory Medicine: Interpretation and Diagnosis*. Philadelphia: WB Saunders.

8. Schott HC II. 1998. Chronic renal failure. In: Reed SM, Bayly WM, eds. *Equine Internal Medicine*, 856–875. Philadelphia: WB Saunders.

9. Breidenbach A, Schlumbohm C, Harmeyer J. 1998. Peculiarities of vitamin D and of the calcium and phosphate homeostatic system in horses. Vet Res 29:173–186.

10. Rosol TJ, Capen CC. 1997. Calcium-regulating hormones and diseases of abnormal mineral (calcium, phosphorus, magnesium) metabolism. In: Kaneko JJ, Harvey JW, Bruss ML, eds. *Clinical Biochemistry of Domestic Animals*, 5th edition, 619–702. San Diego: Academic.

11. Guyton AC, Hall JE. 2000. *Textbook of Medical Physiology*, 10th edition. Philadelphia: WB Saunders.

12. Nap RC, Hazewinkel HA. 1994. Growth and skeletal development in the dog in relation to nutrition: A review. Vet Q 16:50–59.

13. Rose BD. 1994. *Clinical Physiology of Acid-Base and Electrolyte Disorders*, 4th edition. New York: McGraw-Hill.

14. Guyton AC, Hall JE. 1996. *Textbook of Medical Physiology*, 9th edition. Philadelphia: WB Saunders.

15. Lundberg GD, Iverson C, Radulescu G. 1986. Now read this: The SI units are here. J Am Med Assoc 255:2329–2339.

16. Bienzle D, Jacobs RM, Lumsden JH. 1993. Relationship of serum total calcium to serum albumin in dogs, cats, horses and cattle. Can Vet J 34:360–364.

17. Flanders JA, Scarlett JM, Blue JT, Neth S. 1989. Adjustment of total serum calcium concentration for binding to albumin and protein in cats: 291 cases (1986–1987). J Am Vet Med Assoc 194:1609–1611.

18. Schenck PA, Chew DJ. 2005. Prediction of serum ionized calcium concentration by use of serum total calcium concentration in dogs. Am J Vet Res 66:1330–1336.

19. Berger B, Feldman EC. 1987. Primary hyperparathyroidism in dogs: 21 cases (1976–1986). J Am Vet Med Assoc 191:350–356.

20. Kallet AJ, Richter KP, Feldman EC, Brum DE. 1991. Primary hyperparathyroidism in cats: Seven cases (1984–1989). J Am Vet Med Assoc 199:1767–1771.

21. Frank N, Hawkins JF, Couëtil LL, Raymond JT. 1998. Primary hyperparathyroidism with osteodystrophia fibrosa of the facial bones in a pony. J Am Vet Med Assoc 212:84–86.

22. Feldman EC, Hoar B, Pollard R, Nelson RW. 2005. Pretreatment clinical and laboratory findings in dogs with primary hyperparathyroidism: 210 cases (1987–2004). J Am Vet Med Assoc 227:756–761.

23. Rosol TJ, Capen CC. 1996. Pathophysiology of calcium, phosphorus, and magnesium metabolism in animals. Vet Clin North Am Small Anim Pract 26:1155–1184.

24. Rosol TJ, Nagode LA, Couto CG, Hammer AS, Chew DJ, Peterson JL, Ayl RD, Steinmeyer CL, Capen CC. 1992. Parathyroid hormone (PTH)–related protein, PTH, and 1,25-dihydroxyvitamin D in dogs with cancer-associated hypercalcemia. Endocrinology 131:1157–1164.

25. Pressler BM, Rotstein DS, Law JM, Rosol TJ, LeRoy B, Keene BW, Jackson MW. 2002. Hypercalcemia and high parathyroid hormone–related protein concentration associated with malignant melanoma in a dog. J Am Vet Med Assoc 221:263–265.

26. Bolliger AP, Graham PA, Richard V, Rosol TJ, Nachreiner RF, Refsal KR. 2002. Detection of parathyroid hormone–related protein in cats with humoral hypercalcemia of malignancy. Vet Clin Pathol 31:3–8.

27. Barton MH, Sharma P, LeRoy BE, Howerth EW. 2004. Hypercalcemia and high serum parathyroid hormone–related protein concentration in a horse with multiple myeloma. J Am Vet Med Assoc 225:409–413.

28. Nafe LA, Patnaik AK, Lyman R. 1980. Hypercalcemia associated with epidermoid carcinoma in a dog. J Am Vet Med Assoc 176:1253–1254.

29. Zenoble RD, Crowell WA, Rowland GN. 1979. Adenocarcinoma and hypercalcemia in a dog. Vet Pathol 16:122–123.

30. Engelman RW, Tyler RD, Good RA, Day NK. 1985. Hypercalcemia in cats with feline-leukemia virus–associated leukemia-lymphoma. Cancer 56:777–781.

31. Klausner JS, Bell FW, Hayden DW, Hegstad RL, Johnston SD. 1990. Hypercalcemia in two cats with squamous cell carcinomas. J Am Vet Med Assoc 196:103–105.

32. Meuten DJ, Price SM, Seiler RM, Krook L. 1978. Gastric carcinoma with pseudohyperparathyroidism in a horse. Cornell Vet 68:179–195.

33. Marr CM, Love S, Pirie HM. 1989. Clinical, ultrasonographic and pathological findings in a horse with splenic lymphosarcoma and pseudohyperparathyroidism. Equine Vet J 21:221–226.

34. Esplin DG, Taylor JL. 1977. Hypercalcemia in a horse with lymphosarcoma. J Am Vet Med Assoc 170:180–182.

35. Mair TS, Yeo SP, Lucke VM. 1990. Hypercalcaemia and soft tissue mineralisation associated with lymphosarcoma in two horses. Vet Rec 126:99–101.

36. Fix AS, Miller LD. 1987. Equine adrenocortical carcinoma with hypercalcemia. Vet Pathol 24:190–192.

37. Knecht TP, Behling CA, Burton DW, Glass CK, Deftos LJ. 1996. The humoral hypercalcemia of benignancy: A newly appreciated syndrome. Am J Clin Pathol 105:487–492.

38. Fradkin JM, Braniecki AM, Craig TM, Ramiro-Ibanez F, Rogers KS, Zoran DL. 2001. Elevated parathyroid hormone–related protein and hypercalcemia in two dogs with schistosomiasis. J Am Anim Hosp Assoc 37:349–355.

39. Christakos S, Gabrielides C, Rhoten WB. 1989. Vitamin D–dependent calcium binding proteins: Chemistry, distribution, functional considerations, and molecular biology. Endocr Rev 10:3–26.

40. Carothers MA, Chew DJ, Nagode LA. 1994. 25(OH)-cholecalciferol intoxication in dogs. In: Proceedings of the 12th ACVIM Forum, San Francisco, 822–825.

41. Hilbe M, Sydler T, Fischer L, Naegeli H. 2000. Metastatic calcification in a dog attributable to ingestion of a tacalcitol ointment. Vet Pathol 37:490–492.

42. Campbell A. 1997. Calcipotriol poisoning in dogs. Vet Rec 141:27–28.

43. Fan TM, Simpson KW, Trasti S, Birnbaum N, Center SA, Yeager A. 1998. Calcipotriol toxicity in a dog. J Small Anim Pract 39:581–586.

44. Harrington DD. 1982. Acute vitamin D_2 (ergocalciferol) toxicosis in horses: Case report and experimental studies. J Am Vet Med Assoc 180:867–873.

45. Harrington DD, Page EH. 1983. Acute vitamin D_3 toxicosis in horses: Case reports and experimental studies of the comparative toxicity of vitamins D_2 and D_3. J Am Vet Med Assoc 182:1358–1369.

46. Wasserman RH, Carradino RA, Krook LP. 1975. *Cestrum diurnum*: A domestic plant with 1,25-dihydroxycholecalciferol-like activity. Biochem Biophys Res Commun 62:85–91.

47. Muylle E, Oyaert W, De Roose P, van den Hende C. 1974. Hypercalcaemia and mineralisation of non-osseous tissues in horses due to vitamin-D toxicity. Zentralbl Veterinarmed [A] 21:638–643.

48. Spangler WL, Gribble DH, Lee TC. 1979. Vitamin D intoxication and the pathogenesis of vitamin D nephropathy in the dog. Am J Vet Res 40:73–83.

49. Mellanby RJ, Mee AP, Berry JL, Herrtage ME. 2005. Hypercalcaemia in two dogs caused by excessive dietary supplementation of vitamin D. J Small Anim Pract 46:334–338.

50. Dow SW, Legendre AM, Stiff M, Greene C. 1986. Hypercalcemia associated with blastomycosis in dogs. J Am Vet Med Assoc 188:706–709.

51. Hodges RD, Legendre AM, Adams LG, Willard MD, Pitts RP, Monce K, Needels CC, Ward H. 1994. Itraconazole for the treatment of histoplasmosis in cats. J Vet Intern Med 8:409–413.

52. Savary KCM, Price GS, Vaden SL. 2000. Hypercalcemia in cats: A retrospective study of 71 cases (1991–1997). J Vet Intern Med 14:184–189.

53. Boag AK, Murphy KF, Connolly DJ. 2005. Hypercalcaemia associated with *Angiostrongylus vasorum* in three dogs. J Small Anim Pract 46:79–84.

54. Elfers RS, Bayly WM, Brobst DF, Reed SM, Liggitt HD, Hawker CD, Baylink DJ. 1986. Alterations in calcium, phosphorus and C-terminal parathyroid hormone levels in equine acute renal disease. Cornell Vet 76:317–329.

55. Bertone JJ, Traub-Dargatz JL, Fettman MJ, Wilke L, Wrigley RH, Jaenke R, Paulsen ME. 1987. Monitoring the progression of renal failure in a horse with polycystic kidney disease: Use of the reciprocal of serum creatinine concentration and sodium sulfanilate clearance half-time. J Am Vet Med Assoc 191:565–568.

56. National Research Council. 1989. *Nutrient Requirements of Horses*, 5th edition. Washington, DC: National Academy Press.

57. Brobst DF, Bayly WM, Reed SM, Howard GA, Torbeck RL. 1982. Parathyroid hormone evaluation in normal horses and horses with renal failure. Equine Vet Sci 2:150–157.

58. Eubig PA, Brady MS, Gwaltney-Brant SM, Khan SA, Mazzaferro EM, Morrow CM. 2005. Acute renal failure in dogs after the ingestion of grapes or raisins: A retrospective evaluation of 43 dogs (1992–2002). J Vet Intern Med 19:663–674.

59. Schenck PA, Chew DJ. 2003. Determination of calcium fractionation in dogs with chronic renal failure. Am J Vet Res 64:1181–1184.

60. Peterson MA, Feinman JM. 1982. Hypercalcemia associated with hypoadrenocorticism in 16 dogs. J Am Vet Med Assoc 181:802–804.

61. Smith SA, Freeman LC, Bagladi-Swanson M. 2002. Hypercalcemia due to iatrogenic secondary hypoadrenocorticism and diabetes mellitus in a cat. J Am Anim Hosp Assoc 38:41–44.

62. Peterson ME, Greco DS, Orth DN. 1989. Primary hypoadrenocorticism in ten cats. J Vet Intern Med 3:55–58.

63. Walser M, Robinson BHB, Duckett JW Jr. 1963. The hypercalcemia of adrenal insufficiency. J Clin Invest 42:456–465.

64. Osborne CA, Poffenbarger EM, Klausner JS, Johnston SD, Griffith DP. 1986. Etiopathogenesis, clinical manifestations, and management of canine calcium oxalate urolithiasis. Vet Clin North Am Small Anim Pract 16:133–170.

65. Greco DS, Peterson ME, Cho DY, Markovits JE. 1985. Juvenile-onset hypothyroidism in a dog. J Am Vet Med Assoc 187:948–950.

66. Hirt RA, Kneissl S, Teinfalt M. 2000. Severe hypercalcemia in a dog with a retained fetus and endometritis. J Am Vet Med Assoc 216:1423–1425.

67. Midkiff AM, Chew DJ, Randolph JF, Center SA, DiBartola SP. 2000. Idiopathic hypercalcemia in cats. J Vet Intern Med 14:619–626.

68. Oldham SB, Rude RK, Molloy CT, Lipson LG. 1984. The effects of magnesium on calcium inhibition of parathyroid adenylate cyclase. Endocrinology 115:1883–1890.

69. Bush WW, Kimmel SE, Wosar MA, Jackson MW. 2001. Secondary hypoparathyroidism attributed to hypomagnesemia in a dog with protein-losing enteropathy. J Am Vet Med Assoc 219:1732–1734.

70. Mellanby RJ, Mellor PJ, Roulois A, Baines EA, Mee AP, Berry JL, Herrtage ME. 2005. Hypocalcaemia associated with low serum vitamin D metabolite concentrations in two dogs with protein-losing enteropathies. J Small Anim Pract 46:345–351.

71. Hendy GN, Stotland MA, Grunbaum D, Fraher LJ, Loveridge N, Goltzman D. 1989. Characteristics of secondary hyperparathyroidism in vitamin D–deficient dogs. Am J Physiol 256:E765–E772.

72. Wong KM, Klein L, Hollis B. 1985. Effects of parathyroid hormone on puppies during development of Ca and vitamin D deficiency. Am J Physiol 249:E568–E576.

73. Schreiner CA, Nagode LA. 2003. Vitamin D–dependent rickets type 2 in a four-month-old cat. J Am Vet Med Assoc 222:337–336.

74. Horst RL, Jorgensen NA, DeLuca HF. 1978. Plasma 1,25-dihydroxyvitamin D and parathyroid hormone levels in paretic dairy cows. Am J Physiol 235:E634–E637.

75. Mayer GP, Ramberg CF Jr, Kronfeld DS, Buckle RM, Sherwood LM, Aurbach GD, Potts JT Jr. 1969. Plasma parathyroid hormone concentration in hypocalcemic parturient cows. Am J Vet Res 30:1587–1597.

76. Goff JP, Horst RL. 2003. Role of acid-base physiology on the pathogenesis of parturient hypocalcaemia (milk fever): The DCAD theory in principal and practice. Acta Vet Scand Suppl 97:51–56.

77. Baird JD. 1971. Lactation tetany (eclampsia) in a Shetland pony mare. Aust Vet J 47:402–404.

78. Fascetti AJ, Hickman MA. 1999. Preparturient hypocalcemia in four cats. J Am Vet Med Assoc 215:1127–1129.

79. Young DM, Capen CC, Black HE. 1971. Calcitonin activity in ultimobranchial neoplasms from bulls. Vet Pathol 8:19–27.

80. Fenger CK. 1998. Disorders of calcium metabolism. In: Reed SM, Bayly WM, eds. *Equine Internal Medicine*, 1st edition, 925–934. Philadelphia: WB Saunders.

81. James LF. 1999. Halogeton poisoning in livestock. J Nat Toxins 8:395–403.

82. Crowell WA, Whitlock RH, Stout RC, Tyler DE. 1979. Ethylene glycol toxicosis in cattle. Cornell Vet 69:272–279.

83. Grauer GF, Thrall MA. 1982. Ethylene glycol (antifreeze) poisoning in the dog and cat. J Am Anim Hosp Assoc 18:492–497.

84. Grauer GF, Thrall MA, Henre BA, Grauer RM, Hamar DW. 1984. Early clinicopathologic findings in dogs ingesting ethylene glycol. Am J Vet Res 45:2299–2303.

85. Chew DJ, Leonard M, Muir W III. 1989. Effect of sodium bicarbonate infusions on ionized calcium and total calcium concentrations in serum of clinically normal cats. Am J Vet Res 50:145–150.

86. Freestone JF, Carlson GP, Harrold DR, Church G. 1988. Influence of furosemide treatment on fluid and electrolyte balance in horses. Am J Vet Res 49:1899–1902.

87. Komnenou A, Karayannopoulou M, Polizopoulou ZS, Constantinidis TC, Dessiris A. 2005. Correlation of serum alkaline phosphatase activity with the healing process of long bone fractures in dogs. Vet Clin Pathol 34:35–38.

88. Kimmel SE, Washabau RJ, Drobatz KJ. 2001. Incidence and prognostic value of low plasma ionized calcium concentration in cats with acute pancreatitis: 46 cases (1996–1998). J Am Vet Med Assoc 219:1105–1109.

89. Agarwal N, Pitchumoni CS. 1993. Acute pancreatitis: A multisystem disease. Gastroenterologist 1:115–128.

90. Warshaw AL, Lee KH, Napier TW, Fournier PO, Duchainey D, Axelrod L. 1985. Depression of serum calcium by increased plasma free fatty acids in the rat: A mechanism for hypocalcemia in acute pancreatitis. Gastroenterology 89:814–820.

91. Bhattacharya SK, Crawford AJ, Pate JW, Clemens MG, Chaudry IH. 1988. Mechanism of calcium and magnesium translocation in acute pancreatitis: A temporal correlation between hypocalcemia and membrane-mediated excessive intracellular calcium accumulation in soft tissues. Magnesium 7:91–102.

92. Drobatz KJ, Hughes D. 1997. Concentration of ionized calcium in plasma from cats with urethral obstruction. J Am Vet Med Assoc 211:1392–1395.

93. Vaden SL, Levine J, Breitschwerdt EB. 1997. A retrospective case-control of acute renal failure in 99 dogs. J Vet Intern Med 11:58–64.

94. Schaer M, Cavanagh P, Hause W, Wilkins R. 1977. Iatrogenic hyperphosphatemia, hypocalcemia and hypernatremia in a cat. J Am Anim Hosp Assoc 13:39–41.

95. Garcia-Lopez JM, Provost PJ, Rush JE, Zicker SC, Burmaster H, Freeman LM. 2001. Prevalence and prognostic importance of hypomagnesemia and hypocalcemia in horses that have colic surgery. Am J Vet Res 62:7–12.

96. Delesalle C, Dewulf J, Lefebvre RA, Schuurkes JA, Van VB, Deprez P. 2005. Use of plasma ionized calcium levels and Ca^{2+} substitution response patterns as prognostic parameters for ileus and survival in colic horses. Vet Q 27:157–172.

97. Ray AC, Kyle ALG, Murphy MJ, Reagor JC. 1989. Etiologic agents, incidence, and improved diagnostic methods of cantharidin toxicosis in horses. Am J Vet Res 50:187–191.

98. Helman RG, Edwards WC. 1997. Clinical features of blister beetle poisoning in equids: 70 cases (1983–1996). J Am Vet Med Assoc 211:1018–1021.

99. Harris PA. 1998. Musculoskeletal disease. In: Reed SM, Bayly WM, eds. *Equine Internal Medicine*, 1st edition, 371–426. Philadelphia: WB Saunders.

100. Waldron-Mease E, Klein LV, Rosenberg H, Leitch M. 1981. Malignant hyperthermia in a halothane-anesthetized horse. J Am Vet Med Assoc 179:896–898.

101. Gaschen F, Gaschen L, Seiler G, Welle M, Bornand Jaunin V, Gonin Jmaa D, Neiger-Aeschbacher G, Adé-Damilano M. 1998. Lethal peracute rhabdomyolysis associated with stress and general anesthesia in three dystrophin-deficient cats. Vet Pathol 35:117–123.

102. Perkins G, Valberg SJ, Madigan JM, Carlson GP, Jones SL. 1998. Electrolyte disturbances in foals with severe rhabdomyolysis. J Vet Intern Med 12:173–177.

103. Kerr MG, Snow DH. 1983. Composition of sweat of the horse during prolonged epinephrine (adrenaline) infusion, heat exposure, and exercise. Am J Vet Res 44:1571–1577.

104. Brooks DG. 1995. Acute tumor lysis syndrome in dogs. Compend Contin Educ Pract Vet 17:1103–1106.

105. Blood DC, Radostits OM. 1983. Diseases of the alimentary tract: II. In: Blood DC, Radostits OM, eds. *Veterinary Medicine*, 203–259. London: Baillière Tindall.

106. Ramsey IK, Tebb A, Harris E, Evans H, Herrtage ME. 2005. Hyperparathyroidism in dogs with hyperadrenocorticism. J Small Anim Pract 46:531–536.

107. Lopez I, Aguilera-Tejero E, Estepa JC, Bas S, Mayer-Valor R, Jimenez A, Rodriguez M. 2005. Diurnal variations in the plasma concentration of parathyroid hormone in dogs. Vet Rec 157:344–347.

108. Rosol TJ, Chew DJ, Nagode LA, Schenck P. 2000. Disorders of calcium. In: DiBartola SP, ed. *Fluid Therapy in Small Animal Practice*, 2nd edition, 108–162. Philadelphia: WB Saunders.

109. Larsson L, Ohman S. 1985. Effect of silicone-separator tubes and storage time on ionized calcium in serum. Clin Chem 31:169–170.

110. Boink ABTJ, Buckley BM, Christiansen TF, Covington AK, Maas AHJ, Müller-Plathe O, Sachs C, Siggaard-Andersen O. 1991. International Federation of Clinical Chemistry (IFCC) Scientific Division. IFCC recommendation: Recommendation on sampling, transport and storage for the determination of concentration of ionized calcium in whole blood, plasma and serum. Clin Chim Acta 202:S13–S21.

111. Schenck PA, Chew DJ, Brooks CL. 1995. Effects of storage on normal canine serum ionized calcium and pH. Am J Vet Res 56:304–307.

112. Sachs C, Rabouine P, Chaneac M, Kindermans C, Dechaux M, Falch-Christiansen T. 1991. Preanalytical errors in ionized calcium measurements induced by the use of liquid heparin. Ann Clin Biochem 28:167–173.

113. Hopper K, Rezende ML, Haskins SC. 2005. Assessment of the effect of dilution of blood samples with sodium heparin on blood gas, electrolyte, and lactate measurements in dogs. Am J Vet Res 66:656–660.

114. Lyon ME, Guajardo M, Laha T, Malik S, Henderson PJ, Kenny MA. 1995. Zinc heparin introduces a preanalytical error in the measurement of ionized calcium concentration. Scand J Clin Lab Invest 55:61–65.

115. Barber PJ, Elliott J. 1996. Study of calcium homeostasis in feline hyperthyroidism. J Small Anim Pract 37:575–582.

116. Geiser DR, Andrews FM, Rohrbach BW, White SL, Maykuth PL, Green EM, Provenza MK. 1995. Blood ionized calcium concentrations in horses before and after the cross-country phase of three-day event competition. Am J Vet Res 56:1502–1505.

117. Aguilera-Tejero E, Estepa JC, Lopez I, Bas S, Garfia B, Rodriguez M. 2001. Plasma ionized calcium and parathyroid hormone concentrations in horses after endurance rides. J Am Vet Med Assoc 219:488–490.

118. Jutkowitz LA, Rozanski EA, Moreau JA, Rush JE. 2002. Massive transfusion in dogs: 15 cases (1997–2001). J Am Vet Med Assoc 220:1664–1669.

119. Grove-White DH, Michell AR. 2001. Iatrogenic hypocalcaemia during parenteral fluid therapy of diarrhoeic calves. Vet Rec 149:203–207.

120. Lopez I, Aguilera-Tejero E, Estepa JC, Rodriguez M, Felsenfeld AJ. 2004. Role of acidosis-induced increases in calcium on PTH secretion in acute metabolic and respiratory acidosis in the dog. Am J Physiol Endocrinol Metab 286:E780–E785.

121. Lopez I, Rodriguez M, Felsenfeld AJ, Estepa JC, Aguilera-Tejero E. 2003. Direct suppressive effect of acute metabolic and respiratory alkalosis on parathyroid hormone secretion in the dog. J Bone Miner Res 18:1478–1485.

122. Hulter HN. 1985. Effects and interrelationships of PTH, Ca^{2+}, vitamin D, and Pi in acid-base homeostasis. Am J Physiol 248:F739–F752.

123. Corvilain J, Abramow M. 1964. Effect of growth hormone on tubular transport of phosphate in normal and parathyroidectomized dogs. J Clin Invest 43:1608–1612.

124. Harkin KR, Braselton WE, Tvedten H. 1998. Pseudohypophosphatemia in two dogs with immune-mediated hemolytic anemia. J Vet Intern Med 12:178–181.

125. Bakker AJ, Bosma H, Christen PJ. 1990. Influence of monoclonal immunoglobulins in three different methods for inorganic phosphorus. Ann Clin Biochem 27(Pt 3):227–231.

126. Jorgensen LS, Center SA, Randolph JF, Brum D. 1985. Electrolyte abnormalities induced by hypertonic phosphate enemas in two cats. J Am Vet Med Assoc 187:1367–1368.

127. Atkins CE, Tyler R, Greenlee P. 1985. Clinical, biochemical, acid-base, and electrolyte abnormalities in cats after hypertonic sodium phosphate enema administration. Am J Vet Res 46:980–988.

128. Fulton RB Jr, Fruechte LK. 1991. Poisoning induced by administration of a phosphate-containing urinary acidifier in a cat. J Am Vet Med Assoc 198:883–885.

129. Arden WA, Stick JA. 1988. Serum and peritoneal fluid phosphate concentrations as predictors of major intestinal injury associated with equine colic. J Am Vet Med Assoc 193:927–931.

130. Carlson GP, Mansmann RA. 1974. Serum electrolyte and plasma protein alterations in horses used in endurance rides. J Am Vet Med Assoc 165:262–264.

131. Oster JR, Alpert HC, Vaamonde CA. 1984. Effect of acid-base status on plasma phosphorus response to lactate. Can J Physiol Pharmacol 62:939–942.

132. Dennis SC, Gevers W, Opie LH. 1991. Protons in ischemia: Where do they come from; where do they go to? J Mol Cell Cardiol 23:1077–1086.

133. Darrigrand-Haag RA, Center SA, Randolph JF, Lewis RM, Wood PA. 1996. Congenital Fanconi syndrome associated with renal dysplasia in two border terriers. J Vet Intern Med 10:412–419.

134. Easley JR, Breitschwerdt EB. 1976. Glucosuria associated with renal tubular dysfunction in three Basenji dogs. J Am Vet Med Assoc 168:938–943.

135. Bovée KC, Joyce T, Blazer-Yost B, Goldschmidt MS, Segal S. 1979. Characterization of renal defects in dogs with a syndrome similar to the Fanconi syndrome in man. J Am Vet Med Assoc 174:1094–1104.

136. Roussel AJ, Cohen ND, Ruoff WW, Brumbaugh GW, Schmitz DG, Kuesis BS. 1993. Urinary indices of horses after intravenous administration of crystalloid solutions. J Vet Intern Med 7:241–246.

137. Brautbar N, Leibovici H, Massry SG. 1983. On the mechanism of hypophosphatemia during acute hyperventilation: Evidence for increased muscle glycolysis. Miner Electrolyte Metab 9:45–50.

138. Bayly WM, Brobst DF, Elfers RS, Reed SM. 1986. Serum and urinary biochemistry and enzyme changes in ponies with acute renal failure. Cornell Vet 76:306–316.

139. Steffey EP, Giri SN, Dunlop CI, Cullen LK, Hodgson DS, Willits N. 1993. Biochemical and haematological changes following prolonged halothane anaesthesia in horses. Res Vet Sci 55:338–345.

140. Fontenot JP, Allen VG, Bunce GE, Goff JP. 1989. Factors influencing magnesium absorption and metabolism in ruminants. J Anim Sci 67:3445–3455.

141. Simesen MG. 1980. Calcium, phosphorus, and magnesium metabolism. In: Kaneko JJ, ed. *Clinical Biochemistry of Domestic Animals*, 3rd edition, 575–648. New York: Academic.

142. Martens H, Hammer U. 1981. Resorption von Natrium und Magnesium aus dem forübergehend isolierten Pansen von Schafen während intravenöser Infusion von Aldosteron. Dtsch Tieraerztl Wochenschr 88:404–407.

143. McCoy MA. 2004. Hypomagnesaemia and new data on vitreous humour magnesium concentration as a post-mortem marker in ruminants. Magnes Res 17:137–145.

144. Kasari TR, Woodbury AH, Morcom-Karsari E. 1990. Adverse effect of orally administered magnesium hydroxide on serum magnesium concentration and systemic acid-base balance in adult cattle. J Am Vet Med Assoc 196:735–742.

145. Henninger RW, Horst J. 1997. Magnesium toxicosis in two horses. J Am Vet Med Assoc 211:82–85.

146. Riond JL, Kocabagli N, Spichiger UE, Wanner M. 1995. The concentration of ionized magnesium in serum during the periparturient period of non-paretic dairy cows. Vet Res Commun 19:195–203.

147. Donovan GA, Steenholdt C, McGehee K, Lundquist R. 2004. Hypomagnesemia among cows in a confinement-housed dairy herd. J Am Vet Med Assoc 224:96–99.

148. Kimmel SE, Waddell LS, Michel KE. 2000. Hypomagnesemia and hypocalcemia associated with protein-losing enteropathy in Yorkshire terriers: Five cases (1992–1998). J Am Vet Med Assoc 217:703–706.

149. Martin LG, Matteson VL, Wingfield WE, Van Pelt DR, Hackett TB. 1994. Abnormalities of serum magnesium in critically ill dogs: Incidence and implications. J Vet Emerg Crit Care 4:15–20.

150. Toribio RE, Kohn CW, Chew DJ, Sams RA, Rosol TJ. 2001. Comparison of serum parathyroid hormone and ionized calcium and magnesium concentrations and fractional urinary clearance of calcium and phosphorus in healthy horses and horses with enterocolitis. Am J Vet Res 62:938–947.

151. Johansson AM, Gardner SY, Jones SL, Fuquay LR, Reagan VH, Levine JF. 2003. Hypomagnesemia in hospitalized horses. J Vet Intern Med 17:860–867.

152. Norris CR, Nelson RW, Christopher MM. 1999. Serum total and ionized magnesium concentrations and urinary fractional excretion of magnesium in cats with diabetes mellitus and diabetic ketoacidosis. J Am Vet Med Assoc 215:1455–1459.

153. Shawley RV, Rolf LL Jr. 1984. Experimental cantharidiasis in the horse. Am J Vet Res 45:2261–2266.

154. Toribio RE, Kohn CW, Hardy J, Rosol TJ. 2005. Alterations in serum parathyroid hormone and electrolyte concentrations and urinary excretion of electrolytes in horses with induced endotoxemia. J Vet Intern Med 19:223–231.

155. Fincham SC, Drobatz KJ, Gillespie TN, Hess RS. 2004. Evaluation of plasma-ionized magnesium concentration in 122 dogs with diabetes mellitus: A retrospective study. J Vet Intern Med 18:612–617.

156. Mann FA, Boon GD, Wagner-Mann CC, Ruben DS. 1998. Ionized and total magnesium concentrations in blood from dogs with naturally acquired parvoviral enteritis. J Am Vet Med Assoc 212:1398–1401.

157. Stewart AJ, Hardy J, Kohn CW, Toribio RE, Hinchcliff KW, Silver B. 2004. Validation of diagnostic tests for determination of magnesium status in horses with reduced magnesium intake. Am J Vet Res 65:422–430.

158. Norris CR, Christopher MM, Howard KA, Nelson RW. 1999. Effect of a magnesium-deficient diet on serum and urine magnesium concentrations in healthy cats. Am J Vet Res 60:1159–1163.

159. Chen RA, Goodman WG. 2004. Role of the calcium-sensing receptor in parathyroid gland physiology. Am J Physiol Renal Physiol 286:F1005–F1011.

160. Ramasamy I. 2006. Recent advances in physiological calcium homeostasis. Clin Chem Lab Med 44:237–273.

161. Estepa JC, Garfia B, Gao PR, Cantor T, Rodriguez M, Aguilera-Tejero E. 2003. Validation and clinical utility of a novel immunoradiometric assay exclusively for biologically active whole parathyroid hormone in the horse. Equine Vet J 35:291–295.

162. Estepa JC, Lopez I, Felsenfeld AJ, Gao P, Cantor T, Rodriguez M, Aguilera-Tejero E. 2003. Dynamics of secretion and metabolism of PTH during hypo- and hypercalcaemia in the dog as determined by the "intact" and "whole" PTH assays. Nephrol Dial Transplant 18:1101–1107.

163. Sislak M, Nachreiner RF, Refsal KR, Graham P, Provencher A. 2001. Comparison of protease inhibitors for stabilizing parathyroid hormone and free T4 by dialysis in serum samples. In: Proceedings of the 19th ACVIM Forum, Seattle, Washington, 875.

164. Estepa JC, Aguilera-Tejero E, Mayer-Valor R, Alamaden Y, Felsenfeld AJ, Rodriguez M. 1998. Measurement of parathyroid hormone in horses. Equine Vet J 30:476–481.

165. Pandian MR, Morgan CH, Carlton E, Segre GV. 1992. Modified immunoradiometric assay of parathyroid hormone–related protein: Clinical application in the differential diagnosis of hypercalcemia. Clin Chem 38:282–288.

166. Nykjaer A, Fyfe JC, Kozyraki R, Leheste JR, Jacobsen C, Nielsen MS, Verroust PJ, Aminoff M, de la CA, Moestrup SK, Ray R, Gliemann J, Willnow TE, Christensen EI. 2001. Cubilin dysfunction causes abnormal metabolism of the steroid hormone 25(OH) vitamin D(3). Proc Natl Acad Sci USA 98:13895–13900.

167. Hulter HN, Halloran BP, Toto RD, Peterson JC. 1985. Long-term control of plasma calcitriol concentration in dogs and humans: Dominant role of plasma calcium concentration in experimental hyperparathyroidism. J Clin Invest 76:695–702.

168. Lissner D, Mason RS, Posen S. 1981. Stability of vitamin D metabolites in human blood serum and plasma. Clin Chem 27:773–774.

169. Hollis BW. 1986. Assay of circulating 1,25-dihydroxyvitamin D involving a novel single-cartridge extraction and purification procedure. Clin Chem 32:2060–2063.

170. Gerber B, Hauser B, Reusch CE. 2004. Serum levels of 25-hydroxycholecalciferol and 1,25-dihydroxycholecalciferol in dogs with hypercalcaemia. Vet Res Commun 28:669–680.

171. Gerber B, Hassig M, Reusch CE. 2003. Serum concentrations of 1,25-dihydroxycholecalciferol and 25-hydroxycholecalciferol in clinically normal dogs and dogs with acute and chronic renal failure. Am J Vet Res 64:1161–1166.

172. Rumbeiha WK, Kruger JM, Fitzgerald SF, Nachreiner RF, Kaneene JB, Braselton WE, Chiapuzio CL. 1999. Use of pamidronate to reverse vitamin D_3–induced toxicosis in dogs. Am J Vet Res 60:1092–1097.

173. Mol JA, Kwant MM, Arnold ICJ, Hazewinkel HAW. 1991. Elucidation of the sequence of canine (pro)-calcitonin: A molecular biological and protein chemical approach. Regul Pept 35:189–195.

174. Hazewinkel HAW, Hackeng WHL, Bosch R, Goedegebuure SA, Voorhout G, van den Brom WE, Bevers MM. 1987. Influences of different calcium intakes on calciotropic hormones and skeletal development in young growing dogs. Front Horm Res 17:221–232.

175. Peterson ME, Randolph JF, Zaki FA, Heath H III. 1982. Multiple endocrine neoplasia in a dog. J Am Vet Med Assoc 180:1476–1478.

Chapter 12

ENZYMES

Basic Principles in Clinical Enzymology. 640
Alanine Transaminase (ALT) (Synonym Abbreviation: GPT) 650
Aspartate Transaminase (AST) (Synonym Abbreviation: GOT) 652
Lactate Dehydrogenase (LD) (Also Abbreviated LDH) 653
Iditol Dehydrogenase (ID) (Synonym Abbreviation: SDH). 654
Glutamate Dehydrogenase (GMD) (Also Abbreviated GDH, GLD, and GLDH) 654
Alkaline Phosphatase (ALP). 655
γ-Glutamyltransferase (GGT) (Synonym Abbreviation: GGTP) 659
Creatine Kinase (CK) 661
Amylase (AMS). 663
Lipase (LPS) 665
Other Serum Enzymes. 669

Table 12.1. Abbreviations and symbols in this chapter

(GGT:Crt)$_u$	Urine γ-glutamyltransferase activity to creatinine concentration
[x]	x concentration (x = analyte)
ALP	Alkaline phosphatase
ALT	Alanine transaminase[a]
AMS	α-Amylase
AST	Aspartate transaminase[a]
ATP	Adenosine triphosphate
B-ALP	Bone alkaline phosphatase
C-ALP	Corticosteroid-induced alkaline phosphatase
CK	Creatine kinase
cPLI	Canine pancreatic lipase immunoreactivity
ELISA	Enzyme-linked immunosorbent assay
fPLI	Feline pancreatic lipase immunoreactivity
GFR	Glomerular filtration rate
GGT	γ-Glutamyltransferase[b]
GMD	Glutamate dehydrogenase
GOT	Glutamate oxaloacetate transaminase[a]
GPT	Glutamate pyruvate transaminase[a]
I-ALP	Intestinal alkaline phosphatase
ID	Iditol dehydrogenase (sorbitol dehydrogenase)
L-ALP	Liver alkaline phosphatase
LD	Lactate dehydrogenase
LPS	Lipase
NAD	Nicotinamide adenine dinucleotide
NADH	Reduced nicotinamide adenine dinucleotide
NADPH	Reduced nicotinamide adenine dinucleotide phosphate
P-5-P	Pyridoxal-5′-phosphate
PLI	Pancreatic lipase immunoreactivity
SI	Système International d'Unités
TG	Triglyceride
TLI	Trypsin-like immunoreactivity
U	International unit
URL	Upper reference limit
WRI	Within reference interval

[a] The NC-IUBMB[c] recommended transaminase but considered aminotransferase acceptable.

[b] The NC-IUBMB[c] recommended γ-glutamyltransferase but considered γ-glutamyltranspeptidase (GGTP) acceptable.

[c] NC-IUBMB, Nomenclature Committee of the International Union of Biochemistry and Molecular Biology

BASIC PRINCIPLES IN CLINICAL ENZYMOLOGY

Enzymes are proteins that catalyze chemical reactions. Proteins that have different polypeptide structure but catalyze the same chemical reaction are *isoenzymes* (or isozymes). If the different enzyme structure is created by a posttranslational modification of an original gene product, then the proteins are *isoforms*. Many enzymes require nonprotein cofactors to assist catalysis, converting them from *apoenzymes* (without cofactor) to *holoenzymes* (with cofactor). These are often from

Table 12.2. Cellular or tissue sources and half-lives of common serum enzymes

Enzyme	Major mechanisms that lead to increased serum activity	Cellular sources of increased serum enzyme activity	Half-lives[a]
ALP	Induction (Ingestion)	*Hepatocytes (L-ALP) (C-ALP in dogs) *Biliary epithelium (L-ALP) Osteoblasts (B-ALP) Mammary epithelium	≈ 3 d (canine L-ALP)[126] ≈ 6 min (canine I-ALP)[126] < 8 h (feline L-ALP)[127] ≈ 2 min (feline I-ALP)[127]
ALT	Cell damage	*Hepatocytes Skeletal myocytes	2–3 d (canine)[20]
AMS	Cell damage Decreased renal clearance	*Pancreatic acinar cells	≈ 5 h (canine)[104]
AST	Cell damage	*Hepatocytes *Skeletal myocytes Cardiac myocytes Erythrocytes	7–8 d (equine)[128,129] < 1 d (canine)[21,130]
CK	Cell damage	*Skeletal myocytes Cardiac myocytes Smooth muscle myocytes (minor)	≈ 2 h (equine)[128,129] < 2 h (canine)[131]
GGT	Induction Cell proliferation (Ingestion)	*Biliary epithelial cells *Hepatocytes Mammary epithelium	≈ 3 d (equine)[132]
GMD	Cell damage	Hepatocytes	≈ 14 h (bovine)[133]
ID	Cell damage	*Hepatocytes	≈ 4 h (canine)[134]
LD	Cell damage	*Hepatocytes *Skeletal myocytes Cardiac myocytes Erythrocytes	< 6 h (canine)[135]
LPS	Cell damage Decreased renal clearance Cell proliferation	*Pancreatic acinar cells Liver neoplasms Gastric mucosa	≈ 2 h (canine)[104]

* Major cellular sources of plasma enzyme activity

[a] Data from available but limited sources

a vitamin source (e.g., P-5-P from vitamin B_6, and NAD from niacin) but also may be ions (e.g., Ca^{2+}, and Mg^{2+}).

I.   Sources of serum enzymes (Table 12.2 and Fig. 12.1)
   A. Serum enzymes described in this chapter originate from cells (exogenous to serum) and do not have recognized functions in blood. Before their release from the cells, the serum enzymes may be in a cell's cytoplasm, mitochondria, or membrane. Serum enzyme activity in healthy animals is typically assumed to result from physiologic processes.

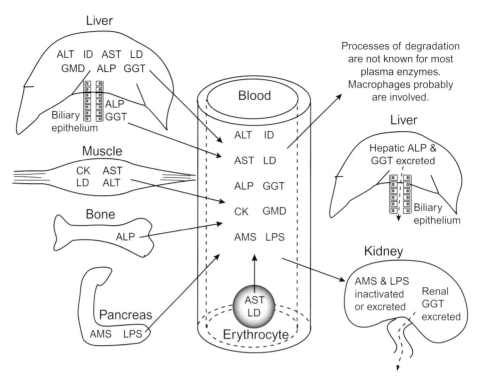

Fig. 12.1. Sources and routes of removal of common serum enzymes. Major sources of serum enzymes that contribute to increased serum activities are hepatocytes (ALT, AST, GGT, GMD, ID, LD, and ALP), biliary epithelial cells (ALP and GGT), skeletal and cardiac muscle fibers (CK, AST, LD, and ALT), osteoblasts (ALP), and pancreatic acinar cells (AMS and LPS). In vitro release of AST and LD from erythrocytes can increase serum activities. Kidneys either inactivate or excrete AMS and LPS. The biliary system is a route of excretion of hepatic ALP and GGT. GGT released from damaged renal tubular cells is excreted in urine. Macrophages probably are involved in removal of damaged or degraded enzymes and enzyme-antiprotease complexes.

      B. Tissue-specific enzymes come from only one cell type. Enzymes with poor tissue specificity may originate from many tissues and thus different cell types.

      C. The presence of an enzyme in a particular tissue does not necessarily mean that damage to that tissue will increase the serum activities of the enzyme.

II.   Serum enzyme activity increases when the rate an enzyme enters plasma exceeds the rate of enzyme inactivation or removal from plasma.[1] In general, there are five mechanisms by which serum enzyme activity may increase: (1) increased release from damaged cells, (2) induction of enzyme synthesis, (3) cell proliferation (hyperplastic or neoplastic), (4) decreased enzyme clearance, and (5) ingestion and absorption.

      A. Increased release of enzymes from damaged cells (major mechanism for cytoplasmic enzymes) (Fig. 12.2)

          1. Enzymes may escape from a cell because of damage caused by minor cell injury (reversible damage) or when enzymes are released with cell death (necrosis). If intracellular enzyme concentrations (cytosolic or mitochondrial) are greater than

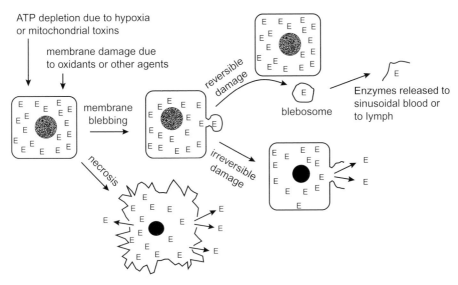

Fig. 12.2. Release of cytosolic enzymes by blebbing or necrosis. Blebbing and necrosis may increase serum activity of ALT, AST, LD, ID, GMD, CK, AMS, LPS, and, to a mild degree, ALP and GGT. A variety of insults to cells may cause direct necrosis or membrane blebbing (irreversible or reversible damage). If irreversible cell damage occurs, cellular enzymes are released with or without bleb formation. If reversible damage occurs, blebosomes form and later lyse, thus releasing their enzymes. E, enzyme.

    extracellular concentrations, and if the enzymes are active in plasma, then enzymes from cells increase enzyme activity in extracellular fluid and thus plasma (or serum).

2. Enzymes may be released from cells by the formation of membrane blebs that form after cell injury.[2,3] Blebs form because of cytoskeletal disruption caused by ATP depletion (because of hypoxia, mitochondrial damage, or substrate depletion), toxicants binding to cytoskeletal proteins, or a variety of agents (proteases, lipases, etc.) that cause membrane damage. Once membrane blebs form, the cell may:
   a. Release blebosomes containing cytoplasmic enzymes to plasma or lymph, where they eventually lyse and cause increased plasma enzyme activity (reversible injury).
   b. Rupture at the site of bleb formation, releasing cytoplasmic enzymes to plasma (irreversible injury).
   c. Repair itself without blebosome release or bleb rupture.

3. Factors that affect the rate of enzyme loss from cells include severity of tissue damage, intracellular enzyme concentration, and intracellular enzyme location (i.e., cytoplasm, mitochondria, or cell membrane). The route of access to plasma also influences the magnitude and rate of increase.
   a. Damage to blood cells and hepatocytes rapidly increases plasma enzyme activity.
   b. Enzymes released from muscle fibers enter plasma via lymph and thus the rate of entry into blood is slower.
   c. Enzymes released from intestinal mucosal cells or renal epithelial cells may not enter plasma but enter the intestinal lumen or urine, respectively.

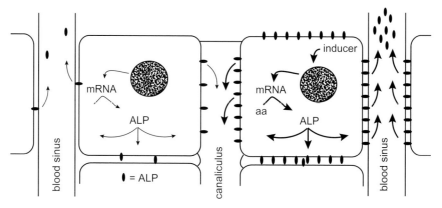

Fig. 12.3. Increased production of ALP by induction. In healthy animals (the *left* half of the drawing), ALP is attached to hepatocyte membranes; more is located on the canalicular than the sinusoidal membrane. In sick animals (the *right* half of the drawing), drugs or metabolites (e.g., bile acid) induce the synthesis of more ALP that accumulates both on the canalicular and sinusoidal hepatocyte membranes. When more ALP is released from the sinusoidal membrane, serum ALP activity increases. aa, amino acid.

      d. Enzymes released from neurons may not cross the blood-brain barrier and thus may not increase plasma enzyme activity.

    4. It is commonly stated that damage to cells allows enzymes to "leak" from cells because of altered cell membrane permeability. When damage is sufficient to allow an enzyme, a large protein, to leak through a porous membrane, then many other intracellular solutes (e.g., K^+ and Ca^{2+}) will leak out and the cell will die. When there is reversible cell damage that increases serum enzyme activity, this "leakage through holes" concept is not applicable unless the cells are capable of quick repair to limit the loss of contents.

  B. Increased enzyme production by individual cells because of induced synthesis

    1. This is the primary mechanism for membrane enzymes and may be a mechanism for mitochondrial and cytoplasmic enzymes.

    2. *Induction* refers to a stimulated increase in production of the enzyme protein via modified transcription, translation, or other processes. Endogenous substances (e.g., bile acids) or drugs such as phenobarbital, prednisolone, or prednisone may trigger induction. Increases in serum ALP activity result mostly from induction (Fig. 12.3).

  C. More enzyme produced by a tissue because of cell proliferation, particularly for membrane-associated enzymes

    1. Neoplasia of the enzyme's cell of origin (e.g., increased ALP and B-ALP with osteosarcoma, or increased LPS with pancreatic or extrapancreatic neoplasia)

    2. Hyperplasia of the enzyme's cell of origin (e.g., increased GGT with bile duct hyperplasia, or increased B-ALP with bone growth or repair)

    3. Conversely, decreased tissue mass may be associated with decreased serum enzyme activity or concentration (e.g., TLI with pancreatic atrophy).

  D. Enzyme removal from plasma is decreased (enzyme has an increased half-life).

    1. Some enzymes (e.g., AMS and LPS) are inactivated or excreted by kidneys. Decreased renal blood flow leads to decreased inactivation of AMS and LPS.

2. Some enzymes form complexes with immunoglobulins or other proteins, and these so-called macroenzymes (e.g., AMS) may have increased survival in the circulation.

3. Other processes of enzyme inactivation include binding to circulating plasma antiproteases with subsequent uptake by macrophages or hepatocytes, and nonspecific proteolysis and then uptake by macrophages. If these processes were inhibited, removal of enzymes from plasma would be decreased.

E. Colostral enzymes (GGT and ALP) are ingested and absorbed in some species concurrently with passive transfer of immunoglobulins.

III. Decreased activity of most enzymes assessed in routine serum chemistry profiles does not have diagnostic importance. Measured enzyme activity may be reduced because of poor sample handling (enzyme degraded), the presence of an inhibitor (e.g., anticoagulants), a reference interval that is not appropriate for the patient, or a decreased mass of origin tissue.

IV. Measurement of serum enzymes
A. Activity per unit volume
1. *Enzymes* are proteins that catalyze chemical reactions. Routine assays measure enzyme *activity* by detecting how fast a substrate is consumed or how fast a product forms.
   a. Enzyme assay theory: In the presence of excess substrate (S), the reaction rate depends on the quantity of enzyme (E). More specifically, the reaction rate depends on the rate of reaction from the enzyme-substrate complex to the product (P) + enzyme: E + S → E-S → P + E.
   b. Nearly all serum enzyme assays are spectrophotometric. They may be either end-point assays or kinetic assays.
      (1) *End-point assays*: The reaction is stopped at a specified time, and enzyme activity is determined from the quantity of product formed or the quantity of substrate used.
      (2) *Kinetic assays*: Multiple readings are taken during a specified time period, and enzyme activity is determined by the rate of the reaction (or rate at which product is being formed). Most current enzyme assays are kinetic assays.
2. Enzyme reactions for common clinical serum enzyme assays
   a. Figure 12.4 contains the initial chemical reactions catalyzed by the common serum enzymes. The initial reactions are usually coupled to other reactions that cause the formation or disappearance of a colored indicator that can be detected by photometry.
   b. Knowledge of the enzyme reactions promotes an understanding of enzyme nomenclature and physiologic roles of enzymes.
3. Units used to express enzyme activity
   a. U = international unit = amount of enzyme that catalyzes conversion of 1 micromole of substrate per minute under defined conditions (1 U = 1 μmol/min). In this context, substrate includes substances such as NADH or NADPH that are also called coenzymes or cosubstrates. Units are usually expressed as U/L but occasionally as mU/mL.
   b. Unit conversion
      (1) SI unit = 1 katal = 1 mol/s
      (2) 1 U = 16.67 nanokatal (SI unit rarely used in medical laboratories)

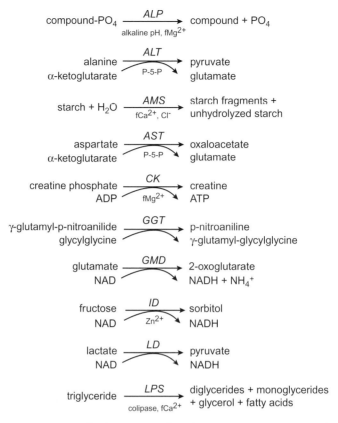

Fig. 12.4. Initial reactions in assays for the common clinical serum enzymes. Assays are designed so that the rate-limiting factor is the catalytic activity of a serum enzyme. Methods of monitoring the chemical reactions that are catalyzed by the enzymes vary but typically involve absorption or reflectance photometry. LD activity can be assessed in reactions that are driven from lactate to pyruvate or pyruvate to lactate. mRNA, messenger ribonucleic acid; and NH_4^+, ammonium.

   c. Arbitrary units: Some enzyme units are named after people who developed the assays. Examples include Somogyi units (AMS), Sigma-Frankel and Karman units (ALT and AST assays), Rose-Byler units (LPS), and King-Armstrong and Bodansky units (ALP). Values expressed in arbitrary units may be much different from values expressed in international units, because arbitrary units may be defined by markedly different assay conditions. It is difficult to impossible to convert the arbitrary units to international units accurately. Fortunately, most current methods have been defined in international units (U).

4. The international unit does not normalize methods. Different assays may measure different amounts of enzyme activity in the same sample.

   a. Because of variations in some assay methods, enzyme activities measured by two different assays may be markedly different. Figure 1.5 illustrates the marked differences that can be found when one sample is analyzed by different methods. Thus, accurate interpretation of serum enzyme activity requires that patient

Table 12.3. Approximate changes in enzyme activities if the same sample is analyzed at different assay temperatures

	Relative enzyme activity at			
	25 °C	30 °C	32 °C	37 °C
Common enzymes[a]	60–80 %	100 %	110–125 %	130–210 %

[a] Including ALP, CK, LD, ID, ALT, and AST

Note: Changes are based on reported conversion factors.[136] In 2002, the International Federation of Clinical Chemistry published serum enzyme reference methods by using a 37 °C reaction temperature. Previous reference methods were designed for 30 °C.[137] Most clinical enzyme activities are measured at 37 °C.

values be compared with reference intervals established for the assay used to measure the patient's enzyme activity.

b. Differences in assay methods that cause different measured values include differences in the following:
(1) Reactions (forward and reverse) and reagent concentrations
(2) Substrates (especially AMS, LPS, and ALP assays)
(3) pH of assay reactions (especially ALP assays)
(4) Incubation or reaction temperatures, although most current automated analyzers assay enzymes at 37 °C
(5) Use of cofactors (e.g., P-5-P)
(6) Use of activators (e.g., N-acetylcysteine for CK)
(7) Use of inhibitors (e.g., AMP and diadenosine pentaphosphate to inhibit adenylate kinase for CK assays)
(8) Measurement times and calculations

c. Most serum enzymes used diagnostically have near maximal activity at normal body temperatures (37–39 °C), but some deteriorate rapidly at 37 °C in sera. Table 12.3 shows the relative enzyme activity at different assay temperatures. For some enzymes, enzyme activity measured at 37 °C may be three times as great as the activity measured at 25 °C.

B. Mass per unit volume
1. Enzymes are proteins, and immunologic assays have been developed to measure their concentration in terms of mass per unit volume.
2. The concentrations of PLI (this chapter) and TLI (Chapter 15) are reported as µg/L. These protein concentrations are relatively small when compared to other common serum protein analytes such as albumin at 3 g/dL or fibrinogen at 0.3 g/dL.
3. Proteins detected by immunologic assays for enzymes may include active forms and inactive forms or precursor forms.

V. Enzyme nomenclature
A. The recommendations of the Nomenclature Committee of the International Union of Biochemistry and Molecular Biology are used for naming enzymes.[4] Most enzymes were named by the reaction substrate first (e.g, alanine and creatine) followed by one of six types of reaction the enzyme catalyzes (e.g., transfer amino group = transaminase; transfer phosphate group = kinase; and oxidize or reduce = oxidoreductases, including dehydrogenase). Each enzyme is also identified by a unique Enzyme Commission

number that describes the specific reaction the enzyme catalyzes (e.g., EC 1.1.1.14 for iditol dehydrogenase).

B. In the conventional system, there was not a systematic method of naming enzymes. Conventional names are still used by some laboratories and authors.

C. Enzyme abbreviations
   1. An international system for abbreviations has not been adopted. Abbreviations in this textbook were recommended by a group of chemists in 1975.[5]
   2. For the conventional system, most abbreviations are "hand-me-downs" from one "school" or another.

VI. Sample processing, handling, and storage for common clinical serum enzymes
   A. Sample type
      1. A clot tube from a fasted animal is preferred (ruminants are not fasted). Harvest serum within 1 h of blood collection but allow time for clot formation and retraction. Prolonged contact with the clot will allow some enzymes to escape from erythrocytes (e.g., AST and LD).
      2. Plasma can be used for some enzymes but not others.
         a. Most anticoagulants tie up divalent cations (Ca^{2+}, Mg^{2+}, Cu^{2+}, and Zn^{2+}) and some enzymes require divalent cations as cofactors for them to have catalytic activity (Mg^{2+} for ALP and CK, Ca^{2+} for LPS, and Zn^{2+} for ID).
         b. In rat samples, heparinized plasma or serum with added heparin had greater GGT activity than did serum samples.[6] To confirm positive interference, similar work needs to be done in domestic animal samples with other GGT assays.
   B. Sample handling
      1. Enzyme activity depends on a protein's conformation. Changes in conformation may alter cofactor or catalytic sites and thus change activity.
      2. There is considerable variation in published data regarding enzyme stability in serum or plasma. For a general guideline, most enzymes are stable for 24 h in sera at 24 °C and 4 °C. The degree of deterioration that occurs after 24 h (at 24 °C, 4 °C, −20 °C, or −70 °C) varies among enzymes and in some cases among species. Rate of deterioration might be different in certain pathologic states (e.g., inflammation) compared to health.
         a. ALT in serum is very susceptible to deterioration during freezing and thawing; it may lose 60 % of original activity.[7] In a study involving bovine samples, ALT at −20 °C was stable in heparinized plasma for 6 wk but was not stable in frozen serum overnight; ALT at 20 °C was stable for 2 and 4 d in sera and plasma, respectively.[8]
         b. ID is stable (>90 % activity remains) in equine serum for up to 5 h at 21 °C, 24 h at 4 °C, and 48 h at −30 °C; 73 % of ID activity was lost by 24 h at 21 °C and 28 % was lost by 72 h at 4 °C.[9]
         c. Isoenzyme LD-5 is heat labile, whereas LD-1 is cold labile. It is best to leave a sample for LD analysis at room temperature and analyze it within 24 h.
         d. Some ALP isoforms are heat labile (B-ALP), whereas others are heat stable (I-ALP and C-ALP). Thawed sera may have greater ALP activities than fresh sera.
         e. GGT activity in heparinized equine plasma was stable for 1 mo at −20 °C.[10]
   C. Sample quality
      1. Sera or plasma with hemolysis may yield erroneous results for three reasons.
         a. Enzymes of erythrocytes may be added to sera or plasma to increase activities; for example, increased AST, LD, and possibly ALT activity.

b. Chemical constituents of erythrocytes may participate in the enzyme assay; for example, glucose-6-phosphate, ATP, or adenylate cyclase for CK activity.

c. Hemoglobin may interfere with light transmission in spectrophotometric assays and yield false increases or decreases, depending on assay design.

2. Sera with elevated bilirubin (icteric sera): Bilirubin may interfere with light transmission.

3. Sera with increased visible lipoproteins (lipemic sera)
    a. Lipid molecules may interfere with light transmission.
    b. Lipid molecules cause unpredictable results because light transmission is hindered not only by number but also by size of molecules.

VII. Interpretation of increased serum enzyme activity
   A. Because of the variations in enzyme activity measured by different assays, patients' enzyme activities need to be compared to appropriate reference intervals. If increased, the degree of increase is usually determined by dividing the patient's enzyme value by the *URL* (the highest value of the reference interval); for example, if a patient's ALT activity = 500 U/L with a reference interval of 10–50 U/L, then the ALT value is 10 times the URL ($10 \times$ URL). The absolute values for enzyme activities may vary considerably between assay methods, but the degree of increase above the URL should be nearly the same.

   B. The magnitude of increased enzyme activity may limit the possible explanations. For example, an ALT activity of $15 \times$ URL is probably caused by hepatocyte damage, not severe muscle damage. Similarly, an ALP activity of $10 \times$ URL is typically considered too great for B-ALP activity in adult dogs, but the ALP activity could be due to either L-ALP or C-ALP.

   C. Consider the half-life of the serum enzymes. For example, CK has a shorter half-life than AST. Thus, after a single insult to muscle, CK activity may return to the reference interval sooner than AST activity.

   D. Integrate potential pathologic processes with other patient information to form ideas or explanations for an animal's illness.

VIII. Significance of increased serum enzyme activities
   A. Serum enzyme activities are markers or indicators of pathologic processes (e.g., hepatocyte injury or cholestasis) and not specific diseases. Many types of diseases may cause common pathologic processes.

   B. For the cytoplasmic enzymes (ALT, AMS, AST, CK, ID, LD, and LPS), the magnitude of increase may relate to the severity of damage; that is, slight damage may cause values $< 2 \times$ URL, whereas severe damage might cause values $> 50 \times$ URL. However, magnitude of increase does not differentiate reversible damage from irreversible damage, or local damage from diffuse damage.

   C. A mild increase (e.g., $2 \times$ URL) might not be very important in one animal because other findings clearly indicate a definite diagnosis. However, in some cases, the same serum enzyme activity might provide the only clue of active disease.

   D. Because of the method of characterizing a patient's enzyme activity (i.e., comparing it to the URL), the magnitude of increase is not accurately described for most animals. For example, if a dog's ALT activity prior to disease was 20 U/L, and it rose to 200 U/L after the onset of disease, then it rose to ten times the baseline value. However, if the ALT reference interval was 20–70 U/L, then the patient's 200 U/L value would represent an increase of only about $3 \times$ URL and might be considered a mild increase.

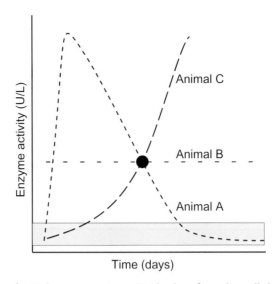

Fig. 12.5. Interpretation of a single enzyme activity. On the day of sampling, all three patients' enzyme activities (●) were about 3× URL (*shaded* area). For animal A (- - -), the 3× value occurred during the disappearance phase after an acute increase. For animal B (– – –), the 3 × value reflects a persistent pathologic process. For animal C (— — —), the 3 × value occurred during a progressive pathologic process. Thus, the clinical significance of the single measurement of enzyme activity may vary from animal to animal.

Because predisease values are usually not available for individual animals, we must consider variations among animals when interpreting serum enzyme activity.

E. Enzyme activity from a single sampling may not reflect the dynamic changes that may be occurring in a patient (Fig. 12.5). Sampling again in 2–3 d may provide a truer image of the pathologic processes.

ALANINE TRANSAMINASE (ALT) (SYNONYM ABBREVIATION: GPT)

I. Physiologic processes, concepts, and facts: *ALT* is a cytoplasmic enzyme that catalyzes a reversible reaction that is involved in the deamination of alanine to form pyruvate, which can enter the gluconeogenesis pathway or the Krebs cycle.

II. Tissue sources of increased serum ALT activity and ALT half-life are listed in Table 12.2.

III. Analytical concepts: Other than variations in assay temperatures, the major factor affecting serum ALT activity among assay systems is the presence or absence of the cofactor P-5-P.

A. Conversion of apoenzymes to holoenzymes with cofactor addition is recommended, although the effect is variable and often not of diagnostic concern.

B. In dogs and cats, the use of P-5-P was associated with a median increased ALT activity of about 10 % (− 27 to 114 %), but, in rare cases, markedly increased activity (336 % and > 14,000 %) was noted with the addition of P-5-P.[11,12]

C. Depending on the degree of hemolysis and the assay, in vitro hemolysis might cause falsely increased ALT activity. In one assay in which marked hemolysis increased the

Table 12.4. Disorders or conditions that cause increased ALT activity

Hepatocyte damage (dogs and cats)
   *Degenerative: hypoxia caused by anemia or congestion
   Anomalous: portosystemic shunt (typically mild)
   *Metabolic: lipidosis, diabetes mellitus, feline hyperthyroidism
   *Neoplastic: lymphoma, metastatic neoplasia, hepatocellular carcinoma
   Nutritional: copper toxicosis, hemochromatosis
   Inflammatory
      *Infectious: leptospirosis, histoplasmosis, feline infectious peritonitis, bacterial
         cholangiohepatitis
      *Noninfectious: chronic hepatitis, cirrhosis
   Inherited: copper storage disease, lysosomal storage diseases
   *Toxic: steroid hepatopathy, anesthetic agents, tetracycline, carprofen, phenobarbital
   *Traumatic: hit by car
Skeletal muscle damage (mild relative to CK changes)
   Inherited: canine musculodystrophy
   Traumatic: hit by car

  * A relatively common disease or condition
  Note: Lists of specific disorders or conditions are not complete but are provided to give examples.

ALT from ≈ 30 U/L to ≈ 60 U/L in equine sera, the interference was considered to be caused by both spectral interference and the addition of ALT from the erythrocytes.[13] In another study using canine sera, marked hemolysis had no effect in some assays and a moderate effect in others.[14]

IV.   Increased serum ALT activity (Table 12.4)
   A. Hepatocyte damage (reversible or irreversible) may occur because of a variety of insults (inflammation, hypoxia, toxicants, trauma, etc.). ALT may be released from hepatocytes also during reparative stages of liver disease.
   B. Increases in canine serum ALT activity that are associated with glucocorticoid therapy may be caused by glucocorticoid-induced hepatopathy instead of true enzyme induction. Glucocorticoids did not increase ALT synthesis in cultured hepatocytes.[15]
   C. Canine serum ALT activity may be increased in dogs treated with phenobarbital. In a study involving 12 phenobarbital-treated dogs, data from the histopathologic examination of liver and chemical analysis of liver homogenates indicated that induction did not cause the increased ALT activity.[16]
   D. Spontaneous muscle damage typically is not associated with increased serum ALT activity, but increased ALT activity does occur with some muscle diseases in dogs and cats.
      1. Young dogs with muscular dystrophy may have markedly increased serum CK activity ($> 500 \times$ URL) and have mild to moderate increases in serum ALT activity ($< 7 \times$ URL).[17,18] Some dystrophic dogs occasionally have extreme ALT increases (values 20 times as great as those in nondystrophic dogs in the same colony).
      2. Dystrophin-deficient cats with acute rhabdomyolysis had markedly increased CK activity ($89–2000 \times$ URL) and increased ALT activity ($6–19 \times$ URL).[19]

V. Species differences
    A. In dogs and cats, ALT is a major marker of hepatocyte damage, but its serum activity is also increased by severe muscle disease.
    B. Hepatocytes of horses and cattle have so little ALT that it is not a useful marker of hepatocyte damage in these species.

ASPARTATE TRANSAMINASE (AST) (SYNONYM ABBREVIATION: GOT)

I. Physiologic processes, concepts, and facts: *AST* is a cytoplasmic and mitochondrial enzyme that catalyzes a reversible reaction involved in the deamination of aspartate to form oxaloacetate, which can enter the Krebs cycle.

II. Tissue sources of increased serum AST activity and AST half-life are listed in Table 12.2.

III. Analytical concepts: Other than variations in assay temperatures, variations in serum AST activity are minimal among assay systems if results are reported in U/L. However, as for ALT, assay methods including the cofactor P-5-P may generate different results from those lacking P-5-P.

IV. Increased serum AST activity (Table 12.5)
    A. Hepatocyte damage (reversible or irreversible) may occur because of a variety of insults (inflammation, hypoxia, toxicants, trauma, etc.). AST also may be released from hepatocytes during reparative stages of liver disease.
    B. Muscle damage (reversible or irreversible) may be caused by a variety of insults.
    C. Hemolysis (in vitro) or delayed removal of serum from clot may cause mild to moderate increases.

Table 12.5. Disorders or conditions that cause increased AST and LD activity

Hepatocyte damage
    *Dogs and cats (see hepatocyte damage conditions listed for increased ALT in Table 12.4)
    Horses and cattle
       *Degenerative: hypoxia caused by anemia, congestion, cholelithiasis
       *Metabolic: lipidosis or fat cow syndrome, diabetes mellitus, equine hyperlipidemia
       Neoplastic: lymphoma, metastatic neoplasia, hepatocellular carcinoma
       Inflammatory
          *Infectious: bacterial hepatitis (Tyzzer's disease), bacterial cholangiohepatitis, infectious necrotic hepatitis, hepatic abscess
          Noninfectious: Theiler's disease, chronic hepatitis, cirrhosis
     Toxic: iron toxicity, pyrrolizidine alkaloid–containing plants, aflatoxins, alsike clover toxicity
  *Skeletal or cardiac muscle damage (see muscle damage conditions listed for increased CK in Table 12.8)

---

  * A relatively common disease or condition

  Note: Lists of specific diseases are not complete but are provided to give examples. Hemolysis (in vitro) or prolonged serum contact with erythrocytes will allow AST and LD from erythrocytes to increase serum AST and LD activities.

V. Species differences
  A. In horses and cattle, AST is a common marker of hepatocyte damage, but muscle damage, hemolysis, and other processes also increase serum AST activity.
  B. AST can also be used as an indicator of hepatocyte damage in dogs and cats. However, it is not as tissue specific as ALT and thus is not as valuable diagnostically. Because canine AST is reported to have a shorter half-life than canine ALT (< 1 d compared to 2–3 d),[20,21] AST might provide a better indication of active hepatocyte damage.

LACTATE DEHYDROGENASE (LD) (ALSO ABBREVIATED LDH)

I. Physiologic processes, concepts, and facts
  A. *LD* is a cytoplasmic enzyme that catalyzes a reversible reaction that converts pyruvate to lactate at the end of anaerobic glycolysis.
  B. *LD isoenzymes* are tetramers of either heart subunits (H) or muscle subunits (M): LD-1 = HHHH, LD-2 = HHHM, LD-3 = HHMM, LD-4 = HMMM, and LD-5 = MMMM. Identification of isoenzymes that are causing the increase in total serum LD activity could increase the diagnostic value of LD activity. However, isoenzyme analysis requires special assays that are not widely available, and species variations in tissue distributions make interpretations difficult.

II. Tissue sources of increased serum LD activity and LD half-life are listed in Table 12.2.

III. Analytical concepts
  A. Variations in assay temperatures can alter LD activity.
  B. Some assays measure LD activity in a pyruvate to lactate reaction, whereas others measure LD activity in a lactate to pyruvate reaction. The LD activity in the two types of reactions can vary considerably,[22] perhaps because LD-1 is inhibited by high pyruvate concentrations and LD-5 maintains activity at high pyruvate concentrations.[23]

IV. Increased serum LD activity (Table 12.5)
  A. In all species, LD is a marker of hepatocyte damage, but serum LD activity is also increased by muscle damage and hemolysis (even mild).
  B. Increased LD activity may be caused by reversible or irreversible, focal or diffuse cell damage.
  C. By itself, serum LD activity is a screening test for hepatocyte or muscle damage. In a group of tests, LD activity provides additional information that may help explain activities of more tissue-specific enzymes (i.e., ALT, ID, and CK).
  D. Alterations in LD isoenzyme patterns in dogs with lymphoma:[24] The percentages of LD isoenzymes were determined in four groups of dogs with lymphoma: Group A had no treatment, group B was treated with steroids, group C was in remission, and group D had recurrent disease. The dogs in groups A, B, and D had greater percentages of LD-2 and LD-3 and lower percentages of LD-5 than healthy dogs and dogs in group C. Also, dogs with lower total LD activity at the time of diagnosis survived longer. LD isoenzyme percentages were determined by agar gel electrophoresis.

IDITOL DEHYDROGENASE (ID) (SYNONYM ABBREVIATION: SDH)

I.   Physiologic processes, concepts, and facts
A.   *ID* is a cytoplasmic enzyme that catalyzes a reversible reaction involving conversion of fructose to sorbitol (or glucitol).
B.   The established name for the enzyme is iditol dehydrogenase, but iditol is not a substrate or product in clinical assays. The enzyme is frequently referred to as *sorbitol dehydrogenase* (SDH). In the clinical assay, fructose is the substrate.

II.   Tissue sources of increased serum ID activity and ID half-life are listed in Table 12.2.

III.   Analytical concepts
A.   Other than variations caused by differences in assay temperatures, variations in serum ID activity are minimal among assay systems if results are reported in U/L.
B.   ID assays are not consistently included in serum chemical profiles, in part because the enzyme's stability is a concern for routine handling of mail-in samples.

IV.   Increased serum ID activity
A.   This indicates hepatocyte damage and may be reversible or irreversible, focal or diffuse. It is unusual to find ID activity > 10 × URL.
B.   ID activity is used primarily in horses and cattle because other common hepatic cytosolic enzymes (AST and LD) are not liver specific, and ALT is not a useful marker of hepatocyte damage in horses and cattle.
C.   ID activity is sometimes used as a marker of hepatocyte damage in dogs and cats, but ALT assays are more commonly available and ALT is more stable.

GLUTAMATE DEHYDROGENASE (GMD) (ALSO ABBREVIATED GDH, GLD, and GLDH)

I.   Physiologic processes, concepts, and facts
A.   *GMD* is a mitochondrial enzyme[1] that catalyzes a reversible reaction involving conversion of glutamate to 2-oxoglutarate. In people, centrilobular hepatocytes have relatively more GMD activity than do the periportal hepatocytes.
B.   GMD is not a common abbreviation for this enzyme, but it is a recommended abbreviation.[5] Two more common abbreviations are GDH and GLDH. GDH is also used as an abbreviation for glycerate dehydrogenase and glucose dehydrogenase.

II.   Tissue sources of increased serum GMD activity and GMD half-life (Table 12.2.): Serum GMD activity is mostly from hepatocytes, but GMD is also found in many other tissues (e.g., kidney, intestine, and muscle). However, damage to those tissues does not increase serum GMD activity, because the enzyme does not enter plasma (e.g., kidney and intestine) or there is too little in the tissues (e.g., muscle and salivary glands).

III.   Analytical concepts: GMD assays have not been available in the United States but have been widely applied in other parts of the world.

IV.   Increased GMD activity
    A. This typically indicates hepatocyte damage that may be reversible or irreversible, focal
        or diffuse. Disorders or conditions (listed in Tables 12.4 and 12.5) that cause hepato-
        cyte damage may increase serum GMD activity.
    B. Based on results of liver biopsies, the diagnostic sensitivity of increased GMD activity
        for differentiating the presence of liver disease from the absence of liver disease in
        horses was not as good as that of GGT activity, but GMD had a better positive
        predictive value.[25] However, this may vary with the types of hepatic diseases encoun-
        tered. The diagnostic value of GMD for specific liver diseases was not reported.
    C. GMD activity appears to be very sensitive indicator of hepatic disease in dogs;
        that is, more sensitive than ALT, AST, ALP, and GGT activity.[26] GMD activity
        was increased in about 15 % of dogs that received anticonvulsant phenobarbitone
        therapy; it is not known whether the increase was caused by hepatocyte damage or
        induction.[27]

ALKALINE PHOSPHATASE (ALP)

I.   Physiologic processes, concepts, and facts
    A. *ALP* includes a family of phosphatases that have phosphatase activity in an alkaline
        environment. Another family has phosphatase activity in an acid environment (the acid
        phosphatases).
    B. Many cell membranes have ALP activity, but only a few produce enough ALP to
        increase serum ALP activity. Physiologic roles of ALP are not clearly established and
        might vary from tissue to tissue. L-ALP may be involved in the degradation of endotox-
        ins,[28] and B-ALP is involved in the mineralization of bone.[29]
    C. Serum ALP activity may be up to 30 × URL in postsuckling pups; the increased ALP
        activity might be due to colostral ALP or increased ALP production induced by
        ingestion of colostrum.[30] Serum ALP activity returned to presuckling values within
        10 d. Increased ALP activity in older pups (compared to adult values) is due to
        B-ALP.[31]
    D. Serum ALP activity in presuckling foals can be 20 × URL for healthy adult horses but
        decreases to about 5 × URL by 3 wk of age.[32] The increase in total ALP activity is due
        to B-ALP.[32] Total serum ALP activity does not increase after colostrum ingestion by
        foals.[32]
    E. Serum ALP activity in calves increases up to three times above presuckling values 1–2 d
        after nursing. At least part of this increase is caused by the ingestion of colostrum. The
        ALP activity nearly returned to presuckling values by the day 3.[33]

II.   Tissue sources of increased serum ALP activity and ALP half-life (Table 12.2)
    A. In domestic mammals, there appear to be two genes for the production of two isoen-
        zymes: (1) I-ALP and (2) tissue-nonspecific ALP. Posttranslational modification of the
        nonspecific ALP creates different isoforms of ALP: L-ALP of hepatocytes and biliary
        epithelium, and B-ALP of osteoblasts. I-ALP has not been shown to increase serum
        ALP activity.[7]
    B. *C-ALP* is a unique canine enzyme that is produced by hepatocytes when stimulated by
        corticosteroids. Chemically, its amino acid sequence is the same as I-ALP, but it is more
        highly glycosylated.

III.   Analytical concepts: Besides variations in assay temperatures, variations in substrates and pH may cause marked differences in serum ALP activity among assay systems.

A.   In routine assays, measured ALP activity represents total ALP activity and typically includes activity from L-ALP and B-ALP (also C-ALP in dogs). The relative contributions to total ALP activity vary with age.

B.   In healthy dogs, C-ALP contributes about 10–30 % of total ALP activity; it contributes more in older dogs than in younger dogs.[34] Although often not routinely measured separately, it is helpful to consider the different isoforms of ALP when interpreting ALP activity.

C.   The relative contributions of the different ALP isoforms to total ALP activity can be determined by enzyme electrophoresis, selective inhibition, thermal stability, or selective precipitation.[31,35–37]

1.   Affinity electrophoresis is the conventional or standard method but requires special equipment and is time and labor intensive.[38] L-ALP, C-ALP, and B-ALP can be identified in canine serum.

2.   Levamisole selectively inhibits L-ALP and B-ALP activity, but C-ALP is relatively resistant. Measurement of serum ALP activity with and without the addition of levamisole can help determine whether much of the serum ALP activity is due to C-ALP.

3.   C-ALP is relatively heat stable at 56 °C and 65 °C, whereas L-ALP and B-ALP are heat labile. Measurement of serum ALP activity prior to and after incubating serum in a heated water bath can help determine whether much of the serum ALP activity is due to C-ALP.

4.   B-ALP and C-ALP are selectively precipitated by wheat germ lectin, whereas L-ALP is not. ALP activity before and after the precipitation can be used to estimate B-ALP activity when combined with determination of C-ALP activity by levamisole inhibition.

IV.   Increased serum ALP activity (Table 12.6)

A.   Cholestasis (intrahepatic or posthepatic)

1.   Increased ALP activity appears to be primarily caused by increased production of L-ALP by hepatocytes and biliary epithelium during obstructive cholestasis. It is not known whether ALP production is increased in functional cholestasis (see Chapter 13).

2.   Many diseases lead to impaired bile flow, which leads to an accumulation of bile acids in hepatocytes. Increased bile acid concentrations stimulate L-ALP production, promote accumulation of L-ALP on sinusoidal hepatocyte membranes, and are linked to increased serum ALP activity (Fig. 12.3).[37,39] Bile acids may promote L-ALP release from the hepatocyte membranes by promoting activity of glycosylphosphatidylinositol phospholipase D.[40,41]

3.   In cholestatic disorders, other substances or factors might also induce L-ALP production, or there might be decreased biliary excretion of ALP. In the absence of cholestasis, there appears to be too little ALP associated with hepatocytes and biliary epithelium for hepatic necrosis to cause large increases in serum ALP activity.

B.   Induction by drugs or hormones

1.   Many drugs have the potential to increase L-ALP activity. Corticosteroids (prednisone and prednisolone), phenobarbital, and primidone are commonly reported to induce L-ALP production. The degree of induction typically depends on dose and

Table 12.6. Disorders or conditions that cause increased ALP activity (the isoform produced is in parentheses)

Cholestasis, either intrahepatic or posthepatic (L-ALP)
  *Degenerative: necrosis or hepatocyte swelling that leads to impaired bile flow
  *Metabolic: lipidosis, diabetes mellitus, hyperadrenocorticism, cholelithiasis
  *Neoplastic: bile duct carcinoma, pancreatic carcinoma, lymphoma
  *Inflammatory: periportal hepatitis, cholangitis, cholangiohepatitis, pancreatitis
   Toxic: pyrrolizidine alkaloid–containing plants, alsike clover toxicity, sporodesmin
     toxicosis
Induction by drugs or hormones
  *Phenobarbital, dilantin, primidone (L-ALP)
  *Corticosteroids (L-ALP and canine C-ALP): endogenous or exogenous
  *Thyroxine (B-ALP): feline hyperthyroidism
Increased osteoblastic activity (B-ALP): osteosarcoma, fracture repair, rickets
Canine mammary neoplasms, benign and malignant
Benign familial hyperphosphatasemia in Siberian huskies

* A relatively common disease or condition
Note: Lists of specific diseases are not complete but are provided to give examples. Young growing animals have serum ALP activities up to three times the activities expected in mature animals. Ingestion and absorption of colostrum by neonatal foals and pups may increase serum ALP activity.

duration of administration of the compound. It takes hours for hepatocytes to increase L-ALP production (it may take days for clinical evidence of increased production), and increased serum ALP activity may persist for 2–4 wk after removal of the drug.[42,43]

a. In a study involving 12 phenobarbital-treated dogs, data from the histopathologic examination of liver and chemical analysis of liver homogenates indicated that the increased ALP activity was not caused by induction.[16]

b. Data from hepatic tissue homogenates analyzed after 32 d of prednisone injections indicate that the steroid treatment increased L-ALP production by increasing gene transcription in hepatocytes.[44]

2. C-ALP

a. In canids, corticosteroids (e.g., endogenous cortisol or exogenous prednisone or prednisolone) induce the production of a unique ALP isoform of I-ALP called *C-ALP* (also called *CI-ALP* for corticosteroid-induced ALP, *SI-ALP* for steroid-induced ALP, and *CAP* for corticosteroid alkaline phosphatase). The increase in serum C-ALP activity begins about a week after initiation of steroid therapy. Most experimental evidence supports that corticosteroids up-regulate a specific gene in canine hepatocytes to produce this unique enzyme.[45]

b. Measuring C-ALP activity can be a screening test for canine hyperadrenocorticism because most dogs (83–100 %) with spontaneous hyperadrenocorticism have increased serum C-ALP activity.[46] However, increased C-ALP activity is not specific for hyperadrenocorticism, because there are physiologic and therapeutic reasons for increased glucocorticoid hormones and thus increased C-ALP activity.

C. Increased osteoblastic activity
  1. Bone lesions that cause increased osteoblastic activity may cause increased serum activity of B-ALP and thus increased total ALP activity. Generally, the magnitude of increase in total ALP is mild (< 4 × URL) but has been reported to be as much as 12 times the average ALP activity in sera of two healthy dogs.[36]
  2. Increased total ALP and B-ALP activities in frozen sera from dogs with osteosarcoma have been associated with reduced patient survival. The degrees of increases in ALP and B-ALP were not reported.[47]
  3. Total ALP activity increased (about 2–3 times the baseline by day 10) during fracture healing in dogs.[48] The return to baseline activity corresponded with cessation of callus formation. In contrast, dogs with nonunion fractures did not have increased ALP activity during a 2 mo evaluation.
  4. Cats with hyperthyroidism have increased B-ALP (and L-ALP) activity that contributes to increased total ALP activity.[49]
D. Dogs with malignant and benign mammary neoplasms may have increased serum ALP activity (typically < 8 × URL) in the absence of detectable hepatic or bone metastasis.[50,51] The source of the ALP was not firmly established, but myoepithelial cells in mammary neoplasms do have ALP activity.[52] Serum ALP activity in dogs with other neoplasms was not assessed.
E. Benign familial hyperphosphatasemia in Siberian huskies[53]
  1. Of 42 pups in eight related litters of Siberian huskies, 17 pups had serum ALP activities about six times the activities found in other age-matched Siberian huskies. B-ALP was the isoform causing increased total ALP activity in all five of the puppies for which isoforms were assessed.
  2. The cause of the increased ALP was not determined. Serum concentrations of total calcium, inorganic phosphorus, and parathyroid hormone were not different from those of matched pups.
F. Pregnant women may have an increased serum ALP activity because of increased placental ALP. ALP activity did not increase in pregnant mares.[54] The increase in serum ALP during pregnancy in bitches is too small to affect ALP interpretation.[55] Placental ALP may contribute to serum ALP activity in the late-term pregnancy of cats.[56]

V. Species and breed differences
  A. Dogs
    1. ALP has high diagnostic sensitivity for detecting cholestasis. ALP activity may be increased before icterus appears. ALP values may range from < 2 × URL to > 20 × URL.
    2. Increased ALP activity induced by corticosteroids results from induced synthesis of L-ALP and C-ALP. ALP values may range from < 2 × URL to > 20 × URL.[43]
    3. Phenobarbital, primidone, and phenytoin are described in clinical studies as either inducing the synthesis of L-ALP or causing hepatic damage that increases serum L-ALP in dogs.[57]
    4. Increased ALP activity caused by increased osteoblastic activity in growing dogs (production of B-ALP) is typically mild (< 4 × URL).[58]
    5. At least some Scottish terriers have greater serum ALP activities than other dogs, and the difference was greater in dogs more than 6 yr old. Part of the increase may be caused by a higher incidence in the breed of diseases that cause increased ALP. However, Scottish terriers without these diseases had a mean ALP activity near

1350 U/L, whereas age-matched dogs without the diseases had a mean ALP near 230 U/L.[59]

B. Cats
  1. ALP has poor diagnostic sensitivity for detecting cholestasis. Cats typically are icteric before ALP activity increases. ALP values may range from < 2 × URL to > 10 × URL.
  2. In 12 (80 %) of 15 of cats with lipidosis, the ALP : GGT ratio was increased (i.e., ALP activity increased more than GGT activity).[60] Only 4 (10 %) of 39 of the cats with liver diseases other than lipidosis (i.e., bile duct obstruction, cholangitis, cholangiohepatitis, neoplasia, hepatic necrosis, and cirrhosis) had increased ALP : GGT ratios (magnitudes of change not reported).
  3. It has been reported that from 43 % to 75 % of hyperthyroid cats have increased serum ALP activities. ALP activities typically are < 4 × URL. In such cats, the increased ALP activity is caused by L-ALP and B-ALP, whereas ALP activity in healthy mature cats is due to L-ALP. Some hyperthyroid cats have increased B-ALP activity in serum without a concurrent increase in total ALP activity.[61]

C. Horses
  1. ALP has poor diagnostic sensitivity for detecting cholestasis. Horses typically are icteric before ALP activity increases. ALP values may range from < 2 × URL to > 10 × URL.
  2. There is no evidence that glucocorticoid treatments increase serum L-ALP activity in horses, nor that horses produce C-ALP.[62] In two reported cases of steroid hepatopathy in horses, ALP activity was not measured.[63,64]
  3. In horses with colic or intestinal lesions, ALP activity may increase in the peritoneal fluid predominantly because of increased granulocytic ALP activity,[65] but other data suggest that intestinal ALP may contribute (see Chapter 19).[66]

D. Cattle: ALP has moderate diagnostic sensitivity for detecting cholestasis, but cholestasis disorders are uncommon in cattle.

γ-GLUTAMYLTRANSFERASE (GGT) (SYNONYM ABBREVIATION: GGTP)

I. Physiologic processes, concepts, and facts
  A. GGT is associated with cell membranes. It catalyzes the transfer of glutamyl groups between peptides and is involved in glutathione reactions. Many cells have GGT activity, but biliary epithelial cells, pancreatic acinar cells, and renal tubular epithelial cells are classically considered to have the greatest activity. In some species, mammary glands also have high GGT activity. In these species, GGT is associated with mammary glandular epithelial membranes and milk membranes in milk.[67,68]
  B. Colostrum of cows has high GGT activity, and the GGT molecules may be absorbed from the calf intestine after colostral intake. Postsuckling calves may have GGT activities as high as 20 × URL (using adult reference intervals) and up to 16 times the presuckling values.[33,69–71] This physiologic change can be used as evidence of suckling and thus as an indication of successful passive transfer.
  C. Mare colostrum contains relatively little GGT activity, and GGT activity in neonatal foals does not increase after suckling. However, serum GGT activity in foals less than 1 mo old is about 1.5–3.0 times as great as the GGT activity in adult horses.[72]
  D. Because of high colostral GGT, serum GGT activity in 1- to 3-d-old pups is up to 100 × URL (using adult reference intervals) but returns to presuckle values within 10 d after suckling.[30]

Table 12.7. Disorders or conditions that cause increased GGT activity

*Cholestasis (see cholestasis conditions listed for increased ALP in Table 12.6)
 Biliary hyperplasia: pyrrolizidine alkaloid–containing plants, sporodesmin toxicity, alsike
   clover toxicity
Drugs or hormones
   Phenobarbital, dilantin, primidone
   Corticosteroids: endogenous or exogenous

*A relatively common disease or condition.
Note: Ingestion and absorption of colostrum by neonatal calves and pups may increase serum GGT
activity.

II. Tissue sources of increased serum GGT activity and GGT half-life are listed in Table 12.2.

III. Analytical concepts
   A. Serum GGT activity varies minimally among assay systems if results are reported in U/L
      and assay temperatures are the same.
   B. In a study involving rat samples, heparin was shown to nearly double the GGT activity
      in an assay that used γ-glutamyl-p-nitroanilide as a substrate.[6,73] Heparin also can cause
      turbidity in the reaction fluid, which would interfere with transmission photometry.[22]
      There were no differences in GGT activities between canine serum and heparinized
      plasma samples when using the dry-slide method (Vitros) that uses the same substrate
      (authors' unpublished data).

IV. Increased serum GGT activity (Table 12.7)
   A. Cholestasis or biliary hyperplasia
      1. Increased hepatic and plasma bile acid concentrations are expected with cholestasis.
         Increased bile acids or other constituents of bile may stimulate the synthesis and
         release of GGT similarly to ALP, but mechanisms of increase are not completely
         established.[39] Disorders that cause cholestasis may also induce biliary hyperplasia and
         a resultant increase in GGT activity.
      2. Experimental data from rat studies indicate that increased serum GGT activity
         primarily depends on the degree of hyperplasia of biliary epithelial cells and not on
         induction of GGT synthesis, hepatocyte damage, or cholestasis.[74]
   B. Associated with drugs or hormones
      1. Serum GGT activities transiently increased to 2–3 times the baseline values from
         weeks 13 to 17 in dogs given phenobarbital for 27 wk, but mean activity did not
         exceed reference intervals.[75]
      2. Induction may not increase serum GGT activity in dogs being treated with gluco-
         corticoid hormones, since glucocorticoids did not induce GGT synthesis in cultured
         hepatocytes.[15] However, in prednisone-treated dogs, both hepatic and serum GGT
         activities increased, which suggested induction or the effects of steroid
         hepatopathy.[43]
   C. Hepatocyte damage in horses: Experimental data indicate that acute hepatocellular
      necrosis may cause mild increases (< 4 × baseline) in GGT activity.[76] It is not known
      whether the increased GGT represented hepatocyte necrosis or release of GGT from
      cells because of secondary cholestasis.

V. Species differences
    A. Horses
        1. Increased GGT activity has better diagnostic sensitivity than does ALP for detecting cholestasis or other biliary disorders in horses. In experimental cholestasis, both GGT and ALP activities increased, but the GGT increase ($\approx 7\times$) was greater than the ALP increase ($\approx 2\times$).[76]
        2. Neonatal foals have greater serum GGT activity than do their mares, but not because of GGT uptake in colostrum as occurs in other species.[72]
    B. Cattle
        1. Increased GGT activity is generally considered to have better diagnostic sensitivity than does ALP for detecting cholestasis or other biliary disorders in cattle. Experimentally, GGT activity is increased in acute hepatic necrosis, but the increase may reflect secondary cholestasis.[77]
        2. Disorders associated with increased GGT activity include bile duct obstruction, cholangitis, cholecystitis, copper toxicosis, hepatic mycotoxicosis, and fascioliasis.[78–81] GGT activity may be increased with hepatic lipidosis, but the magnitude is frequently mild.[82,83]
    C. In dogs, increased GGT activity tends to parallel increases in ALP activity caused by cholestatic disorders, but ALP probably has more diagnostic sensitivity. GGT values can be increased in dogs with steroid hepatopathy.
    D. In 54 cats with liver diseases, disorders associated with increased GGT activity included bile duct obstruction, cholangitis, cholangiohepatitis, lipidosis, neoplasia, hepatic necrosis, and cirrhosis. GGT activity in nine (17 %) of the cats was WRI.[60]

VI. GGT activity in urine
    A. Damage to renal epithelial cells increased the urinary excretion of renal GGT without increasing the serum GGT activity.
    B. Because the urinary GGT activity depends on the amount of H_2O excreted by the kidneys, the measured urine GGT activity is difficult to interpret. The $(GGT:Crt)_u$ ratio reduces the variations caused by variable degrees of renal tubular resorption of H_2O (see Chapter 8).
        1. An increased $(GGT:Crt)_u$ ratio should indicate that the rate of GGT excretion is increased relative to the rate of creatinine excretion. Such an increased $(GGT:Crt)_u$ ratio has occurred with renal diseases in dogs and ponies.[84]
        2. Because Crt clearance depends almost entirely on GFR, but GGT excretion does not, an increased $(GGT:Crt)_u$ ratio might be caused by decreased GFR and not increased release of GGT by tubules.
        3. The units for reported $(GGT:Crt)_u$ ratios have been mixed volume units; that is, calculated from GGT in U/L and Crt in mg/dL.

CREATINE KINASE (CK)

I. Physiologic processes, concepts, and facts
    A. *CK* is a cytoplasmic enzyme that catalyzes a reversible reaction involved in the transfer of phosphate (PO_4) from creatine-PO_4 to adenosine diphosphate (ADP) to form ATP. Creatine phosphokinase (CPK) is not an acceptable name for the enzyme.

B. CK is a dimer. There are four isoenzymes that have variable cell distributions: CK-1 dominates in brain, CK-2 and CK-3 in cardiac and skeletal muscle, and CK-Mt in mitochondria of many tissues.

C. Puppies and young dogs have greater serum CK activity than adult dogs. Compared to adult dogs (> 1 yr old), the mean CK activity was about 60 % greater in the 6- to 12-mo-old dogs, 280 % greater in the 1- to 6-mo-old puppies, and 410 % greater in puppies less than 1 mo old.[85] Also, the mean CK activity in small-breed dogs (< 10 kg) was about 70 % greater than activity in large-breed dogs (> 25 kg).[85] Physiologic explanations for the age and body size differences were not found.

II. Tissue sources of increased serum CK activity and CK half-life are listed in Table 12.2.

III. Analytical concepts
   A. Other than variations caused by differences in assay temperatures, serum CK activity has minimal variation among assay systems if results are reported in U/L. The analytical ranges of some commercial assays are too narrow for some domestic mammals, and thus sera frequently may need to be diluted to obtain numeric results when CK activity is increased.
   B. In samples from healthy dogs, the CK activity in serum samples is about 2.5 times that of plasma samples.[85] The difference may be caused by the release of CK from platelets during clotting, as canine platelets have been reported to contain CK activity.[86] This difference may not be clinically relevant when the increase in CK activity is moderate to marked. Incomplete removal of platelets from plasma could lead to mildly increased CK activity.
   C. Canine CK activity in plasma was stable for 1 wk at −4 °C and for 1 mo at −20 °C.[85]

IV. Increased serum CK activity (Table 12.8)
   A. A variety of insults (pathologic and iatrogenic) may damage muscle fibers and cause the release of CK from muscle fibers. CK may be released because of necrosis or reversible cell damage.

Table 12.8. Disorders or conditions that cause increased CK activity

Muscle damage (mostly skeletal, occasionally cardiac, rarely smooth)
   *Degenerative: hypoxia caused by exertion or seizures, exertional rhabdomyolysis, saddle thrombus
   Neoplastic: metastatic neoplasia
   Nutritional: vitamin E or selenium deficiency
   Inherited: musculodystrophy, hyperkalemic myopathy
   Inflammatory: myositis caused by *Neospora*, *Toxoplasma*, bacteria or other agents; bovine endometritis
   Toxic: monensin, castor bean, gossypol
   *Traumatic: intramuscular injections, hit by car, recumbency in horses and cattle, seizures, exertion

---

* A relatively common disease or condition

Note: Lists of specific diseases or conditions are not complete but are provided to give examples. In vitro hemolysis may cause a falsely increased CK activity in some CK assays. Young dogs and dogs of small breeds may have greater values than those on which reference intervals are based.

1. The magnitude of increase can be mild to extreme ($< 2 \times$ URL to $> 100 \times$ URL) and is somewhat proportional to the degree of muscle damage.
2. From a single insult (e.g., recumbency or other trauma), there can be very rapid increase (hours) and a rapid decline (hours to days) because of the short CK half-life.

B. Mild to marked increases in serum CK activity were reported in anorectic cats with nasoesophageal tubes.[87] The exact pathogenesis of the increased activity is not known but probably involves muscle damage. The method of placing the tubes was not described.

C. Hypothyroidism in dogs is reported to cause increased CK activity, sometimes marked, but a pathophysiologic explanation of the increased activity is not established.[88] Whereas some hypothyroid dogs have increased serum CK activity, other hypothyroid dogs have decreased serum CK activity.

D. In vitro hemolysis may cause falsely increased CK activity. Erythrocytes do not contain CK but do contain glucose-6-phosphate, adenylate kinase, and ATP, which may interfere with the coupled reactions of CK assays.

E. Injury to organs and tissues containing smooth muscle may cause increased serum CK activity but to a lesser extent than with striated muscle damage. There is sufficient CK in the bovine uterus that endometritis can cause increased serum CK activity.[89] Four cows with moderate or severe endometritis had greater CK values (≈ 7 or 15 times as high, respectively) than values in found in five healthy cows. There was a concurrent, but relatively minimal, increase in AST activity.

V. CK activity in animals with neurologic disease
A. Brain and other tissues of the central nervous system contain high CK activity. Necrosis or demyelination of neural tissues may cause increased CK activity in cerebrospinal fluid samples, but neither is known to cause increases in serum CK activity.
B. Increased serum CK activity in domestic mammals with neurologic disease appears to result from the release of muscle CK secondary to convulsions or recumbency.

AMYLASE (AMS)

I. Physiologic processes, concepts, and facts
A. *AMS* is a cytoplasmic enzyme that requires Ca^{2+} and Cl^- as cofactors and catalyzes the hydrolysis of complex starches.
B. Via electrophoresis, four AMS isoenzymes (I–IV) are classified in dogs; isoenzyme IV includes macroamylases. Macroamylases are protein complexes that contain AMS bound to other proteins (immunoglobulins or other proteins).
C. People and pigs have salivary α-amylase, whereas dogs, cats, horses, and cattle do not.
D. AMS activity in sera of healthy dogs includes pancreatic AMS, intestinal AMS, and macroamylase activities. The liver may also contribute.
   1. Compared to presurgical measurements, serum AMS activity in two of five dogs did not decrease by 7 d after pancreatectomy. In three of five dogs, serum AMS activity decreased by about 50 %. Therefore, in healthy dogs, serum AMS activity may be from pancreatic and nonpancreatic tissues.[90]
   2. Up to 70 % of the plasma AMS in healthy dogs was of intestinal origin;[91] however, intestine is not considered to be a source of increased serum AMS activity. In another group of healthy dogs, about 14 % of total amylase was bound to immuno-globulins (macroamylase).[92]

E. Some investigators have found AMS activity and mRNA for AMS in canine liver,[91,93–96] so the liver might contribute to baseline serum AMS activity without storing appreciable amounts of the enzyme. Further observations support this idea: (1) serum AMS activity is sometimes less than the reference interval in dogs with portosystemic shunts (authors' observation), and (2) serum AMS activity decreased in rats after liver damage or inhibition of hepatic AMS synthesis. However, there is not good evidence that hepatic disease increases serum AMS activity.

F. The kidneys are a route of plasma AMS excretion or inactivation (see Amylase, sect. IV.B).

II. Tissue sources of increased serum AMS activity and AMS half-life are listed in Table 12.2.

III. Analytical concepts
  A. Besides variations in assay temperatures, variations in substrates may cause marked differences in serum AMS activity among assay systems.
  B. There are three major types of assays that measure AMS activity.
    1. In saccharogenic assays (*saccharo-* means "sugar" and *-geny* means "produce"), AMS catalyzes the degradation of starch to produce glucose and maltose. These assays are typically coupled with other reactions to measure the glucose produced by the AMS reaction. Canine serum contains glucoamylase and maltase (synonym: α-glucosidase). Both may produce falsely increased AMS activity by reacting with the maltose produced by the AMS reaction.[97]
    2. In amyloclastic assays (*amylo-* means "starch" and *-clast* means "broke"), a dye binds to the available starch. If there is less bound dye at the end of the assay, then there was more AMS activity. These assays were the preferred canine AMS assays because glucoamylase did not interfere, but they are not easily automated.
    3. In chromogenic assays, AMS catalyzes the cleavage of a dye bound to a synthetic substrate. Some of these assays are acceptable for measuring canine AMS activity, whereas others are not.[98]
  C. Specific AMS isoenzymes can be measured, but their clinical value is limited.

IV. Increased serum AMS activity (Table 12.9)
  A. Pancreatic acinar cell damage
    1. Acute pancreatitis is the most common cause of damage to pancreatic acinar cells, and it may result in the release of AMS, especially in dogs. The damage may lead to

---

Table 12.9. Disorders or conditions that cause increased AMS and LPS activities

*Pancreatic acinar cell damage: inflammation, neoplasia (AMS and LPS)
Decreased renal clearance
    Prerenal disorders: dehydration, shock (AMS and LPS)
    *Renal disorders: acute or chronic renal diseases (AMS and LPS)
    Postrenal disorders: urinary tract obstruction (AMS and LPS)
    Macroamylasemia (AMS)
Other or unknown mechanism
    Dexamethasone treatment (LPS)
    Pancreatic or hepatic neoplasia (LPS)

* A relatively common disease or condition

acinar cell necrosis. The AMS may gain access to blood via veins draining the pancreas and via lymphatic vessels.[99] In experimental canine pancreatitis, serum AMS activity peaks within 12–48 h and persists for 8–14 d.[100]

2. Species variations

   a. Serum AMS activities in dogs with acute pancreatitis range from WRI to extremely increased (> 10× URL).

   b. In cats with spontaneous pancreatitis, serum AMS activities range from WRI to mildly increased (< 3× URL).[101,102] In experimental pancreatitis in six cats, serum AMS activity did not increase.[103]

   c. Measurement of serum AMS activity has not been useful for diagnosing pancreatitis or other diseases in horses or cattle.

3. Pancreatic neoplasia can also lead to increased serum AMS activity.

B. Decreased renal inactivation or excretion

1. In dogs, clinical and experimental data indicate that the half-life of plasma AMS increases when renal blood flow or functional renal tissue decreases.[104,105] Experimentally, the increased half-life may lead to hyperamylasemia (mean increase, 2.5–4.0 times the baseline values). Clinically, the increased AMS activity is expected to be < 3× URL in conditions that cause decreased GFR without pancreatic acinar cell damage.

2. Exactly how renal functions influence serum AMS activity has not been established.

   a. Very little to no AMS activity is found in the urine of healthy dogs, perhaps because AMS does not pass through the glomerular filtration barrier or because it is inactivated or resorbed by tubular cells after it passes through the barrier.

   b. There is a correlation between amylasuria and proteinuria, especially glomerular proteinuria. Thus, it appears in health that the glomerular filtration barrier limits the amount of AMS that reaches the tubular lumen, or perhaps a large amount of luminal protein resulting from glomerular disease interferes with AMS inactivation by the tubular epithelial cells.[92,106,107]

   c. Experimental damage to proximal renal tubular cells increased urinary loss of AMS, but relatively not as much as urinary loss of LPS or lysozyme. Proximal tubular epithelial cells have some capability of inactivating or resorbing AMS if AMS does pass through the glomerular filtration barrier.[108]

   d. Formation of macroamylase molecules in blood also influences serum AMS activity. *Macroamylase*, a complex between AMS and an immunoglobulin or other protein, is too large to pass through a healthy glomerular filtration barrier and thus may have a longer half-life than noncomplexed AMS. Macroamylasemia contributes to the hyperamylasemia in some proteinuric and azotemic dogs; however, hyperamylasemia was still present in some sera after the macroamylase molecules were removed.[92]

3. The importance of renal inactivation or excretion of AMS by feline kidneys has not been established. Of 32 cats with renal failure, 10 had hyperamylasemia (slight to 3× URL).[109]

C. Intestinal AMS has not been shown to increase total serum AMS activity.

LIPASE (LPS)

I. Physiologic processes, concepts, and facts

A. *Pancreatic LPS* is a cytoplasmic enzyme that requires Ca^{2+}, colipase, and bile salts as cofactors. It catalyzes the hydrolysis of triglycerides. The pancreatic LPS molecule

(M_r = 48,000) and colipase are small enough to pass through the glomerular filtration barrier to be inactivated or excreted.

B. Several lipases are in the body, and each has specific roles in lipid metabolism. More information about lipid metabolism is in Chapter 16.

1. *Gastric LPS* is produced by gastric mucosal cells[110] and degrades ingested triglyceride (TG).
2. *Pancreatic LPS* (triacylglycerol LPS) is produced by pancreatic acinar cells[110] and catalyzes the hydrolysis of dietary TG in the intestine.
3. Many extrahepatic cells, including adipocytes and myocytes, produce *lipoprotein LPS*, which migrates to the luminal surface of endothelial cells, where it catalyzes the hydrolysis of TG in plasma lipoproteins.
4. *Hepatic LPS* is produced by hepatocytes, is present on endothelial cells of hepatic sinusoids, and hydrolyzes TG in low-density lipoprotein molecules.
5. *Hormone-sensitive LPS* in adipocytes catalyzes the hydrolysis of stored TG and the liberation of fatty acids; it is stimulated by epinephrine and glucagon.
6. *Lysosomal acid LPS* is an intracellular LPS that catalyzes the hydrolysis of cholesterol esters.

C. Compared to presurgical measurements, serum LPS activity in four of five dogs decreased by 50–75 % by day 7 after pancreatectomy. However, LPS activity increased by 40 % for one dog in the same study. Data indicated that the pancreas was a contributor to serum LPS activity, but there were other tissue sources in some dogs.[90] The nonpancreatic LPS in serum might be gastric LPS or hepatic LPS.

II. Tissue sources of increased serum LPS activity and LPS half-life are listed in Table 12.2.

III. Analytical concepts

A. Clinical LPS assay methods have varied greatly, yielding disparate results caused partly by variations in analytical specificity for pancreatic LPS.

1. Besides variations in assay temperatures, variations in substrates may cause marked differences in serum LPS activity among assay systems.[111]
2. Exogenous colipase is required for an assay to measure total pancreatic LPS activity, and colipase is not always included in LPS assays.
3. Exogenous Ca^{2+} enhances LPS activity.
4. In some assays, heparin may enhance serum lipoprotein LPS activity sufficiently to increase serum LPS activity,[112] and other lipases may be detected.[22] This is especially true for assays that use 1,2-diglyceride as a substrate.

B. A newer enzymatic LPS assay has been purported to have greater analytical specificity for pancreatic LPS and better diagnostic sensitivity for pancreatitis than a 1,2-diglyceride assay, but the evidence for greater analytical specificity was indirect.[111]

C. Immunologic assays for pancreatic LPS have been developed for dogs[113,114] (cPLI assay) and cats[115] (fPLI assay). These assays measure the actual concentration of the pancreatic LPS protein, not the activity of the enzyme. An assay for canine gastric LPS has also been developed,[116] but its clinical value has not been established.

IV. Increased serum LPS activity (Table 12.9)

A. Interpretation of published data regarding serum LPS is complicated by the wide variation in assay methods used. The following are general conclusions:

B. Pancreatic acinar cell damage
   1. Acute pancreatitis is the most common cause of damage to pancreatic acinar cells and will result in the release of LPS, especially in dogs. The damage may or may not cause acinar cell necrosis. The LPS may gain access to blood via veins draining the pancreas and via lymphatic vessels.[99]
   2. Species variations
      a. Serum LPS activity in dogs with acute pancreatitis ranges from WRI to extremely increased (> 10× URL).
      b. In spontaneous feline pancreatitis, serum LPS activity ranges from WRI to moderately increased (< 5× URL).[101,102] In experimental pancreatitis in six cats, serum LPS activity was increased up to six times the baseline values for the first day and then reduced to about two times the baseline values for 1 wk.[103]
      c. Measurement of serum LPS activity has not been useful for diagnosing pancreatitis or other diseases in horses or cattle.
   3. The reported diagnostic sensitivity of LPS for canine pancreatitis has varied from 39 % to 100 %, and the reported diagnostic specificity of LPS for canine pancreatitis has varied from 50 % to 93 %. These values vary for many reasons, including use of different assays, different diagnostic criteria, and different populations of dogs.
C. Proliferation of cells containing LPS activity: Pancreatic neoplasia and extrapancreatic neoplasia (e.g., cholangiocarcinoma) can also lead to increased serum LPS activity.[117] Some of the serum activity may stem from enzyme release from damaged cells.
D. Decreased renal inactivation or excretion
   1. Serum LPS activity tends to parallel serum AMS activity when renal blood flow or functional renal tissue is decreased.[104,105] Experimentally, the decreased clearance may lead to hyperlipasemia (mean increase, 2.5–4.0 times the baseline values). Clinically, the increased LPS activity is expected to be < 4× URL in conditions that cause a decreased GFR without pancreatic acinar cell damage. However, greater LPS activity (6–8× URL) has been reported with some renal cases that did not have evidence of pancreatic disease,[118] and a LPS activity 10× URL was reported in a case of spontaneous primary renal failure.[105]
   2. Hyperlipasemia associated with renal disease may be caused by decreased renal inactivation of LPS.
E. Associated with pancreatic or hepatic neoplasia in dogs: In five of six cases, histochemical and immunohistochemical findings indicated that pancreatic and hepatic neoplasms were potential sources of mild to marked increased serum LPS activity.[119] The same dogs did not have significant increases in serum AMS activity.
F. Associated with dexamethasone treatments in dogs[120]
   1. Hyperlipasemia (< 2× URL) was found in 24 healthy dogs by day 8 of treatment with dexamethasone either at 2 mg/kg or 0.2 mg/kg. In dogs with neurologic disease, hyperlipasemia of increasing severity (mean value, 4.6× URL) occurred by day 10 of treatment (initial dose at 2 mg/kg and then reduced doses). The number of dogs sampled varied from two to eight on different days.
   2. Microscopic evidence of pancreatic damage was not found, and concurrent hyperamylasemia was not found.
G. Marked hyperlipasemia may be associated with widespread steatitis caused by LPS effects on adipose tissue. Panniculitis may be detected as firm subcutaneous masses consisting of fat with a mild inflammatory component.[121]

Table 12.10. Other serum enzymes

Serum enzyme	Disorder causes	Diagnostic value
5′-Nucleotidase	↑	Hepatobiliary disease
Aldolase	↑	Muscle fiber damage
Arginase	↑	Hepatocyte damage
Cholinesterase[a]	↓	Organophosphate toxicosis, infections, chronic liver disease
Isocitrate dehydrogenase	↑	Hepatocyte damage
Leucyl aminopeptidase[b]	↑	Hepatobiliary disease
Maltase	↑	Intestinal mucosa damage
Muramidase (lysozyme)	↑	Neoplasia (histiocytic)
Malate dehydrogenase	↑	Hepatocyte damage
Ornithine carbamoyltransferase	↑	Hepatocyte damage
Trypsin-like immunoreactivity (TLI) (see Chapter 15)	↑	Pancreatitis or decreased GFR
	↓	Exocrine pancreatic insufficiency in dogs and cats

[a] Plasma pseudocholinesterase or butyrylcholinesterase; not acetylcholinesterase of the myoneural junction
[b] Also called leucine aminopeptidase

V. Pancreatic lipase immunoreactivity (PLI)
  A. To improve the analytical specificity of LPS assays, immunoassays were developed by using an antibody specific for canine pancreatic LPS (M_r = 51,000). A similar feline assay has also been developed.
  B. Dogs
    1. A cPLI radioimmunoassay[113] and a cPLI ELISA[114] have been used, and the lower and upper reference limits for the ELISA were about half of those values for the radioimmunoassay. The ELISA detected only about 55 % of LPS activity added to test samples, indicating a problem with analytical accuracy.
    2. PLI was usually decreased in dogs with exocrine pancreatic insufficiency.
    3. PLI had greater diagnostic sensitivity for pancreatitis than did LPS or TLI.[122]
    4. When the ELISA was used, the [PLI] values were mildly increased in dogs with chronic renal failure, but not enough to suggest acute pancreatitis.[123] In a study in which renal failure was created via 15/16th nephrectomy, 16 dogs became azotemic ([creatinine] 4.3 ± 1.5 mg/dL; mean ± sd), but both serum LPS activity and serum [PLI] remained within reference intervals. The lack of increased serum LPS activity suggests that the model may not have been appropriate for assessing the effects of renal failure on [PLI].[124]
  C. Cats
    1. In experimental pancreatitis, PLI increased more (50 × baseline versus 35 × baseline) and was more persistently increased (10 d vs 3 d) than was TLI.
    2. In spontaneous pancreatitis, when a fPLI assay and a decision threshold of 10 μg/L (reference interval, 2.0–6.8 μg/L) were used, the diagnostic sensitivity of the [PLI] was 100 % for cats with moderate to severe pancreatitis (six cats) and 54 % for cats with mild pancreatitis (eight cats).[125] PLI measurements had more diagnostic sensitivity than did TLI measurements or abdominal ultrasound.

OTHER SERUM ENZYMES

Many serum enzymes have been assessed in an attempt to find better indicators of pathologic states involving hepatocytes or other cells (Table 12.10). For a variety of reasons, most have failed to be as clinically valuable as those described earlier in this chapter.

Decreased TLI has been shown to be valuable in diagnosing exocrine pancreatic insufficiency. Increased TLI has been found in active pancreatitis (see Chapter 15).

References

1. Boyd JW. 1983. The mechanisms relating to increases in plasma enzymes and isoenzymes in diseases of animals. Vet Clin Pathol 12:9–24.
2. Gores GJ, Herman B, Lemasters JJ. 1990. Plasma membrane bleb formation and rupture: A common feature of hepatocellular injury. Hepatology 11:690–698.
3. Kamiike W, Fujikawa M, Koseki M, Sumimura J, Miyata M, Kawashima Y, Wada H, Tagawa K. 1989. Different patterns of leakage of cytosolic and mitochondrial enzymes. Clin Chim Acta 185:265–270.
4. Webb EC, ed, for the International Union of Biochemistry and Molecular Biology. Nomenclature Committee. 1992. *Enzyme Nomenclature 1992: Recommendations of the Nomenclature Committee of the International Union of Biochemistry and Molecular Biology on the Nomenclature and Classification of Enzymes.* San Diego, Academic.
5. Baron DN, Moss DW, Walker PG, Wilkinson JH. 1975. Revised list of abbreviations for names of enzymes of diagnostic importance. J Clin Pathol 28:592–593.
6. Castro-e-Silva O Jr, Franco CFF, Picinato MANC, Souza MEJ, Mazzetto SA, Ceneviva R. 1989. Heparin-induced increase in plasma and serum γ-glutamyl transpeptidase activity. Braz J Med Biol Res 22:1333–1335.
7. Kramer JW, Hoffmann WE. 1997. Clinical enzymology. In: Kaneko JJ, Harvey JW, Bruss ML, eds. *Clinical Biochemistry of Domestic Animals*, 5th edition, 303–325. San Diego: Academic.
8. Jones DG. 1985. Stability and storage characteristics of enzymes in cattle blood. Res Vet Sci 38:301–306.
9. Horney BS, Honor DJ, MacKenzie A, Burton S. 1993. Stability of sorbitol dehydrogenase activity in bovine and equine sera. Vet Clin Pathol 22:5–9.
10. West HJ. 1989. Observations on γ-glutamyl transferase, 5′-nucleotidase and leucine aminopeptidase activities in the plasma of the horse. Res Vet Sci 46:301–306.
11. Mesher CI, Rej R, Stokol T. 1998. Alanine aminotransferase apoenzyme in dogs. Vet Clin Pathol 27:26–30.
12. Stokol T, Erb H. 1998. The apo-enzyme content of aminotransferases in healthy and diseased domestic animals. Vet Clin Pathol 27:71–78.
13. Allen HS, Steiner J, Broussard J, Mansfield C, Williams DA, Jones B. 2006. Serum and urine concentrations of trypsinogen-activation peptide as markers for acute pancreatitis in cats. Can J Vet Res 70:313–316.
14. O'Neill SL, Feldman BF. 1989. Hemolysis as a factor in clinical chemistry and hematology of the dog. Vet Clin Pathol 18:58–68.
15. Hadley SP, Hoffmann WE, Kuhlenschmidt MS, Sanecki RK, Dorner JL. 1990. Effect of glucocorticoids on alkaline phosphatase, alanine aminotransferase, and gamma-glutamyltransferase in cultured dog hepatocytes. Enzyme 43:89–98.
16. Gaskill CL, Miller LM, Mattoon JS, Hoffmann WE, Burton SA, Gelens HC, Ihle SL, Miller JB, Shaw DH, Cribb AE. 2005. Liver histopathology and liver and serum alanine aminotransferase and alkaline phosphatase activities in epileptic dogs receiving phenobarbital. Vet Pathol 42:147–160.
17. Kornegay JN, Tuler SM, Miller DM, Levesque DC. 1988. Muscular dystrophy in a litter of golden retriever dogs. Muscle Nerve 11:1056–1064.
18. Valentine BA, Blue JT, Shelley SM, Cooper BJ. 1990. Increased serum alanine aminotransferase activity associated with muscle necrosis in the dog. J Vet Intern Med 4:140–143.
19. Gaschen F, Gaschen L, Seiler G, Welle M, Bornand Jaunin V, Gonin Jmaa D, Neiger-Aeschbacher G, Adæ-Damilano M. 1998. Lethal peracute rhabdomyolysis associated with stress and general anesthesia in three dystrophin-deficient cats. Vet Pathol 35:117–123.
20. Fleisher GA, Wakim KG. 1963. The fate of enzymes in body fluids: An experimental study. I. Disappearance rates of glutamic-pyruvic transaminase under various conditions. J Lab Clin Med 61:76–85.
21. Fleisher GA, Wakim KG. 1963. The fate of enzymes in body fluids: An experimental study. III. Disappearance rates of glutamic-oxalacetic transaminase II under various conditions. J Lab Clin Med 61:98–106.

22. Moss DW, Henderson AR. 1999. Clinical enzymology. In: Burtis CA, Ashwood ER, eds. *Tietz Textbook of Clinical Chemistry*, 3rd edition, 617–721. Philadelphia: WB Saunders.
23. Cardinet GH III. 1989. Skeletal muscle function. In: Kaneko JJ ed. *Clinical Biochemistry of Domestic Animals*, 4th edition, 462–495. San Diego: Academic.
24. Zanatta R, Abate O, D'Angelo A, Miniscalco B, Mannelli A. 2003. Diagnostic and prognostic value of serum lactate dehydrogenase (LDH) and LDH isoenzymes in canine lymphoma. Vet Res Commun 27(Suppl 1): 449–452.
25. Durham AE, Smith KC, Newton JR. 2003. An evaluation of diagnostic data in comparison to the results of liver biopsies in mature horses. Equine Vet J 35:554–559.
26. Mühlberger N, Kraft W. 1994. Diagnostic value of glutamate dehydrogenase determination in the dog [in German]. Tierarztl Prax 22:567–573.
27. Aitken MM, Hall E, Scott L, Davot JL, Allen WM. 2003. Liver-related biochemical changes in the serum of dogs being treated with phenobarbitone. Vet Rec 153:13–16.
28. Poelstra K, Bakker WW, Klok PA, Hardonk MJ, Meijer DK. 1997. A physiologic function for alkaline phosphatase: Endotoxin detoxification. Lab Invest 76:319–327.
29. Balcerzak M, Hamade E, Zhang L, Pikula S, Azzar G, Radisson J, Bandorowicz-Pikula J, Buchet R. 2003. The roles of annexins and alkaline phosphatase in mineralization process. Acta Biochim Pol 50:1019–1038.
30. Center SA, Randolph JF, ManWarren T, Slater M. 1991. Effect of colostrum ingestion on gamma-glutamyltransferase and alkaline phosphatase activities in neonatal pups. Am J Vet Res 52:499–504.
31. Sanecki RK, Hoffmann WE, Hansen R, Schaeffer DJ. 1993. Quantification of bone alkaline phosphatase in canine serum. Vet Clin Pathol 22:17–23.
32. Hank AM, Hoffmann WE, Sanecki RK, Schaeffer DJ, Dorner JL. 1993. Quantitative determination of equine alkaline phosphatase isoenzymes in foal and adult serum. J Vet Intern Med 7:20–24.
33. Zanker IA, Hammon HM, Blum JW. 2001. Activities of gamma-glutamyltransferase, alkaline phosphatase and aspartate-aminotransferase in colostrum, milk and blood plasma of calves fed first colostrum at 0–2, 6–7, 12–13 and 24–25 h after birth. J Vet Med [A] 48:179–185.
34. Syakalima M, Takiguchi M, Yasuda J, Hashimoto A. 1997. The age dependent levels of serum ALP isoenzymes and the diagnostic significance of corticosteroid-induced ALP during long-term glucocorticoid treatment. J Vet Med Sci 59:905–909.
35. Mahaffey EA, Lago MP. 1991. Comparison of techniques for quantifying alkaline phosphatase isoenzymes in canine serum. Vet Clin Pathol 20:51–55.
36. Syakalima M, Takiguchi M, Yasuda J, Hashimoto A. 1997. Separation and quantification of corticosteroid-induced, bone and liver alkaline phosphatase isoenzymes in canine serum. J Vet Med [A] 44:603–610.
37. Syakalima M, Takiguchi M, Yasuda J, Hashimoto A. 1998. The canine alkaline phosphatases: A review of the isoenzymes in serum, analytical methods and their diagnostic application. Jpn J Vet Res 46:3–11.
38. Kidney BA, Jackson ML. 1988. Diagnostic value of alkaline phosphatase isoenzyme separation by affinity electrophoresis in the dog. Can J Vet Res 52:106–110.
39. Putzki H, Reichert B, Heymann H. 1989. The serum activities of AP, gamma-GT, GLDH, GPT and CHE after complete biliary obstruction and choledochocaval fistula in the rat. Clin Chim Acta 181:81–86.
40. Solter PF, Hoffmann WE. 1995. Canine corticosteroid-induced alkaline phosphatase in serum was solubilized by phospholipase activity in vivo. Am J Physiol 269:G278–G286.
41. Solter PF, Hoffmann WE. 1999. Solubilization of liver alkaline phosphatase isoenzyme during cholestasis in dogs. Am J Vet Res 60:1010–1015.
42. Meyer DJ, Noonan NE. 1981. Liver tests in dogs receiving anticonvulsant drugs (diphenylhydantoin and primidone). J Am Anim Hosp Assoc 17:261–264.
43. Solter PF, Hoffmann WE, Chambers MD, Schaeffer DJ, Kuhlenschmidt MS. 1994. Hepatic total 3α-hydroxy bile acids concentration and enzyme activities in prednisone-treated dogs. Am J Vet Res 55:1086–1092.
44. Wiedmeyer CE, Solter PF, Hoffmann WE. 2002. Alkaline phosphatase expression in tissues from glucocorticoid-treated dogs. Am J Vet Res 63:1083–1088.
45. Wiedmeyer CE, Solter PF, Hoffmann WE. 2002. Kinetics of mRNA expression of alkaline phosphatase isoenzymes in hepatic tissues from glucocorticoid-treated dogs. Am J Vet Res 63:1089–1095.
46. Solter PF, Hoffmann WE, Hungerford LL, Peterson ME, Dorner JL. 1993. Assessment of corticosteroid-induced alkaline phosphatase isoenzyme as a screening test for hyperadrenocorticism in dogs. J Am Vet Med Assoc 203:534–538.
47. Ehrhart N, Dernell WS, Hoffmann WE, Weigel RM, Powers BE, Withrow SJ. 1998. Prognostic importance of alkaline phosphatase activity in serum from dogs with appendicular osteosarcoma: 75 cases (1990–1996). J Am Vet Med Assoc 213:1002–1006.

48. Komnenou A, Karayannopoulou M, Polizopoulou ZS, Constantinidis TC, Dessiris A. 2005. Correlation of serum alkaline phosphatase activity with the healing process of long bone fractures in dogs. Vet Clin Pathol 34:35–38.
49. Archer FJ, Taylor SM. 1996. Alkaline phosphatase bone isoenzyme and osteocalcin in the serum of hyperthyroid cats. Can Vet J 37:735–739.
50. Karayannopoulou M, Koutinas AF, Polizopoulou ZS, Roubies N, Fytianou A, Saridomichelakis MN, Kaldrymidou E. 2003. Total serum alkaline phosphatase activity in dogs with mammary neoplasms: A prospective study on 79 natural cases. J Vet Med [A] 50:501–505.
51. Hamilton JM, Wright J, Kight D. 1973. Alkaline phosphatase levels in canine mammary neoplasia. Vet Rec 93:121–123.
52. Tateyama S, Cotchin E. 1977. Alkaline phosphatase reaction of canine mammary mixed tumours: A light and electron microscopic study. Res Vet Sci 23:356–364.
53. Lawler DF, Keltner DG, Hoffmann WE, Nachreiner RF, Hegstad RL, Herndon PA, Fischer BJ. 1996. Benign familial hyperphosphatasemia in Siberian huskies. Am J Vet Res 57:612–617.
54. Meuten DJ, Kociba G, Threlfall WR, Nagode LA. 1980. Serum alkaline phosphatase in pregnant mares. Vet Clin Pathol 9:27–30.
55. Bebiak DM, Lawler DF, Reutzel LF. 1987. Nutrition and management of the dog. Vet Clin North Am Small Anim Pract 17:505–533.
56. Leveille-Webster CR. 2000. Laboratory diagnosis of hepatobiliary disease. In: Ettinger SJ, Feldman EC, eds. *Textbook of Veterinary Internal Medicine: Diseases of the Dog and Cat*, 5th edition, 1277–1293. Philadelphia: WB Saunders.
57. Bunch SE. 1993. Hepatotoxicity associated with pharmacologic agents in dogs and cats. Vet Clin North Am Small Anim Pract 23:659–670.
58. Harper EJ, Hackett RM, Wilkinson J, Heaton PR. 2003. Age-related variations in hematologic and plasma biochemical test results in beagles and Labrador retrievers. J Am Vet Med Assoc 223:1436–1442.
59. Nestor DD, Holan KM, Johnson CA, Schall W, Kaneene JB. 2006. Serum alkaline phosphatase activity in Scottish Terriers versus dogs of other breeds. J Am Vet Med Assoc 228:222–224.
60. Center SA, Baldwin BH, Dillingham S, Erb HN, Tennant BC. 1986. Diagnostic value of serum γ-glutamyl transferase and alkaline phosphatase activities in hepatobiliary disease in the cat. J Am Vet Med Assoc 188:507–510.
61. Foster DJ, Thoday KL. 2000. Tissue sources of serum alkaline phosphatase in 34 hyperthyroid cats: A qualitative and quantitative study. Res Vet Sci 68:89–94.
62. van der Kolk JH, Klein WR, van der Putten SW, Mol JA. 1991. A horse with Cushing's disease [in Dutch]. Tijdschr Diergeneeskd 116:670–675.
63. Cohen ND, Carter GK. 1992. Steroid hepatopathy in a horse with glucocorticoid-induced hyperadrenocorticism. J Am Vet Med Assoc 200:1682–1684.
64. Ryu SH, Kim BS, Lee CW, Yoon J, Lee YL. 2004. Glucocorticoid-induced laminitis with hepatopathy in a thoroughbred filly. J Vet Sci 5:271–274.
65. Froscher BG, Nagode LA. 1981. Origin and importance of increased alkaline phosphatase activity in peritoneal fluids of horses with colic. Am J Vet Res 42:888–891.
66. Davies JV, Gerring EL, Goodburn R, Manderville P. 1984. Experimental ischaemia of the ileum and concentrations of the intestinal isoenzyme of alkaline phosphatase in plasma and peritoneal fluid. Equine Vet J 16:215–217.
67. Baumrucker CR. 1980. Purification and identification of γ-glutamyl transpeptidase of milk membranes. J Dairy Sci 63:49–54.
68. Baumrucker CR, Pocius PA. 1978. γ-Glutamyl transpeptidase in lactating mammary secretory tissue of cow and rat. J Dairy Sci 61:309–314.
69. Perino LJ, Sutherland RL, Woollen NE. 1993. Serum γ-glutamyltransferase activity and protein concentration at birth and after suckling in calves with adequate and inadequate passive transfer of immunoglobulin G. Am J Vet Res 54:56–59.
70. Thompson JC, Pauli JV. 1981. Colostral transfer of gamma glutamyl transpeptidase in calves. NZ Vet J 29:223–226.
71. Bouda J, Dvorák V, Minksová E, Dvorák R. 1980. The activities of GOT, gamma-GT, alkaline phosphatase in blood plasma of cows and their calves fed from buckets. Acta Vet Brno 49:193–198.
72. Patterson WH, Brown CM. 1986. Increase of serum γ-glutamyltransferase in neonatal standardbred foals. Am J Vet Res 47:2461–2463.
73. Szasz G. 1969. A kinetic photometric method for serum γ-glutamyl transpeptidase. Clin Chem 15:124–136.
74. Bulle F, Mavier P, Zafrani ES, Preaux AM, Lescs MC, Siegrist S, Dhumeaux D, Guellaën G. 1990. Mechanism of γ-glutamyl transpeptidase release in serum during intrahepatic and extrahepatic cholestasis in the rat: A histochemical, biochemical and molecular approach. Hepatology 11:545–550.

75. Müller PB, Taboada J, Hosgood G, Partington BP, VanSteenhouse JL, Taylor HW, Wolfsheimer KJ. 2000. Effects of long-term phenobarbital treatment on the liver in dogs. J Vet Intern Med 14:165–171.

76. Hoffmann WE, Baker G, Rieser S, Dorner JL. 1987. Alterations in selected serum biochemical constituents in equids after induced hepatic disease. Am J Vet Res 48:1343–1347.

77. Yonezawa LA, Kitamura SS, Mirandola RM, Antonelli AC, Ortolani EL. 2005. Preventive treatment with vitamin E alleviates the poisoning effects of carbon tetrachloride in cattle. J Vet Med [A] 52:292–297.

78. Cable CS, Rebhun WC, Fortier LA. 1997. Cholelithiasis and cholecystitis in a dairy cow. J Am Vet Med Assoc 211:899–900.

79. Auza NJ, Olson WG, Murphy MJ, Linn JG. 1999. Diagnosis and treatment of copper toxicosis in ruminants. J Am Vet Med Assoc 214:1624–1628.

80. Putnam MR, Qualls CW, Rice LE, Dawson LJ, Edwards WC. 1986. Hepatic enzyme changes in bovine hepatogenous photosensitivity caused by water-damaged alfalfa hay. J Am Vet Med Assoc 189:77–82.

81. Molina EC, Lozano SP, Barraca AP. 2006. The relationship between haematological indices, serum gamma-glutamyl transferase and glutamate dehydrogenase, visual hepatic damage and worm burden in cattle infected with *Fasciola gigantica*. J Helminthol 80:277–279.

82. Cebra CK, Garry FB, Getzy DM, Fettman MJ. 1997. Hepatic lipidosis in anorectic, lactating Holstein cattle: A retrospective study of serum biochemical abnormalities. J Vet Intern Med 11:231–237.

83. Komatsu Y, Itoh N, Taniyama H, Kitazawa T, Yokota H, Koiwa M, Ohtsuka H, Terasaki N, Maeno K, Mizoguchi M, Takeuchi Y, Tanigawa M, Nakamura T, Watanabe H, Matsuguchi Y, Kukino T, Honma A. 2002. Classification of abomasal displacement in cows according to histopathology of the liver and clinical chemistry. J Vet Med [A] 49:482–486.

84. Gossett KA, Turnwald GH, Kearney MT, Greco DS, Cleghorn B. 1987. Evaluation of γ-glutamyl transpeptidase-to-creatinine ratio from spot samples of urine supernatant, as an indicator of urinary enzyme excretion in dogs. Am J Vet Res 48:455–457.

85. Aktas M, Auguste D, Concordet D, Vinclair P, Lefebvre H, Toutain PL, Braun JP. 1994. Creatine kinase in dog plasma: Preanalytical factors of variation, reference values and diagnostic significance. Res Vet Sci 56:30–36.

86. Lindena J, Sommerfeld U, Hopfel C, Wolkersdorfer R, Trautschold I. 1983. Enzyme activities in blood cells of man and dogs after separation on a discontinuous Percoll gradient. Enzyme 29:100–108.

87. Fascetti AJ, Mauldin GE, Mauldin GN. 1997. Correlation between serum creatine kinase activities and anorexia in cats. J Vet Intern Med 11:9–13.

88. Dixon RM, Reid SW, Mooney CT. 1999. Epidemiological, clinical, haematological and biochemical characteristics of canine hypothyroidism. Vet Rec 145:481–487.

89. Sattler T, Furll M. 2004. Creatine kinase and aspartate aminotransferase in cows as indicators for endometritis. J Vet Med [A] 51:132–137.

90. Simpson KW, Simpson JW, Lake S, Morton DB, Batt RM. 1991. Effect of pancreatectomy on plasma activities of amylase, isoamylase, lipase and trypsin-like immunoreactivity in dogs. Res Vet Sci 51:78–82.

91. Stickle JE, Carlton WW, Boon GD. 1980. Isoamylases in clinically normal dogs. Am J Vet Res 41:506–509.

92. Corazza M, Tognetti R, Guidi G, Buonaccorsi A. 1994. Urinary α-amylase and serum macroamylase activities in dogs with proteinuria. J Am Vet Med Assoc 205:438–440.

93. Moore WE, Cunningham BA. 1976. Comparative properties of canine hepatic and pancreatic amylase. Bull Am Soc Vet Clin Pathol 5:11–12 (abstract).

94. Nothman MM, Callow AD. 1971. Investigations on the origin of amylase in serum and urine. Gastroenterology 60:82–89.

95. Keller P. 1981. Enzyme activities in the dog: Tissue analyses, plasma values, and intracellular distribution. Am J Vet Res 42:575–582.

96. Mocharla H, Mocharla R, Hodes ME. 1990. Alpha-amylase gene transcription in tissues of normal dog. Nucleic Acids Res 18:1031–1036.

97. O'Donnell MD, McGeeney KF. 1975. α-Amylase and glucoamylase activities of canine serum. Comp Biochem Physiol 50:269–274.

98. Braun JP, Ouedraogo G, Thorel B, Mædaille C, Rico AG. 1990. Determination of plasma α-amylase in the dog: A test of the specificity of new methods. J Clin Chem Clin Biochem 28:493–495.

99. Mayer AD, Airey M, Hodgson J, McMahon MJ. 1985. Enzyme transfer from pancreas to plasma during acute pancreatitis: The contribution of ascitic fluid and lymphatic drainage of the pancreas. Gut 26:876–881.

100. Brobst D, Ferguson AB, Carter JM. 1970. Evaluation of serum amylase and lipase activity in experimentally induced pancreatitis in the dog. J Am Vet Med Assoc 157:1697–1702.

101. Schaer M, Holloway S. 1991. Diagnosing acute pancreatitis in the cat. Vet Med 86:782–795.

102. Hill RC, Van Winkle TJ. 1993. Acute necrotizing pancreatitis and acute suppurative pancreatitis in the cat: A retrospective study of 40 cases (1976–1989). J Vet Intern Med 7:25–33.

103. Kitchell BE, Strombeck DR, Cullen J, Harrold D. 1986. Clinical and pathologic changes in experimentally induced acute pancreatitis in cats. Am J Vet Res 47:1170–1173.

104. Hudson EB, Strombeck DR. 1978. Effects of functional nephrectomy on the disappearance rates of canine serum amylase and lipase. Am J Vet Res 39:1316–1321.

105. Polzin DJ, Osborne CA, Stevens JB, Hayden DW. 1983. Serum amylase and lipase activities in dogs with chronic primary renal failure. Am J Vet Res 44:404–410.

106. Jacobs RM. 1989. Relationship of urinary amylase activity and proteinuria in the dog. Vet Pathol 26:349–350.

107. de Schepper J, Capiau E, van Bree H, de Cock I. 1989. The diagnostic significance of increased urinary and serum amylase activity in bitches with pyometra. J Vet Med [A] 36:431–437.

108. Jacobs RM. 1988. Renal disposition of amylase, lipase, and lysozyme in the dog. Vet Pathol 25:443–449.

109. Lulich JP, Osborne CA, O'Brien TD, Polzin DJ. 1992. Feline renal failure: Questions, answers, questions. Compend Contin Educ Small Anim Pract 14:127–153.

110. Steiner JM, Berridge BR, Wojcieszyn J, Williams DA. 2002. Cellular immunolocalization of gastric and pancreatic lipase in various tissues obtained from dogs. Am J Vet Res 63:722–727.

111. Graca R, Messick J, McCullough S, Barger A, Hoffmann W. 2005. Validation and diagnostic efficacy of a lipase assay using the substrate 1,2-*o*-dilauryl-*rac*-glycero glutaric acid-(6′ methyl resorufin)-ester for the diagnosis of acute pancreatitis in dogs. Vet Clin Pathol 34:39–43.

112. Greten H, Levy RI, Fredrickson DS. 1968. A further characterization of lipoprotein lipase. Biochim Biophys Acta 164:185–194.

113. Steiner JM, Williams DA. 2003. Development and validation of a radioimmunoassay for the measurement of canine pancreatic lipase immunoreactivity in serum of dogs. Am J Vet Res 64:1237–1241.

114. Steiner JM, Teague SR, Williams DA. 2003. Development and analytic validation of an enzyme-linked immunosorbent assay for the measurement of canine pancreatic lipase immunoreactivity in serum. Can J Vet Res 67:175–182.

115. Steiner JM, Wilson BG, Williams DA. 2004. Development and analytical validation of a radioimmunoassay for the measurement of feline pancreatic lipase immunoreactivity in serum. Can J Vet Res 68:309–314.

116. Steiner JM, Williams DA. 2004. Development and analytical validation of an enzyme linked immunosorbent assay for the measurement of canine gastric lipase immunoreactivity in serum. Can J Vet Res 68:161–168.

117. Quigley K, Jackson M, Haines D. 2000. Canine hyperlipasemia in association with pancreatic and/or hepatic neoplasia: A case series. Vet Pathol 37:527 (abstract).

118. Strombeck DR, Farver T, Kaneko JJ. 1981. Serum amylase and lipase activities in the diagnosis of pancreatitis in dogs. Am J Vet Res 42:1966–1970.

119. Quigley KA, Jackson ML, Haines DM. 2001. Hyperlipasemia in six dogs with pancreatic or hepatic neoplasia: Evidence for tumor lipase production. Vet Clin Pathol 30:114–120.

120. Parent J. 1982. Effects of dexamethasone on pancreatic tissue and on serum amylase and lipase activities in dogs. J Am Vet Med Assoc 180:743–746.

121. Mellanby RJ, Stell A, Baines E, Chantrey JC, Herrtage ME. 2003. Panniculitis associated with pancreatitis in a cocker spaniel. J Small Anim Pract 44:24–28.

122. Steiner JM, Broussard J, Mansfield CS, Gumminger SR, Williams DA. 2001. Serum canine pancreatic lipase immunoreactivity (cPLI) concentrations in dogs with spontaneous pancreatitis. J Vet Intern Med 15:274 (abstract).

123. Williams DA. 2003. Diagnosis of canine and feline pancreatitis. In: 38th Annual Meeting of the American Society of Veterinary Clinical Pathologists, Banff, Canada, 6–12.

124. Steiner JM, Finco DR, Gumminger SR, Williams DA. 2001. Serum canine pancreatic lipase immunoreactivity (cPLI) in dogs with experimentally induced chronic renal failure. J Vet Intern Med 15:311 (abstract).

125. Forman MA, Marks SL, De Cock HE, Hergesell EJ, Wisner ER, Baker TW, Kass PH, Steiner JM, Williams DA. 2004. Evaluation of serum feline pancreatic lipase immunoreactivity and helical computed tomography versus conventional testing for the diagnosis of feline pancreatitis. J Vet Intern Med 18:807–815.

126. Hoffmann WE, Dorner JL. 1977. Disappearance rates of intravenously injected canine alkaline phosphatase isoenzymes. Am J Vet Res 38:1553–1556.

127. Hoffmann WE, Renegar WE, Dorner JL. 1977. Serum half-life of intravenously injected intestinal and hepatic alkaline phosphatase isoenzymes in the cat. Am J Vet Res 38:1637–1639.

128. Harris P. 1997. Equine rhabdomyolysis syndrome. In: Robinson NE, ed. *Current Therapy in Equine Medicine 4*, 115–121. Philadelphia: WB Saunders.

129. Cardinet GH, Littrell JF, Freedland RA. 1967. Comparative investigations of serum creatine phosphokinase and glutamic-oxaloacetic transaminase activities in equine paralytic myoglobinuria. Res Vet Sci 8:219–226.

130. Wakim KG, Fleisher GA. 1963. The fate of enzymes in body fluids: An experimental study. II. Disappearance rates of glutamic-oxalacetic transaminase I under various conditions. J Lab Clin Med 61:86–97.

131. Rapaport E. 1975. The fractional disappearance rate of the separate isoenzymes of creatine phosphokinase in the dog. Cardiovasc Res 9:473–477.

132. Barton MH, Morris DD. 1998. Disease of the liver. In: Reed SM, Bayly WM, eds. *Equine Internal Medicine*, 707–738. Philadelphia: WB Saunders.

133. Collis KA, Symonds HW, Sansom BF. 1979. The half-life of glutamate dehydrogenase in plasma of dry and lactating dairy cows. Res Vet Sci 27:267–268.

134. Freedland RA, Kramer JW. 1970. Use of serum enzymes as aids to diagnosis. Adv Vet Sci Comp Med 14:61–103.

135. Bär U, Friedel R, Heine H, Mayer D, Ohlendorf S, Schmidt FW, Trautschold I. 1972. Studies on enzyme elimination: III. Distribution, transport, and elimination of cell enzymes in the extracellular space. Enzyme 14:133–156.

136. Kaneko JJ, Harvey JW, Bruss ML. 1997. *Clinical Biochemistry of Domestic Animals*, 5th edition. San Diego: Academic.

137. Siekmann L, Bonora R, Burtis CA, Ceriotti F, Clerc-Renaud P, Færard G, Ferrero CA, Forest JC, Franck PF, Gella FJ, Hoelzel W, Jørgensen PJ, Kanno T, Kessner A, Klauke R, Kristiansen N, Lessinger JM, Linsinger TP, Misaki H, Mueller MM, Panteghini M, Pauwels J, Schiele F, Schimmel HG, Vialle A, Weidemann G, Schumann G. 2002. IFCC primary reference procedures for the measurement of catalytic activity concentrations of enzymes at 37 °C. Part 1. The concept of reference procedures for the measurement of catalytic activity concentrations of enzymes. Clin Chem Lab Med 40:631–634.

Chapter 13

LIVER FUNCTION

Physiologic Functions of the Liver 676
Abnormal Results of Routine Laboratory Tests Because of Hepatic Insufficiency
  or Disease 677
Bilirubin Concentration 681
    I.   Physiologic Processes 681
    II. Analytical Concepts 683
    III. Hyperbilirubinemia 684
    IV. Bilirubinuria 689
    V. Icterus Index 689
Bile Acid (BA) Concentration. 690
    I.   Physiologic Processes 690
    II. Analytical Concepts 691
    III. Increased Bile Acid (BA) Concentration in Serum or Plasma 691
    IV. Bile Acid Challenge Test for Dogs and Cats 693
    V. Urine Bile Acid to Creatinine (BA : Crt) Ratios 696
Ammonium (NH_4^+) Concentration in Plasma. 697
    I.   Physiologic Processes 697
    II. Analytical Concepts 697
    III. Hyperammonemia 699
    IV. NH_4^+ Tolerance Test 702
    V. Postprandial Venous NH_4^+ Tolerance Test for Dogs 702
Dye-Excretion Tests 703

Table 13.1. Abbreviations and symbols in this chapter

[x]	Concentration of x (x = analyte)
ALP	Alkaline phosphatase
ALT	Alanine transaminase
AST	Aspartate transaminase
Bδ	δ-Bilirubin
BA	Bile acid
BA:Crt	Bile acid to creatinine
Bc	Conjugated bilirubin
Bd	Direct bilirubin
Bi	Indirect bilirubin
Bt	Total bilirubin
Bu	Unconjugated bilirubin
Bu/Alb	Unconjugated bilirubin bound to albumin (noncovalent)
Crt	Creatinine
GGT	γ-Glutamyltransferase
GMD	Glutamate dehydrogenase
HCO_3^-	Bicarbonate
Hgb	Hemoglobin
ID	Iditol dehydrogenase
LD	Lactate dehydrogenase
NH_3	Ammonia
NH_4^+	Ammonium
SI	Système International d'Unités
TNFα	Tumor necrosis factor α
UNSBA	Urine nonsulfated bile acid
URL	Upper reference limit
USBA	Urine sulfated bile acid
USG_{ref}	Refractometric urine specific gravity
WRI	Within reference interval

PHYSIOLOGIC FUNCTIONS OF THE LIVER

The liver has many vital physiologic functions involving synthesis, excretion, and storage. When a disease process damages cells within a liver, changes in hepatic function may alter the composition of body fluids, and the resulting abnormalities may be detected by laboratory assays.

I.   Functions involving body fuels
       A. Protein metabolism: Hepatocytes synthesize most plasma proteins (over 1000 proteins), including albumin and most globulins (except immunoglobulins). Most synthesis is *de novo* ("from new"), either from essential (dietary) amino acids or from nonessential amino acids made by hepatocytes.
       B. Carbohydrate metabolism: Hepatocytes remove most dietary glucose from portal blood and store glucose as glycogen for emergency needs. Glucose from hepatic gluconeogenesis is the major source of glucose in the blood of fasting animals.

C. Lipid metabolism: Hepatocytes make fatty acids, triglycerides, cholesterol, and apolipo-proteins for lipoproteins, and esterify cholesterol for phospholipids. Hepatocytes degrade chylomicrons from portal and systemic blood and remove lipoprotein remnants from systemic blood.

II. Storage functions: Hepatocytes store glycogen, triglyceride, and a variety of elements, including iron and copper.

III. Detoxification: Hepatocytes modify or degrade endogenous compounds (e.g., uric acid, steroidal hormones, polypeptide hormones, and hemoglobin) and exogenous compounds (e.g., steroidal hormones) via a wide range of chemical reactions, including conjugations, oxidations, reductions, and hydrolysis. Hepatocytes are a major site of NH_4^+ fixation (i.e., NH_4^+ incorporation into urea or amino acids).

IV. Actions of mononuclear phagocytic system: The liver filters blood (systemic and portal; capability second only to spleen) through the actions of Kupffer cells. The macrophages remove damaged cells (erythrocytes, leukocytes, and platelets), inflammatory mediators, organisms, and endotoxins from the blood (and thus also detoxifies).

V. Excretory function: Hepatocytes change compounds to H_2O-soluble forms for excretion via the biliary system, urinary system, or intestines. Hepatocytes degrade cholesterol to bile acids for excretion in bile.
   A. Bile is formed by three processes. In a BA-dependent pathway, the active secretion of BA produces an osmotic gradient that increases H_2O excretion. In a BA-independent pathway, active transport of Na^+, glutathione, and HCO_3^- promotes bile formation via Na^+-K^+-adenosine 5'-triphosphatase. Third, secretin promotes bile formation by stimulating HCO_3^- and Cl^- secretion into bile.[1]
   B. Components of hepatic bile include H_2O, BA (at least 50 % of bile solids), Bc, lecithin, cholesterol, fatty acids, electrolytes (Na^+, K^+, Ca^{2+}, Cl^-, and HCO_3^-), and a variety of H_2O-soluble wastes. In the biliary ducts and gallbladder, BA-rich bile is formed by resorption of H_2O and some electrolytes.

ABNORMAL RESULTS OF ROUTINE LABORATORY TESTS BECAUSE OF HEPATIC INSUFFICIENCY OR DISEASE

I. Routine laboratory test results may suggest the presence of liver disease or decreased hepatic function (Tables 13.2 and 13.3). However, individual results are not specific for hepatic insufficiency or disease; that is, other disorders may cause the abnormalities.

II. It is important to recognize the difference between abnormalities that indicate hepatocellular disease, biliary disease, or hepatobiliary disease, because some pathologic processes affect mostly hepatocytes, whereas others affect mostly biliary cells. Also, it is important to recognize data that indicate hepatic insufficiency.
   A. Hepatocellular disease may result from a wide variety of pathologic states (i.e., degenerative, autoimmune, anomalous, metabolic, nutritional, neoplastic, inflammatory, infectious, inherited, toxic, or traumatic).
   B. Biliary disease may also result from a variety of insults. It is most often the result of inflammatory, neoplastic, or toxic disorders.

Table 13.2. Complete blood count (CBC) and chemistry test results (pathologic findings) that suggest or indicate hepatic disease or dysfunction

Pathologic finding	Hepatic lesion suggested	Pathogenesis of finding[a]
CBC results		
Acanthocytosis	Hemangiosarcoma	Possibly vascular trauma
	Lipid metabolism defect	Altered lipid composition of erythrocyte membrane
Anemia	Hepatitis (chronic)	Anemia of inflammatory disease
	↓ Functional mass[b]	Possibly ↓ erythropoietin or abnormal protein or amino acid metabolism
Codocytosis	↓ Functional mass	Altered lipid composition of erythrocyte membrane
Microcytosis	↓ Functional mass	Possibly ↓ transferrin production and thus ↓ delivery of iron to erythrocyte precursors
	Portosystemic shunt	
Chemistry assay results		
Decreased UN	↓ Functional mass	↓ Urea production
Hyperammonemia	↓ Functional mass	Inadequate fixing of NH_4^+ into urea
	Portosystemic shunt	
Hyperbilirubinemia	Cholestasis	Inadequate biliary excretion of bilirubin
	↓ Bc transport	
Hypercholesterolemia	Cholestasis	↑ Production of cholesterol
		↓ Clearance of lipoproteins
Hyperglycemia	Cirrhosis	Hyperglucagonemia or increased gluconeogenesis of hepatocutaneous syndrome
	Hepatopathy	
Hyperuricemia	↓ Functional mass	↓ Conversion of uric acid to allantoin by hepatocytes
Hypoalbuminemia	↓ Functional mass	↓ Albumin production
Hypocholesterolemia	↓ Functional mass	↓ Cholesterol synthesis
Hypofibrinogenemia	↓ Functional mass	↓ Fibrinogen production
Hypoglycemia	↓ Functional mass	↓ Gluconeogenesis
Hypoproteinemia	↓ Functional mass	↓ Production of albumin and globulins other than γ-globulins
Increased ALT, AST, ID, LD, or GMD	Damaged hepatocytes	Release of cytoplasmic enzymes due to blebbing or necrosis
Increased ALP	Cholestasis	↑ Production of L-ALP
Increased GGT	Biliary hyperplasia	↑ Production of GGT
	Cholestasis	Release of GGT from damaged cells
	Possibly hepatocyte damage	
Lipemia (gross)	↓ Functional mass	↓ Clearance of lipoproteins

[a] See more complete explanations in chapters for each particular analyte.

[b] Decreased functional mass results from diffuse hepatocyte damage, destruction, atrophy, or hypoplasia.

L-ALP, liver isoform of alkaline phosphatase; and UN, urea nitrogen

Table 13.3. Urinalysis, coagulation, fecal, and peritoneal fluid test results (pathologic findings) that suggest or indicate hepatic disease or dysfunction

Pathologic finding	Hepatic lesion suggested	Pathogenesis of finding[a]
Urinalysis results		
Ammonium (bi)urate crystalluria[b]	↓ Functional mass Urea cycle defect	Inadequate fixing of NH_4^+ into urea and ↓ conversion of uric acid to allantoin
Bilirubinuria[b]	Cholestasis ↓ Bc transport	Inadequate biliary excretion of bilirubin
Hyposthenuria or isosthenuria[b]	↓ Functional mass	↓ Renal medullary tonicity due to decreased urea ↑ NH_4^+ excretion may inhibit concentrating mechanism
Urate crystalluria[b]	↓ Functional mass	↓ Conversion of uric acid to allantoin
Coagulation assay results		
Prolonged partial thromboplastin time or prothrombin time	Cholestasis	↓ Vitamin K–dependent coagulation factors due to impaired intestinal absorption of vitamin K
	↓ Functional mass	↓ Clearance of inhibitors of coagulation factors such as fibrin or fibrinogen degradation products (fibrin fragments + fibrinogen fragments) ↓ Production of most coagulation factors
Fecal exam results		
Steatorrhea	Cholestasis	Defective lipid digestion because bile acids are not delivered to intestine
Peritoneal fluid analysis		
Transudate	↓ Functional mass Cirrhosis	↑ Na^+ and H_2O retention, ↓ plasma oncotic pressure, portal hypertension, ↓ lymph drainage

[a] See more complete explanations in the chapters for each particular analyte.

[b] Finding may occur in clinically healthy animals; for example, ammonium bi(urate) crystalluria in Dalmatians, urate crystalluria in English bulldogs, bilirubinuria in dogs, and hyposthenuria or isosthenuria as a physiologic response to excess water intake.

    C. *Hepatic insufficiency* is a pathophysiologic state in which the number of functioning hepatocytes is markedly reduced. Hepatic insufficiency and hepatic failure are usually considered synonyms. Disorders that cause hepatic insufficiency fall into two groups:
        1. Disorders that destroy hepatocytes (hepatocellular disease) may progress slowly, recur episodically, or involve rapid, extensive necrosis.

    2. Portosystemic shunts (congenital or acquired) cause either hypoplasia or atrophy of the liver because of decreased nutrients reaching hepatocytes from portal blood.

  D. All animals with hepatic insufficiency have too few functioning hepatocytes, but many animals with hepatocellular disease do not have hepatic insufficiency. Most animals with primary biliary disease will develop secondary hepatocellular disease. Many animals with primary hepatocellular disease develop secondary biliary disorders. Either hepatocellular or biliary diseases may cause hepatic insufficiency.

  E. Laboratory test results that indicate hepatic insufficiency do not tell us which hepatocellular or hepatobiliary disease the animal has or whether the disease process is reversible or irreversible.

III. In clinical jargon, some people refer to hepatic enzyme assays (ALT, AST, ALP, GGT, and ID) as liver function tests. However, these enzymes are not solely hepatic in origin, increased activities of these enzymes do not directly indicate loss of any liver function, and liver function can be greatly reduced without increased serum enzyme activities. To emphasize the last concept, would the serum activity of a hepatic enzyme increase if one removed an animal's liver?

IV. Decreased functional hepatic mass

  A. Hepatic insufficiency occurs when hepatic functional mass has decreased enough to cause a pathophysiologic state. The decreased functional mass typically results from too few hepatocytes (and thus a small liver). Evidence of hepatic dysfunction is expected with loss of 70–80 % of liver mass. However, hepatic insufficiency also may result from dysfunction of existing hepatocytes and occur with hepatomegaly or a normal-sized liver.

  B. Many diseases and conditions may decrease an animal's functional hepatic mass. Examples are listed in Table 13.4.

V. Cholestasis

  A. Cholestasis is defined in different ways. In a dictionary definition, *cholestasis* is the "stoppage or suppression of bile flow."[2]

Table 13.4. Examples of diseases and conditions that cause decreased functional hepatic mass (using the *DAMNIT* acronym)

*D*egenerative: hypoxia caused by anemia or congestion
**A*nomalous: portosystemic shunt
*M*etabolic: lipidosis, diabetes mellitus, hyperadrenocorticism
*N*eoplastic: lymphoma, metastatic neoplasia
*I*nflammatory
  Infectious: leptospirosis, histoplasmosis, feline infectious peritonitis
  *Noninfectious: chronic active hepatitis
*I*nherited: copper or lysosomal storage diseases
**T*oxic: steroid hepatopathy, some anesthetic agents, tetracycline, carprofen, copper toxicosis, hemochromatosis, pyrrolizidine alkaloid–containing plants
*T*raumatic: hit by car

  * A relatively common disease or condition
  Note: Lists of specific disorders or conditions are not complete but are provided to give examples.

1. The *stoppage* component of the definition is consistent with the observations of distended bile ducts (grossly) and bile plugs, lakes, or pigments (microscopic) that are caused by extrahepatic or intrahepatic lesions that obstruct bile flow and thus reduce the volume of bile leaving the biliary system.

2. The *suppression* component of the definition is consistent with pathophysiologic states involving impaired BA secretion into bile. As the osmotic effects of secreted BA largely control bile volume, decreased BA secretion may reduce the volume of bile produced by the biliary system and thus reduce bile flow (less bile volume per day).

3. Cholestasis is commonly used in the context of the icterus that occurs because of obstructive biliary lesions. However, Bc is a very small component of bile and contributes little to formation of bile or bile volume. When there is obstructive biliary disease, there probably is decreased bile flow, decreased Bc excretion, and decreased BA excretion.

4. From one perspective, understanding *obstructive cholestasis* is necessary to explain structural consequences of biliary disease. However, from another perspective, understanding *functional cholestasis* is necessary to explain the pathophysiologic consequences of defective bile acid secretion.

B. The different uses of the term cholestasis are mentioned to help clarify statements that may appear to be conflicting. For example, a pathophysiologic state associated with endotoxemia is called either *functional cholestasis* or *sepsis-associated cholestasis*. In this context, there is defective BA secretion from hepatocytes to bile, but there is not an obstructive lesion that impairs bile flow (see additional information on functional cholestasis in Bilirubin Concentration, sect. III.E.2).

C. Bile acid and bilirubin pathways have similarities but also marked differences.[3] These pathways will be covered in more detail in separate sections.

1. Bu is a product of heme degradation, whereas BA is a product of cholesterol degradation. Heme and cholesterol do not share physiologic pathways.

2. Bilirubin (Bc and Bu) and BA enter hepatocytes through sinusoidal membranes but by different membrane transport systems.

3. Bc and BA are secreted from hepatocytes through canalicular membranes but by different membrane transport systems.

4. Pathologic states that damage hepatocyte membranes can impair both bilirubin and BA excretion. These defects may be further linked because accumulation of BA in hepatocytes may cause hepatocyte damage that interferes with bilirubin metabolism. However, pathologic states that selectively interfere with transport systems may impair secretion of one analyte but not the other.

BILIRUBIN CONCENTRATION

I. Physiologic processes (Fig. 13.1)

A. In plasma, there are three fractions of total bilirubin (Bu/Alb, Bc, and Bδ). Bu/Alb is dominant in the absence of disease. Bu is constantly produced from the degradation of heme from senescent erythrocytes and heme-containing proteins. In health, Bu and Bc are rapidly removed from plasma by either liver (Bu and Bc) or kidneys (Bc). The spontaneous and covalent binding of bilirubin glucuronide isomers (Bc) to albumin forms Bδ (Bc-Alb), which, once formed, has the circulating half-life of albumin ($\approx$ 8–20 d).[4] Bc and Bδ concentrations are negligible in health.

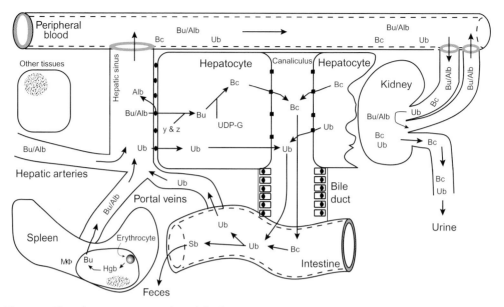

Fig. 13.1. Physiologic processes involving bilirubin.

- In health, erythrocyte destruction within macrophages of the spleen, liver, or bone marrow is followed by the degradation of heme and its conversion to Bu. Small and usually clinically insignificant amounts of Bu are formed from heme degradation associated with ineffective erythropoiesis and degradation of other heme-containing molecules (catalase, peroxidase, and cytochromes). As Bu leaves a macrophage, it forms a noncovalent association with albumin (Alb) and remains associated with Alb until uptake by hepatocytes. Bu is relatively water insoluble prior to binding to Alb.
- When Bu enters the liver and its protein-permeable sinusoids, it enters hepatocytes without albumin and binds to Y-protein (ligandin, glutathione S-transferase B) or Z-protein (fatty acid–binding protein). Bu probably enters hepatocytes by a passive but facilitated process; binding proteins enhance the process by reducing the efflux of Bu back to the sinusoidal plasma.
- Within hepatocytes, Bu is conjugated with glucuronide (also glucose in horses) to form bilirubin monoglucoronide or bilirubin diglucoronide, collectively called Bc.
- Bc is transported from hepatocytes into canaliculi (the rate-limiting step in bilirubin excretion) by an energy-dependent transport system for organic anions other than BAs.
- Bc in bile enters the intestine and is degraded to urobilinogen (colorless). Urobilinogen can be passively absorbed in the intestine and then enter hepatocytes for excretion in bile, or bypass the liver and be excreted in urine. Urobilinogen can also be degraded to stercobilinogen (dark brown) and excreted in feces.
- If Bc escapes hepatocytes and enters the blood, it can pass through the glomerular filtration barrier and be excreted in the urine. Because Alb does not pass through the glomerular filtration barrier of most mammals, Bu/Alb does not enter the urine in those animals.

Bu/Alb, Bu associated with albumin; Mφ, macrophage; Sb, stercobilinogen; Ub, urobilinogen; and UDP-G, uridine diphosphoglucuronide.

B. Small amounts of bilirubin are commonly found in the urine of healthy dogs. It has not been established whether the bilirubin is Bc or Bu/Alb. It is frequently assumed to be Bc because Bc is H_2O soluble and passes freely through the glomerular filtration barrier. However, small amounts of albumin are also commonly present in the urine of healthy dogs, so some bilirubin may be in the form of Bu/Alb.

C. Healthy horses have greater serum [Bt] than other domestic animals: about 0.7–2.0 mg/dL in horses versus < 0.5 mg/dL in other animals.

II. Analytical concepts
   A. Unit conversion: mg/dL × 17.10 = μmol/L (SI unit, nearest 2 μmol/L)[5]
   B. Conventional spectrophotometric methods (wet chemical assays)
      1. Several bilirubin assays are used to measure all bilirubin fractions (Bt) or only the non-Bu fractions (Bd). The classic bilirubin assay was the van den Bergh method, but it has been replaced by other assays (e.g., Malloy-Evelyn and Jendrassik-Gróf methods) for several decades.
         a. Bu reacts slower than Bc in most bilirubin reactions, so substances are added to accelerate its participation in Bt assays. When the accelerant factors are not present, only the non-Bu fractions are measured (called *direct bilirubin reaction*).
         b. From the measured [Bt] and [Bd], [Bi] is calculated by subtraction: [Bt] − [Bd] = [Bi].
      2. If these assays are used, laboratories may report the following concentrations that should represent the bilirubin fractions listed below. [Bδ] is not specifically measured and cannot be calculated by these methods.
         a. [Bt] (measured) = [Bc] + [Bδ] + [Bu]
         b. [Bd] (measured) = [Bc] + [Bδ]
         c. [Bi] (calculated) = [Bt] − [Bd] = [Bu]
   C. Dry-chemical methods using thin-layer reagent slides (Kodak or Vitros instruments)
      1. The assays use modified bilirubin diazo reactions in thin-layer reagent films and are designed to measure the following:
         a. [Bt] = [Bc] + [Bδ] + [Bu]
         b. [Bu]
         c. [Bc]
      2. From those measured concentrations, the following are calculated:
         a. [Bδ] = [Bt] − [Bc] − [Bu]
         b. [Bd] = [Bc] + [Bδ]
   D. Procedural notes
      1. Hgb interferes with azo reactions and produces falsely low [Bt] with the Malloy-Evelyn and Jendrassik-Gróf methods. However, in the thin-layer reagent slides, Hgb falsely increases the [Bt] and [Bc] and falsely decreases [Bu].
      2. Ultraviolet light degrades bilirubin. In direct sunlight, [Bt] may decrease up to 50 % in 1 h.
      3. Immunoglobulins may precipitate after the addition of acidic bilirubin reagents, and this precipitant interferes with light transmission and causes a falsely increased [Bt].[6] The interference occurs primarily when there is an increased γ-globulin concentration (e.g., paraproteinemia). A clearly increased [Bt] (e.g., > 5 mg/dL) can be easily recognized as a false value when the serum is visually not icteric. In one case, the [Bt] was "measured" to be > 20 mg/dL, but the sample was not icteric (observation by S.L.S.). Minor interferences, however, may not be detected via this comparison.
      4. Using thin-layer slide assays, the sum of [Bc] and [Bu] may exceed the measured [Bt] (especially in horses). It has not been established whether the [Bt] is falsely decreased or whether the sum of [Bc] and [Bu] is falsely increased.

Table 13.5. Diseases and conditions that cause hyperbilirubinemia

Increased Bu production
    *Hemolytic disorders, especially extravascular hemolysis (see Table 3.10)
Decreased Bu uptake by hepatocytes
    *Fasting or anorexia (especially in horses)
    Decreased functional mass (diffuse hepatocellular disease; see the text for examples)
Decreased Bu conjugation
    Decreased functional mass (diffuse hepatocellular disease; see the text for examples)
Decreased Bc excretion in bile
    Obstructive cholestasis
        *Hepatic cholestasis: lipidosis, diabetes mellitus, steroid hepatopathy, lymphoma, histoplasmosis, cytauxzoonosis, cirrhosis, cholangitis, cholangiohepatitis, periportal hepatitis, pyrrolizidine alkaloid toxicosis, sporodesmin toxicosis, and alsike clover (*Trifolium hybridum*) toxicosis
        *Posthepatic cholestasis: cholangitis, bile duct carcinoma, liver flukes, cholelithiasis, cholecystitis, pancreatitis, and pancreatic carcinoma
    Functional cholestasis (sepsis-associated cholestasis)
Persistence of Bδ in plasma

    * A relatively common disease or condition
    Notes: Lists of specific disorders or conditions are not complete but are provided to give examples. Depending on the assay method, hemolysis may cause either positive or negative interference with bilirubin assays.

III. Hyperbilirubinemia (Table 13.5)
    A. Hyperbilirubinemia occurs when the rate of Bu production exceeds the rate of Bu uptake by hepatocytes, or the rate of Bc formation in hepatocytes exceeds the rate of Bc excretion in bile. Hyperbilirubinemia may persist after removal of the cause (e.g., obstruction) because of the long half-life of Bδ.
    B. Increased Bu production
        1. Hemolytic (prehepatic) icterus (Fig. 3.10)
            a. Disorders
                (1) Hemolytic disorders that may cause icterus are listed in Table 3.10. Animals with acute intravascular hemolytic disorders are less likely to be icteric initially but will typically develop icterus within 2–3 d.
                (2) If the rate of extravascular hemolysis is low, the hepatobiliary system may be able to eliminate Bu so it does not accumulate in plasma.
            b. Pathogenesis
                (1) An animal that has a hemolytic anemia may develop icterus if the rate of Bu formation exceeds the hepatobiliary system's capacity for Bu uptake or Bc excretion (Fig. 3.10).
                (2) Pathogeneses of hemolytic diseases are described in Chapter 3.
            c. Results of serum bilirubin profile (Table 13.6)
                (1) [Bt] may be mildly to markedly increased.
                (2) Initially, [Bu] >> [Bc]. If persistent, then [Bu] may approximate [Bc]. Secondary (e.g., hypoxic hepatocellular degeneration) or concurrent hepatobiliary disease may complicate the pattern.

Table 13.6. Bilirubin profiles in common pathophysiologic states that cause icterus

[Bt][a]	[Bd]	[Bi]	[Bc]	[Bu]	[Bδ]	Pathophysiologic state
↑↑	WRI–↑[bc]	↑↑	WRI–↑[c]	↑↑	WRI–↑	Hemolytic disorders
↑↑	WRI–↑	↑↑	WRI–↑	↑↑	WRI–↑	Fasting hyperbilirubinemia (horse)
↑↑	↑↑	↑–↑↑	↑–↑↑	↑–↑↑	↑–↑↑	Hepatocellular dysfunction and concurrent cholestasis
↑↑	↑↑	WRI–↑	↑↑	WRI–↑	WRI–↑↑	Obstructive cholestasis[d]
↑↑	↑↑	WRI–↑	↑↑	WRI–↑	WRI–↑↑	Functional cholestasis

[a] The [Bt] may be mildly to markedly increased.

[b] The number of arrows for the bilirubin fractions in the table indicates the relative concentrations to illustrate the fractions that typically contribute most to the hyperbilirubinemia.

[c] Excretion of Bc from hepatocytes is considered the rate-limiting step. Thus, when there is increased Bu and Bc formation in hemolytic disorders, Bc may accumulate in hepatocytes and then be regurgitated to blood.

[d] In horses, the [Bu] may be greater than the [Bc].

Note: Depending on the assay method, hemolysis may cause either positive or negative interference with bilirubin assays.

(3)   It has been written that bilirubin fractions do not help differentiate hemolytic and hepatobiliary icterus because [Bc] is always greater than [Bu].[7] This conclusion appears to be supported by findings in a group of eight dogs that had concurrent hemolytic anemia and liver disease,[8] but it is inconsistent with the authors' experiences.

(4)   [Bu] is often greater than [Bc] in animals with hemolytic anemias, but it will not always be greater. When [Bu] > [Bc], it supports the concept that the icterus is directly related to extravascular hemolysis. When clinical data indicate a hemolytic anemia and [Bu] < [Bc], concurrent hepatobiliary disease should be considered.

d. Other expected laboratory findings with hemolytic icterus
(1)   Anemia, regenerative if of sufficient duration, moderate to marked severity
(2)   Hemoglobinuria and hemoglobinemia if there is sufficient intravascular hemolysis
(3)   Bilirubinuria if sufficient Bc escapes from hepatocytes or, with intravascular hemolysis, if there is sufficient renal tubular heme degradation and bilirubin excretion into urine
(4)   If plasma hepatic enzyme activities are increased, hepatocyte damage or cholestasis could be due to anemic hypoxia.

2. Increased Bu production not associated with hemolysis
a. Besides Bu from erythrocyte destruction, heme degradation also occurs with destruction of erythrocyte precursors (ineffective erythropoiesis) and degradation of other heme proteins (myoglobin, cytochromes, and peroxidases).
b. By themselves, these processes are not considered to cause increased [Bt]. However, they could contribute to an increased [Bu] if there are other reasons for increased [Bt].

C. Decreased Bu uptake by hepatocytes
1. Fasting hyperbilirubinemia
a. Disorders

(1) Horses that are off feed (either feed withheld or anorexia) typically develop hyperbilirubinemia (increased [Bu]).[9] The hyperbilirubinemia can be detected as early as 12–15 h after feed is withheld and usually reaches a steady concentration in 2–3 d.

(2) Sick cattle with anorexia and rumen stasis may have hyperbilirubinemia (increased [Bu] not associated with hemolytic or hepatic disease).[10] Fasting healthy cattle also develop mild hyperbilirubinemia ([Bt] < 1.4 mg/dL).[11]

(3) Lack of colostrum intake was considered a contributing factor to icterus in veal calves.[12]

b. Pathogenesis: The fasting state leads to increased mobilization of fat (lipolysis in adipocytes) and thus increased [fatty acids] in the blood. The fatty acids interfere with Bu uptake by hepatocytes, and thus plasma [Bu] increases.[11]

(1) The interference may be competitive because fatty acids and Bu bind to the same cytoplasmic receptor proteins; that is, Z-protein (fatty acid–binding protein) and Y-protein (ligandin, also known as glutathione S-transferase B).[3,13]

(2) Experimental data clearly indicate that fasting reduces the hepatic clearance rate of bilirubin and that the reduction is greater than the reduction in the hepatic clearance of bile acids.[9]

c. Comments on species differences

(1) Horses might be more prone to this form of icterus because they use primarily glucose (> 60 %) to conjugate bilirubin.[14] Fasting may make less glucose available in hepatocytes for Bu conjugation. Administration of glucose to horses with fasting hyperbilirubinemia lowered plasma concentrations of bilirubin and fatty acids.[15] It was not established whether the lower [Bt] was due to availability of glucose or reduced [fatty acids].

(2) Similar interferences in bilirubin excretion likely occur in other animals, but changes in [Bt] are minimal. Anorectic cats occasionally have slight hyperbilirubinemias (increased [Bu]), and thus it is easy to speculate that fatty acids are contributing to defective Bu clearance.

(3) Increased [Bu] may also occur in horses that are not anorectic or anemic and are not diagnosed with hepatic disease. The pathogenesis of hyperbilirubinemia in these instances is not understood.

d. Results of serum bilirubin profile (Table 13.6)

(1) In horses, the [Bt] is typically < 8 mg/dL and nearly all is [Bu] or [Bi].

(2) Minor increases in [Bc] or [Bd] may occur because Bu and Bc compete for uptake by hepatocytes.

e. Other expected laboratory findings

(1) In horses, fasting or anorexia does not produce abnormalities in other routine laboratory tests. Thus, plasma or serum hepatic enzyme activities are expected to be WRI if hepatobiliary disease is not present. Hematocrit is expected to be WRI unless anemia is produced by the disorder that is causing the anorexia.

(2) In cattle and horses with hepatic lipidosis, the accumulation of lipid leads to hepatocyte swelling and damage. Thus, serum activities of hepatic enzymes may be increased.

2. Decreased functional hepatic mass

a. A marked reduction in functional hepatocytes can result in decreased Bu uptake by hepatocytes, decreased Bu conjugation, and decreased Bc excretion. However, if a disease is causing only decreased functional mass and not obstructive cholestasis, then clinical icterus is not expected.

     b. Disorders that may cause decreased functional mass are listed in Table 13.4.

  3. Hereditary deficiencies in the hepatic uptake of Bu may cause hyperbilirubinemia and have been recognized in Southdown sheep[16] and Corriedale sheep.[17]

D. Decreased Bu conjugation

  1. As mentioned in the preceding section 2.a, a marked reduction in functional mass would reduce Bu conjugation. When cytoplasmic receptor proteins are saturated, the uptake of Bu by hepatocytes decreases.

  2. Hereditary deficiencies of enzymes that catalyze conjugation reactions occur in people and laboratory animals but have not been confirmed in our common domestic mammals. A persistent hyperbilirubinemia in an otherwise healthy Thoroughbred was probably caused by a defective conjugation pathway, but the exact defect was not established.[18] The [Bt] ranged from 9.4 to 12.7 mg/dL during a 2 yr evaluation, and about 90 % of the bilirubin was Bu.

E. Decreased Bc excretion

  1. *Obstructive cholestasis* is caused by a pathologic state that obstructs bile flow through bile canaliculi or bile ducts (hepatic or posthepatic). Lesions that impair bile flow include hepatocellular swelling that compresses canaliculi, periportal lesions that compress bile ducts, infections and other processes that damage bile ducts, and blockage of bile ducts by stones, parasites, or neoplasms.

     a. Pathogenesis (Fig. 13.2)

        (1) Increased [Bc] in systemic and thus sinusoidal blood saturates bilirubin receptors on hepatocytes, and thus Bu uptake is impaired.

        (2) With time, increased [Bc] leads to increased [Bu], but the [Bc] is expected to remain greater than the [Bu].

     b. Results of a serum bilirubin profile (Table 13.6)

        (1) The [Bt] may be mildly to extremely increased.

        (2) Typically, [Bc] > [Bu] ([Bd] > [Bi]) except in horses and cattle.

           (a) Concurrent hepatocellular disease may complicate patterns by decreasing functional mass and therefore decreasing uptake and conjugation of Bu.

           (b) In horses with cholestasis, the [Bd] is typically < 30 % of [Bt]. The increased [Bd] in horses strongly suggests cholestasis.

           (c) In cattle with cholestasis, the [Bd] may be greater than or less than the [Bi].

     c. Other expected laboratory findings

        (1) Anemia may or may not be present. If present, it typically is nonregenerative.

        (2) Increased serum activities of enzymes associated with cholestasis (ALP and GGT)

           (a) ALP and GGT activities may be increased in dogs before icterus develops.

           (b) ALP and GGT activities typically are not increased in cats until there is marked obstructive icterus.

           (c) Biliary obstruction is uncommon in horses and cattle. When present, ALP and GGT activities may be substantially increased.

        (3) Serum activities of hepatocellular enzymes (ALT, AST, LD, ID, and GMD) may be increased because of hepatocyte damage.

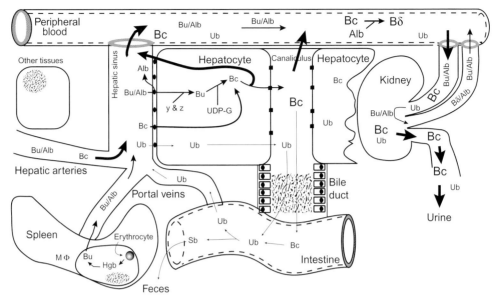

Fig. 13.2. Obstructive cholestatic icterus: Lesions of bile canaliculi or bile ducts (hepatic or posthepatic) inhibit bile flow, and thus less or no Bc is excreted to the intestine. Bc enters systemic blood because of (1) increased permeability of canalicular tight junctions and leakage to the space of Disse and the central vein, (2) hepatocyte necrosis allowing Bc entry to hepatic sinusoids, or (3) concurrent increased BA content that inhibits excretion of Bc to canaliculi and thus Bc is "regurgitated" to hepatic sinusoids. A persistently increased plasma [Bc] results in increased formation of Bδ and increased urinary excretion of Bc (bilirubinuria). Bu/Alb, Bu associated with albumin; Bδ, Bc covalently bound to albumin; Mφ, macrophage; Sb, stercobilinogen; Ub, urobilinogen; and UDP-G, uridine diphosphoglucuronide.

(4) Hypercholesterolemia occurs in some cholestatic conditions and can be marked, but is not a consistent finding (see Chapter 16).

2. *Functional cholestasis* (*sepsis-associated cholestasis*) is impaired excretion of Bc from hepatocytes to canaliculi in the absence of biliary obstruction. A functional cholestasis was reported in dogs with *Escherichia coli* and *Staphylococcus intermedius* infections causing pneumonia, peritonitis, urinary tract infection, endocarditis, and soft tissue infection.[19] This type of icterus is more commonly recognized in people and may be more common in domestic mammals than has been recognized.

a. Pathogenesis

(1) Increased [tumor necrosis factor alpha] (directly or with endotoxins) results in decreased BA transport proteins in hepatocyte canalicular membranes.[20,21] Interleukin 6 also interferes with bile salt transport.[22]

(2) It is not clear whether the impaired Bc excretion is a direct defect or whether it occurs secondary to canalicular membrane damage caused by retained BA.

b. Results of a serum bilirubin profile (Table 13.6)

c. Other expected laboratory findings

(1) Inflammatory changes in blood leukocytes (e.g., neutrophilia, neutropenia, left shift, toxic change, or lymphopenia)

(2) Other changes would depend on the duration and the location of the bacterial infection.

   3. Hereditary deficiencies in the hepatocellular excretion of Bc may cause a hyperbiliru-
      binemia and have been recognized in Corriedale sheep. The sheep also have a defect
      in Bu uptake by hepatocytes.[17]
 F. Persistence of Bδ in plasma
   1. Since Bδ has the plasma half-life of albumin (8–20 d), an increased [Bt] may persist
      for more than 1–2 wk after correction of the pathologic defect in bilirubin excretion
      (e.g., surgical removal of a biliary tract obstruction).
   2. The persistent increase in [Bδ] and thus persistent increase in [Bt] is not commonly
      recognized. In most animals with cholestatic icterus, the half-life of Bδ may actually
      be shorter than the time required for the [Bc] to decrease if there is slow recovery
      from an obstructive cholestatic disease. Also, there is limited use of the dry-chemical
      method that enables calculation of the [Bδ].

IV. Bilirubinuria
 A. Excessive bilirubin formation (in hemolytic states) or impaired hepatobiliary excretion
    of Bc may increase plasma [Bc]. Bc easily passes through the glomerular filtration
    barrier and is then excreted in the urine.
 B. Because of the low renal threshold for Bc, bilirubinuria may be detected before
    hyperbilirubinemia is detected. If hyperbilirubinemia (from Bc) is present, then
    bilirubinuria is expected.
 C. As explained in Chapter 8, a positive bilirubin reaction in a urinalysis should be
    interpreted with knowledge of USG_{ref}, especially in dogs. Moderately concentrated
    urine (USG_{ref} = 1.025–1.040) of healthy dogs frequently gives a 1+ bilirubin reaction;
    2+ reactions occasionally occur with more concentrated urine (USG_{ref} > 1.040).

V. Icterus index
 A. Definition: a value that represents an estimation of the yellow discoloration of plasma
    caused by hyperbilirubinemia
 B. Methods
   1. Potassium dichromate method[23]
      a. Icterus index is determined by comparing the color of a patient's plasma to a set
         of standard solutions containing potassium dichromate. The degree of icterus is
         recorded in units from 0 to 100. The plasma of healthy herbivores is expected to
         be more yellow because carotenoid pigments from plants may impart a yellow
         discoloration.
      b. Hemolyzed or lipemic plasma can falsely elevate the icterus index.
   2. Icterus index determination by chemistry analyzers
      a. The Hitachi chemistry analyzers estimate the bilirubin concentration by spectro-
         photometric assessment of absorbance changes caused by the presence of biliru-
         bin. The method involves consideration of absorbance changes caused by
         hemoglobin or lipids, if present. This icterus index is reported as a numerical
         value (e.g., 10) that corresponds to absorbance changes expected by a [Bt] of the
         same numeric value (e.g., 10 mg/dL).
      b. Olympus chemistry analyzers have a similar spectrophotometric system in which
         absorbance readings at different wavelengths are used to assess degrees of icterus,
         lipemia, and hemolysis.
      c. Plant carotenoids (e.g., β-carotene and lycopene) may interfere with these
         methods.

C. Clinical laboratories may subjectively grade the severity of icterus (mild, moderate, or marked) by assessing the degree of yellow to orange discoloration of plasma or serum. Serum [Bt] typically exceeds 1.5 mg/dL before visible icterus (in sera or mucous membranes) is detected. This depends somewhat on the species and the observer's experience.

BILE ACID (BA) CONCENTRATION[24]

I. Physiologic processes (Fig. 13.3)
A. In health, the enterohepatic circulation of bile acids is highly efficient, and nearly all bile salts excreted in bile are returned to the liver via intestinal absorption and portal blood flow.

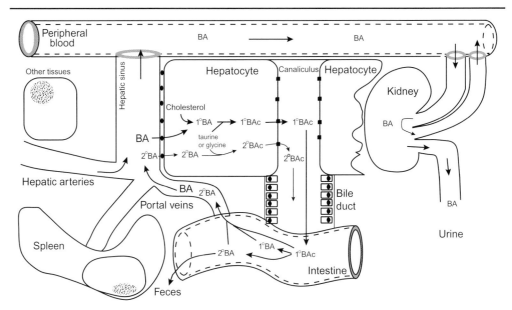

Fig. 13.3. Physiologic processes of bile acids: Cholesterol is degraded in hepatocytes to a 1°BA, either cholic or chenodeoxycholic acid. A 1°BA becomes conjugated (usually with taurine or glycine, but sometimes with sulfate or gluconate) in hepatocytes to form a 1°BAc. A 1°BAc is secreted into the biliary system and transported via the bile ducts to the intestine. In the intestine, a 1°BAc has three possible fates: (1) absorption by the intestinal mucosa and entrance into the portal blood, (2) deconjugation by enteric bacteria to a 1°BA and then absorption by the intestinal mucosa and entrance into the portal blood, or (3) degradation to a 2°BA (either deoxycholic acid or lithocholic acid), which may have two fates—excretion in the feces or absorption by the intestinal mucosa and entrance into the portal blood. If conjugated with sulfate, BAs are poorly absorbed by the intestinal mucosa. When returned to the liver via the portal blood, conjugated BAs, deconjugated BAs, and 2°BAs are efficiently removed from the blood by the hepatocytes. The deconjugated BAs and 2°BAs are conjugated by hepatocytes and returned to the biliary system to complete the enterohepatic circulation. In health, nearly all BA molecules are within the enterohepatic circulation; very few are in the systemic blood. BA molecules that escape the enterohepatic circulation can be cleared from the plasma via glomerular filtration and excreted in the urine. 1°BA, primary bile acid; 1°BAc, conjugated primary bile acid; and 2°BA, secondary bile acid.

B. Bile salts are the major solids in bile that enter the intestine after gallbladder contraction. After intestinal absorption of BAs, the resulting higher [BA] in portal blood may exceed the liver's ability to extract BAs, and thus there is a postprandial increase in [BA] in systemic blood. Typically, gallbladder contraction results from actions of cholecystokinin that is released after ingestion of a meal. However, gallbladder contraction may occur at other times.

C. BA secretion from hepatocytes to canaliculi occurs through two processes; one is Na^+ dependent and one is not.

II.   Analytical concepts
   A. Terms and units
      1. In common use, the term *bile acids* refers to a group of cholesterol-derived anionic acids and their dissociated anions. The bile acids include cholic acid, chenodeoxycholic acid, deoxycholic acid, and lithocholic acid, all of which are 3α-hydroxylated bile acids. At a pH of 7.4, the dissociated anionic forms of the molecules dominate (e.g., cholate and lithocholate). Collectively, the anionic forms are called *bile salts*.
      2. Unit conversion[5]
         a. Total bile acid: mg/L $\times$ 2.547 = μmol/L (SI unit, nearest 0.2 μmol/L)
         b. Cholic acid: mg/L $\times$ 2.448 = μmol/L (SI unit, nearest 0.2 μmol/L)
         c. Chenodeoxycholic acid: mg/L $\times$ 2.547 = μmol/L (SI unit, nearest 0.2 μmol/L)
         d. Deoxycholic acid: mg/L $\times$ 2.547 = μmol/L (SI unit, nearest 0.2 μmol/L)
         e. Lithocholic acid: mg/L $\times$ 2.656 = μmol/L (SI unit, nearest 0.2 μmol/L)
         f. Occasionally, other units are used (i.e., mg/mL and mmol/L). See Table 1.6 for the conversion factors.
   B. Assays
      1. The [BA] is measured in clinical laboratories by a spectrophotometric assay that uses 3α-hydroxysteroid dehydrogenase in reactions with primary and secondary bile acids or their anions (either conjugated or deconjugated). Free Hgb in a hemolyzed sample will cause a negative interference in the assay. Lipids in a lipemic sample create unacceptable errors according to the assay's manufacturer.
      2. The concentration of conjugated bile acids can be measured by either radioimmunoassays or enzyme immunoassays. These assays may be more economical in reference laboratories.
      3. Clinically, abnormalities in total bile acid concentration and conjugated bile acid concentration tend to parallel each other, and thus either type of assay can be used.
      4. A IDEXX SNAP bile acid test is available to screen animals for increased [BA].

III. Increased bile acid (BA) concentration in serum or plasma (Table 13.7)
   A. An increased [BA] can be called *hypercholemia*, but the term is not commonly used. It should not be confused with hyperchloremia or hypercholesterolemia.
   B. There are two major pathologic processes that increase serum [BA] in fasting dogs and cats: (1) decreased BA clearance from portal blood and (2) decreased biliary excretion of BA (Fig. 13.4). Accordingly, increased serum [BA] supports the conclusion that an animal has decreased hepatobiliary function. Increased serum [BA] has high diagnostic sensitivity for hepatobiliary dysfunction. However, many primary and secondary liver diseases can cause the dysfunction, and the dysfunctional state may or may not be reversible.

Table 13.7. Diseases and conditions that cause an increased fasting [BA]

Decreased BA clearance from portal blood
   *Decreased functional hepatic mass: diffuse hepatocellular disease
   *Decreased portal blood flow to liver: congenital and acquired portosystemic shunts
Decreased BA excretion in bile
  Obstructive cholestasis
    *Hepatic cholestasis: lipidosis, diabetes mellitus, steroid hepatopathy, lymphoma,
      histoplasmosis, cytauxzoonosis, cirrhosis, cholangitis, cholangiohepatitis, periportal
      hepatitis, pyrrolizidine alkaloid toxicosis, sporodesmin toxicosis, alsike clover
      (*Trifolium hybridum*) toxicosis
    *Posthepatic cholestasis: cholangitis, bile duct carcinoma, liver flukes, cholelithiasis,
      cholecystitis, pancreatitis, pancreatic carcinoma
  Functional cholestasis (sepsis-associated cholestasis)

* A relatively common disease or condition
Note: Lists of specific disorders or conditions are not complete but are provided to give examples.
Serum bile acid concentrations are increased postprandially.

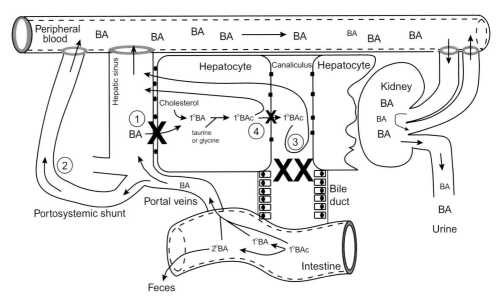

Fig. 13.4. Pathologic processes that increase serum [BA] (hypercholemia). Two major pathologic processes cause hypercholemia:
• Decreased clearance from the portal blood: The defect may occur because of (1) decreased uptake of BA from the sinusoidal blood because of a decreased functional hepatic mass or because (2) there is a portosystemic shunt.
• Decreased biliary BA excretion: When there is obstructive cholestasis (3) or functional cholestasis (4), the BAs are regurgitated to the sinusoidal blood instead of passing through the biliary ducts to the intestine.

1. Decreased BA clearance from portal blood
    a. Many pathologic states (e.g., inflammatory, metabolic, and degenerative) involving hepatocytes cause sufficient damage to reduce functional hepatic mass enough to impair BA clearance.[25–29]
    b. Congenital and acquired portosystemic shunts enable bile salts absorbed in the intestine to bypass the liver, escape the enterohepatic circulation, and enter the systemic blood.[30]
    c. Mild increases in [BA] may occur when feed is withheld from horses.[31] The increase is probably caused by a decreased hepatic clearance rate of bile acids.[9]
2. Decreased biliary BA excretion
    a. A variety of hepatic and posthepatic disorders can impair bile flow and thus impair excretion of bile acids. Concurrent impairment of Bc excretion is expected, but it may not be enough to cause hyperbilirubinemia. Similarly, when hepatic or posthepatic hyperbilirubinemia is present, increased serum [BA] is expected.
    b. During obstructive cholestasis, there is a down-regulation of canalicular BA transport proteins, and hepatocytes may pump BA into sinusoidal blood instead of into canaliculi. This process may explain the "regurgitation" concept of BA leaving hepatocytes.[32]
    c. BAs are toxic to cells. Thus, accumulation of BAs in the liver may lead to cell damage and release of BAs and other substances from canaliculi and hepatocytes.
    d. Cytokines (notably tumor necrosis factor alpha) have been shown to decrease BA transport proteins in hepatocyte canalicular membranes and thus impair BA secretion.[20,21] The resultant impairment in BA excretion is called *functional cholestasis* (see Bilirubin Concentation, sect. III.E.2).
C. Mild increases in serum [BA] occur in healthy animals after meals. Postprandial increases are also exaggerated in some hepatobiliary disorders. These findings are the basis of the bile acid challenge test (see sect. IV).
D. In horses, increased serum [BA] was found in nearly all horses (36 of 38) with hepatic necrosis, lipidosis, neoplasia, or cirrhosis. In contrast, only 2 of 78 sick horses without liver disease had increased serum [BA] (reference interval not stated but upper limit estimated from a graph to be 18 µmol/L).[27]
E. In cattle, the diagnostic sensitivity of serum [BA] varied among liver disorders: fascioliasis (100 %, n = 11), biliary calculi (100 %, n = 2), hepatic abscesses (53 %, n = 15), leptospirosis (71 %, n = 7), and hepatic lipidosis (86 %, n = 36) (reference interval not stated but upper limit estimated from a graph to be 40 µmol/L).[26] In another report, values for serum [BA] were increased in cattle with hepatic lipidosis, hepatic abscesses, leptospirosis, and fascioliasis with mean concentrations of 90–225 µmol/L at initial evaluation.[33]

IV. Bile acid challenge test for dogs and cats
    A. Principle: A 12 h fasting [BA] provides a baseline assessment of the amount of BA that escapes the enterohepatic circulation and enters the systemic blood. After ingestion of a standardized meal, gallbladder contraction releases bile salts to the intestine, from which they are absorbed and then enter the portal blood. This influx of endogenous bile acids challenges the ability of the hepatocytes to keep bile acids within the enterohepatic circulation.

Table 13.8. Results of the bile acid challenge test in dogs

Group	n	Percentage with fasting [BA] > 5 μmol/L	Percentage with 2-h postprandial [BA] > 15.5 μmol/L
Healthy	66	2.5[a]	2.5
Severe liver disease[b]	62	86.9	78.7
All liver disease[c]	101	82.5	77.7
Portosystemic shunt[d]	29	100	100
Ill, liver disease not detected[e]	40	17.5[f]	12.5[g]

[a] Because the upper limit of the reference interval (5.0 μmol/L fasting and 15.5 μmol/L postprandially) was determined as the value 2 standard deviations above the mean, the 2.5 % assumes that reference values had a Gaussian distribution.

[b] Disorders (followed by median fasting/postprandial concentrations) included cirrhosis (62/149 μmol/L), chronic hepatitis (12/74 μmol/L), hepatic necrosis (40/78 μmol/L), and cholestasis (111/111 μmol/L).

[c] Disorders (followed by median fasting/postprandial concentrations) included those for the severe liver disease groups and hepatic neoplasia (10/29 μmol/L), glucocorticoid hepatopathy (12/19 μmol/L), and passive congestion (5/5 μmol/L).

[d] The median fasting/postprandial bile acid concentrations in the portosystemic shunt dogs were 114/221 μmol/L.

[e] Disorders included idiopathic epilepsy, inflammatory intestinal disease, metastatic neoplasia without hepatic involvement, disseminated intravascular coagulation, brain neoplasia, hypoadrenocorticism, glomerulonephritis, peritonitis, meningoencephalitis, endocarditis, congestive heart failure, and cystitis. Each dog lacked histologic evidence of hepatobiliary disease. The median [BA] in fasting and postprandial samples were 3 and 6 μmol/L, respectively.

[f] None exceeded 17.1 μmol/L.

[g] None exceeded 21.9 μmol/L.

Source: Center et al.[28]

    B. Procedure

        1. A fasting sample is collected from the dog or cat after a 12 h fast. Then, the animal is observed while it ingests food containing protein and fat (e.g., 2 teaspoons of a canned food for those < 10 lb, and 2 tablespoons for large dogs). A 2 h postprandial sample is collected.

        2. Sample hemolysis should be avoided during blood collection and processing because Hgb interferes with the spectrophotometric BA assay. Postprandial lipemia should be avoided by first collecting a fasting sample and then limiting the amount of ingested food.

    C. Published data

        1. Dogs[28] (Table 13.8)

            a. Fasting and postprandial samples had high diagnostic sensitivity for liver disease and portosystemic shunts, but the samples did not consistently differentiate the type or severity of the disease. Some dogs with nonhepatic diseases may have an increased fasting and postprandial [BA], but increases are typically minor.

            b. When decision thresholds of 20 μmol/L for fasting samples and 25 μmol/L for postprandial samples were used, the diagnostic specificity of the bile acid concentration approached 100 % and the diagnostic sensitivity values were about 60 % and 75 %, respectively (data from a total BA enzymatic assay; different decision thresholds may be needed for different assays).

Table 13.9. Results of the bile acid challenge test in cats

Group	n	Percentage with fasting [BA] > 5 μmol/L	Percentage with 2-h postprandial [BA] > 10.0 μmol/L
Healthy	?	2.5[a]	2.5
All liver disease	82	73	98
Portosystemic shunt[b]	24	79	100
Liver disease but not shunt[c]	58	71	97
Ill, liver disease not detected[d]	26	11.5[e]	30.8[f]

[a] The method of establishing reference interval was not reported. For the purpose of comparison, the 2.5 % assumes that reference values had a Gaussian distribution. Upper reference limits were 5.0 μmol/L for fasting samples and 10.0 μmol/L for postprandial samples.

[b] The median fasting/postprandial bile acid concentrations in the portosystemic shunt cats were 32/140 μmol/L.

[c] Diagnoses (number of cats [n] followed by the median fasting/postprandial [BA]) included hepatic lipidosis (n = 20; 28/142 μmol/L), hepatic necrosis (n = 13; 15/29 μmol/L), hepatic neoplasia (n = 8; 8/26 μmol/L), and cholestasis disorders (n = 17; 40/140 μmol/L).

[d] Diagnoses included a variety of nonhepatic disorders. Each cat lacked histologic evidence of hepatobiliary disease.

[e] None exceeded 16.0 μmol/L.

[f] Maximal value was not reported.

Source: Center et al.[29]

2. Cats[29] (Table 13.9)
   a. Fasting and postprandial [BA] values had high diagnostic sensitivity for hepatobiliary disease when the respective URLs were used, but the [BA] did not differentiate the type or severity of the diseases.
   b. The diagnostic specificity for the absence of liver disease approached 100 % when values > 4 × URL and 2 × URL were considered abnormal for fasting or postprandial samples, respectively, but the diagnostic sensitivity for hepatobiliary disease was only 49 % (fasting) and 81 % (postprandial) when these decision thresholds were used (data from a total BA enzymatic assay).
D. Factors other than hepatobiliary and portal systems that influence results
   1. Fasting [BA]
      a. Spontaneous contraction of the gallbladder may increase fasting [BA] unexpectedly.
      b. Fasting serum [BA] depends on the enterohepatic cycle; for example, intestinal diseases may impair intestinal absorption of BA and thus lower a serum [BA].
   2. 2 h postprandial [BA]
      a. The peak [BA] may not occur 2 h postprandially because of variations in gastric emptying, intestinal transit time, intestinal absorption, or other factors.
      b. The animal may not have eaten the food provided, or it may have a poor cholecystokinin response.
      c. The gallbladder may have contracted prior to feeding.
   3. The aforementioned factors may contribute to the relatively common finding that the fasting [BA] is greater than the 2 h postprandial [BA]. The lower [BA] in the 2 h postprandial sample is not of diagnostic value.

E. Conclusions
1. The diagnostic value of a serum [BA] is primarily for detecting hepatobiliary disease or portosystemic shunts.
2. The highest serum [BA] occurs when there is a disease process that enables BA molecules to escape enterohepatic circulation. However, many diseases or pathologic states can cause the dysfunction.
3. The popularity of the bile acid test (compared to other liver function tests, such as plasma [NH_4^+] or dye-excretion tests) is probably due to its simplicity; that is, it does not require special patient preparation, sample collection, or sample handling.

V. Urine Bile Acid to Creatinine (BA:Crt) Ratios
A. Principle
1. As shown in Fig. 13.3 and 13.4, BA molecules that escape the enterohepatic circulation are excreted in the urine. Whenever there is defective clearance of BA from the portal blood or decreased biliary excretion of BA that leads to BA entering the peripheral blood, there will be increased BA excretion via the kidneys. The BA conjugated with sulfate (sulfated bile acids) are more water soluble than nonsulfated BA.
2. The amount of BA excreted via urine should reflect plasma [BA] during the time the collected urine was formed. In the published studies, dogs and cats were not fasted prior to collection of the analyzed urine samples.[34,35]
B. Procedure
1. The [BA] and the [Crt] are measured in a randomly collected urine sample. The urine concentrations of sulfated BA, nonsulfated BA, or sulfated plus nonsulfated BA are measured using enzymatic colorimetric assays.
2. A ratio of their concentrations is calculated. The reported ratios represent a mixture of units; that is, μmol of BA/mg of Crt.[34–36] Unitless ratios could be calculated by converting the [Crt] of mg/L to μmol/L before dividing the BA concentration (also in μmol/L) by the [Crt].
3. The relative ease of a one-time collection of urine compared to fasting and postprandial blood collections makes this assay attractive for assessing bile acids.
C. UNSBA:Crt and (USBA + UNSBA):Crt have been shown to have diagnostic properties similar to serum [BA] in dogs and cats when ratios were compared to the greatest serum [BA] found in fasting or postprandial samples (Tables 13.10 and 13.11)
1. With use of the selected decision thresholds in the population studied, the ratios for canine urine had excellent diagnostic specificity and positive predictive values for

Table 13.10. Results of BA:Crt ratios in dogs and cats

Group	n	USBA:Crt μmol/mg	UNSBA:Crt μmol/mg	(USBA + UNSBA):Crt μmol/mg
Dogs				
Healthy	15	0.0–0.9	0.0–6.0	0.4–6.6
Hepatic disorders	120	0.0–42.6	0.3–2377.0	0.0–2377.0
Cats				
Healthy	8	0.0–1.9	0.7–1.2	0.2–3.9
Hepatic disorders	54	0.0–14.4	2.0–12.9	0.4–35.7

Note: Reported ratios included a multiplication factor of 100.
Sources: Trainor et al.[35] and Balkman et al.[34,36]

Table 13.11. Diagnostic properties of BA:Crt ratios in dogs and cats

	Diagnostic sensitivity (%)	Diagnostic specificity (%)	Positive predictive value (%)	Negative predictive value (%)
Dogs				
BA (serum)	78	67	96	23
USBA:Crt	17	100	100	10
UNSBA:Crt	63	100	100	18
(USBA + UNSBA):Crt	61	100	100	18
Cats				
BA (serum)	87	88	96	68
USBA:Crt	78	94	98	57
UNSBA:Crt	87	88	96	68
(USBA + UNSBA):Crt	85	88	96	65

Note: The reported ratios included a multiplication factor of 100. The decision threshold for SBA was the URL. The decision thresholds for the ratio values were calculated (mean + 2 standard deviations; 15 dogs and 8 cats). The predictive values may differ considerably with different prevalences of hepatic disease.
Sources: Trainor et al.[35] and Balkman et al.[34,36]

liver disease because there were no false positives. However, the decision thresholds yielded only fair diagnostic sensitivity values and poor negative predictive values because of frequent false negatives.

2. With use of the selected decision thresholds in the population studied, the ratios for feline urine had very good diagnostic specificity and positive predictive values because there were few false positives. The decision thresholds yielded good diagnostic sensitivity values and fair negative predictive values.

3. Predictive values may vary considerably with variations in the prevalence of hepatic diseases in populations of interest.

D. Establishing the diagnostic value of the urine BA:Crt ratios will depend on the use of appropriate decision thresholds and comparing the results with other methods of detecting liver disease.

AMMONIUM (NH_4^+) CONCENTRATION IN PLASMA

I. Physiologic processes (Fig. 13.5)

II. Analytical concepts
 A. Units and terms
  1. The analyte is commonly called *blood ammonia* (NH_3), but the dominant form in plasma is *ammonium* (NH_4^+). At a pH of 7.4 and a pK_a of 9.25, the $NH_4^+ : NH_3$ ratio is about 70, and thus there is relatively little NH_3 in plasma. At body temperature and pressures, NH_3 is a gas. Routine clinical assays use plasma and not whole blood as a sample.
  2. Unit conversion[5]
   a. NH_3: μg/dL × 0.5871 = μmol/L (SI unit, nearest 5 μmol/L)
   b. NH_4^+: μg/dL × 0.5543 = μmol/L (SI unit, nearest 5 μmol/L)

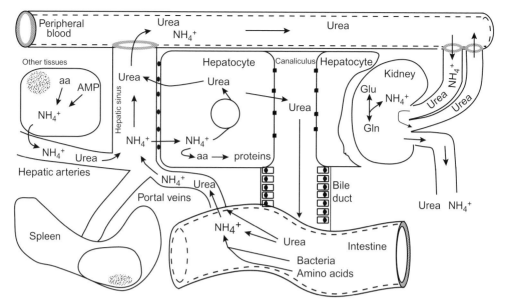

Fig. 13.5. Physiologic processes of ammonium.

- Most NH_4^+ is produced in intestines by digestion of dietary proteins or by the metabolism of bacteria. Some NH_4^+ is produced by the deamination of amino acids (in many cells) and adenosine monophosphate (especially in muscle fibers).
- After NH_4^+ enters the liver (via the portal vein or the hepatic artery), it enters hepatocytes and is used for the synthesis of urea (in urea cycle), amino acids, and proteins. Urea diffuses from hepatocytes to the sinusoidal blood or the bile canaliculi, from which it may be excreted via the kidneys or the intestine, respectively. Urea that enters the intestine (from diet, bile, or blood) may be reabsorbed as part of an enterohepatic circulation (also see Fig. 8.5).
- Renal excretion of NH_4^+ may occur by NH_4^+ passing through the glomerular filtration barrier and being excreted in the urine. NH_4^+ is also fixed into urea in the hepatocytes or into glutamine (Gln) in the renal tubular cells. In response to acidemia, deamination of Gln to glutamate (Glu) in the renal tubules results in NH_4^+ excretion (see Fig. 9.6).
- NH_4^+ is the molecular form that is present in most aqueous body fluids at a pH of 7.4, but it does not diffuse through cell membranes. NH_3 is relatively lipid soluble and rapidly diffuses across cell membranes, but very little is present in body fluids.

B. Assays for NH_4^+ concentration
   1. Methods
      a. Enzymatic method: $NH_4^+ + \alpha\text{-ketoglutarate} + NADPH \rightarrow glutamate + NADP$
      b. If an alkalinizing agent is used to convert NH_4^+ to NH_3, NH_3 can be measured by a dye-binding method.
      c. Other assays measure NH_4^+ via colorimetric or ion-selective electrode methods.
   2. When [NH_4^+] values from two commercial analyzers were compared with values generated by the generally accepted enzymatic assay, there was good agreement between the Blood Ammonia Checker and the enzymatic assays but poor agreement between the VetTest and enzymatic assays.[37]

C. Samples
1. In healthy fasting dogs, the $[NH_4^+]$ in arterial and venous plasma samples were not significantly different. However, in dogs with liver disease, the arterial samples had greater $[NH_4^+]$ (see Ammonium Concentration, sect. III.A.5).[38]
2. The $[NH_4^+]$ in serum samples is greater than in paired plasma samples.[1]
3. Hemolysis causes false increases of $[NH_4^+]$ in some assays because the heme pigment interferes with light transmittance or because erythrocytes contain NH_4^+.[39]
4. Sample handling
   a. Ideal: EDTA- or heparin-anticoagulated blood is delivered to a laboratory immediately after collection. The plasma is harvested immediately after arrival and cooled to 4 °C (in an ice bath), and chemical analysis is completed within 1 h. All steps should be completed with minimal exposure to air.
   b. The plasma $[NH_4^+]$ is usually considered to be stable for up to 4 h at 4 °C and adequately stable for 1–2 d at −20 °C.
   c. Suboptimal handling and instability problems can lead to highly variable results.[40]
      (1) Within hours of storage at room temperature, the $[NH_4^+]$ will be up to 2–3 times the starting value because of the generation of NH_4^+ from the degradation of labile proteins and amino acids (e.g., glutamine).
      (2) Delayed collection of plasma from the blood enables NH_4^+ to be produced by erythrocytes and leukocytes, thus increasing the measured $[NH_4^+]$.
      (3) Delayed analysis of plasma enables $NH_{3(g)}$ to escape from plasma particularly if the sample is not stoppered or if an evacuated tube is incompletely filled. Loss of $NH_{3(g)}$ will cause a decrease in the plasma $[NH_4^+]$.

III. Hyperammonemia (Table 13.12)
A. Decreased clearance of NH_4^+ from portal blood
1. Diseases or conditions that reduce the removal of NH_4^+ from portal blood may cause hyperammonemia because intestinal bacteria produce large quantities of NH_4^+. Two major types of diseases have this pathologic defect:
   a. Diffuse hepatocellular diseases that reduce functional mass (e.g., cirrhosis, necrosis, and lipidosis)[25]
   b. Portosystemic shunts, either congenital or acquired[30,41]
2. Decreased NH_4^+ clearance can potentially be caused by congenital deficiencies that directly or indirectly involve the urea cycle (Fig. 13.6). These disorders are rare.
   a. Argininosuccinate synthetase deficiency has been reported in dogs.[42]
   b. A probable case of ornithine carbamoyltransferase (ornithine transcarbamylase) deficiency caused hyperammonemia in a cat.[43]
   c. Defective mitochondrial transport of ornithine, a substance that is transported from cytosol to mitochondria in the urea cycle, probably caused hyperammonemia, hyperornithinemia, and homocitrullinuria syndrome in Morgan fillies.[44]
   d. Congenital cystinuria is caused by defective renal tubular resorption of cystine; concurrently, there is defective resorption of arginine and ornithine. A cystinuric cat had multiple episodes of hyperammonemic encephalopathy during its life.[45] The authors concluded that if dietary sources did not maintain sufficient amounts of arginine and ornithine for a functional urea cycle (Fig. 13.6), then argininuria and ornithinuria caused a depletion of those amino acids, and the cat was then prone to hyperammonemia.

Table 13.12. Diseases and conditions that cause hyperammonemia

*Decreased NH_4^+ clearance from portal blood
 *Decreased functional mass: diffuse hepatocellular disease
 *Decreased portal blood flow to liver: congenital and acquired portosystemic shunts
 Urea cycle enzyme deficiencies (congenital)
 Cystinuria with concurrent arginuria and ornithinuria (cat)
 Cobalamin deficiency
Increased NH_4^+ production
 Postprandial
 Urea toxicosis in cattle
 Strenuous exercise (racehorses and dogs)
 Urinary infection with urease-containing bacteria and concurrent urethral obstruction
 Intestinal disease in horses
Increased NH_4^+ intake
 NH_4Cl administration per os or per rectum
 Ammoniated forage toxicosis in cattle
 Exposure to NH_3 from anhydrous NH_3

 * A relatively common disease or condition
 Note: Lists of specific disorders or conditions are not complete but are provided to give examples. A falsely increased $[NH_4^+]$ may occur if delayed analysis of the sample results in proteolysis or NH_4^+ production by the blood cells.

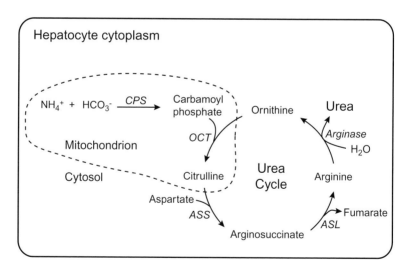

Fig. 13.6. The urea cycle (Krebs-Henseleit cycle) in hepatocytes: The dashed structure represents a mitochondrion; the other reactions occur in a hepatocyte's cytoplasm. The roles of adenosine triphosphate (ATP) and phosphate are not shown.

- Carbamoyl phosphate synthetase (CPS) catalyzes the reaction in which NH_4^+ and HCO_3^- are used to produce carbamoyl phosphate. Ornithine carbamoyltransferase (OCT) catalyzes the combination of carbamoyl phosphate and ornithine to produce citrulline. Argininosuccinate synthetase (ASS) catalyzes the combination of citrulline with aspartate to form argininosuccinate (a link between the urea cycle and the citric acid cycle). Argininosuccinate lyase (ASL) catalyzes the generation of arginine and fumarate from argininosuccinate. Arginase catalyzes the combination of arginine and H_2O to urea and ornithine; ornithine is then available to begin the urea cycle again.
- Congenital deficiencies in ASS or OCT cause a defective urea cycle and hyperammonemia because NH_4^+ is not incorporated into urea.

3. Decreased NH_4^+ clearance can also occur with acquired disorders that cause a defective urea cycle (Fig. 13.6). A cobalamin deficiency (see Chapter 15) may cause methylmalonic acid to accumulate, which decreases the concentrations of N-acetyl glutamate. A decreased N-acetyl glutamate concentration causes decreased activity of carbamoyl phosphate synthetase and thus less fixation of NH_4^+ into urea.[46]

4. The ammonium concentrations of Irish wolfhound puppies that were 7–8 wk old were 47–115 μmol/L compared to 6–27 μmol/L for adults. The pathogenesis of the hyperammonemia in these pups was not determined, but Irish wolfhounds do have a high incidence of portosystemic shunts.[47]

5. In 69 dogs with hepatic encephalopathy caused by several liver diseases (including 14 congenital and 29 acquired shunts), the $[NH_4^+]$ in arterial plasma averaged 1.5 times the $[NH_4^+]$ of venous plasma. The venous concentrations may be lower because of enhanced NH_4^+ clearance from arterial blood by kidneys, muscle, or other tissues. Because of the difference, some investigators recommend that arterial samples should be collected for measurement of plasma $[NH_4^+]$.[38] However, collecting an arterial sample is not as easy as collecting a venous sample. Also, based on the graphed data provided by the investigators, nearly all dogs that were hyperammonemic based on fasting arterial samples were also hyperammonemic based on fasting venous samples.

B. Increased NH_4^+ production

1. Postprandial: Increased NH_4^+ production during the digestion of a meal may cause temporary hyperammonemia. This condition should not be considered if the animal was appropriately fasted prior to sample collection.

2. Urea toxicosis in cattle: Hydrolysis of urea in the rumen liberates NH_3 that combines with H^+ to form NH_4^+. This makes ruminal fluid more alkaline. When the rumen pH is > 8.0, the NH_3:NH_4^+ ratio shifts toward NH_3, which diffuses from the rumen to plasma, where it combines with H^+ to increase the plasma $[NH_4^+]$.[48]

3. Strenuous exercise: During exercise, two adenosine diphosphate (ADP) molecules combine to form adenosine monophosphate (AMP) and adenosine triphosphate (ATP) via the myokinase reaction of myocytes. The deamination of adenosine monophosphate produces inosine monophosphate and NH_3. The NH_3 diffuses to blood and increases the plasma $[NH_4^+]$ and pH.[49]

   a. In greyhounds, the plasma $[NH_4^+]$ increased from a mean of 82 μmol/L before the race to a mean of 256 μmol/L immediately after the run.[50]

   b. In quarter horses, the plasma $[NH_4^+]$ increased from a mean of 67 μmol/L before exercise (treadmill) to a mean of 137 μmol/L immediately after exercise.[51] In another study, the mean NH_4^+ concentrations before and after exercise were 37 and 113 μmol/L, respectively.[49]

4. Urinary infection with urease-containing bacteria and concurrent urethral obstruction: An azotemic dog with staphylococcal urinary tract infection and urethral calculi had a fasting $[NH_4^+]$ of 258 μg/dL. The hyperammonemia may have been caused by increased NH_4^+ production in the urinary tract, decreased renal excretion due to obstruction, and perhaps decreased urea cycle activity due to acidosis.[52]

5. Intestinal disease in horses: Horses with certain intestinal disorders may have a markedly increased plasma $[NH_4^+]$ and clinical signs of colic and encephalopathy without evidence of hepatic disease. An increased plasma $[NH_4^+]$ is thought to be caused by increased generation of NH_4^+ by abnormal proliferations of colonic bacteria and/or by increased intestinal absorption of NH_4^+. No single type of

bacteria has been cultured consistently in these cases. Diagnosis requires measurement of blood [NH_4^+].[53–56]

C. Increased NH_4^+ intake or absorption
  1. NH_4Cl administration per os or via the colon (see the next sect. IV, NH_4^+ Tolerance Test)
  2. Ammoniated forage toxicosis in calves: A 30-d-old calf had a plasma [NH_4^+] that was considered increased while nursing a cow that had ingested hay treated with anhydrous NH_3.[57]
  3. Cattle dying after exposure to anhydrous NH_3 presumably would have increased plasma [NH_4^+]. Cattle exposure occurs with the malicious release of anhydrous NH_3 from storage tanks.[58]

IV. NH_4^+ tolerance test
  A. Principle: By administration of NH_4Cl either orally or rectally, a challenge dose of NH_4^+ is presented to the liver via the portal veins. Either decreased hepatic functional mass or a portosystemic shunt will enable NH_4^+ to escape the enterohepatic circulation and cause an excessive increase in the plasma [NH_4^+].
  B. The NH_4^+ tolerance test may be used when decreased hepatic function is suspected but other laboratory results do not strongly support hepatic insufficiency or a portosystemic shunt. Typically, an NH_4^+ tolerance test is not indicated if there is a fasting hyperammonemia. Also, an excessively high plasma [NH_4^+] might contribute to hepatic encephalopathy.
  C. Basics of procedures in dogs
    1. *Oral NH_4^+ tolerance test*: After a 12 h fast and collection of a fasting sample, NH_4Cl is administered orally (0.1 g/kg but not more than 3 g) in 20–50 mL H_2O. A 30 min post-NH_4Cl blood sample is collected.
    2. *Rectal NH_4^+ tolerance test*: After a 12 h fast and collection of a fasting sample, NH_4Cl is administered (5 % solution; 2 mL/kg) via a catheter inserted 20–35 cm into the colon. Blood samples are collected 20 and 40 min later. Both 20 min and 40 min samples have been recommended because peak [NH_4^+] occurred before 30 min in some dogs and after 30 min in others.[59]
  D. Interpretation of results
    1. Fasting [NH_4^+]
      a. WRI: There is no evidence of hepatic insufficiency or a portosystemic shunt. These conditions could be present, but the production of NH_4^+ is not enough to overwhelm the weakened system. There is no evidence of a rare congenital urea cycle enzyme deficiency.
      b. Hyperammonemia: See Table 13.12 for potential pathogeneses.
    2. Postchallenge [NH_4^+]
      a. WRI: There is no evidence of hepatic insufficiency, portosystemic shunt, or a rare congenital urea cycle enzyme deficiency.
      b. Increased above reference interval: The functional hepatic mass, portosystemic shunt, or both are decreased. Rarely, a congenital or acquired urea cycle enzyme deficiency is present.
  E. Example results for dogs with portosystemic shunts are listed in Table 13.13.

V. Postprandial venous NH_4^+ tolerance test for dogs[60]
  A. This procedure is similar to the NH_4^+ tolerance test (see the preceding sect. IV) except digested food provides the NH_4^+ for the tolerance testing. The major advantage over

Table 13.13. Ammonia tolerance test results for six dogs with portosystemic shunts

Results for assay 1	10 Healthy dogs	Dog 1[a]	Dog 2[b]	Dog 3[b]
Fasting $[NH_4^+]$ (µg/dL)	88 ± 36[c]	100	370	260
30 min $[NH_4^+]$ (µg/dL)	155 ± 71	1000	1400	850
Results for assay 2	10 healthy dogs	Dog 4[d]	Dog 5[b]	Dog 6[b]
Fasting $[NH_4^+]$ (µg/dL)	56 ± 14	100	250	125
30 min $[NH_4^+]$ (µg/dL)	76 ± 30	550	900	650

[a] The fasting $[NH_4^+]$ was WRI, and thus hepatic function was sufficient to handle the NH_4^+ load during the fasting state. The marked hyperammonemia in the 30 min sample is consistent with a portosystemic shunt or hepatic insufficiency.

[b] The fasting hyperammonemia revealed the defective NH_4^+ clearance. The marked hyperammonemia in the 30 min sample would be expected because of influx of NH_4^+ into the system.

[c] All data for healthy dogs are expressed as mean ± standard deviation. The data may not have had normal distributions.

[d] The fasting $[NH_4^+]$ was slightly increased and thus not strong evidence of hepatic insufficiency or a portosystemic shunt. However, the $[NH_4^+]$ in the 30 min sample was definitely increased and thus supportive of hepatic insufficiency or a portosystemic shunt.

Note: Two sets of data are reported because of the lack of analytical agreement of the two NH_4^+ assays (note the different values in the healthy dog groups).

Source: Meyer et al.[61]

the NH_4^+ tolerance test is that the administration of NH_4Cl solution is considered stressful, and some dogs may vomit the solution if it is administered orally.

B. Basics of the procedure
  1. Withhold food for 24 h and then feed a commercial diet containing about 30 % protein to provide 33 kcal/kg ($\approx$ 25 % of the estimated daily metabolizable energy requirement). This estimate is adjusted for growing dogs.
  2. Heparinized blood is collected prior to feeding and at 2 h intervals (2, 4, 6, and 8 h) after feeding. Blood is chilled during processing, and the plasma $[NH_4^+]$ is measured immediately after plasma is harvested.

C. In the published study, the postprandial $[NH_4^+]$ did not exceed 16 µmol/L in samples from healthy dogs. Dogs with hepatocellular disease frequently had a preprandial $[NH_4^+]$ and a postprandial $[NH_4^+]$ above 16 µmol/L without significant change between preprandial and postprandial values; the maximum concentrations occurred 6 h postprandially. Dogs with portosystemic shunts had preprandial ammonium concentrations up to 250 µmol/L (90th percentile near 150 µmol/L) and postprandial ammonium concentrations up to 400 µmol/L (90th percentile near 250 µmol/L) in the 2, 4, or 6 h samples.

D. The data support the use of this tolerance test to detect portosystemic shunts and that a 6 h sampling may be beneficial. This tolerance test had poor diagnostic sensitivity for hepatocellular disease. Appropriate laboratory-specific decision thresholds should be used for diagnostic investigations.

DYE-EXCRETION TESTS

Prior to availability of spectrophotometric assays for bile acids, hepatic function was clinically assessed by excretion tests involving two organic anions or dyes: BSP (bromosulfophthalein or sulfobromophthalein) and ICG (indocyanine green).

Excretion of these dyes depends on hepatic blood flow, hepatocyte uptake, conjugation (BSP but not ICG), excretion to the biliary system, and enterohepatic circulation (BSP but not ICG). Impaired excretion (caused by a defect in any step of the pathway) was detected as either an increased percent retention of the dye or an increased plasma half-life of the dye.

The use of dye-excretion tests is limited in clinical diagnostic testing because BSP is no longer commercially available, ICG is expensive, and assessment of [BA] and [Bt] provides essentially the same information about hepatic function.

References

1. Tolman KG, Rej R. 1999. Liver function. In: Burtis CA, Ashwood ER, eds. *Tietz Textbook of Clinical Chemistry*, 3rd edition, 1125–1177. Philadelphia: WB Saunders.
2. 1988. *Dorland's Illustrated Medical Dictionary*, 27th edition. Philadelphia: WB Saunders.
3. Berk PD, Noyer C. 1994. Bilirubin metabolism and the hereditary hyperbilirubinemias. 2. Hepatic uptake, binding, conjugation, and excretion of bilirubin. Semin Liver Dis 14:331–343.
4. McDonagh AF, Palma LA, Lauff JJ, Wu TW. 1984. Origin of mammalian biliprotein and rearrangement of bilirubin glucuronides in vivo in the rat. J Clin Invest 74:763–770.
5. Lundberg GD, Iverson C, Radulescu G. 1986. Now read this: The SI units are here. J Am Med Assoc 255:2329–2339.
6. Pantanowitz L, Horowitz GL, Upalakalin JN, Beckwith BA. 2003. Artifactual hyperbilirubinemia due to paraprotein interference. Arch Pathol Lab Med 127:55–59.
7. Rothuizen J. 2000. Jaundice. In: Ettinger SJ, Feldman EC, eds. *Textbook of Veterinary Internal Medicine: Diseases of the Dog and Cat*, 5th edition, 210–212. Philadelphia: WB Saunders.
8. Rothuizen J, van den Brom WE. 1987. Bilirubin metabolism in canine hepatobiliary and haemolytic disease. Vet Q 9:235–240.
9. Engelking LR. 1993. Equine fasting hyperbilirubinemia. Adv Vet Sci Comp Med 37:115–125.
10. McSherry BJ, Lumsden JH, Valli VE, Baird JD. 1984. Hyperbilirubinemia in sick cattle. Can J Comp Med 48:237–240.
11. Reid IM, Harrison RD, Collins RA. 1977. Fasting and refeeding in the lactating dairy cow. 2. The recovery of liver cell structure and function following a six-day fast. J Comp Pathol 87:253–265.
12. Gray ML, Bounous DI, Kelley LC, Almazan P, Brown J. 1995. Icterus in bob veal calves and its association with lack of colostrum intake and high serum creatine kinase activity. Am J Vet Res 56:1506–1512.
13. Naylor JM, Kronfeld DS, Johnson K. 1980. Fasting hyperbilirubinemia and its relationship to free fatty acids and triglycerides in the horse. Proc Soc Exp Biol Med 165:86–90.
14. Cornelius CE, Kelley KC, Himes JA. 1975. Heterogeneity of bilirubin conjugates in several animal species. Cornell Vet 65:90–99.
15. Gronwall R, Engelking LR. 1982. Effect of glucose administration on equine fasting hyperbilirubinemia. Am J Vet Res 43:801–803.
16. Mia AS, Gronwall RR, Cornelius CE. 1970. Bilirubin-^{14}C turnover studies in normal and mutant Southdown sheep with congenital hyperbilirubinemia. Proc Soc Exp Biol Med 133:955–959.
17. Mia AS, Gronwall RR, Cornelius CE. 1970. Unconjugated bilirubin transport in normal and mutant Corriedale sheep with Dubin-Johnson syndrome. Proc Soc Exp Biol Med 135:33–37.
18. Divers TJ, Schappel KA, Sweeney RW, Tennant BC. 1993. Persistent hyperbilirubinemia in a healthy thoroughbred horse. Cornell Vet 83:237–242.
19. Taboada J, Meyer DJ. 1989. Cholestasis associated with extrahepatic bacterial infection in five dogs. J Vet Intern Med 3:216–221.
20. Moseley RH, Wang W, Takeda H, Lown K, Shick L, Ananthanarayanan M, Suchy FJ. 1996. Effect of endotoxin on bile acid transport in rat liver: A potential model for sepsis-associated cholestasis. Am J Physiol 271:G137–G146.
21. Whiting JF, Green RM, Rosenbluth AB, Gollan JL. 1995. Tumor necrosis factor-alpha decreases hepatocyte bile salt uptake and mediates endotoxin-induced cholestasis. Hepatology 22:1273–1278.
22. Green RM, Whiting JF, Rosenbluth AB, Beier D, Gollan JL. 1994. Interleukin-6 inhibits hepatocyte taurocholate uptake and sodium-potassium-adenosinetriphoshatase activity. Am J Physiol 267:G1094–G1100.
23. Jain NC. 1986. *Schalm's Veterinary Hematology*, 4th edition. Philadelphia: Lea & Febiger.
24. Center SA. 1993. Serum bile acids in companion animal medicine. Vet Clin North Am Small Anim Pract 23:625–657.

25. West HJ. 1996. Clinical and pathological studies in horses with hepatic disease. Equine Vet J 28:146–156.

26. West HJ. 1991. Evaluation of total serum bile acid concentrations for the diagnosis of hepatobiliary disease in cattle. Res Vet Sci 51:133–140.

27. West HJ. 1989. Evaluation of total plasma bile acid concentrations for the diagnosis of hepatobiliary disease in horses. Res Vet Sci 46:264–270.

28. Center SA, ManWarren T, Slater MR, Wilentz E. 1991. Evaluation of twelve-hour preprandial and two-hour postprandial serum bile acids concentrations for diagnosis of hepatobiliary disease in dogs. J Am Vet Med Assoc 199:217–226.

29. Center SA, Erb HN, Joseph SA. 1995. Measurement of serum bile acids concentrations for diagnosis of hepatobiliary disease in cats. J Am Vet Med Assoc 207:1048–1054.

30. Buonanno AM, Carlson GP, Kantrowitz B. 1988. Clinical and diagnostic features of portosystemic shunt in a foal. J Am Vet Med Assoc 192:387–389.

31. Hoffmann WE, Baker G, Rieser S, Dorner JL. 1987. Alterations in selected serum biochemical constituents in equids after induced hepatic disease. Am J Vet Res 48:1343–1347.

32. Fricker G, Landmann L, Meier PJ. 1989. Extrahepatic obstructive cholestasis reverses the bile salt secretory polarity of rat hepatocytes. J Clin Invest 84:876–885.

33. West HJ. 1997. Clinical and pathological studies in cattle with hepatic disease. Vet Res Commun 21:169–185.

34. Balkman CE, Center SA, Randolph JF, Trainor D, Warner KL, Crawford MA, Adachi K, Erb HN. 2003. Evaluation of urine sulfated and nonsulfated bile acids as a diagnostic test for liver disease in dogs. J Am Vet Med Assoc 222:1368–1375.

35. Trainor D, Center SA, Randolph F, Balkman CE, Warner KL, Crawford MA, Adachi K, Erb HN. 2003. Urine sulfated and nonsulfated bile acids as a diagnostic test for liver disease in cats. J Vet Intern Med 17:145–153.

36. Balkman CE, Center SA, Randolph JF, Trainor D, Warner KL, Crawford MA, Adachi K, Erb HN. 2003. Evaluation of urine sulfated and nonsulfated bile acids as a diagnostic test for liver disease in dogs. J Am Vet Med Assoc 223:339 (erratum).

37. Sterczer A, Meyer HP, Boswijk HC, Rothuizen J. 1999. Evaluation of ammonia measurements in dogs with two analysers for use in veterinary practice. Vet Rec 144:523–526.

38. Rothuizen J, van den Ingh TSGAM. 1982. Arterial and venous ammonia concentrations in the diagnosis of canine hepato-encephalopathy. Res Vet Sci 33:17–21.

39. Seligson D, Hirahara K. 1957. The measurement of ammonia in whole blood, erythrocytes, and plasma. J Lab Clin Med 49:962–974.

40. Hitt ME, Jones BD. 1986. Effects of storage temperature and time on canine plasma ammonia concentrations. Am J Vet Res 47:363–364.

41. Beech J, Dubielzig R, Bester R. 1977. Portal vein anomaly and hepatic encephalopathy in a horse. J Am Vet Med Assoc 170:164–166.

42. Strombeck DR, Meyer DJ, Freedland RA. 1975. Hyperammonemia due to a urea cycle enzyme deficiency in two dogs. J Am Vet Med Assoc 166:1109–1111.

43. Washizu T, Washizu M, Zhang C, Matsumoto I, Sawamura M, Suzuki T. 2004. A suspected case of ornithine transcarbamylase deficiency in a cat. J Vet Med Sci 66:701–703.

44. McConnico RS, Duckett WM, Wood PA. 1997. Persistent hyperammonemia in two related Morgan weanlings. J Vet Intern Med 11:264–266.

45. Osborne CA, Lulich JP, Lehkcharoensuk C, Ross SJ, Rogers QR, Koehler LA, Ulrich LK, Carpenter KA, Swanson LL, Pedersen LA. 2006. Hyperammonemic encephalopathy in cystinuric cats. In: Proceedings of the 19th ACVIM Forum, Denver, 794–795.

46. Battersby IA, Giger U, Hall EJ. 2005. Hyperammonaemic encephalopathy secondary to selective cobalamin deficiency in a juvenile Border collie. J Small Anim Pract 46:339–344.

47. Meyer HP, Rothuizen J, Tiemessen I, van den Brom WE, van den Ingh TSGAM. 1996. Transient metabolic hyperammonaemia in young Irish wolfhounds. Vet Rec 138:105–107.

48. Haliburton JC, Morgan SE. 1989. Nonprotein nitrogen-induced ammonia toxicosis and ammoniated feed toxicity syndrome. Vet Clin North Am Food Anim Pract 5:237–249.

49. Miller PA, Lawrence LM. 1987. The effect of submaximal treadmill training on heart rate, lactate and ammonia in quarter horses. In: Gillespie JR, Robinson NE, eds. Equine Exercise Physiology 2, 476–484. Davis, CA: ICEEP.

50. Snow DH, Harris RC, Stuttard E. 1988. Changes in haematology and plasma biochemistry during maximal exercise in greyhounds. Vet Rec 123:487–489.

51. Miller PA, Lawrence LM. 1986. Changes in equine metabolic characteristics due to exercise fatigue. Am J Vet Res 47:2184–2186.

52. Hall JA, Allen TA, Fettman MJ. 1987. Hyperammonemia associated with urethral obstruction in a dog. J Am Vet Med Assoc 191:1116–1118.

53. Hasel KM, Summers BA, de Lahunta A. 1999. Encephalopathy with idiopathic hyperammonaemia and Alzheimer type II astrocytes in equidae. Equine Vet J 31:478–482.

54. Peek SF, Divers TJ, Jackson CJ. 1997. Hyperammonaemia associated with encephalopathy and abdominal pain without evidence of liver disease in four mature horses. Equine Vet J 29:70–74.

55. Stickle JE, McKnight CA, Williams KJ, Carr EA. 2006. Diarrhea and hyperammonemia in a horse with progressive neurologic signs. Vet Clin Pathol 35:250–253.

56. Sharkey LC, DeWitt S, Stockman C. 2006. Neurologic signs and hyperammonemia in a horse with colic. Vet Clin Pathol 35:254–258.

57. Kerr LA, Groce AW, Kersting KW. 1987. Ammoniated forage toxicosis in calves. J Am Vet Med Assoc 191:551–552.

58. Fitzgerald SD, Grooms DL, Scott MA, Clarke KR, Rumbeiha WK. 2006. Acute anhydrous ammonia intoxication in cattle. J Vet Diagn Invest 18:485–489.

59. Rothuizen J, van den Ingh TSGAM. 1982. Rectal ammonia tolerance test in the evaluation of portal circulation in dogs with liver disease. Res Vet Sci 33:22–25.

60. Walker MC, Hill RC, Guilford WG, Scott KC, Jones GL, Buergelt CD. 2001. Postprandial venous ammonia concentrations in the diagnosis of hepatobiliary disease in dogs. J Vet Intern Med 15:463–466.

61. Meyer DJ, Strombeck DR, Stone EA, Zenoble RD, Buss DD. 1978. Ammonia tolerance test in clinically normal dogs and in dogs with portosystemic shunts. J Am Vet Med Assoc 173:377–379.

Chapter 14

GLUCOSE, KETOAMINES, AND RELATED REGULATORY HORMONES

Glucose Concentration in Serum, Plasma, or Whole Blood 708
   I. Physiologic Processes 708
   II. Analytical Concepts 709
   III. Hyperglycemia 713
   IV. Hypoglycemia 719
   V. [Glucose] During Insulin Therapy 722
Ketoamines: Fructosamine and Glycated Hemoglobin 723
   I. Physiologic Processes 723
   II. Analytical Concepts 724
   III. Increased [Fructosamine] and Increased Glycated Hemoglobin
      Percentage or Concentration 724
   IV. Decreased [Fructosamine] and Decreased Glycated Hemoglobin
      Percentage or Concentration 725
   V. Correction of the [Fructosamine] for Abnormal Protein Concentrations 726
Immunoreactive Insulin (IRI) Concentration in Serum or Plasma 726
   I. Physiologic Processes 726
   II. Analytical Concepts 727
   III. Hyperinsulinemia 728
   IV. Hypoinsulinemia 728
   V. Immunoreactive Insulin to Glucose (IRI : G) Ratio 729
Immunoreactive Glucagon (IRG) Concentration in Plasma 730
   I. Physiologic Processes 730
   II. Analytical Concepts 730
   III. Hyperglucagonemia Associated with Glucagonomas 731

Table 14.1. Abbreviations and symbols in this chapter

[x]	x concentration (x = analyte)
ACTH	Adrenocorticotropic hormone (corticotropin)
DM	Diabetes mellitus
EDTA	Ethylenediaminetetraacetic acid
GH	Growth hormone
GLP	Glucagon-like peptide
GLUT	Facilitative hexose transporter
Hct	Hematocrit
Hgb	Hemoglobin
IRG	Immunoreactive glucagon
IRI	Immunoreactive insulin
IRI:G	Immunoreactive insulin to glucose
NaF	Sodium fluoride
SI	Système International d'Unités

GLUCOSE CONCENTRATION IN SERUM, PLASMA, OR WHOLE BLOOD

I.   Physiologic processes (Fig. 14.1)

    A. Blood [glucose] is regulated and influenced by several hormones. For the hormones to influence metabolism, there must be appropriate receptors and transport systems in the target cells.

        1. Insulin activity lowers blood [glucose] by promoting the uptake, utilization, or storage of glucose by hepatocytes, myocytes, and adipocytes. Insulin is not needed for glucose transport into neurons, leukocytes, erythrocytes, platelets, or hepatocytes. Insulin does influence hepatocyte glucose uptake by altering activities of hepatic enzymes that promote glycolysis or glycogen synthesis, or by reducing gluconeogenesis.

        2. Glucose entry into most cells is modulated by a family of proteins called facilitative hexose transporters (GLUT-1 to GLUT-7). Insulin promotes glucose entry into myocytes and adipocytes via GLUT-4; insulin is not needed for the other carriers (e.g., GLUT-2 in hepatocytes).

        3. Glucagon activity increases blood [glucose] by stimulating gluconeogenesis and glycogenolysis.

        4. Catecholamine activity alters blood [glucose] by several mechanisms.[1,2]

            a. An α_2-adrenergic stimulus of pancreatic β-cells decreases insulin release and thus reduces glucose utilization by hepatocytes, myocytes, and adipocytes.[3]

            b. A β-adrenergic stimulus of pancreatic β-cells increases insulin release. However, α_2-adrenergic receptors predominate on pancreatic β-cells, so catecholamines primarily inhibit insulin secretion.

            c. A β_2-adrenergic stimulus of hepatocytes increases glycogenolysis.[4]

            d. An α_2-adrenergic stimulus of the pituitary gland increases the release of GH-releasing hormone, which then causes GH release.[5]

5. GH (somatotropin) activity increases blood [glucose] by reducing glucose uptake by myocytes and adipocytes.

6. Cortisol activity increases blood [glucose] by stimulating gluconeogenesis and creating a state of insulin resistance (see Glucose Concetration in Serum, sect. III.B).

B. In monogastric animals, fasting blood [glucose] is maintained by gluconeogenesis by using products of protein and lipid catabolism. In ruminants, propionate from rumen fermentation is used for hepatic gluconeogenesis. In horses, colonic propionate contributes to gluconeogenesis.[6]

C. Fasting normoglycemia represents a balance between the actions of insulin (promoting storage and utilization of fuels) and glucagon (promoting mobilization of fuels). When there is an imbalance and fuel mobilization dominates, then the animal will be hyperglycemic and potentially glucosuric; glucosuria reduces the magnitude of the hyperglycemia. If fuel storage and utilization are dominant, then the animal will be hypoglycemic. Even though the balance of insulin and glucagon actions is assessed by a blood [glucose], these hormones also influence lipid and protein metabolism.

II. Analytical concepts

A. Terms and units

1. As explained in the following section C, the [glucose] in whole blood may not be equal to its concentration in plasma or serum harvested from the same blood. Assuming similar contact times with blood cells, [glucose] in serum and plasma will be nearly equal to each other.

2. Unit conversion: mg/dL $\times$ 0.05551 = mmol/L (SI unit, nearest 0.1 mmol/L)[7]

B. Sample for [glucose]

1. For most clinical laboratory methods, serum is recommended and plasma (especially heparinized) can be used. Serum and plasma should be removed from cells within 1 h of blood collection because glycolysis continues in blood cells in vitro, thus lowering [glucose].

a. If plasma or serum has contact with cells at room temperature prior to centrifugation of blood, [glucose] typically decreases about 5–10 % per hour; marked leukocytosis and erythrocytosis will accelerate the process. The rate of glucose consumption can be decreased by placing the blood sample in a cool environment, but clot formation and contraction are also reduced.

b. Serum separator tubes (tubes with gold or red/black stoppers) contain an activator (silica) that enhances clot formation and gel that enables easier separation of a blood clot and serum. After centrifugation, the serum [glucose] remains stable in a refrigerator for at least 48 h if the gel barrier is intact.[8,9] The gel barrier may break down in transit.

2. Special collection tubes containing NaF (tubes with grey stoppers) can be used to block glycolysis. However, they are not routinely used in clinical medicine.

a. F^- complexes with Mg^{2+}, which is a cofactor for phosphopyruvate hydratase (synonym: enolase) in the glycolytic pathway. The NaF tubes may also contain anticoagulants (oxalate or EDTA). F^- will also inhibit glucose oxidase activity (and other enzymes), and thus NaF plasma should not be used in glucose assays that use glucose oxidase.

b. Plasma [glucose] decreased by 5–10 % during the first hour after blood collection into NaF tubes.[10] The decrease may result from the osmotic movement of H_2O from erythrocytes to plasma when the blood is mixed with the hyperosmotic salts

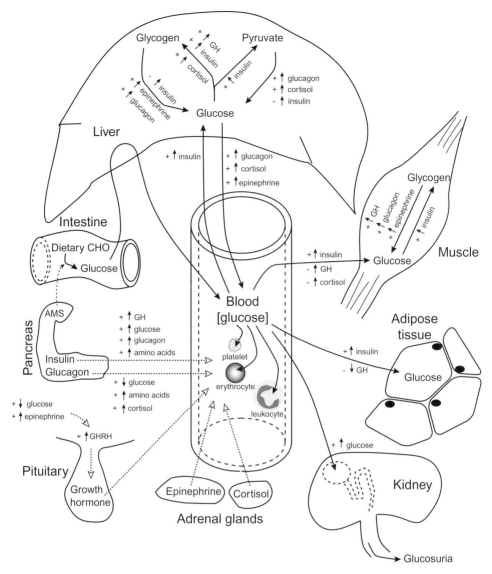

Fig. 14.1. Physiologic factors that influence blood [glucose].

- Intestine: Dietary carbohydrates (CHO) are broken down to monosaccharides (including glucose) that are absorbed in the small intestine, from which they enter portal blood and then systemic blood if not removed by hepatocytes.

- Pancreas: Insulin and glucagon are released from pancreatic islet β-cells and α-cells, respectively. Insulin secretion is stimulated by increased blood concentrations of glucose, GH, glucagon, or amino acids. Glucagon secretion is stimulated by increased blood concentrations of amino acids and cortisol, or by decreased blood [glucose]. Amylase (AMS) is released from the pancreas and catalyzes the breakdown of ingested starches to form glucose.

- Liver: Hepatocytes are the primary source of blood glucose during fasting. Glucose can be obtained from glycogenolysis (stimulated by epinephrine and glucagon but inhibited by insulin) or gluconeogenesis (stimulated by glucagon and cortisol but inhibited by insulin). Insulin also promotes glycolysis. Increased glucose release from hepatocytes is promoted by increased glucagon, cortisol, or epinephrine. Insulin promotes the hepatic uptake of glucose by promoting glucokinase activity, but this glucose uptake does not require insulin.

(NaF and potassium oxalate). Other data indicate that it takes about 1 h for the F^- to inhibit glycolysis completely, but then [glucose] remains stable for at least 3 d.[11] The antiglycolytic effect of F^- depends on its concentration in the blood sample.[12]

    c. Erythrocytes are prone to lysis when exposed to NaF and potassium oxalate, especially if there is not an optimal amount of blood drawn into the evacuated blood tube. The release of erythrocyte contents (e.g., Hgb, inorganic phosphates, and K^+) may lead to erroneous results in some clinical chemistry assays.

  3. Many point-of-care instruments are available that can be used for measuring blood [glucose]. Several are designed for use by people who are monitoring the control of their diabetic states. The instruments typically will provide useful results if the unit is operating correctly, if the sample is collected properly, and if manufacturer's directions are followed precisely.

  4. [Glucose] in arterial or capillary blood is greater than in venous blood because peripheral tissues consume glucose. The difference in normoglycemic and normoinsulinemic states is probably < 10 mg/dL.

C. What is measured: whole blood or plasma [glucose]?

  1. When an assay uses whole blood for a sample, it is important to know whether the result represents a whole blood [glucose], a plasma [glucose], or a calculated plasma [glucose]. Some instruments measure and report whole blood [glucose]. Other instruments measure a whole blood [glucose] and calculate a plasma [glucose]. Of these, some assume a normal Hct value, and thus the calculated value will not be correct in anemic or erythrocytotic samples.[13] Some whole blood assays measure molality and not molarity, and thus variations in the H_2O content of blood (e.g., due to displacement of H_2O by proteins or lipids) will influence measured [glucose].[14,15] There have been several reports of comparisons of [glucose] measured by different blood glucose instruments or assays. Some of these studies are difficult to interpret because the types of [glucose] (i.e., blood, plasma, or serum) were not specified and differences due to different Hct values were not considered.

  2. Whole blood versus plasma or serum [glucose]

    a. Glucose is uniformly distributed in H_2O components of whole blood (glucose freely diffuses between plasma and erythrocytes), but there are about 71 mL of

---

Fig. 14.1. *continued*

• Muscle: Glucose uptake by myocytes is promoted by insulin through specific insulin receptors and glucose transporters; GH and cortisol inhibit the uptake of glucose. Insulin promotes glycogen synthesis in myocytes, whereas GH, glucagon, and epinephrine promote glycogenolysis to provide glucose for glycolysis.

• Adipose tissue: Insulin promotes the uptake of glucose by adipocytes; GH reduces glucose uptake.

• Kidney: If the renal threshold for tubular resorption of glucose is exceeded, then hyperglycemic glucosuria will develop.

• Pituitary: GH release from the pituitary is stimulated by growth hormone–releasing hormone, which is released from the hypothalamus during hypoglycemia or after epinephrine stimulation.

• Blood cells: Glucose enters erythrocytes, leukocytes, and platelets through insulin-independent processes and is used in glycolysis and the hexose monophosphate shunt.

Note: The *solid arrows* indicate the movement of glucose, and the *dashed arrows* represent the movement of hormones or amylase.

H$_2$O per 100 mL of erythrocytes and about 93 mL of H$_2$O per 100 mL of plasma. Thus, the H$_2$O content of whole blood varies with its Hct. Because there is less H$_2$O in erythrocytes than in plasma, the [glucose] in erythrocytes is about 76 % of that in plasma, and therefore whole blood [glucose] measured by some methods are lower than those of serum or plasma. Whole blood [glucose] can be converted to plasma [glucose] (Eq. 14.1).[13]

$$\text{Plasma}\left[\text{glucose}\right] = \frac{\text{Whole blood}\left[\text{glucose}\right]}{\left(1.0 - \left(0.0024 \times \text{Hct in \%}\right)\right)} \tag{14.1.}$$

    b. The differences that may occur between whole blood [glucose] and plasma or serum [glucose] are listed in Table 14.2. When severe anemia is present, whole blood [glucose] and plasma [glucose] will be nearly equal.

D. Methods of measuring [glucose]
    1. Photometric assays: Most current methods use glucose oxidase (specific enzyme for glucose), glucose dehydrogenase, or hexokinase (enzyme for all hexoses) for the initial reaction. In other assays, glucose (and other monosaccharides) reacts with *o*-toluidine or glucose reduces reagents such as copper or ferricyanide. Color changes can be detected by spectrophotometry or reflectance photometry. Lipemia, hemolysis, and icterus can interfere with the light transmission, but the degree of interference varies among assays. Isopropyl alcohol can produce a positive interference with reagent pad methods (e.g., Dextrostix) when blood is contaminated with isopropyl alcohol during blood collection; the resulting [glucose] can be greatly increased (change from 100 mg/dL to nearly 300 mg/dL).[16]
    2. Nonphotometric assays: These modifications of the glucose oxidase methods have an advantage over photometric assays in that there are fewer chemical and photometric interferences. In the glucose oxidase reaction, O$_2$ is consumed and hydrogen peroxide is produced. Some instruments measure the rate of O$_2$ consumption with oxygen electrodes, and others measure the rate of hydrogen peroxide generation with hydrogen peroxide electrodes. Some of the glucose oxidase methods are inhibited by

Table 14.2. Calculated plasma [glucose] in a blood sample with given whole blood concentration and Hct value

	If whole blood [glucose] (mg/dL) is:				Increase above whole blood [glucose] (%)
	50	100	400	800	
	Calculated plasma [glucose] (mg/dL) is:				
If Hct is: 10 %	51	102	410	820	2
45 %	56	112	448	897	12
60 %	58	117	467	935	17

Note: Concentrations of plasma glucose were calculated by using Eq. 14.1 and assuming variables in sample handling, and in vitro glycolysis were not present. Agreement between calculated and measured plasma concentrations depends on the analytical properties (accuracy, precision, specificity, and sensitivity) of the assays. Conversion using Eq. 14.1 is applicable when the glucose assay result is a whole blood [glucose] in mg/dL or mmol/L. Other conversion factors are needed if the glucose assay measures molal concentration (mmol/kg) instead of molar concentration (mmol/L).

F^- or bromide; false decreases in [glucose] can be marked in samples from patients receiving potassium bromide for neurologic disease.

E. Artifactual hypoglycemia from cellular consumption

1. Extreme leukocytosis: Some leukemias and inflammatory states (see Chapter 2) have been reported to cause hypoglycemia because of increased glycolysis. Depending on sample handling, the hypoglycemia could be partially caused by in vitro glycolysis. Increased glucose consumption may occur because of increased numbers of leukocytes or because of increased metabolic activity in leukocytes (e.g., malignant blast cells or after stimulation by granulocyte colony–stimulating factor).[17]

2. Erythrocytosis (same concepts as with extreme leukocytosis): A leukocyte needs more glucose than an erythrocyte, but typically there are about 1000 times as many erythrocytes as leukocytes. Marked rubricytosis would also probably cause increased glucose consumption.[18]

III. Hyperglycemia

A. As in summarized in the preceding Physiologic Processes section, plasma [glucose] is influenced by many factors, so it should not be surprising that there are many causes of hyperglycemia.

1. The definitions, diagnostic criteria, and classifications of DM used in this chapter were described in a report from a committee organized by the American Diabetes Association.[19]

a. Definition of DM: "Diabetes mellitus is a group of metabolic diseases characterized by hyperglycemia resulting from defects in insulin secretion, insulin action, or both."

b. Diagnostic criteria for human DM (Table 14.3)[19]

(1) To adapt these criteria to domestic mammals, veterinarians will need to establish appropriate decision values for [glucose] in each animal species (see Table 14.3 for suggested decision thresholds for dogs, cats, horses, and cattle).

(2) The expert committee recommended that the classifications of "insulin-dependent" and "non–insulin-dependent" DM be dropped because of the confusion generated by their use.

2. A proposed classification system for canine DM[20] is similar to the classifications of pathologic hyperglycemia in Table 14.4. It consists of two major groups: (1) insulin-deficiency diabetes (IDD) includes those disorders that cause a progressive loss of β-cells (e.g., type 1 DM, and pancreatitis), and (2) insulin-resistance diabetes (IRD) includes those disorders in which there is insulin antagonism by hormones (e.g., type 2 DM and endocrine DM).

3. For the pathologic hyperglycemic disorders, several other abnormal laboratory findings may be present and can be used to help characterize the diabetic states.

a. Glucosuria and associated polyuria (Chapter 8)

b. Ketonemia and ketonuria (Chapters 9 and 8, respectively)

c. Metabolic acidosis (Chapters 9 and 10)

d. Lipemia (Chapter 16)

e. Increased [ketoamine] or ketoamine percentage (see the Ketoamines: Fructosamine and Glycated Hemoglobin section)

Table 14.3. Criteria for the diagnosis of diabetes mellitus in people

1. Symptoms of diabetes plus casual plasma [glucose] ≥ 200 mg/dL (11.1 mmol/L).[a] *Casual* is defined as any time of day without regard to time since last meal. The classic symptoms of diabetes include polyuria, polydipsia, and unexplained weight loss.

Or

2. Fasting plasma [glucose] ≥ 126 mg/dL (7.0 mmol/L).[b] *Fasting* is defined as no caloric intake for at least 8 h.

Or

3. 2-h plasma [glucose] ≥ 200 mg/dL (11.1 mmol/L) during an oral glucose tolerance test.[c] The test should be performed as described by the World Health Organization, using a glucose load containing an equivalent of 75 g anhydrous glucose dissolved in water.

In the absence of unequivocal hyperglycemia with acute metabolic decompensation, these criteria should be confirmed by repeat testing on a different day. The oral glucose tolerance test is not recommended for routine clinical use.

[a] The > 200 mg/dL criterion should work for dogs and horses; > 250 mg/dL is proposed for cats and >150 mg/dL is proposed for cattle.

[b] The decision limit of 126 mg/dL (7.0 mmol/L) was based on several factors, including correlation with results of glucose tolerance tests and complications of persistent hyperglycemia (e.g., retinopathy or arterial disease). Until similar studies are done in domestic species, similar decision limits cannot be established for them.

[c] It is unlikely that veterinarians will need such a criterion in clinical medicine.

Sources: WHO Study Group[148] and Gavin[19]

B. Disorders and conditions (Table 14.4)
1. Physiologic hyperglycemia
   a. Postprandial hyperglycemia: Glucose absorbed after carbohydrate (starch) digestion increases glucose entry into blood. Also, amino acids absorbed after protein digestion stimulate the release of glucagon which then promotes hyperglycemia via gluconeogenesis. [Glucose] in a monogastric animal should return to fasting values within 4 h.
   b. Excitement or fright: Catecholamines (epinephrine and norepinephrine) stimulate glycogenolysis (β_2-adrenergic response) and promote GH release (α_2-adrenergic response).[5] GH then interferes with glucose uptake by myocytes and adipocytes. An α_2-adrenergic stimulus of pancreatic β-cells decreases insulin release and thus reduces glucose utilization by hepatocytes, myocytes, and adipocytes. Also, epinephrine may stimulate ACTH secretion, which would promote hypercortisolemia and associated hyperglycemic effects.[21] The magnitude of the hyperglycemia varies among species and is probably greatest in cats (peak values near 300 mg/dL).[22]
   c. Steroid-associated hyperglycemia: Glucocorticoids produced by "stressed" patients stimulate gluconeogenesis and create a state of insulin resistance by decreasing the number or efficiency of glucose membrane transporters (GLUT-4) and indirectly by increasing glucagon and fatty-acid concentrations.[23,24] However, the number of insulin receptors in target cell membranes may actually be increased because glucocorticoids stimulate their formation.[25]
   d. Diestrus: Progesterone released from the corpus luteum promotes release of GH, which decreases uptake of glucose by myocytes and adipocytes.[26] In dogs, this

Table 14.4. Diseases and conditions that cause hyperglycemia

*Physiologic hyperglycemia: postprandial, excitement, fright, steroid-associated, diestrus
Pathologic hyperglycemia
 Type 1 DM: targeted β-cell destruction, usually leading to absolute insulin deficiency
   (major form in dogs)
  *Idiopathic DM
  Immune-mediated DM
 Type 2 DM: insulin resistance with inadequate compensatory insulin secretory
   response
  *Pancreatic insular amyloidosis (major form in cats)
  Obesity
Other specific types of DM
 *Pancreatic DM: pancreatitis, pancreatic carcinoma
 *Endocrine (nonpancreatic) DM: acromegaly, glucagonoma, hyperadrenocorticism,
   hyperpituitarism, hyperthyroidism, hypothyroidism, pheochromocytoma, bovine
   milk fever, canine hepatocutaneous syndrome
 Drug-induced DM: steroids (glucocorticoids), thyroid hormone, megestrol acetate
 Infectious DM: sepsis, bovine virus diarrhea
 Hyperammonemia: horses and cattle
 Genetic DM: keeshonds, possibly Samoyed dogs
 Anti-insulin antibodies
Pharmacologic or toxicologic hyperglycemia (transient)
 *Oral or intravenous glucose, steroids (glucocorticoids), megestrol acetate, ketamine,
   glucagon, thyroxine, ethylene glycol, xylazine, detomidine, propranolol, insulin
   (Somogyi effect), morphine, progestins

* A relatively common disease or condition

Note: A whole blood [glucose] is lower than serum or plasma [glucose], and thus appropriate reference intervals should be used to determine whether hyperglycemia exists (see the text). The classification system of an Expert Committee of the American Diabetes Association (2000) served as the basis of the DM categories (see the text). The World Health Organization classification (2002) is similar to the above.

  GH is produced by ductal epithelial cells of mammary glands and not by the pituitary gland.[27]

 2. Pathologic hyperglycemia
  a. Type 1 DM (β-cell destruction, usually leading to absolute insulin deficiency); previously called insulin-dependent DM, type I DM, or juvenile-onset DM
   (1) This form of DM is caused by specific destruction of pancreatic β-cells. The destruction is typically considered immune mediated.
   (2) This may be the most common form of canine DM, but documentation of an immune-mediated pathogenesis is uncommon.[28] Investigators have shown that some diabetic dogs have anti-β-cell antibodies.[29]
  b. Type 2 DM (insulin resistance with inadequate compensatory insulin secretory response); previously called non–insulin-dependent DM, type II DM, or adult-onset DM
   (1) This form of DM is most common in cats and is caused by defects in insulin secretion and postinsulin receptor defects in target cells, the two major criteria for type 2 DM.[28]

(2) In cats, evidence indicates that amylin (amyloid polypeptide) that normally is produced by pancreatic β-cells is often involved in the disorder.[30] When amylin is overproduced, it accumulates in pancreatic islets (pancreatic amyloidosis) and damages β-cells. Also, amylin may mediate the insulin resistance in target cells.[31]

(3) Persistent hyperglycemia may lead to glucose toxicosis, a state in which there is down-regulation of glucose transporters on the β-cells. If there are fewer transporters, hyperglycemia is not recognized by β-cells, and thus there is not appropriate insulin secretion.[31,32] Glucose toxicosis may play a role in several types of DM.

(4) Obesity is associated with an increased incidence of DM in cats (and people). As cats changed from a lean state to an obese state, they developed glucose intolerance and a lower GLUT4 expression.[33] The results suggest that decreased GLUT4 expression occurs in obese cats before they develop clinical DM. Alterations in blood nonesterified fatty-acid, leptin, and glucagon concentrations may also be contributing factors to the feline diabetic state.[28] Even though there are alterations in glucose tolerance and insulin secretion in obese dogs, obesity does not appear to cause clinical DM in dogs.[28]

c. Other specific types of DM

(1) Pancreatic DM: Any pancreatic disease (e.g., pancreatitis) may damage enough β-cells to cause DM. In one study, 13 % of the canine diabetic cases were diagnosed as having pancreatitis.[34]

(2) Endocrine (nonpancreatic) DM

(a) Acromegaly in dogs and cats: Excess GH creates insulin resistance by causing insulin receptor and postreceptor defects.[35,36]

(b) Glucagonoma: Excess glucagon antagonizes insulin activity by stimulating gluconeogenesis and inhibiting glucose utilization and storage.

(c) Hyperadrenocorticism: Excess cortisol antagonizes insulin activity by stimulating gluconeogenesis and creating insulin resistance (see Glucose Concentration in Serum, sect. III.B.1.b). In one study, 23 % of the diabetic dogs were diagnosed as having hyperadrenocorticism.[34]

(d) Hyperpituitarism: A diabetic state can be created through excess secretion of GH or ACTH (which stimulates cortisol production).

(i) A pituitary adenoma that was producing ACTH created an insulin-resistant diabetic state in a cat. The adenoma also produced α-melanocyte–stimulating hormone.[37]

(ii) Pituitary adenomas (one producing ACTH and one producing GH) were found in a cat that had clinical signs and laboratory data indicative of hyperadrenocorticism and DM.[38]

(iii) Horses with pituitary adenomas may be hyperglycemic because of secretion of ACTH and the resultant excess production of glucocorticoid hormones.[39,40]

(e) Hyperthyroidism: Studies in cats suggest that hyperthyroidism creates a state of insulin resistance. The mechanism is not known.[41,42]

(f) Hypothyroidism: Some dogs with untreated hypothyroidism are hyperglycemic, but some euthyroid dogs suspected of having hypothyroidism are also hyperglycemic.[43] In another study of hypothyroid dogs that had increased [fructosamine], the hypothyroid dogs were not hyperglycemic.[44] The concurrent finding of hypothyroidism and hyperglycemia may, in some cases, be because of a genetic predisposition to both thyroid disease and DM.[45,46]

(g) Pheochromocytoma: In one study, about 15 % of dogs with pheochromocytomas had mild to moderate hyperglycemia.[47] Catecholamines (epinephrine and norepinephrine) secreted in excess by a pheochromocytoma stimulate glycogenolysis and promote GH release (see Glucose Concentration in Serum, sect. III.B.1.b). Available glycogen stores may limit the severity of hyperglycemia.

(h) Bovine milk fever: The hyperglycemia may be partially caused by Ca^{2+} deficiency; Ca^{2+} is involved in the cleavage of proinsulin to insulin.[48–50] Other physiologic responses in stressed cows may contribute to the hyperglycemia via catecholamines and/or cortisol.

(i) Canine hepatocutaneous syndrome: Hyperglycemia is a common finding in the hepatocutaneous syndrome of dogs. Most of the affected dogs have cirrhosis or other hepatic lesions.[51–53] The syndrome's dermatopathy has been called diabetic dermatopathy, necrolytic migratory erythema, and superficial necrolytic dermatitis. The pathogenesis of the hyperglycemia is not established but may involve insulin resistance, glucagon, GH, or alterations in amino acid, fatty acid, or zinc metabolism. It appears that the diabetic state develops after the onset of hepatic disease, but it has not yet been established if the liver disease causes the diabetic state.

(3) Drug-induced DM: persistent hyperglycemia (2 or more days) associated with use of a drug

(a) Steroids (glucocorticoids) (see Glucose Concentration in Serum, sect. III.B.1.c)

(b) Thyroid hormones: Studies in cats suggest that hyperthyroidism creates a state of insulin resistance, but the mechanism is not known.[41,42] In a study in which thyroxine was given to create experimental hyperthyroidism in dogs, data indicated that the glucose-induced hyperglycemia was prolonged because of defective insulin secretion.[54]

(c) Megestrol acetate: As a steroid, it promotes gluconeogenesis; as a progestin, it stimulates release of GH. Both mechanisms probably occur in dogs, but perhaps only the latter occurs in cats.[55]

(4) Infectious DM

(a) Cattle infected with BVD virus can develop DM that appears to result from damage to β-cells.[56,57]

(b) Sepsis: An early response to endotoxemia is insulin resistance and resultant hyperglycemia. Hypoglycemia may develop later. There are several hormonal and cellular responses in sepsis that alter glucose metabolism.[58] Because animals with DM are considered more susceptible to infections (especially urinary), sepsis could be the cause or result of DM.

(5) Hyperammonemia (horses and cattle): Hyperammonemia occurs in horses and cattle for a variety of reasons (Chapter 13), and hyperglycemia may be a concurrent finding.[59–62] The hyperglycemia may develop because NH_4^+ (ammonium) stimulates the release of glucagon, which then promotes

gluconeogenesis and reduces glucose utilization by tissues.[63] If that is the mechanism, hyperglycemia would depend on glucose production by hepatocytes, and thus hyperglycemia would be more likely when the hyperammonemia is caused by disorders other than hepatic insufficiency (e.g., excess NH_4^+ production in intestine, urea toxicosis, and ammonia forage toxicosis).

    (6) Genetic DM
        (a) An inherited form of DM occurred in keeshonds. The onset of the disorder was frequently before 6 mo of age and was caused by β-cell hypoplasia.[64]
        (b) A probable familial insulin-dependent DM was reported in a group of adult Samoyed dogs. The pathogenesis of the diabetic state was not established.[65]
        (c) Certain breeds of dogs (e.g., Alaskan malamute, Finish spitz, miniature schnauzer, miniature poodle, and English springer spaniel) have a higher incidence of DM, but a genetic pathogenesis is not established in those breeds.[28]
    (7) Anti-insulin antibodies: Dogs with anti-insulin antibodies prior to insulin treatments have been reported, but without case details.[28,66] (Note: Diabetic dogs treated with bovine insulin may develop anti-insulin antibodies.)[67]

3. Pharmacologic or toxicologic hyperglycemia: hyperglycemia associated with occasional or sporadic administration or ingestion of a drug or toxicant (persistent use of some agents may produce a disorder that fulfills diagnostic criteria for DM; see Table 14.3)
    a. Oral or intravenous glucose (dextrose) enters plasma faster than it is utilized, stored, or excreted.
    b. Steroids (glucocorticoids) (see Glucose Concentration in Serum, sect. III.B.1.c)
    c. Megestrol acetate: As a steroid, it promotes gluconeogenesis; as a progestin, it stimulates release of GH. Both mechanisms probably occur in dogs, but perhaps only the latter in cats.[55]
    d. Ketamine stimulates release of epinephrine, which promotes glycogenolysis, reduced uptake and utilization of glucose, and therefore hyperglycemia.[68]
    e. Glucagon antagonizes insulin activity by stimulating gluconeogenesis and inhibiting glucose utilization and storage.
    f. Thyroxine: In a study in which thyroxine was given to create experimental hyperthyroidism in dogs, data indicated that the duration of the hyperglycemia after intravenous glucose infusion was prolonged because of defective insulin secretion.[54]
    g. Ethylene glycol[69] may inhibit glycolysis and the Krebs cycle, and thus may indirectly stimulate gluconeogenesis in "starved" cells.
    h. Xylazine and detomidine[3] bind to α_2-adrenergic receptors on β-cells, resulting in the inhibition of insulin release and thus reduction in glucose utilization by hepatocytes, myocytes, and adipocytes.
    i. Propranolol and other β-adrenergic blockers inhibit insulin release from β-cells.[49] Additionally, propranolol may create a state of insulin resistance.[70]
    j. Insulin (Somogyi effect): In response to excess injected insulin, an animal develops hypoglycemia that stimulates the release of glucagon, epinephrine, cortisol, and GH. Together, these hormones promote hyperglycemia. In a normal

animal, the hyperglycemia is minimized by insulin release. In a diabetic, insulin release does not compensate, and thus the animal develops hyperglycemia that might be misinterpreted as evidence that not enough insulin was given.

k. In humans, thiazides, diazoxide, phenytoin, phenothiazine, and nicotinic acid are reported to produce hyperglycemia by inhibiting insulin release.

l. Progestins stimulate GH release from mammary glands in dogs. GH is also produced by feline mammary glands, but it does not appear to enter blood.[26]

m. Morphine may stimulate the release of GH and ACTH, which could lead to hyperglycemia through multiple processes.[71]

IV. Hypoglycemia

A. Hypoglycemic disorders are caused by increased glucose utilization by tissues, decreased glucose production, or both.

B. A diagnostician should always be alert to the possibility of a mild to extreme spurious hypoglycemia created by the following: (1) in vitro glycolysis in leukocytes, erythrocytes, platelets, and possibly bacteria (see Glucose Concentration in Serum, sect. II.E) or (2) the bromide interference in glucose oxidase assays.

C. Disorders and pathogeneses (Table 14.5)

1. Pathologic hypoglycemia

a. Increased insulin secretion

(1) Functional pancreatic β-cell neoplasia (insulinoma)

(a) Hyperinsulinism will cause both increased glucose utilization by hepatocytes, myocytes, and adipocytes and decreased glucose production by hepatocytes. Insulinomas may cause persistent or sporadic hypoglycemia of sufficient severity to cause weakness and seizures. With sporadic hypoglycemia, a prolonged fast (up to 72 h) may be needed to document hypoglycemia.

(b) Insulinomas have been recognized in dogs for many years. More recently, an insulinoma was reported in a cat.[72] They also occur in ferrets. An insulin-secreting neoplasm can be part of multiple endocrine neoplasia type 1.[73]

(c) Documentation of hyperinsulinism requires a measured [IRI] and increased IRI:G ratio (see Immunoreactive Insulin Concentration in Serum, sect. V).

(2) Xylitol toxicosis

(a) *Xylitol* is a 5-carbon sugar alcohol (polyol) that is used as a sugar substitute (alone or with aspartame) in candy, chewing gum, and some toothpastes. In dogs, it is a potent stimulant for release of insulin, which then promotes increased glucose uptake and utilization and thus hypoglycemia.[74,75] When it is given per os, xylitol causes a greater release of insulin than when glucose is given per os. Xylitol stimulates insulin release in cattle and goats, but not in people and horses.

(b) A dog that ingested xylitol-containing gum (Atkins sugar-free gum) quickly developed hypoglycemia secondary to the stimulated release of insulin.[76,77]

b. Decreased insulin antagonists

(1) Hypoadrenocorticism: When hypoglycemia is present in this disorder, it is probably because of the hypocortisolemia (thus, decreased gluconeogenesis and increased insulin sensitivity in target cells).[78]

Table 14.5. Diseases and conditions that cause hypoglycemia

Pathologic hypoglycemia
  Increased insulin secretion
    *Pancreatic β-cell neoplasia (insulinoma)
    Xylitol toxicosis (dogs)
  Decreased insulin antagonists
    *Hypoadrenocorticism (decreased cortisol)
    Growth hormone deficiency
    Hypopituitarism (decreased cortisol and GH)
  Decreased gluconeogenesis
    *Hepatic insufficiency/failure: acquired, congenital
    *Hypoadrenocorticism (decreased cortisol)
    Neonatal or juvenile hypoglycemia
    Starvation and severe malnutrition
  Decreased glycogenolysis
    Glycogen storage diseases (rare)
  Increased glucose utilization
    *Lactational hypoglycemia (spontaneous bovine ketosis)
    Exertional hypoglycemia (hunting dogs, endurance horses)
  Other pathologic hypoglycemias with uncertain or unknown pathogeneses
    Non–β-cell neoplasms: epithelial and nonepithelial
    *Sepsis, especially with endotoxemia
    Pregnancy hypoglycemia
    Malonic aciduria in Maltese dogs
Pharmacologic or toxicologic hypoglycemia
  Insulin
  Sulfonylurea compounds (glipizide, glyburide)
  Ethanol

* A relatively common disease or condition
Note: Delayed analysis of blood samples or failure to remove serum or plasma from blood cells appropriately will result in falsely low [glucose] because of cell utilization. Bromide ions will cause a falsely low [glucose] when using the i-STAT instrument, and marked leukocytosis and erythrocytosis may accelerate glucose consumption in vitro as cells utilize glucose. Whole blood [glucose] is lower than serum or plasma [glucose], and thus appropriate reference intervals should be used to determine if hypoglycemia exists (see the text).

   (2) GH deficiency: Reduced GH activity promotes increased insulin sensitivity and thus has the potential to cause hypoglycemia, but reports of hypoglycemia in animals with a GH deficiency were not found.

   (3) Hypopituitarism: Hypoglycemia could be caused by decreased secretion of GH or ACTH (and thus less cortisol production), but hypoglycemia is not a common problem in animals with hypopituitarism.

  c. Decreased gluconeogenesis

   (1) Hepatic insufficiency: With marked reduction in functional hepatic mass because of congenital or acquired diseases, there are too few hepatocytes to maintain fasting normoglycemia. Other evidence of hepatic disease or

insufficiency is expected (e.g., increased hepatic enzyme activities, hypoalbu-minemia, decreased [urea nitrogen], and increased [bile acid]).

(2) Hypoadrenocorticism (see the preceding section on hypoadrenocorticism)

(3) Neonatal or juvenile hypoglycemia: This neonatal canine disorder occurs in toy and miniature breeds and may be caused by hepatic immaturity and insufficient gluconeogenesis relative to metabolic rate and glucose consumption.[79]

(4) Starvation: With chronic depletion of body fuels (including proteins and fats), gluconeogenesis may not be able to maintain normoglycemia. A starved state may be caused by lack of food intake, maldigestion, or intestinal malabsorption. Generally, physiologic pathways will attempt to maintain blood glucose at the expense of other body fuels, and thus animals with this form of hypoglycemia are expected to be markedly underweight or emaciated.

d. Decreased glycogenolysis: Congenital deficiencies of enzymes needed for glycoge-nolysis may contribute to hypoglycemia and accumulation of glycogen in cells (glycogen storage diseases).[80]

e. Increased glucose utilization

(1) Lactational hypoglycemia (spontaneous bovine ketosis): During marked milk production (especially in very productive cows), there is a huge need for glucose in mammary glands. The cows will become hypoglycemic if gluconeogenesis cannot meet demand. Ketosis develops secondarily because of enhanced fatty-acid catabolism.[81]

(2) Exertional hypoglycemia: Hunting dogs and endurance horses may become hypoglycemic because glycolysis consumes glucose faster than it is replaced by either glycogenolysis or gluconeogenesis. In contrast, catecholamine and catecholamine-independent factors tend to cause hyperglycemia in exercised animals.

f. Other Pathologic states causing hypoglycemia through unknown mechanisms

(1) Non–β-cell neoplasms (epithelial and nonepithelial): Several non–β-cell neoplasms have been associated with hypoglycemia. Most were leiomyomas, leiomyosarcomas, hepatocellular carcinomas, or renal carcinomas.[82–87] The hypoglycemia might result from secretion of an insulin-like substance, excessive glucose utilization by neoplastic cells, liver dysfunction, or a combination of factors.

(2) Sepsis (especially endotoxemia)

(a) Hypoglycemia is probably due to both increased utilization by tissue and decreased glucose production. Glucose consumption by organisms is an unlikely explanation in most infections. Endotoxins have been shown to produce hypoglycemia, possibly by increasing glucose utiliza-tion.[88] The complex interactions of endotoxins and cytokines result in a decreased perfusion of tissues. Consequently, the target cells switch to anaerobic glycolysis, which requires more glucose to generate energy for the cells; also, leukocytes of the inflammatory response consume more glucose. Concurrently, hepatic production of glucose is reduced because of acidosis and decreased delivery of precursors for gluconeogenesis.[89]

(b) If there are numerous organisms, they might contribute to the hypoglycemia.[90]

(3) Pregnancy hypoglycemia: A ketotic hypoglycemia occurs in late pregnancy in dogs. The pathogenesis of the disorder is not established.[91]

(4) Malonic aciduria in Maltese dogs: Dogs with this metabolic disorder had marked hypoglycemia, but the specific enzymatic defect was not established. The dogs did not have malonyl-coenzyme A (CoA) decarboxylase deficiency.[92] Decreased gluconeogenesis probably contributed to the hypoglycemia, because increased [malonyl-CoA] inhibits pyruvate carboxylase, an enzyme of a gluconeogenesis pathway.

2. Pharmacologic or toxicologic hypoglycemia
   a. Insulin
      (1) An overdose of insulin in a diabetic animal may cause hypoglycemia because of the excess utilization of glucose and decreased gluconeogenesis. The amount of insulin that a diabetic needs will depend on food intake, physical activity, and other factors.
      (2) Surreptitious insulin injections: Malicious administration of insulin to a horse has been reported.[93]
   b. Sulfonylurea compounds (glipizide and glyburide): These drugs, sometimes referred to as oral hypoglycemic agents, directly stimulate insulin secretion and may also improve cellular responses to insulin.[94]
   c. Ethanol: Ethanol oxidation generates reduced nicotinamide adenine dinucleotide (NADH). When there is an acute excess of ethanol, an increased ratio of reduced nicotinamide adenine dinucleotide to nicotinamide adenine dinucleotide (NADH:NAD) blocks gluconeogenesis and may cause hypoglycemia.[95]

V. [Glucose] during insulin therapy
   A. Serial blood [glucose] curve
      1. Data from this procedure may be useful for initial regulation of a diabetic state, for suspected hypoglycemia during therapy, or for poorly controlled DM.
      2. In dogs, the serial blood [glucose] curve is created by measuring blood [glucose] in the following samples from hospitalized patients that are fed and exercised as similarly as possible to their normal routine:[96]
         a. An 8 a.m. sample, just before morning insulin injection
         b. Samples collected at 2 h intervals for 8–12 h (insulin administered q12h) and at 16 h and 24 h if receiving insulin q24h
         c. An 8 p.m. sample, just before evening insulin injection (insulin q12h)
      3. One set of recommendations for altering insulin dose (porcine lente insulin, subcutaneous, q12h) in diabetic dogs is as follows:[96]
         a. Increase the insulin dose if the nadir [glucose] is > 145 mg/dL and the 8 a.m. and 8 p.m. samples had [glucose] > 180 mg/dL.
         b. Do not change the insulin dose if the nadir [glucose] is between 90 and 145 mg/dL and the 8 a.m. and 8 p.m. samples had [glucose] > 180 mg/dL.
         c. Decrease the insulin dose if nadir [glucose] is < 90 mg/dL or if either the 8 a.m. or the 8 p.m. sample had [glucose] < 180 mg/dL.
      4. Guidelines for cats are similar but with greater decision thresholds (e.g., nadir values between 100 and 150 mg/dL).[97]
      5. Because there can be marked variation in the serial blood [glucose] curves from one day to the next, especially during hospitalization, a decision to alter an insulin dose should consider other clinical information.[96]

6. Problems that may be revealed by serial blood [glucose] curves include the following:
    a. Insufficient insulin dose: If so, increase the dose.
    b. Too short an insulin effect: If so, use longer-acting insulin or give q12h.
    c. Overlap of insulin effect between insulin doses: If so, use shorter-acting insulin.
    d. The Somogyi effect (see Glucose Concentration in Serum, sect. III.B.3.j): If so, reduce the insulin dose and repeat the curve in 1 wk.
B. Unexpected hyperglycemia: There are several possible reasons for inadequate response to insulin treatments.
    1. There may be an insufficient insulin dosage, the insulin may have deteriorated, or the owner may be having problems injecting the insulin.
    2. The caloric intake in the diet may have increased.
    3. A state of insulin resistance may have developed because of stress, hyperadrenocorticism, infections, hypothyroidism, pancreatitis, or acromegaly.
C. Unexpected hypoglycemia
    1. As previously indicated (Glucose Concentration in Serum, sect. IV.C.2.a), an insulin overdose may cause hypoglycemia.
    2. Other reasons for hypoglycemia in treated diabetic animals include decreased caloric intake (e.g., anorexia, vomiting, exocrine pancreatic insufficiency, and inflammatory intestinal disease) and excess glucose utilization by tissues (e.g., excess physical activity and increased metabolic state). The diabetic state might also be due to a transient disorder that decreased in severity or resolved itself.

KETOAMINES: FRUCTOSAMINE AND GLYCATED HEMOGLOBIN (Hgb)

I.   Physiologic processes
     A. When glucose reacts nonenzymatically with a protein's amino groups, mostly at lysine sites, a Schiff base is formed that then converts to a more stable ketoamine adduct.
        1. Generally speaking, fructosamines are glycated proteins. In clinical chemistry, *fructosamine* refers to ketoamines that are formed by the posttranslational irreversible nonenzymatic linking of glucose to albumin or other plasma proteins (mostly IgG); glycated albumin accounts for about 80 % of human serum ketoamines.[98] The carbon backbone of these ketoamines is identical to fructose (hence the name "fructosamine"). The half-life of fructosamine molecules is generally stated to be near 2–3 wk, but the half-life varies among species and can be altered during pathologic states.
        2. Glycated (glycosylated) Hgb is a ketoamine formed by the nonenzymatic addition of glucose to Hgb. The half-life of glycated Hgb is generally stated to be 2–3 mo but varies with the circulating life span of erythrocytes (e.g., dogs ≈ 100 d, cats ≈ 70 d, and cattle ≈ 150 d). Hemoglobin A_{1c} is the major subset of human glycated Hgb, representing glycation of the amino terminus of the β-globin chain.
     B. The formation of ketoamines in blood is positively correlated with the magnitude and duration of hyperglycemia, whereas the removal of ketoamines depends on the degradation or loss of the parent molecules (e.g., albumin or Hgb). Transient hyperglycemia, as may occur after intravenous glucose administration or in physiologic responses, does not significantly affect the concentrations of the ketoamines in dogs (nitroblue tetrazolium assay)[99] or cattle (nitroblue tetrazolium assay)[100] and should not affect ketoamine concentrations in any species.

II.   Analytical concepts
   A. [Fructosamine]
       1. In the nitroblue tetrazolium assay, fructosamine acts as a reducing agent in an
           alkaline medium to generate formazane, which is detected spectrophotometrically.
           Nonspecific reduction occurs within the first 10 min, so measurements are taken
           after that time. However, other reducing agents in serum could cause false-positive
           results. In contrast, the fructosyl lysine oxidase assay is considered to be specific for
           fructosyl lysine, a specific glycated amino acid.
           a. In a comparison study, the fructosamine concentrations in canine sera deter-
               mined by the nitroblue tetrazolium assay were about 3–4 times those determined
               by the enzymatic assay (about 100 µmol/L).[101] This study raises a concern about
               the validity of the [fructosamine] reported from the nitroblue tetrazolium assay.
           b. Modifications of the nitroblue tetrazolium assay to remove actions of reducing
               substances other than fructosamine reportedly resulted in [fructosamine] of about
               10 % that of the original nitroblue tetrazolium assays.[102]
       2. When measured by spectrophotometric assays, hemolyzed and icteric samples can
           cause erroneous results.
   B. Glycated Hgb concentrations or percentages
       1. Glycated Hgb has been measured by chromatographic, immunoturbidimetric, and
           chemical assays, each with its own limitations. Some assays were designed to
           specifically detect human hemoglobin A_{1c}, whereas others (e.g., chemical methods)
           detect multiple forms of glycated Hgb.
       2. Results are usually reported as the percentage of total Hgb that is glycated.
       3. If lipemia is present, the assay should be completed after washing the erythrocytes;
           lipemia will falsely increase percentages in some assays.[103]
       4. There was good agreement between a colorimetric assay and a chromatographic
           method with canine blood.[104]
       5. An immunoturbidimetric assay, manufactured for measuring human [glycated Hgb],
           has been used to measure canine [glycated Hgb].[99,105]

III.   Increased [fructosamine] and increased glycated hemoglobin percentage or concentration
       (Table 14.6)
   A. Diabetes mellitus: Increased concentrations of fructosamine or glycated hemoglobin
       occur in animals with DM. Concentrations of these glycated proteins can be used to
       monitor the effectiveness of controlling the diabetic state. [Ketoamine] has been
       measured in diabetic dogs[102,106–108] and cats.[109–113]
   B. Hypothyroidism
       1. Mildly increased [fructosamine] (assay type not reported) was found in hypothyroid
           dogs that were not considered to have DM.[43] In another study of normoglycemic

Table 14.6. Diseases and conditions that increase [ketoamine]

Fructosamine	Glycated hemoglobin
*Hyperglycemia (persistent)[a]	*Hyperglycemia (persistent)
Hypothyroidism	

* A relatively common disease or condition
[a] See Table 14.4 for causes of hyperglycemia.

Table 14.7. Diseases and conditions that decrease [ketoamine]

Fructosamine	Glycated hemoglobin
*Hypoglycemia (persistent)[a]	*Hypoglycemia (persistent)
Hypoproteinemia	Anemia (see the text for variables)
Hyperthyroidism	

* A relatively common disease or condition
[a] See Table 14.5 for causes of hypoglycemia.

    normoproteinemic hypothyroid dogs, 9 of 11 had an increased [fructosamine] (nitroblue tetrazolium assay), and the concentrations decreased after initiation of thyroid hormone supplementation.[44]

2. Based on studies in people, the increased [fructosamine] is the result of an increased albumin half-life (reduced protein turnover).[114]

C. Hyperproteinemia

    1. In theory, hyperproteinemia could cause increased [fructosamine]. However, variations in the duration of the hyperproteinemia and variations in albumin to globulin ratios result in variable fructosamine concentrations in hyperproteinemic samples.[115,116]

    2. In one study, corrected [fructosamine] in hyperproteinemic animals did not improve the diagnostic value of [fructosamine].[115]

IV. Decreased [fructosamine] and decreased glycated hemoglobin percentage or concentration (Table 14.7)

A. Decreased [fructosamine]

    1. Insulinoma in dogs: Persistent hypoglycemia caused by an inappropriate release of insulin can lead to a decreased serum [fructosamine].[117,118]

    2. Hypoproteinemia and hypoalbuminemia

        a. Normoglycemic dogs with hypoalbuminemia had decreased fructosamine concentrations.[116,119]

        b. About 67 % of normoglycemic cats with hypoproteinemia had decreased serum [fructosamine].[116] The [fructosamine] was better correlated with [total protein] than with [albumin].

    3. Decreased [fructosamine] has been associated with azotemia and hyperlipidemia in normoglycemic dogs.[116] However, the report did not describe whether the azotemic or hyperlipidemic dogs had dysproteinemias.

    4. Cats with hyperthyroidism have significantly lower serum fructosamine concentrations than healthy cats.[120,121] Similar findings are found in people with thyrotoxicosis.[122]

B. Decreased glycated Hgb percentage or concentration

    1. Insulinoma: Persistent hypoglycemia caused by an inappropriate release of insulin can lead to a decreased glycated Hgb percentage or concentration.[107,108]

    2. Anemia: If [erythrocyte] is stable, then the degree of glycated Hgb formation will primarily depend on blood [glucose] during the life span of the erythrocytes.

        a. If there is an acute anemia (e.g., because of hemorrhage or hemolysis) and a subsequent regenerative response, then the glycated Hgb concentration and percentage will be reduced because young erythrocytes have less glycated Hgb and blood [Hgb] is decreased.

  b. If there is anemia of any origin and the animal has not been hyperglycemic, then the [glycated Hgb] will be decreased because the blood [Hgb] is decreased.[108]

  c. The glycated Hgb percentages in dogs with acute and chronic anemias were similar to those in dogs with hypoglycemias caused by β-cell neoplasia.[108]

V. Correction of the [fructosamine] for abnormal protein concentrations

  A. Because dysproteinemias affect [fructosamine] independently of blood [glucose], some authors have recommended correction formulas to adjust for the dysproteinemia (Eq. 14.2). The formulas suggest the relationships are completely linear and depend only on albumin or total protein concentrations, but the degree of glycation per mole of albumin depends also on the half-lives of the proteins. At a lower [albumin], the catabolism of albumin is decreased, so its half-life is increased. This results in greater glycation per mole of albumin, thus somewhat counteracting the decrease in fructosamine caused by hypoalbuminemia.[123] Consequently, the correlation between albumin and fructosamine concentrations is poor to moderate.

$$\text{Corrected canine [fructosamine]} = \text{observed [fructosamine]} \times \frac{\text{median [albumin] for healthy dogs}}{\text{observed [albumin]}}$$
$$(14.2a.)$$

$$\text{Example: corrected canine [fructosamine]} = 180 \ \mu\text{mol/L} \times \frac{3.3 \ \text{g/dL}}{2.0 \ \text{g/dL}} = 297 \ \mu\text{mol/L}$$

$$\text{Corrected feline [fructosamine]} = \text{observed [fructosamine]} \times \frac{\text{median [total protein] for healthy cats}}{\text{observed [total protein]}}$$
$$(14.2b.)$$

  B. A canine correction formula using serum [albumin] was recommended because of a greater correlation coefficient (r) for serum [albumin] (r = 0.79) than for [total protein] (r = 0.54).[116] However, in one study involving diabetic and nondiabetic dogs, use of the corrected concentrations did not substantially increase the diagnostic sensitivity or diagnostic specificity of the [fructosamine] (nitroblue tetrazolium assay) for DM.[115]

  C. A feline correction formula using serum [total protein] was recommended because of a greater correlation coefficient for serum [total protein] (r = 0.68) than for [albumin].[116] Because there was very poor correlation with serum [albumin], the authors suggested that a greater proportion of the glycated proteins were globulins.

IMMUNOREACTIVE INSULIN (IRI) CONCENTRATION IN SERUM OR PLASMA

I. Physiologic processes

  A. Insulin is a polypeptide hormone ($M_r \approx 6000$) with 51 amino acids in two chains (A and B) linked by disulfide bridges. The amino acid sequences of insulin molecules of dogs and pigs are identical and have one amino acid difference from human insulin. Equine insulin has one amino acid difference from porcine insulin. Feline and bovine insulin molecules are similar but have minor differences from the molecules of canine, porcine, and human insulin.[94,124]

B. Physiologic stimuli for insulin secretion include increased concentrations of glucose, xylitol, amino acids, and several hormones (glucagon, gastrin, secretin, pancreozymin, gastrointestinal polypeptide, and β-adrenergic hormones).

C. Inhibitors of insulin secretion include somatostatin, α_2-adrenergic agonists, and β-adrenergic antagonists.[70]

D. Preproinsulin is made by ribosomes of pancreatic β-cells and is quickly cleaved to proinsulin that is stored in secretory granules of the Golgi complex. Insulin is formed after cleavage enzymes (some Ca^{2+} regulated) break peptide bonds to form insulin, C-peptide, and split peptides. [Glucose] regulates synthesis of proinsulin and one cleavage enzyme. Insulin and C-peptide secretions are equimolar; small amounts of proinsulin and split peptides are also released.[49]

E. The major actions of insulin are illustrated in Fig. 14.1.

II. Analytical concepts

A. Terms and units

1. IRI is the preferred term for immunoassay measurements of serum or plasma insulin for two reasons: (1) measurements may include proinsulin, and (2) measurements of insulin are in immunoreactive units, not biologic activity units of injectable insulin.

2. Units: $\mu U/mL = mU/L$; $\mu U/mL \times 7.175 = pmol/L$; and $\mu g/L \times 172.2 = pmol/L$ (SI unit, nearest 5 pmol/L)[7]

B. Assays

1. Most measurements of IRI are made using commercial radioimmunoassay kits and therefore anti-insulin antibody reagents. Chemiluminescent assays and enzyme-linked immunosorbent assays (ELISAs) are also available.

2. The antibody in commercial assays may have been developed to react with porcine or human insulin. There is sufficient cross-immunoreactivity that commercial assays have been validated for canine insulin. Commercial assays may not be valid for feline insulin.[125]

3. Wide ranges of [IRI] have been reported for canine, feline, and human samples assessed with commercial insulin assays.[49,125,126] The variation may partially be due to differences in standard or calibrator solutions, but unacceptable variation persisted after laboratories used a common calibrator.[49] Because of this variation:

a. A patient's [IRI] should be compared against reference intervals established for the assay used to measure the patient's [IRI], and the assay should have been validated for the species being tested. Diagnostic decision limits for [IRI] or IRI : G ratios need to be established for each validated insulin assay.

b. Laboratories offering quantitation of [IRI] should thoroughly evaluate their insulin assays for performance characteristics with varying lots of reagents.

4. Samples

a. An [IRI] may be determined in serum or heparinized plasma. EDTA-plasma can give falsely increased values in some assays.[49]

b. IRI is stable in whole blood at room temperature for at least 5 h. In serum, it is stable for 7 d at 4 °C and for several months at −20 °C. Thawing and refreezing should be avoided.[49]

c. Because glucose, amino acids, and several gastric, intestinal, and pancreatic hormones influence insulin secretion, it is very important that samples be collected from fasted animals to reduce the effects of these physiologic factors.

Table 14.8. Diseases and conditions that cause hyperinsulinemia

Increased insulin production and release
   *Functional pancreatic β-cell neoplasia (insulinoma)
   Xylitol toxicosis
   Hyperglycemic disorders not caused by decreased insulin production (see the text)

* A relatively common disease or condition
Note: Anti-insulin antibodies may produce a positive interference in some assays.

III.   Hyperinsulinemia
   A.   The major reason for measuring [IRI] is to document the inappropriate release of insulin from neoplastic β-cells; that is, too much insulin released for the animal's plasma or serum [glucose].
   B.   Disorders and pathogeneses (Table 14.8)
       1.   Increased insulin production and release
           a.   Functional pancreatic β-cell neoplasia (insulinoma): Neoplastic β-cells may consistently or sporadically produce insulin, which causes hypoglycemia because of enhanced glycolysis, reduced gluconeogenesis, and increased glucose uptake by myocytes and adipocytes.
           b.   Hyperglycemia not caused by decreased insulin production
               (1)   Hyperinsulinemia is expected with physiologic hyperglycemia because hyperglycemia stimulates the production and release of insulin.
               (2)   Hyperinsulinemia is expected with pathologic and pharmacologic hyperglycemias if insulin release from β-cells is not defective. Also, a state of insulin resistance may initiate or augment a hyperglycemic state and concurrent hyperinsulinemia.
       2.   Anti-insulin antibodies: The presence of anti-insulin antibodies may result in a falsely increased [IRI] in some assays (see Fig. 17.2 for the concept). Anti-insulin antibodies may arise from spontaneous pathologic processes or insulin therapy.

IV.   Hypoinsulinemia
   A.   Documenting hypoinsulinemia could help in classifying or characterizing DM states; for example, confirming type 1 DM, staging type 2 DM, or assessing insulin status in other diabetic states.
       1.   Measuring [IRI] in hyperglycemic animals is not common. The infrequent measurement of [IRI] in DM cases is probably due to many factors, such as cost, lack of standardized assays, and lack of diagnostic or prognostic criteria associated with variations in [IRI] in different types of DM.
       2.   A deficiency in insulin can be defined in two ways: (1) an absolute deficiency in which [IRI] is below an appropriate reference interval, and (2) a relative deficiency in which the amount of insulin is insufficient to maintain a normal carbohydrate metabolism. Fasting plasma [IRI] has been used as a method of detecting insulin resistance in cats fitting the second definition.[127]
   B.   Disorders or conditions where [IRI] is expected to decrease
       1.   Pathologic hypoinsulinemia
           a.   *Type 1 DM*: Insulin production is decreased because of the destruction of β-cells.
           b.   *Type 2 DM*: Advanced stages of pancreatic amyloidosis involve β-cell damage and thus decreased insulin production.

2. Physiologic hypoinsulinemia: Animals with a variety of hypoglycemic states (see Table 14.5) would be expected to have hypoinsulinemia if the hypoglycemic state was not caused by increased insulin secretion.

3. In some assays, the presence of anti-insulin antibodies can cause falsely decreased values.

V. Immunoreactive insulin to glucose (IRI : G) ratio

A. Because insulin production and release from β-cells depend on plasma [glucose], an IRI : G ratio should indicate whether the measured [IRI] is appropriate for the degree of glucose stimulation. When used, the ratio is typically calculated by using conventional units for both IRI and glucose concentrations (Eq. 14.3).

$$IRI{:}G = \frac{[IRI] \times 100}{[glucose]} \qquad\qquad \textbf{(14.3.)}$$

with [IRI] in μU/mL and glucose in mg/dL; thus IRI:G ratio unit is μU/mg glucose

B. The lack of analytical agreement among insulin assays requires that reference intervals for IRI : G ratios be established for each assay, which is a task that is not commonly accomplished.

C. Interpretation of the fasting IRI : G ratio (assuming valid concentrations of IRI and glucose and comparison to an appropriate reference interval for IRI : G ratio)

1. Increased
   a. If associated with hypoglycemia, then insulin is contributing to the hypoglycemia.
   b. If associated with normoglycemia or hyperglycemia, then an increased IRI : G ratio may indicate insulin resistance. When this ratio was calculated from values measured in samples from fasted cats, it was shown to be a relatively reliable method for assessing insulin sensitivity compared to several other methods.[127]

2. Within the reference interval
   a. If associated with hypoglycemia, then a pathologic state other than hyperinsulinemia is causing the hypoglycemia.
   b. If associated with hyperglycemia, then a factor other than insulin deficiency is causing the hyperglycemia.

3. Decreased: If associated with hyperglycemia, then an absolute insulin deficiency is present that could be due to β-cell damage or glucose toxicosis.[31]

D. The IRI : G ratio may be difficult to interpret for reasons other than the variations created by different assays.

1. Substances other than glucose influence insulin release from β-cells.

2. Much of the released insulin is removed from portal blood by hepatocytes and thus does not appear in peripheral blood.

E. Amended insulin to glucose ratio and the "< 30 mg/dL theory"

1. In 1971, Turner and associates reported an "observation that the plasma insulin levels of normal subjects [humans] are near zero if the plasma glucose is 30 mg/dL or less"[128] and referenced an article by Turner, Oakley, and Nabarro that was in press. Based on the observation, they proposed that [glucose] above 30 mg/dL would result in insulin entry into peripheral blood. To evaluate [IRI] in hypoglycemic people, they modified the IRI : G ratio by subtracting 30 mg/dL from the measured

[glucose]. If the modification was valid, there would be a direct relationship between insulin and glucose concentrations over 30 mg/dL; that is, x µU of insulin for every y mg of glucose > 30.

2. In 1973, Turner, Oakley, and Nabarro reported changes in plasma [insulin] during ethanol-induced hypoglycemia in obese and nonobese people.[129]

   a. They did not mention their "< 30 mg/dL" theory or proposed amended IRI:G ratio of 1971, and their published data were not consistent with the theory. Insulin was not detected in several samples with a [glucose] of 40–65 mg/dL. There were only three samples with a [glucose] < 30 mg/dL; insulin values in those samples ranged from 0–2.0 µU/mL.

   b. They did write, "The fall in plasma insulin was a function of the fall, rather than of the absolute values of the plasma glucose."

   c. Another variable not considered was the difference between insulin concentrations in portal and peripheral blood. Because much of the secreted insulin is removed from portal blood by hepatocytes, assessment of insulin secretion stimulated by glucose is better evaluated by measuring portal blood concentrations, which is a technique generally limited to experimental investigations.

3. Many veterinary publications have included the use of the amended IRI:G ratio to evaluate [IRI] and [glucose] in domestic and nondomestic animals. There have also been several attempts to squelch the use of the amended IRI:G ratio, but it seems to have a life of its own.[130–134] The amended IRI:G ratio should not be used.

IMMUNOREACTIVE GLUCAGON (IRG) CONCENTRATION IN PLASMA

I. Physiologic processes

A. *Pancreatic glucagon* (M_r = 3485) is a 29-amino-acid polypeptide hormone that is secreted by the α-cells of the pancreas. Glucagon is a member of a superfamily of peptide hormones (collectively called GLPs) that influence or regulate several digestive and metabolic processes. Other than glucagon, the major GLP involved in glucose metabolism is GLP-1.[135]

   1. The major role of glucagon is to maintain blood [glucose] during fasting. Stimuli for pancreatic glucagon secretion include hypoglycemia (which may be induced by exercise), increased amino acids, hypercortisolemia, and probably hypoinsulinemia.

   2. *GLP-1*, which is released from L cells (large granule cells) of the intestinal mucosa after feeding, stimulates the release of insulin and reduces postprandial hyperglycemia. Prior to the identification of GLP-1, the hormone was referred to as gut glucagon, which cross-reacted with glucagon in some immunoassays.

B. Proglucagon is produced by pancreatic α-cells, intestinal L cells, and the parasympathetic nucleus of the vagus nerve.[135] A variety of factors control the cleavage of proglucagon into glucagon (primarily in the pancreas), GLP-1 (primarily in intestine), and other GLPs.

C. The major actions of glucagon are illustrated in Fig. 14.1.

II. Analytical concepts

A. Terms and units

   1. The term *IRG* should be reserved for the glucagon that is measured by immunoassays that are specific for pancreatic glucagon. Unfortunately, some

radioimmunoassay antibodies also detect other GLPs, especially GLP-1 or gut glucagon. Some authors refer to IRG as *glucagon-like immunoreactivity*.

   2. Unit conversion: pg/mL = ng/L (SI unit, nearest 10 ng/L)[7]

B. Assays

   1. For many years, the gold standard assay for canine IRG was a radioimmunoassay with Unger's 30K antibody, an antibody that was considered specific for the C terminus of glucagon.[136] Other investigators have shown varying degrees of antibody specificity for pancreatic glucagon and glucagon-like immunoreactivity.[137]

   2. One group of investigators described validation studies using an anti-(bovine glucagon) antibody to assess [glucagon] in dogs, cats, sheep, cows, and horses. In the fasting state, about 30 % of the glucagon-like immunoreactivity was pancreatic glucagon. Their antibody did cross-react with larger molecular forms that had glucagon-like immunoreactivity.[138]

   3. Some investigators use commercial glucagon assays.[139] Results from two commercial glucagon assays differed considerably (> 10-fold in some plasma samples) in a screening evaluation.[140]

C. Samples

   1. Most investigators consider IRG to be very unstable in blood, and thus special handling is recommended.[49] Immediately after collection, EDTA-blood is immersed in an ice bath and a protease inhibitor (aprotinin) is added. Plasma is separated from erythrocytes in a 4 °C centrifuge and then frozen at −20 °C. Samples should be protected from light.

   2. Serum has been used in some studies.[141] There is evidence that the stability of radiolabeled glucagon is not the same in all species.[142] In some assay systems, degradation of radiolabeled glucagon will cause falsely increased measured values.[143]

   3. The presence of arginine can lead to an overestimation of measured [IRG].[144] This finding must be considered when interpreting results of the arginine stimulation tests that have been used to validate IRG assays; that is, an increased [IRG] after arginine stimulation was used as evidence that the assay was measuring glucagon released from the α-cells.

III. Hyperglucagonemia associated with glucagonomas

A. Because glucagon is a hormone involved in carbohydrate and lipid metabolism, there are many reports of immunoreactive glucagon concentrations in various physiologic and pathologic states. However, [IRG] has very limited use in veterinary diagnostic efforts.

B. Some dogs with pancreatic glucagonomas have a characteristic superficial necrolytic dermatitis, but not all dogs with the dermatologic disorder have glucagonomas.

   1. Increased plasma [IRG] has been reported in some dogs with the disorder.[53,139,145,146]

   2. In a study involving 22 dogs with superficial necrolytic dermatitis, pancreatic neoplasms were not found (19 of 22 had histologic pancreatic examinations), and immunoreactive glucagon concentrations were within the reference interval in the five dogs that were evaluated.[147]

References

1. Adams HR. 1995. Adrenergic agonists and antagonists. In: Adams HR, ed. *Veterinary Pharmacology and Therapeutics*, 7th edition, 91–116. Ames: Iowa State University Press.
2. Rizza RA, Cryer PE, Haymond MW, Gerich JE. 1980. Adrenergic mechanisms of catecholamine action on glucose homeostasis in man. Metabolism 29:1155–1163.

3. Thurmon JC, Tranquilli WJ, Benson GJ. 1996. Preanesthetics and anesthetic adjuncts. In: Thurmon JC, Tranquilli WJ, Benson GJ, eds. *Lumb and Jones' Veterinary Anesthesia*, 3rd edition, 183–209. Baltimore: Williams & Wilkins.

4. Adams HR. 2001. Introduction to neurohormonal transmission and the autonomic nervous system. In: Adams HR, ed. *Veterinary Pharmacology and Therapeutics*, 8th edition, 69–90. Ames: Iowa State University Press.

5. McMahon CD, Radcliff RP, Lookingland KJ, Tucker HA. 2001. Neuroregulation of growth hormone secretion in domestic animals. Domest Anim Endocrinol 20:65–87.

6. Simmons HA, Ford EJH. 1991. Gluconeogenesis from propionate produced in the colon of the horse. Br Vet J 147:340–345.

7. Lundberg GD, Iverson C, Radulescu G. 1986. Now read this: The SI units are here. J Am Med Assoc 255:2329–2339.

8. Laessig RH, Hassemer DJ, Westgard JO, Carey RN, Feldbruegge DH, Schwartz TH. 1976. Assessment of the serum separator tube as an intermediate storage device within the laboratory. Am J Clin Pathol 66:653–657.

9. Bush VJ, Janu MR, Bathur F, Wells A, Dasgupta A. 2001. Comparison of BD Vacutainer SST Plus Tubes with BD SST II Plus Tubes for common analytes. Clin Chim Acta 306:139–143.

10. Christopher MM, O'Neill S. 2000. Effect of specimen collection and storage on blood glucose and lactate concentrations in healthy, hyperthyroid and diabetic cats. Vet Clin Pathol 29:22–28.

11. Chan AY, Swaminathan R, Cockram CS. 1989. Effectiveness of sodium fluoride as a preservative of glucose in blood. Clin Chem 35:315–317.

12. Chan AY, Ho CS, Cockram CS, Swaminathan R. 1990. Handling of blood specimens for glucose analysis. J Clin Chem Clin Biochem 28:185–186.

13. Astles JR, Sedor FA, Toffaletti JG. 1996. Evaluation of the YSI 2300 glucose analyzer: Algorithm-corrected results are accurate and specific. Clin Biochem 29:27–31.

14. Fogh-Andersen N, D'Orazio P. 1998. Proposal for standardizing direct-reading biosensors for blood glucose. Clin Chem 44:655–659.

15. Fogh-Andersen N, Wimberley PD, Thode J, Siggaard-Andersen O. 1990. Direct reading glucose electrodes detect the molality of glucose in plasma and whole blood. Clin Chim Acta 189:33–38.

16. Grazaitis DM, Sexson WR. 1980. Erroneously high Dextrostix values caused by isopropyl alcohol. Pediatrics 66:221–223.

17. Astles JR, Petros WP, Peters WP, Sedor FA. 1995. Artifactual hypoglycemia associated with hematopoietic cytokines. Arch Pathol Lab Med 119:713–716.

18. Macaron CI, Kadri A, Macaron Z. 1981. Nucleated red blood cells and artifactual hypoglycemia. Diabetes Care 4:113–115.

19. Gavin JR III. 2000. Report of the Expert Committee on the Diagnosis and Classification of Diabetes Mellitus. Diabetes Care 23(Suppl 1):S4–S19.

20. Catchpole B, Ristic JM, Fleeman LM, Davison LJ. 2005. Canine diabetes mellitus: Can old dogs teach us new tricks? Diabetologia 48:1948–1956.

21. Labrie F, Giguere V, Proulx L, Lefevre G. 1984. Interactions between CRF, epinephrine, vasopressin and glucocorticoids in the control of ACTH secretion. J Steroid Biochem 20:153–160.

22. Rand JS, Kinnaird E, Baglioni A, Blackshaw J, Priest J. 2002. Acute stress hyperglycemia in cats is associated with struggling and increased concentrations of lactate and norepinephrine. J Vet Intern Med 16:123–132.

23. Munck A, Náray-Fejes-Tóth A. 2001. Glucocorticoid action: Physiology. In: DeGroot LJ, Jameson JL, eds. *Endocrinology*, 4th edition, 1632–1646. Philadelphia: WB Saunders.

24. Drucker DJ. 2001. Glucagon secretion, a cell metabolism, and glucagon action. In: DeGroot LJ, Jameson JL, eds. *Endocrinology*, 4th edition, 728–736. Philadelphia: WB Saunders.

25. Moller DE, Flier JS. 1991. Insulin resistance: Mechanisms, syndromes, and implications. N Engl J Med 325:938–948.

26. Eigenmann JE, Eigenmann RY, Rijnberk A, van der Gaag I, Zapf J, Froesch ER. 1983. Progesterone-controlled growth hormone overproduction and naturally occurring canine diabetes and acromegaly. Acta Endocrinol 104:167–176.

27. Rijnberk A, Mol JA. 1997. Progestin-induced hypersecretion of growth hormone: An introductory review. J Reprod Fertil Suppl 51:335–338.

28. Hoenig M. 2002. Comparative aspects of diabetes mellitus in dogs and cats. Mol Cell Endocrinol 197:221–229.

29. Hoenig M, Dawe DL. 1992. A qualitative assay for beta cell antibodies: Preliminary results in dogs with diabetes mellitus. Vet Immunol Immunopathol 32:195–203.

30. O'Brien TD. 2002. Pathogenesis of feline diabetes mellitus. Mol Cell Endocrinol 197:213–219.

31. Lutz TA, Rand JS. 1995. Pathogenesis of feline diabetes mellitus. Vet Clin North Am Small Anim Pract 25:527–552.

32. Hostettler-Allen RL, Tappy L, Blum JW. 1994. Insulin resistance, hyperglycemia, and glucosuria in intensively milk-fed calves. J Anim Sci 72:160–173.

33. Brennan CL, Hoenig M, Ferguson DC. 2004. GLUT4 but not GLUT1 expression decreases early in the development of feline obesity. Domest Anim Endocrinol 26:291–301.

34. Hess RS, Saunders M, Van Winkle TJ, Ward CR. 2000. Concurrent disorders in dogs with diabetes mellitus: 221 cases (1993–1998). J Am Vet Med Assoc 217:1166–1173.

35. Peterson ME, Taylor RS, Greco DS, Nelson RW, Randolph JF, Foodman MS, Moroff SD, Morrison SA, Lothrop CD. 1990. Acromegaly in 14 cats. J Vet Intern Med 4:192–201.

36. Hurty CA, Flatland B. 2005. Feline acromegaly: A review of the syndrome. J Am Anim Hosp Assoc 41:292–297.

37. Meij BP, van der Vlugt-Meijer RH, van den Ingh TSGAM, Flik G, Rijnberk A. 2005. Melanotroph pituitary adenoma in a cat with diabetes mellitus. Vet Pathol 42:92–97.

38. Meij BP, van der Vlugt-Meijer RH, van den Ingh TSGAM, Rijnberk A. 2004. Somatotroph and corticotroph pituitary adenoma (double adenoma) in a cat with diabetes mellitus and hyperadrenocorticism. J Comp Pathol 130:209–215.

39. Reed SM. 1998. Pituitary adenomas: Equine Cushing's disease. In: Reed SM, Bayly WM, eds. *Equine Internal Medicine*, 912–916. Philadelphia: WB Saunders.

40. Keen JA, McLaren M, Chandler KJ, McGorum BC. 2004. Biochemical indices of vascular function, glucose metabolism and oxidative stress in horses with equine Cushing's disease. Equine Vet J 36:226–229.

41. Hoenig M, Peterson ME, Ferguson DC. 1992. Glucose tolerance and insulin secretion in spontaneously hyperthyroid cats. Res Vet Sci 53:338–341.

42. Hoenig M, Ferguson DC. 1989. Impairment of glucose tolerance in hyperthyroid cats. J Endocrinol 121:249–251.

43. Dixon RM, Reid SW, Mooney CT. 1999. Epidemiological, clinical, haematological and biochemical characteristics of canine hypothyroidism. Vet Rec 145:481–487.

44. Reusch CE, Gerber B, Boretti FS. 2002. Serum fructosamine concentrations in dogs with hypothyroidism. Vet Res Commun 26:531–536.

45. Hargis AM, Stephens LC, Benjamin SA, Brewster RD, Brooks RK. 1981. Relationship of hypothyroidism to diabetes mellitus, renal amyloidosis, and thrombosis in purebred beagles. Am J Vet Res 42:1077–1081.

46. Feldman EC, Nelson RW. 1996. Hypothyroidism. In: *Canine and Feline Endocrinology and Reproduction*, 2nd edition, 68–117. Philadelphia: WB Saunders.

47. Barthez PY, Marks SL, Woo J, Feldman EC, Matteucci M. 1997. Pheochromocytoma in dogs: 61 cases (1984–1995). J Vet Intern Med 11:272–278.

48. Witzel DA, Littledike ET. 1973. Suppression of insulin secretion during induced hypocalcemia. Endocrinology 93:761–766.

49. Sacks DB. 1999. Carbohydrates. In: Burtis CA, Ashwood ER, eds. *Tietz Textbook of Clinical Chemistry*, 3rd edition, 750–808. Philadelphia: WB Saunders.

50. Steiner DF, Bell GI, Rubenstein AH, Chan SJ. 2001. Chemistry and biosynthesis of the islet hormones: Insulin, islet amyloid peptide (amylin), glucagon, somatostatin, and pancreatic polypeptide. In: DeGroot LJ, Jameson JL, eds. *Endocrinology*, 4th edition, 667–696. Philadelphia: WB Saunders.

51. McNeil PE. 1992. The underlying pathology of the hepatocutaneous syndrome: A report of 18 cases. In: Ihrke PJ, Mason IS, White SD, eds. *Advances in Veterinary Dermatology*, 113–129. Oxford: Pergamon.

52. Miller WH Jr, Scott DW, Buerger RG, Shanley KJ, Paradis M, McMurdy MA, Angarano DW. 1990. Necrolytic migratory erythema in dogs: A hepatocutaneous syndrome. J Am Anim Hosp Assoc 26:573–581.

53. Turnwald GH, Foil CS, Wolfsheimer KJ, WIlliams MD, Rougeau BL. 1989. Failure to document hyperglucagone-mia in a dog with diabetic dermatopathy resembling necrolytic migratory erythema. J Am Anim Hosp Assoc 25:363–369.

54. Renauld A, Sverdlik RC. 1989. Influence of exogenous ATP on blood sugar, serum insulin and serum free fatty acids in short-term experimental hyperthyroid dogs and in euthyroid controls. Acta Diabetol Lat 26: 301–307.

55. Peterson ME. 1987. Effects of megestrol acetate on glucose tolerance and growth hormone secretion in the cat. Res Vet Sci 42:354–357.

56. Taniyama H, Ushiki T, Tajima M, Kurosawa T, Kitamura N, Takahashi K, Matsukawa K, Itakura C. 1995. Spontaneous diabetes mellitus associated with persistent bovine viral diarrhea (BVD) virus infection in young cattle. Vet Pathol 32:221–229.

57. Murondoti A, van der Kolk JH, van der Linde-Sipman JS. 1999. Type 1 diabetes mellitus in a pregnant heifer persistently infected with bovine viral diarrhoea virus. Vet Rec 144:268–269.

58. Michie HR. 1996. Metabolism of sepsis and multiple organ failure. World J Surg 20:460–464.

59. Hintz HF, Lowe JE, Clifford AJ, Visek WJ. 1970. Ammonia intoxication resulting from urea ingestion by ponies. J Am Vet Med Assoc 157:963–966.

60. Kitamura SS, Antonelli AC, Maruta CA, Soares PC, Sucupira MC, Mori CS, Mirandola RM, Ortolani EL. 2003. A model for ammonia poisoning in cattle. Vet Hum Toxicol 45:274–277.

61. Stickle JE, McKnight CA, Williams KJ, Carr EA. 2006. Diarrhea and hyperammonemia in a horse with progressive neurologic signs. Vet Clin Pathol 35:250–253.

62. Peek SF, Divers TJ, Jackson CJ. 1997. Hyperammonaemia associated with encephalopathy and abdominal pain without evidence of liver disease in four mature horses. Equine Vet J 29:70–74.

63. Roller MH, Riedemann GS, Romkema GE, Swanson RN. 1982. Ovine blood chemistry values measured during ammonia toxicosis. Am J Vet Res 43:1068–1071.

64. Kramer JW, Klaassen JK, Baskin DG, Prieur DJ, Rantanen NW, Robinette JD, Graber WR, Rashti L. 1988. Inheritance of diabetes mellitus in Keeshond dogs. Am J Vet Res 49:428–431.

65. Kimmel SE, Ward CR, Henthorn PS, Hess RS. 2002. Familial insulin-dependent diabetes mellitus in Samoyed dogs. J Am Anim Hosp Assoc 38:235–238.

66. Hoenig M. 1995. Pathophysiology of canine diabetes. Vet Clin North Am Small Anim Pract 25:553–561.

67. Davison LJ, Ristic JM, Herrtage ME, Ramsey IK, Catchpole B. 2003. Anti-insulin antibodies in dogs with naturally occurring diabetes mellitus. Vet Immunol Immunopathol 91:53–60.

68. Lin HC. 1996. Dissociative anesthetics. In: Thurmon JC, Tranquilli WJ, Benson GJ, eds. *Lumb and Jones' Veterinary Anesthesia*, 3rd edition, 241–296. Baltimore: Williams & Wilkins.

69. Thrall MA, Grauer GF, Mero KN. 1984. Clinicopathologic findings in dogs and cats with ethylene glycol intoxication. J Am Vet Med Assoc 184:37–41.

70. Dornhorst A, Powell SH, Pensky J. 1985. Aggravation by propranolol of hyperglycaemic effect of hydrochlorothiazide in type II diabetics without alteration of insulin secretion. Lancet 1:123–126.

71. Branson KR, Gross ME, Booth NH. 1995. Opioid agonists and antagonists. In: Adams HR, ed. *Veterinary Pharmacology and Therapeutics*, 7th edition, 274–310. Ames: Iowa State University Press.

72. Kraje AC. 2003. Hypoglycemia and irreversible neurologic complications in a cat with insulinoma. J Am Vet Med Assoc 223:812–814.

73. Reimer SB, Pelosi A, Frank JD, Steficek BA, Kiupel M, Hauptman JG. 2005. Multiple endocrine neoplasia type I in a cat. J Am Vet Med Assoc 227:101–104.

74. Hirata Y, Fujisawa M, Sato H, Asano T, Katsuki S. 1966. Blood glucose and plasma insulin responses to xylitol administrated intravenously in dogs. Biochem Biophys Res Commun 24:471–475.

75. Kuzuya T, Kanazawa Y, Kosaka K. 1969. Stimulation of insulin secretion by xylitol in dogs. Endocrinology 84:200–207.

76. Dunayer EK. 2004. Hypoglycemia following canine ingestion of xylitol-containing gum. Vet Hum Toxicol 46:87–88.

77. Dunayer EK, Gwaltney-Brant SM. 2006. Acute hepatic failure and coagulopathy associated with xylitol ingestion in eight dogs. J Am Vet Med Assoc 229:1113–1117.

78. Syme HM, Scott-Moncrieff JC. 1998. Chronic hypoglycaemia in a hunting dog due to secondary hypoadrenocorticism. J Small Anim Pract 39:348–351.

79. Vroom MW, Slappendel RJ. 1987. Transient juvenile hypoglycaemia in a Yorkshire terrier and in a Chihuahua. Vet Q 9:172–176.

80. Johnson SE. 2000. Chronic hepatic disorders. In: Ettinger SJ, Feldman EC, eds. *Textbook of Veterinary Internal Medicine: Diseases of the Dog and Cat*, 5th edition, 1298–1325. Philadelphia: WB Saunders.

81. Bruss ML. 1997. Lipids and ketones. In: Kaneko JJ, Harvey JW, Bruss ML, eds. *Clinical Biochemistry of Domestic Animals*, 5th edition, 83–115. San Diego: Academic.

82. Leifer CE, Peterson ME, Matus RE, Patnaik AK. 1985. Hypoglycemia associated with nonislet cell tumor in 13 dogs. J Am Vet Med Assoc 186:53–55.

83. Bagley RS, Levy JK, Malarkey DE. 1996. Hypoglycemia associated with intra-abdominal leiomyoma and leiomyosarcoma in six dogs. J Am Vet Med Assoc 208:69–71.

84. Roby KAW, Beech J, Bloom JC, Black M. 1990. Hepatocellular carcinoma associated with erythrocytosis and hypoglycemia in a yearling filly. J Am Vet Med Assoc 196:465–467.

85. Bellah JR, Ginn PE. 1996. Gastric leiomyosarcoma associated with hypoglycemia in a dog. J Am Anim Hosp Assoc 32:283–286.

86. Thompson JC, Hickson PC, Johnstone AC, Jones BR. 1995. Observations on hypoglycaemia associated with a hepatoma in a cat. NZ Vet J 43:186–189.

87. Swain JM, Pirie RS, Hudson NP, Else RW, Evans H, McGorum BC. 2005. Insulin-like growth factors and recurrent hypoglycemia associated with renal cell carcinoma in a horse. J Vet Intern Med 19:613–616.
88. Bieniek K, Szuster-Ciesielska A, Kaminska T, Kondracki M, Witek M, Kandefer-Szerszen M. 1998. Tumor necrosis factor and interferon activity in the circulation of calves after repeated injection of low doses of lipopolysaccharide. Vet Immunol Immunopathol 62:297–307.
89. Gerich JE. 2001. Hypoglycemia. In: DeGroot LJ, Jameson JL, eds. *Endocrinology*, 4th edition, 921–940. Philadelphia: WB Saunders.
90. Smith JE, Cipriano JE, Hall SM. 1990. In vitro and in vivo glucose consumption in swine eperythrozoonosis. Zentralbl Veterinarmed [B] 37:587–592.
91. Jackson RF, Bruss ML, Growney PJ, Seymour WG. 1980. Hypoglycemia-ketonemia in a pregnant bitch. J Am Vet Med Assoc 177:1123–1127.
92. O'Brien DP, Barshop BA, Faunt KK, Johnson GC, Gibson KM, Shelton GD. 1999. Malonic aciduria in Maltese dogs: Normal methylmalonic acid concentrations and malonyl-CoA decarboxylase activity in fibroblasts. J Inherit Metab Dis 22:883–890.
93. Given BD, Mostrom MS, Tully R, Ditkowsky N, Rubenstein AH. 1988. Severe hypoglycemia attributable to surreptitious injection of insulin in a mare. J Am Vet Med Assoc 193:224–226.
94. Feldman EC, Nelson RW. 1996. Diabetes mellitus. In: *Canine and Feline Endocrinology and Reproduction*, 2nd edition, 339–391. Philadelphia: WB Saunders.
95. Madison LL, Lochner A, Wulff J. 1967. Ethanol-induced hypoglycemia. II. Mechanism of suppression of hepatic gluconeogenesis. Diabetes 16:252–258.
96. Fleeman LM, Rand JS. 2003. Evaluation of day-to-day variability of serial blood glucose concentration curves in diabetic dogs. J Am Vet Med Assoc 222:317–321.
97. Stein JE, Greco DS. 2002. Portable blood glucose meters as a means of monitoring blood glucose concentrations in dogs and cats with diabetes mellitus. Clin Tech Small Anim Pract 17:70–72.
98. Armbruster DA. 1987. Fructosamine: Structure, analysis, and clinical usefulness. Clin Chem 33:2153–2163.
99. Marca MC, Loste A, Ramos JJ. 2000. Effect of acute hyperglycaemia on the serum fructosamine and blood glycated haemoglobin concentrations in canine samples. Vet Res Commun 24:11–16.
100. Jensen AL, Petersen MB, Houe H. 1993. Determination of the fructosamine concentration in bovine serum samples. Zentralbl Veterinarmed [A] 40:111–117.
101. Watanabe D, Nakara H, Akagi K, Ishii T, Mizuguchi H, Nagashima Y, Okaniwa A. 2004. Oral glucose tolerance test and determination of serum fructosamine level in beagle dogs. J Toxicol Sci 29:33–36.
102. Jensen AL. 1995. Glycated blood proteins in canine diabetes mellitus. Vet Rec 137:401–405.
103. Mahaffey EA, Cornelius LM. 1981. Evaluation of a commercial kit for measurement of glycosylated hemoglobin in canine blood. Vet Clin Pathol 10:21–24.
104. Smith JE, Wood PA, Moore K. 1982. Evaluation of a colorimetric method for canine glycosylated hemoglobin. Am J Vet Res 43:700–701.
105. Marca MC, Loste A. 2000. Glycosylated haemoglobin assay of canine blood samples. J Small Anim Pract 41:189–192.
106. Loste A, Marca MC. 2001. Fructosamine and glycated hemoglobin in the assessment of glycaemic control in dogs. Vet Res 32:55–62.
107. Marca MC, Loste A, Unzueta A, Perez M. 2000. Blood glycated hemoglobin evaluation in sick dogs. Can J Vet Res 64:141–144.
108. Elliott DA, Nelson RW, Feldman EC, Neal LA. 1997. Glycosylated hemoglobin concentrations in the blood of healthy dogs and dogs with naturally developing diabetes mellitus, pancreatic B-cell neoplasia, hyperadrenocorticism, and anemia. J Am Vet Med Assoc 211:723–727.
109. Elliott DA, Nelson RW, Reusch CE, Feldman EC, Neal LA. 1999. Comparison of serum fructosamine and blood glycosylated hemoglobin concentrations for assessment of glycemic control in cats with diabetes mellitus. J Am Vet Med Assoc 214:1794–1798.
110. Hoenig M, Ferguson DC. 1999. Diagnostic utility of glycosylated hemoglobin concentrations in the cat. Domest Anim Endocrinol 16:11–17.
111. Kaneko JJ, Kawamoto M, Heusner AA, Feldman EC, Koizumi I. 1992. Evaluation of serum fructosamine concentration as an index of blood glucose control in cats with diabetes mellitus. Am J Vet Res 53:1797–1801.
112. Crenshaw KL, Peterson ME, Heeb LA, Moroff SD, Nichols R. 1996. Serum fructosamine concentration as an index of glycemia in cats with diabetes mellitus and stress hyperglycemia. J Vet Intern Med 10:360–364.
113. Elliott DA, Nelson RW, Feldman EC, Neal LA. 1997. Glycosylated hemoglobin concentration for assessment of glycemic control in diabetic cats. J Vet Intern Med 11:161–165.

114. Waterson MJ, Mills RJ. 1988. Serum fructosamine in patients with overt and treated thyroid disease. Ann Clin Biochem 25(Pt 5):587–588.

115. Jensen AL. 1993. Various protein and albumin corrections of the serum fructosamine concentration in the diagnosis of canine diabetes mellitus. Vet Res Commun 17:13–23.

116. Reusch CE, Haberer B. 2001. Evaluation of fructosamine in dogs and cats with hypo- or hyperproteinaemia, azotaemia, hyperlipidaemia and hyperbilirubinaemia. Vet Rec 148:370–376.

117. Thoresen SI, Aleksandersen M, Lonaas L, Bredal WP, Grondalen J, Berthelsen K. 1995. Pancreatic insulin-secreting carcinoma in a dog: Fructosamine for determining persistent hypoglycaemia. J Small Anim Pract 36:282–286.

118. Mellanby RJ, Herrtage ME. 2002. Insulinoma in a normoglycaemic dog with low serum fructosamine. J Small Anim Pract 43:506–508.

119. Loste A, Marca MC. 1999. Study of the effect of total serum protein and albumin concentrations on canine fructosamine concentration. Can J Vet Res 63:138–141.

120. Graham PA, Mooney CT, Murray M. 1999. Serum fructosamine concentrations in hyperthyroid cats. Res Vet Sci 67:171–175.

121. Reusch CE, Tomsa K. 1999. Serum fructosamine concentration in cats with overt hyperthyroidism. J Am Vet Med Assoc 215:1297–1300.

122. Lloyd D, Marples J. 1986. Serum fructosamine and thyroid function. Clin Chem 32:1985.

123. Schleicher ED, Olgemoller B, Wiedenmann E, Gerbitz KD. 1993. Specific glycation of albumin depends on its half-life. Clin Chem 39:625–628.

124. Kaneko JJ. 1997. Carbohydrate metabolism and its diseases. In: Kaneko JJ, Harvey JW, Bruss ML, eds. *Clinical Biochemistry of Domestic Animals*, 5th edition, 45–81. San Diego: Academic.

125. Lutz TA, Rand JS. 1993. Comparison of five commercial radioimmunoassay kits for the measurement of feline insulin. Res Vet Sci 55:64–69.

126. Stockham SL, Nachreiner RF, Krehbiel JD. 1983. Canine immunoreactive insulin quantitation using five commercial radioimmunoassay kits. Am J Vet Res 44:2179–2183.

127. Appleton DJ, Rand JS, Sunvold GD. 2005. Basal plasma insulin and homeostasis model assessment (HOMA) are indicators of insulin sensitivity in cats. J Feline Med Surg 7:183–193.

128. Turner RC, Oakley NW, Nabarro JDN. 1971. Control of basal insulin secretion, with special reference to the diagnosis of insulinomas. Br Med J 2:132–135.

129. Turner RC, Oakley NW, Nabarro JDN. 1973. Changes in plasma insulin during ethanol-induced hypoglycemia. Metabolism 22:111–121.

130. Edwards DF. 1986. It's time to unamend the insulin-glucose ratio. J Am Vet Med Assoc 188:951–953.

131. Knowlen GG, Schall WD. 1984. The amended insulin-glucose ratio: Is it really better? J Am Vet Med Assoc 185:397–399.

132. McCaw D. 1979. Pancreatic adenocarcinoma. J Am Vet Med Assoc 175:247–248 (letter).

133. Brown SA, Edwards DF. 1986. Final comments on amended insulin-glucose ratio. J Am Vet Med Assoc 189:408–409.

134. Schaer M. 1986. Winding down on the amended insulin:glucose ratio. J Am Vet Med Assoc 189:259.

135. Kieffer TJ, Habener JF. 1999. The glucagon-like peptides. Endocr Rev 20:876–913.

136. Conlon JM, Ipp E, Unger RH. 1978. The molecular forms of immunoreactive glucagon secreted by the isolated, perfused dog pancreas. Life Sci 23:1655–1658.

137. Heding LG, Frandsen EK, Jacobsen H. 1976. Structure-function relationship: Immunologic. Metabolism 25(Suppl 11):1327–1329.

138. McCann JP, Bergman EN, Aalseth DL. 1989. Validation of radioimmunoassay (RIA) for glucagon in domestic animals. J Anim Sci 67:220 (abstract).

139. Bond R, McNeil PE, Evans H, Srebernik N. 1995. Metabolic epidermal necrosis in two dogs with different underlying diseases. Vet Rec 136:466–471.

140. Stockham SL, Nachreiner RF, Krehbiel JD. 1980. Radioimmunoassay of canine insulin, glucagon and C-peptide: A comparison and evaluation of commercial assays. Vet Clin Pathol 9:41 (abstract).

141. O'Brien TD, Hayden DW, Johnson KH, Stevens JB. 1985. High dose intravenous glucose tolerance test and serum insulin and glucagon levels in diabetic and non-diabetic cats: Relationships to insular amyloidosis. Vet Pathol 22:250–261.

142. Mirsky IA, Perisutti G, Davis NC. 1959. The destruction of glucagon by the blood plasma from various species. Endocrinology 64:992–1001.

143. Eisentraut AM, Whissen N, Unger RH. 1968. Incubation damage in the radioimmunoassay for human plasma glucagon and its prevention with "Trasylol." Am J Med Sci 235:137–142.

144. Lacey RJ, Scarpello JHB, Morgan NG. 1992. Evidence that the presence of arginine can lead to overestimation of glucagon levels measured by radioimmunoassay. Clin Chim Acta 210:211–219.
145. Torres S, Johnson K, McKeever P, Hardy R. 1997. Superficial necrolytic dermatitis and a pancreatic endocrine tumour in a dog. J Small Anim Pract 38:246–250.
146. Miller WH Jr, Anderson WI, McCann JP. 1991. Necrolytic migratory erythema in a dog with a glucagon-secreting endocrine tumor. Vet Dermatol 2:179–182.
147. Gross TL, Song MD, Havel PJ, Ihrke PJ. 1993. Superficial necrolytic dermatitis (necrolytic migratory erythema) in dogs. Vet Pathol 30:75–81.
148. WHO Study Group. 1985. Diabetes mellitus. WHO Tech Rep Ser 727:1–113.

Chapter 15

EXOCRINE PANCREAS AND INTESTINE

Exocrine Pancreatic and Intestinal Absorptive Malfunctions 740
Trypsin-like Immunoreactivity (TLI) Concentration in Dogs, Cats, and Horses 741
Pancreatic Lipase Immunoreactivity (PLI) Concentration in Dogs and Cats 745
Trypsinogen Activation Peptide (TAP) in Dogs 746
Cobalamin (Vitamin B_{12}) Concentration in Dogs, Cats, and Cattle 747
Folate Concentration in Dogs and Cats 750
Fecal α_1-Protease Inhibitor (α_1-PI) Concentration in Dogs and Cats 753
D-Xylose Absorption Test in Dogs, Cats, and Horses 754
Glucose Absorption Test in Horses 755
Lactose Tolerance Test in Horses 756
Urine Sucrose Concentration in Horses 757
Other Methods of Evaluating Digestive or Absorptive Functions 758

Table 15.1. Abbreviations and symbols in this chapter

[x]	Concentration of x (x = analyte)
AMS	Amylase
EDTA	Ethylenediaminetetraacetic acid
ELISA	Enzyme-linked immunosorbent assay
EPI	Exocrine pancreatic insufficiency
GFR	Glomerular filtration rate
HCO_3^-	Bicarbonate
LPS	Lipase
PLI	Pancreatic lipase immunoreactivity
RIA	Radioimmunoassay
SI	Système International d'Unités
TAP	Trypsinogen activation peptide
TAP:Crt	Trypsinogen activation peptide to creatinine
TLI	Trypsin-like immunoreactivity
URL	Upper reference limit
α_1-PI	α_1-Protease inhibitor

EXOCRINE PANCREATIC AND INTESTINAL ABSORPTIVE MALFUNCTIONS

I.   Exocrine pancreatic insufficiency (maldigestion)

    A. *Exocrine pancreatic insufficiency* (EPI) is a pathophysiologic state in which inadequate pancreatic secretions (enzyme rich or HCO_3^- rich) cause incomplete digestion of food (maldigestion) and, secondarily, inadequate absorption of nutrients.

        1. Dogs and cats with EPI typically have lost weight and produce malformed feces. Pancreatic maldigestion may result from inadequate secretion of LPS, AMS, trypsinogen, chymotrypsinogen, carboxypeptidases, or combinations of these zymogens and enzymes.

        2. Three pancreatic conditions are recognized as causes of EPI in dogs and cats. EPI is not recognized in cattle or horses. There must be extensive loss of acinar cells before there is clinical evidence of maldigestion caused by EPI.

            a. *Pancreatic acinar atrophy* (or juvenile pancreatic atrophy) in dogs: Current evidence indicates this condition is caused by a hereditary immune-mediated lymphocytic pancreatitis (atrophic lymphocytic pancreatitis) in German shepherds and rough-coated collies.[1,2] When presented for weight loss, there is nearly a complete absence of pancreatic acinar cells. Using a decreased serum [TLI] value as a marker of affected dogs, a study involving 134 German shepherds indicated an autosomal recessive inheritance pattern.[3]

            b. Chronic pancreatitis in dogs[4] and cats:[5] This disorder is typically an idiopathic, recurring pancreatitis that causes extensive destruction of acinar cells. If there is concurrent destruction of islet cells, the dog or cat can develop diabetes mellitus.

            c. Pancreatic duct obstruction in dogs and cats: Impaired secretion of pancreatic enzymes into the intestine could cause maldigestion. However, the obstructive lesion would probably lead to acute inflammation, and thus the animal would be presented for an acute illness and may not develop a maldigestive state that causes chronic weight loss or chronic diarrhea.

B. Dogs and cats with EPI may develop secondary intestinal abnormalities, such as increased mucosal maltase and sucrase activities, increased microvillar membrane proteins, or bacterial overgrowth. The latter could lead to mucosal changes that cause malabsorption.[6]

II. Pancreatitis
    A. Even though the initiating factors for pancreatic inflammation are not thoroughly understood, it is known that pancreatic acinar cell damage is a major consequence of the inflammation.
    B. In acute pancreatitis (from mild edematous to severe necrotizing or hemorrhagic), the release of cytoplasmic enzymes from the damaged acinar cells can result in increased serum activities of AMS and LPS (see Chapter 12), increased serum [TLI] and [PLI] (see Chapter 12), and increased urine and plasma [TAP] (see Trypsinogen Activation Peptide (TAP) in Dogs, sect. III.A). Among domestic mammals, acute pancreatitis is most common in dogs. Affected dogs frequently have an acute onset of clinical signs such as vomiting and anterior abdominal pain.
    C. Chronic pancreatitis may result from recurrent episodes of acute pancreatitis or slowly progressive destruction of pancreatic acinar cells. When severe, the pancreas may not be able to secrete sufficient enzymes to digest food, and the animal may develop EPI. Chronic pancreatitis occurs in cats and less commonly in dogs, and may result in EPI with clinical signs such as progressive weight loss and soft or malformed feces. Endocrine pancreatic dysfunction may also arise.

III. Intestinal malabsorption
    A. Several small intestinal diseases cause inadequate absorption of nutrients and thus intestinal malabsorption. The malabsorptive state could be localized (e.g., proximal small intestine or ileum) or diffuse; it could involve malabsorption of many nutrients (e.g., sugars, proteins, and fats) or be very specific (e.g., cobalamin). When intestinal malabsorption is not caused by a specific absorption defect, the animal is presented because of weight loss or malformed feces. Acute enteric diseases that cause diarrhea for a few days probably cause a temporary malabsorptive state, but such disorders are not typically considered in discussions of malabsorptive disorders because there is not a concurrent malnourished state.
    B. Intestinal diseases that lead to malabsorption occur in most animal species, but laboratory tests are used mostly to evaluate the disorders of dogs and occasionally of cats and horses. Specific diagnosis of suspected primary intestinal disease usually requires histologic examination of intestinal tissue. Examples of intestinal diseases that cause malabsorption include the following:
        1. Inflammatory: histoplasmosis, lymphocytic enteritis, lymphocytic-plasmacytic enteritis, eosinophilic enteritis, granulomatous enteritis, pythiosis, giardiasis, and protothecosis
        2. Neoplastic: lymphoma
        3. Lymphangiectasia

TRYPSIN-LIKE IMMUNOREACTIVITY (TLI) CONCENTRATION IN DOGS, CATS, AND HORSES

I. Physiologic processes (Fig. 15.1)

II. Analytical concepts
    A. Terms and units

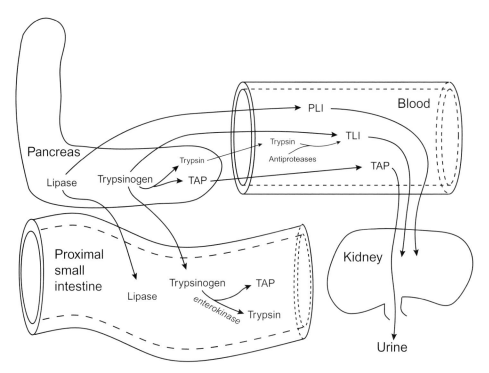

Fig. 15.1. Physiologic processes that influence plasma or serum concentrations of TLI, PLI, or TAP.

- TLI: Most trypsinogen is secreted in enzyme-rich pancreatic secretions into the intestine, where it is converted to trypsin, a potent digestive protease. In health, a small amount of trypsinogen escapes the pancreas and enters the blood, in which it can be measured as TLI. Also, small amounts of trypsin may be formed in the pancreas (see TAP); this trypsin may enter the blood, bind to antiproteases, and contribute to [TLI]. Plasma trypsinogen and trypsin are degraded in the kidneys and by the mononuclear phagocyte system.

- TAP: In health, small amounts of trypsinogen are cleaved to form trypsin and TAP within the pancreas; this TAP enters the plasma (probably via lymph), and some of it is cleared via the kidneys and is excreted in the urine. Activation of trypsinogen to trypsin by enterokinase in the intestine also results in the formation of TAP, but this TAP is not absorbed and thus does not enter the plasma.

- PLI: Most pancreatic LPS is secreted in enzyme-rich pancreatic secretions into the intestine, where it catalyzes the lipolysis of dietary triglycerides. In health, a small amount of pancreatic LPS escapes the pancreas and enters the blood, in which it can be measured as PLI. The kidneys are involved in the removal of LPS from the plasma.

1. Immunologic assays detect cationic trypsinogen, trypsin, and trypsin bound to protease inhibitors (probably α_1-antitrypsin); thus the name TLI. In healthy animals, nearly all TLI is trypsinogen.
2. TLI is reportedly pancreas specific, and values were markedly decreased after pancreas removal; however, TLI was still measurable. Trypsin is present in the human small intestine (Paneth cells), in bile epithelium, and in ovarian and hepato-biliary neoplasms.
3. Units: µg/L (SI units not found)

Table 15.2. Diseases and conditions that cause increased [TLI], [PLI], or [TAP] in dogs and cats

Increased release of trypsinogen (or trypsin), LPS, or TAP[a] from pancreatic acinar cells
  *Acinar cell damage caused by pancreatitis or other disorders
   Stimulated by food intake[b] or cholecystokinin and secretin administration
Decreased GFR (see prerenal, renal, and postrenal azotemia in Chap. 8)
Cobalamin deficiency in cats ([TLI])

  * A relatively common disease or condition
  [a] Increased urinary excretion of TAP is also found with damage to pancreatic acinar cells (see the text).
  [b] The [TLI] has been shown to increase after food intake. The same change has not been documented for [PLI] or [TAP] yet.

    B. Assays
       1. Canine, feline, and equine [TLI] are measured by species-specific immunoassays. Trypsin's enzymatic activity is not measured because of the presence of trypsin inhibitors in serum.
       2. In cats, reference intervals for [TLI] measured by a RIA (17–49 µg/L) were different from those measured by an ELISA (12–82 µg/L).[7]
    C. Sample: Serum is the preferred sample, but EDTA plasma or heparinized plasma can be used. Samples should be stored at 4 °C or −20 °C.[8]

  III.   Increased [trypsin-like immunoreactivity] [TLI] (Table 15.2)
    A. Increased release from pancreatic acinar cells
       1. Acinar cell damage caused by pancreatitis[9,10]
         a. Trypsinogen or trypsin released from damaged acinar cells enters blood, probably via lymph and peritoneal fluid.[11]
         b. Dogs
           (1) In an experimental canine pancreatitis study, serum [TLI] tended to parallel serum AMS and LPS activities; that is, all started to increase within 1 d, remained increased through day 5, and had returned to near baseline values at 2 wk. However, the peak in [TLI] occurred 1–2 d prior to the peak activities of AMS and LPS.[12] Using decision thresholds based on receiver operating characteristic (ROC) analysis (not URLs), diagnostic specificity for severe pancreatitis was about 90 %, but diagnostic sensitivities for pancreatitis have been reported to be about 33–50 % (less than those for serum LPS activity).
           (2) Dexamethasone (0.25 mg/kg per os daily) was associated with increased [TLI] by day 7 of treatment and was within the reference interval again 7 d after withdrawal. The mean increase was three times baseline mean, but only 2 of 12 dogs had [TLI] > the URL. The authors suggested that the [TLI] was increased because of toxic effects of dexamethasone on the pancreas.[13]
         c. Cats
           (1) In a prospective study involving 28 cats with clinical signs compatible with pancreatitis, there were not significant differences in serum [TLI] found in cats without pancreatic lesions (10), cats with pancreatitis and fibrosis (9), cats with pancreatic fibrosis but without active inflammation (4), and cats

with acute necrotizing pancreatitis (5).[14] These conclusions were questioned by other investigators who wrote that increased [TLI] is specific for feline pancreatitis.[7]

    (2) Other studies described that [TLI] has an 80–86 % diagnostic sensitivity for moderate to severe pancreatitis in cats when empirical decision thresholds greater than the URL are used.[15,16]

  d. Horses

    (1) Horses that have strangulating intestinal obstruction and endotoxic shock can have increased plasma [trypsin] (as measured by an activity assay).[17] The trypsin is probably released from pancreatic acinar cells because of poor perfusion of splanchnic tissues.

    (2) In a study involving ten horses, some with strangulating intestinal obstructions had increased plasma [TLI], but those with nonstrangulating intestinal obstructions did not.[18] It is not known whether the increased plasma [TLI] was due to increased release of pancreatic TLI molecules, whether more TLI molecules were bound to proteins (e.g., acute-phase proteins), or whether trypsin gained access to plasma via damaged intestines.

  2. Stimulated by food intake or cholecystokinin and secretin administration[19]

B. Decreased renal clearance in disorders that cause decreased GFR

  1. Trypsinogen is cleared from plasma by kidneys. Disorders that cause a decreased GFR cause an increased [TLI].[20]

  2. Prerenal, renal, or postrenal disorders (see Chapter 8) can decrease GFR, and thus concurrent azotemia is expected.

C. Cobalamin deficiency in cats

  1. Of 19 cats with severe cobalamin deficiencies associated with gastrointestinal disease, 15 had increased serum [TLI] at the time of diagnosis; 10 had a [TLI] > 100 µg/L (reference interval = 12–82 µg/L). The reasons for the increased [TLI] in these cats were not determined. Serum [TLI] decreased in 9 of 19 cats when they were given parenteral cobalamin therapy.[21]

  2. Of nine cats with various types of inflammatory bowel disease, five had mild to moderate decreases in [cobalamin]. One of those five had a greatly increased [TLI] of undetermined origin.[22]

D. Associated with higher protein diets in dogs: Serum [TLI] was greater in dogs on a high-protein diet when compared to dogs on a low-protein diet, but the mean concentrations for all groups were within common canine reference intervals.[23]

IV. Decreased [trypsin-like immunoreactivity] [TLI] (Table 15.3)

A. Decreased release from pancreatic acinar cells

  1. Chronic pancreatitis that leads to destruction of most acinar cells[4]

  2. Pancreatic acinar atrophy in dogs

B. In dogs with clinical signs of maldigestion (due to EPI) or malabsorption (due to small intestinal disease), the diagnostic sensitivity, specificity, and accuracy of a fasting serum [TLI] for EPI are very high (approaching 100 %).[24] The presence of active pancreatitis[9] or a disorder that is causing decreased GFR may increase [TLI] enough to mask a deficient state.

C. A decrease in serum [TLI] was found in 20 German shepherds and rough-coated collies in the absence of clinical disease.[25] Of these dogs, seven later developed clinical EPI (within 6–46 mo) and were treated with enzyme supplementation. The results indicated

Table 15.3. Diseases and conditions that cause decreased [TLI] or [PLI] in dogs and cats

Decreased release of trypsinogen (or trypsin) or pancreatic LPS from pancreas
    Chronic pancreatitis
    *Pancreatic acinar atrophy

* A relatively common disease or condition
Note: The [TLI] has been shown to decrease in these disorders in both dogs and cats. A decreased [PLI] has not been documented yet in cats.

that decreased [TLI] may represent subclinical immune-mediated lymphocytic pancreatitis (atrophic lymphocytic pancreatitis).

D. In a group of 20 cats with clinical signs suggestive of EPI (e.g., weight loss, soft or voluminous stool, and polyphagia), 17 had decreased serum [TLI] values.[5] Additional diagnostic evaluations and/or response to enzyme replacement treatments supported the conclusion that the cats did have EPI.

PANCREATIC LIPASE IMMUNOREACTIVITY (PLI) CONCENTRATION IN DOGS AND CATS

I.   Physiologic processes (Fig. 15.1)

II.   Analytical concepts
      A. Terms and units
         1. Because the immunoassays are designed to measure the pancreatic LPS protein (M_r = 51,000 in dogs) and not its activity, the analyte is called *pancreatic lipase immunoreactivity* (PLI).
         2. Units: µg/L
      B. Assays
         1. Species-specific immunoassays for pancreatic LPS have been developed for dogs (RIA and ELISA)[26,27] and cats (RIA).[28] These assays measure the actual concentration of the lipase protein, not the activity of the enzyme. The polyclonal antibodies localized only to pancreatic acinar cells in immunohistochemical studies of canine tissues.
         2. The sources of the standard solutions for the assays were not specified but assumed to be LPS isolated from canine and feline pancreatic tissue, respectively, by the investigators.
         3. Reference intervals vary with the methods used and among laboratories.
      C. Sample: Serum is the preferred sample.

III. Increased [pancreatic lipase immunoreactivity] [PLI] (Table 15.2)
      A. Increased release from damaged pancreatic acinar cells
         1. During experimental and spontaneous pancreatitis, LPS is released from damaged pancreatic acinar cells and enters the blood (probably via lymphatic vessels).
         2. PLI testing has the advantage over most routine serum LPS assays of being specific for pancreatic lipase, and testing is offered by some large veterinary referral laboratories. However, results may be too delayed to be useful for diagnosing and managing patients with acute pancreatitis.

      3. Dogs: When decision thresholds of the URL or of an empirical value greater than the URL were used, the [PLI] had a diagnostic sensitivity for acute pancreatitis of 100 % and 82 %, respectively.[29] Diagnostic sensitivities of LPS and TLI were less.

      4. Cats: The [PLI] (with decision threshold of 10 µg/L) is reported to have better diagnostic sensitivity for pancreatitis than does the [TLI] in cats.[15] After experimental initiation of pancreatitis in cats, the [PLI] had greater increases (50× baseline vs 35× baseline) and more persistent increases (10 d vs 3 d) than did the [TLI].[30]

  B. Decreased renal clearance in disorders that cause decreased GFR

      1. The kidneys are involved in the removal of pancreatic LPS from plasma (see Chapter 12). When there are disorders that result in decreased blood flow through the kidneys (i.e., prerenal, renal, or postrenal disorders), then LPS has a longer circulating half-life and thus can accumulate in plasma.

      2. Using the canine PLI ELISA, the [PLI] was mildly increased in dogs with experimentally induced chronic renal failure, but not above the suggested diagnostic threshold for pancreatitis.[31,32] Lack of increased serum LPS activity in this study suggests that the model may not have been appropriate for assessing changes in [PLI] caused by renal failure.

IV.   Decreased [pancreatic lipase immunoreactivity] [PLI] (Table 15.3)

  A. Release of LPS from pancreatic acinar cells may be decreased in disorders associated with reduced functional pancreatic acinar tissue, and therefore serum pancreatic lipase immunoreactivity concentrations may be decreased. The primary disorders in dogs and cats are chronic pancreatitis (which leads to destruction of most acinar cells) and, in dogs, pancreatic acinar atrophy (an immune-mediated disorder of German shepherds and rough-coated collies).

  B. In a study using an ELISA, all 25 dogs with EPI (as defined by having a decreased [TLI]) had decreased [PLI].[33] However, TLI is preferred over PLI for diagnosis of EPI because TLI appears to differentiate affected dogs from healthy dogs more clearly, and it may have greater diagnostic sensitivity for EPI.

TRYPSINOGEN ACTIVATION PEPTIDE (TAP) IN DOGS

I.   Physiologic processes: After ingestion of a meal, trypsinogen from pancreatic acinar cells enters the intestinal lumen and is cleaved by the action of enterokinase to produce trypsin and TAP, an eight-amino-acid N-terminal cleavage peptide. In theory, the TAP is not absorbed and thus does not enter plasma. A minute [TAP] can be found in plasma and urine of healthy dogs, presumably from activation within the pancreas.[34]

II.   Analytical concepts

  A. Units

      1. Plasma: nmol/L

      2. Urine: nmol/L; also reported as a TAP:Crt ratio

  B. Assays: An immunoassay (either enzyme immunoassay or RIA) detects TAP; five highly conserved amino acids allow for cross-species testing with a single assay. The analytical detection limit of the enzyme immunoassay is near the lower plasma concentrations found in healthy dogs and thus cannot be used to detect decreased plasma [TAP]. Assays are not widely available.

    C. Sample
      1. EDTA blood is collected and centrifuged at 4 °C, and plasma is separated within 1 h. EDTA plasma is frozen (at −20 °C) until just prior to analysis.
      2. Urine is collected into EDTA-containing vacuum tubes and frozen (at −20 °C) until just prior to analysis.

III.   Increased plasma [TAP] or increased urinary TAP:Crt ratio[34,35] (Table 15.2)
    A. Acinar cell damage caused by pancreatitis: During pancreatitis, trypsinogen is cleaved to form trypsin and TAP within the pancreas through actions of cathepsin B or through autoactivation. TAP probably enters plasma via lymph, and some of it is cleared via kidneys.
      1. In dogs with increased plasma [TAP] because of pancreatitis, most had an increased urine [TAP] and an increased urinary TAP:Crt ratio. In a study involving 22 dogs with a histopathologic diagnosis of pancreatitis and using receiver operating characteristic curve analysis (see Chapter 1) to determine decision thresholds, the urinary TAP:Crt ratio had the best capability of differentiating mild pancreatitis from severe pancreatitis (compared to TLI, plasma [TAP], serum LPS activity, and serum AMS activity) based on the stated classification for severity. Diagnostic sensitivity and specificity for severe pancreatitis were 86 % and 100 %, respectively. In comparison, serum LPS activity had diagnostic sensitivity and specificity for severe pancreatitis of 64 % and 100 % in the same study.[35]
      2. In a study of ten cats with spontaneous pancreatitis, plasma TAP was increased in all cats, but the urinary TAP:Crt ratios were not significantly increased when compared to those of healthy cats.[36]
      3. In experimentally induced pancreatitis in cats, there was increased urinary excretion of TAP during the 24 h of the study. Serum LPS activity also increased.[37]
    B. Decreased renal clearance in disorders that cause decreased GFR: Dogs with renal disease may have increased plasma [TAP]. In four dogs with plasma [TAP] increased by renal disease, the urine [TAP] was decreased. In two of these dogs, the urinary TAP:Crt was within the reference interval.

COBALAMIN (VITAMIN B_{12}) CONCENTRATION IN DOGS, CATS, AND CATTLE

I.   Physiologic processes (Fig. 15.1)
    A. Cobalamin is a required cofactor in the metabolic pathways involving folate (Fig. 15.2).[38]
    B. Cobalamin is also a required cofactor for the conversion of methylmalonyl coenzyme A to succinyl coenzyme A. Without this conversion, plasma [methylmalonic acid] accumulates (methylmalonic acidemia and aciduria), and a neurologic disease develops because of defective formation of neuronal lipids.

II.   Analytical concepts
    A. Terms and units
      1. *Cobalamins* are a group of compounds that have a corrin (porphyrin-like) ring and side chains bound to cobalt. One cobalamin is *cyanocobalamin* (vitamin B_{12}) that has a cyanide side chain; other side chains include methyl and hydroxyl groups. In common clinical use, cyanocobalamin is simply called cobalamin.

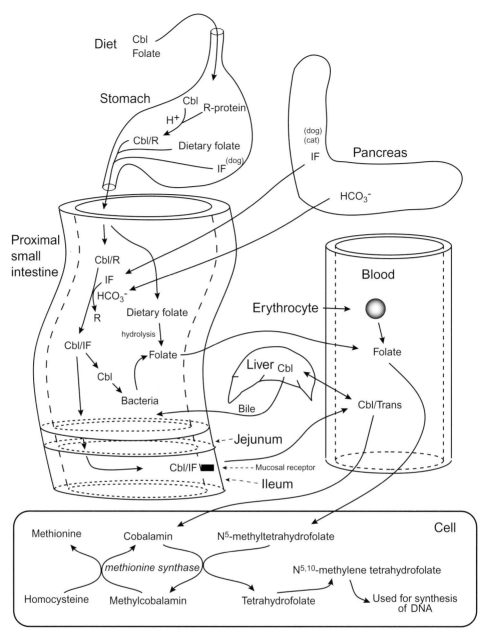

Fig. 15.2. Physiologic processes that influence plasma or serum concentrations of cobalamin or folate and the cellular relationship of cobalamin and folate.

- Cobalamin: Cobalamin (Cbl) enters the stomach via ingested foods. In the acidic environment, it binds with R protein (cobalophilin or haptocorrin; R for rapid electrophoretic migration) that is produced by the gastric mucosa. Cobalamin enters the intestine bound to R protein (R), but when it enters the alkaline environment, it detaches from R protein and binds to intrinsic factor (IF) that is secreted by the pancreatic cells (dogs and cats) and the gastric mucosa (dogs). Enteric bacteria use some of the cobalamin as it moves through the small intestine. When it reaches the ileum, the cobalamin/intrinsic factor complex binds to specific mucosal receptors involving cubam (cubilin and amnionless) and megalin, and enters enterocytes. When cobalamin enters the portal blood, it binds to transcobalamin 2 (Trans), a transport protein. From the blood, cobalamin may be used in tissues, stored in the liver, or excreted in bile.

748

2. Unit conversion for cyanocobalamin: pg/mL × 0.7378 = pmol/L; and ng/dL × 7.378 = pmol/L (SI unit, nearest 10 pmol/L)[39]

B. Assays
1. The assays are designed to measure [cyanocobalamin]. Competitive protein-binding assays are more common than bioassays that are technically difficult.
2. Assays designed for human sera may not be reliable for other species because of cobalamin-binding proteins in canine and feline sera. Some commercial assays designed for analysis of human samples use porcine gastric intrinsic factor as the binding agent. If the binding reagent contains contaminant R proteins, they can bind to inactive cobalamin metabolites and give falsely increased values.[40]

C. Sample[8]
1. Serum is the preferred sample. The use of heparinized or hemolyzed plasma should be avoided.
2. Samples are stable at 8 °C overnight and up to 8 wk at −20 °C.
3. Falsely low concentrations may occur when cobalamin is degraded by excess exposure to light.

III. Increased serum [cobalamin]
A. Increased serum [cobalamin] is uncommon. However, disorders or conditions that could increase [cobalamin] should be considered when interpreting concentrations that are decreased or within the reference interval.
B. Diseases or conditions that cause increased serum [cobalamin]
1. Cobalamin supplementation: parenteral or oral
2. Release from damaged hepatocytes: Because hepatocytes are a storage site for cobalamin, hepatic necrosis could increase serum [cobalamin]. The magnitude or duration of the increase is not known.

IV. Decreased serum [cobalamin] (Table 15.4)
A. Serum [cobalamin] will not be decreased until the body reserve is depleted. Depletion typically occurs because of decreased ileal absorption of cobalamin, but the primary defect may be preabsorptive (i.e., before cobalamin absorption by the ileum).

Fig. 15.2. *continued*

• Folate: Folate is present in food (e.g., green leafy plants) in a polyglutamate form. After digestion releases it from food, the polyglutamate folate is hydrolyzed to monoglutamate folate at the brush border of the proximal small intestine. After cellular uptake, it is converted to N^5-methyltetrahydrofolate (commonly called *folate*), which enters the blood and is transported to tissues for biochemical reactions. Enteric bacteria can also produce folate. Folate from erythrocytes lysed during sample collection can increase measured serum [folate].

• Relationship of cobalamin and folate. Cobalamin is a required cofactor for methionine synthase, which catalyzes the conversion of N^5-methyltetrahydrofolate (the primary molecule in plasma) to tetrahydrofolate, which is then available for DNA synthesis in cells. If there is a cobalamin deficiency, the methyl group of N^5-methyltetrahydrofolate is not transferred to cobalamin (methyl trapped), and thus a cellular deficiency in tetrahydrofolate occurs.

Table 15.4. Diseases and conditions that cause decreased serum [cobalamin]

Cobalt deficiency in cattle
Preabsorptive defect in dogs and cats
    EPI: pancreatic atrophy, chronic pancreatitis
    Intestinal bacterial overgrowth: EPI, impaired gastric acid secretion, enteric disorders
      (see the text)
Defective absorption of cobalamin in ileum of dogs and cats
    *Ileal disease: inflammation, resection, villous atrophy (viral, hypersensitivity, cytotoxic
      drugs)
    Congenital deficiency of receptor in giant schnauzers and Border collies
Severe cobalamin deficiency in a cat (probable congenital malabsorption defect)

    * A relatively common disease or condition
    Note: Lists of specific disorders or conditions are not complete but are provided to give examples.
Falsely low concentrations may occur when cobalamin is degraded by excess exposure to light.

    B. Diseases or conditions that reduce cobalamin absorption in the intestine
        1. Cobalt deficiency: A dietary cobalt deficiency in cattle can cause a decreased serum
           [cobalamin]; cobalt is needed for synthesis of cobalamin by ruminal bacteria.[43] The
           cobalamin deficiency leads to an increased plasma [homocysteine] because methylco-
           balamin is needed for the methylation of homocysteine to form methionine (Fig.
           15.2).
        2. Preabsorptive defect
           a. EPI[41]
               (1) Failure to secrete HCO_3^--rich fluid into the duodenum results in cobalamin
                    not being released from R proteins (a pH-dependent event).
               (2) The production of intrinsic factor may be decreased (especially in cats
                    because they apparently lack gastric intrinsic factor). Thus, there is less
                    cobalamin/intrinsic factor complex formation for absorption.
           b. Intestinal bacterial overgrowth ($> 10^5$ colony-forming units/mL of duodenal
              juice),[42] especially involving obligate anaerobes, can lower serum [cobalamin] by
              increasing the amount of cobalamin bound to intestinal bacteria and thereby
              decreasing the amount of cobalamin that is free for absorption.
        3. Defective absorption of cobalamin in the ileum of dogs and cats
           a. Diseases that damage the ileal mucosa: inflammation, villous atrophy, cytotoxic
              drugs, and resection
           b. Congenital deficiency of the cobalamin/intrinsic factor complex receptor has
              been reported in giant schnauzers.[44,45] This receptor appears to involve *cubam* (a
              complex of cubilin and amnionless) and megalin. A similar disorder occurs in
              Border collies, Australian shepherds, beagles, and komondors.[46]
        4. Severe cobalamin deficiency in a cat with methylmalonic acidemia:[47] The cause of
           the cobalamin deficiency was not established, but clinical evidence supported a
           congenital defect in cobalamin absorption.

FOLATE CONCENTRATION IN DOGS AND CATS

I. Physiologic processes
    A. See Figs. 15.1 and 15.2 for basic processes.
    B. Cobalamin and folate metabolism are linked in a reaction in which a methyl group is
       transferred from N^5-methyltetrahydrofolate to cobalamin in one-carbon pathways. In

the absence of cobalamin, the methyl group is trapped in N^5-methyltetrahydrofolate, and the result is a functional folate deficiency. Because N^5-methyltetrahydrofolate contributes to the total measured [folate], serum [folate] may not be decreased even though there is a functional folate deficiency (i.e., the manifestations of a folate deficiency are present).

II. Analytical concepts[40]
  A. Terms and units
    1. Specifically, folate is the anionic form of folic acid, which is composed of pteroic acid and glutamic acid. Several derivatives of folic acid are formed by the addition of substitution groups (e.g., methyl, formyl, glutamyl, and pteridine) to three positions in the molecule. The clinical serum assay detects primarily N^5-methyltetrahydrofolate, but the assay is commonly considered a test for folate.
    2. Unit conversion: ng/mL $\times$ 2.266 = nmol/L; and µg/dL $\times$ 22.66 = nmol/L (SI unit, nearest 2 nmol/L)[39]
  B. Assays
    1. Competitive-binding assays (sometimes combined with cobalamin assay) are most common. The competitive-binding agent in folate assays is β-lactoglobulin (milk folate binder), which binds principally with N^5-methyltetrahydrofolate.[40] Assays may involve denaturation of endogenous binding proteins (by boiling or high pH) to release folate.
    2. Bioassays have been used[48] but have been replaced by more convenient assays. Immunometric assays using ferromagnetic particles or charcoal are also used to measure [folate].
  C. Sample[8]
    1. Serum is the preferred sample. An erythrocyte has high [folate], and thus hemolysis will give falsely increased values. EDTA-plasma may be used in some assays.
    2. Serum [folate] are stable at 4 °C for 1 d and at −20 °C for 6–8 wk. Repeated thawing and freezing should be avoided.

III. Increased serum [folate] (Table 15.5)
  A. Increased absorption of folate in the small intestine
    1. Small intestinal bacterial overgrowth: Excessive folate produced by enteric bacteria is absorbed in the small intestine. The overgrowth could be secondary to EPI or caused

---

Table 15.5. Diseases and conditions that cause increased serum [folate]

Increased absorption of folate in small intestine
  Intestinal bacterial overgrowth: EPI, impaired gastric acid secretion, enteric disorders (see text)
  Low intestinal pH: EPI, excessive gastric acid production
  High dietary intake
Parenteral supplementation
Cobalamin deficiency in cats

---

* A relatively common disease or condition
Note: Lists of specific disorders or conditions are not complete but are provided to give examples. Hemolysis may give falsely increased values.

Table 15.6. Diseases and conditions that cause decreased serum [folate]

Decreased absorption of folate in small intestine

    *Small intestinal mucosal disease (proximal or diffuse)

    Dietary deficiency

   * A relatively common disease or condition

      by impaired gastric acid secretion, decreased intestinal peristalsis, a defective mucus barrier, or decreased production of immunoglobulin by intestinal lymphoid cells.[49] A relative IgA deficiency has been associated with intestinal bacterial overgrowth in German shepherds.[50]

    2. Low intestinal pH: Maximal folate absorption occurs in an acidic environment. Decreased intestinal pH (increased absorption) may occur with EPI (impaired HCO_3^- secretion) or excessive gastric acid production.

    3. High dietary intake: Folate absorption usually occurs by a facilitated transport system, but, at high intestinal concentrations, absorption occurs by passive diffusion.[51]

  B. Parenteral supplementation: The magnitude and duration of increased serum [folate] would depend on dosage. A complete history should indicate whether this process is a potential cause of the abnormality.

  C. Cobalamin deficiency in cats: Five of 19 cats with severe cobalamin deficiencies had increased serum [folate]. When given parenteral cobalamin therapy, the [folate] decreased significantly in the 19 cats. The authors suggested that the cobalamin deficiency decreased the utilization of folate (see Fig. 15.2), which resulted in the accumulation of folate in plasma.[21]

  D. As indicated in the preceding section II.C.1, in vitro hemolysis can cause falsely increased serum [folate] because erythrocytes contain folate.

IV.   Decreased serum [folate] (Table 15.6)

  A. Decreased absorption of folate in the small intestine

    1. Diseases of the proximal small intestinal mucosa can cause impaired absorption of folate.

    2. Dietary deficiency: Commercial diets should have more than minimum folate requirements, and thus folate-deficient diets are uncommon. Feeding an all-cheese diet to dogs created a folate deficiency.[52]

  B. Other concepts

    1. Prolonged phenytoin (Dilantin) treatment is known to lower serum [folate] in people. [Folate] was not significantly different in phenytoin-treated and nontreated dogs that were fed a folate-deficient diet.[52] The effects of phenytoin on [folate] is not known for dogs fed a folate-adequate diet.

    2. Sulfasalazine also is reported to lower [folate] in people, but similar findings have not been reported for dogs or cats.[53]

    3. In theory, sterilization of the intestine with antibiotics may lower serum [folate] because a major source of folate (intestinal flora) would be removed. Also, folate is involved in DNA synthesis, so extensive neoplastic cell growth could potentially deplete folate levels.

FECAL α_1-PROTEASE INHIBITOR (α_1-PI) CONCENTRATION IN DOGS AND CATS

I. Physiologic processes

    A. *α_1-PI* is a protein that inhibits the activity of proteases (e.g., trypsin) in feces. It is reported to have nearly the same molecular mass as albumin. α_1-PI is normally present in plasma, interstitial fluid, and lymph but not in the intestinal lumen.[54]

    B. The exact identity of this protein has not been found. Because it is considered to be of blood (plasma) origin, the antiprotease activity may be due to α_1-antitrypsin (human $M_r = 54,000$) or α_1-antichymotrypsin (human $M_r = 68,000$). The reported molecular mass of domestic mammal α_1-PI molecules varies slightly with the species: canine $M_r = 59,000$, feline $M_r = 57,000$, and equine $M_r = 58,000$.[55]

II. Analytical concepts

    A. Units: $\mu g/g$ of feces

    B. Sample

        1. Because of the variations in [α_1-PI] fecal samples, three separate voided fecal samples are collected. Collection of feces by digital or mechanical removal of feces may introduce blood into the sample, which will result in falsely increased [α_1-PI].[56]

        2. After collection, the fecal samples should be immediately frozen and shipped with dry ice to the reference laboratory. When kept at 37 °C for 72 h, the [α_1-PI] decreased by about 30 %; when kept at 4 °C for 72 h, the concentration decreased about 5 %.[57]

    C. Currently, there is one ELISA for measuring immunoreactivity for [α_1-PI] at Texas A&M's Gastrointestinal Laboratory (College Station, TX).[57]

    D. An assay for feline [α_1-PI] in serum has been developed, but documented evidence of clinical application was not found.[55]

III. Increased fecal [α_1-PI]

    A. Increased plasma protein loss into intestines

        1. Protein-losing enteropathies caused by extensive intestinal disease such as lymphangiectasia, idiopathic inflammatory bowel disease (including lymphocytic, plasmacytic, or eosinophilic disorders), intestinal lymphoma, intestinal carcinoma, histoplasmosis, intestinal parasitism, and parvoviral enteritis.[54,58]

        2. Blood loss into the alimentary tract: Blood loss may be associated with protein-losing enteropathies (e.g., ulceration or carcinoma), but it may also be due to hemorrhage from nonenteric disease (i.e., thrombocytopenia, coagulopathy, or gastric ulceration).

    B. Contamination of feces with blood or plasma during collection of the fecal sample.

    C. Increased fecal [α_1-PI] may be more sensitive to early protein-losing enteropathy than are serum albumin, globulin, and total protein concentrations.

IV. In a study involving seven dogs that were being treated with the nonsteroidal anti-inflammatory agents meloxicam or carprofen, fecal [α_1-PI] did not increase.[59]

D-XYLOSE ABSORPTION TEST IN DOGS, CATS, AND HORSES

I. Physiologic processes
    A. *D-Xylose* is a simple pentose that is not commonly ingested, and very little is present in blood or liver. If ingested, it is passively absorbed in the duodenum and proximal jejunum, from which it enters portal blood. After bypassing the liver, it passes through the glomerular filtration barrier and is excreted in urine.
    B. In people, xylose enters the glucuronic acid–xylulose pathway in hepatocytes. It is usually assumed that very little of the absorbed xylose is degraded by hepatocytes of domestic mammals.

II. Analytical concepts
    A. Unit conversion: mg/dL $\times$ 0.06661 = mmol/L (SI unit, nearest 0.1 mmol/L)[39]
    B. Assays
        1. Multiple xylose assays are available, but clinical laboratories do not commonly offer them.
        2. A colorimetric assay using phyloroglucinol has been used for equine and feline sera.[60] There also are assays that involve deproteination of whole blood, gas chromatography, or enzymatic methods.[61] An *o*-toluidine assay can measure [xylose] based on differences in absorbances of the reaction products produced by hexoses (e.g., glucose) and pentoses (e.g., xylose).[62]
        3. The capability of the intestine to absorb sugars other than just xylose (e.g., methyl glucose, rhamnose, and lactulose) can be determined by quantitation using high-performance liquid chromatography.[63,64]
    C. Sample
        1. The preferred sample varies with the assay system. Serum is generally preferred.
        2. Information on xylose stability was not found.

III. Xylose absorption tests
    A. Basics of procedure
        1. The *D-xylose absorption test* consists of administering D-xylose orally and then collecting multiple timed blood samples to assess the intestinal ability to absorb D-xylose. Most of the absorbed xylose passes through the liver and enters systemic blood. The peak blood [xylose] should reflect the amount of xylose absorbed by the intestine.
        2. Xylose is cleared from plasma by passing through the glomerular filtration barrier. The amount of xylose in urine is related to the amount of xylose absorbed in the intestine.
    B. In dogs and cats
        1. Xylose absorption tests have been used to evaluate the small intestinal function of dogs and cats.[65–69] In some animals with small intestinal disease, xylose was poorly absorbed and thus the absorption curves were flat.
        2. In most of the current textbooks, small animal internists no longer recommend xylose absorption tests, perhaps because of the limited availability of xylose assays or because other methods of characterizing intestinal disease are more fruitful.
    C. In horses: Xylose absorption tests have been used to evaluate the function of the small intestine.[70–74]

IV. Diseases and conditions that alter xylose absorption curves (Table 15.7)

Table 15.7. Diseases and conditions that alter xylose absorption curves

Flat xylose absorption curve (decreased absorption)
   *Reduced absorption because of small intestinal mucosal disease
    Incomplete delivery of xylose to intestine: vomiting, delayed gastric emptying
    Rapid transit time: diarrhea
Persistent [xylose] (decreased elimination)
    Decreased GFR

  * A relatively common disease or condition

GLUCOSE ABSORPTION TEST IN HORSES

I. Physiologic processes and introductory concepts
   A. The glucose absorption test is used primarily in horses that are presented because of chronic weight loss. The horses may be passing malformed feces (e.g., cow-pie). If the mucosal disease is limited to the small intestine, feces may have normal consistency.
   B. Glucose is a simple hexose that is absorbed in the duodenum and proximal jejunum, from which it enters portal blood. A large portion of the absorbed glucose is removed from the portal blood by hepatocytes, and the remainder enters the peripheral blood. From the peripheral blood, glucose may enter metabolic pathways of cells (e.g., glycolysis or glycogen synthesis) or be excreted by kidneys if the renal resorptive maximum for glucose is exceeded.
   C. In horses, microbes of the large intestine digest carbohydrates and produce volatile fatty acids that are absorbed by the mucosa. Therefore, disorders of the large intestine in horses can cause clinical states in which ingested carbohydrates are malassimilated.
   D. Whereas the results of the xylose absorption test depend primarily on the intestinal absorption of xylose, the results of the glucose absorption test depend on intestinal absorption and glucose utilization by hepatocytes and peripheral tissues (primarily muscle and adipose tissue). There are three major advantages of the glucose absorption test compared to the xylose absorption test: (1) glucose is more readily available, (2) glucose is less expensive, and (3) assays are more readily available for measuring serum [glucose].
   E. The glucose absorption test can be used to assess the intestinal absorption of monosaccharides in monogastric mammals, but cannot be used to assess intestinal absorption in ruminants. It is rarely used in the evaluation of dogs and cats, probably for two reasons: (1) other diagnostic methods are available (e.g., those using folate and cobalamin), and (2) disorders that cause glucose intolerance are more common. When used to assess carbohydrate tolerance, the procedure is called the *oral glucose tolerance test*.

II. Analytical concepts (see the Glucose Concentration, sect. II in Chapter 14)

III. Oral glucose absorption test
   A. Basics of procedure: Glucose is administered via a stomach tube, and then multiple blood samples are collected to assess the intestinal ability to absorb it. Assuming normal glucose metabolism, the peak blood [glucose] should reflect the amount of glucose absorbed by the intestine.

Table 15.8. Diseases and conditions that alter oral glucose absorption curves

Failure to meet criteria of adequate absorption
    *Malabsorption caused by small intestinal mucosal disease (inflammation, neoplasia, villous atrophy)
    Incomplete delivery of glucose to intestine (delayed gastric emptying, prolonged intestinal transit time)
    Rapid transit time associated with diarrhea
    Increased utilization of glucose by hepatocyte or peripheral tissues
Peak concentrations unexpectedly high or prolonged
    *Diabetes mellitus

* A relatively common disease or condition

  B. Procedure[75]
    1. Feed is withheld overnight prior to the procedure.
    2. A blood sample is collected for a baseline (or 0 time) [glucose].
    3. Glucose (1 g/kg body weight as a 20 % solution, weight/volume) is administered via stomach tube.
    4. Blood samples are collected at 30, 60, 90, 120, and 180 min after glucose is administered.
    5. Blood samples are processed appropriately, and glucose concentrations are measured in the serum or plasma samples.
  C. Expected values in healthy horses
    1. Two criteria are used as evidence of adequate intestinal absorption of glucose: [glucose] at 120 min is greater than either 85 %[76] or 100 %[77] above the baseline [glucose]
    2. The guidelines are based on data from 11 healthy horses. The peak [glucose] at 120 min was approximately twice the concentration in the baseline sample; that is, 178 ± 29 mg/dL at 120 min and 83 ± 11 mg/dL at 0 min (mean $\pm$ sd).[75]

IV.   Diseases and conditions that alter oral glucose absorption curves (Table 15.8)

LACTOSE TOLERANCE TEST IN HORSES

I.   Physiologic processes and introductory concepts
  A. The lactose tolerance test is used primarily in foals to detect a lactase deficiency that typically is secondary to intestinal mucosal damage.
  B. Lactose is a disaccharide composed of glucose and galactose. Lactase is typically present in the brush border of the small intestine in foals and young adult horses (< 3 yr old). Older horses lack the enzyme.[78]
  C. Lactase catalyzes the splitting of monosaccharides from lactose. The fate of the glucose is described in the Glucose Absorption Test in Horses section.

II.   Analytical concepts (see the Glucose Concentration, sect. II in Chapter 14)

III. Lactose tolerance test
  A. Basics of procedure: Lactose is administered via a stomach tube, and then multiple blood samples are collected to assess the intestinal mucosa's ability to digest lactose to

glucose and galactose. Assuming normal glucose absorption and metabolism, the peak blood [glucose] should reflect the amount of lactase activity in the intestine.

B. Procedure[79]
   1. Feed is withheld for 4 h prior to the procedure.
   2. A blood sample is collected for a baseline (or 0 time) [glucose].
   3. Lactose monohydrate (1 g/kg body weight as a 20 % solution, weight/volume) is administered via stomach tube.
   4. Blood samples are collected at 30, 60, and 90 min after lactose is administered.
   5. Blood samples are processed appropriately, and glucose concentrations are measured in the serum or plasma samples.
C. Criteria for adequate lactase activity
   1. [Glucose] is 150–250 % of baseline concentrations at 60 or 90 min.[77]
   2. A peak [glucose] is at least 35 mg/dL above the baseline concentration.[79]

IV. Diseases and conditions that alter the results of the oral lactose tolerance test
   A. Maldigestion caused by lactase deficiency
      1. Viral enteritis (e.g., rotavirus)
      2. *Clostridium difficile* enterocolitis[80]
   B. Malabsorption of glucose because of disease of the small intestine.
   C. Excessive cellular utilization of absorbed glucose

URINE SUCROSE CONCENTRATION IN HORSES[81]

I. Physiologic processes
   A. Sucrose is a disaccharide that is split into glucose and fructose by sucrase in the proximal small intestine.
   B. Sucrose is typically not absorbed by either gastric mucosa (impermeable) or enteric mucosa (degraded before absorption can occur).

II. Analytical concepts
   A. Assays
      1. For the equine study cited, high-performance liquid chromatography was used to separate sucrose from other sugars, and pulsed amperometric detection was used to quantify the separated sugars.[81]
      2. A spectrophotometric sucrose assay is available,[82] but reports of its use in domestic mammals were not found.
   B. Sample: Urine samples were collected, immediately mixed with sodium azide, and then frozen (at −80 °C) until analysis.
   C. Urine osmolality was also measured so that sucrose to osmolality ratios could be calculated.

III. Sucrose absorption tests
   A. Basics of procedure: The urinary bladder was emptied, and then horses were fed 1 kg of Omolene and then given 454 g of sucrose (10 % solution in H_2O) via a nasogastric tube. Urine samples were collected 2 and 4 h later.
   B. Horses with gastric ulcers had increased urine [sucrose] and increased sucrose to osmolality ratios. Those horses with more severe gastric ulcers excreted more sucrose in urine.

Table 15.9. Other laboratory methods used to evaluate for exocrine pancreatic insufficiency

Laboratory method	Abnormal result	Suggested pathologic state
Azocasein digestion test	Feces failed to digest azocasein	Decreased fecal proteolytic activity
Fecal fat excretion	Increased fecal fat excreted in 24 h sample	Maldigestion of ingested lipids
Fecal fat, microscopic exam	↑ Sudanophilic droplets in feces	Maldigestion of ingested lipids
Fecal starch, microscopic exam	↑ Starch granules stained by Lugol's iodine	Maldigestion of ingested starch
Gelatin tube digestion	Feces failed to liquefy gelatin adequately	Decreased fecal protease activity
Muscle fibers, microscopic exam	Undigested muscle fibers present	Maldigestion of dietary muscle (protein)
PABA[a]	Decreased plasma [PABA] or decreased urinary PABA excretion	Decreased chymotrypsin released from pancreas
Plasma turbidity test	Absence of plasma turbidity after ingesting lipid meal, but turbidity present after ingesting predigested lipids	Decreased pancreatic LPS activity in intestine
Radiographic film digestion	Feces failed to clear gelatin from film	Decreased fecal proteolytic activity
Starch digestion test	Flat glucose absorption curve	Maldigestion of starch or malabsorption of glucose

[a] PABA: N-benzoyl-L-tyrosyl-para-aminobenzoic acid (bentiromide)

Note: Increases in serum AMS and LPS activities can be indicators of active or recent pancreatic acinar cell damage. Serum AMS and LPS activities should not be used to detect EPI, because there are extrapancreatic sources of AMS and LPS that can keep serum activity within the reference interval in EPI cases. Serum AMS and LPS activity can be decreased when an animal does not have EPI.

OTHER METHODS OF EVALUATING DIGESTIVE OR ABSORPTIVE FUNCTIONS

I.   Many other laboratory assays or methods are used to evaluate animals with potential exocrine pancreatic or intestinal diseases (Tables 15.9 and 15.10). Most of the assays listed in the tables are no longer or only rarely used, often because of unacceptably high rates of false-negative and false-positive results.
   A. The measurement of [TLI] has generally replaced other tests that were used to evaluate potential maldigestive disorders.
   B. Most of the absorption tests have not been found to be clinically valuable. If malabsorption is suspected, histologic examination of biopsy samples is frequently used to establish a diagnosis so that appropriate therapy can be recommended or initiated.

II. Fecal assays used to detect intestinal parasitism are common in veterinary medicine, but discussion of the procedures is beyond the scope of this textbook. The reader is referred to diagnostic parasitology resources.

Table 15.10. Other laboratory methods used to evaluate intestinal diseases

Laboratory method	Abnormal result	Suggested pathologic state
Bacterial culture (isolation)	Specific isolate (e.g., *Salmonella* sp.)	Bacterial enteritis
Bacterial culture (quantitative)	> 10^5 colony-forming units/mL of duodenal juice	Small intestinal bacterial overgrowth
Biopsy procedures (incision or excision)	Abnormal cell populations or abnormal tissue structure	Varies with the histologic lesion; typically inflammation or neoplasia
Direct fecal exam	Motile parasites	Giardiasis or amebiasis
Fecal flotation test	Parasitic ova, oocytes, or larvae	Parasitism
Fecal occult blood	Positive reaction for heme	Blood in alimentary tract
Fecal sedimentation test	Fluke ova	Parasitism
Hydrogen breath test	Increased hydrogen production	Bacterial overgrowth or carbohydrate malabsorption
Plasma turbidity test with predigested fat	Absence of plasma turbidity	Malabsorption of digested lipids
Stained feces, microscopic exam	Acid-fast organisms	*Cryptosporidia* oocysts or *Mycobacterium* bacilli
	Giardia trophozoites	Giardiasis
	Histoplasma organisms	Histoplasmosis
	Increased leukocytes	Enteritis
	Neoplastic cells	Neoplasia
	Uniform bacilli	Bacterial overgrowth
Starch digestion test	Flat glucose absorption curve	Malabsorption of glucose
Unconjugated bile acids	Increased serum concentrations	Increased deconjugation of bile acids by an overgrowth of intestinal bacteria
Urine indican test	Positive for indican	Increased degradation of tryptophan by enteric bacteria
Urine nitrosonaphthol test	Positive nitrosonaphthol test	Increased bacterial degradation of tyrosine by enteric bacteria

Note: This is not a complete list. Other special assays are used for specific organisms or pathologic states.

References

1. Wiberg ME, Saari SA, Westermarck E. 1999. Exocrine pancreatic atrophy in German shepherd dogs and rough-coated collies: An end result of lymphocytic pancreatitis. Vet Pathol 36:530–541.
2. Wiberg ME. 2004. Pancreatic acinar atrophy in German shepherd dogs and rough-coated collies: Etiopathogenesis, diagnosis and treatment—A review. Vet Q 26:61–75.
3. Moeller EM, Steiner JM, Clark LA, Murphy KE, Famula TR, Williams DA, Stankovics ME, Vose AS. 2002. Inheritance of pancreatic acinar atrophy in German shepherd dogs. Am J Vet Res 63:1429–1434.
4. Watson PJ. 2003. Exocrine pancreatic insufficiency as an end stage of pancreatitis in four dogs. J Small Anim Pract 44:306–312.

5. Steiner JM, Williams DA. 2000. Serum feline trypsin-like immunoreactivity in cats with exocrine pancreatic insufficiency. J Vet Intern Med 14:627–629.

6. Williams DA. 2000. Exocrine pancreatic disease. In: Ettinger SJ, Feldman EC, eds. *Textbook of Veterinary Internal Medicine: Diseases of the Dog and Cat*, 5th edition, 1345–1367. Philadelphia: WB Saunders.

7. Steiner JM, Williams DA. 2000. Disagrees with criteria for diagnosing pancreatitis in cats. J Am Vet Med Assoc 217:816–817.

8. Tietz NW. 1995. *Clinical Guide to Laboratory Tests*, 3rd edition. Philadelphia: WB Saunders.

9. Keller ET. 1990. High serum trypsin-like immunoreactivity secondary to pancreatitis in a dog with exocrine pancreatic insufficiency. J Am Vet Med Assoc 196:623–626.

10. Steiner JM. 2003. Diagnosis of pancreatitis. Vet Clin North Am Small Anim Pract 33:1181–1195.

11. Hayakawa T, Kondo T, Shibata T, Naruse S. 1992. Peritoneal absorption of pancreatic enzymes in dogs. Gastroenterol Jpn 27:230–233.

12. Simpson KW, Batt RM, McLean L, Morton DB. 1989. Circulating concentrations of trypsin-like immunoreactivity and activities of lipase and amylase after pancreatic duct ligation in dogs. Am J Vet Res 50:629–632.

13. Lucena R, Ginel PJ, Novales M, Molleda JM. 1999. Effects of dexamethasone administration on serum trypsin-like immunoreactivity in healthy dogs. Am J Vet Res 1357–1359.

14. Swift NC, Marks SL, MacLachlan NJ, Norris CR. 2000. Evaluation of serum feline trypsin-like immunoreactivity for the diagnosis of pancreatitis in cats. J Am Vet Med Assoc 217:37–42.

15. Forman MA, Marks SL, De Cock HE, Hergesell EJ, Wisner ER, Baker TW, Kass PH, Steiner JM, Williams DA. 2004. Evaluation of serum feline pancreatic lipase immunoreactivity and helical computed tomography versus conventional testing for the diagnosis of feline pancreatitis. J Vet Intern Med 18:807–815.

16. Gerhardt A, Steiner JM, Williams DA, Kramer S, Fuchs C, Janthur M, Hewicker-Trautwein M, Nolte I. 2001. Comparison of the sensitivity of different diagnostic tests for pancreatitis in cats. J Vet Intern Med 15:329–333.

17. Grulke S, Gangl M, Deby-Dupont G, Caudron I, Deby C, Serteyn D. 2002. Plasma trypsin level in horses suffering from acute intestinal obstruction. Vet J 163:283–291.

18. Grulke S, Deby-Dupont G, Gangl M, Franck T, Deby C, Serteyn D. 2003. Equine trypsin: Purification and development of a radio-immunoassay. Vet Res 34:317–330.

19. Reidelberger RD, O'Rourke M, Durie PR, Geokas MC, Largman C. 1984. Effects of food intake and cholecystokinin on plasma trypsinogen levels in dogs. Am J Physiol 246:G543–G549.

20. Geokas MC, Reidelberger R, O'Rourke M, Passaro E Jr, Largman C. 1982. Plasma pancreatic trypsinogens in chronic renal failure and after nephrectomy. Am J Physiol 242:G177–G182.

21. Ruaux CG, Steiner JM, Williams DA. 2005. Early biochemical and clinical responses to cobalamin supplementation in cats with signs of gastrointestinal disease and severe hypocobalaminemia. J Vet Intern Med 19:155–160.

22. Meneses F, Ehinger B, Gerhardt A, Meyer-Lindenberg A, Hewicker-Trautwein M, Amtsberg G, Nolte I. 2003. Chronic-idiopathic enteropathy in cats: A case control study. Berl Munch Tierarztl Wochenschr 116:340–345.

23. Carro T, Williams DA. 1989. Relationship between dietary protein concentration and serum trypsin-like immunoreactivity in dogs. Am J Vet Res 50:2105–2107.

24. Williams DA, Batt RM. 1988. Sensitivity and specificity of radioimmunoassay of serum trypsin-like immunoreactivity for the diagnosis of canine exocrine pancreatic insufficiency. J Am Vet Med Assoc 192:195–201.

25. Wiberg ME, Westermarck E. 2002. Subclinical exocrine pancreatic insufficiency in dogs. J Am Vet Med Assoc 220:1183–1187.

26. Steiner JM, Williams DA. 2003. Development and validation of a radioimmunoassay for the measurement of canine pancreatic lipase immunoreactivity in serum of dogs. Am J Vet Res 64:1237–1241.

27. Steiner JM, Teague SR, Williams DA. 2003. Development and analytic validation of an enzyme-linked immunosorbent assay for the measurement of canine pancreatic lipase immunoreactivity in serum. Can J Vet Res 67:175–182.

28. Steiner JM, Wilson BG, Williams DA. 2004. Development and analytical validation of a radioimmunoassay for the measurement of feline pancreatic lipase immunoreactivity in serum. Can J Vet Res 68:309–314.

29. Steiner JM, Broussard J, Mansfield CS, Gumminger SR, Williams DA. 2001. Serum canine pancreatic lipase immunoreactivity (cPLI) concentrations in dogs with spontaneous pancreatitis. J Vet Intern Med 15:274 (abstract).

30. Williams DA, Steiner JM, Ruaux CG, Zavros N. 2003. Increases in serum pancreatic lipase immunoreactivity (PLI) are greater and of longer duration than those of trypsin-like immunoreactivity (TLI) in cats with experimental pancreatitis. J Vet Intern Med 17:445–446 (abstract).

31. Williams DA. 2003. Diagnosis of canine and feline pancreatitis. In: 38th Annual Meeting of the American Society of Veterinary Clinical Pathologists, Banff, Alberta, 6–12.

32. Steiner JM, Finco DR, Gumminger SR, Williams DA. 2001. Serum canine pancreatic lipase immunoreactivity (cPLI) in dogs with experimentally induced chronic renal failure. J Vet Intern Med 15:311 (abstract).

33. Steiner JM, Rutz GM, Williams DA. 2006. Serum lipase activities and pancreatic lipase immunoreactivity concentrations in dogs with exocrine pancreatic insufficiency. Am J Vet Res 67:84–87.

34. Mansfield CS, Jones BR. 2000. Plasma and urinary trypsinogen activation peptide in healthy dogs, dogs with pancreatitis and dogs with other systemic diseases. Aust Vet J 78:416–422.

35. Mansfield CS, Jones BR, Spillman T. 2003. Assessing the severity of canine pancreatitis. Res Vet Sci 74:137–144.

36. Allen HS, Steiner J, Broussard J, Mansfield C, Williams DA, Jones B. 2006. Serum and urine concentrations of trypsinogen-activation peptide as markers for acute pancreatitis in cats. Can J Vet Res 70:313–316.

37. Karanjia ND, Widdison AL, Jehanli A, Hermon-Taylor J, Reber HA. 1993. Assay of trypsinogen activation in the cat experimental model of acute pancreatitis. Pancreas 8:189–195.

38. Rucker RB, Morris JG. 1997. The vitamins. In: Kaneko JJ, Harvey JW, Bruss ML, eds. *Clinical Biochemistry of Domestic Animals*, 5th edition, 703–739. San Diego: Academic.

39. Lundberg GD, Iverson C, Radulescu G. 1986. Now read this: The SI units are here. J Am Med Assoc 255:2329–2339.

40. Fairbanks VF, Klee GG. 1999. Biochemical aspects of hematology. In: Burtis CA, Ashwood ER, eds. *Tietz Textbook of Clinical Chemistry*, 3rd edition, 1642–1710. Philadelphia: WB Saunders.

41. Simpson KW, Morton DB, Batt RM. 1989. Effect of exocrine pancreatic insufficiency on cobalamin absorption in dogs. Am J Vet Res 50:1233–1236.

42. Williams DA, Batt RM, McLean L. 1987. Bacterial overgrowth in the duodenum of dogs with exocrine pancreatic insufficiency. J Am Vet Med Assoc 191:201–206.

43. Stangl GI, Schwarz FJ, Jahn B, Kirchgessner M. 2000. Cobalt-deficiency–induced hyperhomocysteinaemia and oxidative status of cattle. Br J Nutr 83:3–6.

44. Fyfe JC, Giger U, Hall CA, Jezyk PF, Klumpp SA, Levine JS, Patterson DF. 1991. Inherited selective intestinal cobalamin malabsorption and cobalamin deficiency in dogs. Pediatr Res 29:24–31.

45. Fyfe JC, Jezyk PF, Giger U, Patterson DF. 1989. Inherited selective malabsorption of vitamin B_{12} in giant schnauzers. J Am Anim Hosp Assoc 25:533–539.

46. Outerbridge CA, Myers SL, Giger U. 1996. Hereditary cobalamin deficiency in Border collie dogs. J Vet Intern Med 10:169 (abstract).

47. Vaden SL, Wood PA, Ledley FD, Cornwell PE, Miller RT, Page R. 1992. Cobalamin deficiency associated with methylmalonic acidemia in a cat. J Am Vet Med Assoc 200:1101–1103.

48. Batt RM, Morgan JO. 1982. Role of serum folate and vitamin B_{12} concentrations in the differentiation of small intestinal abnormalities in the dog. Res Vet Sci 32:17–22.

49. Rutgers HC, Batt RM, Elwood CM, Lamport A. 1995. Small intestinal bacterial overgrowth in dogs with chronic intestinal disease. J Am Vet Med Assoc 206:187–193.

50. Batt RM, Barnes A, Rutgers HC, Carter SD. 1991. Relative IgA deficiency and small intestinal bacterial overgrowth in German shepherd dogs. Res Vet Sci 50:106–111.

51. Hall EJ, Simpson KW. 2000. Diseases of the small intestine. In: Ettinger SJ, Feldman EC, eds. *Textbook of Veterinary Internal Medicine: Diseases of the Dog and Cat*, 5th edition, 1182–1238. Philadelphia: WB Saunders.

52. Bunch SE, Easley JR, Cullen JM. 1990. Hematologic values and plasma and tissue folate concentrations in dogs given phenytoin on a long-term basis. Am J Vet Res 51:1865–1868.

53. Williams DA. 1999. Defining small intestinal disease. In: Proceedings of the 17th ACVIM Forum, Chicago, 466–468.

54. Murphy KF, German AJ, Ruaux CG, Steiner JM, Williams DA, Hall EJ. 2003. Fecal α_1-proteinase inhibitor concentration in dogs with chronic gastrointestinal disease. Vet Clin Pathol 32:67–72.

55. Fetz K, Ruaux CG, Steiner JM, Suchodolski JS, Williams DA. 2004. Purification and partial characterization of feline α_1-proteinase inhibitor ($f\alpha_1$-PI) and the development and validation of a radioimmunoassay for the measurement of $f\alpha_1$-PI in serum. Biochimie 86:67–75.

56. Koenig A, Slater M, Ruaux CG, Steiner JM, Williams D. 2002. Comparison of fecal α_1-proteinase inhibitor concentrations in fecal samples obtained via spontaneous defecation and rectal palpation. J Vet Intern Med 16:329 (abstract).

57. Melgarejo T, Williams DA, Asem EK. 1998. Enzyme-linked immunosorbent assay for canine α_1-protease inhibitor. Am J Vet Res 59:127–130.

58. Mohr AJ, Leisewitz AL, Jacobson LS, Steiner JM, Ruaux CG, Williams DA. 2003. Effect of early enteral nutrition on intestinal permeability, intestinal protein loss, and outcome in dogs with severe parvoviral enteritis. J Vet Intern Med 17:791–798.

59. Murphy KF, German AJ, Ruaux CG, Steiner JM, Williams DA, Hall EJ. 2003. Fecal α_1-proteinase inhibitor concentration in dogs receiving long-term nonsteroidal anti-inflammatory drug therapy. Vet Clin Pathol 32:136–139.

60. Eberts TJ, Sample RH, Glick MR, Ellis GH. 1979. A simplified, colorimetric micromethod for xylose in serum or urine, with phloroglucinol. Clin Chem 25:1440–1443.

61. Henderson AR, Rinker AD. 1999. Gastric, pancreatic, and intestinal function. In: Burtis CA, Ashwood ER, eds. *Tietz Textbook of Clinical Chemistry*, 3rd edition, 1271–1327. Philadelphia: WB Saunders.

62. Bauer JD, Ackermann PG, Toro G. 1974. *Clinical Laboratory Methods*, 8th edition. St Louis: CV Mosby.

63. Sørensen SH, Proud FJ, Rutgers HC, Markwell P, Adam A, Batt RM. 1997. A blood test for intestinal permeability and function: A new tool for the diagnosis of chronic intestinal disease in dogs. Clin Chim Acta 264:103–115.

64. Rutgers HC, Batt RM, Proud FJ, Sørensen SH, Elwood CM, Petrie G, Matthewman LA, Forster-van Hijfte MA, Boswood A, Entwistle M, Fensome RH. 1996. Intestinal permeability and function in dogs with small intestinal bacterial overgrowth. J Small Anim Pract 37:428–434.

65. Hill FWG, Kidder DE, Frew J. 1970. A xylose absorption test for the dog. Vet Rec 87:250–255.

66. Hill FWG. 1972. Malabsorption syndrome in the dog: A study of thirty-eight cases. J Small Anim Pract 13:575–594.

67. Burrows CF, Merritt AM, Chiapella AM. 1979. Determination of fecal fat and trypsin output in the evaluation of chronic canine diarrhea. J Am Vet Med Assoc 174:62–66.

68. Sherding RG, Stradley RP, Rogers WA, Johnson SE. 1982. Bentiromide:xylose test in healthy cats. Am J Vet Res 43:2272–2273.

69. Hawkins EC, Meric SM, Washabau RJ, Feldman EC, Turrel JM. 1986. Digestion of bentiromide and absorption of xylose in healthy cats and absorption of xylose in cats with infiltrative intestinal disease. Am J Vet Res 47:567–569.

70. Jacobs KA, Norman P, Hodgson DRG, Cymbaluk N. 1982. Effect of diet on the oral D-xylose absorption test in the horse. Am J Vet Res 43:1856–1858.

71. Bolton JR, Merritt AM, Cimprich RE, Ramberg CF, Streett W. 1976. Normal and abnormal xylose absorption in the horse. Cornell Vet 66:183–197.

72. Tate LP Jr, Ralston SL, Koch CM, Everitt JI. 1983. Effects of extensive resection of the small intestine in the pony. Am J Vet Res 44:1187–1191.

73. Roberts MC. 1974. The D (+) xylose absorption test in the horse. Equine Vet J 6:28–30.

74. Roberts MC, Norman P. 1979. A re-evaluation of the D (+) xylose absorption test in the horse. Equine Vet J 11:239–243.

75. Roberts MC, Hill FWG. 1973. The oral glucose tolerance test in the horse. Equine Vet J 5:171–173.

76. Mair TS, Hillyer MH, Taylor FG, Pearson GR. 1991. Small intestinal malabsorption in the horse: An assessment of the specificity of the oral glucose tolerance test. Equine Vet J 23:344–346.

77. Sweeney RW. 1987. Laboratory evaluation of malassimilation in horses. Vet Clin North Am Equine Pract 3:507–514.

78. Roberts MC. 1975. Carbohydrate digestion and absorption in the equine small intestine. J S Afr Vet Assoc 46:19–27.

79. Martens RJ, Malone PS, Brust DM. 1985. Oral lactose tolerance test in foals: Technique and normal values. Am J Vet Res 46:2163–2165.

80. Weese JS, Parsons DA, Staempfli HR. 1999. Association of *Clostridium difficile* with enterocolitis and lactose intolerance in a foal. J Am Vet Med Assoc 214:229–232.

81. O'Conner MS, Steiner JM, Roussel AJ, Williams DA, Meddings JB, Pipers F, Cohen ND. 2004. Evaluation of urine sucrose concentration for detection of gastric ulcers in horses. Am J Vet Res 65:31–39.

82. Hessels J, Snoeyink EJ, Platenkamp AJ, Voortman G, Steggink J, Eidhof HH. 2003. Assessment of intestinal permeability: Enzymatic determination of urinary mannitol, raffinose, sucrose and lactose on Hitachi analyzer. Clin Chem Lab Med 41:33–38.

Chapter 16

LIPIDS

Lipids 764
Overview of Lipoproteins 764
    I.   Lipoprotein Classification, Content, and Properties 764
    II. Lipoprotein Metabolism 766
    III. Lipases 767
Cholesterol Concentration of Serum 767
    I.   Physiologic Processes 767
    II. Analytical Concepts 769
    III. Hypercholesterolemia 770
    IV. Hypocholesterolemia 770
Triglyceride (TG) (Triacylglycerol) Concentration of Serum 771
    I.   Physiologic Processes 771
    II. Analytical Concepts 771
    III. Hypertriglyceridemia 772
    IV. Hypotriglyceridemia 772
Hyperlipemia, Hyperlipidemia, and Hyperlipoproteinemia Disorders 773
    I.   Terms 773
    II. Classification of Hyperlipoproteinemia Conditions and Disorders 773
    III. Physiologic (Postprandial) Hyperlipidemia 773
    IV. Primary or Possible Primary Hyperlipidemia Disorders in Domestic
        Mammals 773
    V. Secondary Hyperlipidemia Disorders 775
Other Assessments of Lipids 778
    I.   Lipoprotein Electrophoresis 778
    II. Nonesterified Fatty Acids (NEFA, Free Fatty Acids, and Fatty Acids) 778
    III. Standing Plasma Test for Chylomicrons 780

Table 16.1. Abbreviations and symbols in this chapter

[x]	Concentration of x (x = analyte)
CoA	Coenzyme A
EDTA	Ethylenediaminetetraacetic acid
HDL	High-density lipoprotein
IDL	Intermediate-density lipoprotein
LCAT	Lecithin-cholesterol acyltransferase
LDL	Low-density lipoprotein
LPL	Lipoprotein lipase
LPS	Lipase
NEFA	Nonesterified fatty acid, free fatty acid, fatty acid
SI	Système International d'Unités
TG	Triglyceride (also called triacylglycerol)
TNF	Tumor necrosis factor
VLDL	Very low-density lipoprotein

LIPIDS

I.   A *lipid* is a compound that is soluble in organic solvents and relatively insoluble in H_2O. Of the lipid compounds in blood or other body fluids, serum [cholesterol] and [TG] are the most frequently measured and thus are the focus of this chapter.

II.   Lipids found in mammals[1]
    A. Sterols: cholesterol, cholesterol esters, bile acids, steroid hormones, and vitamin D
    B. Glycerol esters: phosphoglycerides (phospholipids), monoglycerides, diglycerides, and triglycerides
    C. Fatty acids: short-, medium-, and long-chain fatty acids, and prostaglandins (fatty-acid derivatives)
    D. Sphingosines: sphingomyelin (phospholipids), and glycosphingolipids
    E. Terpenes: vitamins A, E, and K

III.   Lipids have many functions in the body but are particularly important as an energy source (triglycerides and fatty acids), as structural components of all cell membranes (phospholipids and cholesterol), and as substrates for hormones and second messengers.

OVERVIEW OF LIPOPROTEINS

I.   Lipoprotein Classification, Content, and Properties
    A. A basic understanding of lipoprotein composition and properties is needed to understand serum [TG] and [cholesterol] because all TG and most cholesterol molecules are transported in serum within lipoproteins. Formation of lipoproteins enables lipids to form small particles that can circulate through the vasculature without coalescing into large lipid masses that would obstruct blood flow.
    B. Lipoproteins are classified either by their electrophoretic mobility or by their density relative to H_2O. Their properties depend on composition (Table 16.2).

Table 16.2. Lipoprotein classification, content, and properties of human lipoproteins

Property		Lipoproteins			
	Chylomicron	VLDL	IDL	LDL	HDL
Density (g/mL)	< 0.95	< 1.006	1.006–1.019	1.019–1.063	1.063–1.210
Major lipid	Dietary TG	Hepatic TG, phospholipid, & cholesterol ester	Hepatic TG & cholesterol ester	Phospholipid & cholesterol ester	Phospholipid & cholesterol ester
Lipid to protein ratio	40:1 to 70:1	10:1 to 15:1	5:1 to 10:1	3:1 to 4:1	1:1
Apolipoproteins	A, B, C, E	B, C, E	B, C, E	B	A, C, D, E
Electrophoretic migration	Origin	Pre-β	β to pre-β	β	α
Diameter (nm)	> 70 (often 500–1000)	25–70	22–24	19–23	4–10
Contribute to serum lactescence	Yes, floats with time	Yes	Maybe	No	No
Major site of formation	Small intestine enterocytes	Hepatocyte	Plasma (from VLDLs)	Plasma (from IDLs and VLDLs)	Hepatocytes, enterocytes
Major sites of degradation or transformation	Plasma and hepatocytes	Plasma	Plasma	Nonhepatic cells, hepatocytes, macrophages	Hepatocytes

Source (modified): Rifai et al.[1]

1. The general composition of lipoproteins in domestic mammals is similar to the composition of human lipoproteins.[2,3]
    a. The outside surface of lipoprotein particles contains phospholipids, nonesterified cholesterol molecules, and apolipoproteins. The hydrophilic aspects of the molecules are on the plasma surface; the hydrophobic aspects are adjacent to a core of mostly TG and cholesterol ester molecules. Fatty acids may be present in the core but also circulate outside of lipoproteins bound to albumin.
    b. *Apolipoproteins* (apoproteins) are the specific protein and polypeptide components of lipoproteins. They are separated into five major classes (A, B, C, D, and E), some with subclasses (e.g., C-1, C-II, and C-III).
    c. Lipoprotein density increases with increased percentage of protein content (chylomicrons < VLDL < IDL < LDL < HDL), whereas the ratios of lipid to protein and triglyceride to cholesterol decrease with increasing lipoprotein density.
2. There are also significant variations in the relative amounts, content, and electrophoretic migration of lipoprotein fractions and subfractions among species.
    a. Dogs, cats, and horses have predominantly HDL cholesterol rather than LDL cholesterol. LDL cholesterol predominates in people.
    b. Predominance of HDL cholesterol is associated with decreased or absent cholesterol ester transfer activity (transferring cholesterol from HDL to LDL) and decreased susceptibility to atherogenesis. Most domestic mammals have little or no cholesterol ester transfer activity.
C. In veterinary medicine, TG and cholesterol are the routine screening tests to assess lipoproteins, whereas in human medicine, a routine lipoprotein profile also includes measurement of HDL cholesterol ("good cholesterol"), a calculation of LDL cholesterol ("bad cholesterol"), and sometimes a calculation of VLDL cholesterol.
D. More complete lipoprotein analysis includes qualitative and quantitative lipoprotein subfraction analysis by various electrophoretic and density separations, and assessment of apolipoproteins by immunoassays or genetic tests. Such assays are used to assess lipoprotein metabolism in people but are rarely used in clinical veterinary medicine.

II. Lipoprotein metabolism (Fig. 16.1)
A. In the context of serum [cholesterol] and [TG], disorders involving lipoprotein metabolism involve excess synthesis, defective lipolysis, or defective clearance or cellular uptake of lipoproteins.
    1. Nascent (newly made) lipoproteins are produced in small intestinal enterocytes (chylomicrons) and in hepatocytes (VLDL and discoid HDL).
    2. Lipolysis of lipoproteins (chylomicrons, VLDL, and IDL) occurs on the luminal surface of capillary endothelial cells and is catalyzed by LPL. LPL production and activity depend on insulin. Insulin enables LPL to "float" from the inner surface of the cell membrane to the outer surface, where it can contact plasma lipoproteins and thus facilitate the removal of TG from lipoproteins.[2,4]
    3. Intravenous heparin promotes the release of LPL from endothelial cells and thus an increased plasma LPL activity.[1] Heparin also promotes release of hepatic lipase from the sinusoidal endothelial cells to plasma.[5,6] Because of its actions, heparin is sometimes called *lipemia clearing factor.*
    4. Lipoprotein remnants are cleared from plasma by hepatocytes. LDL molecules are removed from plasma by many types of cells. LPL increases LDL uptake by promoting LDL binding to cell receptors.[7]

B. Apolipoproteins are critical for normal lipoprotein metabolism, influencing lipoprotein structure, acting as cofactors for enzymes involved in lipid metabolism, and acting as ligands for receptor-mediated cellular interactions.
   1. The A class, from intestine and liver, is associated mostly with HDL. Apolipoprotein A-I is an activator of lecithin-cholesterol acyltransferase (LCAT) and is a structural protein.
   2. The B class, from intestine and liver, is involved in synthesis and secretion of chylomicrons and VLDL and in the endocytosis of lipoprotein particles from VLDL, IDL, LDL, and chylomicron remnants.
   3. The C class, from liver, is mostly in VLDL, HDL, and chylomicrons. Apolipoprotein C-II is a cofactor for LPL.
   4. Apolipoprotein D is associated with LCAT in HDL.
   5. The E class, from liver and macrophages, is in all lipoproteins and may be involved in ligand binding and conversion of VLDL to IDL.
C. There are many other aspects of lipoprotein metabolism (e.g., mobilization and oxidation of lipids, and apolipoprotein receptor regulation) that will not be considered here. For more detailed information about control and processes of lipoproteins, the reader is referred to textbooks or review articles.[1,2,5] A detailed understanding of lipoprotein metabolism is needed to understand coronary heart disease and some primary lipoprotein disorders. Because such disorders are uncommon in domestic mammals, lipoprotein information will be limited.

III. Of the several lipases in the body, the major ones that pertain to lipid disorders are LPL and hepatic lipase. More information about lipases is in Chapter 12.
A. Hepatic lipase is produced by hepatocytes, is present on endothelial cells of hepatic sinusoids, and hydrolyzes TG in LDL.
B. Many extrahepatic cells, including adipocytes and myocytes, produce LPL. It migrates from these cells to the luminal surface of endothelial cells, where it catalyzes the hydrolysis of TG in chylomicrons, VLDL, and IDL. Its activity is enhanced by insulin, thyroxine, and heparin.

CHOLESTEROL CONCENTRATION OF SERUM

I. Physiologic processes
A. Nearly all cholesterol in a fasting serum sample is within lipoproteins, and most was produced in hepatocytes. However, essentially all cells can synthesize cholesterol. Particularly significant nonhepatic sources are intestinal mucosal cells, which synthesize cholesterol that is packaged into chylomicrons, and gonads and adrenal glands.
B. In the healthy state, cholesterol synthesis begins with acetyl-CoA and is a regulated process that depends on cellular [cholesterol]. The major rate-limiting enzyme is 3-hydroxy-3-methylglutaryl-coenzyme A reductase.
C. The potential toxic effects of free cholesterol are prevented by cholesterol esterification involving two enzymes: plasma LCAT and cellular acylcholesterol acyltransferase. Esterification also increases the lipid-carrying capacity of lipoproteins.
D. In general, LDL delivers cholesterol produced in the liver to other cells in the body, and HDL scavenges excess cholesterol from cells throughout the body and delivers it to the liver.

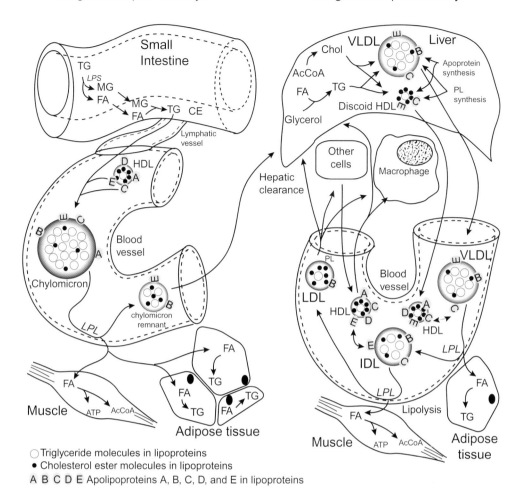

Exogenous Lipid Pathways

Endogenous Lipid Pathways

○ Triglyceride molecules in lipoproteins
● Cholesterol ester molecules in lipoproteins
A B C D E Apolipoproteins A, B, C, D, and E in lipoproteins

Fig. 16.1. Basic physiologic processes in lipoprotein metabolism. The three major processes that affect [lipoprotein] and thus [TG] and [cholesterol] are (1) synthesis of chylomicrons in enterocytes and VLDL in hepatocytes, (2) LPL-catalyzed lipolysis on endothelial cell membranes, and (3) hepatocyte clearance of lipoprotein remnants. There are two major metabolic pathways for lipids, one for endogenous and one for exogenous lipids.

- Exogenous or dietary lipids: Ingested TG in the presence of bile acids and LPS undergoes lipolysis to form MG and FA. After absorption by enterocytes, MG and FA are reassembled into TG. Enterocytes also produce CE, phospholipids, and apolipoproteins A and B and then assemble the molecules into TG-rich lipoproteins called *chylomicrons*. The chylomicrons are secreted into lymphatic vessels and then enter blood via the thoracic duct. In blood, chylomicrons obtain C and E apolipoproteins from circulating HDL. In the presence of insulin, apolipoprotein C-II activates LPL (on endothelial cell membranes) that catalyzes the lipolysis of TG to generate FA. The FA enters adipocytes to be stored in TG or enters muscle fibers (or other cells) to undergo oxidation to generate energy. After removal of most TG molecules, the chylomicron remnants are cleared from plasma by hepatocytes in a process involving B apolipoproteins.

E. Cholesterol esters enter cells by receptor-mediated endocytosis of lipoprotein fragments. They are delivered to lysosomes, where acid lipase promotes their hydrolysis. Cholesterol can then be released for use by the cell.

F. When cholesterol reaches hepatocytes via lipoprotein remnants, it may be reused for lipoprotein synthesis, excreted unchanged in bile, or degraded to bile acids.

II. Analytical concepts

   A. Terms and units

      1. Serum [cholesterol] represents the total [cholesterol], including cholesterol and cholesterol esters that are hydrolyzed during analysis. The reacting cholesterol molecules are within lipoproteins, typically in cholesterol-rich LDL and HDL molecules.

      2. Units: mg/dL × 0.02586 = mmol/L (SI unit, nearest 0.05 mmol/L)[8]

   B. Sample

      1. Serum is the preferred sample. Total [cholesterol] is stable at 4 °C for 5–7 d, at −20 °C for 3 mo, and at −70 °C for years. Repeated thawing and refreezing should be avoided.[9]

      2. Dogs and cats should be fasted overnight or for about 12 h to avoid postprandial hyperlipidemia, which may affect [cholesterol].

   C. Methods

      1. Most automated assays are enzymatic methods that hydrolyze cholesterol esters and then use cholesterol oxidase to oxidize cholesterol and generate hydrogen peroxide, which then reacts with an indicator dye. Some assays use an O_2-sensing electrode to measure O_2 consumption.

Fig. 16.1. *continued*

- Endogenous lipids produced by hepatocytes: Hepatocytes produce TG, phospholipids, apolipoproteins, and CE that may form from dietary cholesterol or de novo synthesis.
  - TG-rich VLDL is assembled in hepatocytes and secreted into sinusoidal blood. In the presence of insulin, apolipoproteins C-II on the VLDL activate LPL on endothelial cells to initiate lipolysis and liberation of FA from TG. As VLDL loses TG, it becomes denser to form IDL, which may also undergo additional lipolysis to form LDL. LDL delivers cholesterol to many cells for maintenance of cell membranes or steroid hormone synthesis. Hepatocyte clearance of LDL involves the action of hepatic lipase and the binding of a cholesterol-rich remnant to a B-apolipoprotein receptor on hepatocytes. LDL is also removed by macrophages in either receptor or non–receptor-mediated processes.
  - Discoid HDL particles consisting primarily of apolipoproteins and phospholipid are produced by hepatocytes and have two major functions: (1) they serve as a source of C and E apolipoproteins for other lipoproteins, and (2) they accept cholesterol from plasma membranes or lipoproteins and transport it for reutilization (in hepatocytes) or degradation (in hepatocytes or macrophages). Cholesterol is captured by the LCAT-catalyzed formation of cholesterol ester and lysolecithin from lecithin and cholesterol. This is supported by apolipoprotein A. As HDL accumulates cholesterol in circulation, they become larger and acquire their spherical form.
- The outer surfaces of lipoproteins contain phospholipids, nonesterified cholesterol, and apolipoproteins. Shaded letters A, B, C, and E are A, B, C, and E apolipoproteins; AcCoA, acetyl-coenzyme A; ATP, adenosine 5′-triphosphate; CE, cholesterol ester; Chol, cholesterol; FA, fatty acid; LPL, lipoprotein lipase; LPS, pancreatic lipase; MG, monoglyceride; PL, phospholipid; and TG, triglyceride.

Table 16.3. Diseases and conditions that cause hypercholesterolemia

Increased cholesterol production
    By hepatocytes
        *Nephrotic syndrome or protein-losing nephropathy
    By enterocytes
        *Postprandial hyperlipidemia
Decreased lipolysis or intravascular processing of lipoproteins
    *Hypothyroidism
    *Nephrotic syndrome or protein-losing nephropathy
    Lipoprotein lipase deficiency (very rare in dogs)
Other, unknown, or multiple mechanisms
    Acute pancreatitis
    *Cholestasis (obstructive)
    *Diabetes mellitus
    Hyperadrenocorticism or excess glucocorticoids
    Hypercholesterolemia in briards
    Idiopathic hyperlipidemia of miniature schnauzers or other breeds

* A relatively common disease or condition

    2. High [bilirubin] and [ascorbic acid] may cause negative interference with the enzymatic assays.[1,10] Ascorbic oxidase may be included in an assay's reagents to remove the effect of ascorbic acid.

III.   Hypercholesterolemia
    A. Increased serum [cholesterol] indicates there are increased concentrations of lipoproteins that contain cholesterol.
    B. Disorders or conditions (Table 16.3)
    C. The pathologic processes that cause hypercholesterolemia are described in a later section on lipoprotein disorders (Hyperlipemia, Hyperlipidemia, and Hyperlipoproteinemia Disorders).

IV.   Hypocholesterolemia
    A. Hypocholesterolemia is an uncommon finding in clinical cases.
    B. Disorders or conditions that cause hypocholesterolemia (Table 16.4)
        1. Portosystemic shunts: It is reported that about 60–70 % of dogs and cats with portosystemic shunts have hypocholesterolemia.[11] Two pathogeneses are proposed for the hypocholesterolemia: (1) decreased cholesterol production because of decreased functional hepatic mass, and (2) inhibition of cholesterol synthesis by bile acids.
        2. Protein-losing enteropathy (especially because of intestinal lymphangiectasia):[12–14] The pathogenesis of the hypocholesterolemia may include decreased lipoprotein production because of the catabolic state or, in the case of lymphangiectasia, loss of lipids that are normally produced by enterocytes.
        3. Hypoadrenocorticism
            a. In one study involving 17 dogs with hypoadrenocorticism, 13 had hypocholesterolemia.[15] In another study involving 201 dogs, 14 were hypocholesterolemic, but 29 had hypercholesterolemia.[16]

Table 16.4. Diseases and conditions that cause hypocholesterolemia

Decreased cholesterol production
    Portosystemic shunts in dogs and cats
    Protein-losing enteropathy
Other, unknown, or multiple mechanisms
    Hypoadrenocorticism

      b. As explained in the section on hyperadrenocorticism in dogs (Hyperlipemia, Hyperlipidemia, and Hyperlipoproteinemia Disorders, sect. V.E), cortisol does influence lipoprotein metabolism, but how hypocortisolemia is associated with hypocholesterolemia is not established.

TRIGLYCERIDE (TG) (TRIACYLGLYCEROL) CONCENTRATION OF SERUM

I.   Physiologic processes
    A. In general, lipoproteins transport TG from intestines and liver to muscle for energy or to adipose tissue for storage.
    B. Nearly all TG in a fasting serum sample is within lipoproteins that were produced in hepatocytes. Much of the TG in a postprandial sample is in chylomicrons that were assembled in enterocytes from dietary lipids.
    C. TG synthesis begins with fatty acids (short, medium, or long chain) and glycerol from carbohydrate metabolism. TG synthesis for lipoproteins occurs in hepatocytes and enterocytes.
    D. When lipoproteins containing apolipoprotein C-II bind to LPL on endothelial cells, fatty acids are cleaved from TG molecules and enter cells (e.g., adipocytes and myocytes). With repeated processing, the lipoproteins become TG depleted and thus serum [TG] decreases.

II. Analytical concepts
    A. Terms and units
       1. *Triglyceride* is the more common term for a group of lipids that contain three fatty acids attached to a glycerol backbone. The more correct term for the molecules is *triacylglycerol*, but it is not used as frequently in medical communication.
       2. Serum [TG] represents the total [TG]; the reacting TG molecules were mostly within TG-rich lipoprotein (i.e., chylomicrons, VLDL, and IDL). TG molecules are a highly variable population of molecules because of the varied fatty acids that are attached to the glycerol backbone.
       3. Units: mg/dL $\times$ 0.01129 = mmol/L (SI unit, nearest 0.05 mmol/L)[8]
    B. Sample
       1. Serum is the preferred sample. Total [TG] is stable at 4 °C for 5–7 d, at −20 °C for 3 mo, and at −70 °C for years. Repeated thawing and refreezing should be avoided.[9]
       2. Vacuum tubes with silicone-coated stoppers have not been recommended for TG analysis because glycerin from glycerin-coated stoppers may be detected in assays that measure glycerol released from TG. However, in a pilot study with the Vitros TG assay, exposure of serum to glycerin-coated stoppers did not increase the measured [TG] (authors' unpublished data).

3. Increased concentrations of chylomicrons, VLDL, and possibly IDL may cause lactescence or turbid serum and may interfere with spectrophotometric assays. Thus, laboratory personnel may clear the serum (by centrifugation or addition of clearing agents) prior to chemical analysis. When the serum is cleared of the TG-rich lipoproteins, the [TG] in the sample will be decreased.

4. Harvesting serum below a superficial "cream" layer after routine centrifugation may also falsely decrease serum [TG].

5. Dogs and cats should be fasted overnight or for about 12 h to avoid physiologic postprandial hyperlipidemia. Prolonged postprandial hyperlipidemia indicates the presence of a pathologic state.

C. Methods

1. In most automated assays, the initial reaction involves a lipase that liberates glycerol from TG. The liberated glycerol is then measured in coupled reactions that result in products that can be detected by spectrophotometry.

2. High [free glycerol] in serum would produce falsely elevated [TG], but such conditions are rarely recognized.

3. [TG] in a grossly lipemic sample may exceed an assay's analytical range, and thus the sample may need to be diluted prior to analysis.

III. Hypertriglyceridemia

A. Increased serum [TG] indicates there are increased concentrations of lipoproteins that contain TG.

B. Disorders or conditions (Table 16.5)

C. The pathologic processes that cause hypertriglyceridemia are described in the next section: Hyperlipemia, Hyperlipidemia, and Hyperlipoproteinemia Disorders.

IV. Hypotriglyceridemia: no significant pathologic states

Table 16.5. Diseases and conditions that cause hypertriglyceridemia

Increased triglyceride (triacylglycerol) production
    By hepatocytes
      *Equine hyperlipemia or hyperlipidemia
    By enterocytes
      *Postprandial hyperlipidemia
Decreased lipolysis or intravascular processing of lipoproteins
    Hypothyroidism
    Nephrotic syndrome
    Lipoprotein lipase deficiency (rare in cats, very rare in dogs)
Other, unknown, or multiple mechanisms
    *Acute pancreatitis
    *Diabetes mellitus (see different types in Chapter 14)
    High-lipid diet
    Hyperadrenocorticism or excess glucocorticoids
    Hyperlipidemia in a Brittany dog
    Idiopathic hyperlipidemia of miniature schnauzers or other breeds

* A relatively common disease or condition

HYPERLIPEMIA, HYPERLIPIDEMIA, AND HYPERLIPOPROTEINEMIA DISORDERS

I. Terms
   A. Hyperlipemia, hyperlipidemia, and hyperlipoproteinemia are nearly synonyms.
      1. *Hyperlipemia* and *hyperlipidemia* refer to an increased [lipid] in blood, whether it is from hyperlipoproteinemia, hypercholesterolemia, hypertriglyceridemia, or even increased [fatty acids].
      2. *Hyperlipoproteinemia* is an increased concentration of one or more lipoproteins in blood. It is the preferred term when a measured concentration of a lipoprotein (e.g., LDL or HDL) is increased.
      3. The terms are sometimes used to identify clinical disorders (e.g., equine hyperlipidemia or equine hyperlipoproteinemia).
   B. *Lipemia* (also lipidemia), by most dictionary definitions, is a synonym for both hyperlipidemia and hyperlipoproteinemia. In routine clinical use, lipemia is usually defined as the turbid or opaque appearance of serum or plasma as seen by the naked eye. The lactescence is primarily caused by increased concentrations of the large lipoprotein particles (i.e., chylomicrons and VLDLs).

II. Classification of hyperlipoproteinemia conditions and disorders
   A. *Physiologic* (postprandial) *hyperlipidemia* is the hyperlipidemia that occurs after ingestion of a meal containing TG.
   B. *Primary* (or familial) *hyperlipoproteinemia* disorders, which are caused by congenital defects in lipoprotein metabolism, are relatively uncommon in domestic mammals. The defects involve three major processes:[1]
      1. Increased production of lipoproteins by hepatocytes
      2. Defective intravascular processing of lipoproteins, including defective lipolysis
      3. Defective cellular uptake of lipoproteins or lipoprotein remnants
   C. *Secondary hyperlipoproteinemia* disorders are acquired disorders involving damaged cells or abnormal hormonal activity. They are relatively common in domestic mammals (see Tables 16.3 and 16.5).

III. Physiologic (postprandial) hyperlipidemia
   A. The hyperlipidemia occurs in monogastric mammals and is caused by a hyperchylomicronemia that occurs after intestinal absorption of monoglycerides and fatty acids that have formed from digestion of ingested triglycerides (Fig. 16.1). Hypertriglyceridemia will be present; hypercholesterolemia may not be present.
   B. In dogs and cats, the hyperchylomicronemia peaks by 2–6 h after a meal, and the chylomicrons are usually cleared by 8–16 h.[5] Delayed clearing of chylomicrons indicates defective lipoprotein metabolism, either a primary or secondary hyperlipidemia.
   C. The presence of postprandial hyperlipidemia with and without addition of pancreatic extracts to food has been used to assess for exocrine pancreatic insufficiency (plasma turbidity test; see Table 15.9). However, variations in gastrointestinal function cause variations in the development and clearing of the postprandial hyperlipidemia, thus complicating interpretation of the test, which has been largely replaced by measurement of serum trypsin-like immunoreactivity (see Chapter 15).

IV. Primary and possible primary hyperlipidemia disorders in domestic mammals
   A. Idiopathic hyperlipidemia of miniature schnauzers[2,3]

1. The pathogenesis of the hyperlipoproteinemia is not established. It may be caused by a deficiency in LPL activity or an apolipoprotein C-II deficiency.
2. There is hypertriglyceridemia with or without hypercholesterolemia. There may be concurrent glucose intolerance due to insulin resistance.

B. Hyperlipidemia in a Brittany dog[17]
   1. A 9-yr-old male Brittany dog was suspected to have "hyperlipemia due to a progressive inactivation of lipoprotein lipase with aging." Hypertriglyceridemia was found at 5, 7, and 9 yr of age, and hypercholesterolemia was not present. Serum [TG] did not decrease after heparin administration.
   2. The hyperlipidemia was considered a primary disorder because a secondary cause was not found and the dog's son (3 years younger) also had a fasting hypertriglyceridemia. However, response to heparin in the son was similar to a control dog's response.

C. Idiopathic hyperlipidemia occurring in dogs of other breeds (e.g., Shetland sheepdogs) may have a similar or different pathogeneses from hyperlipidemias in Brittany and miniature schnauzer breeds.

D. Congenital LPL deficiency in a mixed-breed pup[18]
   1. A 1-mo-old mixed-breed dog had marked hypertriglyceridemia (830 mg/dL), hypercholesterolemia (312 mg/dL), and normoglycemia in a serum sample that looked like cream-of-tomato soup. The pup was the smallest dog of the litter and died a few days after initial presentation.
   2. LPL deficiency was diagnosed by the failure of intravenous heparin (3000 units) to produce fatty-acid changes consistent with lipolytic activity.

E. Primary hyperchylomicronemia in cats, type III LPL deficiency[19–21]
   1. Affected cats have a mutated LPL gene resulting in lack of plasma LPL activity (prior to and after heparin) but increased concentrations of the LPL protein (type III LPL defect). This autosomal recessive hereditary defect causes defective lipolysis of plasma lipoproteins.
   2. Cats with this disorder have marked hypertriglyceridemia. Concentrations of cholesterol were not statistically significantly different from those in unaffected cats in published reports. The persistent hyperlipidemia causes lipemia retinalis and subcutaneous xanthomas that sometimes appeared to compress nerves.

F. Hypercholesterolemia in briards[22]
   1. The mean [cholesterol] in sera from 15 clinically healthy briards was 309 mg/dL compared to an age-matched and gender-matched group of nonbriards that had a mean [cholesterol] of 159 mg/dL. The briards had increased α_2-lipoprotein concentrations that suggested increased concentrations of HDL in the samples. The hyperlipoproteinemia appears to be familial, but until the defect is known, classification as a primary disorder is premature. Note that the mean [cholesterol] was only slightly above common cholesterol reference intervals, so many affected briards were not hypercholesterolemic if compared to most dogs. TG concentrations were not abnormal.
   2. The healthy briards were evaluated to explore the cause of lipid droplet accumulation associated with retinal pigment epithelial dystrophy in the breed. The results of the study suggested a possible relationship. The genetic defect in the retinal lesion has been established, but the relationship to hypercholesterolemia (if any) is still not understood.

V.   Secondary hyperlipidemia disorders
   A.   Acute pancreatitis[23,24]
      1.   Dogs with acute pancreatitis frequently have hypertriglyceridemia with or without hypercholesterolemia. The hypertriglyceridemia may be either an initiating factor or a consequence of the pancreatitis.
      2.   The pathogenesis of the hyperlipoproteinemia is not firmly established but appears to be a defect in the intravascular processing of chylomicrons and VLDL.
         a.   One theory is that decreased [insulin] causes defective LPL activity because movement of LPL to the luminal surface of endothelial cells is dependent on insulin.[4] However, in the early stages of experimental canine pancreatitis, there were parallel increases in [insulin] and [glucose].[25]
         b.   TNF and other cytokines have been shown to alter lipoprotein metabolism and result in increased [VLDL].[26,27] Thus, the lipemia of pancreatitis could be associated with release of cytokines during inflammation.
         c.   Because pancreatitis may cause obstructive cholestasis, part of the hyperlipidemia may relate to defects in lipid metabolism caused by cholestasis.
   B.   Cholestasis in dogs and cats
      1.   Dogs and cats with obstructive cholestatic disorders frequently but inconsistently have hypercholesterolemia without concurrent hypertriglyceridemia.
      2.   The hypercholesterolemia of cholestasis is associated with increased cholesterol content of hepatocytes, and it appears to result from multiple processes.
         a.   Cholestasis reduces biliary excretion of cholesterol from hepatocytes.
         b.   Experimental bile duct obstruction in rats causes increased 3-hydroxy-3-methylglutaryl-coenzyme A reductase activity, which results in increased cholesterol synthesis.[28] Because bile acid synthesis is concurrently increased, it has been speculated that a common positive effector induces synthesis of cholesterol and bile acids.
         c.   In experimental cholestasis in dogs, increased [LDL] suggests a defective uptake of LDL by hepatocytes.[29]
      3.   Cholestasis has been associated with the appearance of unique lipoproteins called lipoprotein X1, X2, and X3 that have cathodal electrophoretic migrations.
         a.   These lipoproteins have a similar density to LDL but have a characteristic lipid content predominated by phospholipids and nonesterified cholesterol, and a protein content dominated by albumin within the core and apolipoprotein C on the surface.
         b.   Lipoprotein X may form from a physicochemical, nonmetabolic interaction of plasma lipids with bile acids. Another theory is that reduced LCAT activity from hepatic disease may play a role; this is consistent with the presence of lipoprotein X in human familial LCAT deficiency.
         c.   Some investigators have reported the presence of lipoprotein X in cholestatic dogs, but in other studies of experimental cholestasis in dogs, none of the increased lipoprotein fractions had a composition characteristic of human lipoprotein X.[29,30]
   C.   Diabetes mellitus
      1.   Diabetic dogs and cats frequently have hypertriglyceridemia, typically with hypercholesterolemia. The pathogenesis and severity of the hyperlipoproteinemia may vary with the type of diabetes mellitus (see Chapter 14).

2. The hyperlipoproteinemia may be caused by multiple mechanisms:
    a. Defective intravascular processing of chylomicrons and VLDL may occur because of low [insulin] and thus defective LPL activity.
    b. Increased VLDL synthesis by hepatocytes may occur due to mobilization of body lipids that is caused by increased hormone-sensitive lipase activity in adipocytes. The influx of fatty acids into hepatocytes and their oxidation causes excess formation of acetyl-CoA that promotes TG, cholesterol, and ketone production.
    c. There is increased synthesis of HDL cholesterol by intestinal mucosa cells in experimental canine diabetes mellitus.[31]
D. Hypothyroidism in dogs
    1. About 75 % of dogs with hypothyroidism have a fasting hypercholesterolemia; hypertriglyceridemia may or may not be present.[32,33] Because some forms of hypothyroidism are familial, the associated hyperlipoproteinemia is familial.[34] However, the lipid metabolism defect is a secondary hyperlipoproteinemia because it is caused by decreased thyroid hormone activity. One of the first reports of hyperlipoproteinemia in beagles[35] is sometimes cited as a form of primary hyperlipoproteinemia, but the investigators did not exclude hypothyroidism as a cause.
    2. In human hypothyroidism, the hyperlipidemia appears to be related primarily to decreased expression of hepatic LDL receptors and decreased activities of hepatic lipase and LPL.[36,37]
       a. Decreased clearance of LDL causes hypercholesterolemia.[38] Data in people have shown a correlation between serum [triiodothyronine] and hepatic lipase activity.
       b. Low [thyroxine] is associated with low LPL activity. Thus, reduced intravascular processing of chylomicrons and VLDL may cause hypertriglyceridemia.
E. Hyperadrenocorticism in dogs
    1. About 90 % of dogs with hyperadrenocorticism have a fasting hypercholesterolemia; hypertriglyceridemia may or may not be present.[39] Because increased glucocorticoid activity may lead to diabetes mellitus or a steroid hepatopathy, it may be difficult to determine which pathologic state is causing the hyperlipidemia.
    2. Glucocorticoid hormones (endogenous and exogenous) may promote hyperlipoproteinemia through multiple mechanisms:
       a. They stimulate VLDL synthesis in hepatocytes.[40]
       b. They stimulate hormone-sensitive lipase and thus increased liberation of fatty acids from adipose tissue. The influx of fatty acids into hepatocytes will stimulate TG and cholesterol synthesis and thus increased production of VLDL.
       c. They antagonize the actions of insulin, which thus may cause decreased LPL activity.[41]
F. Nephrotic syndrome and protein-losing nephropathy in dogs and cats
    1. The cause of the hypercholesterolemia (sometimes accompanied by hypertriglyceridemia) is typically considered to be increased hepatic production of VLDL, defective lipolysis of lipoproteins due to deficiencies of lipases and some lipoprotein receptors, and defective conversion of cholesterol to bile acids.[42]
       a. There is good evidence that there is defective lipolysis of lipoproteins that contain apolipoprotein B; that is, chylomicrons, VLDL, IDL, and LDL. It is possible that a protein needed for LPL binding to endothelial cells or the action of LPL is lost with other proteins in the urine.[43] There also are several reported alterations in lipoprotein-receptor proteins and enzymes involved in lipid metabolism.[42]

b. The possible increased production of cholesterol has been questioned in people because cholesterol synthesis did not appear to be increased in nephrotic patients.[44]

c. Experimental data in rats indicate that there is not a down-regulation of the LDL receptor–related protein.[42]

2. Dogs and cats with protein-losing nephropathy may have hypoalbuminemia and hypercholesterolemia but not enough sodium and H_2O retention to cause the ascites and edema of the nephrotic syndrome.

G. Equine hyperlipemia of horses, ponies, and donkeys

1. These secondary equine hyperlipidemic disorders or syndromes have been given the name *hyperlipemia*, which occurs secondarily in several metabolic disorders that alter lipoprotein metabolism.

2. Some authors divide the condition into two forms:[45,46]

a. Hyperlipidemia: Plasma lipids are increased but with little clinical significance. Serum [TG] is usually < 500 mg/dL.

b. Hyperlipidemic syndrome: Increased plasma lipids are associated with hepatic lipidosis and marked clinical changes. Serum [TG] is usually > 500 mg/dL.

3. The disorders that produce changes in lipoprotein metabolism are varied, but the changes are similar.

a. Physiologic or pathologic processes result in mobilization of fatty acids from the TG molecules of adipose tissue.

b. Hepatocytes increase the synthesis of TG-rich VLDL molecules that enter blood to cause hypertriglyceridemia. These VLDL molecules have altered apolipoprotein content.

c. If the condition is severe enough, then TG accumulation in hepatocytes causes hepatic lipidosis and subsequent damage to hepatocytes.

4. Conditions that are associated with equine hyperlipidemia include anorexia, obesity, pregnancy, lactation, renal failure, endotoxemia, and other states that create a negative energy balance. Hormones or other substances can contribute to the defective metabolic pathways.[47]

a. Catecholamines and glucagon stimulate hormone-sensitive lipase in adipocytes to increase release of fatty acids. Insulin typically inhibits this enzyme, and thus decreased insulin activity may remove a negative effector and promote fatty-acid release.

b. Glucocorticoid hormones also stimulate hormone-sensitive lipase.

c. Insulin stimulates LPL for hydrolysis of TG in most lipoproteins, especially the TG-rich chylomicrons and VLDL. Decreased insulin activity reduces the activity of LPL, and thus the intravascular processing of lipoproteins is reduced.

d. Progesterone (when increased in pregnancy or lactation) stimulates growth hormone, which creates insulin resistance by causing insulin receptor and postreceptor defects.[48]

e. Hypoglycemia, when present, stimulates glucagon release. Glucagon stimulates hormone-sensitive lipase in adipocytes and thus promotes the liberation of fatty acids.

f. Either directly or through cytokine release, endotoxins stimulate TG and VLDL synthesis by hepatocytes, and they also can inhibit lipoprotein catabolism.[27,49]

g. Rats in renal failure (created by partial nephrectomy) had defective lipolysis of VLDL molecules and thus hypertriglyceridemia. The agent or agents that produce the defective lipolysis were not identified.[50] It is not known whether a similar defect occurs in horses with renal failure.

5. Congenital hyperlipemia in a Shetland pony foal[51]
   a. A Shetland pony neonate had visually lipemic sera, increased total [lipid], and hypercholesterolemia. By definition, the foal had a congenital hyperlipidemia, but it may not have been hereditary.
   b. The mare was hyperlipidemic (perhaps associated with pregnancy), so the foal's lipemia may have been caused by the placental transfer of fatty acids from the mare. The influx of fatty acids may have stimulated VLDL synthesis sufficiently to cause hyperlipemia in the foal.

H. High dietary fat intake in dogs
   1. Excessive dietary lipid would result in storage of lipids and potentially obesity. Such dogs may have prolonged postprandial hyperlipidemia because of insulin resistance or other factors.
   2. Extremely elevated fat intake and concurrent inadequate protein intake can lead to defective lipoprotein metabolism and hepatic lipidosis.

OTHER ASSESSMENTS OF LIPIDS

I. Lipoprotein electrophoresis
   A. Lipoprotein electrophoresis has been used as an adjunct qualitative assessment of lipoprotein abnormalities in clinical veterinary samples. However, methods vary, and test availability and interpretive expertise are limited. The following is a brief summary of the procedure:
      1. EDTA plasma (or serum) is applied to a gel (usually agarose).
      2. An electric current causes lipoproteins to migrate through the gel based on their charge, size, shape, and interaction with the gel.
      3. After separation, lipid stains are applied to visualize the lipoprotein bands, which are named according to serum α- and β-protein bands of corresponding mobility.
         a. Chylomicrons, if present, remain at the application origin.
         b. HDL molecules migrate furthest toward the anode (α-bands).
         c. LDL and VLDL molecules migrate intermediately (β- or pre-β-bands).
      4. The gel should be examined qualitatively for dyslipoproteinemic patterns. In dogs, increased α_2-migrating lipoproteins are associated with hypercholesterolemia, and increased pre-β-bands, β-bands, or application site bands are associated with hypertriglyceridemia.[52]
   B. Although gel banding patterns can provide useful information about lipoprotein subfractions, bands are not consistently associated with certain classes of lipoproteins as defined by their densities. Therefore, lipoprotein electrophoresis is most useful when combined with density fractionation studies or to monitor response to therapy.

II. Nonesterified fatty acids (NEFA, free fatty acids, and fatty acids)
   A. Physiologic processes
      1. NEFAs and glycerol form from hydrolysis of triacylglycerol in adipose tissue, liver, and mammary gland.
      2. Hydrolysis in adipocytes is mediated by hormone-sensitive lipase, which is stimulated by epinephrine and glucagon. Insulin is inhibitory.

3. After hydrolysis, NEFAs are released to blood, where they bind to albumin and are transported to other tissues. Major target organs are muscle and liver.

4. After passive uptake, NEFAs are activated and then undergo β-oxidation in mitochondria to form acetyl-CoA.

5. Acetyl-CoA enters the tricarboxylic acid cycle for generation of energy or conversion to amino acids. In liver, acetyl-CoA may be used for ketogenesis.

6. Glycerol enters hepatocytes and is converted to glyceraldehyde 3-phosphate, an intermediate in glycolysis and gluconeogenesis.

7. NEFAs may be incorporated into TG and VLDL in hepatocytes.

B. Analytical methods

1. Terms and units

a. NEFAs are commonly called free fatty acids because they are outside of lipoprotein particles, but most circulate bound to albumin and are not free. The International Union of Pure and Applied Chemistry (IUPAC) recommended term is *fatty acids*.

b. Units: mEq/L × 1 = mmol/L

2. Sample

a. Serum or plasma from EDTA-anticoagulated blood (not heparin or collection from heparinized patients) should be used.[53]

b. Serum or plasma should be separated from cells as soon as possible and be frozen or maintained at 4 °C before testing. Frozen samples should yield valid results for at least 1 mo, and refrigerated samples are best tested within 24 h. Values may be falsely increased if serum separator tubes are used, if samples are not kept cool, or if testing of samples kept at 4 °C is delayed beyond 24 h.[53]

c. Significant false increases also occur with moderate to severe hemolysis.[54]

d. For monitoring prepartum cattle, samples should be collected shortly before feeding time and 2–14 d before calving. They can be processed and stored frozen until calving occurs, at which time it will be known whether the samples were collected in the desired 2–14 d precalving window.

3. Methods

a. NEFAs may be measured in automated systems with an enzymatic colorimetric assay in which they are enzymatically acylated and then oxidized to hydrogen peroxide linked to a reaction that generates a colored product.

(1) This assay detects medium- to long-chain (6–26 carbon) fatty acids.

(2) Volatile fatty acids (e.g., propionic acid and butyric acid) are not measured.

b. Enzymatic methods replace more time-consuming nonenzymatic methods that rely on extraction of NEFAs by organic solvents after converting them to copper salts.

4. Increased [NEFA]

a. Increases occur with increased fat mobilization in response to a negative energy balance from any cause.

b. NEFAs are usually assessed in ruminants, particularly to monitor transition cows in the last 1–2 wk prepartum, when there are high energy demands for the fetus and milk production (see Herd-based Testing for Cattle in Chapter 1).

(1) When a certain proportion of prepartum cows in a dairy herd have values above a decision threshold, it is evidence that too many cows are in a negative energy balance, and management changes are needed.

        (2) Increased prepartum [NEFA] is associated with more postparturient ketosis, fatty liver, and displaced abomasums.

    c. [NEFA] may also be increased with diabetes mellitus, hepatic lipidosis, overfeeding and obesity, food deprivation, and after exercise.

III. Standing plasma test for chylomicrons (also called a refrigeration test)

    A. Because of their high TG content and thus low density, chylomicrons will float to the surface of a serum or plasma sample if the sample is undisturbed.

    B. A 16 h–standing test has been used to detect chylomicrons. In the procedure, 2 mL of plasma is placed in a small glass tube and then examined after 16 h of refrigeration at 4 °C.

      1. The presence of a creamy layer on the plasma sample indicates the presence of chylomicrons. Chylomicrons indicate postprandial hyperlipidemia (which could be pathologic if it represents delayed clearing).

      2. Turbidity below or without a surface creamy layer suggests that other causes of hyperlipidemia may need to be considered.

    C. However, the 16 h–standing test has a relatively poor capability of detecting chylomicrons when compared to lipoprotein electrophoresis and ultracentrifugation. In one study, only about 20 % of the chylomicron-positive samples (as detected by electrophoresis) had a positive 16 h–standing test.[55] Similar results were found when the standing test was compared to ultracentrifugation.[56] The presence of a creamy layer in the standing test is specific for chylomicrons, but many samples that contain chylomicrons do not have a detectable lipid layer.

References

1. Rifai N, Bachorik PS, Albers JJ. 1999. Lipids, lipoproteins, and apolipoproteins. In: Burtis CA, Ashwood ER, eds. *Tietz Textbook of Clinical Chemistry*, 3rd edition, 809–861. Philadelphia: WB Saunders.
2. Bauer JE. 2000. Hyperlipidemias. In: Ettinger SJ, Feldman EC, eds. *Textbook of Veterinary Internal Medicine: Diseases of the Dog and Cat*, 5th edition, 283–292. Philadelphia: WB Saunders.
3. Bruss ML. 1997. Lipids and ketones. In: Kaneko JJ, Harvey JW, Bruss ML, eds. *Clinical Biochemistry of Domestic Animals*, 5th edition, 83–115. San Diego: Academic.
4. Gross KL, Wedekind KJ, Cowell CS, Schoenherr WD, Jewell DE, Zicker SC, Debraekeleer J, Frey RA. 2000. Nutrients. In: Hand MS, Thatcher CD, Remillard RL, Roudebush P, eds. *Small Animal Clinical Nutrition*, 4th edition, 21–107. Topeka, KS: Mark Morris Institute.
5. Watson TDG, Barrie J. 1993. Lipoprotein metabolism and hyperlipidaemia in the dog and cat: A review. J Small Anim Pract 34:479–487.
6. Baginsky ML. 1981. Measurement of lipoprotein lipase and hepatic triglyceride lipase in human postheparin plasma. Methods Enzymol 72:325–338.
7. Williams KJ, Fless GM, Petrie KA, Snyder ML, Brocia RW, Swenson TL. 1992. Mechanisms by which lipoprotein lipase alters cellular metabolism of lipoprotein(a), low density lipoprotein, and nascent lipoproteins: Roles for low density lipoprotein receptors and heparan sulfate proteoglycans. J Biol Chem 267:13284–13292.
8. Lundberg GD, Iverson C, Radulescu G. 1986. Now read this: The SI units are here. J Am Med Assoc 255:2329–2339.
9. Tietz NW, with Druden EL, McPherson RA, Fuhrman SA, eds. 1995. *Clinical Guide to Laboratory Tests*, 3rd edition. Philadelphia: WB Saunders.
10. Young DS, Pestaner LC, Gibberman V. 1975. Effects of drugs on clinical laboratory tests. Clin Chem 21:1D–432D (special issue).
11. Center SA, Magne ML. 1990. Historical, physical examination, and clinicopathologic features of portosystemic vascular anomalies in the dog and cat. Semin Vet Med Surg (Small Anim) 5:83–93.
12. Fossum TW. 1989. Protein-losing enteropathy. Semin Vet Med Surg (Small Anim) 4:219–225.

13. Littman MP, Dambach DM, Vaden SL, Giger U. 2000. Familial protein-losing enteropathy and protein-losing nephropathy in soft coated Wheaten terriers: 222 cases (1983–1997). J Vet Intern Med 14:68–80.
14. Willard MD, Helman G, Fradkin JM, Becker T, Brown RM, Lewis BC, Weeks BR. 2000. Intestinal crypt lesions associated with protein-losing enteropathy in the dog. J Vet Intern Med 14:298–307.
15. Lifton SJ, King LG, Zerbe CA. 1996. Glucocorticoid deficient hypoadrenocorticism in dogs: 18 cases (1986–1995). J Am Vet Med Assoc 209:2076–2081.
16. Peterson ME, Kintzer PP, Kass PH. 1996. Pretreatment clinical and laboratory findings in dogs with hypoadrenocorticism: 225 cases (1979–1993). J Am Vet Med Assoc 208:85–91.
17. Hubert B, de La Farge F, Braun JP, Magnol JP. 1987. Hypertriglyceridemia in two related dogs. Companion Anim Pract 1:33–35.
18. Baum D, Schweid AI, Porte D Jr, Bierman EL. 1969. Congenital lipoprotein lipase deficiency and hyperlipemia in the young puppy. Proc Soc Exp Biol Med 131:183–185.
19. Peritz LN, Brunzell JD, Harvey-Clarke C, Pritchard PH, Jones BR, Hayden MR. 1990. Characterization of a lipoprotein lipase class III type defect in hypertriglyceridemic cats. Clin Invest Med 13:259–263.
20. Jones BR, Johnstone AC, Hancock WS, Wallace A. 1986. Inherited hyperchylomicronemia in the cat. Feline Pract 16:7–12.
21. Ginzinger DG, Lewis ME, Ma Y, Jones BR, Liu G, Jones SD. 1996. A mutation in the lipoprotein lipase gene is the molecular basis of chylomicronemia in a colony of domestic cats. J Clin Invest 97:1257–1266.
22. Watson P, Simpson KW, Bedford PGC. 1993. Hypercholesterolaemia in briards in the United Kingdom. Res Vet Sci 54:80–85.
23. Whitney MS. 1992. Evaluation of hyperlipidemias in dogs and cats. Semin Vet Med Surg (Small Anim) 7:292–300.
24. Whitney MS, Boon GD, Rebar AH, Ford RB. 1987. Effects of acute pancreatitis on circulating lipids in dogs. Am J Vet Res 48:1492–1497.
25. Satake K, Carballo J, Appert HE, Howard JM. 1973. Insulin levels in acute experimental pancreatitis in dogs. Surg Gynecol Obstet 137:467–471.
26. Krauss RM, Grunfeld C, Doerrler WT, Feingold KR. 1990. Tumor necrosis factor acutely increases plasma levels of very low density lipoproteins of normal size and composition. Endocrinology 127:1016–1021.
27. Feingold KR, Grunfeld C. 1992. Role of cytokines in inducing hyperlipidemia. Diabetes 41(Suppl 2):97–101.
28. Dueland S, Reichen J, Everson GT, Davis RA. 1991. Regulation of cholesterol and bile acid homoeostasis in bile-obstructed rats. Biochem J 280:373–377.
29. Danielsson B, Ekman R, Johansson BG, Petersson BG. 1977. Plasma lipoprotein changes in experimental cholestasis in the dog. Clin Chim Acta 80:157–170.
30. Ritland S, Bergan A. 1975. Plasma concentration of lipoprotein-X (LP-X) in experimental bile duct obstruction. Scand J Gastroenterol 10:17–24.
31. Kwong LK, Feingold KR, Peric-Golia L, Le T, Karkas JD, Alberts AW, Wilson DE. 1991. Intestinal and hepatic cholesterogenesis in hypercholesterolemic dyslipidemia of experimental diabetes in dogs. Diabetes 40:1630–1639.
32. Feldman EC, Nelson RW. 1996. Hypothyroidism. *Canine and Feline Endocrinology and Reproduction*, 2nd edition, 68–117. Philadelphia: WB Saunders.
33. Scott-Moncrieff JCR, Guptill-Yoran L. 2000. Hypothyroidism. In: Ettinger SJ, Feldman EC, eds. *Textbook of Veterinary Internal Medicine: Diseases of the Dog and Cat*, 5th edition, 1419–1429. Philadelphia: WB Saunders.
34. Manning PJ. 1979. Thyroid gland and arterial lesions of beagles with familial hypothyroidism and hyperlipoproteinemia. Am J Vet Res 40:820–828.
35. Wada M, Minamisono T, Ehrhart LA, Naito HK, Mise J. 1977. Familial hyperlipoproteinemia in beagles. Life Sci 20:999–1008.
36. Valdemarsson S, Hansson P, Hedner P, Nilsson-Ehle P. 1983. Relations between thyroid function, hepatic and lipoprotein lipase activities, and plasma lipoprotein concentrations. Acta Endocrinol 104:50–56.
37. Valdemarsson S. 1983. Plasma lipoprotein alterations in thyroid dysfunction: Roles of lipoprotein lipase, hepatic lipase and LCAT. Acta Endocrinol 103(Suppl 255):1–52.
38. Duntas LH. 2002. Thyroid disease and lipids. Thyroid 12:287–293.
39. Feldman EC. 2000. Hyperadrenocorticism. In: Ettinger SJ, Feldman EC, eds. *Textbook of Veterinary Internal Medicine: Diseases of the Dog and Cat*, 5th edition, 1460–1488. Philadelphia: WB Saunders.
40. Gibbons GF. 1990. Assembly and secretion of hepatic very-low-density lipoprotein. Biochem J 268:1–13.
41. Bagdade JD, Yee E, Albers J, Pykalisto OJ. 1976. Glucocorticoids and triglyceride transport: Effects on triglyceride secretion rates, lipoprotein lipase, and plasma lipoproteins in the rat. Metabolism 25:533–542.
42. Kim S, Kim CH, Vaziri ND. 2005. Upregulation of hepatic LDL receptor–related protein in nephrotic syndrome: Response to statin therapy. Am J Physiol Endocrinol Metab 288:E813–E817.
43. Orth SR, Ritz E. 1998. The nephrotic syndrome. N Engl J Med 338:1202–1211.

44. Dullaart RPF, Gansevoort RT, Sluiter WJ, de Zeeuw D, de Jong PE. 1996. The serum lathosterol to cholesterol ratio, an index of cholesterol synthesis, is not elevated in patients with glomerular proteinuria and is not associated with improvement of hyperlipidemia in response to antiproteinuric treatment. Metabolism 45:723–730.

45. Naylor JM. 1982. Hyperlipemia and hyperlipidemia in horses, ponies, and donkeys. Compend Contin Educ Pract Vet 4:S321–S326.

46. Jeffcott LB, Field JR. 1985. Current concepts of hyperlipaemia in horses and ponies. Vet Rec 116:461–466.

47. Barton MH, Morris DD. 1998. Disease of the liver. In: Reed SM, Bayly WM, eds. *Equine Internal Medicine*, 707–738. Philadelphia: WB Saunders.

48. Peterson ME, Taylor RS, Greco DS, Nelson RW, Randolph JF, Foodman MS, Moroff SD, Morrison SA, Lothrop CD. 1990. Acromegaly in 14 cats. J Vet Intern Med 4:192–201.

49. Feingold KR, Staprans I, Memon RA, Moser AH, Shigenaga JK, Doerrler W, Dinarello CA, Grunfeld C. 1992. Endotoxin rapidly induces changes in lipid metabolism that produce hypertriglyceridemia: Low doses stimulate hepatic triglyceride production while high doses inhibit clearance. J Lipid Res 33:1765–1776.

50. Gregg RC, Diamond A, Mondon CE, Reaven GM. 1977. The effects of chronic uremia and dexamethasone on triglyceride kinetics in the rat. Metabolism 26:875–882.

51. Gilbert RO. 1986. Congenital hyperlipaemia in a Shetland pony foal. Equine Vet J 18:498–500.

52. Rogers WA, Donovan EF, Kociba GJ. 1975. Lipids and lipoproteins in normal dogs and in dogs with secondary hyperlipoproteinemia. J Am Vet Med Assoc 166:1092–1100.

53. Stokol T, Nydam DV. 2005. Effect of anticoagulant and storage conditions on bovine nonesterified fatty acid and beta-hydroxybutyrate concentrations in blood. J Dairy Sci 88:3139–3144.

54. Stokol T, Nydam D. 2005. Effect of hemolysis on bovine non-esterified fatty acid and beta-hydroxybutyrate concentrations. Vet Clin Pathol 34:288–289 (abstract).

55. McNeely S, Seatter K, Yuhaniak J, Kashyap ML. 1981. The 16-hour-standing test and lipoprotein electrophoresis compared for detection of chylomicrons in plasma. Clin Chem 27:731–732.

56. Luley C, Prellwitz W. 1988. Qualitative detection of chylomicrons with a high-speed laboratory centrifuge compared with 16-h-standing test, lipoprotein electrophoresis, and preparative ultracentrifugation. Clin Chem 34:1362–1363.

Chapter 17

THYROID FUNCTION

Physiologic Processes 784
Analytical Concepts 785
Thyroxine (T_4) Concentration 789
    I.   [Total Thyroxine] (tT_4). 789
        A. Hyperthyroxemia. 789
        B. Hypothyroxemia. 790
    II. [Free Thyroxine]$_{ed}$ ([fT_4]$_{ed}$) 793
        A. Increased [fT_4]$_{ed}$ (Free Thyroxine Concentration by
           Equilibrium Dialysis) 793
        B. Decreased [fT_4]$_{ed}$ (Free Thyroxine Concentration by
           Equilibrium Dialysis) 793
Total Triiodothyronine (tT_3) and Free Triiodothyronine (fT_3) Concentrations 793
Thyroid-Stimulating Hormone (TSH) Concentration 794
Autoantibodies 794
    I.   Thyroglobulin Autoantibodies (TgAA) 794
    II. Thyroxine Autoantibodies (T_4AA) and Triiodothyronine
        Autoantibodies (T_3AA) 795
    III. Thyroid Peroxidase Autoantibodies (TpAA). 795
Response and Suppression Tests. 795
    I.   Thyroid-Stimulating Hormone (TSH) Response Test 795
    II. Thyrotropin-Releasing Hormone (TRH) Response Test 796
    III. Triiodothyronine (T_3) Suppression Test 796
Total Thyroxine to Thyroid-Stimulating Hormone (tT_4:TSH) and Free
   Thyroxine to Thyroid-Stimulating Hormone (fT_4:TSH) Ratios in Dogs 798
Interpretation of Thyroid Hormone Concentrations and Profiles 799

Table 17.1. Abbreviations and symbols in this chapter

$[fT_4]_{ed}$	Free thyroxine concentration by equilibrium dialysis
$[x]$	Concentration of x (x = analyte)
fT_3	Free triiodothyronine
fT_4	Free thyroxine
RIA	Radioimmunoassay
SI	Système International d'Unités
T_3	Triiodothyronine
T_3AA	Triiodothyronine autoantibodies
T_4	Thyroxine
T_4AA	Thyroxine autoantibodies
TgAA	Thyroglobulin autoantibodies
TpAA	Thyroid peroxidase autoantibodies
TRH	Thyrotropin-releasing hormone
TSH	Thyroid-stimulating hormone (thyrotropin)
tT_3	Total triiodothyronine
tT_4	Total thyroxine
WRI	Within reference interval

PHYSIOLOGIC PROCESSES

I. Hormonal control of thyroid glands (Fig. 17.1)
    A. TRH from the hypothalamus stimulates the production and release of pituitary TSH. Factors that influence the secretion of TRH are poorly understood.
    B. TSH binds to thyroid TSH receptors and stimulates the production and release of T_4 and T_3 from the thyroid glands. All circulating T_4 is produced by the thyroid glands, but a minority (10–40 %) of circulating T_3 is produced by the thyroid glands.[1-3] The rest of T_3 is generated from T_4 in cells throughout the body; in this context, T_4 is a prohormone. In the pituitary gland, T_3 produced by the deiodination of T_4 inhibits secretion of TSH.
        1. Synthesis of T_4 and T_3 is also influenced by intrathyroidal factors, including availability of iodide, sensitivity to TSH, and the ratio of T_3 to T_4.[2]
        2. Thyroglobulin is produced by luminal thyroid cells and is stored in follicular lumina. Thyroglobulin acts as an acceptor protein and is involved in the synthesis and later release of T_4 and T_3.
        3. Daily variations in $[tT_4]$ have been reported.
            a. In horses, the highest concentrations are in the late afternoon, and the lowest concentrations are in the early morning.[4]
            b. In dogs, some authors report that there is not a predictable diurnal variation, and there can be confusing fluctuations in random baseline $[tT_4]$.[2] However, based on a study of a small group of dogs, $[tT_4]$ was significantly lower at 8 a.m. (mean, 1.75 µg/dL) than at 11 a.m., 2 p.m., 5 p.m., and 10 p.m. The highest mean $[tT_4]$ was at 2 p.m. (3.54 µg/dL).[5] A similar pattern (but with less change) was found in 8 a.m., 2 p.m., and 8 p.m. samples.[6] Thus, the time of sampling may influence the interpretation of $[tT_4]$. Similar patterns were seen in $[fT_4]_{ed}$.

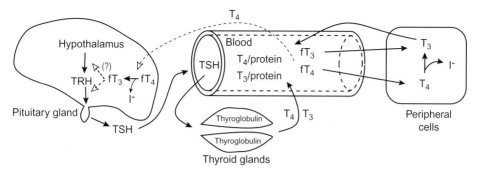

Fig. 17.1. Hormonal control of thyroid glands. TRH released from the hypothalamus stimulates the release of TSH from the pituitary. TSH stimulates the production and release of T_4 and T_3 in pathways involving thyroglobulin in the thyroid glands. In blood, most T_4 and T_3 molecules are protein bound. fT_4 and fT_3 may enter peripheral cells in which some of the T_4 is converted to T_3. T_3 has more activity than T_4. In the negative-feedback system (dashed lines), fT_4 and fT_3 (produced locally) inhibit the secretion of TSH and possibly TRH.

    C. In blood, most tT_4 and tT_3 molecules are protein bound.
        1. Nearly all T_4 released from the thyroid glands becomes bound to plasma proteins.[1,7] Factors that influence protein binding are not clearly established. In dogs, about 99 % of T_4 is bound to thyroid hormone–binding globulin, transthyretin, albumin, and apolipoproteins. The binding proteins in cats are not established. In horses, T_4 is bound to thyroid hormone–binding globulin (61 %), T_4-binding prealbumin (22 %), and albumin (17 %).
        2. T_4 not bound to plasma proteins is called fT_4 and is the biologically active form of T_4. fT_4 enters most cells of the body and is converted to either T_3 or reverse-T_3 by the actions of deiodinase enzymes.[3] Reverse-T_3 is biologically insignificant.
        3. Like T_4, most T_3 (99 %) is protein bound (specific globulins and albumin). fT_3 is about 3–5 times as potent as fT_4.[7]
    D. T_3 and T_4 dissociate from plasma proteins and enter cells, where they bind to receptors, including nuclear receptor proteins.[8] The hormone-receptor complexes initiate changes to cause or promote increased metabolic rate, increased O_2 consumption, increased heart rate, enhanced response to catecholamines, bone formation and resorption, increased catabolism of muscle and adipose tissue, protein synthesis, erythropoiesis, and alterations in lipoprotein metabolism.
    E. T_3 and T_4 are excreted in bile and urine.

ANALYTICAL CONCEPTS

I.   Terms and units
    A. Thyroxine and triiodothyronine are commonly referred to as T_4 and T_3, respectively. It is important to differentiate tT_4 from fT_4.
    B. Unit conversion[9]
        1. tT_4: µg/dL × 10 = ng/mL; µg/dL × 12.87 = nmol/L; and ng/mL × 1.287 = nmol/L (SI unit, nearest 1 nmol/L)
        2. fT_4: ng/dL × 12.87 = pmol/L (SI unit, nearest 1 pmol/L)

3. T_3: ng/dL $\times$ 10 = pg/mL; ng/dL $\times$ 0.01536 = nmol/L; and pg/dL $\times$ 15.4 = nmol/L (SI unit, nearest 0.1 nmol/L)
4. TSH: μg/dL $\times$ 10 = ng/mL; also reported as mU/L (or μU/mL)
5. TgAA: positive or negative result or percentage of a known positive sample

II. Sample
   A. Canine [tT_4] is stable in EDTA-plasma and serum when stored in plastic tubes for 5 d at 25 °C, 8 d at 22 °C, and months at −20 °C; [tT_4] increased in serum samples stored at 37 °C for 5 d but remained stable in EDTA-plasma samples.[10] Stability of canine [tT_4] (serum or plasma) is similar in glass tubes at 22 °C and −20 °C for 5 d; [tT_4] increased when stored in glass tubes at 37 °C for reasons that are not established. Similar stability is expected in sera from other species.
   B. Stability of [fT_4] is similar to that described for [tT_4].[10] As for [tT_4], [fT_4] increased in both EDTA-plasma and serum samples stored in glass at 37 °C for 5 d.
   C. TSH and TgAA are stable at 4 °C for a few days, or longer if frozen.
   D. To reach reliable conclusions about the endogenous thyroid status of an animal receiving thyroid medication, a 4 wk medication withdrawal period is recommended prior to testing.
   E. Increased plasma [fatty acid] can result in falsely increased [fT_4] in people; the fatty acids displace T_4 on binding proteins. The increased [fatty acid] and falsely increased [fT_4] have been shown to occur when people were given either intravenous or subcutaneous heparin.[11,12]

III. Assay principles and procedures
   A. [tT_4]
      1. [tT_4] is the concentration of free and bound T_4.
      2. [tT_4] is usually measured by RIA, but enzyme immunoassays (enzyme-linked immunosorbent assay and chemiluminescent enzyme immunoassay) are also used. However, results from the different assays do not always agree,[13–15] and there can be good agreement for [tT_4] for one species but not another.[16] Comparisons of results have detected sufficient biases so that reference intervals for different assays would be different.
      3. [tT_4] in healthy dogs is much lower than [tT_4] in healthy cats, horses, and people. Thus, assays for canine [tT_4] must have lower detection limits to measure normal and decreased [tT_4] correctly. Assays that have an analytical range appropriate for human [tT_4] should not be used to evaluate canine [tT_4].
      4. In the common solid-phase RIA systems, T_4AA in serum will cause falsely elevated measured [tT_4] (Fig. 17.2). In less common assays, a falsely low [tT_4] will be measured if the assay detects all antibody-bound radiolabeled T_4 (bound to either reagent antibody or autoantibody). TgAA do not interfere with these assays, but sera that have TgAA may have T_4AA.[17,18]
   B. [fT_4]
      1. Equilibrium dialysis
         a. [fT_4] is best measured by an assay that involves equilibrium dialysis. In equilibrium dialysis procedures, fT_4 is allowed to diffuse through a membrane that does not allow diffusion of protein-bound T_4. After sufficient time has passed, [T_4] is measured in the protein-poor dialysate, or ratios between predialysis and postdialysis values are used to determine a sample's [fT_4].[19]

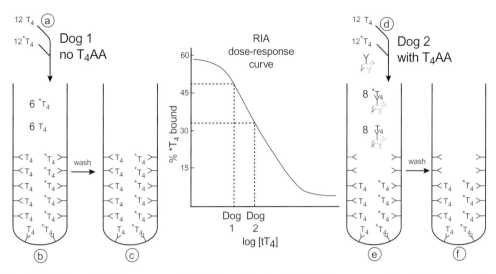

Fig. 17.2. Effects of T_4AA on measured $[tT_4]$ in a solid-phase RIA. RIAs are competitive-binding assays in which the patient's T_4 competes with a known amount of radioactive T_4 ($*T_4$) for a limited number of antibody-binding sites (e.g., in a tube coated with anti-T4 antibodies). Thus, a greater concentration of patient T_4 results in less bound $*T_4$.

- In the analysis of dog 1's serum, its serum (containing T_4) and a $*T_4$ reagent are added to an antibody-coated tube (step a). During incubation (step b), some of the patient T_4 and $*T_4$ bind competitively to anti-T_4 antibodies on the tubes; other T_4 molecules remain unbound. After incubation, the unbound T_4 is rinsed from the tube, and the bound T_4 stays in the tube (step c). The tube's radioactivity is then measured, and the percentage of added $*T_4$ that remained bound is determined (in this simplified version, 6 of 12 added $*T_4$ were bound, or 50 % bound). Using a standard dose-response curve, dog 1's $[tT_4]$ is determined (see the graph).
- In the analysis of dog 2's serum, its serum (containing T_4 and T_4AA) and $*T_4$ reagent are added to an antibody-coated tube (step d). During incubation, $*T_4$ binds to the anti-T_4 antibodies coating the tube and to the T_4AA, and thus less $*T_4$ is bound to the tube (step e). After rinsing out T_4 not bound to the tube (step f), the tube's radioactivity is measured, and the percentage of added $*T_4$ that remained bound to the tube is determined (in this simplified version, 4 of 12 added $*T_4$ were bound, or 33 % bound). Using a standard dose-response curve, dog 2's $[tT_4]$ is determined (see the graph). The lower % $*T_4$ bound translates to a greater $[tT_4]$ on the standard dose-response curve.

In this schematic assay, the $[T_4]$ in the sera of dogs 1 and 2 were the same (each had 12). However, the T_4AA in dog 2's serum interfered with binding of $*T_4$ to the tube and resulted in a falsely increased measured $[tT_4]$.

---

    b. Anti-T_4 antibodies do not interfere with the equilibrium dialysis assay because the antibodies do not diffuse through the semipermeable membrane.

    c. The major disadvantage of determining $[fT_4]$ by equilibrium dialysis is the expense.

  2. Nondialysis fT_4 RIAs

    a. Nondialysis RIAs designed for quantitation of human $[fT_4]$ are not reliable for canine serum fT_4 because they tend to underestimate the canine $[fT_4]$. In a comparison of an equilibrium dialysis fT_4 assay and five nondialysis fT_4 assays, all five nondialysis assays produced falsely low $[fT_4]$ in sera of healthy dogs and sick dogs with nonthyroidal illness.[19]

b. In a comparison study of the Nichols equilibrium dialysis assay and nine nondialysis assays using sera from euthyroid people, the concordance percentages varied from 59 % to 96 % when serum T_4-binding capacity was within the reference interval, from 66 % to 90 % when serum T_4-binding capacity increased, but from only 31 % to 69 % when serum T_4-binding capacity decreased.[20] As shown in bias plots, poor agreements were found when the serum T_4-binding capacity was in the lower part of the reference interval or poorest agreements were found when the serum T_4-binding capacity was decreased.

3. Chemiluminescence assay: Results from a chemiluminescence assay for [fT_4] were lower than results from the equilibrium dialysis assay. They were about 50 % lower for cat sera.[21] The degree of difference was not reported for dog sera.[22]

C. [tT_3] and [fT_3]

1. Generally, the same basic principles for T_4 assays (tT_4 and fT_4) apply to T_3 (tT_3 and fT_3) assays. Unlike tT_4 assays, assays designed for measuring [tT_3] in human sera have adequate analytical ranges to measure [tT_3] in dogs and cats.

2. RIAs have the analytical specificity to differentiate T_4 and T_3 molecules. Because of lower concentrations, assays that measure [tT_3] tend to be less reproducible than assays that measure [tT_4].

D. TSH

1. Canine TSH

a. There are commercial assays (immunoradiometric and chemiluminescent immunometric) for canine [TSH], but it is not known whether they detect all glycosylated forms of TSH.[23] The canine TSH assays lack sufficient analytical range to enable documentation of decreased [TSH].[24] There was good agreement between two immunoassays when the measured [TSH] was ≥ 0.5 ng/mL and fair agreement when the [TSH] was between 0.1 and 0.5 ng/mL.[24]

b. The reference intervals for canine [TSH] and the methods used to generate reference intervals have differed among investigators. Thus, a [TSH] considered WRI by one investigator might be considered an increased [TSH] by another investigator. Such differences make comparison of reports difficult.

c. There is sufficient antigenic variation between human and canine TSH molecules that the human TSH assay does not measure canine [TSH] accurately.

d. The presence of T_3AA or T_4AA does not interfere with TSH measurement.

2. Feline TSH

a. Hypothyroidism is an uncommon disorder in cats, and thus there is little need to measure feline [TSH].

b. However, it appears that feline [TSH] can be assessed with assays designed for other species. There is evidence that the canine TSH assay can be used to measure feline [TSH].[25] Also, results from a human TSH assay indicated that [TSH] in a group of hypothyroid kittens were, as expected with primary hypothyroidism, at least twice the concentration found in healthy cats.[26]

3. Equine TSH: A RIA for equine TSH has been developed by using a noncommercial source of anti-TSH antibody as the ligand and purified equine TSH as the standard.[27]

E. TgAA

1. A commercial enzyme immunoassay (EIA) for TgAA was developed during the 1990s (produced by Oxford Biomedical Research). Prior to its availability, there was

a lack of assay standardization. Thus, results from different laboratories were difficult to interpret. Another EIA for TgAA was developed, and its results were in good agreement with the commercial assay.[28]

2. For the commercial assay, TgAA results are reported as a percentage of the result obtained for a known positive sample, with percentages above a certain decision threshold considered positive for TgAA. Prior to 2005, a positive result was an optical density value greater than 2 standard deviations above the optical density value in a negative control serum.

3. As with any diagnostic assay, establishing the decision threshold that separates positive and negative results affects the diagnostic sensitivity and specificity of the assay. A lower decision threshold for a TgAA result led to frequent false positives. A higher decision threshold would cause more false-negative results.

4. Because nonspecific binding of immunoglobulins to assay plates can falsely increase TgAA values, testing with and without assessing and subtracting the nonspecific binding yields different results that must be interpreted with different decision thresholds. Some laboratories have labeled the assay *sTgAA* (specific TgAA) to differentiate from *NSB TgAA* (nonspecific binding TgAA) when nonspecific binding is assessed and excluded from the result.

F. T_4AA and T_3AA: Assays for T_4AA and T_3AA have been used in special laboratories for many years. The diagnostic sensitivity of the TgAA values for canine lymphocytic thyroiditis is greater than diagnostic sensitivity values of T_4AA and T_3AA,[17,28] but these assays help identify false T_3 and T_4 results caused by interference from T_4AA and T_3AA.

G. TpAA: Canine TpAA have been detected in sera by using an immunoblot assay.[18]

THYROXINE (T_4) CONCENTRATION

I.   [Total thyroxine] ($[tT_4]$)
   A. Hyperthyroxemia (Table 17.2)
      1. Increased production of T_4 by thyroid neoplasia
         a. Thyroid adenoma (or "adenomatous thyroid hyperplasia") in cats
            (1) When presented with the clinical signs of hyperthyroidism, about 90 % of hyperthyroid cats will have increased $[tT_4]$.[29] The most common presenting problems include weight loss and polyphagia. Others include alopecia, polyuria, polydipsia, and nonspecific gastrointestinal or nervous system findings. Laboratory data may include the following: erythrocytosis;

Table 17.2. Diseases and conditions that cause hyperthyroxemia (increased $[tT_4]$)

Increased production by thyroid neoplasia
  *Thyroid adenoma (common in cats, uncommon in dogs, rare in horses)
  Thyroid adenocarcinoma (dogs, cats, horses)
  Multiple endocrine neoplasia (type II)
Administration of T_4, TSH, or TRH
Administration of compounds containing iodide

  * Relatively common disease or condition
  Note: During diestrus and pregnancy, dogs have greater $[tT_4]$.[65] Pregnant horses have greater $[tT_4]$ than nonpregnant horses.[4] T_4AA may cause positive interference in some tT_4 assays.

increased alanine transaminase (ALT), alkaline phosphatase (ALP), or creatine kinase (CK) activity; azotemia; hyperglycemia; and decreased [fructosamine].

(2) [tT$_4$] may fluctuate sufficiently in hyperthyroid cats so that the [tT$_4$] may be WRI on a random sample.[30] Also, nonthyroidal illness may lower the [tT$_4$] in hyperthyroid cats so that the [tT$_4$] is WRI.[31] A T$_3$ suppression test may confirm the presence of hyperfunctional thyroid tissue, and a subsequent [tT$_4$] may be increased.

(3) Mutations in the TSH receptor causing constitutive activation and thyroid hormone production may cause hyperthyroidism in cats.[32]

(4) Thyroid carcinomas have been reported to occur in about 2 % of hyperthyroid cats.[33]

b. Thyroid adenoma or adenocarcinoma in dogs: About 25 % of canine thyroid neoplasms produce sufficient T$_4$ to cause hyperthyroxemia and clinical signs of hyperthyroidism.[1]

c. Thyroid adenoma or adenocarcinoma in horses: Hyperthyroxemia is rarely reported in horses with thyroid neoplasia. In one horse, the [tT$_4$] was about double the upper reference limit.[34]

d. Multiple endocrine neoplasia (type II) in dogs: This rare disorder involves neoplasia of APUD (amine precursor uptake and decarboxylation) cells and is characterized by thyroid medullary carcinoma, pheochromocytoma, and parathyroid hyperplasia or neoplasia.[35]

2. Administration of T$_4$, TSH, or TRH

3. Administration of compounds containing iodide: Horses may have temporarily increased [tT$_4$] because of increased production of T$_4$ after exposure to iodide in expectorants, counterirritants, contrast media, leg paints, or shampoos.[4]

4. T$_4$AA may cause positive interference in some tT$_4$ assays (Fig. 17.2).

B. Hypothyroxemia (Table 17.3)

1. Decreased production of T$_4$

a. Primary hypothyroidism (caused by thyroid gland disease)

(1) Primary hypothyroidism is a common disorder in dogs.

(2) The most common presenting problems include weight gain, lethargy, and symmetric alopecia. The more common abnormal laboratory data include mild anemia (nonregenerative), codocytosis, hypercholesterolemia, and hypertriglyceridemia.

(3) A basal [tT$_4$] is the standard screening test for hypothyroidism in dogs. Decreased values support hypothyroidism, but there are several reasons for hypothyroxemia other than hypothyroidism. Conversely, it is very unlikely that a dog with a [tT$_4$] that is WRI has primary hypothyroidism (if the [tT$_4$] is valid; see Fig. 17.2).

(4) Lymphocytic thyroiditis, considered an inheritable autoimmune disorder in many dog breeds, is a common cause of thyroid gland destruction and primary hypothyroidism in dogs (at least 50 % of cases).[36] The damaged thyroid gland exposes antigens from immunologically privileged sites so that the immune system produces autoantibodies such as TgAA, T$_4$AA, T$_3$AA, and TpAA. Idiopathic thyroid gland atrophy is another common finding in dogs with hypothyroidism. It may be the terminal stages of lymphocytic thyroiditis.

Table 17.3. Diseases and conditions that cause hypothyroxemia (decreased [tT$_4$])

Decreased production of T$_4$
    *Primary hypothyroidism: lymphocytic thyroiditis, idiopathic thyroid atrophy, congenital thyroid gland dysgenesis, destruction of thyroid gland (neoplasia, surgery, radioactive iodide treatments, or other means)
    Secondary hypothyroidism: TSH deficiency caused by pituitary malformation or destruction by neoplasia, radiation, or other means
    Defective thyroxine production
        Iodine organification defect
        Congenital thyroid peroxidase deficiency in toy fox terriers
        Iodine deficiency
Multifactorial (may include decreased T$_4$ production) or unknown mechanisms
    *Nonthyroidal diseases: hyperadrenocorticism, inflammatory diseases
    *Drugs: glucocorticoids, trimethoprim-sulfadiazine, trimethoprim-sulfamethoxazole, phenobarbital, phenylbutazone, clomipramine
    Diets high in energy, protein, copper, zinc, endophyte-infected fescue grass (horses)
    Food deprivation for 4 d (horses)
    Diet high in *Leucaena leucocephala* (cattle)

* A relatively common disease or condition
Note: Healthy large-breed and medium-breed dogs tend to have lower [tT$_4$] than small-breed dogs.[61] Healthy greyhounds (and possibly other sighthound breeds) have lower [tT$_4$] than other dogs of other breeds.[62]

    (5) Thyroid neoplasia may destroy enough functional follicular cells to create a hypothyroid state. Conversely, old, untreated, hypothyroid beagles had a relatively high incidence of developing thyroid neoplasia, possibly because of chronic TSH stimulation.[37]
    (6) Thyroid glands can also be damaged during surgery, during radioactive iodide treatments, and by other physical means.
    (7) Congenital thyroid gland dysgenesis with hypothyroidism has been reported in dogs.[38]
    (8) Nongoitrous hypothyroidism was found in two Scottish deerhound puppies. The congenital disorder was caused either by primary thyroid hypoplasia or by thyroid-unresponsiveness to TSH.[39]
    (9) Congenital hypothyroidism has been reported in kittens of Abyssinian cats, Japanese cats, and a domestic shorthair cat.[26,40,41] Because healthy 5- to 6-wk-old kittens have [tT$_4$] that are 2–3 times greater than adult cat concentrations, a hypothyroid kitten may have [tT$_4$] within the adult reference interval.[42]
  b. Secondary hypothyroidism (caused by TSH deficiency) is one form of central hypothyroidism.
    (1) Rare cases caused by pituitary neoplasia or malformation are reported in dogs and cats. It may also occur because of pituitary gland damage caused by surgery, radiation, or trauma.[43]
    (2) Thyroid neoplasms may produce abnormal hormones that do not stimulate physiologic responses (therefore hyperthyroidism does not develop) but do suppress TSH release (therefore hypothyroidism develops).[44]

(3) Lack of TSH secretion causes atrophy of thyroidal follicular cells and thus decreased T_4 and T_3 production.

   c. Tertiary hypothyroidism (caused by TRH deficiency) (one form of central hypothyroidism): The authors are not aware of documented cases in domestic mammals.

   d. Defective T_4 production

(1) In dogs, iodine organification defect[2,45] or congenital thyroid peroxidase deficiency in toy fox terriers[46]

(2) In foals, iodine deficiency from decreased dietary intake (foal and dam)[47]

(3) Defective thyroglobulin synthesis in Merino sheep, Dutch goats, and mice produced hypothyroidism. However, defective thyroglobulin synthesis in Afrikaner (Afrikander) cattle and Bongo antelope produced euthyroid congenital goiters.[48]

2. Multifactorial (may include decreased T_4 production) or unknown mechanisms

   a. Nonthyroidal diseases

(1) Many inflammatory, neoplastic, metabolic (e.g., renal failure), and endocrine disorders (especially hyperadrenocorticism) are known to decrease $[tT_4]$. Sick euthyroidism (*eu* from Greek, meaning "well") is the condition in which a disease outside of the thyroid hormonal system creates hypothyroxemia.

(2) Nonthyroidal diseases may lower $[tT_4]$ by one or more of the following processes:

   (a) Decreased protein-bound T_4 because of decreased concentration or affinity of binding proteins

   (b) Inhibition of TSH secretion

   (c) Inhibition of T_4 production

(2) Assessment of TSH and $[fT_4]_{ed}$ may help differentiate nonthyroidal illness from hypothyroidism when $[tT_4]$ is decreased in dogs with clinical signs of hypothyroidism.

   b. Many drugs (especially glucocorticoids) are known to lower $[tT_4]$.

(1) Dogs with hyperadrenocorticism frequently have decreased $[tT_4]$,[49] but changes in $[tT_4]$ in dogs receiving glucocorticoid therapy are variable. The $[tT_4]$ did not change in one study,[50] whereas the $[tT_4]$ decreased in another study.[6] There is evidence that the changes in $[tT_4]$ are caused by multiple factors, including reduced TSH secretion,[49] and that the thyroid glands are less responsive to TSH.[6] There is also evidence that glucocorticoids reduce the conversion of T_4 to T_3 in peripheral tissues.[49] Increased [TSH] is not expected.

(2) In dogs, prednisolone,[6] trimethoprim-sulfadiazine,[51] trimethoprim-sulfamethoxazole,[52] and phenobarbital[53,54] treatments have been shown to cause hypothyroxemia. Sulfonamides interfere with the iodination of thyroid hormones by inhibiting thyroid peroxidase activity,[55,56] so [TSH] may be increased.

(3) In horses, phenylbutazone and glucocorticoid treatments have been shown to cause hypothyroxemia.[57]

(4) Clomipramine (ClomiCalm) administered to dogs for nearly 4 mo decreased $[tT_4]$ and $[fT_4]_{ed}$. The decrease in $[tT_4]$ was detectable after 1 mo of treatment, persisted for the duration of the experiment, but did not drop below

the lower reference limit.[58] Clomipramine is used for a variety of behavioral disorders.

    c. The following have been shown to produce lower $[tT_4]$ in horses:

        (1) Diets high in energy, protein, copper, or zinc

        (2) Ingestion of endophyte-infected fescue grass[57]

        (3) Food deprivation for 4 d (mean $[tT_4]$ decreased from 19.9 nmol/L to 7.6 nmol/L)[59]

    d. Cattle fed foliage from *Leucaena leucocephala* (common names: miracle tree, ipil-ipil, uazin, yaje, and kubabule) developed hypothyroxemia and hypothyroidism.[60]

  3. Certain dog breeds tend to have lower $[tT_4]$ than other breeds. In one study, the mean $[tT_4]$ in large-breed and medium-breed dogs was about 0.5 µg/dL lower than the $[tT_4]$ in the small-breed dogs.[61] Greyhounds, and possibly dogs in other sight-hound breeds, have lower reference values for $[tT_4]$ and $[fT_4]$ than most other dogs.[62] The diagnosis of hypothyroidism in sighthound dogs may require data other than $[tT_4]$ (e.g., increased [TSH]). Unpublished data for dogs in the sighthound breeds indicate that different reference intervals are needed for $[tT_4]$ and $[fT_4]$, but not for $[tT_3]$ or [TSH].

II. $[Free\ thyroxine]_{ed}$ $([fT_4]_{ed})$

  A. Increased $[fT_4]_{ed}$ (free thyroxine concentration by equilibrium dialysis)

    1. The same disorders that cause a truly increased $[tT_4]$ (Table 17.2) are expected to cause a concurrently increased $[fT_4]_{ed}$. About 98 % of hyperthyroid cats have increased $[fT_4]_{ed}$ when tested.[29]

    2. $[fT_4]_{ed}$ does not always mirror $[tT_4]$.

      a. A horse with clinical hyperthyroidism had a normal $[tT_4]$ but an increased $[fT_4]_{ed}$.[63]

      b. Concurrently finding decreased $[tT_4]$ and increased $[fT_4]_{ed}$ in cats suggests the presence of a sick euthyroid state.[64] For unknown reasons, sick cats occasionally have an increased $[fT_4]_{ed}$ but a $[tT_4]$ that is WRI.

    3. T_4AA may cause positive interference in some fT_4 assays, but values for $[fT_4]_{ed}$ are not affected.

  B. Decreased $[fT_4]_{ed}$[65] (free thyroxine concentration by equilibrium dialysis)

    1. Thyroidal disorders that cause decreased $[tT_4]$ by decreasing production of T_4 are expected to have concurrently decreased $[fT_4]_{ed}$.

    2. Other disorders or conditions that may cause decreased $[fT_4]_{ed}$ include hyperadreno-corticism, inflammation (interleukin 1, interleukin 2, interferon γ, and tumor necrosis factor may cause decreased $[fT_4]_{ed}$), and treatments with prednisolone, sulfonamides, or phenobarbital.

    3. Decreased $[fT_4]_{ed}$ was found in horses with experimentally induced hypothyroidism and in horses with a variety of illnesses (especially with severe disorders).[66]

TOTAL TRIIODOTHYRONINE (tT3) AND FREE TRIIODOTHYRONINE (fT3) CONCENTRATIONS

I. Basal $[tT_3]$ and $[fT_3]$ assess conversion of T_4 to T_3 but have less diagnostic sensitivity for hypothyroidism and provide little useful additional information over $[tT_4]$ and $[fT_4]$. In dogs, diurnal variations in $[tT_3]$ were less than the variations found in $[tT_4]$.[5]

II. $[tT_3]$ is measured to monitor therapeutic concentrations and to assess owner compliance in the T_3 suppression test.

III. If a solid-phase RIA is used to measure $[tT_3]$, then T_3AA can cause erroneously increased values just like T_4AA in tT_4 assays (Fig. 17.2). In some assays, T_3AA falsely decrease $[tT_3]$ and falsely increase $[fT_3]$.

THYROID-STIMULATING HORMONE (TSH) CONCENTRATION

I. Dogs
   A. Increased canine [TSH]
      1. Primary hypothyroidism: Lack of negative feedback because of decreased $[fT_4]$ and decreased $[fT_3]$ should increase pituitary synthesis and release of TSH and thus cause an increased [TSH]. Studies indicate that about 60–75 % of hypothyroid dogs have increased [TSH].[67,68]
      2. Compensated hypothyroidism: It appears that some dogs with thyroiditis can maintain $[tT_4]$ or $[tT_3]$ WRI but only with greater stimulation of remaining thyroid cells by TSH.
      3. [TSH] is expected to increase during the TRH response test (see Response and Suppression Tests, sect. II).
   B. Because [TSH] in euthyroid dogs can be at the detection limit of the canine TSH assay, a decreased [TSH] cannot be reliably differentiated from a [TSH] that is WRI. Therefore, [TSH] will be WRI in dogs with secondary hypothyroidism. The hypothyroid dogs without increased [TSH] may have secondary hypothyroidism or primary hypothyroidism. Dogs with sick euthyroidism or drug-induced changes in thyroidal hormone concentrations also may have [TSH] values that are WRI.[67,69]

II. Cats
   A. By using the canine TSH assay to attempt to measure feline TSH, the feline [TSH] in 50 healthy cats was 0.00–0.32 ng/mL (note: canine TSH used as standards).[25] Increased concentrations of feline [TSH] were found in cats after thyroidectomies or after chronic methimazole therapy. Because the lower reference limit is 0.00 ng/mL, this assay cannot document decreased feline [TSH].
   B. If there is not 100 % cross-reactivity between canine and feline TSH, then the use of purified feline TSH in the assay would produce different results. However, the analytical inaccuracy would be reflected in the reference interval, so interpretations may not be affected.

III. Horses: Equine [TSH] was increased in horses after experimental production of hypothyroidism and as a response to TRH administration.[27] Additional studies are needed to assess the diagnostic value of [TSH] in horses.

AUTOANTIBODIES

I. Thyroglobulin autoantibodies (TgAA)
   A. The reported prevalence of TgAA in dogs with hypothyroidism varies, but the percentages are relatively large; that is, 36 % of 42 dogs[70] and 55 % of 31 dogs.[28] With marked

thyroid atrophy or end-stage lymphocytic thyroiditis, the amount of circulating TgAA may diminish.[71]

B. In one study, all eight dogs with a positive TgAA result had lymphocytic thyroiditis.[72] TgAA probably form when thyroglobulin is released from a damaged thyroid gland and the body reacts to the "foreign" protein. A positive TgAA result is evidence of thyroid disease and not evidence of thyroid dysfunction.

C. Predictive values of TgAA results for thyroidal disease have varied among investigators, at least partially because of different methods of establishing a decision threshold between positive and negative reactions.[72,73] Positive results were also found in dogs with hypercalcemia, hypocalcemia, hypoadrenocorticism, hyperadrenocorticism, or diabetes mellitus. It was not determined whether the positive reactions were true or false-positive results in these cases.[72]

II. Thyroxine autoantibodies (T_4AA) and triiodothyronine autoantibodies (T_3AA)

A. Many dogs with lymphocytic thyroiditis also have autoantibodies against T_4 (T_4AA) and T_3 (T_3AA). In a study of nearly 300,000 dogs with clinical signs of hypothyroidism, thyroid hormone autoantibodies were found in about 6 % of the dogs' sera.[71]

B. When autoantibodies are detected, TgAA are more common than either T_4AA or T_3AA. However, some dogs have a negative TgAA result and a positive T_4AA or T_3AA result.[17]

III. Thyroid peroxidase autoantibodies (TpAA)

A. Thyroid peroxidase catalyzes the iodination of tyrosine molecules that are attached to thyroglobulin in thyroidal colloid. The iodination leads to the formation of T_4 and T_3 bound to thyroglobulin. The hormones are cleaved from the thyroglobulin in thyroid epithelial cells and are released to blood.

B. The diagnostic value of the canine TpAA assay has not been established. In canine sera that contained TgAA, T_4AA, or T_3AA, 17 % contained TpAA.[18] TpAA may be involved in the pathogenesis of lymphocytic thyroiditis, but there are also other proposed theories for the immune-mediated destruction of thyrocytes.[74]

RESPONSE AND SUPPRESSION TESTS

I. Thyroid-stimulating hormone (TSH) response test

A. Poor or inadequate response to TSH stimulation was the gold standard for establishing thyroid hypoplasia (hypothyroidism) for many years. Because an approved pharmacologic form of bovine TSH is no longer available, the TSH response test is rarely used for clinical investigations. Recombinant human TSH is available but is expensive.[75] Basic aspects of the TSH response test are provided to assist in the understanding of published reports on canine hypothyroidism.

B. A TSH response test assesses the ability of the thyroid gland to produce T_4 after being stimulated by TSH. Several protocols have been recommended. The amount of administered TSH and the sample collection times vary among feline, canine, and equine protocols.

C. Example of a canine TSH response test

1. Procedure: A blood sample for a basal [tT_4] is collected, bovine TSH is administered intravenously (0.1 units/kg body weight with a maximum of 5 units), and a blood sample is collected 6 h after TSH administration.

2. Interpretation guidelines (expected values may vary among assays)[65]
   a. Euthyroid dogs
      (1) Basal [tT$_4$] in healthy dogs is expected to be 1.0–4.0 µg/dL. In nonthyroidal illness, it may be < 1.0 µg/dL.
      (2) Post-TSH [tT$_4$] > 3.0 µg/dL
   b. Borderline results: post-TSH [tT$_4$] = 1.5–3.0 µg/dL
   c. Hypothyroid dogs: basal and post-TSH [tT$_4$] < 1.5 µg/dL

II. Thyrotropin-releasing hormone (TRH) response test
   A. The TRH response test indirectly assesses thyroid function by causing the release of TSH that stimulates release of T$_4$.
   B. In dogs, the TRH response test is not as good as the TSH response test in detecting hypothyroidism.[76,77] Some euthyroid dogs (as classified by the TSH response test and clinical signs) appear to be hypothyroid by the TRH response test (positive predictive value of 50 %).[78] The TRH response test does not reliably differentiate primary from secondary hypothyroidism, because TRH-induced TSH release is diminished in secondary hypothyroidism and in most primary hypothyroid dogs.[65]
   C. TRH is not approved for use in horses.
   D. The TRH response test is not needed to diagnose hyperthyroidism in cats but has been used.[79]
      1. In hyperthyroid cats, TRH is expected to have little or no effect on TSH and [tT$_4$] because of feedback inhibition on the pituitary gland. Serum [tT$_4$] in a healthy euthyroid cat is expected to double in the post-TRH sample.
      2. Advantages of the TRH response test over the T$_3$ suppression test are that it is shorter (4 h versus 3 d) and does not require owners to administer pills to their cats. Disadvantages are the side effects of TRH administration (salivation, vomiting, tachypnea, and defecation).

III. Triiodothyronine (T$_3$) suppression test
   A. Cats
      1. Most cats with clinical hyperthyroidism have hyperthyroxemia, and thus additional diagnostic testing is not needed. However, some cats with hyperthyroidism have a basal [tT$_4$] that is WRI or only slightly increased, perhaps because of variable secretion of T$_4$ from hyperfunctional thyroid glands, a nonthyroidal disease that is lowering [tT$_4$], or other reasons. For these animals, a T$_3$ suppression test should differentiate the hyperthyroid cats (those with defective hypothalamus-pituitary-thyroid regulation) from euthyroid cats.[80,81]
      2. Basics of the procedure
         a. Collect serum for basal [tT$_4$] and basal [tT$_3$] and freeze it for submission with later serum samples.
         b. Owners administer T$_3$ (liothyronine) per os starting the next morning at 25 µg q8h for 2 d.
         c. Within 2–4 h of the final and seventh dosage of T$_3$, the cat is returned to the clinic, and serum is collected for post-T$_3$ [tT$_4$] and [tT$_3$].
         d. Basal and post-T$_3$ sera are submitted to a laboratory for determination of [tT$_4$] and [tT$_3$].

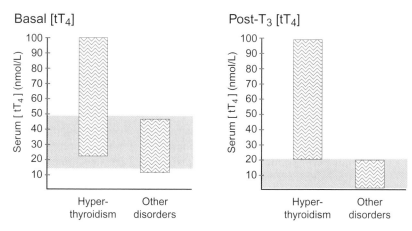

Fig. 17.3. T_3 suppression test results in cats; liothyronine, 25 µg per os, q8h for seven doses. In cats with hyperthyroidism, there was a failure to suppress $[tT_4]$ below 20 nmol/L. In cats with other disorders, the $[tT_4]$ in post-T_3 samples was < 20 nmol/L. Hyperthyroidism was diagnosed in 77 cats, based on clinical signs, palpable thyroid nodules, high-normal to increased $[tT_4]$, and response to treatment for hyperthyroidism. Cats (n = 22) with other disorders had clinical signs suggestive of hyperthyroidism. Their disorders included gastrointestinal diseases, chronic renal disease, cardiomyopathy, and behavioral disorders. The *grey-shaded area* represents the $[tT_4]$ found in 44 clinically healthy cats. The graph was constructed from published data.[80]

      3. Expected results
         a. The post-T_3 $[tT_3]$ should be greater than the basal $[tT_3]$. If it is not, then failure of suppression may be due to failure to administer T_3 to the cat.
         b. Interpretation guidelines of post-T_3 $[tT_4]$ (Fig. 17.3): Values may vary with the assay and laboratory. Using an absolute decision threshold is considered a better method of interpreting results than using a percent decrease,[29,80] but at least a 50 % decrease in $[tT_4]$ typically excludes hyperthyroidism.
           (1) Post-T_3 $[tT_4]$ > 20 nmol/L (> 1.6 µg/dL) indicates a lack of suppression of T_4 secretion and thus supports the presence of a thyroid adenoma.
           (2) Post-T_3 $[tT_4]$ < 20 nmol/L (< 1.6 µg/dL) demonstrates a suppression of T_4 secretion and thus indicates that the cat does not have a thyroid adenoma.
    B. Horses
      1. Hyperthyroidism is uncommon in horses, and thus the need for a T_3 suppression test is limited. Interpretive guidelines and optimal sampling times are not firmly established.
      2. Basics of the procedure[34]
         a. EDTA-plasma is collected for basal $[tT_4]$ and basal $[tT_3]$ for 2 consecutive days prior to administration of T_3. Samples are frozen for submission with later samples.

b. T_3 (2.5 mg diluted in 5 mL saline) is administered at 8:30 a.m. and 6 p.m. for 3 d and at 8:30 a.m. on day 4.

c. EDTA-plasma is collected at 6 p.m. on day 4 and at 8:30 a.m. on days 6, 7, and 9.

d. Basal and post-T_3 plasma are submitted to a laboratory for determination of $[tT_4]$ and $[tT_3]$.

3. Expected results[34]

a. In three clinically healthy horses, plasma $[tT_4]$ values were suppressed (< 4 ng/mL) for at least 5 d after the last dose of T_3.

b. In a horse with a thyroid adenoma, plasma $[tT_4]$ remained increased (> 24 ng/mL) during and after administration of T_3.

c. $[tT_3]$ should be increased in samples collected on days 4 and 6.

TOTAL THYROXINE TO THYROID-STIMULATING HORMONE (tT_4:TSH) AND FREE THYROXINE TO THYROID-STIMULATING HORMONE (fT_4:TSH) RATIOS IN DOGS

I. Because of the physiologic relationships among tT_4, fT_4, and TSH secretion, tT_4:TSH and fT_4:TSH ratios have the potential to differentiate hypothyroid from euthyroid states. Lower ratios suggest that the thyroid glands are not responding to endogenous TSH (primary hypothyroidism). However, the tT_4:TSH ratio may also decrease in secondary hypothyroidism because the $[tT_4]$ decreases more than the detectable decrease in [TSH].

II. Reported results

A. Reported ratios have been calculated directly from the numerical value of reported concentrations; for example, $[tT_4]$ of 10 nmol/L, $[fT_4]$ of 5 pmol/L, and a [TSH] of 0.5 ng/mL would result in a ratio of 20 nmol tT_4:μg TSH (20 mmol tT_4:g TSH) and 10 pmol fT_4:μg TSH (10 μmol fT_4:g TSH). It would be better if analyte concentrations were converted to similar units before a ratio is calculated so that the ratios were unitless.

B. tT_4:TSH ratios (as nmol : μg) in one study showed that hypothyroid dogs usually had lower ratios (values of 1–66; 10 of 11 ratios < 30) than healthy euthyroid dogs (values of 36–173) and sick euthyroid dogs (values of 45–2114; a ratio > 4000 was an obvious outlier).[82]

C. tT_4:TSH and fT_4:TSH ratios in a 1999 study[83]

1. tT_4:TSH ratio: Using a decision threshold of 17.3 nmol tT_4:μg TSH, the tT4:TSH ratio had a diagnostic sensitivity for hypothyroidism of 86.7 % and a diagnostic specificity of 92.2 %.

2. fT4:TSH ratio: Using a decision threshold of 7.5 pmol fT_4:μg TSH, the fT4:TSH ratio had a diagnostic sensitivity for hypothyroidism of 80.0 % and a diagnostic specificity of 97.4 %.

3. Ratios and diagnostic performance will vary with specific assays, laboratories, and decision threshold values.

D. The ratios have not been widely used, and their diagnostic value compared to other assessments is not firmly established. Inaccurate [TSH] at very low concentrations (the assay's detection limit is near concentrations found in euthyroid dogs) could result in inaccurate and perhaps misleading ratios.

Table 17.4. Interpretation of thyroid profile results in dogs

[tT$_4$]	[fT$_4$]$_{ed}$	[TSH]	TgAA	Interpretation
WRI	—	—	—	Rules out hypothyroidism unless [tT$_4$] is falsely increased by T$_4$AA
↓	↓	↑	Positive	Primary hypothyroidism caused by lymphocytic thyroiditis
↓	↓	↑	Negative	Primary hypothyroidism caused by thyroid atrophy or possibly end-stage immune thyroiditis
↓	↓	WRI[a]	Negative	Secondary hypothyroidism caused by pituitary gland dysfunction Sick euthyroidism, nonthyroidal illness[69] Hypothyroxemia caused by effects of drugs[b]
↓	WRI–↑[c]	WRI–↑	Negative	Nonthyroidal illness (sick euthyroidism)
WRI–↑	↓	↑	Positive	Primary hypothyroidism (lymphocytic thyroiditis) with T$_4$AA increasing the [tT$_4$] (see Fig. 17.2)
WRI	WRI	WRI	Positive	Thyroiditis without thyroid dysfunction or false positive (e.g., nonspecific binding)
WRI	WRI	↑	Positive	Thyroiditis with compensatory increase in TSH production
WRI	WRI	↑	Negative	Potentially responding after withdrawal of suppressive drugs or after a nonthyroidal illness[23]

[a] The canine TSH assay lacks an adequate analytical range to measure decreased [TSH] accurately. Therefore, the lower limit of a TSH reference interval cannot be reliably established.

[b] Sulfamethoxazole-trimethoprim, prednisolone, or phenobarbital

[c] [fT$_4$]$_{ed}$ will vary. Results depend on where the illnesses or drugs interfere with thyroid hormone production (see the text).

Note: [tT$_4$] and [fT$_4$]$_{ed}$ near respective reference limits (borderline results) should be interpreted cautiously.

INTERPRETATION OF THYROID HORMONE CONCENTRATIONS AND PROFILES

I.   Dogs
    A. Major patterns of thyroid profile results in dogs (Table 17.4)[49,52,67,69,72,82–87]
    B. [tT$_4$] can be used to help monitor thyroxine therapy. For dogs receiving appropriate thyroxine supplementation, [tT$_4$] is expected to be high-normal to increased 4–6 h after thyroxine administration and [TSH] should be WRI.[65]
    C. To reassess a diagnosis of hypothyroidism via hormone assays in a dog receiving thyroxine supplementation, thyroxine should be discontinued for at least 4 wk prior to testing, in order to remove the influence of treatments on thyroid profile results.[2]

II. Major patterns of [tT$_4$] and [fT$_4$] in cats (Table 17.5)

Table 17.5. Interpretation of [tT$_4$] and [fT$_4$]$_{ed}$ in cats

Clinical history & signs suggest	[tT$_4$]	[fT$_4$]$_{ed}$	Interpretation
Hyperthyroidism	↑	—	Strong evidence of hyperthyroidism (a concurrent ↑ [fT$_4$] provides additional evidence but is typically not needed)
	↓-WRI	WRI-↑	May be hyperthyroidism and/or nonthyroidal illness; T$_3$ suppression test recommended
Euthyroidism	WRI	WRI	No evidence of thyroid dysfunction
	↑	—	Could be early hyperthyroidism, normal random variation, or inappropriate reference interval; a confirmatory ↑ [tT$_4$] or a positive T$_3$ suppression test is needed before diagnosing hyperthyroidism
	↓	—	Probably nonthyroidal illness altering [tT$_4$] or [fT$_4$]
	↓-WRI	↑	
	↓	WRI	
Hypothyroidism	↓	WRI-↑	Nonthyroidal illness causing sick euthyroidism
	↓	↓	Probable primary hypothyroidism; could be secondary hypothyroidism or changes due to nonthyroidal illness or drug therapy

Note: [tT$_4$] and [fT$_4$]$_{ed}$ near respective reference limits (borderline results) should be interpreted cautiously.

References

1. Chastain CB, Ganjam VK. 1986. *Clinical Endocrinology of Companion Animals*, Philadelphia: Lea & Febiger.
2. Feldman EC, Nelson RW. 1996. Hypothyroidism. *Canine and Feline Endocrinology and Reproduction*, 2nd edition, 68–117. Philadelphia: WB Saunders.
3. Bianco AC, Salvatore D, Gereben B, Berry MJ, Larsen PR. 2002. Biochemistry, cellular and molecular biology, and physiological roles of the iodothyronine selenodeiodinases. Endocr Rev 23:38–89.
4. Duckett WM. 1998. Thyroid gland. In: Reed SM, Bayly WM, eds. *Equine Internal Medicine*, 916–925. Philadelphia: WB Saunders.
5. Hoh WP, Oh TH. 2006. Circadian variations of serum thyroxine, free thyroxine and 3,5,3'triiodothyronine concentrations in healthy dogs. J Vet Sci 7:25–29.
6. Torres SMF, McKeever PJ, Johnston SD. 1991. Effect of oral administration of prednisolone on thyroid function in dogs. Am J Vet Res 52:416–421.
7. Larsson M, Pettersson T, Carlström A. 1985. Thyroid hormone binding in serum of 15 vertebrate species: Isolation of thyroxine-binding globulin and prealbumin analogs. Gen Comp Endocrinol 58:360–375.
8. Bassett JH, Harvey CB, Williams GR. 2003. Mechanisms of thyroid hormone receptor-specific nuclear and extra nuclear actions. Mol Cell Endocrinol 213:1–11.
9. Lundberg GD, Iverson C, Radulescu G. 1986. Now read this: The SI units are here. J Am Med Assoc 255:2329–2339.
10. Behrend EN, Kemppainen RJ, Young DW. 1998. Effect of storage conditions on cortisol, total thyroxine, and free thyroxine concentrations in serum and plasma of dogs. J Am Vet Med Assoc 212:1564–1568.

11. Stevenson HP, Archbold GP, Johnston P, Young IS, Sheridan B. 1998. Misleading serum free thyroxine results during low molecular weight heparin treatment. Clin Chem 44:1002–1007.
12. Vermaak WJ, Kalk WJ, Kuyl JM, Smit AM. 1986. Fatty acid induced changes in circulating total and free thyroid hormones: In vivo effects and methodological artefacts. J Endocrinol Invest 9:121–126.
13. Kemppainen RJ, Birchfield JR. 2006. Measurement of total thyroxine concentration in serum from dogs and cats by use of various methods. Am J Vet Res 67:259–265.
14. Lurye JC, Behrend EN, Kemppainen RJ. 2002. Evaluation of an in-house enzyme-linked immunosorbent assay for quantitative measurement of serum total thyroxine concentration in dogs and cats. J Am Vet Med Assoc 221:243–249.
15. Peterson ME, DeMarco CL, Sheldon KM. 2003. Total thyroxine testing: Comparison of an in-house test kit with radioimmuno- and chemiluminescent assays. J Vet Intern Med 17:396 (abstract).
16. Singh AK, Jiang Y, White T, Spassova D. 1997. Validation of nonradioactive chemiluminescent immunoassay methods for the analysis of thyroxine and cortisol in blood samples obtained from dogs, cats, and horses. J Vet Diagn Invest 9:261–268.
17. Thacker EL, Refsal KR, Bull RW. 1992. Prevalence of autoantibodies to thyroglobulin, thyroxine, or triiodo-thyronine and relationship of autoantibodies and serum concentrations of iodothyronines in dogs. Am J Vet Res 53:449–453.
18. Skopek E, Patzl M, Nachreiner RF. 2006. Detection of autoantibodies against thyroid peroxidase in serum samples of hypothyroid dogs. Am J Vet Res 67:809–814.
19. Schachter S, Nelson RW, Scott-Moncrieff C, Ferguson DC, Montgomery T, Feldman EC, Neal L, Kass PH. 2004. Comparison of serum-free thyroxine concentrations determined by standard equilibrium dialysis, modified equilibrium dialysis, and 5 radioimmunoassays in dogs. J Vet Intern Med 18:259–264.
20. Sapin R, d'Herbomez M. 2003. Free thyroxine measured by equilibrium dialysis and nine immunoassays in sera with various serum thyroxine-binding capacities. Clin Chem 49:1531–1535.
21. Paradis M, Pagé N. 1996. Serum free thyroxine concentrations measured by chemiluminescence in hyperthyroid and euthyroid cats. J Am Anim Hosp Assoc 32:489–494.
22. Paradis M, Pagé N, Larivière N, Fontaine M. 1996. Serum-free thyroxine concentrations, measured by chemilumines-cence assay before and after thyrotropin administration in healthy dogs, hypothyroid dogs, and euthyroid dogs with dermatopathies. Can Vet J 37:289–294.
23. Mooney CT. 1999. Canine TSH: A help or a hindrance? In: Proceedings of the 17th ACVIM Forum, Chicago, 456–457.
24. Marca MC, Loste A, Orden I, Gonzalez JM, Marsella JA. 2001. Evaluation of canine serum thyrotropin (TSH) concentration: Comparison of three analytical procedures. J Vet Diagn Invest 13:106–110.
25. Graham PA, Refsal KR, Nachreiner RF, Provencher-Bolliger AL. 2000. The measurement of feline thyrotropin (TSH) using a commercial canine immunoradiometric assay. J Vet Intern Med 14:342 (abstract).
26. Tanase H, Kudo K, Horikoshi H, Mizushima H, Okazaki T, Ogata E. 1991. Inherited primary hypothyroidism with thyrotrophin resistance in Japanese cats. J Endocrinol 129:245–251.
27. Breuhaus BA. 2002. Thyroid-stimulating hormone in adult euthyroid and hypothyroid horses. J Vet Intern Med 16:109–115.
28. Patzl M, Mostl E. 2003. Determination of autoantibodies to thyroglobulin, thyroxine and triiodothyronine in canine serum. J Vet Med [A] 50:72–78.
29. Peterson ME. 2006. Diagnostic tests for hyperthyroidism in cats. Clin Tech Small Anim Pract 21:2–9.
30. Peterson ME, Graves TK, Cavanagh I. 1987. Serum thyroid hormone concentrations fluctuate in cats with hyperthyroidism. J Vet Intern Med 1:142–146.
31. Peterson ME, Gamble DA. 1990. Effect of nonthyroidal illness on serum thyroxine concentrations in cats: 494 cases (1988). J Am Vet Med Assoc 197:1203–1208.
32. Peeters ME, Timmermans-Sprang EP, Mol JA. 2002. Feline thyroid adenomas are in part associated with mutations in the $G_{s\alpha}$ gene and not with polymorphisms found in the thyrotropin receptor. Thyroid 12:571–575.
33. Turrel JM, Feldman EC, Nelson RW, Cain GR. 1988. Thyroid carcinoma causing hyperthyroidism in cats: 14 cases (1981–1986). J Am Vet Med Assoc 193:359–364.
34. Alberts MK, McCann JP, Woods PR. 2000. Hemithyroidectomy in a horse with confirmed hyperthyroidism. J Am Vet Med Assoc 217:1051–1054.
35. Peterson ME, Randolph JF, Zaki FA, Heath H III. 1982. Multiple endocrine neoplasia in a dog. J Am Vet Med Assoc 180:1476–1478.
36. Graham PA, Nachreiner RF, Refsal KR, Provencher-Bolliger AL. 2001. Lymphocytic thyroiditis. Vet Clin North Am Small Anim Pract 31:915–933.

37. Benjamin SA, Stephens LC, Hamilton BF, Saunders WJ, Lee AC, Angleton GM, Mallinckrodt CH. 1996. Associations between lymphocytic thyroiditis, hypothyroidism, and thyroid neoplasia in beagles. Vet Pathol 33:486–494.

38. Greco DS, Peterson ME, Cho DY, Markovits JE. 1985. Juvenile-onset hypothyroidism in a dog. J Am Vet Med Assoc 187:948–950.

39. Robinson WF, Shaw SE, Stanley B, Wyburn RS. 1988. Congenital hypothyroidism in Scottish Deerhound puppies. Aust Vet J 65:386–389.

40. Jones BR, Gruffydd-Jones TJ, Sparkes AH, Lucke VM. 1992. Preliminary studies on congenital hypothyroidism in a family of Abyssinian cats. Vet Rec 131:145–148.

41. Crowe A. 2004. Congenital hypothyroidism in a cat. Can Vet J 45:168, 170.

42. Greco DS. 2006. Diagnosis of congenital and adult-onset hypothyroidism in cats. Clin Tech Small Anim Pract 21:40–44.

43. Mellanby RJ, Jeffery ND, Gopal MS, Herrtage ME. 2005. Secondary hypothyroidism following head trauma in a cat. J Feline Med Surg 7:135–139.

44. Branam JE, Leighton RL, Hornof WJ. 1982. Radioisotope imaging for the evaluation of thyroid neoplasia and hypothyroidism in a dog. J Am Vet Med Assoc 180:1077–1079.

45. Chastain CB, McNeel SV, Graham CL, Pezzanite SC. 1983. Congenital hypothyroidism in a dog due to an iodide organification defect. Am J Vet Res 44:1257–1265.

46. Fyfe JC, Kampschmidt K, Dang V, Poteet BA, He Q, Lowrie C, Graham PA, Fetro VM. 2003. Congenital hypothyroidism with goiter in toy fox terriers. J Vet Intern Med 17:50–57.

47. Osame S, Ichijo S. 1994. Clinicopathological observations on thoroughbred foals with enlarged thyroid gland. J Vet Med Sci 56:771–772.

48. Medeiros-Neto G, Targovnik HM, Vassart G. 1993. Defective thyroglobulin synthesis and secretion causing goiter and hypothyroidism. Endocr Rev 14:165–183.

49. Ferguson DC, Peterson ME. 1992. Serum free and total iodothyronine concentrations in dogs with hyperadrenocorticism. Am J Vet Res 53:1636–1640.

50. Moore GE, Ferguson DC, Hoenig M. 1993. Effects of oral administration of anti-inflammatory doses of prednisone on thyroid hormone response to thyrotropin-releasing hormone and thyrotropin in clinically normal dogs. Am J Vet Res 54:130–135.

51. Gookin JL, Trepanier LA, Bunch SE. 1999. Clinical hypothyroidism associated with trimethoprim-sulfadiazine administration in a dog. J Am Vet Med Assoc 214:1028–1031.

52. Hall IA, Campbell KL, Chambers MD, Davis CN. 1993. Effect of trimethoprim/sulfamethoxazole on thyroid function in dogs with pyoderma. J Am Vet Med Assoc 202:1959–1962.

53. Gaskill CL, Burton SA, Gelens HCJ, Ihle SL, Miller JB, Shaw DH, Brimacombe MB, Cribb AE. 1999. Effects of phenobarbital treatment on serum thyroxine and thyroid-stimulating hormone concentrations in epileptic dogs. J Am Vet Med Assoc 215:489–496.

54. Müller PB, Wolfsheimer KJ, Taboada J, Hosgood G, Partington BP, Gaschen FP. 2000. Effects of long-term phenobarbital treatment on the thyroid and adrenal axis and adrenal function tests in dogs. J Vet Intern Med 14:157–164.

55. Doerge DR, Decker CJ. 1994. Inhibition of peroxidase-catalyzed reactions by arylamines: Mechanism for the antithyroid action of sulfamethazine. Chem Res Toxicol 7:164–169.

56. Gupta A, Eggo MC, Uetrecht JP, Cribb AE, Daneman D, Rieder MJ, Shear NH, Cannon M, Spielberg SP. 1992. Drug-induced hypothyroidism: The thyroid as a target organ in hypersensitivity reactions to anticonvulsants and sulfonamides. Clin Pharmacol Ther 51:56–67.

57. Messer NT, IV. 1997. Thyroid disease (dysfunction). In: Robinson NE, ed. *Current Therapy in Equine Medicine 4*, 502–503. Philadelphia: WB Saunders.

58. Gulikers KP, Panciera DL. 2003. Evaluation of the effects of clomipramine on canine thyroid function tests. J Vet Intern Med 17:44–49.

59. Messer NT, Johnson PJ, Refsal KR, Nachreiner RF, Ganjam VK, Krause GF. 1995. Effect of food deprivation on baseline iodothyronine and cortisol concentrations in healthy, adult horses. Am J Vet Res 56:116–121.

60. Jones RJ, Blunt CG, Nurnberg BI. 1978. Toxicity of *Leucaena leucocephala*: The effect of iodine and mineral supplements on penned steers fed a sole diet of *Leucaena*. Aust Vet J 54:387–392.

61. Reimers TJ, Lawler DF, Sutaria PM, Correa MT, Erb HN. 1990. Effects of age, sex, and body size on serum concentrations of thyroid and adrenocortical hormones in dogs. Am J Vet Res 51:454–457.

62. Gaughan KR, Bruyette DS. 2001. Thyroid function testing in greyhounds. Am J Vet Res 62:1130–1133.

63. Ramirez S, McClure JJ, Moore RM, Wolfsheimer KJ, Gaunt SD, Mirza MH, Taylor W. 1998. Hyperthyroidism associated with a thyroid adenocarcinoma in a 21-year-old gelding. J Vet Intern Med 12:475–477.

64. Peterson ME. 2000. Hyperthyroidism. In: Ettinger SJ, Feldman EC, eds. *Textbook of Veterinary Internal Medicine: Diseases of the Dog and Cat*, 5th edition, 1400–1419. Philadelphia: WB Saunders.

65. Scott-Moncrieff JCR, Guptill-Yoran L. 2000. Hypothyroidism. In: Ettinger SJ, Feldman EC, eds. *Textbook of Veterinary Internal Medicine: Diseases of the Dog and Cat*, 5th edition, 1419–1429. Philadelphia: WB Saunders.

66. Breuhaus BA, Refsal KR, Beyerlein SL. 2006. Measurement of free thyroxine concentration in horses by equilibrium dialysis. J Vet Intern Med 20:371–376.

67. Peterson ME, Melián C, Nichols R. 1997. Measurement of serum total thyroxine, triiodothyronine, free thyroxine, and thyrotropin concentrations for diagnosis of hypothyroidism in dogs. J Am Vet Med Assoc 211:1396–1402.

68. Boretti FS, Reusch CE. 2004. Endogenous TSH in the diagnosis of hypothyroidism in dogs. Schweiz Arch Tierheilkd 146:183–188.

69. Scott-Moncrieff JCR, Nelson RW, Bruner JM, Williams DA. 1998. Comparison of serum concentrations of thyroid-stimulating hormone in healthy dogs, hypothyroid dogs, and euthyroid dogs with concurrent disease. J Am Vet Med Assoc 212:387–391.

70. Dixon RM, Mooney CT. 1999. Canine serum thyroglobulin autoantibodies in health, hypothyroidism and non-thyroidal illness. Res Vet Sci 66:243–246.

71. Nachreiner RF, Refsal KR, Graham PA, Bowman MM. 2002. Prevalence of serum thyroid hormone autoantibodies in dogs with clinical signs of hypothyroidism. J Am Vet Med Assoc 220:466–471.

72. Nachreiner RF, Refsal KR, Graham PA, Hauptman J, Watson GL. 1998. Prevalence of autoantibodies to thyroglobulin in dogs with nonthyroidal illness. Am J Vet Res 59:951–955.

73. Haines DM, Lording PM, Penhale WJ. 1984. Survey of thyroglobulin autoantibodies in dogs. Am J Vet Res 45:1493–1497.

74. Stassi G, De Maria R. 2002. Autoimmune thyroid disease: New models of cell death in autoimmunity. Nat Rev Immunol 2:195–204.

75. Stegeman JR, Graham PA, Hauptman JG. 2003. Use of recombinant human thyroid-stimulating hormone for thyrotropin-stimulation testing of euthyroid cats. Am J Vet Res 64:149–152.

76. Ramsey I, Herrtage M. 1997. Distinguishing normal, sick, and hypothyroid dogs using total thyroxine and thyrotropin concentrations. Canine Pract 22:43–44.

77. Scott-Moncrieff JC. 1997. Serum canine thyrotropin concentrations in experimental and spontaneous canine hypothyroidism. Canine Pract 22:41–42.

78. Frank LA. 1996. Comparison of thyrotropin-releasing hormone (TRH) to thyrotropin (TSH) stimulation for evaluating thyroid function in dogs. J Am Anim Hosp Assoc 32:481–487.

79. Peterson ME, Broussard JD, Gamble DA. 1994. Use of the thyrotropin releasing hormone stimulation test to diagnose mild hyperthyroidism in cats. J Vet Intern Med 8:279–286.

80. Peterson ME, Graves TK, Gamble DA. 1990. Triiodothyronine (T3) suppression test: An aid in the diagnosis of mild hyperthyroidism in cats. J Vet Intern Med 4:233–238.

81. Refsal KR, Nachreiner RF, Stein BE, Currigan CE, Zendel AN, Thacker EL. 1991. Use of the triiodothyronine suppression test for diagnosis of hyperthyroidism in ill cats that have serum concentration of iodothyronines within normal range. J Am Vet Med Assoc 199:1594–1601.

82. Dixon RM, Graham PA, Mooney CT. 1996. Serum thyrotropin concentrations: A new diagnostic test for canine hypothyroidism. Vet Rec 138:594–595.

83. Dixon RM, Mooney CT. 1999. Evaluation of serum free thyroxine and thyrotropin concentrations in the diagnosis of canine hypothyroidism. J Small Anim Pract 40:72–78.

84. Panciera DL. 1999. Is it possible to diagnose canine hypothyroidism? J Small Anim Pract 40:152–157.

85. Kantrowitz LB, Peterson ME, Trepanier LA, Melián C, Nichols R. 1999. Serum total thyroxine, total triiodothyronine, free thyroxine, and thyrotropin concentrations in epileptic dogs treated with anticonvulsants. J Am Vet Med Assoc 214:1804–1808.

86. Beale KM, Halliwell RE, Chen CL. 1990. Prevalence of antithyroglobulin antibodies detected by enzyme-linked immunosorbent assay of canine serum. J Am Vet Med Assoc 196:745–748.

87. Dixon RM, Mooney CT. 1999. New diagnostic methods in the evaluation of canine thyroid disease. Comp Haematol Intl 9:232–233 (abstract).

Chapter 18

ADRENOCORTICAL FUNCTION

Physiologic Processes 806
Analytical Concepts 807
Cortisol Concentration 808
    I. Diseases and Conditions That Cause Hypercortisolemia 808
    II. Diseases and Conditions That Cause Hypocortisolemia 810
Urine Cortisol to Creatinine (Cort:Crt)$_u$ Ratio 812
Adrenocorticotropic Hormone (ACTH) Concentration 813
Plasma Cortisol to ACTH Ratio 814
Suppression and Stimulation Tests 815
    I. Dogs 815
        A. Low-dose Dexamethasone Suppression Test (LDDST) 815
        B. High-dose Dexamethasone Suppression Test (HDDST) 817
        C. Interpretation of Dexamethasone Suppression Tests 818
        D. Adrenocorticotropic Hormone (ACTH) Stimulation (Response) Test 818
    II. Cats 821
        A. Low-dose Dexamethasone Suppression Test (LDDST) 821
        B. High-dose Dexamethasone Suppression Test (HDDST) 821
        C. Adrenocorticotropic Hormone (ACTH) Stimulation (Response) Test 821
    III. Horses 822
        A. Dexamethasone Suppression Test 822
        B. Adrenocorticotropic Hormone (ACTH) Stimulation (Response) Test 822
Combined Dexamethasone Suppression–Adrenocorticotropic Hormone (ACTH)
  Stimulation (Response) Test 823
Aldosterone Concentration 824
Other Assessments of Adrenocortical Function 826
    I. Thorn Test and Modified Thorn Test 826
    II. Concentrations of Other Steroid Hormones 827

Table 18.1. Abbreviations and symbols in this chapter

(Cort:Crt)$_u$	Urine cortisol to creatinine
[x]	Concentration of x (x = analyte)
ACTH	Adrenocorticotropic hormone (corticotropin)
CRH	Corticotropin-releasing hormone
EDTA	Ethylenediaminetetraacetic acid
ELISA	Enzyme-linked immunosorbent assay
FAN	Functional adrenal neoplasia
HDDST	High-dose dexamethasone suppression test
LDDST	Low-dose dexamethasone suppression test
*op'*DDD	1,1-Dichloro-2-(*o*-chlorophenyl)-2-(*p*-chlorophenyl)ethane
PDH	Pituitary-dependent hyperadrenocorticism
PPID	Pituitary pars intermedia dysfunction
RIA	Radioimmunoassay
SI	Système International d'Unités
WRI	Within reference interval

PHYSIOLOGIC PROCESSES

I.   Regulation of cortisol and aldosterone secretion (Fig. 18.1)

      A. CRH from the hypothalamus stimulates the production and release of pituitary ACTH and other hormones. Low [cortisol] promotes secretion of CRH and ACTH. High [cortisol] inhibits secretion of CRH and ACTH.

      B. ACTH stimulates the production and release of cortisol, aldosterone, and other steroid compounds from the adrenal glands. The adrenal gland cortices produce most circulating cortisol.

      C. Aldosterone secretion is also stimulated by angiotensin II, hyperkalemia, and hyponatremia but is inhibited by atrial natriuretic peptide. The secreted aldosterone stimulates the renal retention of Na^+ and Cl^- and excretion of K^+ and H^+.

      D. Peak secretion of cortisol occurs in the morning in dogs and horses but in the evening in cats. The degree of daily variation is minimal in domestic mammals[1] but may need to be considered when interpreting diagnostic tests in horses (average about 3.0 μg/dL at midnight; averages 4.5–5.0 μg/dL from 8 a.m. to 4 p.m.).[2]

      E. Nearly all cortisol released from the adrenal glands becomes bound to plasma proteins.[1] In dogs, about 40 % of cortisol is bound to transcortin, 50 % to albumin, and the remainder (5–10 %) is free. The half-life of cortisol is about 1.5 h in dogs and less in cats.

      F. Cortisol binds to receptor proteins in cells. The cortisol-receptor complex initiates synthesis of hormone and cytokine receptors and other proteins involved in gluconeogenesis, protein catabolism, lipolysis, immune responses, and H_2O balance.

      G. Most cortisol is removed from plasma by hepatocytes, but there is also urinary excretion of cortisol and cortisol metabolites.

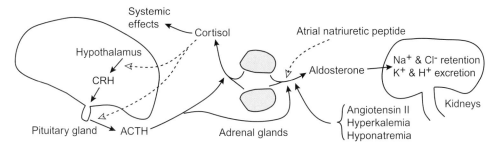

Fig. 18.1. Regulation of cortisol and aldosterone secretion.
- CRH released from the hypothalamus stimulates the production and release of ACTH from the pituitary gland. ACTH stimulates the production and release of cortisol and aldosterone from the adrenal gland cortices. In the negative-feedback system (dashed lines), increasing the [cortisol] inhibits the secretion of CRH and ACTH.
- Increased [angiotensin II], hyperkalemia, hyponatremia, and increased [ACTH] promote the release of aldosterone from adrenal gland cortices. Atrial natriuretic peptide inhibits aldosterone release. The secreted aldosterone stimulates the renal retention of Na^+ and Cl^- and excretion of K^+ and H^+.

ANALYTICAL CONCEPTS

I.   Unit conversion[3]
      A. Cortisol: μg/dL × 10 = ng/mL and μg/dL × 27.6 = nmol/L (SI unit, nearest 10 nmol/L)
      B. Aldosterone: ng/dL × 10 = pg/mL and ng/dL × 27.74 = pmol/L (SI unit, nearest 10 pmol/L)
      C. ACTH: ng/L = pg/mL and pg/mL × 0.2202 = pmol/L (SI unit, nearest 1 pmol/L)

II.   Sample
      A. Cortisol
          1. Serum or EDTA-plasma may be used.
          2. Stability of [cortisol] in EDTA-plasma is better than in sera and better in cold samples (−20 °C best and 4 °C acceptable) than in warm ones (25 °C or 37 °C). Therefore, samples (especially sera) should be shipped with ice packs.[4]
          3. It is occasionally written that serum or plasma should be collected from blood quickly because of the uptake of cortisol by erythrocytes. Erythrocytes do bind cortisol that is added to blood,[5] but cortisol should already be distributed to plasma and erythrocytes in patient blood samples. There was no difference between measured [cortisol] in plasma samples removed from cells either 10 min or 40 h after blood collection.[6]
      B. Aldosterone
          1. Serum or heparinized plasma may be used.
          2. [Aldosterone] is stable for a week at 2–8 °C and for at least 2 mo at −20 °C.[7]
      C. ACTH
          1. EDTA-plasma is preferred (addition of a protease inhibitor such as aprotinin has been recommended to reduce degradation). Plasma should be removed from the erythrocytes immediately, placed in a plastic tube, and chilled. The sample should not have prolonged contact with glass because ACTH adheres to glass.

2. ACTH is very labile, so the plasma requires special handling.[8] If not analyzed the day of collection, then the sample should be frozen and shipped to the reference laboratory in a dry-ice shipment. Equine [ACTH] is stable in EDTA-plasma (without aprotinin) for 3 h at 19 °C.[9]

III. Principles and assay procedures
    A. Cortisol
        1. Several commercial cortisol assays are available. RIAs are the most common and are considered the *gold standard*, but enzyme immunoassays (e.g., enzyme-linked immunosorbent assay and chemiluminescent enzyme immunoassay) are also used.
        2. Anticortisol antibodies in the immunoassays may cross-react with other glucocorticoids. Unless you know the cross-reactivity of an assay, interpret a [cortisol] with caution if an animal has received corticosteroid therapy. The following cross-reactivity percentages are for a common cortisol RIA (manufacturer's data): cortisol (100 %), prednisolone (69 %), 11-deoxycortisol (7.5 %), prednisone (6.4 %), cortisone (4.2 %), corticosterone (3.5 %), spironolactone (< 0.2 %), and dexamethasone (< 0.1 %). Poor cross-reactivity with dexamethasone is an important fact for dexamethasone suppression tests.
        3. Assays designed to measure plasma cortisol are also used to measure urine cortisol for $(Cort:Crt)_u$ ratio.
    B. ACTH
        1. Antibodies in RIA reagents designed for measuring human ACTH tend to cross-react with canine and feline ACTH.
        2. Instability of ACTH is the major concern with ACTH measurement. Samples must be processed appropriately to obtain valid results.
    C. Aldosterone
        1. Aldosterone RIAs are not as common as cortisol assays. A relatively minute [aldosterone] requires assays with high analytical sensitivity and very low detection limits (pg/mL).
        2. Physiologic and dietary factors that influence aldosterone production need to be considered when establishing reference intervals for [aldosterone].

CORTISOL CONCENTRATION

I. Diseases and conditions that cause hypercortisolemia (Table 18.2)
    A. Spontaneous conditions: Basal plasma [cortisol] by itself is of limited value because many patients with hyperadrenocorticism do not have increased basal [cortisol]. However, there is sufficient cortisol production to cause clinical disorders either because of episodic exaggerated secretions or because of a mild but continuously increased production of cortisol. A [cortisol] is best interpreted in either dexamethasone suppression tests or ACTH stimulation tests (see later sections). Historical, physical, and preliminary laboratory data may clearly indicate that an animal has hyperadrenocorticism but may not clearly differentiate the causes of the pathologic state. Adrenal suppression and stimulation tests (covered later in this chapter) can be helpful for this, and diagnostic imaging methods (i.e., radiography, ultrasonography, computed axial tomography, or magnetic resonance imaging) can locate the pituitary or adrenal neoplasms but cannot determine whether the abnormal tissue is producing excessive amounts of hormones.

Table 18.2. Diseases and conditions that cause hypercortisolemia

Increased production of cortisol
    Spontaneous conditions
        *Pituitary-dependent hyperadrenocorticism
        *Functional adrenocortical neoplasia: adenoma, adenocarcinoma
        *Stress-induced hypercortisolemia
        Ectopic production of ACTH by a neoplasm
        Ovarian steroid cell tumor
    Iatrogenic conditions
        Exogenous ACTH administration

* A relatively common disease or condition
Note: Pharmacological doses of some steroid compounds may result in a cross-reaction and give a falsely elevated [cortisol].

1. Pituitary-dependent hyperadrenocorticism (PDH): (Hyperadrenocorticism is commonly referred to as Cushing's disease, the name originally given to the human pituitary disorder described by Dr. Harvey Cushing.)
   a. In PDH, the neoplastic pituitary cells release excess ACTH, which causes bilateral adrenocortical hyperplasia. The ACTH release may or may not be inhibited by exogenous glucocorticoids. Also, individual neoplasms can be inhibited by some steroids but not others.
   b. In dogs, about 80–85 % of clinical hyperadrenocorticism cases are caused by increased release of ACTH from pituitary adenomas. A small percentage are caused by pituitary adenocarcinomas or pituitary hyperplasia.[10]
   c. In cats, about 75–85 % of clinical hyperadrenocorticism cases are caused by increased release of ACTH from pituitary adenomas. A small percentage are caused by pituitary adenocarcinomas.[11] One cat had clinical hyperadrenocorticism and diabetes mellitus because of the secretion of ACTH and growth hormone by two pituitary neoplasms.[12]
   d. In horses, nearly all cases of clinical hyperadrenocorticism are caused by a pituitary adenoma or hyperplasia.[13] The endocrine disorder is common in old horses and referred to as *pituitary pars intermedia dysfunction* (PPID). There is evidence that PPID is secondary to hypothalamic degeneration that decreases dopamine production. Normally, dopamine inhibits the melanotropes of the pars intermedia. Without this inhibition, the melanotropes produce excess pro-opiomelanocortin, which is cleaved into β-melanocyte–stimulating hormone (β-MSH), corticotropin-like intermediate lobe peptide, β-endorphin–related peptide (βEND peptide), and ACTH. The combination of increased β-MSH, βEND peptide, and ACTH causes excess steroidogenesis and clinical hyperadrenocorticism.[14]
2. Functional adrenocortical neoplasia (FAN)
   a. In FAN, cells of the adrenocortical adenoma or adrenocortical carcinoma produce excess cortisol. The neoplastic cells may or may not be responsive to exogenous ACTH. A high [cortisol] is expected to inhibit ACTH release, and the nonneoplastic adrenal gland will atrophy.

     b. In dogs, about 10–20 % of clinical hyperadrenocorticism cases are due to adrenal adenomas or adenocarcinomas.[10]

     c. In cats, about 15–25 % of clinical hyperadrenocorticism cases are due to adrenal adenomas or adenocarcinomas.[11] Clinical hyperadrenocorticism may also be seen when adrenocortical neoplasms produce steroid hormones other than cortisol (such as progesterone).[15]

   3. Stress-induced hypercortisolemia

     a. Stress caused by an illness or environmental changes may stimulate the release of CRH, then ACTH, and thus stimulate the adrenal glands to produce more cortisol.

     b. If persistent, the stress response may lead to bilateral adrenocortical hyperplasia, but it should not cause the clinical manifestations of pathologic hyperadrenocorticism.

   4. Ectopic production of ACTH: Neoplastic tissue other than pituitary neoplasms can produce ACTH that causes bilateral adrenocortical hyperplasia and clinical hyperadrenocorticism.[16] These disorders are rarely recognized in domestic mammals but have been found in people for many years.

   5. Ovarian steroid cell tumor in a dog:[17] Ovarian neoplasms can produce cortisol-like compounds that cause clinical hyperadrenocorticism.

  B. Iatrogenic conditions

   1. Exogenous ACTH administration is expected to cause hypercortisolemia (see Suppression and Stimulation Tests, sect. I.D).

   2. Because the anticortisol antibody in immunoassays may cross-react with other steroids, recent administration of steroids could result in a falsely increased measured concentration. For example, assays that list significant cross-reactivity with prednisolone may have false values if the animal was recently treated with prednisolone (e.g., Prednis-Tab), prednisone (e.g., Meticorten), or prednisolone sodium succinate (e.g., Solu-Delta-Cortef).

  C. Other common routine laboratory findings with hypercortisolemia

   1. Leukogram: steroid leukogram (see Chapter 2)

   2. Chemistry profile: increased serum activity of alkaline phosphatase (ALP) in dogs, hyperglycemia, hypercholesterolemia, and lipemia

   3. Urinalysis: relatively unconcentrated, isosthenuric, or hyposthenuric urine, and glucosuria in horses

II.   Diseases and conditions that cause hypocortisolemia (Table 18.3)

  A. Spontaneous conditions

   1. Primary hypoadrenocorticism (Hypoadrenocorticism is commonly referred to as Addison's disease, the name originally given to the human adrenal disorder described by Dr. Thomas Addison.)

     a. Causes of spontaneous bilateral atrophy or destruction of adrenal glands are usually not known, but they may include immune-mediated disease, adrenalitis, or adrenal hemorrhage.

     b. The disorder is recognized primarily in dogs but also occurs in cats[18] and occasionally in foals.[19]

   2. Secondary hypoadrenocorticism (ACTH deficiency): ACTH deficiency could result from destruction of the pituitary gland by disease processes or surgery, but this is much less common than primary hypoadrenocorticism.

Table 18.3. Diseases and conditions that cause hypocortisolemia

Decreased production of cortisol
   Spontaneous conditions
      *Primary hypoadrenocorticism
      Secondary hypoadrenocorticism (ACTH deficiency)
      Atypical primary hypoadrenocorticism (selective cortisol deficiency)
      Iatrogenic conditions
    *Iatrogenic hyperadrenocorticism[a]
    Iatrogenic hypoadrenocorticism[b]
    Ketoconazole or trilostane treatment

[a] The animal has clinical manifestations (e.g., polyuria or alopecia) of excess glucocorticoid hormonal activity because of prolonged treatment with glucocorticoid compounds.

[b] The animal has clinical manifestations of deficiencies in glucocorticoid and mineralocorticoid hormonal activity (e.g., weakness, azotemia, hyponatremia, hypochloremia, or hyperkalemia) caused by adrenocortical hypoplasia induced by *op′*DDD, trilostane, or sudden withdrawal of prolonged treatment with glucocorticoid compounds (e.g., prednisolone, prednisone, or megestrol acetate).

   3. Atypical primary hypoadrenocorticism (selective cortisol deficiency): Rare spontaneous cases of hypocortisolemia without concurrent hypoaldosteronemia, hyponatremia, or hyperkalemia have been reported.[20] In some of these cases, [aldosterone] was not reported but was only presumed to be WRI because of the absence of electrolyte changes.[21] In another case, the concurrent cortisol and thyroxine deficiencies were considered a polyglandular deficiency syndrome.[22]

B. Iatrogenic conditions
   1. Iatrogenic hyperadrenocorticism
     a. Chronic administration of glucocorticoid drugs (e.g., prednisone or prednisolone) may produce clinical signs consistent with hyperadrenocorticism.
     b. The exogenous glucocorticoids will cause a negative feedback on the release of CRH and ACTH, and thus adrenal glands will atrophy and produce less cortisol. Baseline [cortisol] typically will be decreased ($< 1.0 \ \mu g/dL$), and there will be a diminished response in the ACTH stimulation test. Slow withdrawal of the steroid treatments enables the adrenal glands to recover.
   2. Iatrogenic hypoadrenocorticism
     a. Treatment of dogs with *op′*DDD (mitotane [Lysodren]) for hyperadrenocorticism because of PDH or FAN causes progressive necrosis of the adrenal cortex (zona fasciculata and zona reticularis). Excessive necrosis can decrease adrenal function and clinical hypoadrenocorticism with cortisol deficiency and sometimes mineralocorticoid deficiency.
     b. Sudden withdrawal of glucocorticoid treatments (including megestrol acetate in cats) may cause clinical hypoadrenocorticism because of adrenal gland atrophy that developed while the animal was receiving glucocorticoids.
   3. Treatment of dogs or cats with ketoconazole can cause decreased [cortisol] because ketoconazole inhibits steroid biosynthesis.[23,24] Treatment with trilostane reduces [cortisol] by inhibiting 3β-hydroxysteroid dehydrogenase, an enzyme that catalyzes an intermediate reaction in steroid synthesis.[25]

C. Other common routine laboratory findings with hypocortisolemia (except with iatrogenic hyperadrenocorticism caused by glucocorticoid administration)
   1. Leukogram: absence of steroid leukogram in stressed, ill patients (particularly a lack of lymphopenia; and possible lymphocytosis or eosinophilia)
   2. Chemistry profile: hyponatremia, hypochloremia, hyperkalemia, hypercalcemia, hypoglycemia, and azotemia
   3. Urinalysis: inappropriately low urine specific gravity with azotemia

URINE CORTISOL TO CREATININE (Cort:Crt)$_u$ RATIO

I. As described in Chapter 8, comparison of a urine analyte's concentration to urine [creatinine] will provide a relative rate of urinary excretion of the analyte (such as cortisol) compared to creatinine. In theory, the (Cort:Crt)$_u$ ratio should detect a hyperadrenal state better than a basal [cortisol] because the cortisol that accumulates in urine was produced over a longer period and thus is not as susceptible to variations caused by episodic cortisol secretions. Episodic secretions can cause fluctuations in a random serum [cortisol]. However, the increased urinary cortisol excretion could be either a physiologic or pathologic state.

II. The (Cort:Crt)$_u$ ratio should be calculated by using molar concentrations of urine cortisol and creatinine (Eq. 18.1). A markedly different ratio would result if [cortisol] and [creatinine] were expressed as µg/dL and mg/dL, respectively. Instead of stating the true ratio value (e.g., 20×10^{-6}), sometimes it is shortened to "20" in clinical jargon.

$$\left(\text{Cort:Crt}\right)_u \text{ratio} = \frac{\text{urine cortisol concentration}}{\text{urine creatinine concentration}} \qquad \textbf{(18.1.)}$$

with cortisol in nmol/L & creatinine in mmol/L
Example: urine cortisol concentration = 200 nmol/L
urine creatinine concentration = 10 mmol/L

$$\left(\text{Cort:Crt}\right)_u \text{ratio} = \frac{200\,\text{nmol/L}}{10\,\text{mmol/L}} = \frac{200\,\text{nmol/L}}{10 \times 10^6\,\text{nmol/L}} = 20 \times 10^{-6}$$

III. Conclusions from published reports (Fig. 18.2)
   A. Dogs[26,27]
      1. A (Cort:Crt)$_u$ ratio that is WRI is strong evidence that a dog does not have hyperadrenocorticism, but increased (Cort:Crt)$_u$ ratios are frequently found in dogs without hyperadrenocorticism. In other words, the (Cort:Crt)$_u$ ratio has a high diagnostic sensitivity for canine hyperadrenocorticism (relatively few false negatives) but has a poor positive predictive value and poor diagnostic specificity (relatively frequent false positives) (Fig. 18.2).
      2. Basal (Cort:Crt)$_u$ ratios cannot reliably differentiate PDH from FAN, but the greatest ratios are usually associated with PDH, as is suppression of (Cort:Crt)$_u$ ratio in conjunction with a HDDST.[28]
   B. Cats:[29] The (Cort:Crt)$_u$ ratios in 15 of 32 cats with hyperthyroidism were greater than the upper reference limit of the feline reference interval (8.0×10^{-6} to 42.0×10^{-6}; n = 45). For the hyperthyroid cats, the median ratio value was 37.5×10^{-6}, with two values above 100×10^{-6}. The greater (Cort:Crt)$_u$ ratios may be reflective of the stress

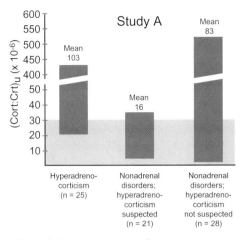
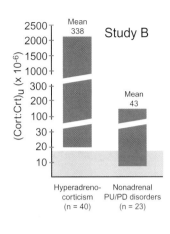

Fig. 18.2. $(Cort:Crt)_u$ ratios in two studies.

- In study A, the $(Cort:Crt)_u$ ratios from three groups of dogs were compared to a group of healthy dogs (background grey region; mean = 13×10^{-6}, n = 31). Of 25 dogs with hyperadrenocorticism (21 PDH and 4 FAN), 23 had increased $(Cort:Crt)_u$ ratios. Of 21 dogs with nonadrenal disorders (renal insufficiency, liver disease, pyelonephritis, hypothyroidism, bronchitis, and diabetes insipidus) but in which hyperadrenocorticism was suspected, only one had an increased $(Cort:Crt)_u$ ratio. However in 28 dogs with moderate to severe nonadrenal disorders (gastrointestinal, renal, lower urinary tract, liver, neurologic, immune-mediated, cardiac, traumatic, and infectious diseases), 22 had increased $(Cort:Crt)_u$ ratios.[26]
- In study B, the $(Cort:Crt)_u$ ratios from dogs with hyperadrenocorticism (36 with PDH and 4 with FAN) and other polyuria/polydipsia disorders (diabetes insipidus, hypercalcemic disorders, liver disease, pyometra, and diabetes mellitus) were compared to the $(Cort:Crt)_u$ ratios found in healthy dogs (background grey region; mean = 6×10^{-6}, n = 20). All 40 dogs with hyperadrenocorticism had an increased $(Cort:Crt)_u$ ratio but so did 18 of the 23 polyuria/polydipsia (PU/PD) dogs that did not have hyperadrenocorticism.[27]

associated with the hyperthyroid state and should not be considered reflective of pathologic hyperadrenocorticism.

ADRENOCORTICOTROPIC HORMONE (ACTH) CONCENTRATION

I. Dogs and cats: Measuring [ACTH] can be very helpful in differentiating PDH from FAN, and primary hypoadrenocorticism from secondary hypoadrenocorticism (Fig. 18.3).
  A. An [ACTH] is expected to be WRI or increased in animals with PDH, primary hypoadrenocorticism, perhaps with ectopic production of ACTH,[16] and perhaps after stressful stimuli. Dogs with primary hypoadrenocorticism may also have an exaggerated increase in [ACTH] after an injection of corticotropin-releasing hormone.[30]
  B. An [ACTH] is expected to be decreased in animals with FAN, secondary hypoadrenocorticism, after dexamethasone injections, and while they are being given therapeutic doses of glucocorticoid steroids (e.g., prednisone or prednisolone). Dogs with secondary hypoadrenocorticism have an inadequate increase in [ACTH] after an injection of CRH.[30]

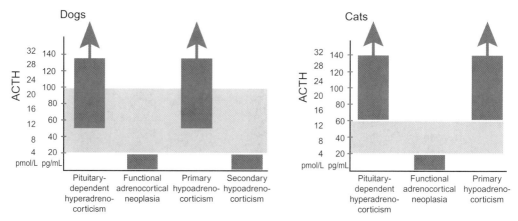

Fig. 18.3. ACTH concentrations in adrenocortical disorders of dogs and cats.

- Dogs with PDH and primary hypoadrenocorticism have ACTH concentrations WRI or increased, whereas dogs with FAN and secondary hypoadrenocorticism have ACTH concentrations below reference intervals. The background grey region represents the canine reference interval. Data for the graph were extracted from published concentrations.[30,66]
- Cats with PDH and primary hypoadrenocorticism have increased ACTH concentrations, whereas cats with FAN have decreased ACTH concentrations. The background grey region represents the feline reference interval. Data for the graph were extracted from published concentrations.[66]

Note: The arrows above the solid bars indicate that concentrations may be much greater than the values shown in the y-axes.

II. Horses

    A. Plasma [ACTH] > 50 pg/mL strongly support the presence of pituitary gland adenoma or hyperplasia. For ponies, an [ACTH] > 27 pg/mL is supportive.[9] Values and diagnostic decision thresholds may vary among assays and laboratories. In another study using chemiluminescent enzyme immunoassay, ACTH concentrations in five healthy horses were 13.4 ± 2.2 pg/mL, whereas a PPID horse with clinical hyperadrenocorticism had an [ACTH] of 155 pg/mL.[31]

    B. The foregoing data must be interpreted with caution because of the seasonal variation in [ACTH] in horses (and ponies).[32] Plasma ACTH concentrations were significantly greater in September than in January or May in horses and ponies. The seasonal variation was also found in the dexamethasone suppression test results (see Suppression and Stimulation Tests sect. III.A). The reason for the seasonal differences is unknown. Also, it is unknown whether differences exist during other months.

III. Clinical use of [ACTH] is hampered by instability of ACTH and expensive dry-ice shipments.

PLASMA CORTISOL TO ACTH RATIO

I. Because of the negative feedback in the hypothalamic-pituitary-adrenal hormonal system, decreased production of cortisol by adrenal glands is expected to result in a high plasma

[ACTH] (thus low cortisol to ACTH ratio). Conversely, increased production of cortisol by an adrenal neoplasm is expected to result in a low plasma [ACTH] (thus a high cortisol to ACTH ratio). These relationships may be used to interpret individual hormone concentrations (i.e., expect a high [cortisol] with a high [ACTH] in PDH), but published attempts to use the ratios in diagnostic decisions have been limited.

II. One published study of 22 dogs with primary hypoadrenocorticism reported that cortisol to ACTH ratios in those dogs (range, 0.003–0.17 nmol/pmol) (or 3–170 as unitless ratios) were consistently lower than the ratios in 60 healthy dogs (0.79–175 nmol/pmol) (or 790–175,000 as unitless ratios).[33] The authors reported the ratios in truncated form (e.g., 0.003–0.17). Examples of the calculations are presented in Eq. 18.2.

Using molar concentrations: **(18.2a.)**

$$\text{Cortisol:ACTH Ratio} = \frac{48\,\text{nmol cortisol/L}}{6.5\,\text{pmol ACTH/L}} = \frac{7.4\,\text{nmol cortisol}}{\text{pmol ACTH}} = \frac{7,400\,\text{pmol cortisol}}{\text{pmol ACTH}} = 7.4 \times 10^3$$

Ratio reported in the article for these data would have been 7.4.

Using weight/volume concentrations: **(18.2b.)**

$$\text{Cortisol:ACTH Ratio} = \frac{17\,\mu\text{g/L cortisol/L}}{30\,\text{pg ACTH/L}} = \frac{0.57\,\mu\text{g cortisol}}{\text{pg ACTH}} = \frac{570,000\,\text{pg cortisol}}{\text{pg ACTH}} = 570 \times 10^3$$

Ratio was not reported in the article for these units.

III. Because of the lack of agreement among some hormone assays, interpretative guidelines may need to be developed for each set of cortisol and ACTH assays. The cortisol to ACTH ratios may be helpful in differentiating primary from secondary hypoadrenocorticism and in differentiating different forms of hyperadrenocorticism. The special sample handling required for ACTH samples and the associated expenses will limit the use of cortisol to ACTH ratios.

SUPPRESSION AND STIMULATION TESTS

I. Dogs[34]
   A. Low-dose dexamethasone suppression test (LDDST): a screening test for PDH and FAN
      1. Procedure
         a. A predexamethasone blood sample is collected and processed.
         b. Dexamethasone is given at 0.01 mg/kg IV (some use IM)
         c. Postdexamethasone samples are processed after collections at 4 h and 8 h (some use 3 h and 8 h, 4–6 h and 8 h, or just 8 h).
         d. Predexamethasone and postdexamethasone plasma or serum samples are submitted for measurement of [cortisol].
      2. Expected results (Fig. 18.4)
         a. In healthy animals, dexamethasone is expected to reduce the secretion of CRH and ACTH for several hours and thus decrease release of cortisol from the adrenal glands. Because the half-life of cortisol is < 2 h, plasma [cortisol] is

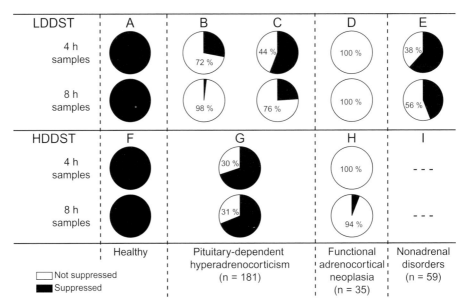

Fig. 18.4. Responses for canine dexamethasone suppression tests.

- Data for A and F are results expected for healthy dogs, based on common decision limits. Suppression was defined as a postdexamethasone [cortisol] < 1.4 μg/dL and < 50 % of predexamethasone concentration.
- Data for B–D, G, and H were extracted from published results.[67] In B and D, suppression was defined as a postdexamethasone [cortisol] < 1.4 μg/dL. In C, suppression was defined as a postdexamethasone [cortisol] < 50 % of the predexamethasone concentration. In G and H, suppression was defined as a postdexamethasone [cortisol] < 1.4 μg/dL or < 50 % of the predexamethasone [cortisol].
- Data for E were extracted from published results;[68] comparative data for HDDST (I) were not found. In the LDDST, suppression was defined as a postdexamethasone [cortisol] < 30 nmol/L (1.1 μg/dL), a decision limit estimated from graphical data. Nonadrenal disorders included hepatic, pancreatic, urinary, gastrointestinal, respiratory, and cardiac diseases and endocrine disorders other than hyperadrenocorticism (e.g., diabetes mellitus, hyperparathyroidism, and insulinoma). Dogs selected for this group were not suspected of having hyperadrenocorticism.
- Using the LDDST, all dogs with FAN (D), most dogs with PDH (B and C), and many dogs with nonadrenal illnesses (E) had inadequate suppression. Using a < 50 % criterion for suppression (C), more dogs with PDH had adequate cortisol suppression than when judged by the < 1.4 μg/dL criterion (B). Using the < 1.4 μg/dL criterion, 48 of 51 (94 %) PDH dogs that had suppression at 4 h had escaped suppression by 8 h. Using the < 50 % criterion, 58 of 102 (57 %) PDH dogs that had suppression at 4 h had escaped suppression by 8 h.
- Using HDDST, nearly all dogs with FAN (H), but a minority of dogs with PDH (G), failed to have adequate suppression at the 4 h and 8 h samplings.
- If results from LDDST and HDDST are examined together,[67] there was inadequate suppression of cortisol concentrations in both tests in nearly all dogs with FAN (D and H; 94 %) but in a minority of dogs with PDH (B, C, and G; 24 %). A few dogs with PDH (14 %) and two dogs with FAN (6 %) had inadequate suppression with the LDDST but had adequate suppression with the HDDST. Two dogs with PDH (1 %) had adequate suppression with the LDDST but inadequate suppression with the HDDST.

HD, high dose; and LD, low dose.

expected to be decreased dramatically at 4 h and 8 h (Fig. 18.4A). Values are usually inadequately suppressed at 8 h with both PDH and FAN.

    (1) Most veterinarians interpret a postdexamethasone [cortisol] < 1.4 μg/dL (< 40 nmol/L) to indicate there was adequate suppression of cortisol secretion. This decision threshold appears to have been calculated from data collected from 22 healthy dogs; it represented the mean concentration (0.5 μg/dL) plus 3 standard deviations (3 × 0.3 = 0.9 μg/dL) at 8 h.[35,36]

    (2) Some authors propose that suppression is present if the postdexamethasone [cortisol] in the 4 h and 8 h samples is < 50 % of the predexamethasone concentration. Such an interpretative guideline is consistent with the half-life of plasma cortisol.

  b. If hyperadrenocorticism is caused by PDH or ectopic production of ACTH, then a low dose of dexamethasone may or may not lead to suppressed release of ACTH by neoplastic pituitary cells, and thus cortisol production from hyperplastic adrenal glands may or may not decrease (Fig. 18.4B and C).

    (1) In some cases, the 4 h postdexamethasone [cortisol] is below the decision threshold, but the 8 h postdexamethasone [cortisol] is above the decision threshold. In such cases, the escaped suppression is highly indicative of PDH if the clinical signs support a hyperadrenocorticism diagnosis. Nonadrenal disorders may also be associated with this pattern (Fig. 18.4E).

    (2) Suppression is demonstrated in more PDH cases if the "< 50 %" criterion (Fig. 18.4C) is used compared to the "< 1.4 μg/dL" (< 40 nmol/L) criterion (Fig. 18.4B).

  c. If hyperadrenocorticism is caused by FAN, then low-dose dexamethasone is not expected to decrease the secretion of cortisol (Fig. 18.4D). Even though suppression criteria are not fulfilled, cortisol concentrations may fluctuate during the testing, because of variations in cortisol secretion by neoplastic cells, binding to proteins, or plasma clearance. The LDDST has high diagnostic sensitivity for FAN.

  d. Suppression may not be adequate in dogs with nonadrenal illness (Fig. 18.4E).

  e. In two dogs receiving phenobarbital therapy, cortisol concentrations were not suppressed adequately, possibly because phenobarbital's effects on clearance of synthetic steroids enhance dexamethasone's clearance rate. However, phenobarbital therapy did not affect results of the LDDST in five other dogs.[37]

  f. Too few cases of ectopic ACTH production have been reported to establish a pattern, but there should be a lack of suppression of cortisol in these animals.

B. High-dose dexamethasone suppression test (HDDST) (Fig. 18.4): a test that may differentiate PDH from FAN after hyperadrenocorticism is diagnosed

  1. Procedure: the same as for the LDDST except that dexamethasone is given at 0.1 mg/kg IV (some use IM)

  2. Expected results

    a. In healthy animals, dexamethasone is expected to dramatically reduce plasma [cortisol] at 4 h, and concentrations should remain decreased in the 8 h samples (Fig. 18.4F).

    b. If hyperadrenocorticism is caused by PDH, then high-dose dexamethasone usually causes suppression of ACTH release by neoplastic pituitary cells and thus reduces cortisol production from hyperplastic adrenal glands (Fig. 18.4G).

    c. If hyperadrenocorticism is caused by FAN, then high-dose dexamethasone is not expected to decrease the secretion of cortisol (Fig. 18.4H). Even though suppression criteria are not fulfilled, cortisol concentrations may fluctuate during the testing, because of variations in cortisol secretion by neoplastic cells, binding to proteins, or plasma clearance.

    d. If a HDDST is done in a dog with nonadrenal illness, then cortisol production is expected to be decreased sufficiently to indicate a suppression of ACTH secretion.

    e. Too few cases of ectopic ACTH production have been reported to establish a pattern, but there should be a lack of suppression of cortisol in these animals.

C. Interpretation of dexamethasone suppression tests

  1. Expected patterns of LDDST and HDDST results for individual dogs

    a. In healthy dogs, [cortisol] will be suppressed to < 1.4 μg/dL (< 40 nmol/L) with both tests (both 4 h and 8 h samples).

    b. If hyperadrenocorticism is caused by PDH, then [cortisol] is usually suppressed to < 1.4 μg/dL (< 40 nmol/L) with the HDDST and often with the LDDST also.

    c. If hyperadrenocorticism is caused by FAN, then [cortisol] is expected to be ≥ 1.4 μg/dL (≥ 40 nmol/L) in nearly all postdexamethasone samples.

    d. If hyperadrenocorticism is caused by ectopic production of ACTH, then [cortisol] is expected to be ≥ 1.4 μg/dL (≥ 40 nmol/L) in nearly all postdexamethasone samples.

    e. In dogs with nonadrenal illnesses, there may or may not be cortisol suppression with the LDDST. The [Cortisol] is expected to be < 1.4 μg/dL (< 40 nmol/L) with the HDDST.

  2. Table 18.4 lists examples of cortisol concentrations from dexamethasone suppression tests.

  3. Interpretations for Table 18.4 were made by using Fig. 18.4 as a guide. Best interpretations are made when results are interpreted in context of historical or physical findings.

D. Adrenocorticotropic hormone (ACTH) stimulation (response) test

  1. Different ACTH products, routes of administration, and doses have been used, and results of some have been directly compared. Results and interpretation are generally similar,[38–40] but some differences are recognized.[41]

  2. Procedure (may begin at any time of day)[42]

    a. A sample for pre-ACTH [cortisol] is collected.

    b. ACTH is administered to stimulate cortisol production.

      (1) Synthetic ACTH (cosyntropin [Cortrosyn]) is usually given IV at 5 μg/kg or IM at 0.25 mg/dog.

      (2) Porcine ACTH gel (Cortigel-40) or bovine ACTH gel (Acthar) is usually given at 2.2 U/kg IM.

      (3) Other ACTH products (e.g., Synacthen) and dosing regimens are also used. Laboratories should be consulted for information about local protocols and preferences.

    c. A post-ACTH sample is collected 1 h later if cosyntropin is given (2 h if porcine or bovine ACTH is used) to assess for a cortisol response.

  3. Expected results (Fig. 18.5) (Specific patient results should be interpreted by using reference intervals and interpretation guidelines provided with results.)

Table 18.4. Example results of dexamethasone suppression tests in dogs

	LDDST			HDDST		
	Cortisol (μg/dL)[a]			Cortisol (μg/dL)		
	Predex.[b]	4 h postdex.[b]	8 h postdex.	Predex.	4 h postdex.	8 h postdex.
Healthy dogs	0.5–6.0	< 1.4	< 1.4	0.5–6.0	< 1.4	< 1.4
Dog 1[c]	4.5	3.0	3.5	3.5	3.3	2.9
Dog 2[d]	7.0	1.0	3.8	6.2	0.8	0.6
Dog 3[e]	5.0	0.9	0.6	5.5	0.5	0.3
Dog 4[f]	6.5	3.2	2.8	4.5	0.8	0.4
Dog 5[g]	0.2	0.1	0.1	—	—	—

[a] Conversion to SI units: μg/dL × 27.6 = nmol/L (round to nearest 10)

[b] Predex., predexamethasone [cortisol]; and postdex, postdexamethasone [cortisol]

[c] Dog 1 had either PDH or FAN. In the LDDST, inadequate suppression indicates PDH, FAN, or nonadrenal disorders. In the HDDST, inadequate suppression is more likely in FAN but can be found with PDH. Adequate suppression is expected in nonadrenal disorders.

[d] Dog 2 had adrenal hyperplasia caused by PDH or a hyperresponsive adrenal gland because of a nonadrenal disorder. In the LDDST, 4 h suppression and then escape at 8 h suggests PDH or nonadrenal disorders. In the HDDST, suppression can be found with PDH and is expected with nonadrenal disorders but is not consistent with FAN.

[e] Dog 3 was healthy or had PDH or a nonadrenal disorder. In the LDDST, suppression can be found with health, PDH, and nonadrenal disorders. In the HDDST, suppression can be found with health, PDH, and nonadrenal disorders. Suppression is not expected with FAN.

[f] Dog 4 had adrenal hyperplasia caused by PDH or a nonadrenal disorder. In the LDDST, failure to suppress the [cortisol] to < 1.4 μg/dL (< 40 nmol/L) could be PDH, FAN, or nonadrenal disorder. In the HDDST, suppression can be found with PDH and is expected with nonadrenal disorders. Suppression is not consistent with FAN.

[g] Dog 5 had a hypoadrenal state. In the LDDST, the predexamethasone hypocortisolemia indicates a hypoadrenal state that could be primary, secondary, or iatrogenic. The HDDST is not needed in such cases.

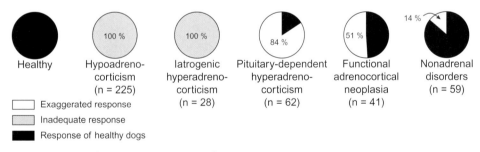

Fig. 18.5. Responses from canine ACTH stimulation tests.

- Criteria used to determine appropriate, inadequate, or exaggerated responses to ACTH stimulation varied among publications. For each set of extracted data, the authors' criteria were used.
- In all hypoadrenocorticism cases, there were inadequate responses to ACTH stimulation. The 225 cases included 220 cases of primary idiopathic hypoadrenocorticism and five cases of secondary hypoadrenocorticism.[69]
- In all cases of iatrogenic hyperadrenocorticism, adrenocortical atrophy resulted in inadequate responses to ACTH stimulation.[70]
- In 84 % of PDH cases and in 51 % of FAN cases, there were exaggerated responses to ACTH stimulation.[35,60,68,71–74]
- In 14 % of dogs with nonadrenal illnesses, there were exaggerated responses to ACTH stimulation.[68]

a. Healthy dogs
   (1) ACTH should stimulate the production and release of cortisol from the adrenal cortices.
   (2) Expected pre-ACTH and post-ACTH concentrations of cortisol are different in published reports and reference laboratories. Usually, the post-ACTH [cortisol] is < 17 µg/dL (470 nmol/L).
b. Hypoadrenocorticism
   (1) Dogs with primary, secondary, or iatrogenic adrenocortical hypoplasia or atrophy are expected to have fewer or no responsive cells, and thus the post-ACTH [cortisol] increases inadequately or not at all.
   (2) Pre-ACTH and post-ACTH cortisol concentrations < 1.0 µg/dL (< 30 nmol/L) indicate adrenocortical atrophy, destruction, or hypoplasia.
c. Hyperadrenocorticism
   (1) From 60 % to 80 % of dogs with PDH and about 50 % of dogs with FAN have exaggerated responses to ACTH that reflect either bilateral adrenocortical hyperplasia or responsive neoplastic cells. It is not clear why exaggerated responses do not occur in all dogs with hyperplastic glands. Some of the adrenocortical neoplasms may not respond because the neoplastic cells have defective receptors or other signaling pathways. Dogs with ectopic production of ACTH would be expected to have an exaggerated cortisol increase because of the presence of bilateral adrenocortical hyperplasia. Dogs with iatrogenic hyperadrenocorticism from chronic glucocorticoid administration have little or no response.
   (2) The decision threshold that represents an exaggerated response varies among studies and usually is near 18–22 µg/dL (500–610 nmol/L).
d. Nonadrenal illnesses
   (1) Some dogs with disorders other than PDH or FAN may have exaggerated responses to ACTH.
   (2) Typically, these animals are thought to have stress-induced hypercortisolemia.
e. After *op'*DDD (mitotane [Lysodren]) treatment
   (1) *op'*DDD is an adrenocorticolytic compound that is used to treat PDH and FAN. The compound damages the zona fasciculata and the zona reticularis.
   (2) ACTH stimulation tests can be used to monitor destruction of adrenocortical tissue. Typically, the goal of *op'*DDD treatment is to get the post-ACTH [cortisol] to be < 5 µg/dL (< 140 nmol/L) but not cause sufficient destruction to create a hypoadrenocortical state.
f. After trilostane (Vetoryl or Modrenal) treatment
   (1) Trilostane, which is an alternative to *op'*DDD for treatment of PDH, reduces steroid synthesis by inhibiting 3β-hydroxysteroid dehydrogenase and thus reduces the synthesis of cortisol, aldosterone, and other steroid hormones. Trilostane reduces [cortisol] in dogs with PDH and also reduces [aldosterone], but to a lesser degree.[25]
   (2) ACTH stimulation tests can be used to monitor the effectiveness of trilostane treatment of PDH. If the dog has continuing clinical signs and the post-ACTH [cortisol] is > 9 µg/dL (> 250 nmol/L), then the dosage is

increased. If the dog has continuing clinical signs suggestive of hypoadreno-corticism and the post-ACTH [cortisol] is < 0.8 µg/dL (< 20 nmol/L), then treatment is discontinued.[43]

II. Cats
  A. Low-dose dexamethasone suppression test (LDDST): not recommended
    1. Procedure: Basically the same procedure as for the canine LDDST except dexameth-asone is given at either 0.01 or 0.015 mg/kg IV. Some people refer to use of a 0.1 mg/kg IV dose as a LDDST in cats, but it is considered a HDDST in this text.
    2. Expected results[34] (Specific patient results should be interpreted by using reference intervals and interpretation guidelines provided with results.)
      a. In healthy cats, the 4 h and 8 h cortisol concentrations are usually < 1.0 µg/dL (< 30 nmol/L), but they are not suppressed this low in about 15–20 % of healthy cats. Cortisol suppression may also fail to occur in cats with nonadrenal illness. Therefore, the LDDST has poorer diagnostic specificity than the HDDST (for which cortical suppression fails to occur in very few cats) and thus is not recommended. A postdexamethasone [cortisol] of 1.0–1.4 µg/dL (30–40 nmol/L) is considered a borderline result.
      b. In cats with hyperadrenocorticism, the 4 h and 8 h cortisol concentrations are expected to be > 1.5 µg/dL (> 40 nmol/L).
  B. High-dose dexamethasone suppression test (HDDST)
    1. Procedure
      a. The initial protocol is the same as with the canine HDDST, but 1 mg/kg dexamethasone is also used. Some people refer to a 0.1 mg/kg dose as a low dose in cats and consider 1 mg/kg a high dose. Others consider the 1 mg/kg an ultra-high dose.
      b. Cats may escape the suppressive effects of dexamethasone faster than dogs, so suppression may be seen only if samples are collected at 2 h, 4 h, and 6 h after dexamethasone.[44]
    2. Expected results for 0.1 mg/kg dosage[34] (Specific patient results should be interpreted by using reference intervals and interpretation guidelines provided with results.)
      a. In almost all healthy cats, the 4 h and 8 h cortisol concentrations are < 1.0 µg/dL (< 30 nmol/L). A postdexamethasone [cortisol] of 1.0–1.4 µg/dL (30–40 nmol/L) is considered a borderline result.
      b. In about 90 % of cats with hyperadrenocorticism, the 4 h and 8 h cortisol concentrations were > 1.5 µg/dL (> 40 nmol/L).
  C. Adrenocorticotropic hormone (ACTH) stimulation (response) test
    1. Procedure (may begin at any time of day)
      a. A sample for pre-ACTH [cortisol] is collected.
      b. Synthetic ACTH (Cortrosyn) is given IV at 5 µg/kg or 0.125 mg/cat. Porcine ACTH gel (Cortigel-40) may be used at 2.2 U/kg IM.
      c. Post-ACTH samples are collected at 30 min and 60 min or just at 1 h.
    2. Expected results[42]
      a. Specific patient results should be interpreted by using reference intervals and interpretation guidelines provided with results.
      b. A healthy cat should have a pre-ACTH [cortisol] of 1.0–6.0 µg/dL (30–170 nmol/L) and a post-ACTH [cortisol] < 13.0 µg/dL (< 360 nmol/L).

    c. Cats with hyperadrenocorticism may have a pre-ACTH [cortisol] WRI or increased, and a 30 min or 60 min post-ACTH [cortisol] > 16 µg/dL (> 440 nmol/L). However, only about 40–50 % of cats with hyperadrenocorticism have an exaggerated response.[34]

III. Horses
  A. Dexamethasone suppression test
    1. Overnight method[2,14]
      a. A sample for predexamethasone [cortisol] is collected between 4 p.m. and 6 p.m.
      b. Dexamethasone is given at 40 µg/kg (about 2 mg/100 lb) IM.
      c. Postdexamethasone samples are collected at noon the next day (about 19 h after dexamethasone), or two samples are collected at 15 h and 19 h.
      d. Expected results[14]
        (1) Specific patient results should be interpreted by using reference intervals and interpretation guidelines provided with results.
        (2) Healthy horses: adequate suppression resulting in a postdexamethasone [cortisol] < 1.0 µg/dL (< 30 nmol/L)
        (3) Hyperadrenocorticism caused by PPID: inadequate suppression resulting in a postdexamethasone [cortisol] > 1.0 µg/dL (> 30 nmol/L)
    2. Cortisol concentrations during a 24 h period after dexamethasone (40 µg/kg)[2]
      a. In 34 healthy horses, cortisol concentrations were decreased 8–24 h after dexamethasone. All had concentrations < 1.0 µg/dL at 20–24 h after dexamethasone.
      b. In 52 horses with PPID, the maximal suppression was seen 8–12 h after dexamethasone. All had cortisol concentrations > 1.0 µg/dL at 20–24 h after dexamethasone.
    3. Seasonal variation: Concurrent with the seasonal variation in [ACTH], results of the equine dexamethasone suppression test were different in January compared with those in September.[32] In a study of 10 healthy horses and 29 ponies, there was no seasonal difference in the predexamethasone [cortisol] (all < 1.0 µg/dL), but the postdexamethasone cortisol concentrations were > 1.0 µg/dL in 26 % of the September samples (some > 2.0 µg/dL). The increased ACTH concentrations and the results of the dexamethasone suppression tests in September samples suggest that a seasonal hyperadrenocortical state is present, but the reason for this variation is unknown.
  B. Adrenocorticotropic hormone (ACTH) stimulation (response) test
    1. Multiple ACTH compounds have been used for stimulation tests, but nearly all studies included a presample and a 2 h post-ACTH sample.
    2. Results expected for healthy and PDH horses if ACTH gel is given (1 U/kg IM)
      a. In healthy horses, the post-ACTH [cortisol] is expected to be 2–3 times the presample's concentration.[2] However, four healthy horses had post-ACTH cortisol concentrations that ranged from 3.7 to 4.7 times the pre-ACTH concentrations.[9]
      b. In most, but not all, PDH horses, the post-ACTH [cortisol] is more than three times the pre-ACTH sample concentration.[9,45]

   c. Because of overlapping findings for healthy horses and horses with PDH, the ACTH gel stimulation test is not recommended as a diagnostic test for equine PDH.[9]
   3. Results expected for healthy and PDH horses if ACTH (cosyntropin) is given (1 mg IV)
      a. In healthy horses, the post-ACTH [cortisol] is expected to be < 1.8 times the presample's [cortisol].[46]
      b. In PDH horses, the post-ACTH [cortisol] is expected to be > 1.8 times the presample's [cortisol].

COMBINED DEXAMETHASONE SUPPRESSION–ADRENOCORTICOTROPIC HORMONE (ACTH) STIMULATION (RESPONSE) TEST

The major advantage of the combined test is that it combines adrenal assessment into one diagnostic procedure, and thus only one set of samples is submitted to a reference laboratory. The major disadvantage in dogs is that it does not have the same diagnostic power as the combination of LDDST and HDDST done individually.

I.   Canine method[36]
     A. A sample for a basal [cortisol] is collected, and then dexamethasone is administered (0.1 mg/kg IV). A 2–4 h postdexamethasone sample is collected, and then the ACTH stimulation test is done as described in Suppression and Stimulation Tests, sect. I.D. All samples are submitted for measurement of [cortisol].
     B. The dexamethasone dose is the same as that used in the HDDST, but the postdexamethasone sample occurs only at 2 h and thus does not assess the possible escape in the 8 h sample of the HDDST.
     C. An exaggerated ACTH response would support hyperadrenocorticism but does not reliably differentiate PDH and FAN.

II. Feline method[47]
     A. A sample for a basal [cortisol] is collected, and then dexamethasone is administered (0.1 mg/kg IV). A 2–4 h postdexamethasone sample is collected, and then the ACTH stimulation test is done as described in Suppression and Stimulation Tests, sect. II.C. All samples are submitted for measurement of [cortisol].
     B. In two cases of feline PDH, there was inadequate suppression after dexamethasone and exaggerated responses to ACTH.[47,48]
     C. In one study involving cats with nonadrenal illnesses (17 diabetic cats and 18 nondiabetic cats) and 19 healthy cats, results were very similar among groups.[49]

III. Equine method[50]
     A. A sample for a basal [cortisol] is collected, and then dexamethasone is administered (10 mg IM at 9 a.m.). A 3 h postdexamethasone sample is collected, and then cosyntropin is administered IV (1 mg = 100 IU). Then, a 2 h post-ACTH sample is collected. All samples are submitted for measurement of [cortisol].
     B. There has been limited use of the procedure in horses. In one study, the combined test did not reliably differentiate six healthy horses from six horses with PDH.[2]

ALDOSTERONE CONCENTRATION

I. An [aldosterone] in clinical hypoadrenocorticism should be decreased except in rare atypical cases. In primary and secondary hyperaldosteronism, aldosterone concentrations are increased. Because ACTH stimulates the release of cortisol and aldosterone, aldosterone concentrations before and after ACTH administration may reflect adrenal function. However, relatively few published data support these concepts.

II. Primary hyperaldosteronism
   A. Dogs
      1. Three cases of primary hyperaldosteronism caused by adrenal neoplasms were described.[42] All three dogs were presented because of episodic weakness, and each had hypokalemia and an [aldosterone] > 3000 pmol/L (reference interval not provided with case information; see pre-ACTH aldosterone concentrations in healthy dogs in Table 18.5).
      2. Another case was described in which the presenting problem was polyuria. Other findings were mild hypokalemia, marked hypophosphatemia, alkalemia, decreased plasma renin activity, and increased plasma [aldosterone] (740 and 840 pmol/L in two samples) compared to 30–210 pmol/L in 12 healthy dogs.[51] Plasma cortisol concentrations during a LDDST were within reference intervals; measurement of other precursor steroid concentrations was not mentioned.
   B. Cats
      1. Cases of primary hyperaldosteronism caused by adrenal neoplasms have been described.[52–54] Problems in each cat included weakness and hypokalemia. Each cat had increased plasma [aldosterone]: > 5000 pmol/L with a reference interval of 540–1080 pmol/L,[52,53] or 877–14,653 pmol/L with a reference interval of 150–430 pmol/L.
      2. Other cases of primary hyperaldosteronism were diagnosed based on high-normal to increased [aldosterone] concurrent with hypokalemia and increased aldosterone to plasma renin activity ratios.[55] The cats were not hypernatremic, and some developed renal lesions consistent with persistent hypertension.
      3. Another cat had an adrenocortical carcinoma that produced excessive amounts of aldosterone and progesterone. The resulting clinical signs were due to the effects of progesterone (i.e., diabetes mellitus) more than to aldosterone effects.[56]

III. Aldosterone concentrations in other canine disorders
   A. There is not a clear separation of pre-ACTH aldosterone concentrations between healthy dogs and dogs with hypoadrenocorticism. However, aldosterone concentrations in the post-ACTH samples were lower in dogs with hypoadrenocorticism than in clinically healthy dogs (Table 18.5).
   B. Dogs with PDH had aldosterone concentrations similar to those of healthy dogs in both pre-ACTH and post-ACTH samples (Table 18.5).
   C. Some dogs with nonadrenal disorders had a very high [aldosterone]. The high concentrations are probably related to hypovolemia or decreased effective blood volume (Table 18.5).
   D. Results of a study of 31 dogs with PDH, 5 dogs with FAN, and 12 healthy dogs:[57]
      1. Aldosterone concentrations were significantly lower in the PDH dogs than in the healthy dogs. The authors suggested that under chronic ACTH stimulation, some of

Table 18.5. Aldosterone concentrations from ACTH stimulation tests in dogs

	Aldosterone concentrations						
	Healthy dogs and dogs with adrenal disorders (mean ± 2 sd) (pg/mL)[64]			Healthy dogs and dogs with nonadrenal disorders (range of observed values) (pg/mL)[65]			
Clinical state	n	Before ACTH	1 h after ACTH[a]	n	Before ACTH	1 h after ACTH[b]	2 h after ACTH
Healthy	7	203 ± 142	397 ± 188	21	5–345	91–634	71–758
Hypoadrenocorticism	5	167 ± 30	162 ± 56	6	0–56	—	0–36
PDH	28	124 ± 120	331 ± 216	—	—	—	—
Iatrogenic hyperadrenocorticism[c]	9	126 ± 118	213 ± 132	—	—	—	—
Various nonadrenal disorders[d]	—	—	—	5	>1200	>1200	—
Diabetes mellitus and mitral insufficiency	—	—	—	1	10	—	20

[a] 0.5 U/kg IV

[b] 2.2 U/kg IM

[c] A diagnosis of iatrogenic hyperadrenocorticism was based on finding reduced cortisol concentrations in pre-ACTH and post-ACTH samples in dogs with appropriate clinical signs and history of exogenous steroid treatments.

[d] Diagnoses included chylothorax (1), lymphocytic gastritis (1), glomerulonephritis and mitral insufficiency (1), acute renal failure (1), and acute renal failure and diabetes mellitus (1). In the chylothorax and gastritis cases, the aldosterone concentrations in 2 h post-ACTH samples were also > 1200 pg/mL.

the aldosterone-secreting cells converted to cortisol-secreting cells as has been described in experimental sheep and rat studies.

2. Aldosterone concentrations were significantly greater in the FAN dogs than in the PDH dogs, but the concentrations are probably related to renin (angiotensinogenase) concentrations via changes in blood volume and electrolyte concentrations.

E. Aldosterone to renin ratio
1. Plasma aldosterone concentrations are related to renin concentrations via changes in blood volume or electrolyte concentrations.
   a. Aldosterone production is stimulated by angiotensin II, which is produced by the renal release of renin in response to renal hypotension or decreased delivery of sodium to the distal tubules.
   b. Renal responses to aldosterone result in retention of Na^+ and Cl^-, which promotes plasma volume expansion and thus decreased stimulation of the renin-angiotensin system.
   c. Aldosterone concentrations are expected to be greater in people on a sodium-restricted diet (i.e., aldosterone is needed to retain Na^+) than in people who are not on a sodium-restricted diet. Similar responses would be expected in domestic mammals.
   d. Interpretation of an increased plasma [aldosterone] should include a consideration of whether the increase is appropriate (e.g., stimulated release because of decreased effective blood volume) or inappropriate (i.e., uncontrolled release from adrenal neoplasia).
2. In a study of 22 dogs with primary hypoadrenocorticism, aldosterone to renin ratios were consistently lower (0.002–0.08 pmol/fmol/s [or 2–80/s]) than the ratios in 60 healthy dogs (0.09–1.6 pmol/fmol/s [or 90–1600/s])[33] (note: the authors reported the ratios without units). Units of the ratios are complex because the authors measured renin activity (rather than concentration) via the generation of angiotensin I; the ratio represents the amount of aldosterone (pmol) related to renin activity (fmol of angiotensin I produced per second).
3. Conceptually, the aldosterone to renin ratio should improve the interpretation of a plasma [aldosterone]. However, it probably will have limited use in clinical medicine because of sample collection requirements and availability of renin assays. As with many other hormone assays, differences in assay methods may also limit the usefulness of the ratio because interpretation guidelines may not apply from one set of assays to another.

OTHER ASSESSMENTS OF ADRENOCORTICAL FUNCTION

I. Thorn test and modified Thorn test[58,59]
   A. Instead of directly measuring [cortisol] after an ACTH injection, changes in [cortisol] can be indirectly and roughly assessed via changes in blood [eosinophil] (Thorn test) or changes in neutrophil to lymphocyte ratios (modified Thorn test). An [eosinophil] is measured directly, whereas the neutrophil to lymphocyte ratio is calculated from leukocyte differential counts determined on blood films.
      1. In a healthy dog, blood [eosinophil] is expected to decrease and the neutrophil to lymphocyte ratio is expected to increase if blood [cortisol] increases.
      2. Failure to see a decrease in [eosinophil] or failure to see an increased neutrophil to lymphocyte ratio after administration of ACTH suggests the presence of hypoplastic or atrophied adrenal glands.

    B. Increased ease of obtaining serum or plasma cortisol concentrations and their superior diagnostic value have made the Thorn test and modified Thorn test nearly obsolete. However, the relationship between blood [cortisol] and blood leukocyte concentrations should be remembered when interpreting routine complete blood count results.

II. Concentrations of other steroid hormones
    A. Adrenal glands produce other steroid hormones, including intermediates in the synthetic pathways.
        1. Increased progesterone concentrations have been reported in dogs and a cat with FAN.[15,60]
        2. In a study of 53 dogs with confirmed hyperadrenocorticism (including PDH and FAN cases), 69 % had an exaggerated increase in [17-hydroxyprogesterone] in the ACTH stimulation test, and 79 % had an exaggerated increase in [cortisol].[61]
        3. Another study included 127 dogs with suspected hyperadrenocorticism. After ACTH stimulation, 59 (46 %) had an exaggerated increase in [cortisol]. Of those 59, 42 (71 %) had an exaggerated increase in [17-hydroxyprogesterone].[62] Also, an exaggerated increase in [17-hydroxyprogesterone] was found in 31 % of dogs that had neoplasms not related to pituitary or adrenal glands. These findings emphasize that adrenocortical hyperplasia may occur secondarily to nonadrenal diseases.
    B. Measurement of other steroid hormone concentrations may help detect adrenal disorders, especially if the synthetic pathways are defective. Some laboratories measure concentrations of the following steroid hormones in pre-ACTH and post-ACTH samples: cortisol, dihydroepiandrostenedione, estradiol, androstenedione, 17-hydroxyprogesterone, progesterone, and testosterone. In some cases, steroid hormones other than cortisol are increased.[63]

References

1. Chastain CB, Ganjam VK. 1986. *Clinical Endocrinology of Companion Animals.* Philadelphia: Lea & Febiger.
2. Dybdal NO, Hargreaves KM, Madigan JE, Gribble DH, Kennedy PC, Stabenfeldt GH. 1994. Diagnostic testing for pituitary pars intermedia dysfunction in horses. J Am Vet Med Assoc 204:627–632.
3. Lundberg GD, Iverson C, Radulescu G. 1986. Now read this: The SI units are here. J Am Med Assoc 255:2329–2339.
4. Behrend EN, Kemppainen RJ, Young DW. 1998. Effect of storage conditions on cortisol, total thyroxine, and free thyroxine concentrations in serum and plasma of dogs. J Am Vet Med Assoc 212:1564–1568.
5. Philip ELI, Marotta SF. 1971. Cellular variation in the uptake and metabolism of cortisol by canine erythrocytes. Acta Endocrinol 68:771–778.
6. Olson PN, Bowen RA, Husted PW, Nett TM. 1981. Effects of storage on concentration of hydrocortisone (cortisol) in canine serum and plasma. Am J Vet Res 42:1618–1620.
7. Feldman EC, Nelson RW. 1996. *Canine and Feline Endocrinology and Reproduction*, 2nd edition. Philadelphia: WB Saunders.
8. Hegstad RL, Johnston SD, Pasternak DM. 1990. Effects of sample handling on adrenocorticotropin concentration measured in canine plasma, using a commercially available radioimmunoassay kit. Am J Vet Res 51:1941–1947.
9. Couëtil L, Paradis MR, Knoll J. 1996. Plasma adrenocorticotropin concentration in healthy horses and in horses with clinical signs of hyperadrenocorticism. J Vet Intern Med 10:1–6.
10. Feldman EC, Nelson RW. 1994. Comparative aspects of Cushing's syndrome in dogs and cats. Endocrinol Metabol Clin North Am 23:671–691.
11. Duesberg C, Peterson ME. 1997. Adrenal disorders in cats. Vet Clin North Am Small Anim Pract 27:321–347.
12. Meij BP, van der Vlugt-Meijer RH, van den Ingh TSGAM, Rijnberk A. 2004. Somatotroph and corticotroph pituitary adenoma (double adenoma) in a cat with diabetes mellitus and hyperadrenocorticism. J Comp Pathol 130:209–215.
13. Schott HC. 2002. Pituitary pars intermedia dysfunction: Equine Cushing's disease. Vet Clin North Am Equine Pract 18:237–270.

14. Messer NT, IV. 1999. How to diagnose equine pituitary pars intermedia dysfunction. In: Proceedings of the 45th Annual Convention of the American Association of Equine Practitioners, Albuquerque, NM, 145–147.

15. Boord M, Griffin C. 1999. Progesterone secreting adrenal mass in a cat with clinical signs of hyperadrenocorticism. J Am Vet Med Assoc 214:666–669.

16. Galac S, Kooistra HS, Voorhout G, van den Ingh TSGAM, Mol JA, van den Berg G, Meij BP. 2005. Hyperadrenocorticism in a dog due to ectopic secretion of adrenocorticotropic hormone. Domest Anim Endocrinol 28:338–348.

17. Yamini B, VanDenBrink PL, Refsal KR. 1997. Ovarian steroid cell tumor resembling luteoma associated with hyperadrenocorticism (Cushing's disease) in a dog. Vet Pathol 34:57–60.

18. Peterson ME, Greco DS, Orth DN. 1989. Primary hypoadrenocorticism in ten cats. J Vet Intern Med 3:55–58.

19. Couëtil LL, Hoffman AM. 1998. Adrenal insufficiency in a neonatal foal. J Am Vet Med Assoc 212:1594–1596.

20. Dunn KJ, Herrtage ME. 1998. Hypocortisolaemia in a Labrador retriever. J Small Anim Pract 39:90–93.

21. Lifton SJ, King LG, Zerbe CA. 1996. Glucocorticoid deficient hypoadrenocorticism in dogs: 18 cases (1986–1995). J Am Vet Med Assoc 209:2076–2081.

22. Kooistra HS, Rijnberk A, van den Ingh TSGAM. 1995. Polyglandular deficiency syndrome in a boxer dog: Thyroid hormone and glucocorticoid deficiency. Vet Q 17:59–63.

23. Feldman EC, Bruyette DS, Nelson RW, Farver TB. 1990. Plasma cortisol response to ketoconazole administration in dogs with hyperadrenocorticism. J Am Vet Med Assoc 157:71–78.

24. Willard MD, Nachreiner R, McDonald R, Roudebush P. 1986. Ketoconazole-induced changes in selected canine hormone concentrations. Am J Vet Res 47:2504–2509.

25. Wenger M, Sieber-Ruckstuhl NS, Müller C, Reusch CE. 2004. Effect of trilostane on serum concentrations of aldosterone, cortisol, and potassium in dogs with pituitary-dependent hyperadrenocorticism. Am J Vet Res 65:1245–1250.

26. Smiley LE, Peterson ME. 1993. Evaluation of a urine cortisol:creatinine ratio as a screening test for hyperadrenocorticism in dogs. J Vet Intern Med 7:163–168.

27. Feldman EC, Mack RE. 1992. Urine cortisol:creatinine ratio as a screening test for hyperadrenocorticism in dogs. J Am Vet Med Assoc 200:1637–1641.

28. Galac S, Kooistra HS, Teske E, Rijnberk A. 1997. Urinary corticoid/creatinine ratios in the differentiation between pituitary-dependent hyperadrenocorticism and hyperadrenocorticism due to adrenocortical tumour in the dog. Vet Q 19:17–20.

29. de Lange MS, Galac S, Trip MR, Kooistra HS. 2004. High urinary corticoid/creatinine ratios in cats with hyperthyroidism. J Vet Intern Med 18:152–155.

30. Peterson ME, Kintzer PP, Kass PH. 1996. Pretreatment clinical and laboratory findings in dogs with hypoadrenocorticism: 225 cases (1979–1993). J Am Vet Med Assoc 208:85–91.

31. Sgorbini M, Panzani D, Maccheroni M, Corazza M. 2004. Equine Cushing-like syndrome: Diagnosis and therapy in two cases. Vet Res Commun 28(Suppl 1):377–380.

32. Donaldson MT, McDonnell SM, Schanbacher BJ, Lamb SV, McFarlane D, Beech J. 2005. Variation in plasma adrenocorticotropic hormone concentration and dexamethasone suppression test results with season, age, and sex in healthy ponies and horses. J Vet Intern Med 19:217–222.

33. Javadi S, Galac S, Boer P, Robben JH, Teske E, Kooistra HS. 2006. Aldosterone-to-renin and cortisol-to-adrenocorticotropic hormone ratios in healthy dogs and dogs with primary hypoadrenocorticism. J Vet Intern Med 20:556–561.

34. Feldman EC. 2000. Hyperadrenocorticism. In: Ettinger SJ, Feldman EC, eds. *Textbook of Veterinary Internal Medicine: Diseases of the Dog and Cat*, 5th edition, 1460–1488. Philadelphia: WB Saunders.

35. Feldman EC. 1983. Comparison of ACTH response and dexamethasone suppression as screening tests in canine hyperadrenocorticism. J Am Vet Med Assoc 182:506–510.

36. Feldman EC. 1985. Evaluation of a combined dexamethasone suppression/ACTH stimulation test in dogs with hyperadrenocorticism. J Am Vet Med Assoc 187:49–53.

37. Chauvet AE, Feldman EC, Kass PH. 1995. Effects of phenobarbital administration on results of serum biochemical analyses and adrenocortical function tests in epileptic dogs. J Am Vet Med Assoc 207:1305–1307.

38. Kerl ME, Peterson ME, Wallace MS, Melián C, Kemppainen RJ. 1999. Evaluation of a low-dose synthetic adrenocorticotropic hormone stimulation test in clinically normal dogs and dogs with naturally developing hyperadrenocorticism. J Am Vet Med Assoc 214:1497–1501.

39. Watson ADJ, Church DB, Emslie DR, Foster SF. 1998. Plasma cortisol responses to three corticotrophic preparations in normal dogs. Aust Vet J 76:255–257.

40. Frank LA, Oliver JW. 1998. Comparison of serum cortisol concentrations in clinically normal dogs after administration of freshly reconstituted versus reconstituted and stored frozen cosyntropin. J Am Vet Med Assoc 212:1569–1571.

41. Kemppainen RJ, Behrend EN, Busch KA. 2005. Use of compounded adrenocorticotropic hormone (ACTH) for adrenal function testing in dogs. J Am Anim Hosp Assoc 41:368–372.

42. Feldman EC, Nelson RW. 1996. Hyperadrenocorticism (Cushing's syndrome). In: *Canine and Feline Endocrinology and Reproduction*, 2nd edition, 187–265. Philadelphia: WB Saunders.

43. Neiger R, Ramsey I, O'Connor J, Hurley KJ, Mooney CT. 2002. Trilostane treatment of 78 dogs with pituitary-dependent hyperadrenocorticism. Vet Rec 150:799–804.

44. Myers NC III, Bruyette DS. 1994. Feline adrenocortical diseases: Part I. Hyperadrenocorticism. Semin Vet Med Surg (Small Anim) 9:137–143.

45. Hillyer MH, Taylor FGR, Mair TS, Murphy D, Watson TDG, Love S. 1992. Diagnosis of hyperadrenocorticism in the horse. Equine Vet Educ 4:131–134.

46. Eiler H, Goble D, Oliver J. 1979. Adrenal gland function in the horse: Effects of cosyntropin (synthetic) and corticotropin (natural) stimulation. Am J Vet Res 40:724–726.

47. Zerbe CA, Nachreiner RF, Dunstan RW, Dalley JB. 1987. Hyperadrenocorticism in a cat. J Am Vet Med Assoc 190:559–563.

48. Peterson ME, Steele P. 1986. Pituitary-dependent hyperadrenocorticism in a cat. J Am Vet Med Assoc 189:680–683.

49. Zerbe CA, Refsal KR, Peterson ME, Armstrong PJ, Nachreiner RF, Schall WD. 1987. Effect of nonadrenal illness on adrenal function in the cat. Am J Vet Res 48:451–454.

50. Eiler H, Oliver J, Goble D. 1980. Combined dexamethasone-suppression cosyntropin-(synthetic ACTH-) stimulation test in the horse: A new approach to testing of adrenal gland function. Am J Vet Res 41:430–434.

51. Rijnberk A, Kooistra HS, van Vonderen IK, Mol JA, Voorhout G, van Sluijs FJ, Ijzer J, van den Ingh TS, Boer P, Boer WH. 2001. Aldosteronoma in a dog with polyuria as the leading symptom. Domest Anim Endocrinol 20:227–240.

52. Flood SM, Randolph JF, Gelzer ARM, Refsal K. 1999. Primary hyperaldosteronism in two cats. J Am Anim Hosp Assoc 35:411–416.

53. Eger CE, Robinson WF, Huxtable CRR. 1983. Primary aldosteronism (Conn's syndrome) in a cat: A case report and review of comparative aspects. J Small Anim Pract 24:293–307.

54. Ash RA, Harvey AM, Tasker S. 2005. Primary hyperaldosteronism in the cat: A series of 13 cases. J Feline Med Surg 7:173–182.

55. Javadi S, Djajadiningrat-Laanen SC, Kooistra HS, van Dongen AM, Voorhout G, van Sluijs FJ, van den Ingh TSGAM, Boer WH, Rijnberk A. 2005. Primary hyperaldosteronism, a mediator of progressive renal disease in cats. Domest Anim Endocrinol 28:85–104.

56. DeClue AE, Breshears LA, Pardo ID, Kerl ME, Perlis J, Cohn LA. 2005. Hyperaldosteronism and hyperprogesteronism in a cat with an adrenal cortical carcinoma. J Vet Intern Med 19:355–358.

57. Javadi S, Kooistra HS, Mol JA, Boer P, Boer WH, Rijnberk A. 2003. Plasma aldosterone concentrations and plasma renin activity in healthy dogs and dogs with hyperadrenocorticism. Vet Rec 153:521–525.

58. Osbaldiston GW, Greve T. 1978. Estimating adrenal cortical function in dogs with ACTH. Cornell Vet 68:308–316.

59. Chastain CB, Madsen RW, Franklin RT. 1989. A screening evaluation for endogenous glucocorticoid deficiency in dogs: A modified Thorn test. J Am Anim Hosp Assoc 25:18–22.

60. Norman EJ, Thompson H, Mooney CT. 1999. Dynamic adrenal function testing in eight dogs with hyperadrenocorticism associated with adrenocortical neoplasia. Vet Rec 144:551–554.

61. Benitah N, Feldman EC, Kass PH, Nelson RW. 2005. Evaluation of serum 17-hydroxyprogesterone concentration after administration of ACTH in dogs with hyperadrenocorticism. J Am Vet Med Assoc 227:1095–1101.

62. Behrend EN, Kemppainen RJ, Boozer AL, Whitley EM, Smith AN, Busch KA. 2005. Serum 17-α-hydroxyprogesterone and corticosterone concentrations in dogs with nonadrenal neoplasia and dogs with suspected hyperadrenocorticism. J Am Vet Med Assoc 227:1762–1767.

63. Scott-Moncrieff JC. 2000. Adrenal tumors in the dog and cat: One disease or many? In: Proceedings of the 18th ACVIM Forum, Seattle, 452–454.

64. Golden DL, Lothrop CD Jr. 1988. A retrospective study of aldosterone secretion in normal and adrenopathic dogs. J Vet Intern Med 2:121–125.

65. Willard MD, Refsal K, Thacker E. 1987. Evaluation of plasma aldosterone concentrations before and after ACTH administration in clinically normal dogs and in dogs with various diseases. Am J Vet Res 48:1713–1718.

66. Nelson RW, Feldman EC. 1992. Indications and interpretation of endocrine tests used in the dog and cat. Semin Vet Med Surg (Small Anim) 7:285–291.

67. Feldman EC, Nelson RW, Feldman MS. 1996. Use of low- and high-dose dexamethasone tests for distinguishing pituitary-dependent from adrenal tumor hyperadrenocorticism in dogs. J Am Vet Med Assoc 209:772–775.

68. Kaplan AJ, Peterson ME, Kemppainen RJ. 1995. Effects of disease on the results of diagnostic tests for use in detecting hyperadrenocorticism in dogs. J Am Vet Med Assoc 207:445–451.

69. Peterson ME, Kintzer PP, Kass PH. 1996. Pretreatment clinical and laboratory findings in dogs with hypoadrenocorticism: 225 cases (1979–1993). J Am Vet Med Assoc 208:85–91.

70. Huang HP, Yang HL, Liang SL, Lien YH, Chen KY. 1999. Iatrogenic hyperadrenocorticism in 28 dogs. J Am Anim Hosp Assoc 35:200–207.

71. Peterson ME, Gilbertson SR, Drucker WD. 1982. Plasma cortisol response to exogenous ACTH in 22 dogs with hyperadrenocorticism caused by adrenocortical neoplasia. J Am Vet Med Assoc 180:542–544.

72. Duesberg CA, Feldman EC, Nelson RW, Bertoy EH, Dublin AB, Reid MH. 1995. Magnetic resonance imaging for diagnosis of pituitary macrotumors in dogs. J Am Vet Med Assoc 206:657–662.

73. Bertoy EH, Feldman EC, Nelson RW, Duesberg CA, Kass PH, Reid MH, Dublin AB. 1995. Magnetic resonance imaging of the brain in dogs with recently diagnosed but untreated pituitary-dependent hyperadrenocorticism. J Am Vet Med Assoc 206:651–656.

74. Lester SJ, Bellamy JEC, MacWilliams PS, Feldman EC. 1981. A rapid radioimmunoassay method for the evaluation of plasma cortisol levels and adrenal function in the dog. J Am Anim Hosp Assoc 17:121–128.

General Concepts and Definitions 832
Pathogeneses of Cavitary Effusions. 837
    I.   Transudates. 841
    II.   Exudates 843
    III.   Hemorrhagic Effusions. 844
    IV.   Lymphorrhagic (Lymphorrheal) Effusions 845
    V.   Effusions Caused by the Rupture of a Hollow Organ or Other Tissue. 846
    VI.   Effusions Caused by Multiple Processes 847
Routine Analysis of Pleural and Peritoneal Fluid 847
    I.   Sample Collection and Processing. 848
    II.   Physical Analysis 849
    III.   Chemical Analysis 850
    IV.   [Erythrocyte] or Hematocrit (Hct) 851
    V.   [Total Nucleated Cell Concentration] (TNCC) 851
    VI.   Microscopic Examination. 851
Selected Analyses for Pleural and Peritoneal Effusions 856
    I.   [Cholesterol] and [TG] 856
    II.   [Urea] and [Crt] 857
    III. $[Na]^+$, $[Cl]^-$, and $[K]^+$ 858
    IV.   [L-lactate] 858
    V.   [Glucose] 859
    VI.   [Bilirubin]. 860
    VII.   [Ammonium]. 861
    VIII.   Protein Concentrations. 861
    IX.   Enzyme Activity 862
    X.   Gram Staining. 862
    XI.   Culturing for Microorganisms. 862
Comments About Specific Effusions 863
    I.   Septic and Nonseptic Exudates 863
    II.   Differentiation of a Bacterial Exudate and Intestinal Contents 863
    III.   Effusions Associated with Neoplasms. 864
    IV.   Lymphocyte-Rich Effusions. 864
    V.   Pericardial Effusions. 865
    VI.   Amniotic Fluid. 865

Table 19.1. Abbreviations and symbols in this chapter

[x]	Concentration of x (x = analyte)
ALP	Alkaline phosphatase
Chol:TG	Cholesterol to triglyceride
Crt	Creatinine
EDTA	Ethylenediaminetetraacetic acid
FIP	Feline infectious peritonitis
Hct	Hematocrit
SG	Specific gravity
TG	Triglyceride
TNCC	Total nucleated cell concentration
TP	Total protein
TP_{ref}	Total protein determination by refractometry

GENERAL CONCEPTS AND DEFINITIONS

I. Effusions accumulate in body cavities because of physiologic or pathologic processes. Results from the analysis of the effusion and other clinical information are used to determine which process or processes are present in a given animal. This chapter provides an introduction to the results of cavitary fluid analyses and how the results relate to pathologic processes. Most of the chapter is directed toward pleural and peritoneal effusions; the last section contains information about pericardial fluid. Any of several excellent textbooks can be consulted for more information about analytical methods and the microscopic features of cells and other structures in effusions.[1–7]

II. The pleural and peritoneal cavities are lined by a layer of mesothelial cells (mesothelium) with two surfaces: the visceral surface that covers viscera (lungs, intestine, etc.) and the parietal surface that covers mediastinum and the pleural and peritoneal walls. In most species, a small amount of clear serous fluid in the cavities provides a lubricant and medium for transport of electrolytes and other substances. The cavities are called *serous* because they contain a clear watery fluid in health. Pleural and peritoneal fluids are formed by similar processes that involve the forces of Starling's law and anatomic structures. Generally, a plasma filtrate leaves the capillaries, enters interstitial space, and diffuses into the serous cavities, from which it is removed by the lymphatic system and returned to plasma. *Pleural fluid* is formed in health by diffusion of fluid through the parietal mesothelium to the pleural cavity (Fig. 19.1).[8] The fluid has a low [protein] and low cellularity. *Peritoneal fluid* is formed similarly, with most of the fluid removed by diaphragmatic lymphatic vessels.[9]

III. Composition of pleural fluid and peritoneal fluid in health.
    A. The chemical composition of a body cavity fluid is primarily determined by permeability of capillaries to H_2O and solutes and, to a lesser extent, permeability of pleural and peritoneal mesothelium.
        1. Capillaries are permeable to H_2O, electrolytes (e.g., Na^+, K^+, Cl^-, Ca^{2+}, bicarbonate, and phosphates) and small nonprotein solutes (e.g., glucose, urea, and Crt). Other than [protein], the interstitial fluid adjacent to most capillaries has electrolyte, urea, glucose, and Crt concentrations similar to plasma.

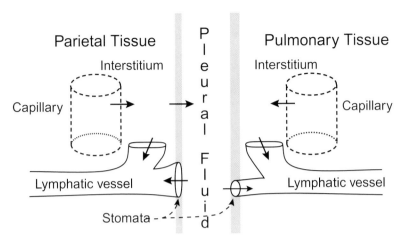

Fig. 19.1. Pleural fluid formation and removal. Forces of Starling's law move protein-poor fluid from capillaries to the parietal and pulmonary interstitial spaces. The parietal capillary beds and parietal pleura are relatively impermeable to proteins, so the fluid that diffuses from the interstitium to the pleural space has a lower [TP] (≈ 1.0 g/dL). Most pleural fluid is drained by the parietal lymphatic vessels, with small amounts entering the pulmonary lymphatic vessels via stomata. The drainage is powered by the lymphatic pump that creates a negative pressure to pull fluid from the interstitium. Evidence indicates the visceral pleural barrier is impermeable to H_2O and solutes in most mammals.

    2. Interstitial fluid is the source of most pleural and peritoneal fluid proteins. Variations in capillary permeability to plasma proteins causes variations in interstitial [TP]. For example, in people, the interstitial fluid [TP] is near 1.5 g/dL in skeletal muscle, near 2.0 g/dL in subcutaneous tissue, near 4 g/dL in intestine, and near 6 g/dL in liver.[10] The [TP] of pleural fluid in health is near 1–2 g/dL.[11]

B. Pleural and peritoneal fluids in healthy animals should not contain erythrocytes and should have low concentrations of nucleated cells (e.g., mesothelial cells, lymphocytes, macrophages, and neutrophils). However, thoracocentesis or abdominocentesis typically damages small blood vessels, and thus a few erythrocytes and rare blood leukocytes are not unusual in collected fluids.

C. Canine pleural and peritoneal fluids.

    1. The amount of pleural and peritoneal fluids in healthy dogs is very small, so it is difficult to collect sufficient fluid for analysis. One source states that healthy dogs have 0–15 mL of peritoneal fluid and about 3 mL of pleural fluid.[12]

    2. There is very little information about the expected features of these fluids in health, but data from multiple sources suggest they should have these features: colorless to slightly yellow, clear, a $[TP_{ref}] < 2.5$ g/dL, a TNCC $< 3.0 \times 10^3/\mu L$, and a mixture of mesothelial cells, neutrophils, lymphocytes, and macrophages.[12] Typically, cavitary fluid is collected when there is an effusion, and the task is determining the cause of the effusion and not whether the fluid is abnormal.

D. Feline pleural and peritoneal fluids: As in dogs, the amounts of pleural and peritoneal fluids in healthy cats are very small, so it is difficult to collect sufficient fluid for analysis. If fluid can be collected, the fluid probably represents an effusion.

E. Equine pleural and peritoneal fluids: Healthy horses do have enough cavitary fluid for collection and analysis, but the reported findings vary considerably (Table 19.2). For

Table 19.2. Reported features of pleural and peritoneal fluids of healthy horses[a]

	Pleural fluid[b]	Peritoneal fluid[c]	Peritoneal fluid[d]	Peritoneal fluid[e]
Number of horses	18	25	20	20
Volume collected (mL)	2–8	10–100	10–100	—
Color	Yellow or red-yellow	Light yellow	Light yellow	—
Clarity	Clear to hazy	Clear to slightly turbid	Clear to slightly turbid	—
TP_{ref} (g/dL)	< 3.4[f] (usually < 2.5)	0.1–3.4[f]	0.1–2.5[f]	0.2–1.5
TNCC ($\times 10^3$/µL)	0.8–12.1	2.0–9.0	0.0–4.6	0.5–10.1
Neutrophils	$0.4–10.3 \times 10^3$/µL	36–78 %	80–98 %	22–82 %
Lymphocytes	$0.0–0.7 \times 10^3$/µL	0–29 %	1–11 %	1–19 %
Monocytes/macrophages	$0.0–2.6 \times 10^3$/µL	3–50 %	1–17 %	19–68 %
Mesothelial cells	—	—	Occasional	—
Eosinophils	$0.0–0.2 \times 10^3$/µL	0–3 %	0–7 %	0–5 %
Mast cell	—	—	Occasional	—
Red blood cells ($\times 10^3$/µL)	22–540	—	0.2–5.4	—

[a] Even though clinically healthy, the $[TP_{ref}] > 2.0$ g/dL and frequent neutrophils suggest that the horses have a subclinical exudative disorder.
[b] *Source:* Wagner and Bennett[80]
[c] *Source:* Bach and Ricketts[81]
[d] *Source:* McGrath[82]
[e] *Source:* Morley and DesNoyers[83]
[f] These data were collected before effective antihelminthic programs were common, so the higher $[TP_{ref}]$ may indicate subclinical parasitic disease.

Table 19.3. Reported features of peritoneal fluids of healthy cattle[a]

	Peritoneal fluid[b]	Peritoneal fluid[c]	Peritoneal fluid[d]
Number of cattle	19	8	?
TP_{ref} (g/dL)	0.1–4.6	2.2–4.0	< 3.0[e]
$Fibrinogen_{ref}$ (g/dL)	0.1–0.4	—	—
TNCC ($\times 10^3/\mu L$)	5.0–30.0	0.4–3.0	< 10.0
Neutrophils	12–58 %	< $2.2 \times 10^3/\mu L$	—[f]
Lymphocytes	1–28 %	< $0.2 \times 10^3/\mu L$	—[f]
Monocytes/macrophages	1–28 %	< $1.0 \times 10^3/\mu L$	—[f]
Eosinophils	25–72 %	< $0.6 \times 10^3/\mu L$	—[f]

[a] Even though clinically healthy, the $[TP_{ref}] > 2.0$ g/dL and frequent neutrophils suggest that the cattle have a subclinical exudative disorder.

[b] *Source* (most data extracted from graphs): Wilson et al.[39]

[c] *Source*: Anderson et al.[84]

[d] *Source*: Kopcha and Schultze[13]

[e] Reported as [total solids] (g/dL)

[f] Described as usually a 1 : 1 ratio of neutrophils and mononuclear cells, but also up to 60 % eosinophils

both the pleural and peritoneal fluids, neutrophil percentages need to be interpreted with knowledge of the fluid's TNCC and the quantity of fluid that is in the cavity.

F. Healthy cattle may have enough peritoneal fluid for collection and analysis. However, pathologic effusions are uncommon, and analysis of effusions is even less common. Reported features of peritoneal fluid in healthy cattle are listed in Table 19.3, but some of the values are much greater than what is expected in healthy animals of most species. Thus, the findings may not truly represent data from healthy cattle. TNCC may be increased during the first 2 wk postpartum.[13]

IV. Definitions

A. *Effusion* is the accumulation of fluid in a body space or cavity, and an *effusion* is the fluid that has accumulated.

B. *Ascites* is the fluid accumulated in a serous cavity (typically peritoneal cavity). It can be a transudate, exudate, or other type of effusion (e.g., hemorrhagic ascites).

C. *Transudation* is the passage of fluid or solute through a membrane because of changes in hydraulic or oncotic pressure gradients.

D. A *transudate* is an effusion produced by changes in mechanical factors such as oncotic or hydraulic pressure within capillary beds. Such changes influence the loss or resorption of fluid.

E. *Hydrostatic pressure* is the energy (pressure) of a fluid at rest.

F. *Hydraulic pressure* is the energy (pressure) of a fluid in motion.

G. *Exudation* is an exuding or oozing out through pores.

H. An *exudate* is an effusion produced by increased vascular permeability to plasma proteins because of inflammation.

I. *Hemorrhage* is the escape or loss of blood from blood vessels or heart.

J. *Lymphorrhage* is the escape or loss of lymph from lymph vessels.

K. A *modified transudate* is a transudate that has been modified by the addition of protein and/or cells. This classification is not recommended by the authors.

1. Pathologic processes that produce these effusions are varied and not consistently described. The origin of *modified transudate* is unknown. It is rarely described in the human literature and was not present in a 1967 veterinary clinical pathology textbook.[14] Benjamin wrote in 1961 that "a typical transudate can usually be readily distinguished from a typical exudate; but many extravascular fluids are modified transudates or modified exudates with some characteristics of both, so that recognition of the etiologic process may be difficult without a more complete examination of the fluid."[15] Modified transudate was listed as one type of effusion in a 1977 veterinary clinical pathology textbook.[16] It is now a common label or classification even though it may not accurately reflect the pathologic process responsible for the effusion.

2. The modified transudate classification is usually based on laboratory data rather than the pathologic process or processes that produced the effusion. Basically, this classification has been used for effusions that had a $[TP_{ref}]$ and/or TNCC in a grey zone between protein-poor transudates and typical exudates.

3. A variety of effusions have been considered to be modified transudates, including hemorrhagic, chylous, congestive, neoplastic, and low-grade inflammatory effusions. Increased hydraulic pressures contribute to transudation in congestive heart failure, but transudation is not the primary mechanism responsible for the fluid that accumulates in hemorrhagic, most chylous, and most neoplastic effusions. In this chapter, effusions are not classified as modified transudates, because the classification does not clearly communicate the pathologic processes that led to the effusions, and many of the so-called *modified transudates* do not accumulate because of transudation and subsequent modification.

V. Basic concepts of Starling's law (Eq. 19.1) are needed to understand the pathogeneses of body cavitary effusions. In the context of most capillary beds, the major variables are illustrated in Fig. 7.3.

$$\text{Net filtration} = LpS[\Delta \text{ hydraulic pressure} - \Delta \text{ oncotic pressure}] \quad \textbf{(19.1.)}$$
$$= LpS[(P_{cap} - P_{if}) - s(\pi_{cap} - \pi_{if})]$$

Net filtration = net flux of fluid from capillary to interstitium
Lp = unit permeability (porosity) of the capillary
S = surface area available for fluid movement
s = reflection coefficient of proteins across the capillary wall
P_{cap} = hydraulic pressure of plasma
P_{if} = hydraulic pressure of interstitial fluid
π_{cap} = oncotic pressure of plasma in capillary
π_{if} = oncotic pressure of interstitial fluid

A. A majority of the fluid that enters the interstitium from plasma returns to the plasma via the permeable venous capillaries (capillaries that open into venules). The remainder enters the lymphatic vessels and returns to the blood via the thoracic duct (most of the body) or the right lymphatic duct (parts of head, neck, and thorax).

B. Most capillary walls have minimal permeability to plasma proteins, but some proteins do enter the interstitium and the resultant lymph. The proteins in the interstitial fluid create an extravascular oncotic pressure (colloidal osmotic pressure) (see Chapter 7).

1. Oncotic pressure in interstitium of skeletal muscle is about 30 % of the plasma oncotic pressure in health.[17]
2. Oncotic pressure in the hepatic interstitium is nearly equal to plasma oncotic pressure because the walls of hepatic sinusoids are permeable to most plasma proteins.[17]
3. Oncotic pressure in the pulmonary interstitium is about 70 % of plasma oncotic pressure. Alveolar capillaries are less permeable to proteins than are the hepatic sinusoids but more than are the skeletal muscle capillaries.[17]

C. The permeability of capillaries is expressed as a reflection coefficient (Eq. 19.1), which ranges from 0 (completely permeable to proteins) to 1 (impermeable to proteins). The reflection coefficient approaches 1 in most capillary beds but is smaller in hepatic and pulmonary capillary beds.

PATHOGENESES OF CAVITARY EFFUSIONS

Effusions accumulate in pleural and peritoneal cavities when one or more pathologic processes (Table 19.4) cause increased entry of fluid into the cavity and/or decreased removal of fluid from the cavity. These processes are illustrated in Fig. 19.2. The composition of the effusion will provide evidence for the type of pathologic process that led to the effusion (Table 19.5). However, frequently the evidence is not diagnostic of a disorder, and thus other information

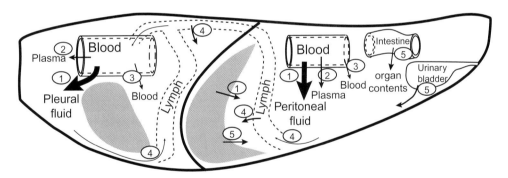

Fig. 19.2. Schematic drawing of the five major pathogeneses of pleural and peritoneal effusions.
1. Transudates form when there is increased vascular hydraulic pressure with or without decreased plasma oncotic pressure. The transudate formed from increased hydraulic pressures in hepatic sinuses and alveolar capillaries (lungs not shown) have relatively higher protein concentrations because the vessels are more permeable to plasma proteins.
2. Exudates form when increased vascular and mesothelial permeability enables protein-rich fluid to escape from the capillaries to the interstitium and then to the cavity.
3. Damage to blood vessels enables blood to escape to create a hemorrhagic effusion.
4. Effusions develop when there is decreased drainage of the fluids by the lymphatic vessels either because of increased pressure within the lymphatic vessel or because cells (e.g., neoplastic) are blocking pathways. Damage to lymphatic vessels enables lymph to escape to create a lymphocyte-rich effusion. If the lymph contains chylomicrons, then a chylous effusion forms.
5. Damage to viscera enables contents of those structures to enter the body cavity (e.g., a uroperitoneum). The contents released from damaged alimentary, biliary, or urinary tissues will initiate an inflammatory reaction and thus exudation.

Table 19.4. Cavitary effusions: Pathologic processes, mechanisms, and conditions or disorders that produce effusions[a]

Pathologic process	Pathologic mechanisms	Effusion	Conditions or disorders
Transudation	Altered hydraulic and oncotic pressures	Transudate, protein poor	*Cirrhosis (dogs) *Protein-losing nephropathies (including nephrotic syndrome) Protein-losing enteropathy Lymphatic obstruction (e.g., lymphangiectasis, lymph node disease)
		Transudate, protein rich	Noncirrhotic portal hypertension (presinusoidal and sinusoidal) *Congestive heart failure Portal hypertension (postsinusoidal)
Exudation	Increased vascular permeability to plasma proteins	Exudate, infectious	*Bacteria (cocci and bacilli), fungi (e.g., *Blastomyces*, *Histoplasma*, *Candida*), viruses (FIP coronavirus), protozoa (e.g., *Leishmania*, *Toxoplasma*), and parasites (*Mesocestoides*)
		Exudate, noninfectious	*Neoplasia, foreign body, bile peritonitis, pancreatitis, steatitis, uroperitoneum, ischemic necrosis of spleen, lung, or other tissues due to torsion or vascular lesions
Hemorrhage	Leakage of blood from vessels	Hemorrhagic effusion, acute	*Trauma to blood vessels, neoplasia, hemostasis defects
		Hemorrhagic effusion, chronic	*Neoplasia, hemostasis defects (vascular damage or factor deficiencies), trauma
Lymphorrhage (lymphorrhea)	Leakage of lymph from lymphatic vessels	Chylous effusion	Cardiac disease, trauma, diaphragmatic lesions or hernia, neoplasms, and mediastinal lesions (see the text)
		Nonchylous lymphatic effusion	Lymphatic obstruction (e.g., lymphangiectasis, lymph node disease)
Rupture of hollow organ or tissue	Leakage of urine from urinary bladder, urethra, or ureter	Uroperitoneum, secondary exudate	*Trauma Urolithiasis Neoplasia of urinary tract
	Leakage of bile from biliary tract	Secondary exudate, noninfectious	Cholelithiasis, cholangitis, bile duct carcinoma, cholecystitis
	Leakage of gastric or intestinal contents	Secondary exudate, infectious or noninfectious	Gastric: perforated ulcer, gastric carcinoma, trauma Intestinal: perforated intestine, intestinal neoplasia, intestinal obstruction, intestinal ischemia

* A relatively common disease or condition

[a] During the development of an effusion, more than one pathologic process may contribute; for example, a persistent chylous effusion elicits an inflammatory process so that exudation contributes to the effusion; bile itself may not cause an effusion but the secondary inflammation will.

Table 19.5. Common features of effusions[a]

	Physical features[b]	TP_ref (g/dL)	TNCC (× 10³/μL)	Predominant nucleated cells	Other findings
Transudate, protein poor	Clear, colorless	< 2.0	< 1.5	Variable	Reactive mesothelial cells may be present
Transudate, protein rich[c]	Clear to cloudy Yellow, orange, red	≥ 2.0	< 5.0	Mostly neutrophils and macrophages	Reactive mesothelial cells are common
Exudate, bacterial	Hazy to cloudy Yellow, tan, cream, orange	≥ 2.0	> 5.0	Neutrophils or neutrophils and macrophages	Bacteria may not be found via microscopy
Exudate, fungal	Hazy to cloudy Yellow, tan, cream, orange	≥ 2.0	> 5.0	Neutrophils or neutrophils and macrophages	Fungus may not be found via microscopy
Exudate, parasitic	Hazy to cloudy Yellow, tan, cream, orange	≥ 2.0	> 5.0	Neutrophils or neutrophils and macrophages	Eosinophil percentages vary; parasite may not be found via microscopy
Exudate, FIP[c]	Clear to hazy Yellow	≥ 2.0	< 5.0	Neutrophils or neutrophils and macrophages	Finely granular pink background, protein crescents, perhaps fibrin particles
Exudate, noninfectious	Hazy to cloudy Yellow, tan, cream, orange, green	≥ 2.0	> 5.0	Neutrophils or neutrophils and macrophages; perhaps lymphocytes	See the text

Continues

Type of effusion	Appearance	TP	Cell count	Predominant cell types	Other findings
Hemorrhagic effusion, acute[c]	Opaque; Red	≥ 2.0	> 2.0	Neutrophils and lymphocytes (most directly from blood)	Platelets if very recent hemorrhage
Hemorrhagic effusion, chronic[c]	Hazy to opaque; Red	≥ 2.0	> 2.0	Neutrophils and macrophages	Erythrophages; Siderophages
Chylous effusion[c]	Hazy to white	≥ 2.0[d]	< 10.0	Small lymphocyte (brief duration); Mixed leukocytes (long duration)	Sudanophilic droplets in fluid and macrophages
Lymphatic effusion[c]	Hazy to cloudy; Yellow to pink	?	< 10.0	Small lymphocytes	
Uroperitoneum (initially)	Yellow	< 2.0	< 1.5	Variable	Urine crystals or sperm occasionally found, and urine odor
Uroperitoneum (persistent)[c]	Variable	Variable	> 1.5	Neutrophils and macrophages	Urine crystals occasionally found

[a] The table contains common features of the effusions. However, the pathologic process that creates an effusion, not the results of fluid analysis, determines the type of effusion.

[b] All effusions may have a pink to red tint because of the presence of erythrocytes or hemoglobin. The erythrocytes or hemoglobin may be present because of the animal's pathologic condition or could be due to blood contamination during sample collection.

[c] Each of these effusions have been classified as *modified transudates*.

[d] The TP$_{ref}$ value will be falsely increased if the fluid is grossly cloudy to opaque because of the lipid. The [TP] after removal of chylomicrons or by a method minimally affected by chylomicrons is expected to be > 2.0 g/dL.

(history, physical examination, imaging findings, or other laboratory data) is needed to interpret the significance of analysis results or establish the pathogenesis of an effusion.

I.   Transudates
   A.   Pathogenesis
      1.   Transudates typically accumulate in pleural and/or peritoneal cavities when there is an excess diffusion of plasma H_2O from the vascular space because of alterations in hydraulic and/or oncotic pressures. They may also accumulate when lymphatic drainage from a cavity is impaired (see Fig. 7.3).
      2.   For most tissues, a transudate is protein poor ($[TP_{ref}] < 2.0$ g/dL), but transudation from a liver can create a protein-rich peritoneal transudate if normoproteinemia is present. If a marked hypoproteinemia is present, then the transudate associated with hepatic transudation will contain a lower [TP] than if formed when the plasma [TP] was not decreased.
      3.   A transudative pleural effusion is caused primarily by increased hydraulic pressure in the alveolar capillaries. Most of the pulmonary transudate remains in the lung (i.e., pulmonary edema), but it may flow into the pleural cavity because of damaged visceral pleura. Concurrently, venous congestion and the resultant increased hydraulic pressure in the posterior vena cava reduce lymphatic drainage from the pleural cavity.
      4.   Portal hypertension is a frequent contributor to the formation of peritoneal transudates and occasionally pleural transudates. *Portal hypertension* is a pathologic state in which the hydraulic pressure in portal blood vessels is increased by either increased portal blood flow or, more likely, increased resistance to portal blood flow.
         a.   Blood enters the abdominal portal venous system from capillary beds in viscera (intestines, spleen, pancreas, stomach, and distal esophagus), travels to the liver via the portal vein and its branches in the portal triad, flows through the hepatic sinusoids (capillaries) of the hepatic lobule to the central vein, exits the liver via the hepatic vein, and enters the vena cava. Lesions within or adjacent to these vessels or the heart may impair portal blood flow and increase hydraulic pressure within the portal system.
         b.   Portal hypertensive disorders can be classified by overlapping systems.[18,19] The *anatomic system* is primarily based on gross anatomy (i.e., prehepatic, intrahepatic, or posthepatic) and relates to the flow of blood to, through, and from the liver. The *vascular system* identifies the location of the lesion relative to the hepatic sinusoids (i.e., presinusoidal, sinusoidal, or postsinusoidal). The disorders that restrict portal blood flow can be classified as luminal (e.g., thrombosis) and extraluminal (e.g., hepatic fibrosis).
            (1)   Portal hypertension caused by right heart failure is posthepatic and postsinusoidal. Because there is increased hydraulic pressure in the hepatic sinusoids, the resulting effusion is protein rich.
            (2)   Portal hypertension caused by hepatic cirrhosis is intrahepatic but may be either presinusoidal or sinusoidal. When the increased hydraulic pressure is presinusoidal, the resulting effusion is protein poor. Sinusoidal hypertension may cause protein-poor transudation when hypoproteinemia is marked.
   B.   Protein-poor transudates (Tables 19.4 and 19.5)
      1.   These tend to form in body cavities when hypoproteinemia (including hypoalbuminemia) is marked. Most mammals with protein-poor transudates have a serum

[albumin] < 1.5 g/dL. However in most disorders, hypoalbuminemia by itself will not cause transudation.

    a. Analbuminemia occurs in people and is characterized by serum [albumin] < 0.1 g/dL; these people typically do not have transudative effusions but may have mild edema. Compensatory processes that prevent transudative effusions include increased synthesis of globulins, reduced intravascular hydraulic pressure, reduced interstitial oncotic pressure, and increased lymphatic drainage. The plasma oncotic pressure in analbuminemic people is about half of that found in healthy people.[20]

    b. The lack of significant transudative effusion in the absence of albumin emphasizes three concepts: (1) globulins contribute to oncotic pressures, (2) increased lymphatic drainage of a cavity may compensate for increased transudation, and (3) factors other than hypoalbuminemia typically contribute to transudative effusions.

    c. An acute onset of marked hypoproteinemia (e.g., marked blood loss followed by intravenous fluid therapy) may lead to transudation because there has been insufficient time for adjustments in the oncotic pressure gradient and lymphatic drainage.

2. The most common disorders that produce protein-poor transudates in dogs are hepatic cirrhosis and protein-losing nephropathy (Table 19.4). Pathologic protein-poor transudates are uncommon in cats, horses, and cattle. In both cirrhosis and protein-losing nephropathies, transudates form because of these two major factors:[17]

    a. Decreased plasma oncotic pressure

        (1) As the plasma [TP] falls, proteins (including albumin) in the interstitial fluid are redistributed to the vascular space. If the plasma [TP] and the interstitial fluid [TP] decrease by the same amount, then the oncotic pressure gradient does not change. Thus, there will not be additional H_2O movement from the vessels. When there is marked hypoproteinemia, less interstitial fluid protein is available for redistribution to the vascular space.

        (2) When the oncotic pressure in plasma decreases more than the interstitial fluid, the oncotic pressure gradient is reduced, and thus more fluid will enter the interstitial space. However, a transudate will not accumulate if increased lymphatic drainage removes the fluid. In people, lymph flow can increase by at least a factor of 10 to compensate for increased rate of fluid leaving plasma.[17]

    b. Increased hydraulic pressure gradient

        (1) In cirrhosis and protein-losing nephropathies, abnormal regulation of blood volume leads to retention of Na^+ and H_2O. The retention of H_2O causes an increased plasma hydraulic pressure and thus a greater rate of fluid leaving plasma and entering interstitium.[21] Portal hypertension also contributes to transudation in cirrhosis.

        (2) The processes that lead to the retention of Na^+ and H_2O involve hormones and renal functions (see Chapters 8 and 9).

3. Occasionally, lymph node diseases, protein-losing enteropathies, and idiopathic noncirrhotic portal hypertension cause the formation of protein-poor effusions.

    a. If a protein-poor effusion is associated with intrathoracic or intra-abdominal lymph node disease, at least part of the reason for the effusion is decreased lymphatic drainage of fluids that normally enter the cavities.

b. If a protein-poor effusion is associated with a protein-losing enteropathy, at least two mechanisms may be contributing to the effusion. If the enteropathy has led to a marked hypoproteinemia, then part of pathogenesis includes a decreased oncotic pressure gradient. Also, some protein-losing enteropathies impair drainage of intestinal lymph (e.g., lymphangiectasia).

c. Idiopathic noncirrhotic portal hypertension in dogs is an uncommonly recognized disorder that may be caused by portal vein hypoplasia. Dogs with this disorder have protein-poor peritoneal transudates and many other laboratory data suggestive of a portosystemic shunt or hepatic insufficiency.[22]

C. Protein-rich transudates (Tables 19.4 and 19.5)

1. Protein-rich transudates typically occur when there is increased plasma hydraulic pressure in the liver or lungs because of venous congestion.

2. The most common disorders that produce protein-rich transudates are congestive heart failure and portal venous hypertension (Table 19.4). In both, transudation occurs because of increased plasma hydraulic pressure.

a. In congestive heart failure, a complex set of events decreases cardiac output, increases hydraulic pressure in veins, and increases Na^+ and H_2O retention (see Chapter 9).

b. In portal venous hypertension (either posthepatic or postsinusoidal), the rate of plasma entering the space of Disse increases because of the increased hydraulic pressure in hepatic sinusoids. If there is not a corresponding increase in lymphatic drainage, the protein-rich fluid may move from the liver to the peritoneal cavity.

c. In people with these disorders, a serum albumin-ascites gradient (serum [albumin] − effusion [albumin]) is used to help differentiate effusions caused by portal hypertension (e.g., cirrhosis and congestive heart failure) from other effusions. This gradient is greater in these congestive disorders than in exudative disorders.[23,24] Very little information about this gradient is available for domestic mammals.

3. The [TP] of a transudate may increase when an animal is given a diuretic agent to reduce edema or the quantity of an effusion.

II. Exudates (Tables 19.4 and 19.5)

A. An exudate forms when inflammation causes increased vascular permeability that allows plasma (and its proteins) to ooze out of the blood. The exudation of protein-rich fluid is usually accompanied by the migration of leukocytes (mostly neutrophils) into the effusion because of chemotactic substances in the fluid.

1. The vascular permeability is typically increased by the effects of inflammatory mediators (e.g., histamine, bradykinin, leukotrienes, and substance P) that were released from inflamed tissue. The inflammatory mediators may also cause selective vasodilation, so that more blood enters the inflamed tissues and thus increases the hydraulic pressure in the capillaries.[25] When associated with sepsis, secondary vascular damage increases the vascular permeability.

2. The inflammation can directly involve blood vessel (vasculitis and phlebitis), and then the vessels become very permeable to plasma proteins.

B. Neutrophils are the most common nucleated cell in most exudates, but nucleated cells in exudates will frequently be predominantly neutrophils and macrophages or a mixture of neutrophils, macrophages, and lymphocytes. Occasionally, nucleated cells of exudates will be predominantly eosinophils or possibly lymphocytes.

C. The leakage of proteins into the interstitium reduces the oncotic pressure gradient between plasma and interstitial fluid, and thus plasma has less ability to retain H_2O. The plasma hydraulic pressure pushes a protein-rich fluid into the interstitium, and less fluid returns in the venous end of the capillary bed. A pleuritis or peritonitis may damage mesothelium so that the protein-rich interstitial fluid easily moves into the cavities.

D. Exudates are caused by infectious and noninfectious agents. The type of exudate (i.e., infectious or noninfectious) cannot be reliably determined until the causative agent or event has been established.

   1. Exudates are frequently caused by an infection with bacteria or other organisms. Some people consider *septic* and *bacterial* to be synonyms, but *sepsis* refers to any microbial infection (e.g., bacterial, fungal, viral, or protozoal). To reduce the possibility of confusion, it may be better to refer to the infectious exudates by the appropriate infectious agent (e.g., bacterial exudate or fungal exudate), when known.

   2. Exudates are also commonly formed during noninfectious inflammatory responses. For example, the inflammatory response may be due to necrotic tissue (e.g., secondary to ischemia or neoplasia), the presence of a sterile foreign body (e.g., surgical sponge or barium), or the presence of an irritating fluid (e.g., bile or urine).

E. When an effusion is protein rich and has a high [neutrophil], it is not difficult to recognize the effusion as an exudate. However, it may be difficult to determine the cause of the exudation.

   1. In bacterial and fungal exudates, a microscopic examination of a fluid may detect bacteria (cocci or bacilli) or fungal structures (yeasts or hyphae) in phagocytes (neutrophils or macrophages) or extracellularly. However, if very few organisms are in the fluid, they may not be detected during the microscopic examination, and the fluid should be placed in appropriate culture media to attempt to grow organisms.

   2. With the exception of the exudate of FIP, viral exudates are uncommon. The types of proteins in the FIP exudate are very similar to the plasma proteins because the FIP vasculitis enables plasma proteins to ooze through the inflamed vessel walls. Compared to most exudates, the FIP exudate tends to have a low nucleated cellularity because the inflammatory process is in the blood vessels and not in the body cavity. Microscopic examination of a stained preparation may reveal a pink granular background reflective of a high [TP].

   3. Protozoal exudates (e.g., *Leishmania* sp.) are uncommon in the United States. Amastigotes can be found in macrophages.

III. Hemorrhagic effusions (Tables 19.4 and 19.5)

A. When the primary reason for an effusion is hemorrhage, the fluid is a *hemorrhagic effusion*. Relatively minor hemorrhage is a component of many exudates because of the vascular damage associated with inflammation. Also, minor hemorrhage commonly occurs during the collection of an effusion; this is commonly called *traumatic tap* or *iatrogenic hemorrhage*. When recent hemorrhage causes an effusion, the collected fluid will have many features of the animal's peripheral blood. Lymphatic vessels attempt to resorb the effusion's H_2O, solutes, and erythrocytes. Thus, the effusion volume and its composition change with time. About 65 % of erythrocytes are resorbed (autotransfused) within 2 d and 80 % within 1–2 wk.[26]

B. When the effusion forms because of frequent but small amounts of hemorrhage, the effusion can have a variety of features.
  1. If collected soon after hemorrhage, it might have features of dilute blood.
  2. With persistent hemorrhage, the extravasation of plasma proteins disrupts the oncotic pressure gradient, and thus H_2O tends to diffuse into the cavity and dilute its contents. Concurrently, H_2O and proteins are returning to plasma via lymphatic vessels.
  3. Some erythrocytes are engulfed by macrophages to form erythrophages, and some degrade hemoglobin to form hematoidin or hemosiderin.
C. It is difficult to set a decision threshold for the classification of hemorrhagic effusion because many factors can alter the effusion's Hct (or hemoglobin or erythrocyte concentrations), and sometimes an effusion develops because of hemorrhage and other processes. If the effusion's Hct is > 3 %, then hemorrhage is contributing to the effusion; for example, an effusion Hct of 5 % and a blood Hct of 25 % suggests that 20 % of the effusion's volume is blood.
D. Occasionally, an abdominal sample is collected from an enlarged spleen. The bloody sample will have a Hct > 3 %, but it does not represent a hemorrhagic effusion. A splenic origin (aspirate or rupture) should be considered when hematopoietic cells are in the collected sample but not the blood.

IV. Lymphorrhagic (lymphorrheal) effusions (Tables 19.4 and 19.5)
A. There is not a common term for the loss of lymph into a body cavity. Two terms that occasionally are used are lymphorrhage and lymphorrhea. For this chapter, *lymphorrhage* will be used similarly to *hemorrhage*; that is, *lymphorrhage* is a process that results in lymph escaping from lymphatic vessels, just as *hemorrhage* is a process that results in blood escaping from blood vessels.
  1. *Lymphorrhage* is sometimes used synonymously with *lymphorrhea* but is also used to refer to a focal accumulation of lymphocytes in tissues.
  2. *Lymphorrhea* more commonly refers to the external loss of lymph from damaged lymphatic vessels. Occasionally, authors also use the term to refer to the process that causes lymphedema or formation of a lymph-rich effusion.
B. Several pathologic states may cause lymphorrhagic effusions. The pathogeneses of these states can be divided into two groups: traumatic and nontraumatic.[27]
  1. In the traumatic group, physical damage to lymphatic vessels allows lymph to enter the body cavity.
  2. In the nontraumatic group, lymphorrhagic effusions occur when one or more of these mechanisms are present: (1) lymph stasis, (2) lymphatic hypertension, (3) defective lymphatic valve function because of dilated lymphatic vessels, and (4) increased permeability of lymphatic vessels.[27] Also, the persistence of a nontraumatic process might weaken a lymphatic vessel and cause lymphorrhage when it ruptures. Clinical findings suggest that many chylous pleural effusions are caused by obstruction of the thoracic duct or cranial vena cava; contrast lymphangiography reveals extensive lymphangiectasia of mediastinal and pleural lymphatic vessels.[28]
  3. Blockage of lymphatic vessels by neoplastic cells can be a major reason for effusions associated with malignancies. However, enhanced vessel proliferation and increased vascular permeability may also contribute to these effusions.[29]
C. Lymphorrhagic effusions can be classified into these two major groups based on the presence or absence of chylomicrons in the effusion:

1. Chylous effusions
    a. A *chylous effusion* is produced when chylomicron-rich lymph leaks from lymphatic vessels and enters the pleural cavity to form a chylothorax or the peritoneal cavity to form a chyloabdomen (chyloperitoneum). Chylomicrons are formed in intestinal mucosal cells, enter intestinal lymphatic vessels, and enter peripheral blood via the thoracic duct. When a chylous effusion is present, it indicates that lymphatic vessels somewhere between the small intestine and the thoracic vena cava are damaged.
    b. Among the domestic mammals, chylothorax is most common in cats. It can be caused by several disorders in cats, dogs, and horses (e.g., neoplasms, cardiomyopathy, heart failure, trauma, lung lobe torsion, and infections) but frequently is idiopathic.[30–35] The leakage of chylomicron-containing lymph may be directly related to damaged lymphatic vessels but also may be secondary to increased hydraulic pressure in the cranial or caudal vena cava. Chyloabdomen occurs rarely.[36,37]
    c. Chylomicrons may be abundant and thus create a creamy white fluid. However, they may be present in low concentrations, requiring chemical assessment of [TG] and [cholesterol] to recognize their presence (see Selected Analyses for Pleural and Peritoneal Effusions, sect. I).
2. Nonchylous lymphatic effusions
    a. A *nonchylous lymphatic effusion* is produced when lymph without chylomicrons leaks from lymphatic vessels and enters the pleural cavity or peritoneal cavity. The lesion may involve lymphatic vessels that are not in the drainage path from intestine to thoracic duct and thus do not contain chyle or chylomicrons. However, the absence of chylomicrons might indicate a lack of dietary intake of lipids (thus, the intestinal lymph did not contain chylomicrons) or that the chylomicrons (or TG) did not persist in the effusion.
    b. These effusions do not have the unique features created by chylomicrons, including the chylous pattern of the [TG] and [cholesterol]. Small lymphocytes may be the predominant nucleated cell if the lymph originated from an efferent lymphatic vessel.
3. Pseudochylous effusions
    a. *Pseudochylous effusions* are fluids that grossly have a similar appearance to chylous effusions (e.g., white to cream colored, and cloudy or turbid) but do not contain chylomicrons and do not have a high [TG]. They have been recognized in people (rarely) but are not described in domestic mammals. Effusions described as "pseudochylous" in older veterinary literature had features of chylous effusions.
    b. Pseudochylous effusions typically have a high [cholesterol] that might result from the degradation of cell membranes or the trapping of cholesterol-rich lipoproteins (e.g., low-density lipoproteins) in the body cavity.

V. Effusions caused by the rupture of a hollow organ or other tissue (Tables 19.4 and 19.5)
    A. Leakage of urine from the urinary bladder, ureter, urethra, or kidney
        1. *Uroperitoneum* occurs when urine enters the peritoneal cavity subsequent to trauma, urolithiasis, or neoplasia. Attempts to expel urine forcefully from a distended urinary bladder can rupture it.

    2. Initially, the peritoneal fluid has features of urine (see Selected Analyses for Pleural and Peritoneal Effusions, sects. II and III), but when the presence of urine in the peritoneal cavity initiates an inflammatory response, the effusion may have features of an exudate. Bacteria may be present when associated with a bacterial infection of the urinary tract, but the TNCC may be quite low because of the relatively large amount of urine entering the cavity.

  B. Leakage of bile from the biliary tract

    1. Several pathologic states may damage the biliary tract sufficiently for bile to enter the peritoneal cavity. The [bilirubin] in the effusion is typically greater than the animal's serum [bilirubin] (see Selected Analyses for Pleural and Peritoneal Effusions, sect. VI).

    2. The bile volume probably is not sufficient to create an excessive amount of peritoneal fluid, but the bile will initiate inflammation (often low to moderate grade), which then creates an exudative effusion.

  C. Leakage of gastric or intestinal contents

    1. Several pathologic states may damage the gastrointestinal tract sufficiently for luminal fluid to enter the peritoneal cavity.

    2. The luminal fluid volume may or may not be sufficient to create an excessive amount of peritoneal fluid. However, the fluid's content (e.g., bacteria and ingesta) will initiate inflammation that then creates an exudative effusion.

VI. Effusions caused by multiple processes

  A. Many cavitary effusions accumulate because of multiple concurrent processes. For example, an abdominal neoplasm may have necrotic areas that result in an inflammatory reaction that causes an exudate. Concurrently, a few blood vessels are damaged sufficiently to cause hemorrhage into the cavity. Also, neoplastic cells may enter lymphatic vessels and impair lymphatic drainage. Therefore, the animal may be presented with an effusion that forms because of exudation, hemorrhage, and impaired lymphatic drainage.

  B. Other examples of multiple pathogeneses include the following:

    1. A persistent protein-rich transudation in heart failure caused by a low-grade inflammatory reaction and exudation

    2. Urine leakage in uroperitoneum and subsequent exudation caused by peritonitis

    3. Gallbladder rupture and subsequent exudation caused by peritonitis

ROUTINE ANALYSIS OF PLEURAL AND PERITONEAL FLUID

Analysis of pleural and peritoneal fluid may yield a cause for the effusion, but, more often, analysis provides information about the fluid's composition so that one or more possible explanations for its excess formation can be considered. The results of the fluid analyses have been used to create effusion classifications. Effusion classifications are not diagnoses, just as classification of an anemia as regenerative is not a diagnosis. Classification schemes provide us with a method to communicate.

    If appropriate historical and physical examination findings are known, results of most fluid analyses can be appropriately interpreted with the following three results: (1) [TP_{ref}], (2) TNCC, and (3) types and percentages of nucleated cells. Other features of an effusion may help clarify the cause of the effusion.

I. Sample collection and processing
    A. Sterile collection methods should be used to ensure that bacteria or other organisms are not introduced into the cavity. The centesis site and method vary among species: dogs and cats,[1,7] horses,[6,38] and cattle.[13,39]
    B. Collected fluid should be placed into two tubes: one tube that contains EDTA, which inhibits fibrin clot formation, and one sterile tube for possible submission for microbiologic testing (e.g., culturing) or chemical analysis. Tubes that are not immediately submitted to a laboratory should be kept cool and delivered to the laboratory within 36 h. Concurrent submission of stained and unstained direct or concentrated preparations made from an aliquot of the fresh fluid can be very helpful. Some EDTA tubes may contain an additive that falsely increases the $[TP_{ref}]$.[40] Heparin may also be used as an anticoagulant, but it alters the staining properties of cells and thus may interfere with microscopic analysis.
    C. Methods of preparing specimens for microscopic examination depend somewhat on the cellularity of the fluid. When possible, the cytopreparations should be made soon after the sample is collected, so that in vitro changes are less likely (e.g., cell deterioration, organism proliferation, or in vitro phagocytosis). The fluid is air-dried prior to staining with routine stains. For all of the film methods, the feathered edge, which frequently contains important cells or structures, should be in the stainable area of the slide.
        1. *Direct smear*: Using the common technique for making a blood film, a small drop of fluid is spread on a glass slide. This method is usually adequate for effusions that have a TNCC $> 5.0 \times 10^3/\mu L$, but an additional concentration method is desirable for fluids with a TNCC of up to at least $20.0 \times 10^3/\mu L$.
        2. *Line preparation*: This method is similar to the direct smear, but the push slide is abruptly stopped and lifted so that cells are concentrated in a terminal line. This method tends to concentrate cells in a line and can be used for fluids with a TNCC $< 10.0 \times 10^3/\mu L$. However, a high [TP] tends to make this area too thick for a microscopic examination. This can be partially resolved by adding a flow-back step: when the spreader slide is lifted to form the terminal line, the slide is tipped up to allow the terminal line to flow back and spread out enough for better cell visibility.
        3. *Sediment smears* are used for effusions with a low TNCC. The concentration method is not needed for effusions that have a TNCC $> 20.0 \times 10^3/\mu L$.
            a. Fluid is centrifuged in a clinical centrifuge by methods similar to preparing urine sediment. After removal of most supernatant, the sediment is resuspended in a small amount of fluid, and then a direct smear method is used to distribute cells on a glass slide.
            b. Another method involves using special devices to allow gravity to form a sediment slowly. This procedure may or may not create a monolayer of cells for microscopic examinations.
        4. *Cytocentrifuge preparation*: Commercial cytocentrifuges are designed to concentrate cells in a fluid on a glass slide and are especially valuable for fluids that have a TNCC $< 1.0 \times 10^3/\mu L$. However, their cost limits their use to larger laboratories that analyze such fluids daily.
        5. Usually, the TNCC is not known prior to preparing the cytopreparations but can be predicted based on the transparency of the fluid. If the fluid is clear or hazy, the TNCC is probably low, and thus a concentrating method is needed. If the fluid is cloudy or opaque, then a concentrating method is probably not needed. When in

doubt, both types of cytopreparations are made, and the microscopist can select the best slide for examination.

II. Physical analysis
    A. Color and transparency of the fluid (noted before centrifugation and, if the effusion is not clear and colorless, also after centrifugation)
        1. A supernatant's color reflects the pigmented solutes in the fluid, such as bilirubin (yellow to orange), hemoglobin (pink to red to brown), stercobilinogen (brown), and chlorophyll (green). A nontransparent white, creamy, or cloudy supernatant typically indicates the presence of lipoproteins (e.g., chylomicrons) in the fluid.
        2. A sediment's color is an indication of the pigments in the suspended cells or particles in the fluid; for example, red for erythrocytes, cream to beige to tan for nucleated cells, and brown for fecal contents. The amount of sediment typically reflects the number of erythrocytes and nucleated cells in the effusion.
    B. Refractometric estimates of [total protein] ([TP_{ref}])
        1. Clinical refractometers measure the refractive index of a fluid, which is then displayed on a TP, SG, or total solids scale; some current refractometers have "TS" in their names but have TP and not total solids scales. Most clinical refractometers are calibrated for the normal constituents of human plasma (TP scale) and human urine (SG scale) A refractometer with a SG scale for domestic mammals is also available (see Chapter 8). To reduce the effects of ambient temperature, temperature-compensated refractometers are recommended.
        2. The [TP] scale is calibrated for plasma [TP] and will approximate the true [TP] in protein-rich fluids because the altered refractive index is mostly due to proteins. Even though the [TP_{ref}] may not be accurate, the estimated [TP] is a differential feature of effusions.
        3. Some clinical refractometers have a total solids (TS) scale. On a g/dL basis, most dissolved solids are proteins; other solids include electrolytes, urea, glucose, and other chemical analytes.
        4. High concentrations of lipids (as seen in chylous effusions) will increase the fluid's refractive index and produce falsely increased values for [TP_{ref}] and SG. High concentrations of solutes other than proteins (e.g., urea in uroperitoneum) will also falsely increase the TP_{ref} value.
        5. Suspended cells typically do not interfere with refractometric values, because the cells do not alter refractive index significantly (see the Physical Examination of Urine section in Chapter 8). However, extremely high cell concentrations (> 100.0 × 10^3/μL) may. Whenever in doubt, the values of fluid with suspended cells can be compared to the fluid's supernatant.
        6. A variety of decision thresholds for [TP_{ref}] have been proposed for differentiating effusions. However, several factors determine an effusion's [TP_{ref}], so such decision thresholds should be considered as suggested guidelines.
            a. A lower [TP_{ref}] (usually < 2.0 g/dL and frequently near 1.0 g/dL) is found primarily in protein-poor transudates and early in uroperitoneal effusions.
            b. A [TP_{ref}] > 2.0 g/dL is found in most other effusions. Typically, the greater the [TP_{ref}] is, the greater is the protein permeability of blood vessels.
        7. One study described a falsely increased [TP_{ref}] (e.g., ≈ 1.5 g/dL increase) when peritoneal fluid was added to an EDTA tube that also contained additives to prevent crystallization of the EDTA.[40] Not all commercial EDTA tubes contain the additive,

Table 19.6. Conversion of refractive indices to [TP$_{ref}$], [total solids], or specific gravity (SG) values[a]

Refractive index	Plasma [TP$_{ref}$] (g/dL)	Plasma [TS] (g/dL)	Urine SG	Plasma SG[b]
1.3368	1.0	2.1	1.011	1.010
1.3376	1.5	2.5	1.013	1.011
1.3386	2.0	3.1	1.017	1.012
1.3396	2.5	3.7	1.019	1.014
1.3406	3.0	4.2	1.021	1.015
1.3416	3.5	4.8	1.024	1.016
1.3426	4.0	5.3	1.027	1.018
1.3436	4.5	5.9	1.029	1.019
1.3444	5.0	6.3	1.031	1.020
1.3454	5.5	6.9	1.033	1.021
1.3464	6.0	7.5	1.035	1.023

[a] The table includes data for [TP$_{ref}$] from 1.0 to 6.0 g/dL at 0.5 g/dL intervals. The table provided by American Optical has TP data for each 0.1 g/dL. Because the relationships are nearly linear, other values can be estimated by interpolation.

[b] Values are rounded to the nearest thousandth so they can more easily be compared with the urine SG values.

and, by itself, the EDTA (at the recommended concentration) had minimal effect on the fluid's refractive index if the EDTA tube was at least one-third full. Refractometry can be used to assess EDTA tubes for their potential to falsely increase [TP$_{ref}$] values (i.e., by assessing the fluid refractometrically prior to and after adding different volumes of it to EDTA tubes).

C. Refractometric estimates of specific gravity (SG)

1. The SG scale is calibrated for urine and will approximate the true SG of a protein-poor and glucose-poor fluid because most of the fluid's refractive index is due to electrolytes (therefore, similar to urine refractive properties).

2. Clinical refractometers do not have a scale for *plasma* SG, but Leica, American Optical, and other refractometer manufacturers provide tables to convert *plasma* refractive index to *plasma* SG.[41] In Table 19.6, note that the difference in the SG values (urine versus plasma) becomes greater as the [TP$_{ref}$] increases. Also note that the total solids (TS) concentration is not equivalent to the [TP$_{ref}$].

3. If a laboratory reports a SG for a body fluid, the value might be a "urine SG" (if taken from refractometer scale) or a "plasma SG" (if taken from a conversion table). Some published methods of classifying effusions use [TP$_{ref}$] and SG values. If a SG of 1.017 or 1.019 is a decision threshold, the SG value was from the urine SG scale. A refractive index of 1.3386 converts to a urine SG of 1.017 and a plasma SG of 1.012 (Table 19.6).

4. Using the refractometer to estimate urine SG is very useful because the SG values typically reflect changes in urine osmolality (see Chapter 8). However, plasma SG or osmolality values typically do not help with the interpretation of effusions.

III. Chemical analysis

A. As described in the previous section, an effusion's [TP] is routinely estimated by measuring its refractive index. A chemical assay to measure [TP] may be used, but additional expense may not be warranted.

B. The concentrations of urea, Crt, cholesterol, TG, electrolytes, and other substances are occasionally measured to characterize some effusions (see the Selected Analyses for Pleural and Peritoneal Effusions section).

IV. [Erythrocyte] or hematocrit (Hct)

A. Either an [erythrocyte] or a Hct should be determined when the effusion is pink to red, so that those values can be compared with peripheral blood [erythrocyte] or Hct. The analytic methods used for measuring [erythrocyte] or Hct in peripheral blood (see Chapter 3) typically can be used for effusions, but the values may be lower than the assay's detection limit.

B. Effusions other than transudates typically contain a few erythrocytes either because the pathologic disorder is causing minor blood vessel damage or because the collected fluid was contaminated with peripheral blood during collection. However, the [erythrocyte] in most pink effusions is typically very low (Hct < 3 %, [erythrocyte] < $0.5 \times 10^{6}/\mu L$); such values do not represent a hemorrhagic effusion.

C. When hemorrhage is a major contributor to the formation of the effusion, the [erythrocyte] (or Hct value) can approach the values found in an animal's peripheral blood. Soon after hemorrhage into a cavity, the [erythrocyte] decreases because of the resorption of erythrocytes via the lymphatic vessels and the altered oncotic pressure gradients that promote fluid movement from interstitium to the body cavity.

V. [Total nucleated cell concentration] (TNCC)

A. Because pleural and peritoneal fluids contain leukocytes, mesothelial cells, and potentially other nucleated cells, it is appropriate to refer to their concentration as a TNCC instead of a [leukocyte]. However, the electronic and manual methods of determining leukocyte concentrations (see Chapter 2) will provide adequate TNCC values for most fluids. If the nucleated cells are present in clumps or tissue fragments, the measured TNCC will be less than the true concentration.

B. The hemocytometer method of measuring TNCC is usually recommended if the fluid is grossly abnormal, because the fluid may contain clumps of cells, debris, or other material that could plug the small tubing or orifices of electronic cell counters.

C. By itself, an effusion's TNCC has limited value for determining the cause of an effusion. The lowest TNCC values (frequently < $1.0 \times 10^{3}/\mu L$) are found in protein-poor transudates. The greatest TNCC values (occasionally > $100.0 \times 10^{3}/\mu L$) are found in exudates and neoplastic lymphoid effusions.

VI. Microscopic examination

A. When cavitary effusions are clear and colorless (i.e., look like H_2O and therefore are protein-poor and cell-poor transudates), a microscopic examination of the fluid typically yields very little useful information. For all other effusions, the microscopic examination of stained cytopreparations is frequently the most important part of the fluid analysis. Part of the microscopic examination is the examination of cells, but examination of other structures and features is frequently important.

1. Stains designed for blood films are frequently used for the routine staining of cytopreparations. One major advantage of using the blood stains is that people are familiar with the staining of blood cells and similar features are found in the nucleated cells of effusions.

    2. The microscopic examination should include all parts of one or more cytoprepara-tions because of the potential uneven distribution of cells and other microscopic structures.

B. Major aspects of the examination are as follows:

    1. Nucleated cell differential count is done to determine percentages of each nucleated cell; the count is completed by either a subjective estimate or an objective enumera-tion. With a measured TNCC and a nucleated cell differential count, approximate concentrations of each cell type can be calculated and interpreted. For example, 60 % neutrophils in a fluid with a TNCC of $1.0 \times 10^3/\mu L$ is interpreted differently than 60 % neutrophils in a fluid with a TNCC of $100.0 \times 10^3/\mu L$. If cell concentra-tions are calculated from the percentages, they probably should be considered crude estimates because of the inaccuracies of TNCC values and the nucleated cell differential counts.

    2. Some people include mesothelial cells in the differential cell count, and others do not. If they are not included, it is more difficult to interpret the TNCC, and concentrations of other nucleated cells cannot be calculated or consistently esti-mated. Mesothelial cells are often in clusters, so their inclusion may lead to increased variability of the differential count, depending on whether clusters of cells were present in the counting region. Variability is also a problem for other cell types when they are clumped.

    3. During the examination, diagnostic features of cells are identified; for example, size, shape, nuclear features, and cytoplasmic features, including inclusions or microorganisms.

    4. If present, extracellular structures such as microorganisms, debris, and other material are identified.

C. Cells that are routinely identified in pleural and peritoneal fluids.

    1. Neutrophils

       a. Generally, an increased [neutrophil] in an effusion indicates that exudation is a component of the effusion formation. However, exudation may be the primary reason for the effusion, or exudation may have occurred after another process created the effusion.

       b. The neutrophils in effusions may have microscopic features that are similar to those seen in blood films; if so, they are called *nondegenerate neutrophils* (Plate 14A and B) [for all plates, see the color section of this book]. The presence of nondegenerate neutrophils in body fluids suggests a nonbacterial cause of the effusion, but such neutrophils can be found in bacterial exudates. For example, neutrophils adjacent to colonies of *Actinomyces* or *Nocardia* may have degenerate features, but other neutrophils in the exudate may not (Plate 14C).

       c. Degenerate neutrophils are cells that have acquired certain structural defects after they have left the blood. Microscopic features of the classic degenerate neutrophil include a swollen and pale-staining nucleus, lack of nuclear chromatin patterns, and variable degrees of cytoplasmic vacuolization (Plate 14C and D).

         (1) There are many variations between the severely degenerate and nondegener-ate cells, so it may be difficult to classify the cells consistently.

         (2) A degenerate neutrophil is not a toxic neutrophil. Toxic neutrophils develop their structural features in bone marrow and typically are seen in blood or marrow samples. Microscopic features of degenerate neutrophils reflect events that occur after neutrophils leave the vascular system.

(3) Nondegenerate neutrophils can deteriorate within hours of sample collection, and thus they may acquire features resembling degenerate neutrophils. Therefore, it may be difficult to differentiate degenerative change from in vitro deterioration if cytopreparations were not made soon after sample collection.

d. Differentiating nondegenerate from degenerate or deteriorated neutrophils is less important than searching for direct evidence of the cause of the inflammation, because degenerate-appearing neutrophils may occur without sepsis and nondegenerate neutrophils may occur with sepsis. However, the presence of degenerate neutrophils suggests that the search for organisms should be more intense.

2. Lymphocytes
   a. The lymphocytes in most effusions resemble the small lymphocytes that are typically seen in peripheral blood films. These cells have small nuclei (with diameters < 10 μm in areas where cells are well spread), clumped chromatin patterns, and small amounts of blue cytoplasm (Plates 14E and 15L).
   b. When they have been stimulated, the lymphocytes may have features of reactive lymphocytes, plasmacytoid lymphocytes, or plasma cells (Plate 14F).
   c. Neoplastic lymphocytes (Plate 14H and I) frequently have nuclei with diameters ≥ 10 μm and finely granular to homogeneous chromatin patterns. Frequently, the cells have moderate amounts of deeply basophilic cytoplasm. The cells may have prominent or large nucleoli.
   d. In some effusions, differentiating neoplastic from reactive (proplastic) lymphocytes can be very difficult or impossible based on their microscopic features. Then, other diagnostic methods (e.g., assessment of associated abnormal solid tissue mass) may be needed to determine whether the lymphocytes are neoplastic.

3. Mesothelial cells
   a. *Mesothelial cells* are of mesodermal origin and occur as individual cells or sheets of squamous-like epithelial cells in health. They have round to oval nuclei and usually moderate amounts of pale blue cytoplasm. Individual cells usually are round to oval; cells in sheets can be polyhedral (Plate 14I and J).
   b. *Reactive mesothelial cells*, which are round to oval, have varying degrees of increased cytoplasmic basophilia and/or hyperchromatic nuclei (Plate 14K and L). These proplastic cells may be multinucleated or have mitotic nuclei. The cells may have small cytoplasmic vacuoles.
   c. Besides their structural functions, mesothelial cells are involved in inflammatory responses of pleural and peritoneal cavities, including antigen presentation, cytokine production, release of oxidants and proteases, and promotion of the migration of neutrophils.[42–44]

4. Macrophages
   a. Outside of the vascular system, monocytes transform into macrophages or histiocytes. Cells with the appearance of monocytes, macrophages, or transition phases occur in fluids, but they may all be lumped into a macrophage category once the cells have left the vasculature.
   b. The cytoplasms of macrophages frequently contain vacuoles, lipid, or cellular debris, and might contain engulfed cells (e.g., erythrocytes and leukocytes), organisms, or foreign material (Plate 14M–O). Cells, organisms, or foreign material may undergo phagocytosis within 30 min in vitro (Plate 14O).

> (1) Erythrophages are relatively common in effusions when blood contaminates a fluid that contains activated macrophages and when cytopreparations are not made soon after sample collection.
>
> (2) Leukophages are relatively common in some fluids, especially in the peritoneal fluid of horses. Frequently, the leukophages contain neutrophils at various stages of degradation (Plate 14B).

5. Mononuclear cells

a. The term is often used collectively for cells that are not granulocytes or mast cells (though they also have only one nucleus). Most so-called mononuclear cells in effusions are lymphocytes, macrophages, or mesothelial cells, and they can be categorized as such in most cases.

b. In well-prepared, well-stained cytopreparations, most small lymphocytes and macrophages that have vacuolated cytoplasms or contain engulfed material are easily recognized. However, some reactive lymphocytes and smaller monocytoid or histiocytic cells are not easily differentiated. Typically, those cells are part of an inflammatory response, and accurate differentiation is probably not needed.

c. Very degenerate neutrophils may be mistaken for macrophages and therefore so-called mononuclear cells. This is most common with bacterial exudates.

d. Some histiocytic cells and reactive mesothelial cells have similar nuclear and cytoplasmic features. If the microscopist is not confident of the cell's lineages, they can be called large mononuclear cells. Such a classification probably will not alter the interpretation of the fluid analysis results because these cells typically are relatively minor contributors to the TNCC.

6. Erythrocytes are found in nearly all samples. Abnormal microscopic features often represent artifacts (e.g., membrane spicules, hypochromia, and refractile membranes) but may reflect pathologic states (e.g., acanthocytes, polychromasia, and associated organisms). Findings suspected to represent a pathologic state should be confirmed by finding the same abnormality in a stained film of fresh blood.

a. If the hemorrhagic effusion has been present for at least a few hours, erythrophages may be found;[45] it may take 2–4 d for siderophages to appear.[45,46] Also, hematoidin crystals may be found in macrophages.

b. Erythrophages, siderophages, and other macrophages become a more prominent feature of effusions the longer the blood has been in a cavity.

c. When the hemorrhage is caused by a nontraumatic event (e.g., hemorrhagic neoplasm), frequently there is either recurring hemorrhage or persistent low-grade hemorrhage. Thus, the effusion may have properties of both an acute hemorrhagic effusion (i.e., high Hct value) and a chronic hemorrhagic effusion (i.e., siderophages).

d. If the making of a cytopreparation was delayed for a few hours or less in some cases, then the presence of erythrophages may represent in vitro phagocytosis.

D. Platelets can be found in collected samples. The presence of platelets suggests ongoing (or very recent) hemorrhage or contamination of fluid with peripheral blood during collection. Clots indicate fibrinogen was in the sample, but the fibrinogen could be present because of exudation, hemorrhage, or blood contamination.

E. Nucleated cells that are less commonly found in pleural and peritoneal fluids.

1. Eosinophils usually have features similar to those seen in peripheral blood (Plate 15A).

2. The presence of relatively few mast cells are not unusual in exudates and are also found in other effusions (e.g., heart failure effusions). Unless the cells have prominent microscopic features of malignancy, neoplastic and nonneoplastic mast cells cannot be reliably differentiated via microscopy.

3. Neoplastic cells are not common in effusions (Plate 15B–D). More information on neoplastic cells is found in Comments About Specific Effusions, sect. III.

4. Occasionally, cells from tissues are found in effusions. Hepatocytes are occasionally found as contaminants in pleural and peritoneal fluids. Squamous epithelial cells from skin may enter the fluid during the collection process, but they may also be present in equine peritoneal effusions because of gastric rupture (Plate 14D) or squamous cell carcinoma (Plate 15D).

F. Noncellular findings.

1. Organisms (primarily bacteria and fungi) can be found in exudates.

   a. Most bacteria stain dark purple, dark grey, or dark blue with a Romanowsky stain (see Chapter 2) and usually can be identified as cocci or bacilli (Plate 15E and F).

   b. *Mycobacterium* spp. do not stain with a Romanowsky stain and therefore appear as white or clear bacilli.

   c. *Actinomyces* and *Nocardia* may not be uniformly distributed in an exudate. Squash preparation of yellow particulates (*sulfur granules*) in an exudate may reveal a colony of filamentous, beaded, branching bacilli consistent with such bacteria (Plate 14C). *Fusobacterium* bacteria may also be beaded and filamentous but do not branch.

   d. Dead or damaged bacteria may stain a variety of colors from red to light grey or light purple. The shapes of the dead organisms may be different from those that were live when the sample was prepared for examination.

   e. Fungi may appear as yeasts (e.g., *Blastomyces* or *Histoplasma*), hyphae (e.g., *Aspergillus* or *Mucor*), or yeasts and pseudohyphae (*Candida*) (Plate 15G). Most yeasts will have a positive staining reaction with a Wright stain (i.e., blues or purples), but hyphae may have negative reactions. Nonstaining hyphae can be detected as delineated linear structures that are displacing cells and other stained material.

   f. Larvae of *Mesocestoides* sp. may be found in dogs with peritoneal cestoidiasis.[47]

   g. Large ciliated protozoa (e.g., *Balantidium* sp., *Polymorphella* sp., and *Cycloposthium* sp.) may be found in equine peritoneal exudates or in intestinal taps (Plate 15H)[48] The protozoa typically are commensal inhabitants of equine intestines but may be secondary invaders of diseased intestinal mucosa.

2. Other material that can be found in exudates and lipid effusions includes urine crystals (Plate 15I), sperm (Plate 15J), bilirubin crystals, bile (Plate 15K), mucus, plant material, barium crystals (Plate 14N), and lipid droplets (Plate 15L). Sudanophilic droplets can be identified in the fluid and in macrophages by using a Sudan stain (Plate 15L). To look for Sudanophilic droplets, Sudan stain is placed on top of an air-dried cytopreparation of the effusion, and then a coverslip is placed on top of the liquid. Via microscopy, the Sudanophilic droplets appear as round, orange to red structures that tend to float (just under the coverslip) or are within macrophages.

3. The staining intensity of the space between cells tends to be greater when the fluid has a high [TP]. A drying artifact may create protein crescents when the [TP] is increased (Plate 15N).

Table 19.7. The [TG], [cholesterol], and Chol:TG ratios in chylous and nonchylous effusions of dogs and cats

	Canine effusions		Feline effusions	
	Chylous	Nonchylous	Chylous	Nonchylous
Fossum study[a]				
Number in group	6	3	4	5
Cholesterol (mg/dL)	37–127	48–139	38–232	65–111
Triglyceride (mg/dL)	45–2,687	8–33	91–4,670	0–59
Chol:TG ratio	0.04–0.15	3.88–6.00	0.05–0.70	1.88–110.00
Waddle study[b]				
Number in group	6	17	13	12
Cholesterol (mg/dL)	23–70	3–119	18–148	16–107
Triglyceride (mg/dL)	110–610	3–83	130–3490	23–93
Chol:TG ratio	0.04–0.64	0.33–27.33	0.01–0.64	0.23–7.64

[a] *Source*: Fossum et al.[49]
[b] *Source*: Waddle and Giger[50]

SELECTED ANALYSES FOR PLEURAL AND PERITONEAL EFFUSIONS

I. [Cholesterol] and [TG]
    A. If a diagnostician suspects an effusion is chylous, but the routine analysis does not provide enough evidence for a firm conclusion, measuring the [cholesterol] and [TG] of the effusion and the animal's serum may provide data to differentiate chylous and nonchylous effusions.
    B. In a study involving dogs and cats,[49] effusions were considered to be chylous if there was microscopic appearance of chylomicrons (i.e., Sudanophilic droplets), the sample could not be cleared with centrifugation, or the fluid did clear after the addition of ether. Effusions were classified as nonchylous if they did not meet the chylous effusion criteria. The results of the study are in Table 19.7.
        1. As would be expected with the presence of Sudanophilic droplets in the chylous effusions but not in the nonchylous effusions, the triglyceride concentrations were greater in the chylous than in the nonchylous. Also the Chol:TG ratios were much smaller in the chylous effusions because of the greater triglyceride concentrations.
        2. The diagnoses for dogs with chylous effusions included thoracic lymphangiectasia, intestinal lymphangiectasia, and aortic body tumor.
        3. The diagnoses for cats with chylous effusions included thoracic lymphangiectasia, diaphragmatic hernia, cardiomyopathy, and metastatic pulmonary adenocarcinoma.
    C. In another study involving dogs and cats,[50] effusions were considered to be chylous effusions if lipoprotein electrophoresis revealed a distinct chylomicron band at the origin of the electrophoretic pattern.
        1. The major findings in this study's laboratory data were as follows (Table 19.7):
            a. Each chylous effusion had a [TG] >100 mg/dL, and each nonchylous effusions had a [TG] < 100 mg/dL.
            b. Each chylous effusions had a Chol:TG ratio < 1, whereas most nonchylous effusions had Chol:TG ratios > 1.

      c. Grossly, nearly all chylous effusions had white, milky appearances after centrifugation, whereas none of the nonchylous effusions had that appearance.

    2. The diagnoses for dogs with chylous effusion included lymphoma, venous thrombosis, cardiomyopathy, and idiopathic chylothorax.

    3. The diagnoses for cats with chylous effusion included cardiomyopathy, diaphragmatic hernia, pericardial effusion, and idiopathic chylothorax.

D. Cholesterol and TG assays that are designed for serum samples (see Chapter 16) typically can be used to analyze the supernatant of suspected chylous effusions. When the sample looks like milk, the sample may need to be diluted before the [TG] is measured.

II. [Urea] and [Crt]

A. When a diagnosis of uroperitoneum is being considered, the measurement of the [urea] and [Crt] in the peritoneal fluid and a time-matched serum sample may help establish a diagnosis. It is important that the effusion concentrations be compared with recent serum concentrations because of the rapid diffusion of urea and Crt from the cavitary fluid to lymph and blood.

B. Urea and Crt are small molecules that diffuse through capillary walls; urea diffuses quicker than Crt. In health and most pathologic states that create effusions, the serum and peritoneal fluid concentrations of urea and Crt are nearly the same.

C. When there is a recent addition of urine to peritoneal fluid, the resulting fluid will have a greater [urea] and [Crt] than plasma concentrations because the [urea] and [Crt] in urine are typically much greater than plasma or serum concentrations. With time and with diffusion of molecules due to concentration gradients, the [urea] and [Crt] in the extravascular and intravascular fluids will become similar again, and both will be increased.

    1. After 45 h of experimentally induced uroperitoneum, the [Crt] in the peritoneal fluid was about twice the serum [Crt]: The mean peritoneal fluid [Crt] was 11.6 mg/dL (range, 5.5–15.6 mg/dL), whereas the mean serum [Crt] was 5.2 mg/dL (range, 1.2–6.7 mg/dL). However, the [urea] in the effusion and serum at 45 h were nearly the same. These data support the fact that urea enters the blood faster than does Crt. Azotemia (either an increased [urea] or [Crt]) was detectable in a few dogs within 5 h but in all 11 dogs by 21 h after "rupture." The serum [urea] and [Crt] continued to increase over the 3 d study.[51]

    2. In a retrospective study of 13 dogs with uroperitoneum, the creatinine concentrations in peritoneal fluid were at least twice the "blood" concentrations in 11 dogs. The durations of the spontaneous conditions were not known. (Note: The authors did not specify whether the "blood" creatinine concentrations were serum or plasma concentrations.)[52] The ratios for eight dogs with other peritoneal effusions were from 0.7 to 1.2.

    3. Ratios of peritoneal fluid [Crt] to serum [Crt] have been reported for other animals with uroperitoneum: foals (mean, 3.5; and range, 2.7–4.6),[53] horses (> 2.0),[54] and cats (mean, 2.0 and range, 0.8–2.4).[55] The ratios can be used as a guideline in the interpretation of data, but other aspects of the case should be carefully considered. For example, a cat with a urinary tract obstruction may have been severely azotemic before the uroperitoneum occurred. Thus, the ratio may not be > 2 when the cat is first examined.

D. Urea (or urea nitrogen) and Crt assays that are designed for serum samples (see Chapter 8) typically can be used to analyze the supernatant of suspected uroperitoneal effusions. For some assays, the sample may need to be diluted before analysis to obtain analyte concentrations within the assay's analytical range.

III.   [Na$^+$], [Cl$^-$], and [K$^+$]

A. Na$^+$, Cl$^-$, and K$^+$ are freely diffusible through most capillary walls, and thus their concentrations in plasma, interstitial fluids, and most pleural and peritoneal effusions are nearly the same. The major exception to this concept occurs in uroperitoneum. Compared to plasma and most extracellular fluids, the urine [Na$^+$] and [Cl$^-$] are less and the urine [K$^+$] are greater. Thus, in the early stages of uroperitoneum, the peritoneal fluid [Na$^+$] and [Cl$^-$] will be less than plasma concentrations, and the peritoneal fluid [K$^+$] will be greater than plasma concentrations. With time, diffusion of electrolytes and H$_2$O will reduce the differences.

B. In a retrospective study of 26 cases of feline uroperitoneum, the [K$^+$] was measured in five cats. The ratios of the peritoneal fluid [K$^+$] to serum [K$^+$] ranged from 0.9 to 2.4, with a mean of 1.2.[55]

C. In a retrospective study of 13 dogs with uroperitoneum, ratios of the peritoneal fluid [K$^+$] to the "blood" [K$^+$] were ≥ 1.4 in all dogs (median, 2.7; and range, 1.4–4.9). (Note: The authors did not specify whether the "blood" [K$^+$] was a serum or plasma concentration.)[52] The ratios for eight dogs with other peritoneal effusions ranged from 0.7 to 1.2.

D. In an experimental production of uroperitoneum in dogs, hyponatremia and hypochloremia were apparent between 1 and 2 d and pronounced by 4 d. Hyperkalemia was apparent in some dogs by 2 d and in nearly all dogs by 4 d.[51]

E. Assays designed for serum [Na$^+$], [K$^+$], and [Cl$^-$] (see Chapter 9) may not provide accurate electrolyte concentrations in the supernatant of cavitary effusions. Some ion-selective electrode methods require a proteinaceous fluid, so urine or a uroperitoneal effusion may not be acceptable. Anions other than Cl$^-$ may react with the electrodes of the Cl$^-$ assay. For cellular samples, measured [K$^+$] might include K$^+$ released from cells either in vivo or in vitro.

IV.   [L-lactate]

A. L-lactate is the product of anaerobic glycolysis, and one reason for hyperlactatemia is tissue hypoxia (see Chapter 9). The L-lactate produced by cells may enter venous blood to cause hyperlactatemia but also may enter interstitial fluids and diffuse into pleural or peritoneal fluids. An increased [L-lactate] in pleural and peritoneal fluids may be a marker of increased anaerobic glycolysis in the body cavities.

B. An increased [L-lactate] in peritoneal fluids has been found in animals with strangulated and nonstrangulated intestinal obstructions, abdominal neoplasms, and bacterial exudates.

1. The [L-lactate] in peritoneal fluids was greater in colicky horses with intestinal ischemia secondary to strangulating obstruction (8.5 ± 5.5 mmol/L, mean ± standard deviation) compared to colicky horses with nonstrangulating obstruction (2.1 ± 2.1 mmol/L) and healthy horses (0.6 ± 0.2 mmol/L).[56] The [L-lactate] in equine peritoneal fluid is used as an indicator of the severity of intestinal ischemia in colicky horses.

2. The [L-lactate] in peritoneal effusions was greater in dogs with intra-abdominal neoplasms (hemangiosarcoma, carcinomatosis, neuroendocrine tumor, metastatic

adenocarcinoma, and pancreatic carcinoma) (3.8 ± 1.7 mmol/L, mean ± standard deviation) than in dogs that did not have abdominal neoplasms (1.7 ± 0.5 mmol/L).[57] The greater [L-lactate] in the neoplastic group could be due to increased anaerobic glycolysis by neoplastic cells or to the neoplasms interfering with blood supply to nonneoplastic tissue.

3. The [L-lactate] in peritoneal effusions was greater in dogs and cats with bacterial exudates than in dogs and cats that had nonbacterial peritoneal effusions caused by a variety of disorders.[58,59]

   a. In the dogs of one study, the [L-lactate] was 4.2 (3.8–8.4) mmol/L (median and range) in the bacterial exudates (n = 3) and 1.9 (1.1–5.7) mmol/L (median and range) in the nonbacterial effusions (n = 4).[58] Similar data were found in another 8 dogs with bacterial exudates and 11 dogs with nonbacterial effusions.[59]

   b. In cats of one study, the [L-lactate] was 6.2 (1.3–10.6) mmol/L (median and range) in the bacterial exudates (n = 5) and 1.4 (1.2–1.6) mmol/L (median and range) in the nonbacterial effusions (n = 2).[58] Similar data were found in another nine cats with bacterial exudates, but a wider range of values was found in nine other cats with nonbacterial effusions.[59]

   c. The differences between peritoneal fluid [L-lactate] and plasma [L-lactate] were usually greater in the bacterial exudate group than in the nonbacterial group. A difference greater than 2 mmol/L was suggested as an indicator of septic peritonitis;[58] the same criterion would have incorrectly classified three of eight dogs and five of nine cats in the second study.[59] The pathogenesis of the increased [L-lactate] in the bacterial exudates was not explained, but at least two explanations are possible:

      (1) Bacteria can produce both L-lactate and D-lactate, and thus bacteria could be a source of the L-lactate in the bacterial exudates.

      (2) L-lactate could also be produced by leukocytes and erythrocytes in the exudate. Cell concentrations in the bacterial effusions tended to be greater than those in the nonbacterial effusions.

4. The [L-lactate] in peritoneal fluid was increased within 2 h of experimental intestinal strangulation in dogs and continued to increase during the 24 h experiment. The plasma [L-lactate] changed very little in the survivor group, but increased rapidly after 8 h in the nonsurvivor group.[60]

C. Assays designed for serum or plasma [L-lactate] (see Chapter 9) typically can be used to analyze the supernatant of effusions. Interpretation of effusion [L-lactate] should also consider that erythrocytes and leukocytes are a potential source of L-lactate. Also, L-lactate could be produced by cells in the effusion after sample collection, and thus samples need to be processed and analyzed quickly. If samples cannot be analyzed quickly, the fluid could be placed in sodium fluoride tubes (see Chapter 9) or the cells removed from the effusion.

V. [Glucose]

A. Because glucose in a peritoneal effusion comes from plasma, it is important to interpret the [glucose] in effusions with knowledge of the plasma or serum [glucose].

B. The glucose concentrations in peritoneal effusions were less in dogs and cats with bacterial exudates than in dogs and cats that had nonbacterial peritoneal effusions caused by a variety of disorders.[58]

1. In dogs, the glucose concentrations were 57 mmol/L (median) in the bacterial exudates (n = 7) and 137 (51–322) mmol/L (median and range) in the nonbacterial effusions (n = 11).

2. In cats, the glucose concentrations were 100 (39–234) mmol/L (median and range) in the bacterial exudates (n = 7) and 141 (107–224) mmol/L (median and range) in the nonbacterial effusions (n = 5).

3. The glucose concentrations in bacterial exudates were less than the corresponding blood glucose concentrations in all dogs and nearly all cats. The authors suggested that a difference of 20 mg/dL or more indicates a bacterial exudate. However, the TNCCs in all nonbacterial effusions were < 13.0 × 10³/μL, and nearly all bacterial exudates had greater TNCC values. Thus, the differences in [glucose] may have been due to differences in nucleated cell concentrations and not due to the presence of bacteria.

C. Glucose assays that are designed for serum or plasma samples (see Chapter 14) typically can be used to analyze the supernatant of effusions. Glucose will be consumed by cells in the effusion, and thus samples should be analyzed soon after collection. If samples cannot be analyzed quickly, the fluid could be placed in sodium fluoride tubes (see Chapter 14) or the cells removed from the effusion.

VI. [Bilirubin]

A. Because conjugated bilirubin is diffusible and plasma proteins are present in most nontransudative effusions, the [bilirubin] in most effusions should be similar to the serum [bilirubin]. The major exception to this concept is seen with bile peritonitis and the formation of a bilious exudate. When damage to bile ducts or gallbladder results in the leakage of bile into the peritoneal cavity, peritonitis will develop and the resultant exudate will have an increased [bilirubin].

B. There are several potential causes of bile entering the peritoneal cavity, including blunt or penetrating trauma, bile duct rupture secondary to manual expression of the gallbladder, necrotizing cholecystitis or cholangitis, cholelithiasis, and neoplasia of the biliary tissues.[61]

C. When the effusion develops secondary to bile leakage, results of fluid analysis reveal the presence of an exudate that typically has a [TP$_{ref}$] > 2.5 g/dL, a TNCC > 5.0 × 10³/μL, and > 80 % neutrophils.[61]

1. Microscopic examination may detect a small to large amount of intracellular or extracellular amorphous yellow to brown bile pigment, or bilirubin crystals, extracellularly or in macrophages.

2. If the bile leakage is secondary to a bacterial infection, the exudate may contain intracellular or extracellular bacteria.

3. Typically, the [bilirubin] in the bile-containing effusions will be at least twice an animal's serum [bilirubin].[61,62]

4. When a gallbladder lesion enables its mucoid secretion (called white bile) to enter the peritoneal cavity, the resultant effusion may contain light basophilic mucinous material when stained with a Romanowsky stain.[62]

D. Results of blood and urine analysis will depend on the cause and duration of the biliary tract leakage; for example, if the animal had obstructive cholestasis prior to bile leakage, hyperbilirubinemia may have preceded the bile peritonitis. However, with trauma-induced bile leakage, the hyperbilirubinemia occurs after the onset of the bile peritonitis. Likewise, an inflammatory leukocytosis may be the result of a bacterial cholangitis that causes bile leakage, or an inflammatory leukocytosis may occur after the onset of acute bile peritonitis.

E. Bilirubin assays that are designed for serum or plasma samples (see Chapter 13) typically can be used to analyze the supernatant of effusions. Bilirubin is degraded by ultraviolet light, and thus effusions should be handled and stored to limit the sample's exposure to light.

VII. [Ammonium]

A. The [ammonium] in peritoneal fluid was increased 24 h after experimental intestinal strangulation in dogs. The increase in the [ammonium] in the effusion may be caused by ammonium passing through devitalized intestinal tissue. The plasma [ammonium] changed very little in the study.[60]

B. Ammonium assays that are designed for plasma samples (see Chapter 13) typically can be used to analyze the supernatant of effusions. In vitro factors can alter the [ammonium] in the collected sample (see Chapter 13).

VIII. Protein concentrations

A. With the possible exception of immunoglobulins, the proteins detected in effusions represent those that leaked through capillary walls. The greater amount of protein and the larger proteins can pass through the more protein-permeable capillaries.

B. Protein electrophoresis

1. Protein electrophoresis of pleural and peritoneal fluid (especially if paired with serum protein electrophoresis) will provide information about the permeability of capillary beds. If the [TP] of the fluid is < 2.0 g/dL, the fluid may need be concentrated before electrophoresis.

2. In FIP exudates, the electrophoretic patterns of the cat's exudative effusion and its serum are very similar because the disorder's vasculitis enables plasma proteins to ooze into the pleural or peritoneal fluid.

C. In people, a pleural effusion [TP] to serum [TP] ratio > 0.5 is indicative of exudation if the effusion does not contain blood.[63]

D. In people, a serum albumin-ascites gradient (serum [albumin] – effusion [albumin]) has been used to help differentiate peritoneal effusions caused by portal hypertension (e.g., cirrhosis and congestive heart failure) from effusions caused by malignancies or inflammatory states; the gradient is greater in the portal hypertension disorders than in the other disorders.[64] Most dogs with transudates caused by hepatic cirrhosis had a serum albumin-ascites gradient > 1.1 g/dL, but so did about half of the dogs that had effusions caused by neoplasia, pancreatitis, congestive heart failure, protein-losing enteropathy, and other disorders.[65]

E. Concentrations of specific proteins can be measured in effusions, but the data available are insufficient to establish the diagnostic value of such concentrations; for example, concentrations of α_1-acid glycoprotein were greater in plasma and peritoneal fluid of cats with FIP than in healthy cats.[66,67] Because α_1-acid glycoprotein is a positive acute-phase protein (see Chapter 7), similar findings would be expected in cats with exudative effusions not caused by FIP, but such documentation is not available.

F. TP and albumin assays that are designed for serum or plasma samples (see Chapter 7) typically can be used to analyze the supernatant of effusions. The [TP] or [albumin] might be below the assays' analytical ranges in some effusions. The bromcresol green assay for [albumin] may not provide an accurate concentration if the dye binds to globulins. Assays for some proteins may need to be species specific.

IX. Enzyme activity
  A. Lipase activity: Peritoneal fluids from dogs with acute pancreatitis had much greater lipase activity than other peritoneal effusions and were at least double the animal's serum lipase activity.[68]
  B. Alkaline phosphatase: In horses with colic or intestinal lesions, ALP activity may increase in the peritoneal fluid predominantly because of increased granulocytic ALP activity,[69] but other data suggest that intestinal ALP may contribute.[70] The magnitude of increased total ALP activity in peritoneal fluid was greater in horses with peritonitis and intestinal rupture than in horses with strangulated and nonstrangulated intestinal disorders; the study's analytical methods did not enable the identification of the ALP isoform that produced the increase.[71,72] The granulocytic and intestinal ALP did not increase total ALP activity in serum.[69,70]
  C. Most enzyme assays that are designed for serum or plasma samples (see Chapter 12) typically can be used to analyze the supernatant of effusions.

X. Gram staining
  A. Gram stain is used to different bacteria into two large groups: Gram-positive bacteria and Gram-negative bacteria. The Gram stain involves two major steps: (1) staining a bacterium's cell wall with a dye (either methyl violet or crystal violet) and iodine, and (2) attempting to decolorize the cell wall by using ethanol or acetone solution. In theory, the dye-iodine complex becomes fixed in the Gram-positive organisms and thus they retain the dark purple stain, whereas the dye-iodine complex is dissolved out of the cell walls of the Gram-negative organisms to produce pink organisms.
  B. The Gram stain is designed for staining of bacteria selected from colonies grown in a variety of culture media, and it is difficult to apply the stain to cellular samples or proteinaceous effusions uniformly and consistently. When the stain is applied to air-dried smears or films of effusions, several factors should be considered:
    1. Dead Gram-positive organisms frequently have a Gram-negative reaction; that is, the stain does not remain in the cell walls of dead Gram-positive bacteria during decolorization.
    2. Using too little ethanol or acetone may produce a false Gram-positive reaction, whereas using too much ethanol or acetone may produce a false Gram-negative reaction.
    3. Cell debris, especially from nuclei, has a Gram-negative reaction, and thus Gram-negative bacteria can be difficult to locate among Gram-negative cellular debris.
    4. If used diagnostically, a set of known Gram-positive and Gram-negative slides prepared from cellular effusions should be stained concurrently to serve as positive and negative control slides.
    5. The use of Gram stains is not necessary to detect the presence of bacteria. Routine Romanowsky stains are excellent for this and offer much more, as well.

XI. Culturing for microorganisms
  A. Whenever an infection is suspected, fluid should be submitted for possible culturing of organisms.
  B. Usually, culturing can better detect organisms than can a microscopic examination of effusions, especially when very few organisms are in the effusion.

COMMENTS ABOUT SPECIFIC EFFUSIONS

I.   Septic and nonseptic exudates
   A. The results of fluid analyses are sometimes classified as either septic exudates or nonseptic exudates.
      1. The term *septic* in this context frequently is used synonymously with *bacterial* and is used when bacteria were found during the microscopic examination of an exudate. However, others use the term *septic* whenever any microbe is found that is considered the cause of the infectious exudate.
      2. The term *nonseptic* in this context frequently is used synonymously with *nonbacterial* and is used when bacteria were not found during the microscopic examination of a stained slide. However, the effusion might be a septic exudate.
         a. Bacteria may have been present but not found via microscopy. This is not uncommon when very few organisms are in a sample.
         b. Bacteria may have been present but not cultured because of inappropriate culture media (e.g., aerobic versus anaerobic organisms) or the animal had been treated with antibiotics prior to collection of an effusion.
         c. The exudation is caused by a microbe other than bacteria but was not found by microscopy or culturing.
      3. Occasionally, bacteria are found in an exudate but are contaminants. In these cases, the exudate with bacteria might be a *nonseptic exudate*.
   B. A classification of *septic exudate* is best applied to an effusion when it is known that the exudation is caused by an infectious agent. Conversely, a classification of *nonseptic exudate* is best applied to an effusion when it is known that the exudation is not caused by an infectious agent; this is typically not known at the time a fluid sample is evaluated, so the term *nonseptic exudate* is not recommended for the interpretation of fluid analyses. When bacteria are not found during the examination of an effusion, it may be better to classify it as an *exudate of unknown cause* than to classify it as a *nonseptic exudate*.

II. Differentiation of a bacterial exudate and intestinal contents
   A. Occasionally, a collected sample will contain numerous and pleomorphic bacteria that are consistent with intestinal flora. The microscopist should consider that the sample might be either a bacterial exudate secondary to intestinal leakage or that the sample inadvertently was collected from an intestine (called an *intestinal tap*).
   B. Both types of samples may contain numerous bacteria and evidence of ingesta (e.g., fragments of plant or muscle fibers, or granular debris) and have odors and a gross appearance of intestinal contents.
      1. The bacterial exudate may have few to numerous leukocytes, often degenerate, and a $[TP_{ref}] > 2.0$ g/dL, whereas the intestinal fluid will not have many leukocytes, and neutrophils, if present, will tend to be nondegenerate if the sample is processed promptly. Rarely, the peritoneal fluid is collected within minutes of an intestinal rupture, and then it will not be possible to differentiate the peritoneal fluid sample from intestinal fluid. However, the resultant inflammatory response will be evident in samples collected a few hours later.
      2. Even though the intestinal bacteria are not pathogens within the intestine, they are recognized as foreign structures in the peritoneal fluid. Accordingly, they will be engulfed by neutrophils and macrophages. Bacteria from an intestinal tap may

undergo phagocytosis in vitro within 15–30 min after collection, further complicating the differentiation of a mixed peritoneal fluid–intestinal tap from a ruptured intestine.

III. Effusions associated with neoplasms
   A. A *neoplastic effusion* is a pleural or peritoneal effusion that contains neoplastic cells. Most intrathoracic and intra-abdominal neoplasms that cause effusions do not slough cells into the fluid; they typically cause an effusion by other processes (exudation, transudation, hemorrhage, or damaged lymphatic system).[73] The features of the effusions can be extremely variable, with only rare neoplastic cells among many inflammatory cells or with an extremely high concentration of neoplastic cells.
   B. A critical examination of the nucleated cells is needed to suggest or confirm the presence of neoplastic cells in an effusion.
      1. Neoplastic lymphocytes are typically recognized when a population of cells has nuclei > 10 μm in diameter and has nuclear and cytoplasmic features of high cellular activity. Smaller neoplastic lymphocytes are more difficult to recognize via microscopy.
      2. Primary carcinomas or adenocarcinomas of abdominal or thoracic organs may exfoliate cells into the effusion (Plate 15B). Metastatic sarcomas typically do not exfoliate cells nor do they cause effusions.
      3. Metastatic mast cell neoplasia may slough cells into the effusion.
      4. Hemangioma or hemangiosarcoma (malignant hemangioendothelioma) of spleen, liver, lung, or heart might rupture and cause a hemorrhagic effusion, but rarely will neoplastic endothelial cells be found in the effusion.
      5. Metastatic melanomas may damage tissues, damage lymphatic vessels, and exfoliate neoplastic cells.
      6. Pleural and peritoneal mesotheliomas can produce effusions with numerous anaplastic cells (Plate 15C). However diagnostically, it may be difficult to differentiate neoplastic mesothelial cells from carcinomatous cells or proplastic mesothelial cells found in nonneoplastic effusions.
      7. Squamous epithelial cells in effusion samples are typically contaminants. However, occasionally they represent neoplastic cells exfoliated from an abdominal neoplasm; for example, gastric squamous cell carcinoma in horses. Poorly differentiated squamous cells may be difficult to differentiate from reactive mesothelial cells. In pregnant animals, squamous cells may be from amniotic fluid (Plate 15O).

IV. Lymphocyte-rich effusions
   A. *Lymphocyte-rich effusions* are those pleural and peritoneal effusions in which the dominant nucleated cell is a lymphocyte (Plates 14E, G, and H and 15L). The two most common causes of a lymphocyte-rich effusion are lymphoid neoplasia (lymphoma) and an accumulation of lymph (Table 19.5). Occasionally, a low-grade inflammatory process may produce a lymphocyte-rich fluid.
   B. Microscopic examination of the lymphocytes may enable a neoplastic lymphoid effusion to be differentiated from a nonneoplastic effusion. The distinguishing features include the following:
      1. Nuclear diameters: If most lymphocyte nuclei are > 10 μm in diameter, then the effusion is probably neoplastic. If most lymphocyte nuclei are <10 μm, lymphoid neoplasia may or may not be present.

2. Chromatin patterns: Dispersed or finely granular chromatin (especially in larger cells) is typical of lymphoid neoplasia.

3. Nucleoli: If many lymphocytes have nucleoli, then they probably are neoplastic; proplastic cells may have similar nucleoli.

C. The [lymphocyte] in nonneoplastic effusions rarely exceeds $10.0 \times 10^3/\mu L$; neoplastic lymphoid effusions occasionally have a TNCC $< 10.0 \times 10^3/\mu L$. The higher the [lymphocyte] is, the more likely the analyzed fluid is a neoplastic lymphoid effusion.

D. The routine analysis of the lymphocyte-rich effusion may not be able to definitively differentiate a neoplastic from a nonneoplastic effusion. Additional diagnostic methods might include clonality studies of the collected lymphocytes or histopathologic examination of excised tissue.

V. Pericardial effusions

A. These are uncommon and mostly detected in radiographs and ultrasonograms (echocardiograms). Disorders associated with pericardial effusions include neoplasia and infections, but they frequently are idiopathic.[74–76]

B. Frequently, the collected pericardial fluid has features of a hemorrhagic effusion. In such samples, erythrophages, siderophages, and hematoidin crystals are frequently found. A chylous pericardial effusion may be secondary to chylothorax or occur alone.[77]

C. Mesothelial cells in pericardial effusion can have marked reactive or proplastic changes, including intense cytoplasmic basophilia, nuclei with distinct nucleoli, and variable nuclear to cytoplasmic ratios. These cells should not be considered neoplastic cells even though their microscopic features are consistent with neoplastic cells. Rarely, mesothelial cells contain hemosiderin granules.

D. Studies have provided data that suggest the pH of pericardial fluid may help differentiate pericardial effusion due to neoplasia from other causes. However, individual cases could not be reliably differentiated by the pH values.[78,79] Like the measurement of blood pH (see Chapter 10), sample handling and processing are critical to obtain accurate pH values.

VI. Amniotic fluid

A. Occasionally, amniotic fluid is inadvertently collected during paracentesis.

B. Unless there is a pathologic state involving a fetus or the amniotic sac, the amniotic fluid is clear and watery, and a microscopic examination reveals numerous nucleated or anucleate cornified squamous epithelial cells (Plate 15O).

References

1. Raskin RE, Meyer DJ. 2001. *Atlas of Canine and Feline Cytology.* Philadelphia: WB Saunders.

2. Cowell RL, Tyler RD. 1992. *Cytology and Hematology of the Horse.* Goleta, CA: American Veterinary.

3. Cowell RL, Tyler RD, Meinkoth JH. 1999. *Diagnostic Cytology and Hematology of the Dog and Cat*, 2nd edition. St Louis: CV Mosby.

4. Baker R, Lumsden JH. 2000. The lymphatic system. In: *Color Atlas of Cytology of the Dog and Cat*, 71–94. St Louis: CV Mosby.

5. Perman V, Alsaker RD, Riis RC. 1979. *Cytology of the Dog and Cat.* South Bend, IN: American Animal Hospital Association.

6. Cowell RL, Tyler RD. 2002. *Diagnostic Cytology and Hematology of the Horse*, 2nd edition. St Louis: CV Mosby.

7. Villiers E, Blackwood L, eds. 2005. *BSAVA Manual of Canine and Feline Clinical Pathology*, 2nd edition. Gloucester: British Small Animal Veterinary Association.
8. Miserocchi G. 1997. Physiology and pathophysiology of pleural fluid turnover. Eur Respir J 10:219–225.
9. Hosgood G, Salisbury SK, Cantwell HD, DeNicola DB. 1989. Intraperitoneal circulation and drainage in the dog. Vet Surg 18:261–268.
10. Guyton AC, Hall JE. 2000. *Textbook of Medical Physiology*, 10th edition. Philadelphia: WB Saunders.
11. Wang NS. 1985. Anatomy and physiology of the pleural space. Clin Chest Med 6:3–16.
12. O'Brien PJ, Lumsden JH. 1988. The cytologic examination of body cavity fluids. Semin Vet Med Surg (Small Anim) 3:140–156.
13. Kopcha M, Schultze AE. 1991. Peritoneal fluid. Part II. Abdominocentesis in cattle and interpretation of nonneoplastic samples. Compend Contin Educ Pract Vet 13:703–709.
14. Coles EH. 1967. *Veterinary Clinical Pathology*, 1st edition. Philadelphia: WB Saunders.
15. Benjamin MM. 1961. *Outline of Veterinary Clinical Pathology*, 2nd edition. Ames: Iowa State University Press.
16. Duncan JR, Prasse KW. 1977. *Veterinary Laboratory Medicine*, 1st edition. Ames: Iowa State University Press.
17. Rose BD, Post TW. 2001. *Clinical Physiology of Acid-Base and Electrolyte Disorders*, 5th edition. New York: McGraw-Hill.
18. Lazaridis KN, Abraham SC, Kamath PS. 2005. Hematological malignancy manifesting as ascites. Nat Clin Pract Gastroenterol Hepatol 2:112–116.
19. Molina E, Reddy KR. 2001. Noncirrhotic portal hypertension. Clin Liver Dis 5:769–787.
20. Koot BG, Houwen R, Pot DJ, Nauta J. 2004. Congenital analbuminaemia: Biochemical and clinical implications—A case report and literature review. Eur J Pediatr 163:664–670.
21. Schrier RW, Ecder T. 2001. Gibbs memorial lecture. Unifying hypothesis of body fluid volume regulation: Implications for cardiac failure and cirrhosis. Mt Sinai J Med 68:350–361.
22. Bunch SE, Johnson SE, Cullen JM. 2001. Idiopathic noncirrhotic portal hypertension in dogs: 33 cases (1982–1998). J Am Vet Med Assoc 218:392–399.
23. Rector WG Jr, Reynolds TB. 1984. Superiority of the serum-ascites albumin difference over the ascites total protein concentration in separation of "transudative" and "exudative" ascites. Am J Med 77:83–85.
24. Runyon BA, Montano AA, Akriviadis EA, Antillon MR, Irving MA, McHutchison JG. 1992. The serum-ascites albumin gradient is superior to the exudate-transudate concept in the differential diagnosis of ascites. Ann Intern Med 117:215–220.
25. Hosgood GL, Salisbury SK. 1989. Pathophysiology and pathogenesis of generalized peritonitis. Probl Vet Med 1:159–167.
26. Clark CH, Woodley CH. 1959. The absorption of red blood cells after parenteral injection at various sites. Am J Vet Res 20:1062–1066.
27. Gorecki R, Zajgner J, Wawrzenczyk B. 1972. Mechanisms of lymphorrhage into the serous cavities with description of a case. Pol Med J 11:1242–1251.
28. Birchard SJ, McLoughlin MA, Smeak DD. 1995. Chylothorax in the dog and cat: A review. Lymphology 28:64–72.
29. Aslam N, Marino CR. 2001. Malignant ascites: New concepts in pathophysiology, diagnosis, and management. Arch Intern Med 161:2733–2737.
30. Birchard SJ, Ware WA, Fossum TW, Fingland RB. 1986. Chylothorax associated with congestive cardiomyopathy in a cat. J Am Vet Med Assoc 189:1462–1464.
31. Fossum TW, Forrester SD, Swenson CL, Miller MW, Cohen ND, Boothe HW, Birchard SJ. 1991. Chylothorax in cats: 37 cases (1969–1989). J Am Vet Med Assoc 198:672–678.
32. Fossum TW, Miller MW, Rogers KS, Bonagura JD, Meurs KM. 1994. Chylothorax associated with right-sided heart failure in five cats. J Am Vet Med Assoc 204:84–89.
33. Fossum TW, Birchard SJ, Jacobs RM. 1986. Chylothorax in 34 dogs. J Am Vet Med Assoc 188:1315–1318.
34. Schumacher J, Brusie R, Spano J. 1989. Chylothorax in an Arabian filly. Equine Vet J 21:132–134.
35. Willard MD, Conroy JD. 1985. Chylothorax associated with blastomycosis in a dog. J Am Vet Med Assoc 186:72–73.
36. Gores BR, Berg J, Carpenter JL, Ullman SL. 1994. Chylous ascites in cats: Nine cases (1978–1993). J Am Vet Med Assoc 205:1161–1164.
37. Mair TS, Lucke VM. 1992. Chyloperitoneum associated with torsion of the large colon in a horse. Vet Rec 131:421.
38. Nelson AW. 1979. Analysis of equine peritoneal fluid. Vet Clin North Am Large Anim Pract 1:267–274.
39. Wilson AD, Hirsch WM, Osborne AD. 1985. Abdominocentesis in cattle: Technique and criteria for diagnosis of peritonitis. Can Vet J 26:74–80.
40. Estepa JC, Lopez I, Mayer-Valor R, Rodriguez M, Aguilera-Tejero E. 2006. The influence of anticoagulants on the measurement of total protein concentration in equine peritoneal fluid. Res Vet Sci 80:5–10.

41. American Optical. 1976. *Instructions for use and care of the AO® TS meter (a Goldberg® refractometer).* Buffalo, NY: American Optical, Scientific Instrument Division.

42. Mutsaers SE. 2004. The mesothelial cell. Int J Biochem Cell Biol 36:9–16.

43. Antony VB, Mohammed KA. 1999. Pathophysiology of pleural space infections. Semin Respir Infect 14:9–17.

44. Yung S, Li FK, Chan TM. 2006. Peritoneal mesothelial cell culture and biology. Perit Dial Int 26:162–173.

45. Kjeldsberg CR, Knight JA. 1986. *Body Fluids: Laboratory Examination of Amniotic, Cerebrospinal, Seminal, Serous & Synovial Fluids—A Textbook Atlas*, 2nd edition. Chicago: American Society of Clinical Pathologists.

46. Ringsrud KM, Linné JJ. 1995. *Urinalysis and Body Fluids: A Colortext and Atlas.* St Louis: CV Mosby.

47. Caruso KJ, James MP, Fisher D, Paulson RL, Christopher MM. 2003. Cytologic diagnosis of peritoneal cestodiasis in dogs caused by *Mesocestoides* sp. Vet Clin Pathol 32:50–60.

48. French RA, Meier WA, Zachary JF. 1996. Eosinophilic colitis and hepatitis in a horse with colonic intramucosal ciliated protozoa. Vet Pathol 33:235–238.

49. Fossum TW, Jacobs RM, Birchard SJ. 1986. Evaluation of cholesterol and triglyceride concentrations in differentiating chylous and nonchylous pleural effusions in dogs and cats. J Am Vet Med Assoc 188:49–51.

50. Waddle JR, Giger U. 1990. Lipoprotein electrophoresis differentiation of chylous and nonchylous pleural effusions in dogs and cats and its correlation with pleural effusion triglyceride concentration. Vet Clin Pathol 19:80–85.

51. Burrows CF, Bovee KC. 1974. Metabolic changes due to experimentally induced rupture of the canine urinary bladder. Am J Vet Res 35:1083–1088.

52. Schmiedt C, Tobias KM, Otto CM. 2001. Evaluation of abdominal fluid: Peripheral blood creatinine and potassium ratios for diagnosis of uroperitoneum in dogs. J Vet Emerg Crit Care 11:275–280.

53. Richardson DW, Kohn CW. 1983. Uroperitoneum in the foal. J Am Vet Med Assoc 182:267–271.

54. Nyrop KA, DeBowes RM, Cox JH, Coffman JR. 1984. Rupture of the urinary bladder in two postparturient mares. Compend Contin Educ Pract Vet 6:S510–S513.

55. Aumann M, Worth LT, Drobatz KJ. 1998. Uroperitoneum in cats: 26 cases (1986–1995). J Am Anim Hosp Assoc 34:315–324.

56. Latson KM, Nieto JE, Beldomenico RM, Snyder JR. 2005. Evaluation of peritoneal fluid lactate as a marker of intestinal ischaemia in equine colic. Equine Vet J 37:342–346.

57. Nestor DD, McCullough SM, Schaeffer DJ. 2004. Biochemical analysis of neoplastic versus nonneoplastic abdominal effusions in dogs. J Am Anim Hosp Assoc 40:372–375.

58. Bonczynski JJ, Ludwig LL, Barton LJ, Loar A, Peterson ME. 2003. Comparison of peritoneal fluid and peripheral blood pH, bicarbonate, glucose, and lactate concentration as a diagnostic tool for septic peritonitis in dogs and cats. Vet Surg 32:161–166.

59. Levin GM, Bonczynski JJ, Ludwig LL, Barton LJ, Loar AS. 2004. Lactate as a diagnostic test for septic peritoneal effusions in dogs and cats. J Am Anim Hosp Assoc 40:364–371.

60. DeLaurier GA, Cannon RM, Johnson RH Jr, Sisley JF, Baisden CR, Mansberger AR Jr. 1989. Increased peritoneal fluid lactic acid values and progressive bowel strangulation in dogs. Am J Surg 158:32–35.

61. Ludwig LL, McLoughlin MA, Graves TK, Crisp MS. 1997. Surgical treatment of bile peritonitis in 24 dogs and 2 cats: A retrospective study (1987–1994). Vet Surg 26:90–98.

62. Owens SD, Gossett R, McElhaney MR, Christopher MM, Shelly SM. 2003. Three cases of canine bile peritonitis with mucinous material in abdominal fluid as the prominent cytologic finding. Vet Clin Pathol 32:114–120.

63. Eid AA, Keddissi JI, Samaha M, Tawk MM, Kimmell K, Kinasewitz GT. 2002. Exudative effusions in congestive heart failure. Chest 122:1518–1523.

64. Han SH, Reynolds TB, Fong TL. 1998. Nephrogenic ascites: Analysis of 16 cases and review of the literature. Medicine (Baltimore) 77:233–245.

65. Pembleton-Corbett JR, Center SA, Schermerhorn T, Yeager AE, Erb HN. 2000. Serum-effusion albumin gradient in dogs with transudative abdominal effusion. J Vet Intern Med 14:613–618.

66. Duthie S, Eckersall PD, Addie DD, Lawrence CE, Jarrett O. 1997. Value of alpha 1-acid glycoprotein in the diagnosis of feline infectious peritonitis. Vet Rec 141:299–303.

67. Bence LM, Addie DD, Eckersall PD. 2005. An immunoturbidimetric assay for rapid quantitative measurement of feline alpha-1-acid glycoprotein in serum and peritoneal fluid. Vet Clin Pathol 34:335–341.

68. Guija de Arespacochaga A, Hittmair KM, Schwendenwein I. 2006. Comparison of lipase activity in peritoneal fluid of dogs with different pathologies: A complementary diagnostic tool in acute pancreatitis? J Vet Med [A] 53:119–122.

69. Froscher BG, Nagode LA. 1981. Origin and importance of increased alkaline phosphatase activity in peritoneal fluids of horses with colic. Am J Vet Res 42:888–891.

70. Davies JV, Gerring EL, Goodburn R, Manderville P. 1984. Experimental ischaemia of the ileum and concentrations of the intestinal isoenzyme of alkaline phosphatase in plasma and peritoneal fluid. Equine Vet J 16:215–217.

71. Saulez MN, Cebra CK, Tornquist SJ. 2004. The diagnostic and prognostic value of alkaline phosphatase activity in serum and peritoneal fluid from horses with acute colic. J Vet Intern Med 18:564–567.

72. Horney B. 2005. The diagnostics and prognostic value of alkaline phosphatase activity in serum and peritoneal fluid from horses with acute colic. J Vet Intern Med 19:783–784.

73. Tamsma JT, Keizer HJ, Meinders AE. 2001. Pathogenesis of malignant ascites: Starling's law of capillary hemodynamics revisited. Ann Oncol 12:1353–1357.

74. Perkins SL, Magdesian KG, Thomas WP, Spier SJ. 2004. Pericarditis and pleuritis caused by *Corynebacterium pseudotuberculosis* in a horse. J Am Vet Med Assoc 224:1133–1138.

75. Sims CS, Tobias AH, Hayden DW, Fine DM, Borjesson DL, Aird B. 2003. Pericardial effusion due to primary cardiac lymphosarcoma in a dog. J Vet Intern Med 17:923–927.

76. MacGregor JM, Faria ML, Moore AS, Tobias AH, Brown DJ, de Morais HSA. 2005. Cardiac lymphoma and pericardial effusion in dogs: 12 cases (1994–2004). J Am Vet Med Assoc 227:1449–1453.

77. Boston SE, Moens NM, Martin DM. 2006. Idiopathic primary chylopericardium in a dog. J Am Vet Med Assoc 229:1930–1933.

78. de Laforcade AM, Freeman LM, Rozanski EA, Rush JE. 2005. Biochemical analysis of pericardial fluid and whole blood in dogs with pericardial effusion. J Vet Intern Med 19:833–836.

79. Fine DM, Tobias AH, Jacob KA. 2003. Use of pericardial fluid pH to distinguish between idiopathic and neoplastic effusions. J Vet Intern Med 17:525–529.

80. Wagner AE, Bennett DG. 1988. Analysis of equine thoracic fluid. Vet Clin Pathol 11:13–17.

81. Bach LG, Ricketts SW. 1974. Paracentesis as an aid to the diagnosis of abdominal disease in the horse. Equine Vet J 6:116–121.

82. McGrath JP. 1975. Exfoliative cytology of equine peritoneal fluid: An adjunct to hematology examination. In: Kitchen H, Krehbiel JD, eds. *Proceedings of the First International Symposium of Equine Hematology*, 408–416. Golden, CO: American Association of Equine Practitioners.

83. Morley PS, DesNoyers M. 1992. Diagnosis of ruptured urinary bladder in a foal by the identification of calcium carbonate crystals in the peritoneal fluid. J Am Vet Med Assoc 200:1515–1517.

84. Anderson DE, Cornwell D, Anderson LS, St-Jean G, Desrochers A. 1995. Comparative analyses of peritoneal fluid from calves and adult cattle. Am J Vet Res 56:973–976.

INDEX

AaDO₂. *See* Arterial alveolar oxygen tension
    gradient
AB system, 119
AcAc. *See* Acetoacetate concentration
Acanthocyte, 143–47, 144t
Accuracy, 37
Acetaminophen, Heinz body formation and, 186
Acetoacetate (AcAc) concentration, 543–45
    analytical concepts in, 544
    physiologic processes, 543–44
Acid-base balance
    abnormalities, 574–81
    Ca^{2+}, free concentration and, 614
    calculated, 567–70
    renal functions related to, 565
    Stewart's method of analysis of, 584–91
Acid-based disorders, 562–65, 562f
    blood gas data in, 578, 578t
    classification, 578, 579f
    compensatory changes in, expected, 578–81
    differences in definitions of, 585–86
    mixed, 578
    simple, 578
Acidemia, 561
    acidosis and, 512
Acidosis, 585
    acidemia and, 512
    compensatory changes in, 578, 581t
    dilutional, 574–75
    HCO_3- and, 532
    inorganic, 574
    K^+, serum and, 509–10, 509f
    lactic, hyperphosphatemia and, 619
    metabolic
        groups of, 574–75
        hyperchloremic, 523
        hypochloremia and, 525, 526f
        physiologic compensation for, 575
    normokalemia and, 516
    organic, 509–10, 574
    renal tubular, 532
    respiratory, 575, 575t
    secretory, 574
    tCO^2 and, 532
    titrational, 574
Aciduria, 456–57, 456t
    paradoxical, 576

ACT. *See* Activated coagulation time
ACTH. *See* Adrenocorticotropic hormone
Activated coagulation time (ACT), 279–80
Acute megakaryocytic leukemia (AML)
    differentiation, 347
    dysplasia, multilineage and, 347–48
    genetic abnormalities and, 347
    MDS and development of, 350
    thrombocytosis and, 245
Acute phase protein (APP)
    analytical concepts, 396–97
    inflammation and, 380
    negative, 372
    positive, 372, 392–98
        fibrinogen as, 393–96
        general concepts of, 392–93
        increased concentrations of, 397–98, 398t
Addison's disease, 83, 515
    in cats, 601–2
    in dogs, 601–2
    $Na^+:K^+$ ratio, decreased and, 519
    USG, refractometric and, 451
Adenosine triphosphate (ATP), 188–90
ADH. *See* Antidiuretic hormone
Adrenocortical function, 805–27
    ACTH and, 813–14, 814f
    aldosterone concentration and, 824–26
    analytical concepts, 807–8
    assessments, 826–27
    cortisol concentration and, 808–12
    cortisol, urine to Crt ratio and, 812–13, 813f
    physiologic processes, 806
    stimulation tests, 815–23
    suppression tests, 815–23
Adrenocorticotropic hormone (ACTH)
    concentration, 813–14, 814f
    cortisol, plasma ratio to, 814–15
    stimulation test
        canine, 818–21, 819f
        dexamethasone suppression test combined
            with, 823
        equine, 822–23
        feline, 821–22
ADVIA, 122
    erythrocyte, 125, 127
    MCHC and evaluation with, 158
Afibrinogenemia, 310

Afibrinogenemia (*continued*)
　BMBT and, 264
　TT, prolonged and, 285
Agglutination
　erythrocyte, 130, 136
　latex, for foal serum, 400
AID. *See* Anemia of inflammatory disease
AIHA. *See* Autoimmune hemolytic anemia
Alanine transaminase (ALT), 650–52
　activity, increased serum, 651, 651t
　analytical concepts, 650–51
　psychologic processes, 650
　serum, 651, 651t
　tissue sources, 650
Albendazole, thrombocytopenia and, 236
Albumin
　analytical principles for total, 372–79
　Ca^{2+} and, 597–98
　concentration, measuring, 374
　Crt to, ratio, 482
　general concepts for total, 370–72
　physiologic processes, 370–71
　renal excretion, 481
　synthesis, decreased, 383
　urine assays, quantitative, 478
Aldosterone
　concentration, 824–26
　　canine, 824–26, 825t
　secretion, 806, 807f
Alkalemia, 561
　hyperventilation and, 563
Alkaline phosphatase (ALP), 655–59
　analytical concepts of, 656
　in cats, 659
　in cattle, 659
　in dogs, 658–59
　in horses, 659
　osteoblastic activity, increased, 658
　physiologic processes, 655
　serum, increased activity of, 655–58, 657t
　　drug/hormone induction of, 656–57
　species/breed differences in, 658–59
Alkalinuria, 456t, 457
Alkaloses, 585
　compensatory changes in, 578
　contraction, 531
　hypochloremic metabolic, 518
　K^+, serum and, 509–10, 509f
　metabolic, 510, 576
　　Ca^{2+} urinary excretion and, 608
　　hypochloremia and, 524–25
　normokalemia and, 516

　respiratory, 523, 576–77
　　diseases/conditions causing, 577, 577t
　　physiologic compensation and, 577
　　PO_4 and, 620
Alkalosis, 561
Alopecia, in Hereford calves, 167
ALP. *See* Alkaline phosphatase
ALT. *See* Alanine transaminase
Altman-Bland bias plot, 32, 32f
American College of Veterinary Pathologists, 5
Amino acids, renal tubule function and, 422
AML. *See* Acute megakaryocytic leukemia
Ammonium
　clearance, decreased, 699–701, 700f
　concentration, plasma, 697–703
　　analytical concepts, 697–99
　　physiologic processes, 697, 698f
　　samples, 699
　effusion analysis with, 861
　intake/absorption, increased, 702
　production, increased, 701–2
　tolerance test, 702
　　in dogs, 702–3, 703t
Amniotic fluid, 866
AMS. *See* Amylase
Amylase (AMS)
　physiologic processes, 663–64
　renal excretion/inactivation and, 665
　serum, increased activity of, 664–65, 664t
Amyloidosis, 385
　systemic, prolonged TT and, 285
Amyloid, serum, 372
Analyte, 5
　analytical accuracy and, 24
　detection limit, 25
　herd-based testing and measuring, 49–50
　urine, to plasma ratios, 476–77
Analytical accuracy, 22f, 24–25
Analytical errors, 21
　reproducibility of random, 22f
　sources of, 37
　Westgard rules and detecting, 26–27
Analytical precision, 21–24
　CV and, 22–24
　variation and need for, 22
Analytical sensitivity, 25
Anaphylaxis, thrombocytopenia and, 243
Anaplasma, leukocyte, 95
Anaplasma platys, 233
　thrombocytopenia and, 242
Anaplasma spp., infectious hemolytic anemia, 182
Anaplasmataceae, leukocyte, 95, 96t

Anemia of inflammatory disease (AID), 160–61
Anemias, 151–59. *See also* Refractory anemia;
    Refractory anemia with excess blasts 1;
    Refractory anemia with excess blasts 2;
    Refractory anemia with ringed sideroblasts
  aplastic, 338
  blood loss, 167–70
    acute, 167–68, 168f
    chronic, 168–70, 169f
  blood-loss, 158
  BMBT and, 264
  CHCM, increased and, 157–58
  classification
    erythrocyte indices, 153–58, 154t
    marrow responsiveness, 151–53
    pathophysiologic, 158–59, 159f
    reticulocytosis and, 151
  cobalamin deficiency and, 165
  copper deficiency and, 165
  erythrocyte production, decreased causing,
    158
  Fe deficiency and, 164–65, 168–70, 169f
  folate deficiency and, 165
  general information, 151
  hemolytic, 158, 170–93
    ATP generation defects and, 188–90
    concepts an classifications of, 170–76
    eccentrocytic, 187–88
    erythrocyte examination and, 171
    Heinz body, 186
    idiopathic, 192
    IMHA as, 177–79
    PFK deficiency, 189
    PK deficiency, 188–89
    porphyria producing, 190
    spherocytic, 192
  hemolytic, erythrocytic metabolic defect, 186–91
    oxidative damage and, 186–88
  hemolytic, immune, 176–81
    disorders of, 177–81
    drug-induced, 179–80
    pathogenesis of, 178f
    vaccine-induced, 180
  hemolytic, infectious, 181–86
    Anaplasma spp., 182
    Babesia spp., 184
    Clostridium spp., 182–83
    EIAV, 183–84
    FeLV, 184
    hemotropic mycoplasma species, 181–82
    Leptospira spp., 182
    Mycoplasma spp., 181

    pathogeneses, 181
    Theileria spp., 185
    Trypanosoma spp., 185–86
  hyperchromic
    macrocytic, 157
    normocytic, 157
  hypochromic
    macrocytic, 155
    microcytic, 156
    normocytic, 157
  of inflammatory disease, 339
  MCHC, increased and, 157–58
  megaloblastic, 201–2
  myelophthisic, 163
  nonregenerative, 151–53, 159–67
    aplasia, pure red cell causing, 163–64
    disorders causing, 160–67, 160t
    endocrine disorders causing, 166
    erythrocyte production and, 159
    erythropoiesis, ineffective causing, 163–67
    general concepts of, 159–60
    hypoplasia, erythroid causing, 163–67
    immune-mediated, 164
    inflammatory disease causing, 160–61, 160t
    marrow hypoplasia/aplasia causing, 162–63
    nutrient deficiencies causing, 164–65
    renal disease causing, 161–62
  normochromic
    macrocytic, 155–56
    microcytic, 156–57
    normocytic, 154–55
  pyridoxine deficiency and, 165
  regenerative, 151, 152
    hyperplasia, erythroid and, 152
  sideroblastic, 143
    in dogs, 202
Anion, 534
  Ca^{2+} binding with diffusible, 608
  charge, 534
  serum, 535, 535t
  strong, 586
Anion gap, 534–38
  analytical concepts, 536–37
  calculating, 535, 536f
  changes, 535
  decreased, 538, 538t
  definitions, 534–35
  increased, 537, 537t
  physiologic processes, 535–36
  serum, 535
  SID and, 589
Anisocytosis, 142

Antibodies
    FDPs and specificity of, 296–97
    fibrin fragment D-dimer and specificity of,
        299–300
    thrombocytopenia and, 239
Anticoagulants
    endogenous
        AT as, 288–91
            anti-(phospholipid-protein) antibodies as,
                292–93
            protein C as, 291
            protein Z as, 291–92
        lupus, 292
Antidiuretic hormone (ADH), 485–87. *See also*
        Syndrome of inappropriate ADH secretion
Anti-(phospholipid-protein) antibodies, 292–93
Antithrombin (AT), 288–91. *See also* Thrombin-
        antithrombin complexes
    activity
        decreased, 289–90, 289t
        increased, 290
    coagulation enzymes inhibited by, 273–74, 275f
    consumption, 290
    heparin therapy and consumption of, 290
    interpretive considerations, 289
    loss, 290
    plasma, 288
    stability, 289
    units, 289
Aplasia
    bone marrow, anemia caused by, 162–63
    lymphoid, protein synthesis/catabolism and, 389
    lymphopenia of lymphoid, 84f, 85
    pure red cell, anemia caused by, 163–64
    red cell, 339
        pure, 163–64
Apoenzymes, 640
Apolipoproteins, 766
APP. *See* Acute phase protein
Arterial alveolar oxygen tension gradient (AaDO$_2$),
        569–70
Ascites
    definition, 835
    hypoalbuminemia and formation of, 505
    hypoproteinemia and formation of, 505
Aspartate transaminase (AST), 652–53
    activity, increased serum, 652, 652t
Aspiration
    bone marrow, 328
        processing samples for, 328–29
    lymph node, 362
AST. *See* Aspartate transaminase
Asynchronous nuclear maturation, 92

AT. *See* Antithrombin
ATP. *See* Adenosine triphosphate
Autoantibodies, 794–95. *See also* Thyroglobulin
        autoantibodies
Autoimmune hemolytic anemia (AIHA), 179
Azotemia, 427, 428f, 429–33
    in cats, 440
    in cattle, 440
    cause, multifactorial, 432–33
    classifications, 429–32
    Crt in serum/plasma and, 437
    differentiation, guidelines for, 432–33, 432t
    disorders, 429–32
    in dogs
        serum chemistry results in, abnormal routine,
            440
        UN:Crt ratio and, 438, 438t
    in horses, 477, 478t
        serum chemistry results in, abnormal routine,
            440
    postrenal, 430t, 431
    prerenal, 429–30
        disorders and, 429, 430t
        renal *v.*, 477, 478t
    renal, 430–31
        prerenal *v.*, 477, 478t
    renal disease and, 433
    renal failure, acute and, 428
    serum chemistry results in, abnormal routine,
        439–40
    UN in serum/plasma and, 435
    urea/Crt urinary excretion and, 429–31
    urea production, increased and, 430t, 431–32

Babesia spp., infectious hemolytic anemia,
        184
Bacteriuria, 472
Base excess in blood (BE$_B$), 567–68
Base excess in ECF (BE$_{ECF}$), 567
Base excess in plasma (BE$_P$), 567
Basopenia, 88
Basophil
    concentrations, abnormal, 88
    kinetics, 59–60
    pools, 59–60
Basophilia, 88
    diffuse cytoplasmic, 92
Basophilic stippling, erythrocyte, 138–41, 140t
Bayer Technicon, 122
Bδ. *See* delta-Bilirubin
BE$_B$. *See* Base excess in blood
Beckman analyzer, 528
BE$_{ECF}$. *See* Base excess in ECF

Bence Jones proteinuria, 385, 460–62
Benzethonium chloride assay, 478
Benzocaine, Heinz body formation and, 186
BE$_P$. *See* Base excess in plasma
BHB. *See* β-Hydroxybutyrate
Bicarbonate (HCO$_3^-$)
  alimentary losses of, 532
  analytical concepts, 527–29
  assays, 528–29
  concentration, 525–34
    decreased, 531–34
    increased, 529–31
    physiologic processes, 525–27
    standard, 567
  decreased
    disorders/pathogeneses and, 531–33, 532t
    hyperchloremia and, 533–34
  increased, 529–31, 529t
  loss, increased, 532–33
  nephron
    distal, 526–27
    proximal, 526, 527f
  quantitation, sample for, 527–28
  renal losses of, 532
  renal tubule function and, 419
  secretion, 527, 528f
Bicarbonaturia, 518
Bile acid
  analytical concepts, 691
  biliary excretion of, 691, 692f
  challenge test, for dogs and cats, 693–96
    factors influencing results of, 695
    procedure in, 694
    published data on, 694–95, 694t, 695t
  cholestasis and, 681
  clearance, decreased, 692f, 693
  concentration, 690–97
    increased, 691–93, 692f, 692t
    physiologic processes, 690–91, 690f
  enterohepatic circulation of, 690
  excretion
    biliary, 691, 692f
    decreased, 693
  secretion, 691
  urine, to Crt ratio, 485, 696–97, 697t
Bile salts, 691
Biliary disease, 677
Bilirubin
  cholestasis and, 681
  concentration, 681–90
    analytical concepts of, 683
    physiologic processes of, 681–83, 682f
  conjugated, decreased excretion of, 687–89

effusion analysis with, 861
  hemolysis and, 684–85, 685t
  hepatocyte uptake of, 685–87, 685t
  hyperbilirubinemia, 684–89, 684t
  icterus, hemolytic and, 684–85, 685t
  metabolism, Hgb degradation and, 114, 114f
  production of, increased, 684–85
  in urine, 466–67
delta-Bilirubin (Bδ), 689
Bilirubinuria, 171–73, 467, 689
Biuret reaction, total proteins measured with, 374
Blast cell, 346
Bleeding disorders, major
  bleeding pattern and, 301
  breed, age and, 301
  diagnosis, 300–304
    clinical findings and, 301
  findings and pathogenesis of, 300–310
  gender and, 301
  hemostasis tests and, 302–4, 302t
    patterns in, 302–4, 303t
  pathogenesis, 304–10
    afibrinogenemia in, 310
    consumptive coagulopathy and, 308–9
    dilutional coagulopathy in, 309–10
    dysfibrinogenemia in, 310
    hepatic disease in, 304–5
    vitamin K antagonism or deficiency and, 305–8, 307t
  types of, 301
Blister beetle poisoning, hypomagnesemia and, 625
Blister cell, 147
Blood. *See also* Base excess in blood; Complete blood count; Nucleated red blood cells
  cells, 6
    staining, 61–62
  crossmatching, 210
  disorders, 301
  erythrocytes, 111, 111t
    data differences and, 129–30
    fragmentation in, 191
  gases, 559–91
    acid-base disorders and, 578, 578t
    analytical concepts in, 565–73
    calculated, 567–70
    compensatory changes in, expected, 580
    erroneous values for, 573, 573t
    exchange, 564–65
    hypoxia and, 582, 583t
    instruments for analyzing, 565–71
    physiologic processes of, 561–65
    pulmonary functions related to, 562–65

Blood (*continued*)
 sample for, 572–73
 temperature and, 570, 570t
 groups, 208–9
  cat, 119
  cattle, 120
  dog, 119
  erythrocytes and, 117–20, 208–10
  horse, 119
 Hgb, 128–29
 impedance cell counter, 63–64
 laboratory assays, 7–8
 leukocytes, 55
  abnormal concentration of, 70–90
  evaluation and, 60–61
 lymphocytes, 58
  processes influencing, 59
 neutrophils, 57
  abnormal concentration of, 70–81
  left shift and, 70–71
  processes influencing measured, 57
  right shift and, 71–72
 oxygenation, 563–65, 564f, 581–82
 pH, 559–91
  analytical concepts in, 565–73
  erroneous values for, 573, 573t
  physiologic processes of, 561–65
  samples for, 572–73
  temperature and, 570, 570t
 plasma, 6–7
 samples, 5–6
  anticoagulants for, 6
  leukocyte evaluation with, 60–61
 serum, 7
 species variations in, 210–11
 typing, 208–10
  cat, 119
  cattle, 120
  dog, 119
  erythrocytes and, 117–20, 208–10
  horse, 119
  methods for, 209–10
 volume, Na^+ and regulation of, 499
 whole
  clotting times for, 279–80
  glucose concentration in, 708–23, 712t
Blood ammonia, 697
Blood films
 examination of stained, 61
 platelet evaluation on, 227, 229–30
  volume and, 247
Blood hemocrit values, 49

Blood loss
 anemias
  acute, 167–68, 168f
  chronic, 168–70, 169f
 causes, 167
 hypoproteinemia and, 385
 platelet survival, decreased and, 240
Blood transfusions
 autologous, 131
 blood groups and, 208–9
 blood species variations and, 210
 Ca^{2+}, free concentration and, 613–14
 incompatible, IMHA secondary to, 180–81
 posttransfusion purpura, 240
Blood vessels (endothelial cells), 300
 disorders, 301
B-lymphocytes, 55
 neoplasia
  hyperproteinemia and, 381–85
  laboratory/clinical problems with, 385
  pathogenesis, 381–82
BMBT. *See* Buccal mucosal bleeding time
Body fluids
 laboratory assays for, 7–8
 samples, 7
Bone
 Ca^{2+}, 596
 neoplasia in, 601
Bone marrow, 54–55, 323–65
 analysis, methods for, 328–34
 anemias
  aplastic, 338
  classification and responsiveness of, 151–53
 aplasia, anemia caused by, 162–63
 aspiration, 328, 334
  processing samples for, 328–29
 biopsy, 328
  processing samples of core, 329
 CBC, 358, 360f
 cell concentrations of, 327
 classifications, 334–37
 collection/processing of, 328–29
 composition, 324
 core samples
  cytologic examination of, 333–34
  histologic examination of, 333
 dyscrasia of poodles, 100
 erythropoiesis and, 334–36
 examination, 329–34
  cytologic, 333–34
  gross, 329
  histologic, 333–34

indications for, 327–28
interpreting results of, 357–58
microscopic, 329–33
Fe, 332–33
flow cytometry, 334
granulopoiesis and, 336–37
hematopoietic cells, 324–27, 329–30
hematopoietic populations, 330–32, 331f
hemic neoplasia, 342–57
classification of, 342–46, 343t
general concepts/terms, 342–46, 344f
hyperplasia, 334–38, 335t
basophilic granulocytic, 337
eosinophilic granulocytic, 337
generalized, 337–38
granulocytic, 336–37
megakaryocytic, 337
monocytic, 337
hypoplasia, 338–40, 338t
anemia caused by, 162–63
erythroid, 339
generalized, 338–39
infections and, 236–37
megakaryocytic, selective, 340
selective granulocytic, 338t, 339–40
lymphocytes, 332
lymphocytosis, 340
major concepts and terms, 324–34
mastocytosis, 340–41
maturation progression, 332
myelitis, 341
myelofibrosis, 341
myelophthisis, 341
necrosis, 341–42
neoplasia
hemic cell, 342–57
histiocytic, 351–52
lymphoid, 351
myeloid, 346–51
neutropenia and, 337
neutrophils, 57
nucleated cell differential count in health and, 327
nutritional deficiencies, 336
postmortem samples of, 334
replacement, thrombocytopenia and, 237
samples, 357–58
Bradypnea, 561
Bromide, L-lactate measurement and, 540
Buccal mucosal bleeding time (BMBT)
analytical concepts, 263
anemia and, 264

platelet function test, 263–64
prolonged, 263
vascular disease and, 264
vWD and, 263
Buffer base, 568
Burmese kittens, hypokalemic myopathy in, 519
Burr cell, 147

Ca²⁺. *See* Calcium
Cachectic states, protein synthesis/catabolism and, 389
Calcitonin concentration, 630–31
Calcium (Ca²⁺), 593–631
anions, diffusible binding of, 608
anticoagulants binding, 611–12
bone, 596
chloride, clotting and, 281
concentration, free, 610–15
abnormal, 613–14
acid-base status affecting, 614
analytical concepts of, 610–13
hormone control of, 613–14
physiologic processes of, 610
samples, 610–11, 612f
true and, 614–15, 615f
concentration, interpreting, 614
concentration, total, 594–610
albumin and, 597–98
analytic concepts of, 596–98
free and, 614–15, 615f
physiologic processes of, 594–96
plasma, 594–95
regulation of, 597–98
serum, 594–95
disorders, major patterns for, 631, 631t
effusion analysis with, 858–59
fracture healing and deposition of, 608
hypercalcemia and, 598–602, 599t
increased protein-bound, 602
mobilization of, 598–601
inadequate, 604–8
PO₄ interaction with, 596
regulatory hormones, 593–631
renal failure/insufficiency and, 601
renal tubule, 596
renal tubule function and, 422
serum, 594–95
factors determining, 595–96, 595f
urinary excretion of
decreased, 601
excess, 608

Canine distemper inclusions
  erythrocytes and, 202
  leukocyte, 95
Carbohydrates metabolism, liver function and,
    676
Casts, urine sediment, 472–73
Cation, 534
  charge
    measured, 534
    total, 534
    unmeasured, 534
  serum, 535, 535t
  strong, 586
Cats
  α_1-PI, fecal in, 753
  ACTH in, 813, 814f
  adrenocortical function tests in, 821–22
  ALP in, 659
  azotemia in, abnormal routine serum chemistry
    results and, 440
  bile acid challenge test for, 693–96, 695t
  blood-groups system, 119
  cobalamin in, 747–50
  cortisol, urine to Crt ratio in, 812–13, 813f
  EPI in, 740
  FeLV in, 164
    infectious hemolytic anemia and, 184
  folate in, 750–52
  GGT in, 661
  Heinz bodies in, 187
    formation of, 186
  hemolytic anemia, idiopathic in, 192
  hyperaldosteronism in, 824
  hyperbilirubinemia, fasting in, 686
  hyperlipidemia disorders, secondary in, 775–78
  hyperparathyroidism in, 452
  hyperthyroidism in, 619
  hypoadrenocorticism in, 601–2
  infectious hemolytic anemia, 181
  leukogram patterns in, 90
  megaloblastic anemia in, 201
  myopathy, hypokalemic in, 519
  PLI and, 668, 745–46
  porphyria, congenital erythropoietic in, 191
  renal disease in, 601
  renal failure, hypokalemic in, 519
  reticulocytes, 117
  reticulocytosis, 117
  TLI in, 741–45, 743t, 745t
  triiodothyronine suppression test in, 796–98,
    797f
  TSH in, 794

UA, 442t, 445
USG, refractometric in, 450
D-xylose absorption tests in, 754
Cattle. *See also* Herd-based testing for cattle
  alopecia in Hereford calves, 167
  ALP in, 659
  azotemia in, abnormal routine serum chemistry
    results and, 440
  bile acid increase in, 693
  blood-group system of, 120
  dyserythropoiesis, congenital in Hereford calves,
    167
  GGT in, 661
  glucocorticoids in, caused by hypoferremia,
    204
  glutaraldehyde testing of calf serum in, 400
  hemoglobinuria, postparturient in, 189
  hereditary band 3 deficiency in Japanese black,
    200
  hypocalcemia, parturient in, 606–7
  Ig
    calf serum and changes of, 402
    deficiencies in, 403
    FPT of, 398–99
    measuring/estimating, 399–402
  leukogram patterns in, 90
  Na_2SO_3 for calf serum in, 401–2
  neutropenia in, 77–79
  porphyria, congenital erythropoietic in, 190–91
  renal failure, 524
  reticulocytosis, 117
  RID testing of calf serum in, 399–400
  Theileria spp. in, 185
  UA, 442t
  USG, refractometric in, 450
  $ZnSO_4$ turbidity testing for calf serum in,
    400–401
Cavalier King Charles spaniel, thrombocytopenia
    in, 235
  idiopathic, 241–42
Cavitary effusions, 831–66
  definitions, 832–37
  general concepts, 832–37
  hemorrhagic, 845–46
  lymphocyte-rich, 865
  lymphorrhagic, 846–47
  neoplasms associated with, 864–65
  pathogenesis of, 837–48, 837t, 840t
  pericardial, 866
  rupture-caused, 847–48
  specific, comments about, 863–66
  Starling's law and, 836–37

Cb_5R deficiency. *See* Cytochrome-b_5 reductase deficiency
CBC. *See* Complete blood count
Cell counting, 63–64, 64f
Cell (corpuscular) hemoglobin concentration mean (CHCM)
   anemia and increased, 157–58
   increased, 157–58
Centrifugation, urine, 455
Cephalosporins, immune hemolytic anemia induced by, 179–80
Ceruloplasmin, 372
CHCM. *See* Cell (corpuscular) hemoglobin concentration mean
Chediak-Higashi syndrome, 99
Chemistry assays, 8
Chloramphenicol, erythroid hypoplasia and, 339
Chloride (Cl⁻)
   alimentary tract functions pertaining to, 521, 521f
   Ca^{2+}, 281
   concentration, 520–25
      analytical concepts, 521–22
      assays, 522
      physiologic processes of, 520–21
      terms/units for, 521
   hyperchloremia, 522–23
   hypochloremia, 523–25
   renal tubule function and, 419
   resorbed, actively/passively, 521
   serum, 520
      control of, 520–21
Cholestasis, 656, 680–81
   functional, 681, 688
   obstructive, 681, 687–88
      laboratory findings for, 687–88
      pathogenesis of, 687, 688f
   stoppage and, 681
   suppression and, 681
Cholesterol
   effusion analysis with, 856–57, 857t
   hypercholesterolemia and, 770, 770t
   hypocholesterolemia and, 770–71, 771t
   serum concentration of, 767–71
Chromogenic assays, 287
Chronic myeloid leukemia, 76
Chylomicrons, standing plasma test for, 780
Chylous thoracic effusions, repeated drainage of, 515
Cl⁻. *See* Chloride
Circulating neutrophil pool (CNP), 57
Cirrhosis, transudation and, 504–5

Citrate, 6
CK. *See* Creatine kinase
Clinical pathology, 4–5
Clinitest. *See* Copper-reduction method
Clomipramine, hypothyroxemia and, 792–93
Clostridium spp., infectious hemolytic anemia, 182–83
Clotting
   assays, coagulation factor, 287
   calcium chloride and, 281
   thrombopathia and, 264–65
   whole blood, times, 279
CNP. *See* Circulating neutrophil pool
Coagulation, 268–93. *See also* Glutaraldehyde coagulation tests
   ACT, 279–80
   analytical concepts, 274–79
      general approach to, 278
      instruments, 278
      samples, 274–78
   assays, 274
   cascade web, 268–69, 270f
   endogenous anticoagulants, 288–92
      AT as, 288–91
      anti-(phospholipid-protein) antibodies as, 292–93
      protein C as, 291
      protein Z as, 291–92
   enzymes, inhibitors of, 273–74, 275f
   factors, 269–71, 272t, 273f
      activities of, 286–87
      antibodies, 292
      clotting assays for specific, 287
      deficiencies in, 286–87, 286t
      inhibition of, 310
      inhibitors, 292
      nonenzymatic, 269–71
   fibrinogen and, 285–86
   hypothermia, hemorrhage and, 278–79
   OSPT, 282–84
   pathways, 269
   physiologic inhibitors of, 271–74
   physiologic processes, 268–74
   PIVKA and, 287–88
   PTT, 280–84
   RVVT, 288
   samples
      citrated, 276–77
      collecting/handling, 274–76
      processing/stability of, 277–78
   TF, 282–83
   whole blood clotting times and, 279–80

Coagulopathy
 consumptive
  hemostatic test results, abnormal in, 309
  recognizing, 308–9
 dilutional, 309–10
Cobalamin (vitamin B$_{12}$)
 concentration, 747–50, 748f
 decreased, 749–50, 750t
 deficiency, anemia and, 165
 increased, 749
Codocyte, 147
Coefficient of variation (CV)
 analytical precision and, 22–24
 between-assay, 23
 determining, 23
 laboratory assay, 22–24
  relevance of, 23–24
 within-assay, 23
Colloidal osmotic pressure (COP), 405–10,
  546–47
 analytical concepts, 407–8, 408f
 decreased, 409–10
 Gibbs-Donnan equilibrium, 405, 407f
 increased, 408–9
 interferences with, 407–8
 osmotic pressure *v.,* 546f
 psychologic processes/concepts and, 405
 Starling's law, 405, 406f
Combs' test, 211, 212f
Complete blood count (CBC), 60–62
 bone marrow, 358, 360f
 components of, 60
 erythrocyte, 120
 platelet, 227
Coomassie brilliant blue assay, 477–78
COP. *See* Colloidal osmotic pressure
Copper deficiency, anemia and, 165
Copper-reduction method (Clinitest), 463
Corrected reticulocyte percentage (CRP), 123,
  134
Cortisol
 ACTH ratio to plasma, 814–15
 concentration, 808–12
 Crt ratio to urine, 812–13, 813f
 hypercortisolemia and, 808–10, 809t
 hypocortisolemia and, 810–12, 811t
 secretion, 806, 807f
Creatine kinase (CK)
 analytical concepts and, 662
 neurological disease and activity of, 663
 physiologic processes, 661–62
 serum, increased activity of, 662–63, 662t

Creatinine (Crt). *See also* Urinary protein to
  creatinine ratio
 albumin to, ratio, 482
 assays, 436–37
 clearance rate, 438–39
 cortisol, urine ratio to, 812–13, 813f
 effusion analysis with, 857–58
 physiologic processes/concepts regarding, 434f
 renal tubule function and, 423
 serum/plasma concentration of, 434f, 436–37
  decreased, 437
  increased, 437
  UN concentration *v.,* 437–38, 438t
 urinary excretion of, 429–31
 urine bile acid to, ratio, 485, 696–97, 697t
Crossmatching, blood, 210
CRP. *See* Corrected reticulocyte percentage
Crt. *See* Creatinine
Crystallography, optical, 489
Crystalluria, 474–75
Crystals, urine sediment, 474–75
Cubic meter, 10
CV. *See* Coefficient of variation
Cyclic hematopoiesis, 80–81
Cylindruria, 473
Cytochemical stains, hemic neoplasia classification
  with, 353, 353t
Cytochrome-b_5 reductase (Cb_5R) deficiency, 199
Cytology, 8
 bone marrow, 333–34
Cytometry, flow, 334
Cytoplasm, foamy, 92

Dacryocyte, 147
DEA. *See* Dog erythrocyte antigen
Decision limits, 20
Decision thresholds, 39–40, 40f
 factors influencing establishing, 48
 reference limits *v.,* 20
 ROC curve establishment of, 45–46, 47f
Dehydration
 causes, net loss of isotonic fluids and, 503–4
 disorders and pathogenesis of, 503–4
 erythrocytosis caused by, 193–96
 hypernatremic, 500
 hyperproteinemia of, 371
 hyponatremic, 500
 normonatremic, 500, 503–5
 pathologic state of, 500
 types, 500
 USG, refractometric and, 450
Deming method comparison, 33–34, 33f

Dendritic cells, 327

Detection limit, 25

Detomidine, hyperglycemia and, 718

Dexamethasone. *See also* High-dose dexamethasone
     suppression test; Low-dose dexamethasone
     suppression test
   glucocorticoid, 204
   LPS and, 667
   suppression tests
      ACTH stimulation tests combined with,
        823
      canine, 815–18, 816f, 819t
      equine, 822
      feline, 821–22
   TLI and, 743

Dextran, biuret reactions for measuring total
     protein and, 364

Diabetes insipidus, nephrogenic, 451

Diabetes mellitus
   diagnostic criteria for, 713, 714t
   drug-induced, 717
   endocrine, 716–17
   genetic, 718
   hyperglycemia and, 713
   infectious, 717
   D-lactate and, 542–43
   $Na^+:K^+$ ratio, decreased and, 520
   pancreatic, 716
   types, 715–18

Diagnostic accuracy, 39

Diagnostic procedures, 5
   ROC curve comparison of, 45–46

Diagnostic properties
   deficiency in theories of, 44
   laboratory assay, 38–45

Diagnostic sensitivity, 38–39

Diagnostic specificity, 39

Diarrhea
   K^+ loss through, 518–19
   $Na^+:K^+$ ratio, decreased and, 520

Diazoxide, hyperglycemia and, 719

DIC. *See* Disseminated intravascular coagulation

Diestrus, 714–15

Direct megakaryocyte immunofluorescence assays,
     249

Discocytes, 136

Disseminated intravascular coagulation (DIC)
   envenomation and, 241
   thrombocytopenia and, 241

Diuresis, prolonged, 506–7

Dog erythrocyte antigen (DEA), 119
   infectious hemolytic anemia, 181

Dogs
   α_1-PI, fecal in, 753
   acidosis in, 581t
   ACTH in, 813, 814f
   adrenocortical function tests in, 815–21, 816f
   aldosterone concentration in, 824–26, 825t
   ALP in, 658–59
   ALT, serum, 651
   ammonium tolerance test in, 702–3, 703t
   azotemia in
      abnormal routine serum chemistry results in,
        440
      UN:Crt ratio and, 438, 438t
   bile acid challenge test for, 693–96, 694t
   bone marrow dyscrasia of poodles, 100
   CK in, 662
   cobalamin in, 747–50
   cortisol, urine to Crt ratio in, 812–13, 813f
   dexamethasone and, 667
   distemper inclusions in, 202
   dyserythropoiesis in English springer spaniels,
      167
   elliptocytosis in, 200–201
      hereditary, 200
   enteropathy, protein-losing in, 604
   EPI in, 740
   exocrine pancreatic insufficiency in, 605–6
   folate in, 750–52
   GGT in, 661
   Heinz body formation in, 186
   hyperadrenocorticism in, 610
   hyperaldosteronism in, 824
   hyperlipidemia disorders, secondary in, 775–78
   hypoadrenocorticism in, 601–2
   hypothyroidism and vWD in, 266
   Ig deficiencies in, 403–4
   IMT, drug-induced in, 238–39
   leukemia, 356
   leukogram patterns in, 90
   LPS and, 667
   microalbuminuria in, 483
   neoplasia in, LPS and, 667
   nonstaining eosinophil granules of, 101–2
   PFK deficiency in English springer spaniels,
      189
   PLI and, 668, 745–46
   portosystemic shunts in, 204
   pyometra in, 451
   renal disease in, 601
   reticulocytosis, 117
   sideroblastic anemia in, 202
   SLE in, 240

Dogs (*continued*)
spectrin deficiency in Dutch golden retrievers
and, 201
TAP in, 746–47
thrombocytopenia in Cavalier King Charles
spaniels, 235, 241–42
thyroid hormone concentrations in, 799, 799t,
800t
thyroxine and TSH in, 798
TLI in, 741–45, 743t, 745t
TSH in, 788, 794
UA, 442t, 445–55
uroliths, 488
USG, refractometric in, 449t, 450
D-xylose absorption tests in, 754
Döhle's inclusion bodies, cytoplasmic, 92
Dutch golden retrievers, spectrin deficiency in,
201
Dye-excretion tests, 703–4
Dyscrasia
bone marrow, of poodles, 100
protein, 371
Dyserythropoiesis, 348
congenital, in Hereford calves, 167
in English springer spaniels, 167
Dysfibrinogenemia, 310
TT, prolonged and, 285
Dyshematopoiesis, acquired secondary, 350
Dysmegakaryopoiesis, 349
Dysmyelopoiesis, 348
Dysplasia, multilineage, 347–48. *See also* Refractory
cytopenia with multilineage dysplasia;
Refractory cytopenia with multilineage
dysplasia and ringed sideroblasts
Dysproteinemia, 371
hyperproteinemia and pattern of, 382–83
patterns, expected, 380–81

Eccentrocyte, 147
ECF. *See* Extracellular fluid
Echinocyte, 147–48
Eclampsia, 607
Edema, isotonic fluid net retention and, 504–5
Edematous animals
hyponatremia and, 507
normonatremia in, 503–4, 503t
EDTA. *See* Ethylenediaminetetraacetic acid
Effusions
definition, 835
peritoneal, 515–16
Ehrlichia, leukocyte, 95
EIAV. *See* Equine infectious anemia virus

Electrolytes
concentrations
abnormal, 498
interpretation of, basic concepts for, 497–98
K^+, 509–19
Na^+, 498–509
plasma, 497–98
serum, 497–98
monovalent, 495–553
weak, 586
Elliptocyte, 148
Elliptocytosis, 148
in dogs, 200–201
hereditary, in dogs, 200
Endocarditis, thrombocytopenia and, 241
Endocrine disorders
anemia caused by, 166
hypoplasia, erythroid caused by, 339
Endomitriosis, 325
Endothelial cells. *See* Blood vessels
Endotoxemia
hypomagnesemia and, 625
neutropenia caused by, 78f, 79
thrombocytopenia and, 242
Endotoxic shock, erythrocytosis caused by, 196
English springer spaniels
dyserythropoiesis in, 167
PFK deficiency in, 189
Enteric diseases, hypomagnesemia and, 624
Enteropathy, protein-losing, 604
Envenomation, 192
thrombocytopenia and, 241
Enzymes, 639–69
activity, 645
effusion analysis with, 862
increased serum, 649–50, 650f
units to express, 645–47, 647t
assays
hepatic, 680
serum, 645–47, 646f, 647t
definition, 640
nomenclature, 647–48
production
cellular, 644
tissue, 644
release of, increased, 643f
cell escape and, 642–43
cellular, 643
rate, factors affecting, 643–44
removal of, plasma, 644–45
serum, 668t
activity, 642–45

activity, increased, 649–50, 650f
assays of, 645–47, 646f, 647t
measurement of, 645–47
samples of, 648–49
sources of, 641–42, 641t, 642f
Enzymology, basic principles in clinical, 640–50
Eosinophilia, 86–88
  causes, 86–87, 87t
  disease states suggested by, 86–87, 87t
  neoplasms linked to, 88
  paraneoplastic, 87–88
Eosinophilic leukemia, 88
Eosinophils
  concentrations, abnormal, 86–88
  kinetics, 59
  nonstaining, granules of dogs, 101–2
  pools, 59
  Pseudo-Pelger-Huët, 101
EPI. See Exocrine pancreatic insufficiency
Epithelial cells, urinary, 473–74
Epo, 110–11
Equine infectious anemia virus (EIAV), 183–84
Erythrocytes, 107–212. See also Dog erythrocyte
      antigen; Wintrobe's erythrocyte indices
  abnormalities, nonregenerative anemia and, 152
  ADVIA, 125, 127
  agglutination, 130, 136
    heparin and, 136
  analysis, graphing data from, 125–26, 126f
  analytical methods
    impedance cell counter, 124–25
    microhematocrit, 124–35
    RC, 131
    RP, 132–34
  anemia, 151–59
  assessment, 135
  blood, 111, 111t
    crossmatching and, 210
    groups/types and, 117–20, 208–10
    species variations and, 210–11
  Cb_5R deficiency and, 199
  CBC, 120
  central pallor, 137
  clinical significance, 135–51
  color, 137–38
  complement, methods for detecting, 211–12
  crenated, 147–48
  data, differences in, 129–31
  discocytes, 136
  distemper inclusions in dogs and, 202
  in dogs, 200–202
  effusions and, 851–52

elliptocytosis in dogs and, 200–201
fragmentation of, in blood, 191
general features, 136–37
ghost cell, 137
Heinz bodies, 141
hemolytic anemia and examination of, 171
hereditary band 3 deficiency in Japanese black
      cattle and, 200
hypochromic, 137–38
inclusions, 138–42, 140t
  basophilic stippling, 138–41, 140t
  Hgb crystals as, 141
  Howell-Jolly bodies as, 141
  refractile artifacts as, 141–42
  siderotic granules as, 142
indices, anemia classification with, 153–58,
      154t
kinetics, 112
megaloblastic anemia and, 201–2
metabolic defect in, hemolytic anemia and,
      186–91
metabolism of mature, 115, 118f
methemoglobinemia and, 198–99
morphologic evaluation, 120
morphologic features of, 135–51
organisms, 138, 139t
osmolality, 130–31
oxidant exposure of, 198–99
pathogenesis, 135–51
physiologic processes, 110–20
polychromatophilic, 138
precursors, 110
production, anemia and, 158–60
QBC analysis of, 127
rouleau, 136
rubricytosis, 136–37
shape, abnormal, 143–51, 144t
sideroblastic anemia in dogs and, 202
small, 130
spectrin deficiency in Dutch golden retrievers
      and, 201
spiculated, 147
splenic, 111–12
stomatocytosis, hereditary and, 199–200
surface antibodies, methods for detecting,
      211–12
urine sediment, 471–72
volume, abnormal, 142–43
Erythrocyte surface-associated immunoglobulin
      (ESAIg)
  disorders with, 212
  flow cytometric detection of, 212

Erythrocytosis, 193–98
  absolute, 193
  hypoxic, 196–97
  idiopathic, 198
  pathogenesis, 195f
  physiologic, 196
  primary, 198, 351
  relative, 193
  secondary appropriate, 196–97
    pathogenesis of, 197
    physiologic processes of, 197
  secondary inappropriate, 197–98
Erythrocytotic disorders/conditions, 193–98, 194f, 194t
  hemoconcentration as, 193–96
  splenic contraction, 196
Erythrogram, 60, 120–23
Erythron, 110–12
Erythrophage, 94
Erythropoiesis
  effective, bone marrow and, 334
  ineffective
    anemia caused by, 163–67
    bone marrow and, 336
ESAIg. *See* Erythrocyte surface-associated immunoglobulin
Ethanol, hypoglycemia and, 722
Ethylenediaminetetraacetic acid (EDTA), 6
Ethylene glycol
  hyperglycemia and, 718
  toxicosis, 608
Euglobulin, 377. *See also* Sia euglobulin test
Evan's syndrome, 240
Exocrine intestine, 739–59
  absorptive malfunctions of, 740–41
  diseases, methods for evaluating, 758, 759t
Exocrine pancreas, 739–59
  absorptive malfunctions of, 740–41
Exocrine pancreatic insufficiency (EPI), 605–6, 740–41
  in cats, 740
  in dogs, 740
  evaluating, methods for, 758, 758t
Extracellular fluid (ECF). *See also* Base excess in ECF
  electrolyte concentrations in, 497
  hyperalbuminemia and, 390
  hyponatremia, 507–8
  hypoproteinemia and, 389–90
Exudates, 844–45
  bacterial, 864
  septic/nonseptic, 863–64
Exudation, 835

Failure of passive transfer (FPT), 389
  immunoglobin, 398–402
    causes of, 399
    physiologic concepts of, 398–99
False negative (FN) results, 38
False positive (FP) results, 38
  ROC curve and rate of, 45
Fanconi syndrome, 620
FDPs. *See* Fibrin or fibrinogen degradation products
Fe. *See* Iron
Feline leukemia virus (FeLV)
  erythroid hypoplasia induced by, 164
  infectious hemolytic anemia and, 184
FeLV. *See* Feline leukemia virus
FE ratios/percentages. *See* Fractional excretion ratios/percentages
Ferritin, 207–8, 372
  hyperferritinemia, 207–8, 207t
  hypoferritinemia, 208
Fibrin fragment D-dimer, 299–300
  analytical concepts, 299–300
  increased, 300
  sample, 299
  theory, 299
Fibrinogen, 271, 285–86, 372, 393–96. *See also* Hyperfibrinogenemia; Plasma protein to fibrinogen ratio
  activity, 285–86
  analytical concepts, 393–94
  antigen, detecting, 286
  heat-precipitant method, 393–94
  heparin and, 285
  hyperfibrinogenemia, 394–96
  hypofibrinogenemia, 396, 396t
  interpretive considerations, 286
  physiologic process, 393
  TT, 394
Fibrinogenolysis, increased, 298
Fibrinolysis, 293–300
  assays, 300
  FDPS and, 293–98
  fibrin fragment D-dimer and, 299–300
  increased, 297–98
  physiologic processes, 293
Fibrinolytic system, 293, 296t
Fibrin or fibrinogen degradation products (FDPs), 293–98
  analytical concepts, 296–97
  antibody specificity and, 296–97
  clearance, decreased, 298
  increased, 297–98, 298t
  interpretive considerations, 297

latex agglutination immunoassays for, 296
measuring, 293
sample, 293–96
unit, 297
Fight-or-flight, 90
FN results. *See* False negative results
Foamy cytoplasm, 92
Folate
concentration, 750–52
decreased, 752, 752t
deficiency, anemia and, 165
increased, 751–52, 751t
FP results. *See* False positive results
FPT. *See* Failure of passive transfer
Fractional excretion (FE) ratios/percentages, 483–85
24 h excretion study *v.,* 484
decreased, 484
increased, 484
interpretive concepts, 484
studies, clinical uses of, 485
theory, 483–84
Fructosamine, 723–26
decreased, 725
increased, 724–25, 724t
protein concentrations, abnormal and, 726
Fucosidosis, 100
Functional hepatic mass, decreased, 680, 680t
bilirubin uptake in hepatocytes and, 686–87
Furosemide
Ca^{2+} urinary excretion and, 608
hypochloremia and, 524–25

Gammopathy, monoclonal, 382
in domestic mammals, 383–84
Gastrointestinal disorders in colicky horses, hypocalcemia and, 609–10
Gaussian distribution, 18, 19f
Genital tract
hemorrhage, 472
inflammation, 471
GFR. *See* Glomerular filtration rate
GGT. *See* γ-Glutamyltransferase
Ghost cell, 137
Gibbs-Donnan equilibrium, 405, 407f
Globulin
analytical principles for total, 372–79
general concepts for total, 370–72
physiologic processes, 370–71
total, measuring, 375
Glomerular filtration, 417–18
concentration/dilution of, 424–25

Glomerular filtration rate (GFR), 417–18
PO_4 and disorders decreasing, 618–19
Glucagon
hyperglycemia and, 718
immunoreactive, concentration of, 730–31
Glucocorticoid therapy
APP, positive concentration increase and, 397
hyperalbuminemia, 390
hypothyroxemia and, 792
Glucose
absorption test, in horses, 755–56, 756t
concentration, 708–23, 712t
analytical concepts for, 709–13
physiologic processes for, 708–9, 710f
effusion analysis with, 860–61
hyperglycemia and, 713–19
hypoglycemia and, 719–23
insulin and, 722–23
immunoreactive ratio to, 729–30
renal tubule function and, 422
in urine, 462–64
analytical concepts of, 463
physiologic processes of, 462–63
Glucose infusion, 620
Glucosuria
disorders, 463–64
hyperglycemic, 463
renal, 463
Glutamate dehydrogenase (GMD), 654–55
activity, increased, 655
serum, 654
γ-Glutamyltransferase (GGT), 659–61
in cats, 661
in cattle, 661
in dogs, 661
in horses, 661
physiologic processes, 659
serum, increased activity of, 659, 659t
species differences, 661
urine activity of, 661
Glutaraldehyde coagulation tests, 400
Glycated hemoglobin, 723–26
decreased, 725–26
increased, 724–25, 724t
Glycogenolysis, 720–21
Glycosuria, disorders, 463–64
GM_1 gangliosidosis, 99
GM_2 gangliosidosis, 99
GMD. *See* Glutamate dehydrogenase
Gold salts, IMT induced by, 238
Gram staining, effusion analysis with, 863
Granules, toxic, 92

Granulocytes, 56
Granulopoiesis, bone marrow and, 336–37
Griseofulvin, myelosuppressive effects of, 236
Group testing, 48–50

H$_2$O
   dehydration and, 500
   electrolyte concentrations and, 498
   hypernatremia and intake of, 501
   hypochloremia and excess, 525
   hyponatremia and excess group of, 507–8
   intake, Na$^+$ excess and, 502
   loss
      Na$^+$ loss and, 502
      pure, 502
   Na$^+$ and, 499, 502
   replacement, 502
   shifting of, 508
H$_2$O deprivation
   in PU/PD, 485–87
   tests for
      abrupt, 486
      gradual, 486–87
      modified, 487
Halothane anesthesia, 621
Haptoglobin, 372
HCO$_3^-$. See Bicarbonate
Hct. See Hematocrit
HDDST. See High-dose dexamethasone
         suppression test
Heat-precipitant method, fibrinogen, 393–94
Heinz bodies
   erythrocyte, 141
   feline, 187
   formation of, 186
   hemolytic anemia, 186
Hematest tablet, 465
Hematocrit (Hct), 120
   conductivity, 131
      determination of, 128
   effusions and, 851–52
   erythrocyte data differences and calculating,
         129–30, 129t
Hematology analyzers, light-scatter patterns
         produced by, 92
Hematology assays, 7–8
Hematopoiesis
   cyclic, 80–81, 86
   extramedullary, 351
Hematopoietic cells, 324–27
   bone marrow nucleated cell differential count in
         health and, 327

dendritic cells and, 327
   erythrocyte lineage, 325, 325t
   lymphocyte lineage, 326
   megakaryocyte lineage, 325
   nonlymphoid leukocyte lineages, 326
   populations, bone marrow, 330–32, 331f
Hematopoietic cellularity, bone marrow, 329–30
Hematuria, 176t, 465–66, 471–72
Heme
   synthesis, porphyria caused by defects in,
         190–91
   in urine, 465–66
Hemic neoplasia, 90–92
   bone marrow, 342–57
      classification of, 342–46, 343t
      general concepts/terms, 342–46, 344f
   cells, methods for characterizing, 92
   classifying, methods of, 352–57
      cytochemical stain, 353, 353t
      immunophenotyping, 353–56, 354t
      microscopic, 352–53
      molecular and cytogenetic studies for, 357
      Wright stain, 352–53
   thrombocytosis and, 244–45
Hemoconcentration, 193–96
   hyperalbuminemia and, 390
   hyperfibrinogemia caused by, 394, 394t
   hyperproteinemia and, 379
Hemocytometer method, 62–63, 63f
   platelet analysis with, 231
Hemodilution
   hypoproteinemia and, 389–90
   thrombocytopenia and, 241
Hemoglobin (Hgb), 112–14. See also Percent
         hemoglobin saturation with oxygen of
         arterial blood by pulse oximetry
   blood, 128–29
   conductivity determination of, 128
   crystals, 141
   degradation, 113f
      bilirubin metabolism and, 114, 114f
   erythrocyte, 120
   function, 112
   glycated, 723–26
   MCHC relationship with, 121–22
   myoglobin differentiation from, 465
   reticulocyte, content/volume of, 208
   structure, 112
   synthesis, 112–13, 113f
      type of, 113
Hemoglobinemia, hemolytic, 174, 175f
Hemoglobinuria, 176t, 466

hemolytic, 174, 175f
postparturient, in cattle, 189
Hemolysis, 170
  alloimmune, 180–81
  bilirubin and, 684–85, 685t
  envenomation and, 192
  extravascular *v.* intravascular, 170–71, 173t
  heparin-induced, 191–92
  hypoosmolar, 191
  intravascular, massive, 513
  pathologic, 170
Hemolytic disorders/conditions, 171, 172t, 176–
    93. *See also specific disorders/conditions*
  idiopathic nonspherocytic, 192
  immune hemolytic anemias as, 176–81
  of unknown pathogenesis, 191–93
Hemolytic hemoglobinemia, 174, 175f
Hemolytic hemoglobinuria, 174, 175f
Hemolytic icterus, 171, 174f
Hemolytic syndrome, in horses, 193
Hemophagocytic histiocytic sarcoma, 192
Hemophilia, gender and, 301
Hemorrhage
  blood loss caused by, 167
  definition, 835
  effusions and, 845–46
  genital tract, 472
  hypothermia and, 278–79
  iatrogenic, 471–72
  proteinuria and, 459–60
  vitamin K and, 306
Hemostasis, 259–311
  abnormal, 261
  bleeding disorders, major, 300–310
    patterns in tests for, 302–4, 303t
    tests for, 302–5, 302t
  blood vessels and, 300
  coagulation and, 268–93
  consumptive coagulopathy tests for, 309
  definition, 261
  fibrinolysis, 293–300
  in health, 261, 261f
  platelets and, 262–65
    concentration of, 262–63
  thrombosis and, 310–11
    abnormalities in, 311
  vitamin K and tests for, abnormal results in,
    305–8
  vWF and, 265–68
Hemotropic mycoplasma species, infectious
    hemolytic anemia, 181–82
Heparin, 6

Ca²⁺ sample anticoagulation with, 611–12
AT consumption and, 290
erythrocyte agglutination and, 136
fibrinogen and, 285
hemolysis induced by, 191–92
IMT induced by, 239
PTT monitoring therapy with, 282
Hepatic disease
  bleeding disorder pathogenesis and, 304–5
  protein catabolism, increased and, 388
  protein synthesis, decreased and, 388
Hepatic enzyme assays, 680
Hepatocellular disease, 677
Hepatocytes, bilirubin uptake by, 685–87, 685t
Hepatocytes, functioning, 680
Hepatozoon americanum, leukocyte, 95–97
Hepatozoon canis, leukocyte, 97
Herd-based testing for cattle, 48–50
  abnormalities in, 50
  analyte measurement in, 49–50
  data evaluation, 50
  metabolic/nutritional status, 49–50
Hereditary band 3 deficiency in Japanese black
    cattle, 200
Hetastarch, increased COP and, 409
Heterobilharzia americana, 600
Heterogeneous nucleation, 489
Hgb. *See* Hemoglobin
HHM. *See* Humoral hypercalcemia of malignancy
High-dose dexamethasone suppression test
    (HDDST)
  canine, 817–18
  feline, 818
Histiocytic neoplasia, 192
Histology, bone marrow, 333–34
Histopathology, surgical, 8
Histoplasma capsulatum, leukocyte, 97
Hitachi analyzers, 528–29
Holoenzymes, 640
Hormones. *See also specific hormones*
  Ca²⁺, free concentration and, 613–14
  Mg²⁺ regulated by, 622
Horses
  ACTH in, 814
  adrenocortical function tests in, 822–23
  ALP in, 659
  azotemia in
    renal/prerenal, 477, 478t
    serum chemistry results in, abnormal routine,
      440
  bile acid increase in, 693
  blood-group system of, 119

Horses (*continued*)
  cobalamin in, 747–50
  EIAV, 183–84
  erythrocyte agglutination in, 136
  gastrointestinal disorders in colicky,
      hypocalcemia and, 609–10
  GGT in, 661
  glucose absorption test in, 755–56
  glutaraldehyde testing of foal serum in, 400
  halothane anesthesia in, 621
  Heinz body formation in, 186
  hemolytic syndrome in, 193
  hyperbilirubinemia, fasting in, 686
  hyperlipemia in, 777–78
  hypomagnesemia and, 625
  idiopathic hypersegmented neutrophils of, 101
  Ig
      deficiencies in, 403
      foal serum and changes of, 402
      FPT of, 398–99
      measuring/estimating, 399–402
  lactose tolerance test in, 756–57
  latex agglutination for foal serum in, 400
  leukogram patterns in, 90
  methemoglobinemia, familial in, 199
  peritoneal fluid in, 833–35, 834t
  pleural fluid in, 833–35, 834t
  renal disease in, 621
  renal failure in, 601
  reticulocytosis, 117
  RID testing of foal serum in, 399–400
  sweat, 507
      K⁺ loss through, 519
  Theileria spp. in, 185
  TLI in, 741–45
  triiodothyronine suppression test in, 797–98
  TSH in, 794
  UA, 442t
  urinary bladder, ruptured in, 602
  urine sucrose concentration in, 757
  USG, refractometric in, 450
  ZnSO₄ turbidity testing for foal serum in,
      400–401
Howell-Jolly bodies, 141
H⁺, renal tubule function and, 421
Humoral hypercalcemia of malignancy (HHM),
      598–600
Hydraulic pressure, 835
Hydrogen peroxide, Heinz body formation and,
      186
Hydrostatic pressure, 835

β-Hydroxybutyrate (BHB)
  concentration, 49, 543–45
      analytical concepts in, 544
      physiologic processes, 543–44
  renal excretion, 544
Hyperadrenocorticism
  hyperphosphatemia and, 619
  USG, refractometric, 450–51
Hyperadrenocorticism, in dogs, 610
Hyperalbuminemia, 390–91
  diseases/conditions causing, 390, 390t
Hyperaldosteronism
  primary, 824
  USG, refractometric and, 451
Hyperammonemia, 699–702, 700t, 717–18
Hyperbilirubinemia, 684–89, 684t
  fasting, 685–86
Hypercalcemia, 385, 598–602, 599t. *See also*
      Humoral hypercalcemia of malignancy
  of benignancy, 600
  Ca²⁺, free concentration and, 613
  diseases/conditions causing, 599t
  USG, refractometric and, 451
Hypercalcitonism, 607
Hypercapnia, 561
Hypercarbia, 561
Hyperchloremia, 522–23
  disorders/pathogeneses and, 522, 522t
  HCO₃⁻, decreased and, 533–34
  metabolic acidosis and, 523
  tCO², decreased and, 533–34
Hypercholesterolemia, 770, 770t, 774
Hypercortisolemia, 808–10, 809t
Hyperestrogenism, anemia and, 166
Hyperferremia, 203, 203t
Hyperferritinemia, 207–8, 207t
Hyperfibrinogenemia, 394–96
  diseases/conditions causing, 394, 394t
  PP : F ratio, 395–96
  TT, prolonged and, 285
Hyperglobulinemia, 392, 404
  hyperproteinemia and, 392
Hyperglucagonemia, 731
Hyperglycemia, 713–19
  classification, 713, 715t
  diabetes mellitus and, 713, 714t
  disorders/conditions, 714–19, 715t
  pathologic, 715–18
  pharmacologic/toxicologic, 718–19
  physiologic, 714–15
  postprandial, 714

steroid-associated, 714
unexpected, 723
Hyperinsulinemia, 728, 728t
Hyperinsulinism, 620
Hyperkalemia. *See also* Pseudo-hyperkalemia
  K^+ and, 511–16
  strenuous exercise causing, 512
Hyperlactatemia, disorders/pathogeneses causing,
    541–42
Hyperlipasemia, LPS and, 667
Hyperlipemia, 773–78
  equine, 777–78
Hyperlipidemia, 773–78
  conditions/disorders, 773–74
  disorders, secondary, 775–78
Hyperlipoproteinemia, 773–78
  conditions/disorders, 773
Hypermagnesemia, 622–23, 623t
Hypernatremia, 501–3
  disorders/pathogenesis of, 501–3, 501t
  H_2O intake and, 501
Hyperosmolality, osmo. gap and serum, 552–53
Hyperparathyroidism
  feline, refractometric USG and, 452
  primary, Ca^{2+} and, 598
Hyperphosphatasemia, 658
Hyperphosphatemia, 618–19, 618t
  pseudo-, 619
Hyperplasia
  basophilic granulocytic, bone marrow and, 337
  bone marrow, 334–38, 335t
    generalized, 337–38
  eosinophilic granulocytic, bone marrow and,
    337
  erythroid
    anemia, regenerative and, 152
    bone marrow, 334–36
  granulocytic
    basophilic, 337
    bone marrow and, 336–37
    eosinophilic, 337
  lymph node, 362
  megakaryocytic, bone marrow and, 337
  monocytic, bone marrow and, 337
  reactive, 362
Hyperproteinemia, 371, 379–85
  diseases/conditions causing, 379, 379t
  dysproteinemia pattern and, 382–83
  hemoconcentration and, 379
  hyperglobulinemia and, 392
  inflammation and, 380–81

neoplasia, B-lymphocyte, 381–85
protein synthesis, increased and, 380–85
Hyperthyroidism
  Ca^{2+}, free concentration and, 613
  hyperphosphatemia and, 619
Hyperthyroxemia, 789–90, 789t
Hypertonicity, 513
Hypertriglyceridemia, 772, 772t
Hyperventilation, 561
  alkalemia and, 563
Hyperviscosity syndrome, 385
Hypoadrenocorticism, 515
  anemia and, 166
  in cats, 601–2
  in dogs, 601–2
  hyponatremia and, 505–6
  lymphocytosis of, 83
  Na^+ : K^+ ratio, decreased and, 519
Hypoadrenocroticism, refractometric USG and, 451
Hypoalbuminemia, 391–92
  albumin synthesis, decrease and, 383
  ascites formation and, 505
  diseases/conditions causing, 391, 391t
  hypocalcemia, 602
  inflammatory, 391
  pathogenesis, 391
Hypoaldosteronism, 515
  hyperreninemic, hyponatremia and, 507
  primary, 518
Hypocalcemia, 602–10, 603t
  Ca^{2+}, free concentration and, 613
  diseases/conditions causing, 603t
  gastrointestinal disorders in colicky horses and,
    609–10
  hypoalbuminemic, 602
  lactational, 606–7
  myopathies, 610
  nutritional, 607
  pancreatis, acute and, 608–9
  parturient, 606–7
  phosphate enemas and, 609
  pregnancy, 606–7
  preparturient, 607
  renal failure, acute and, 609
  tumor lysis syndrome, acute and, 610
  urinary tract obstruction and, 609
Hypocapnia, 561
Hypocarbia, 561
Hypochloremia, 523–25
  acidosis, metabolic and, 525, 526f
  alkaloses, metabolic and, 524–25

Hypochloremia (*continued*)
  diseases/pathogeneses and, 524–25, 524t
  H₂O excess group of, 525
  hyponatremia and, 524–25
Hypocholesterolemia, 770–71, 771t
Hypochromasia, 138
Hypocortisolemia, 810–12, 811t
Hypoferremia, 203–5, 204t
  young animal, 204–5
Hypoferritinemia, 208
Hypofibrinogenemia, 396, 396t
  TT, prolonged and, 285
Hypoglobinemia, 392
Hypoglycemia, 719–22
  disorders/pathogeneses, 719, 720t
  pathologic, 719–22
  pharmacologic/toxicologic, 722
  unexpected, 723
Hypoinsulinemia, 728–29
Hypokalemia, 451–52, 516–19
  alkaloses, metabolic and, 510
  disorders/pathogeneses and, 512–16, 513t, 516,
      517t
  K⁺
      decreased total body and, 516–19
      increased excretion and, 517–19
  myopathy and, in cats, 519
  renal failure and, in cats, 519
Hypomagnesemia, 604, 623–25, 624t
  hypoproteinemia and, 623
Hyponatremia, 505–9
  dilutional, 508
  disorders/pathogeneses and, 505, 506t
  diuresis, prolonged and, 506–7
  ECF, 507–8
  H₂O excess group, 507–8
  hypoaldosteronism, hyperreninemic and, 507
  hypochloremia and, 524–25
  ketonuria and, 507
  Na⁺ deficit group of, 505
  nephropathies, Na⁺-wasting and, 507
  pseudo-, 508–9
  renal loss and, 505–7
Hypoparathyroidism
  pseudo-, 604
  PTH activity, decreased and, 602–4
  USG, refractometric and, 452
Hypophosphatemia, 619–21, 620t
  pseudo-, 621
  thrombocytopenia and, 243
Hypoplasia
  bone marrow, 338–40, 338t

  anemia caused by, 162–63
  generalized, 338–39
  infections and, 236–37
erythroid
  anemia caused by, 163–67
  bone marrow and selective, 339
  drugs and, 339
  endocrine disorders causing, 339
  FeLV-induced, 164
granulocytic
  bone marrow and selective, 338t, 339–40
  selective, 338t, 339–40
lymphoid
  lymphopenia of, 84f, 85
  protein synthesis/catabolism and, 389
megakaryocytic, selective, 340
Hypoproteinemia, 371
  ascites formation and, 505
  COP, decreased and, 409
  diseases/conditions causing, 385, 386t
  FPT and, 389
  hemodilution and, 389–90
  hypomagnesemia and, 623
  plasma loss and, 387–88
  PLE, 387
  PLN, 385–87
  protein catabolism, increased and, 388–89
  protein synthesis, decreased and, 388–89
  in serum/plasma, 385–90
  vascular space protein loss and, 385–88
Hyposthenuria, 424
Hypothermia, hemorrhage and, 278–79
Hypothyroidism
  anemia and, 166
  secondary, 791–92
  vWD and, 266
Hypothyroxemia, 790–93, 791t
  drugs and, 792–93
Hypotriglyceridemia, 772
Hypoventilation, 561
Hypovitaminosis D, 604
Hypoxemia, 561, 581–84
  alkalosis, respiratory and, 577, 577t
  atmospheric, 582
  diseases/conditions causing, 582, 582t
Hypoxia, 561, 581–84
  alveolar, 583
  blood gases and, 582, 583t
  demand, 584
      hyperlactatemia and, 541–42
  hemoglobic, 583–84
  histotoxic, 584

L-lactate production and, 540–41
    stagnant, 584
        hyperlactatemia and, 541
    tidal, 582–83

Icterus
    hemolytic, 684–85, 685t
    index, 689–90
Ictotest, bilirubin in urine and, 467
ID. *See* Iditol dehydrogenase
IDEXX QBC VetAutoread hematology system,
        66–67
Idiopathic hypereosinophilic syndrome, 87
Iditol dehydrogenase (ID), 654
Ig. *See* Immunoglobins
IMHA. *See* Immune-mediated hemolytic anemia
Immune-mediated hemolytic anemia (IMHA),
        177–79
    blood transfusions, incompatible and secondary,
        180
    laboratory features of, 179
Immune-mediated thrombocytopenia (IMT),
        237–38
    drug-induced, 238–39
    idiopathic, 237
    infections associated with, 239
    primary, 237
    secondary, 238
    tests for, 249
Immunodeficiencies, Ig concentrations and
        congenital, 402
Immunoelectrophoresis
    gammopathy, monoclonal, 383–84
    immunofixation sensitivity *v.*, 384
    protein, 377
Immunofixation, immunoelectrophoresis sensitivity
        v., 384
Immunoglobins (Ig), 372, 398–404
    in cattle, 398–402
    deficiencies, 402–4
        analytical concepts in, 404
        in cattle, 403
        in dogs, 403–4
        in horses, 403
    excess, 404
    FPT, 398–402
        causes of, 399
        physiologic concepts of, 398–99
    in horses, 398–402
Immunophenotyping
    hemic neoplasia, 353–56, 354t
    lymphoma, 364–65

Immunoreactive PTH (iPTH)
    assays, analytical concepts for, 626–27
    concentration, 626–27
    plasma, increased/decreased, 627, 627t
    serum, increased/decreased, 627, 627t
Impedance cell counters, 63–64
    basic principles, 63, 64f
    erythrocyte, 124–25
    platelet analysis with, 230
IMT. *See* Immune-mediated thrombocytopenia
Inclusions. *See also* Döhle's inclusion bodies,
            cytoplasmic
    erythrocyte, 138–42, 140t
    leukocyte
        hereditary disorders that have, 99–100
        miscellaneous contained in, 94–95
    platelet, 232–33
Individual testing, 48–50
Induction, 644
Infections
    IMT associated with, 239
    megakaryopoiesis decreased by, 236
    thrombocytopenia and, 236–37, 242
    thrombopoiesis decreased by, 236
Inflammation
    APPs and, 380
    genital tract, 471
    hyperfibrinogemia caused by, 394, 394t
    hyperproteinemia and, 380–81
    monocyte changes and, 94
    neutrophilia and, 74
    proteinuria and, 459–60
    urinary tract, 471
Inflammatory disease, anemias and, 339
    nonregenerative caused by, 160–61, 160t
In-house laboratories, 35–36
INR. *See* International normalized ratio
Insulin
    glucose and, 722–23
    hyperglycemia and, 718–19
    hyperinsulinemia, 728, 728t
    hypoglycemia and, 722
    hypoinsulinemia, 728–29
    immunoreactive
        concentration of, 726–30
        glucose ratio to, 729–30
International normalized ratio (INR), 283–84
Intestine. *See also* Exocrine intestine;
            Gastrointestinal disorders in colicky
            horses, hypocalcemia and
    malabsorption, 741
    PO_4 absorption in, 617

Intestine (*continued*)
  decreased, 620
  increased, 619
Ion difference, 559–91
  analytical concepts in, 565–73
Iron (Fe), 115, 116f
  bone marrow, 332–33
  deficiency, anemia and, 164–65, 168–70, 169f
  percent transferrin saturation and, 206
  profile results, comparative, 208, 209t
  serum, 202–5
    analytical concepts of, 202–3, 207–8
    hyperferremia and, 203, 203t
    hyperferritinemia and, 207–8
    hypoferremia, 203–5, 204t
  stainable, in macrophages, 107
  status, laboratory methods for assessing, 202–8
  TIBC, 205–6
  UIBC, 205–6
Irradiation, thrombocytopenia and, 237
Isoenzymes, 640
Isoforms, 640
Isosthenuria, 424
Isotonic fluids
  dehydration and loss of, 503–4
  edema and net retention of, 504–5
  transudation and retention of, 504–5

K$^+$. *See* Potassium
Kappa agreement, 34, 34f
Keratocyte, 148–49
Ketamine, hyperglycemia and, 718
Ketoacidosis, 465
Ketoamines, 723–26
Ketogenesis, 544
Ketonemia, 544–45
Ketones
  bodies, 543
    concentration of, increased, 544–45
  in urine, 464–65
Ketonuria, 464–65, 517
  hyponatremia and, 507
Ketosis, 465, 544–45
Kidneys
  albumin excretion by, 481
  AMS and, 665
  BHB excretion through, 544
  glomerular filtrate concentration/dilution and, 425
  HCO$_3^-$ losses through, 532
  K$^+$ excretion and, 514–15
    increased, 517–18

LPS and, 667
  PO$_4$ clearance by, 616–17
  urea excretion, disorders increasing, 436

Laboratories in human hospitals, 36–37
Laboratory assays, 7–9. *See also specific assays*
  agreement
    acceptable degree of, 35
    assessing, 32–34
    bias plots and, 32, 32f
    Deming method comparison for, 33–34, 33f
    kappa, 34, 34f
    Passing and Bablok method comparison for, 33f, 34
  amount *v.* concentration in, 12–16
  analytical accuracy, 24–25
  analytical precision in, 21–24
  analytical properties of, 21–25, 22f
  analytical sensitivity, 25
  analytical specificity, 24
  analytical variation for, 23–24
  basic principles/methods, 8–9
  body fluid, 7–8
  chemistry, 8
  chromogenic, 287
  CI$^-$, 522
  clotting, coagulation factor, 287
  coagulation, 274
  comparison of, 31–35
  control solutions and assessing performance of, 22
  Crt, 436–37
  CV, 22–24
    relevance of, 23–24
  detection limit, 25
  diagnostic accuracy, 39
  diagnostic properties, 38–45, 40, 41f
  diagnostic sensitivity, 38–39
  diagnostic specificity, 39
  direct megakaryocyte immunofluorescence assays, IMT, 249
  enzyme
    hepatic, 680
    serum, 645–47, 646f, 647t
  fibrinolysis, 300
  HCO$_3^-$, 528–29
  hematology, 7–8
  hepatic enzyme, 680
  immunologic, microalbuminuria, 481–82
  iPTH, analytical concepts for, 626–27
  K$^+$, 511
  microscopy, 8

Na⁺, 500–501

Na$^+$, 500–501
Pi, 617–18
platelet, IMT, 249
predictive value of, 38–45
quality assurance, 25–29
quantitative urine total protein, 477–78
random error, 37
reference intervals, 16–20
significant figures in, 9–10
  examples of, 10t
  reporting, 9
  rules of, 9–10
substances interfering with, 24–25
systemic error, 37
tCO^2, 528–29
thyroid function, 786–89, 787f
UA, quantitative, 475–76
urea, 435
vitamin D, 629
vWF, 267
Westgard rules for, 26–29
Laboratory methods
  comparing, 44–45
  differences in, 29–31
  evaluating, 44–45
    reasons for, 36–37
  implementing, 37
  validating, 36–37
Laboratory tests, 5
  hepatic insufficiency/disease and, 677–81, 678t,
    679t
  multiples test results, 19–20
  results
    analytical errors in, 21, 22f
    classifications of, 38
    comparing, 31
    differences in, 29–31, 30f
    FN, 38
    FP, 38
    major determinants in, 20–21
    postanalytical errors in, 21
    preanalytical errors in, 21
    quality of, 20–29
    samples and errors in, 21
    terms used for, 16–17
    TN, 38
    TP, 38
Lactate
  chemical structure, 539f
  concentration, 538–43
    analytical concepts of, 540
    physiologic processes, 538, 539f

D-lactate, 538–43
  absorption, 543
  analytical concepts, 540
  concentration, increased plasma, 542–43
  diabetes mellitus and, 542–43
  propylene glycol and, 543
L-lactate, 538–43
  analytical concepts, 540
  concentration, increased plasma, 540–42
  effusion analysis with, 859–60
  hyperlactatemia and, 541–42, 541t
  measuring, 540
  plasma, 540–41
Lactate dehydrogenase (LD), 653
  activity, increased serum, 652t, 653
Lactation tetany, hypomagnesemia and, 625
Lactose tolerance test in horses, 756–57
Lactosuria, 517
LAD. *See* Leukocyte adhesion deficiency
Laser flow cell cytometer, 64–65, 64f
  erythrocyte, 125–27
  platelet analysis with, 230–31
Latex agglutination immunoassays, FDP, 296
LD. *See* Lactate dehydrogenase
LDDST. *See* Low-dose dexamethasone suppression
    test
LE. *See* Lupus erythematosus (LE)
Lee-White method, 279
Left shift
  blood neutrophil concentrations and, 70–71
  classification, blood neutrophil concentrations
    and, 70–71
  degenerative, 71
  neutrophilia and, 72, 73f
  regenerative, 71
Leishmania, leukocyte, 97–98
Leptocyte, 149
Leptospira spp., infectious hemolytic anemia, 182
Leukemia. *See also* Acute megakaryocytic leukemia;
    Feline leukemia virus
  acute, 346
    ambiguous lineage, 348
  canine, 356
  chronic, 346
  chronic myeloid, 76
  definition, 346
  electron microscopy, 356
  eosinophilic, 88
  myelogenous, 326
  myelomonocytic, chronic, 350
Leukemoid response, 74
Leukocyte adhesion deficiency (LAD), 100

Leukocytes, 53–102
  abnormal morphologic features of, 92–100
  agglutination/aggregation, 98–99
  analytical principles and methods, 60–69
  blood, 55
    abnormal concentration of, 70–90
    sample for evaluating, 60–61
  canine distemper inclusions in, 95
  concentrations, principles of determining, 62–69
    hemocytometer method for, 62–63, 63f
    impedance cell counters for, 63–64, 64f
    optical/laser flow cell cytometer, 64–65
    QBC for, 65–67, 66f
  differential, count, 62
    microscopy, 67, 68t
  differentiation, 55
  disorders, nonneoplastic, 100–102
  esterase, in urine, 468
  Hepatozoon americanum in, 95–97
  Hepatozoon canis in, 97
  Histoplasma capsulatum in, 97
  inclusions
    hereditary disorders that have, 99–100
    miscellaneous contained in, 94–95
  Leishmania in, 97–98
  leukogram, 60, 62
  Mycobacterium in, 98
  organisms in, 95–98
  physiologic processes involving, 54–60
  production, 55
  Sarcocystis in, 98
  tissue, 56
  Toxoplasma gondii in, 98
  Trypanosoma cruzi in, 98
  urine sediment, 469–71
Leukocytosis
  inflammatory, 74
  paraneoplastic neutrophilic, 76
Leukogram, 60, 62
  acute inflammatory, 84
  morphologic evaluation, 62
  patterns, 90–92, 91t
    cat, 90
    cattle, 90
    dog, 90
    horse, 90
  results, relative/absolute changes in, 69, 70t
  steroid, 75, 75t
  WBC, 62
Leukon, 54–56
Leukopoiesis, 55, 55f

Levamisole, immune hemolytic anemia induced by, 180
Levey-Jennings control chart, 27, 28f
Light chain identification, neoplasia and, 384
Light chain proteinuria, 462
Lipase (LPS). *See also* Pancreatic lipase immunoreactivity
  analytical concepts of, 666
  pancreatic, 665–66
  physiologic processes, 665–66
  renal excretion/inactivation and, 667
  serum, increased activity of, 664t, 666–67
Lipids, 763–80
  assessments of, 778–80
  cholesterol, 767–71
  definition, 764
  hyperlipemia, 773–78
  hyperlipidemia, 773–78
  hyperlipoproteinemia, 773–78
  metabolism, liver function and, 677
  TG, 771–72
Lipoproteins, 764–67
  classification, 764–66, 765t
  content, 764–66, 765t
  electrophoresis, 778
  metabolism, 766–67, 768f
  properties, 764–66, 765t
Liter, 10
Liver disease/insufficiency
  anemia and, 166–67
  laboratory test results and, 677–81, 678t, 679t
Liver failure, refractometric USG and, 451
Liver function, 675–704
  bilirubin concentration and, 681–90
  body fuels and, 676–77
  carbohydrate metabolism and, 676
  detoxification, 677
  dye-excretion tests, 703–4
  excretory, 677
  lipid metabolism and, 677
  physiologic, 676–77
  protein metabolism and, 676
  storage, 677
Low-dose dexamethasone suppression test (LDDST)
  canine, 815–17, 816f
  feline, 818
LPS. *See* Lipase
L-sorbose intoxication, 190
Lukes-Collins classification, 364
Lupus anticoagulants, 292

Lupus erythematosus (LE), 94–95. *See also* Systemic lupus erythematosus
Lymphadenitis, 363
Lymphadenopathy, 358
Lymph nodes, 58, 323–65
    analysis, methods for, 358–63
    aspiration, 362
    biopsy, 358
        major features of, 359–62
    cells in, of healthy mammals, 362–63
    classification, 363–65
    hyperplasia, 362
    lymphocytes in, 59
    major concepts/terms, 358–63
    neoplasia, 351, 363–65
    reactive, 363
    samples, cytologic, 359–62
Lymphoblasts, 363
Lymphocytes, 56
    blood, 58
        processes influencing, 59
    bone marrow, 332
    concentrations, abnormal, 81–85
    effusions and, 865
    hematopoietic cells and, 326
    kinetics, 58–59, 58f
    life span, 59
    in lymph nodes, 59
    nonlymphoid, 326
    pools, 58–59, 58f
    reactive, 93–94
    in tissues, 59
Lymphocytosis, 81–83
    bone marrow, 340
    causes, 81, 81t
    of hypoadrenocorticism, 83
    physiologic, 81–82, 82f
    of young animals, 83
Lymphomas, 351
    classification systems for, 364
    diagnosis, 364
    evaluation of, 364–65
    immunophenotyping, 364–65
    microscopy, 364
    polymerase chain reaction analysis of, 465
Lymphopenia
    acute inflammatory, 83–85, 84f
    causes, 83–85, 83t
    depletion, 85
    of lymphoid aplasia, 84f, 85
    of lymphoid hypoplasia, 84f, 85
    steroid, 84f, 85

Lymphoproliferative disorders, 82–83, 82f, 346
Lymphorrhage, 835
    effusions and, 846–47

Macrocyte, 142
Macrocytosis, 142
Magnesium (Mg^{2+}), 593–631
    concentration, free, 625–26
        abnormal, 625–26
        analytical concepts in, 625
        measuring, 625
        physiologic processes in, 625
    concentration, total, 621–25
        abnormal, 625
        analytical concepts of, 622
        hormonal regulation of, 622
        physiologic processes and, 621–22
    excretion, 621–22
    hypomagnesemia and, 623–24, 624t
    plasma, 621
    regulatory hormones, 593–631
    renal tubule function and, 422
    serum, 621
        factors determining, 621–22
    urinary excretion of, 624
Marginated neutrophil pool (MNP), 57
Mast cells
    concentrations, abnormal, 88–90
    disease, 351
    kinetics, 60
    precursors, 56
Mastocytemia, 88–90
    disorders causing, 88–89, 89t
Mastocytosis, bone marrow, 340–41
MCHC. *See* Mean cell hemoglobin concentration
MCV. *See* Mean cell volume
MDSs. *See* Myelodysplastic syndromes
MDS-U. *See* Myelodysplastic syndrome, unclassified
Mean cell hemoglobin concentration (MCHC)
    anemia and increased, 157–58
    Hgb relationship with, 121–22
    increased, 157–58
Mean cell volume (MCV), 131
Mean platelet component concentration (MPC), 228
Mean platelet volume (MPV), 228, 246
    decreased, 247
    increased, 246–47
    platelet analysis with, 231–32
Meclofenamic acid, myelosuppressive effects of, 236
Megakaryoblasts, 325

Megakaryocytes, 325. *See also* Direct megakaryocyte
        immunofluorescence assays;
        Promegakaryocytes
    bone marrow, 330
Megakaryopoiesis, 225
    infections decreasing, 236
Megaloblastic anemia, 201–2
Megestrol acetate
    diabetes mellitus induced by, 717
    hyperglycemia and, 718
Metabolic/nutritional status, herd-based testing
        and, 49–50
Methemoglobinemia, 198–99
    acquired, 198–99
    diagnosis, 199
    familial, in horses, 199
Methemoglobinuria, 466
Methimazole, IMT induced by, 239
Methionine, Heinz body formation and, 186
Methylene blue, Heinz body formation and, 186
Mg^{2+}. *See* Magnesium
Microalbuminuria, 480–83
    analytical concepts, 481–83
    canine, 483
    general concepts, 480–81
    immunologic assays, 481–82
Microcyte, 143
Microcytosis, 143
    causes of, 156–57
Microhematocrit, erythrocyte, 124
Microorganisms, culturing for, 863
Microscopy, 8
    electron, leukemia, 356
    hemic neoplasia classification with, 352–53
    leukocyte count, differential, 67
        accuracy of, 67, 68t
    lymphoma, 364
    pleural/peritoneal fluid, 852–56
MNP. *See* Marginated neutrophil pool
Molality, osmolality and, 549
Mole, 545
Monoclonal gammopathy, 382
Monocytes, 56
    concentrations, abnormal, 85–86
    inflammation and changes in, 94
    kinetics, 59
    pools, 59
Monocytopenia, 86
Monocytosis, 85, 86t
    neoplastic, 85–96
    steroid, 85
Morphine, hyperglycemia and, 719

MPC. *See* Mean platelet component concentration
M proteins, 382
MPS. *See* Mucopolysaccharidosis
MPV. *See* Mean platelet volume
Mucopolysaccharidosis (MPS), 99–100
Mycobacterium, leukocyte, 98
Mycoplasma spp., infectious hemolytic anemia, 181
Myelitis, 326
    bone marrow, 341
Myelocytes, 326
Myelodysplastic syndromes (MDSs), 348–51
    AML development and, 350
    classifications, 349
    dyshematopoiesis, acquired secondary and, 350
    dysplastic changes in, 348–49
    thrombocytosis and, 245
Myelodysplastic syndrome, unclassified (MDS-U),
        349
Myelofibrosis
    bone marrow, 341
    chronic idiopathic, 351
Myelogenous leukemia, 326
    chronic, 350
Myeloid cells, 326
Myeloma, plasma cell, 351
Myelonecrosis, thrombocytopenia and, 237
Myelophthisis, bone marrow, 341
Myeloproliferative diseases, 346
    chronic, 346, 350–51
    thrombocytosis and, 245
Myelosis, megakaryocyte, 351
Myoglobin, Hgb differentiation from, 465
Myoglobinuria, 176t, 466
Myopathy
    hypocalcemia, 610
    hypokalemic, in cats, 519

Na$^+$. *See* Sodium
Na$_2$SO$_3$. *See* Sodium sulfite
Na$^+$:K$^+$ ratio, 519–20
Naphthalene, Heinz body formation and, 186
National Institute of Standards and Technology
        (NIST), 11
    unit conventions, 11, 12t
Necrosis
    bone marrow, 341–42
    tissue, massive, 513
NEFA concentration. *See* Nonesterified fatty acid
        concentrations
Neoplasia
    B-lymphocyte
        hyperproteinemia and, 381–85

laboratory/clinical problems with, 385
  pathogenesis, 381–82
bone, 601
histiocytic, 192, 351–52
LPS and, 667
lymphoid, 351, 363–65
lymphoproliferative, 346
myeloid, 346–51
nonlymphoid, 365
thrombocytopenia and, 239–40
Neoplasms
  effusions associated with, 864–65
  thrombocytopenia and, 242–43
Nephrons
  distal, Na$^+$ reabsorption in, 499
  distal, HCO$_3^-$ in, 526–27
  HCO$_3^-$ in, 526–27
  loss of, 427, 428f
  Na$^+$ reabsorption in distal, 499
  proximal, HCO$_3^-$ in, 526, 527f
  urine changes and, 425, 426f
Nephropathies. See also Protein-losing nephropathy
  Na$^+$-wasting, hyponatremia and, 507
  protein-losing, 460, 461f
Nephrotic syndrome, 505
Neurological disease, CK activity and, 663
Neutropenia, 76–81, 77t
  bone marrow and, 337
  causes, 76–77, 77t
  cyclic, 80–81
  endotoxemia-causing, 78f, 79
  granulocytic hypoplasia, 79–80
  ineffective production, 80
  inflammatory, 76–79, 78f
  peripheral destruction, 79
  secondary to immune, 86
Neutrophilia
  diseases and conditions causing, 72, 72f
  inflammatory, 72–74
    acute, 72–74, 73f
    chronic, 73f, 74–75
  kinetics, 73f
  physiologic, 75, 76
  steroid, 75
  stress, 75
Neutrophils. See also Circulating neutrophil pool;
    Marginated neutrophil pool
  blood, 57
    abnormal concentration of, 70–81
    left shift and, 70–71
    processes influencing measured, 57
    right shift and, 71–72

giant, 92, 93
granulation, hereditary anomaly of, 99
hypersegmented, 93
idiopathic hypersegmented, of horses, 101
kinetics, 56–58, 56f
marrow, 57
pools, 56–58, 56f
  blood, 57
Pseudo-Pelger-Huët, 101
structural changes in, 92
tissue, 58
toxic, 92–93
Nicotinic acid, hyperglycemia and, 719
NIST. See National Institute of Standards and
    Technology
Nitrate poisoning, methemoglobinemia and, 198
Nitrite, in urine, 468
Nonesterified fatty acid (NEFA) concentrations, 49,
    778–80
Nonseptic exudates, 863–64
Normochloremia, 523
Normocytes, 136
Normokalemia, 516
Normonatremia, 503–5
  disorders and pathogenesis of, 503–4
nRBCs. See Nucleated red blood cells
Nucleated red blood cells (nRBCs), 122–23
  enumeration of, 123
  WBC correction for, 68–69
Nucleus, asynchronous nuclear maturation, 92
Null-lymphocytes, 55
Nutritional deficiencies, bone marrow, 336

Observed value, 16
Olympus analyzers, 528–29
One-stage prothrombin time (OSPT), 282–84
Optical cell cytometer, 64–65, 64f
  erythrocyte, 125–27
  platelet analysis with, 230–31
Osmo. gap, 545, 550–51
  evaluation of, 551, 551f
  hyperosmolality, serum and, 552–53
Osmolality, 545–53
  analytical concepts, 548–51
  calculated, 549–50
  data, interpretation of, 552–53, 552t
  definition, 545
  effective, 548
    clinical applications of, 548
  erythrocyte, 130–31
  molality and, 549
  physiologic processes, 547

Osmolality (*continued*)
  plasma, Na⁺ and regulation of, 499
  serum, 547–48, 547t
    evaluation of, 551, 551f
  USG, 445–47, 446f
Osmolarity, 545
Osmole, 545
Osmometer, 545
  freezing-point, 549
Osmometry, 545, 548–49
Osmosis, 545
Osmotic pressure, 545
  COP *v.,* 546f
OSPT. *See* One-stage prothrombin time
Ovalocyte, 149
Ovalocytosis, 148
Oxalates, 6
  toxicity, 608
Oxidants, erythrocyte exposure to, 198–99
Oxidative damage, hemolytic anemias and,
    186–88
Oximeter, 571
  C-, 571–72
    blood substitutes interfering with, 572
Oxygen, 581–82. *See also* Arterial alveolar oxygen
    tension gradient; Percent hemoglobin
    saturation with oxygen; Pulse oximetry
Oxygenation
  blood, 563–65, 564f, 581–82
  tissue, 565, 566f

Pancreas. *See* Exocrine pancreas
Pancreatic insufficiency, exocrine and, 605–6
Pancreatic lipase immunoreactivity (PLI), 668
  cats and, 668, 745–46
  concentration, 745–46
  dogs and, 668, 745–46
Pancreatis, acute, 608–9
Pancreatitis, 741
Panhypoproteinemia, 385
Paraneoplastic neutrophilic leukocytosis, 76
Paraproteinemia, prolonged TT and, 285
Parasitism, blood loss caused by, 167
Parasitology, 8
Parathyroid hormone (PTH). *See also*
    Immunoreactive PTH; PTH-related protein
  activity, decreased, 602–4
Partial thromboplastin time (PTT)
  activated, 280–81
  coagulation, 280–84
  heparin therapy monitored by, 282
  interpretive considerations, 281–82

  prolonged, 281t, 282
  shortened, 282
Passing and Bablok method comparison, 33f, 34
PCDW. *See* Platelet component concentration
    distribution width
PDW. *See* Platelet distribution width
Pelger-Huët anomaly, 101
Penicillin
  immune hemolytic anemia induced by, 179
  IMT induced by, 239
Percent hemoglobin saturation with oxygen (SO₂),
    568–69, 568f
Percent hemoglobin saturation with oxygen of
    arterial blood by pulse oximetry (Spo₂), 584
Percent transferrin saturation, 206
Pericardial effusions, 866
Peritoneal effusions, 515–16, 836–39, 839f
  analyses for, selected, 856–63
Peritoneal fluid
  composition, 832–35
  equine, 833–35, 834t
  microscopic examination of, 852–56
  routine analysis of, 848–56, 851t
Peritonitis, hypoproteinemia plasma loss through,
    387–88
PFK deficiency. *See* Phosphofructokinase deficiency
pH
  blood, 559–91
    analytical concepts in, 565–73
    erroneous values for, 573, 573t
    physiologic processes of, 561–65
    samples for, 572–73
    temperature and, 570, 570t
  urine, 455–57
Phagocytic system, mononuclear, 677
Phenazopyridine, Heinz body formation and, 186
Phenobarbital therapy
  APP, positive concentration increase and, 397
  hypothyroxemia and, 792
Phenothiazine, hyperglycemia and, 719
Phenylbutazone
  hypothyroxemia and, 792
  myelosuppressive effects of, 236
Phenylhydrazine, Heinz body formation and, 186
Phenytoin, hyperglycemia and, 719
Phosphate (PO₄)
  absorption of, intestinal, 617
    decreased, 620
    increased, 619
  Ca²⁺ interaction with, 596
  enemas, hypocalcemia and, 609
  renal clearance of, 616–17

renal tubule function and, 422
shift, 617, 619, 620
urinary excretion, 618–19
increased, 619–20
Phosphofructokinase (PFK) deficiency, 189
Phosphorus (Pi), 593–631
analytical concepts of, 617–18
assays, 617–18
concentration, inorganic, 615–21
animal age and, 617
physiologic processes of, 615–17
concentrations, methods of expressing, 618
forms, 615–16
inorganic, major patterns for disorders of, 631, 631t
regulatory hormones, 593–631
sample, 617
serum, factors determining, 616–17, 616f
Physical examination, 5
Pi. *See* Phosphorus
α_1-PI. *See* α_1-Protease inhibitor, fecal
Pincered cell, 149
Pirimicarb, immune hemolytic anemia induced by, 180
PIVKA. *See* Proteins induced by vitamin K antagonism, absence, or deficiency
PK deficiency. *See* Pyruvate kinase deficiency
Plasma, 6–7. *See also* Base excess in plasma; Renal plasma flow
ammonium concentration in, 697–703
Bδ, 689
bile acid concentration, increased in, 691–93, 692t
Ca^{2+} concentration in, 594–95
components, 7
electrolyte concentrations in, 497
abnormal, 498
enzyme removal from, 644–45
glucagon, immunoreactive concentration in, 730–31
glucose concentration in, 708–23, 712t
insulin, immunoreactive, 726–30
iPTH, 627, 627t
K^+, regulation of, 510, 511f, 512f
D-lactate, 542–43
L-lactate, 540–41
Mg^{2+}, 621
osmolality, Na^+ and regulation of, 499
UN, 477
urine analyte to, ratios, 476–77
Plasmacytoma, extramedullary, 351
Plasma protein to fibrinogen (PP:F) ratio, 395–96

Platelet component concentration distribution width (PCDW), 228
Platelet distribution width (PDW), 228
increased, 247
Platelets, 223–49. *See also* Mean platelet component concentration; Mean platelet volume; Platelet component concentration distribution width
analytical principles/methods, 227–32
analyzer, 228–29
blood film evaluation, 227, 229–30
CBC, 227
hemocytometer, 231
impedance cell counter, 230
MPV, 231–32
optical or laser flow cell cytometer, 230–31
QBC, 231
thrombogram, 227–29
Anaplasma platys in, 233
assays, IMT, 249
clumps, 229, 232
concentration, 228, 230–31
hemostasis and, 262–63
consumption, 227
distribution, 229
abnormal, 235
functions, 227
hemostatic, 262
thrombopathia and, 263, 264t
function tests, 263–65
BMBT, 263–64
hemostasis and, 262–65
hemostatic functions of, 262
inclusions, 232–33
kinetics, 225–27, 226f
life spans, 227
microscopic features of, 232–33
general, 232
production, 224–25
adequate, 235
decreased, 235–37
factors affecting, 227
increased, reactive thrombocytosis and, 245–46
psychologic processes, 224–27
redistribution, reactive thrombocytosis and, 245
reticulated, 225, 247–49
assessment method for, 247–48
interpretation of, 248–49
values of, 248–49
shape, 232
size, 232

Platelets (*continued*)
  splenic, 227
  survival, decreased
    blood loss and, 240
    DIC and, 241
    drugs causing, 241
    endocarditis and, 241
    envenomation and, 241
    foreign materials causing, 241
    immunologic causes of, 237–40
    nonimmunologic causes of, 240–41
    platelet activation with accelerated
        consumption and, 240–41
    thrombocytopenia and, 237–41
    vasculitis and, 241
  thrombocytopenia, 233–43
  thrombocytosis, 244–46
  volume, 246–47
    blood film evaluation of, 247
PLE. *See* Protein-losing enteropathy
Pleural effusions, 836–39, 839f
  analyses for, selected, 856–63
Pleural fluid
  composition, 832–35, 833f
  equine, 833–35, 834t
  microscopic examination of, 852–56
  routine analysis of, 848–56, 851t
Pleuritis, hypoproteinemia plasma loss through,
    387–88
PLI. *See* Pancreatic lipase immunoreactivity
PLN. *See* Protein-losing nephropathy
PO_4. *See* Phosphate
Poikilocyte, 143, 144t
Polychromasia, 138
Polychromatophil, 138
Polycythemia, 193–98
Polycythemia vera, 198, 351
Polydipsia, 452. *See also* Polyuria and polydipsia
Polymerase chain reaction analysis, lymphoma, 465
Polyuria, 427
Polyuria and polydipsia (PU/PD)
  ADH response tests in, 485–87
  H_2O deprivation in, 485–87
Porphyria, 113
  congenital erythropoietic
    bovine, 190–91
    feline, 191
  heme synthesis defects causing, 190–91
  hereditary erythropoietic, 191
Porphyrins, 113, 190
Portosystemic shunts in dogs, 204
Postanalytical errors, 21

Posttransfusion purpura, 240
Potassium (K^+). *See also* Na^+K^+ ratio
  alimentary loss of, 518–19
  assays, 510–11, 511
  concentration, 509–19
    analytical concepts of, 510–11
    physiologic processes, 509–10
    terms/units for, 510–11
  decreased
    hypokalemia and, 516–19
    total body, 516–19
  depletion, 508
  effusion analysis with, 858–59
  excretion
    hypokalemia and increased, 517–19
    increased, 517–19
  hyperkalemia and, 511–16
  hypokalemia and, 516–19
  increased, 513
    total body, 514–15
    urinary tract obstruction/leakage and, 514–15
  intake
    decreased, 516–17
    increased, 515
  Na^+ and, 499
  plasma, regulation of, 510, 511f, 512f
  quantitation, sample for, 511
  renal excretion of, 514–15
    decreased, 514–15
    increased, 517–18
  renal tubule function and, 419–21
  retention, trimethoprim-induced, 515
  serum, 509–10, 509f
  shifting of, 512–14
PP:F ratio. *See* Plasma protein to fibrinogen ratio
Preanalytical errors, 21
Predictive value (PV), 41f
  applying concepts of, 40–44
  basic concepts of, 39–40
  deficiency in theories of, 44
  diagnostic value comparison and, 42–44, 43f
  interpreting concepts of, 40–44
  laboratory assay, 38–45
  negative, 39
  positive, 39
Prednisolone, hypothyroxemia and, 792
Prevalence, 39, 40f
Proficiency testing, 29
Progestins, hyperglycemia and, 719
Promegakaryocytes, 325
Propofol, Heinz body formation and, 186

Propranolol, hyperglycemia and, 718

Propylene glycol
Heinz body formation and, 186
D-lactate and, 543

Propylthiouracil
immune hemolytic anemia induced by, 179
IMT induced by, 239

Prot:Crt$_u$ ratio. *See* Urinary protein to creatinine ratio

α_1-Protease inhibitor (α_1-PI), fecal, 753

Protein C
activity, decreased, 291
coagulation inhibited by, 274
as endogenous anticoagulant, 291

Protein-losing dermatopathy, 387

Protein-losing enteropathy (PLE), 387

Protein-losing nephropathy (PLN), 385–87
diseases and, 386
laboratory findings, major of, 386–87

Proteins, 369–410. *See also* Acute phase protein;
Hyperproteinemia; Hypoproteinemia;
Plasma protein to fibrinogen ratio; Urinary
protein to creatinine ratio
analytical principles for total, 372–79
catabolism, increased, 388–89
complement, 372
concentrations, effusion analysis with, 862
COP, 405–10
C-reactive, 372
delayed response, 372
inflammation and, 380
disorders, 371–72
dyscrasia, 371
electrophoretic region contribution of serum,
377, 378t
enteropathy and losing, 604
fractions
calculating concentrations of, 375, 376f
SPE determination of, 375–77
fructosamines and abnormal concentrations of,
726
general concepts for total, 370–72
hyperalbuminemia and, 390–91
hyperglobulinemia and, 392
hypoalbuminemia and, 391–92
hypoglobinemia and, 392
immunoelectrophoresis, 377
immunoglobins, 398–404
loss of
PLE and, 387
PLN and, 385–87
from vascular space, 385–88

M, 382
metabolism, liver function and, 676
nephropathy and loss of, 460, 461f
physiologic processes, 370–71
plasma, 371
loss of, 387–88
renal failure and loss of, 460, 461f
renal tubule function and, 422
Sia euglobulin test, 377–79
synthesis
decreased, 388–89
hyperproteinemia and, 380–85
increased, 380–85
total, 372–74
biuret reaction for measuring, 374
quantitative urine, assays, 477–78
refractometry for measuring, 372–74
transudates and, 842–44
in urine, 457–62
analytical concepts of, 458
assays, 477–78
microalbuminuria and, 482–83
proteinuria and, 458–60, 459f

Proteins induced by vitamin K antagonism,
absence, or deficiency (PIVKA), 287–88

Proteinuria, 458–60, 459f
Bence Jones, 385, 460–62
classifications, 460
glomerular, 458–59
hemorrhagic, 459–60
inflammatory, 459–60
light-chain, 462
prerenal, 458
tubular, 459

Protein Z , as endogenous anticoagulant, 291–92

Protein Z-dependent protease inhibitor (PZI),
291–92

Prothrombin time (PT), 282–84. *See also*
Thrombotest PT
INR and, 284
prolonged, 283, 283t
shortened, 283
warfarin therapy monitored by, 283

Pseudo-hyperkalemia, 514

Pseudo-hyperphosphatemia, hyperphosphatemia
and, 619

Pseudo-hypoparathyroidism, 604

Pseudo- hypophosphatemia, 621

Pseudo-Pelger-Huët eosinophils, 101

Pseudo-Pelger-Huët neutrophils, 101

Pseudo-thrombocytopenia, 233

PT. *See* Prothrombin time

PTH. *See* Parathyroid hormone

PTH-related protein (PTHrp), 628

PTHrp. *See* PTH-related protein

PTT. *See* Partial thromboplastin time

Puerperal tetany, 607

Pulmonary ventilation, 563–65, 564f

Pulse oximetry, 571. *See also* Percent hemoglobin
    saturation with oxygen of arterial blood by
    pulse oximetry

PU/PD. *See* Polyuria and polydipsia

PV. *See* Predictive value

Pyknocyte, 149

Pyometra, canine, 451

Pyridoxine deficiency, anemia and, 165

Pyruvate kinase (PK) deficiency, 188–89

Pyuria, 469, 470t

PZI. *See* Protein Z-dependent protease inhibitor

QBC analysis. *See* Quantitative buffy coat analysis

Quality assurance, 25–29
    concepts, 25–26
    error, acceptable random, 26
    Westgard rules, 26–29

Quantitative buffy coat (QBC) analysis, 65–67,
        66f. *See also* IDEXX QBC VetAutoread
        hematology system
    erythrocyte, 127
    platelet analysis with, 231

RA. *See* Refractory anemia

Radial immunodiffusion (RID), 399–400

RAEB-1. *See* Refractory anemia with excess blasts 1

RAEB-2. *See* Refractory anemia with excess blasts 2

Rappaport classification, 364

RARS. *See* Refractory anemia with ringed
        sideroblasts

RBC. *See* Red blood cell

RC. *See* Reticulocyte concentration

RCDM. *See* Refractory cytopenia with multilineage
        dysplasia

RCMD-RS. *See* Refractory cytopenia with
        multilineage dysplasia and ringed
        sideroblasts

RDW. *See* Red cell distribution width

Reagent strip
    bilirubin in urine and, 467
    glucose in urine and, 463
    heme in urine and, 465
    nitrite in urine and, 468
    protein in urine, 458
    USG estimation and, 447

REAL system. *See* Revised European/American
        Lymphoma system

Receiver operating characteristic (ROC) curves,
        45–46
    assay comparison, 45, 46f
    decision threshold established with, 45–46,
        47f
    diagnostic procedure comparison by, 45–46
    FP rate in, 45
    TP rate in, 45

Red blood cell (RBC), 120
    aplasia, 339
    hemocytometer method, 128

Red cell distribution width (RDW), 122

Reference distribution, 16
    determining, 18
    Gaussian, 18, 19f
    skewed, 18, 19f

Reference individual, 16
    selecting criteria for, 17

Reference intervals, 16–20
    definition of, 16
    determining, 18
    establishment of, 17–18
    expected findings and, 20
    Gaussian distributions and, 18, 19f
    healthy, 19
    herd-based testing, 50
    laboratory results and, 31
    measured values outside of, 19
    multiple test result, 19–20
    skewed distributions and, 18, 19f
    synonymous terms, 16
    use of, 19–20

Reference limits, 16
    decision thresholds *v.*, 20
    determining, 18

Reference population, 16

Reference range, term, 16–17

Reference sample group, 16
    establishing, 17–18

Reference value, 16
    information on, 20
    measuring/determining, 18

Refractile artifacts, erythrocyte, 141–42

Refractometry
    proteins, total measured with, 372–74
    USG, 443–45, 444f, 445f

Refractory anemia (RA), 349

Refractory anemia with excess blasts 1 (RAEB-1),
        349

Refractory anemia with excess blasts 2 (RAEB-2),
        349

Refractory anemia with ringed sideroblasts (RARS),
        349

Refractory cytopenia with multilineage dysplasia (RCMD), 349
Refractory cytopenia with multilineage dysplasia and ringed sideroblasts (RCMD-RS), 349
Regression equation, 33–34
Renal concentrating ability, 423–25, 485–86
  renal failure and loss of, 427
Renal diluting ability, 423–25
Renal disease
  anemia caused by, 161–62
  azotemia and, 433
  in cats, 601
  in dogs, 601
  equine, 621
Renal failure
  acute, 427–29
    azotemia and, 428
    hypocalcemia and, 609
    urine volume and, 429
  bovine, 524
  Ca^{2+} and, 601
  chronic, 425–27
    Ca^{2+}, free concentration and, 613
    evidence of, 427
    polyuria in, 427
    renal concentrating ability and, 427
  in horses, 601
  hypokalemic, in cats, 519
  $Na^+ : K^+$ ratio, decreased and, 520
  protein-losing, 460, 461f
Renal function
  failure/insufficiency, chronic of, 425–27
  impaired, 425–26
  plasma analyte, 416, 417t
Renal insufficiency
  Ca^{2+} and, 601
  chronic, 425–27
    evidence of, 427
    polyuria in, 427
Renal interstitium, 424
Renal loss, hyponatremia and, 505–7
Renal plasma flow (RPF), 423
Renal tubules
  Ca^{2+} and, 596
  functions of, 418
    amino acids and, 422
    Ca^{2+} and, 422
    Cl^- and, 419
    Crt and, 423
    glomerular filtrate concentration/dilution and, 424–25
    glucose and, 422
    H^+ and, 421

HCO_3^- and, 419
K^+ and, 419–21
major solutes and, 418–23, 420f
Mg^{2+} and, 422
Na^+ and, 418–19
PO_4 and, 422
proteins and, 422
urea and, 423
glucosuria and, 463
Reticulocyte concentration (RC), 123
  erythrocyte analysis with, 131
Reticulocyte percentage (RP). *See also* Corrected reticulocyte percentage
  automated techniques for, 132
  erythrocyte analysis with, 132–34
  procedure, basics of, 132
  reticulocytosis and increased, 132, 133t
  RNA fluorescence and, 127
Reticulocyte production index (RPI), 134–35
Reticulocytes, 115–17, 123
  aggregate, 117
  cat, 117
  circulating, life spans of, 115
  erythrocyte appearance and, 138
  punctate, 117
  shift, 134
  types, 115–17
Reticulocytosis, 117, 138
  anemia classification and, 151
  production of, species variation in, 152
  RP, increased and, 132, 133t
Revised European/American Lymphoma (REAL) system, 364
Rhabdomyolysis, K^+ and, 512
Ribonucleic acid (RNA)
  dye staining, 126–27
  RP and fluorescence of, 127
Rickets, 604–5
RID. *See* Radial immunodiffusion
RNA. *See* Ribonucleic acid
ROC curves. *See* Receiver operating characteristic curves
Romanowsky stains, 61
Rouleau/rouleaux, 136
RP. *See* Reticulocyte percentage
RPF. *See* Renal plasma flow
RPI. *See* Reticulocyte production index
Rubricytosis
  appropriate, 137
  erythrocyte, 136–37
  inappropriate, 137
Rumen overload, 610
Ruminants, Heinz body formation in, 186

Russell's viper venom time (RVVT), 288
RVVT. *See* Russell's viper venom time

Salivation, excess, 518–19
Samples, 5–7
    ammonium concentration in plasma, 699
    blood, 5–6
        anticoagulants for, 6
        leukocyte evaluation with, 60–61
    blood gas, 572–73
    blood pH, 572–73
    blood plasma, 6–7
    body fluid, 7
    bone marrow, 357–58
    Ca^{2+}, free concentration, 610–11, 612f
    citrated, coagulation, 276–77
    coagulation, 276–77
        collecting/handling, 274–76
        processing/stability of, 277–78
    collecting, 21
    enzyme, serum, 648–49
    FDPs, 293–96
    fibrin fragment D-dimer, 299
    handling, 21
    laboratory examination of, 5
    laboratory results and, 31
        errors in, 21
    Levy-Jennings control chart for monitoring, 27,
        28f
    lymph node cytologic, 359–62
    Pi, 617
    reference intervals and, 18
    urine, 7
    vitamin D, 629
    vWF, 266
Sarcocystis, leukocyte, 98
Sarcoma, histiocytic, 352
Schizocyte, 149–50
Secondary hemostatic plug, 268
Septic exudates, 863–64
Sequestration, 235
    K^+ loss through, 518–19
Serum
    ALP, increased activity of, 655–58, 657t
        drug/hormone induction of, 656–57
    ALT, increased activity of, 651, 651t
        muscle damage and, 651
    AMS, increased activity of, 664–65, 664t
    anion gap, 535
    AST, increased activity of, 652, 652t
    bile acid concentration, increased in, 691–93,
        692f, 692t

Ca^{2+}
    factors determining, 595–96, 595f
    total concentration, 594–95
cation, 535, 535t
cholesterol concentration in, 767–71
CK, increased activity of, 662–63, 662t
electrolyte concentrations in, 497
    abnormal, 498
enzymes, 668t
    activity, 642–45
    activity, increased, 649–50, 650f
    assays of, 645–47, 646f, 647t
    measurement of, 645–47
    samples of, 648–49
    sources of, 641–42, 641t, 642f
Fe, 202–5
GGT, increased activity of, 659, 659t
glucose concentration in, 708–23, 712t
GMD, 654
hyperosmolality, 552–53
ID, increased activity of, 654
insulin, immunoreactive, 726–30
iPTH, 627, 627t
K^+, 509–10, 509f
LD, increased activity of, 652t, 653
low, 50
LPS, increased activity of, 664t, 666–67
Mg^{2+}, 621
    factors determining, 621–22
osmolality, 547–48, 547t
    evaluation of, 551, 551f
Pi, factors determining, 616–17, 616f
TG concentration of, 771–72
Serum protein electrophoresis (SPE)
    gammopathy, monoclonal, 383
    protein fractions determined with, 375–77
SIADH. *See* Syndrome of inappropriate ADH
        secretion
Sia euglobulin test, 377–79
SID. *See* Strong ion difference
Sideroblastic anemias, 143
Siderocyte, 142
Sideroleukocyte, 94
Siderotic granules, erythrocyte, 142
Sigma, 27
    classification, 27
    theoretical, 28
Significant figures
    laboratory assay, 9–10, 10t
    unit calculations and resultant, 11
SI units, 10–12, 11t
    non-SI unit conversion to, 11–12, 13t

non-SI units, 10–12, 11t
    SI unit conversion of, 11–12, 13t
Six Sigma Quality Management, 27
Skewed distribution, 18, 19f
SLE. *See* Systemic lupus erythematosus
SO$_2$. *See* Percent hemoglobin saturation with
        oxygen
Sodium (Na$^+$). *See also* Na$^+$:K$^+$ ratio
    assay measurement of, 500–501
    blood volume regulation and, 499
    concentrations, 498–509
        analytical concepts of, 500–501
        hyponatremia and, 505–9
        K$^+$ and, 499
        physiologic processes, 498–500
        terms/ units for, 500
    dehydration and, 499
    effusion analysis with, 858–59
    excess group, 502–3
    H$_2$O and, 499
    hypernatremia and, 501–3
    ion activity, 500
    loss
        H$_2$O loss and, 502
        sweating and cutaneous, 507
        third-space, 507
    nephron reabsorption of, 499
    plasma osmolality regulation and, 499
    quantitation, sample for, 500
    renal tubule function and, 418–19
    shifting, 508
    sweating an cutaneous loss of, 507
Sodium sulfite (Na$_2$SO$_3$), 401–2
Solute, 546
Spectrin deficiency in Dutch golden retrievers, 201
Spherocytes, 143, 150
Spleen
    contraction, erythrocytosis caused by, 196
    erythrocytes, 111–12
    platelets in, 227
Spo$_2$. *See* Percent hemoglobin saturation with
        oxygen of arterial blood by pulse oximetry
SSA. *See* Sulfosalicylic acid
Staining
    azurophilic, 62
    basophilic, 62
    blood, 61–62
    eosinophilic, 62
    neutrophilic, 62
Starling's law, 405, 406f
    cavitary effusions and, 836–37
Stem cells, 55

Steroids, hyperglycemia and, 714, 718
Stewart's method of acid-base analysis, 584–91
    definitions, 585–86
Stomatocyte, 150
Stomatocytosis, hereditary, 199–200
Strong ion difference (SID), 538
    anion gap and, 589
    equations, 586–88
    formulas, comparison, 588–89
    Stewart's method of acid-base analysis, 584–91
    theory, 591
    values, interpretation of abnormal, 589–90, 590t
Sulfaquinoxaline, vitamin K antagonism and, 306
Sulfonamides, IMT induced by, 238
Sulfosalicylic acid (SSA), 458
Sweating
    equine, 507
    horse, K$^+$ loss through, 519
    K$^+$ loss through, 519
    Na$^+$ cutaneous loss through, 507
SynBiotics SCA2000 Veterinary Coagulation
        Analyzer, 280
Syndrome of inappropriate ADH secretion
        (SIADH), 507–8
Systemic lupus erythematosus (SLE), 240

Tachypnea, 561
Tamm-Horsfall protein, 457
TAP. *See* Trypsinogen activation peptide
TAT. *See* Thrombin-antithrombin complexes
tCO^2. *See* Total carbon dioxide
TCT. *See* Thrombin clotting time
TF. *See* Tissue factor
TFPI. *See* Tissue factor pathway coagulation
        inhibitor
TG. *See* Triglyceride
TgAA. *See* Thyroglobulin autoantibodies
Theileria spp., infectious hemolytic anemia, 185
Theoretical assays, sigma, 28
Thiazides
    diuretics, 525
    hyperglycemia and, 719
Thrombi
    clinical signs caused by, 311
    formation of, 310–11
Thrombin-antithrombin complexes (TAT), 290–91
Thrombin clotting time (TCT), 284–85
Thrombin time (TT), 284–85
    fibrinogen, 394
    prolonged, 285
    shortened, 285
Thrombocrit, 228

Thrombocytes, 262–65
Thrombocythemia
  essential, 351
  primary, 244–45
Thrombocytopenia, 233–43. *See also* Immune-
      mediated thrombocytopenia
  amegakaryocytic, acquired, 235
  anaphylaxis and, 243
  Anaplasma platys and, 242
  antibodies and, 239
  in Cavalier King Charles spaniels, 235, 241–42
  diseases and conditions, 233–43, 234t
  drugs associated with, 243
  endotoxemia and, 242
  envenomation and, 241
  general concepts, 233
  hemodilution and, 241
  hypophosphatemia and, 243
  idiopathic, 241–43
  infections and, 236–37, 242
  irradiation and, 237
  marrow replacement and, 237
  mechanisms, 243
  MPV and, 246
  multifactorial, 241–43
  myelonecrosis and, 237
  neonatal alloimmune, 239
  neoplasia and, 239–40
  neoplasms and, 242–43
  platelet production, decreased and, 235–37
    drugs causing, 235–36
  platelets and
    distribution, abnormal of, 235
    survival, decreased of, 237–41
  posttransfusion, 240
  pseudo-, 233
Thrombocytosis
  diseases/conditions, 244–46, 244t
  general concepts, 244
  MPV and, 246
  neoplasia, hemic and, 244–45
  reactive, 245
    platelets and, 245–46
Thrombogram, 60
  platelet, 227–29
Thrombopathia, 263, 264t
  clotting and, 264–65
Thrombopoiesis, 225
  infections decreasing, 236
Thrombopoietin (Tpo), 225
Thrombosis
  acquired conditions associated with, 311

clinical signs, 311
  definition, 310
  hemostatic abnormalities, 311
Thrombotest PT, 288
Thyroglobulin autoantibodies (TgAA), 788–89,
      794–95
Thyroid function, 783–800
  analytical concepts, 785–89
  assays, 786–89, 787f
  hormonal control of thyroid glands and, 784–
      85, 785f
  physiologic processes, 784–85, 785f
  response tests, 795–98
  suppression tests, 795–98
  TgAA and, 794–95
  thyroxine and, 789–93, 798
  triiodothyronine concentrations and, 793–94
  TSH concentration and, 794, 798
Thyroid hormone concentrations, 799, 799t, 800t
Thyroiditis, refractometric USG and, 452
Thyroid peroxidase autoantibodies, 795
Thyroid-stimulating hormone (TSH), 788
  in cats, 794
  concentration, 794
  in dogs, 794
  in horses, 794
  response test, 795–96
  thyroxine and, 798
Thyrotropin-releasing hormone (TRH), 796
Thyroxine
  autoantibodies, 795
  concentration, 789–93
  diabetes mellitus induced by, 717
  free, 793
  hyperglycemia and, 718
  hyperthyroxemia, 789–90, 789t
  hypothyroxemia, 790–93, 791t
  TSH and, 798
TIBC. *See* Total iron-binding capacity
Tissue factor (TF)
  coagulation test, 282–83
  PT and, 282–83
Tissue factor pathway coagulation inhibitor (TFPI),
      274
Tissues
  lymphocytes in, 59
  lymphoid, 58
  neutrophils, 58
TLI. *See* Trypsin-like immunoreactivity
T-lymphocytes, 55
TNCC. *See* Total nucleated cell concentration
TN results. *See* True negative results

Tonicity, 546
Torocyte, 150–51
Total carbon dioxide (tCO²)
    analytical concepts, 527–29
    assays, 528–29
    blood collection tube, 528
    concentration, 525–34
        decreased, 531–34
        increased, 529–31
        physiologic processes, 525–27
    decreased, 531–34
        disorders/pathogeneses and, 531–33, 532t
        hyperchloremia and, 533–34
    increased, 529–31
        disorders/pathogeneses and, 529–31, 529t
    vitros enzymatic, 528
Total iron-binding capacity (TIBC)
    analytical concepts, 205
    decreased serum, 206, 206t
    increased serum, 205–6, 206t
Total nucleated cell concentration (TNCC), 852
Toxic granules, 92
Toxic neutrophils, 92–93, 93
Toxoplasma gondii, leukocyte, 98
Tpo. *See* Thrombopoietin
TP results. *See* True positive results
Transferrin, 372
Transudate
    definition, 835
    modified, 835–36
    pathogenesis, 839–42
    protein-poor, 842–43
    protein-rich, 843–44
Transudation
    definition, 835
    hepatic cirrhosis with abdominal, 504
        theories of, 504–5
    isotonic fluid retention and, 504–5
TRH. *See* Thyrotropin-releasing hormone
Trichloroacetic acid method, 477
Triglyceride (TG)
    effusion analysis with, 856–57, 857t
    hypertriglyceridemia, 772, 772t
    hypotriglyceridemia, 772
    serum concentration of, 771–72
Triiodothyronine
    autoantibodies, 795
    concentrations, 793–94
    suppression test, 796–98, 797f
Trimethoprim-sulfadiazine
    hypothyroxemia and, 792
    IMT induced by, 239

K⁺ retention induced by, 515
    myelosuppressive effects of, 236
Trimethoprim-sulfamethoxazole
    hypothyroxemia and, 792
    immune hemolytic anemia induced by, 180
Trimethoprim-sulfonamide, myelosuppressive
    effects of, 236
True negative (TN) results, 38
True positive (TP) results, 38
    ROC curve and rate of, 45
True values, 24
Trypanosoma cruzi, leukocyte, 98
Trypanosoma spp., infectious hemolytic anemia,
    185–86
Trypsin-like immunoreactivity (TLI)
    analytic concepts, 741–43
    concentration, 741–45
    decreased, 744–45, 745t
    increased, 743–44, 743t
    physiologic processes, 741, 742f
Trypsinogen activation peptide (TAP), 746–47
TSH. *See* Thyroid-stimulating hormone
TT. *See* Thrombin time
Tumor lysis syndrome, acute, 610

UA. *See* Urinanalysis
UIBC. *See* Unbound iron-binding capacity
UN. *See* Urea nitrogen
Unbound iron-binding capacity (UIBC), 205–6
Units, 10–16
    abbreviations for major, 12t
    amount *v.* concentration, 12–16
    basic, of measurement, 10, 11t
    calculations and resultant significant figures,
        11
    measured values, 11
    metric system of, 10
    NIST, conventions, 11, 12t
    non-SI unit conversion to SI unit, 11–12, 13t
    SI *v.* non-SI, 10–12
Urea
    assays, 435
    azotemia and production of, 430t, 431–32
    effusion analysis with, 857–58
    physiologic processes/concepts regarding, 434f
    renal excretion, disorders increasing, 436
    renal tubule function and, 423
    urinary excretion of, 429–31
Urea nitrogen (UN)
    plasma, 477
    serum/plasma concentration of, 433–36, 434f
        Crt concentration *v.,* 437–38, 438t

Urea nitrogen (UN) (*continued*)
  decreased, 435–36, 435t
  increased, 435
 urine, 477
Uremia, 429–33
Urinanalysis (UA)
 in cats, 442t, 455
 in cattle, 442t
 components of, 440–41
 in dogs, 442t, 454–55
 in horses, 442t
 major concepts in, 440–41
 procedure, 440
 quantitative, 475–85
  24 h excretion study, 476
  analyte urine to plasma ratios and, 476–77
  assay methods for, 475–76
  basic concepts of, 475–76
  FE ratios/percentages and, 484–85
  interpreting, 476
  microalbuminuria and, 480–83
  Prot:Crt$_u$ ratio and, 478–80
  urine total protein assays and, 477–78
 results
  disorders/conditions causing, 456t
  interpreting, 454–55
Urinary bladder, ruptured, 602
Urinary protein to creatinine (Prot:Crt)$_u$ ratio, 478–80
 analytical concepts, 479
 increased, diagnostic significance of, 479–80
 published data on, 479, 480t
 theory, 478–79
Urinary system, 415–90
 azotemia and, 429–33
  serum chemistry results in, abnormal routine, 439–40
  Crt serum/plasma concentration and, 434f, 436–37
 glomerular filtration, 417–18
 physiologic processes, 416–25
 renal concentrating ability, 423–25
 renal diluting ability, 423–25
 renal failure
  acute, 427–29
  chronic, 425–27
 renal insufficiency, chronic, 425–27
 renal tubule functions in, 418–23, 420f
 UA and, 440–41
  quantitative, 475–84
 UN serum/plasma concentration and, 433–36, 434f
 uremia and, 429–33

urine in, physical examination of, 441–52
urine sediment examination and, 469–75, 470t
urolith analysis, 487–90
Urinary tract
 epithelial cells in, 473–74
 inflammation, urinary sediment examination and, 471
 K^+, increased and obstruction/leakage from, 514–15
 obstruction
  Ca^{2+}, free concentration and, 613
  hypocalcemia and, 609
  $Na^+:K^+$ ratio, decreased and, 520
Urine
 24 h excretion study of, 476
  FE study *v.,* 484
 analyte, to plasma ratios, 476–77
 assays, quantitative
  albumin, 478
  total protein, 477–78
 bilirubin in, 466–67
 Ca^{2+} excretion in, 601
  decreased, 601
  excess, 608
 centrifugation, 455
 chemical examination, 452–68
  major concepts of, 452–55
  semiquantitative, 452–54, 453t
 clarity, 442–43
 collection, 441
 color, 441–42
 composition, 441
 concentration of, 423–24
 cortisol, Crt ratio to, 812–13, 813f
 GGT activity in, 661
 glucose in, 462–64
  analytical concepts of, 463
  physiologic processes of, 462–63
 heme in, 465–66
 ketones in, 464–65
 leukocyte esterase in, 468
 Mg^{2+} excretion in, 624
 nephron and changes in, 425, 426f
 nitrite in, 468
 pH, 455–57
 physical examination of, 441–52
 PO_4 excretion in, 618–20, 618t
 protein assays
  microalbuminuria and, 482–83
  quantitative, 477–78
 protein in, 457–62
  analytical concepts of, 458
  proteinuria and, 458–60, 459f

samples, 7
solute concentration, 443–52
    analytical concepts in, 443–47
    physiologic processes for, 443
UN, 477
urobilinogen in, 467–68
USG and, 443–45
volume
    abnormal, 427, 428f
    renal failure, acute and, 429
    USG, refractometric and, 454
Urine sediment
    analysis, 8
    bacteria in, 472
    casts in, 472–73
    crystals in, 474–75
    epithelial cells in, 473–74
    erythrocytes in, 471–72
    examination, 469–75, 470t
    general concepts, 469
    leukocytes in, 469–71
    organisms in, 475
Urine specific gravity (USG)
    osmolality, 445–47, 446f
    reagent strip for estimating, 447
    refractometric, 445–47, 446f
        in cats, 450
        in cattle, 450
        in dogs, 449t, 450
        expected, 447
        in horses, 450
        hyperadrenocorticism and, 450–51
        hyperaldosteronism and, 451
        hypercalcemia and, 451
        hyperparathyroidism and, 452
        hypoadrenocroticism and, 451
        hypokalemia and, 451–52
        hypoparathyroidism and, 452
        interpreting values of, 447–52, 449t
        liver failure and, 451
        polydipsia, psychogenic and, 452
        pyometra, canine and, 451
        thyroiditis, 452
        urine volume and, 454
        in various disorders/conditions, 448–52
    refractometry, 443–45, 444f, 445f
Urine sucrose concentration in horses, 757
Urobilinogen, in urine, 467–68
Urobilinogenuria, 173–74
    increased, 468
Uroliths, 487–88
    analysis, 487–90
        concepts in, 488–89

calcium oxalate, 489
calcium phosphate, 489
canine, 488
cystine, 490
formation
    factors for, 489–90
    pathogenesis of, 489
inorganic composition of, 488, 488t
silica, 490
struvite, 489
urate, 490
xanthine, 490
Uroperitoneum, 847
USG. See Urine specific gravity

Vascular disease, BMBT and, 264
Vasculitis
    hypoproteinemia plasma loss through, 387–88
    thrombocytopenia and, 241
Veterinary laboratories, 31
    in-house, 35–36
    options, 35–36
Veterinary Laboratory Association (VLA), 29, 30f
Veterinary reference laboratories, 36
Vitamin B$_{12}$. See Cobalamin
Vitamin D
    actions of, 629
    activity, increased of, 600–601
    assays, 629
    concentration, 628–30
        analytical concepts in, 629
        physiologic processes in, 628–29
    endogenous, sources of, 600–601
    exogenous, sources of, 600
    formation, 628–29
    hypervitaminosis, neoplasm-associated, 601
    hypovitaminosis, 604
    rickets and, 604–5
    sample, 629
Vitamin K
    antagonists, 305–6
    bleeding disorders and antagonism or deficiency
        of, 305–8, 307t
    deficiency, 306
    hemorrhage and, 306
    hemostasis tests and, abnormal results in,
        305–8
Vomiting, K$^+$ loss through, 518–19
Von Willebrand disease (vWD), 265–66
    acquired, 265
    BMBT and, 263
    clinical/laboratory signs of, 266
    hypothyroidism and, 266

Von Willebrand disease (vWD) (*continued*)
  physiologic processes, 265
  types, 266
Von Willebrand factor (vWF), 265–68
  analytical concepts, 266–67
    assays and, 267
    sample and, 266
    units and, 266–67
  antigen ratio to, 267–68
    decreased, 267–68, 267t
    interpretive considerations fo, 268
  genetic tests for detecting, 268
vWD. *See* Von Willebrand disease
vWF. *See* Von Willebrand factor

Warfarin therapy, PT monitoring of, 283
WBC. *See* Whole blood count
Westgard rules, 26–29

White cell impedance count (WIC), 65
White cell optical count (WOC), 65
Whole blood count (WBC), 62
  nRBC correction of, 68–69
WIC. *See* White cell impedance count
Wintrobe's erythrocyte indices, 120–23
WOC. *See* White cell optical count
Working Formulation system, 364
Wright stains, 61
  hemic neoplasia classification with, 352–53

X-ray diffraction, 489
Xylazine, hyperglycemia and, 718
Xylitol toxicosis, 719
D-Xylose absorption tests, 754, 755t

Zinc sulfate (ZnSO$_4$), 400–401
ZnSO$_4$. *See* Zinc sulfate